Median Heights and Weights and Recommended Energy Intake

Category	Age (years) or Condition	Weight (kg)	Weight (lb)	Height (cm)	Height (in)	REE[a] (kcal/day)	Multiples of REE	Average Energy Allowance (kcal)[b] Per kg	Average Energy Allowance (kcal)[b] Per day[c]
Infants	0.0-0.5	6	13	60	24	320		108	650
	0.5-1.0	9	20	71	28	500		98	850
Children	1-3	13	29	90	35	740		102	1,300
	4-6	20	44	112	44	950		90	1,800
	7-10	28	62	132	52	1,130		70	2,000
Males	11-14	45	99	157	62	1,440	1.70	55	2,500
	15-18	66	145	176	69	1,760	1.67	45	3,000
	19-24	72	160	177	70	1,780	1.67	40	2,900
	25-50	79	174	176	70	1,800	1.60	37	2,900
	51+	77	170	173	68	1,530	1.50	30	2,300
Females	11-14	46	101	157	62	1,310	1.67	47	2,200
	15-18	55	120	163	64	1,370	1.60	40	2,200
	19-24	58	128	164	65	1,350	1.60	38	2,200
	25-50	63	138	163	64	1,380	1.55	36	2,200
	51+	65	143	160	63	1,280	1.50	30	1,900
Pregnant	1st trimester								+0
	2nd trimester								+300
	3rd trimester								+300
Lactating	1st 6 months								+500
	2nd 6 months								+500

[a]Calculation based on FAO equations, then rounded.
[b]In the range of light to moderate activity, the coefficient of variation is ± 20%.
[c]Figure is rounded.
From Food and Nutrition Board, National Academy of Sciences, National Research Council: *Recommended dietary allowances,* ed 10, Washington, D.C., 1989, National Academy Press.

The Food Guide Pyramid: A Guide to Daily Food Choices

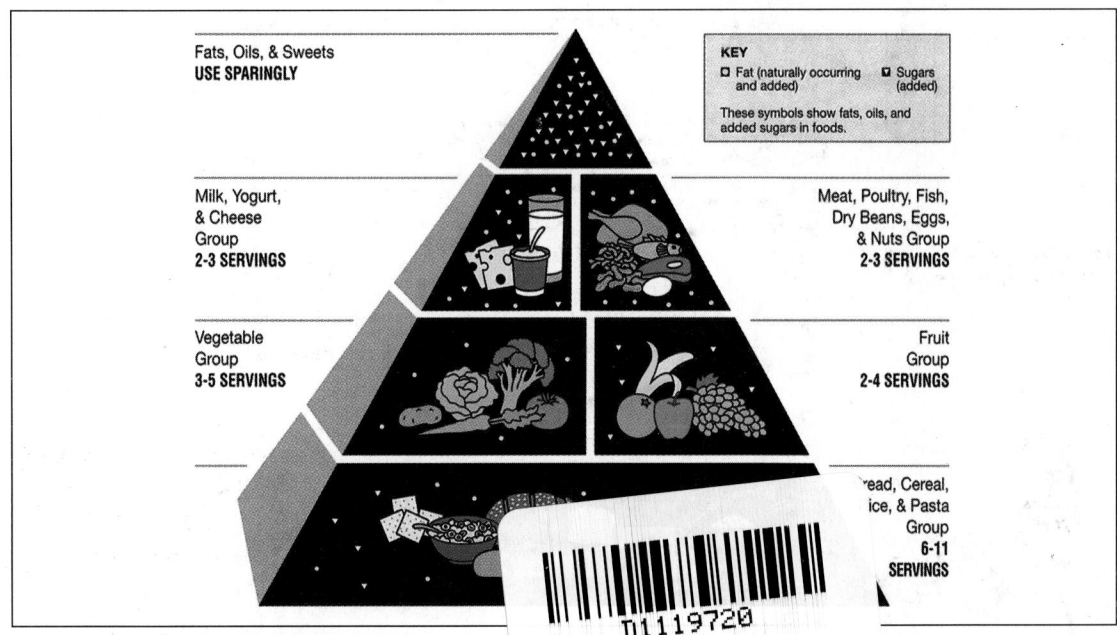

Fats, Oils, & Sweets
USE SPARINGLY

KEY
◻ Fat (naturally occurring and added)   ◼ Sugars (added)
These symbols show fats, oils, and added sugars in foods.

Milk, Yogurt, & Cheese Group
2-3 SERVINGS

Meat, Poultry, Fish, Dry Beans, Eggs, & Nuts Group
2-3 SERVINGS

Vegetable Group
3-5 SERVINGS

Fruit Group
2-4 SERVINGS

Bread, Cereal, Rice, & Pasta Group
6-11 SERVINGS

From USDA: The food guide pyramid, HG252, 1992.

Food and Nutrition Board, National Academy of Sciences—National Research Council
Recommended Dietary Allowances,[a] Revised 1989
Designed for the maintenance of good nutrition of practically all healthy people in the United States

Category	Age (years) or Condition	Weight[b] (kg)	Weight[b] (lb)	Height[b] (cm)	Height[b] (in)	Protein (g)	Fat-Soluble Vitamins — Vitamin A (μg RE)[c]	Vitamin D (μg)[d]	Vitamin E (mg α-TE)[e]	Vitamin K (μg)	Water-Soluble Vitamins — Vitamin C (mg)	Thiamin (mg)	Riboflavin (mg)	Niacin (mg NE)[f]	Vitamin B₆ (mg)	Folate (μg)	Vitamin B₁₂ (μg)	Minerals — Calcium (mg)	Phosphorus (mg)	Magnesium (mg)	Iron (mg)	Zinc (mg)	Iodine (μg)	Selenium (μg)
Infants	0.0-0.5	6	13	60	24	13	375	7.5	3	5	30	0.3	0.4	5	0.3	25	0.3	400	300	40	6	5	40	10
	0.5-1.0	9	20	71	28	14	375	10	4	10	35	0.4	0.5	6	0.6	35	0.5	600	500	60	10	5	50	15
Children	1-3	13	29	90	35	16	400	10	6	15	40	0.7	0.8	9	1.0	50	0.7	800	800	80	10	10	70	20
	4-6	20	44	112	44	24	500	10	7	20	45	0.9	1.1	12	1.1	75	1.0	800	800	120	10	10	90	20
	7-10	28	62	132	52	28	700	10	7	30	45	1.0	1.2	13	1.4	100	1.4	800	800	170	10	10	120	30
Males	11-14	45	99	157	62	45	1,000	10	10	45	50	1.3	1.5	17	1.7	150	2.0	1,200	1,200	270	12	15	150	40
	15-18	66	145	176	69	59	1,000	10	10	65	60	1.5	1.8	20	2.0	200	2.0	1,200	1,200	400	12	15	150	50
	19-24	72	160	177	70	58	1,000	10	10	70	60	1.5	1.7	19	2.0	200	2.0	1,200	1,200	350	10	15	150	70
	25-50	79	174	176	70	63	1,000	5	10	80	60	1.5	1.7	19	2.0	200	2.0	800	800	350	10	15	150	70
	51+	77	170	173	68	63	1,000	5	10	80	60	1.2	1.4	15	2.0	200	2.0	800	800	350	10	15	150	70
Females	11-14	46	101	157	62	46	800	10	8	45	50	1.1	1.3	15	1.4	150	2.0	1,200	1,200	280	15	12	150	45
	15-18	55	120	163	64	44	800	10	8	55	60	1.1	1.3	15	1.5	180	2.0	1,200	1,200	300	15	12	150	50
	19-24	58	128	164	65	46	800	10	8	60	60	1.1	1.3	15	1.6	180	2.0	1,200	1,200	280	15	12	150	55
	25-50	63	138	163	64	50	800	5	8	65	60	1.1	1.3	15	1.6	180	2.0	800	800	280	15	12	150	55
	51+	65	143	160	63	50	800	5	8	65	60	1.0	1.2	13	1.6	180	2.0	800	800	280	10	12	150	55
Pregnant						60	800	10	10	65	70	1.5	1.6	17	2.2	400	2.2	1,200	1,200	320	30	15	175	65
Lactating	1st 6 months					65	1,300	10	12	65	95	1.6	1.8	20	2.1	280	2.6	1,200	1,200	355	15	19	200	75
	2nd 6 months					62	1,200	10	11	65	90	1.6	1.7	20	2.1	260	2.6	1,200	1,200	340	15	16	200	75

[a] The allowances, expressed as average daily intakes over time, are intended to provide for individual variations among most normal persons as they live in the United States under usual environmental stresses. Diets should be based on a variety of common foods in order to provide other nutrients for which human requirements have been less well defined. See text for detailed discussion of allowances and nutrients not tabulated.

[b] Weights and heights of Reference Adults are actual medians for the U.S. population of the designated age, as reported by NHANES II. The use of these figures does not imply that the height-to-weight ratios are ideal.

[c] Retinol equivalents. 1 retinol equivalent = 1 μg retinol or 6 μg β-carotene. See text for calculation of vitamin A activity of diets as retinol equivalents.

[d] As cholecalciferol. 10 μg cholecalciferol = 400 iu of vitamin D.

[e] α-Tocopherol equivalents. 1 mg d-α tocopherol = 1 α-TE. See text for variation in allowances and calculation of vitamin E activity of the diet as α-tocopherol equivalents.

[f] 1 NE (niacin equivalent) is equal to 1 mg of niacin or 60 mg of dietary tryptophan.

From Food and Nutrition Board, National Academy of Sciences, National Research Council: *Recommended dietary allowances*, ed 10, Washington, D.C., 1989, National Academy Press.

Food and Nutrition Board, Institute of Medicine–National Academy of Sciences
Dietary Reference Intakes: Recommended Intakes for Individuals

Life-Stage Group	Calcium (mg/d)	Phosphorus (mg/d)	Magnesium (mg/d)	Vitamin D (µg/d)[a,b]	Fluoride (mg/d)	Thiamin (mg/d)	Riboflavin (mg/d)	Niacin (mg/d)[c]	Vitamin B6 (mg/d)	Folate (µg/d)[d]	Vitamin B12 (µg/d)[d]	Pantothenic Acid (mg/d)	Biotin (µg)	Choline[e] (mg/d)	Vitamin C[†] (mg/d)	Vitamin E[†] (as alpha-Tocopherol) (mg/d)	Selenium[†] (µg/d)
Infants																	
0-6 mo	210*	100*	30*	5*	0.01*	0.2*	0.3*	2*	0.1*	65*	0.4*	1.7*	5*	125*	40*	4*	15*
7-12 mo	270*	275*	75*	5*	0.5*	0.3*	0.4*	4*	0.3*	80*	0.5*	1.8*	6*	150*	50*	6*	20*
Children																	
1-3 yr	500*	460	80	5*	0.7*	0.5	0.5	6	0.5	150	0.9	2*	8*	200*	15	6	20
4-8 yr	800*	500	130	5*	1*	0.6	0.6	8	0.6	200	1.2	3*	12*	250*	25	7	30
Males																	
9-13 yr	1300*	1250	240	5*	2*	0.9	0.9	12	1.0	300	1.8	4*	20*	375*	45	11	40
14-18 yr	1300*	1250	410	5*	3*	1.2	1.3	16	1.3	400	2.4	5*	25*	550*	75	15	55
19-30 yr	1000*	700	400	5*	4*	1.2	1.3	16	1.3	400	2.4	5*	30*	550*	90	15	55
31-50 yr	1000*	700	420	5*	4*	1.2	1.3	16	1.3	400	2.4	5*	30*	550*	90	15	55
51-70 yr	1200*	700	420	10*	4*	1.2	1.3	16	1.7	400	2.4[f]	5*	30*	550*	90	15	55
>70 yr	1200*	700	420	15*	4*	1.2	1.3	16	1.7	400	2.4[f]	5*	30*	550*	90	15	55
Females																	
9-13 yr	1300*	1250	240	5*	2*	0.9	0.9	12	1.0	300	1.8	4*	20*	375*	45	11	40
14-18 yr	1300*	1250	360	5*	3*	1.0	1.0	14	1.2	400[g]	2.4	5*	25*	400*	65	15	55
19-30 yr	1000*	700	310	5*	3*	1.1	1.1	14	1.3	400[g]	2.4	5*	30*	425*	75	15	55
31-50 yr	1000*	700	320	5*	3*	1.1	1.1	14	1.3	400[g]	2.4	5*	30*	425*	75	15	55
51-70 yr	1200*	700	320	10*	3*	1.1	1.1	14	1.5	400	2.4[f]	5*	30*	425*	75	15	55
>70 yr	1200*	700	320	15*	3*	1.1	1.1	14	1.5	400	2.4[f]	5*	30*	425*	75	15	55
Pregnancy																	
≤18 yr	1300*	1250	400	5*	3*	1.4	1.4	18	1.9	600[h]	2.6	6*	30*	450*	80	15	60
19-30 yr	1000*	700	350	5*	3*	1.4	1.4	18	1.9	600[h]	2.6	6*	30*	450*	85	15	60
31-50 yr	1000*	700	360	5*	3*	1.4	1.4	18	1.9	600[h]	2.6	6*	30*	450*	85	15	60
Lactation																	
≤18 yr	1300*	1250	360	5*	3*	1.4	1.6	17	2.0	500	2.8	7*	35*	550*	115	19	70
19-30 yr	1000*	700	310	5*	3*	1.4	1.6	17	2.0	500	2.8	7*	35*	550*	120	19	70
31-50 yr	1000*	700	320	5*	3*	1.4	1.6	17	2.0	500	2.8	7*	35*	550*	120	19	70

NOTE: This table presents Recommended Dietary Allowances (RDAs) in **bold type** and Adequate Intakes (AIs) in ordinary type followed by an asterisk (*). RDAs and AIs may both be used as goals for individual intake. RDAs are set to meet the needs of almost all (97% to 98%) individuals in a group. For healthy breastfed infants, the AI is the mean intake. The AI for other life-stage and gender groups is thought to cover needs of all individuals in the group, but lack of data or uncertainty in the data prevent being able to specify with confidence the percentage of individuals covered by this intake.

[a] As cholecalciferol. 1 µg cholecalciferol = 40 IU vitamin D.

[b] In the absence of adequate exposure to sunlight.

[c] As niacin equivalents (NE). 1 mg of niacin = 60 mg tryptophan; 0-6 months = preformed niacin (not NE).

[d] As dietary folate equivalents (DFE). 1 µg food folate = 0.6 µg of folic acid (from fortified food or supplement) consumed with food = 0.5 µg of synthetic (supplemental) folic acid taken on an empty stomach.

[e] Although AIs have been set for choline, there are few data to assess whether a dietary supply of choline is needed at all stages of the life cycle, and it may be that the choline requirement can be met by endogenous synthesis at some of these stages.

[f] Because 10 to 30 percent of older people may malabsorb food bound B12, it is advisable for those older than 50 years to meet their RDA mainly by consuming foods fortified with B12 or a supplement containing B12.

[g] In view of evidence linking folate intake with neural tube defects in the fetus, it is recommended that all women capable of becoming pregnant consume 400 µg of synthetic folic acid from fortified foods and/or supplements in addition to intake of food folate from a varied diet.

[h] It is assumed that women will continue consuming 400 µg of folic acid until their pregnancy is confirmed and they enter prenatal care, which ordinarily occurs after the end of the periconceptional period—the critical time for formation of the neural tube.

[†] From Food and Nutrition Board, Institute of Medicine: Dietary reference intakes for vitamin C, vitamin E, selenium, and carotenoids, Washington, DC, 2000, National Academy Press.

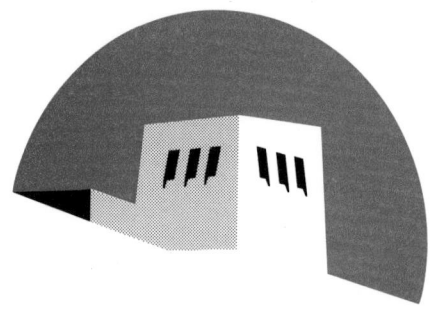
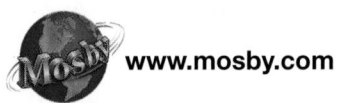

BASIC NUTRITION &
DIET THERAPY

ELEVENTH EDITION

BASIC NUTRITION&
DIET THERAPY

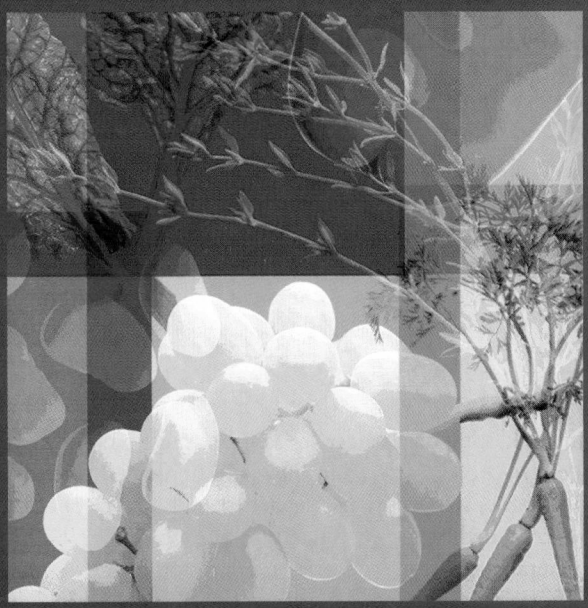

Sue Rodwell Williams, PhD, MPH, RD

President, SRW Productions, Inc.

Clinical Nutrition Consultant

Davis, California

with 73 illustrations

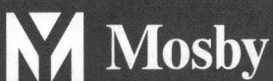 Mosby

An Imprint of Elsevier Science

St. Louis   London   Philadelphia   Sydney   Toronto

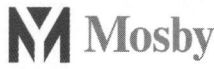
Mosby

An Imprint of Elsevier Science

Vice-President, Nursing Editorial Director: Sally Schrefer
Editor: Yvonne Alexopoulos
Developmental Editor: Melissa K. Boyle
Project Manager: Catherine Jackson
Production Editor: Jodi Everding
Designer: Michael Warrell
Cover Designer: Amy Buxton

Parts 1, 3, and 4 Openers: PhotoDisc. Part 2 Opener: Tony Stone Images.

ELEVENTH EDITION

Mosby, Inc.
An Imprint of Elsevier Science
11830 Westline Industrial Drive
St. Louis, Missouri 63146

Printed in China

International Standard Book Number 0-323-00569-1

02 03 04 GW/KPT 9 8 7 6 5 4 3 2

Reviewers

Linda Bland, RN, MSN
Director, Vocational Nursing Program,
Trinity Valley Community College,
Palestine, Texas

Ruby M. Degener, RN, BS, MS
Assistant Professor of Nursing,
The Community College of Baltimore County—
Catonsville Campus,
Baltimore, Maryland

Kelley DeVane-Hart, MS, RD
Assistant Professor of Nutrition,
School of Nursing,
Troy State University,
Troy, Alabama

Delaine C. Furst, BS, MS, EdS
Associate Professor,
Human Environment Science,
Indian River Community College,
Fort Pierce, Florida

Betty Kenyon, RD, LMNT
Adjunct Faculty,
Western Nebraska Community College
Scottsbluff, Nebraska;
Director of Consultant Services,
Panhandle Community Services,
Gering, Nebraska

Kelly Kohls, PhD, RD, LD
Owner,
Able Weight and Wellness Services,
Lebanon, Ohio

Anne O'Donnell, MS, MPH, RD
Instructor and Department Chair,
Diet Tech Program Coordinator,
Consumer and Family Studies,
Santa Rosa Junior College,
Santa Rosa, California

Sue Smith, RN, BSN
Assistant Professor,
PN Program,
Harlan Center,
Iowa Western Community College,
Harlan, Iowa

Sue G. Thacker, RN, BSN, MS, PhD
Professor,
Nursing,
Wytheville Community College,
Wytheville, Virginia

Janet Willis, RN, BSN, MS
Professor,
Harrisburg Area Community College,
Harrisburg, Pennsylvania

Preface to the Instructor

For many years, through 10 highly successful editions, this compact "little" book has provided a sound learning resource and a handy manual in basic nutrition for support personnel in health care. The new eleventh edition continues this important central focus.

The field of nutrition, however, is a dynamic human endeavor that has expanded and changed since the publication of previous editions. As always, we have tried to capture the excitement of the current, constantly developing nutrition knowledge and its application to human health in the modern format and style of this new edition.

Three main factors continue to change the modern face of nutrition. First, the science of nutrition continues to grow rapidly with exciting basic research. New knowledge in any science always challenges some traditional ideas and develops new ones, which is especially true when current nutritional science is applied to the modern movement in health care for younger populations and to a preventive, early risk-reduction approach to managing chronic disease in our aging population. Second, the rapidly increasing multiethnic diversity of the United States population enriches our food patterns and presents varying health care needs. Third, the public is more aware and concerned about health promotion and the role of nutrition, largely because of media's increasing attention. Clients and patients are raising more questions and seeking intelligent answers. They want sound information to deal with common misinformation and fads, as well as with legitimate controversy. They want to be more involved in their own health care. Nothing, perhaps, is more human a part of that care than food.

This new edition continues to reflect these far-reaching changes. Its guiding principle is my own commitment, along with that of my publisher, to the integrity of the material. Our basic goal is to produce a new book for today's needs, with updated content, to meet the expectations and changing needs of students, faculty, and practitioners of basic health care.

BASIC OBJECTIVES

This text is primarily designed for students and health care workers in beginning, assistance-level programs for practical or licensed vocational nurses (LVNs), as well as for diet technicians or aides. As in previous editions, a limited background in nutrition-related basic sciences is assumed, so basic concepts are carefully explained when introduced. With the changing public health awareness, however, the text also assumes that readers have an expanded general base in nutrition and health. Building on this interest, the general purpose of this text is to introduce some basic principles of scientific nutrition and present their applications in person-centered care in health and disease. In addition, my personal concerns are ever present, as follow: (1) that this introduction to the science and practice I love will continue to lead students and readers to enjoy learning about human nutrition in the lives of people and stimulate further reading in areas of personal interest; (2) that caretakers will be alert to nutrition news and questions raised by their increasingly diverse clients and patients; and (3) that contact and communication with professionals in the field of nutrition helps to build a strong team approach to clinical nutrition problems in all patient care.

FEATURES

In a real sense, the eleventh edition of this classic text is a new book for our changing times and needs. To meet the ever present needs of a rapidly developing science and society, while continuing to use a clearly understood writing style, I have updated content areas and maintained the user-friendly format.

■ **Current chapter materials.** All chapters continue to include materials to help meet practice needs. In Part 1, *Introduction to Basic Principles of Nutritional Science,* Chapter 1 focuses on the directions of health care and health promotion, risk reduction for disease prevention, and community health care delivery systems with emphasis on team care and the active role of clients in educated self-care. A description and illustration accompanies the familiar Food Guide Pyramid. The **Dietary Reference Intakes (DRIs),** the most current dietary recommendations, are introduced and incorporated throughout chapter discussions in Part 1, as well as throughout the rest of the text. Current research updates all of the basic nutrient/ energy chapters in the remainder of Part 1. In Part 2, *Nutrition Throughout the Life Cycle,* Chapters 10, 11, and 12 reflect current material on human growth and development needs in different parts of the life cycle. Current Academy of Science guidelines for positive weight gain to meet the metabolic demands of pregnancy and lactation are reinforced. Positive growth support for infancy, childhood, and adolescence is emphasized. The expanding health-maintenance needs of a growing adult population through the aging process focus on building a healthy lifestyle to reduce disease risks.

In Part 3, *Community Nutrition and Health Care,* a strong focus on community nutrition needs is coordinated with a strong emphasis on weight management and physical fitness as health care benefits and risk reduction. The Nutrition Labeling and Education Act is discussed in terms of its current regulations and helpful label format, as well as effects on food marketing. Highlights of foodborne diseases reinforce concerns about food safety in a changing marketplace. Chapter 14 reinforces information on America's multiethnic cultural food patterns. New information on the topics of obesity and genetics, and the use of diet drugs, is included in Chapter 15. Chapter 16 includes material on athletics to clarify the ongoing practice of glycogen loading for endurance events, the proliferation of sports drinks, and the dangerous illegal use of steroids by athletes and body builders.

In Part 4, *Clinical Nutrition,* chapters are updated to reflect current medical treatment and approaches to nutritional management. Special areas involved include developments in gastrointestinal disease, heart disease, diabetes mellitus, renal disease, surgery, cancer, and AIDS.

■ **Book format and design.** The chapter format and use of color continue to enhance the book's appeal and encourage its use. Basic chapter concepts and overview, use of color, illustrations, tables, boxes, definitions, headings, and subheadings make it easier and more interesting to read.

■ **Learning aids.** Educational aids have been developed to assist both students and instructors in the teaching/learning process. These aids are described later in detail.

■ **Illustrations.** Color illustrations—including artwork, graphs, charts, and photographs—help students and practitioners better understand the concepts and clinical practices presented.

■ **Enhanced readability and student interest.** This eleventh edition is written in a style that not only continues its simple unfolding of the material but also creates new interest and helps students better understand basic concepts through expanded explanations to "flesh out" the topics discussed.

LEARNING AIDS

As indicated, this new edition is especially significant because of its use of many learning aids throughout the text.

✔ **Part openers.** To provide the "big picture" of the book's overall focus on nutrition and health, the four main sections are introduced as successive developing parts of that unifying theme.

✔ **Chapter openers.** To immediately draw students into the topic for study, each chapter opens with a short list of the basic concepts involved and a brief chapter overview leading into the topic to "set the stage."

✔ **Chapter headings.** Throughout each chapter, the major headings and subheadings in special type or color indicate the organization of the chapter material making for easy reading and understanding of the key ideas. Main concepts and terms are also brought out with color or bold type and italics.

✔ **Special boxes.** The inclusion of *For Further Focus* boxes and *Clinical Applications* boxes leads students a step further on a given topic or presents a case study for analysis. These boxes enhance understanding of concepts through further exploration or application.

✔ **Case studies.** In clinical care chapters, case studies are provided in *Clinical Applications* boxes to focus students' attention to related patient care problems. Each case is accompanied by questions for case analysis. Students can use these examples for similar patient care needs in their own clinical assignments.

✔ **Diet therapy guides.** In clinical chapters, various diet therapy guides provide practical help in patient care and education.

✔ **Definitions of terms.** Key terms important to students' understanding and application of the material in patient care are presented in two ways. They are identified in the body of the text—often with interesting derivation and description of the words, and they are listed in a glossary at the back of the book for quick reference.

✔ **Illustrations.** The use of color illustrations throughout the text creates interest and helps students better understand important concepts and applications.

✔ **Summaries.** A brief summary at the end of each chapter reviews chapter highlights and

helps students see how the chapter contributes to the book's "big picture." Students can then return to any part of the material for repeated study and clarification of details as needed.

✔ **Review questions.** To help students understand key parts of the chapter or apply it to patient care problems, questions are given after each chapter summary for review and analysis of the material presented.

✔ **Self-test questions.** In addition, self-test questions in both true-false and multiple-choice formats are provided at the end of each chapter to allow students to check their basic knowledge.

✔ **Suggestions for additional study.** At the end of each chapter, a variety of activities are also suggested for better understanding and application of the text material. These suggestions include projects, surveys, situational problems, and analysis of information gathered.

✔ **References.** Use of background references throughout the text provides more resources for students who may want to probe a particular topic of interest further.

✔ **Further reading.** To encourage further reading of useful materials for expanding knowledge of key concepts or applying material in practical ways for patient care and education, a brief list of annotated resources is provided at the end of each chapter.

✔ **Appendixes.** The numerous appendixes provided include an extensive table of food nutrient values from *Mosby's NutriTrac Nutrition Analysis CD-ROM*, along with information on the cholesterol content of foods, dietary fiber, and sodium and potassium. The *Exchange Lists for Meal Planning* are included, along with the Recommended Dietary Allowances (RDAs) and available Dietary Reference Intakes (DRIs), and the Recommended Nutrient Intakes for Canadians. A new appendix on cultural dietary patterns has been added in this new edition to help students better understand the diet habits of their increasingly diverse client/patient population. These—and all of the appendixes provided—serve as valuable reference tools and guides in learning and practice.

ANCILLARIES

✔ **Instructor's manual and test bank.** This valuable ancillary contains an *Instructor's Manual*, a *Test Bank*, and *Transparency Masters*. The *Instructor's Manual* portion includes detailed chapter outlines, essay questions, and extensive print, audiovisual, and software and website resources that can be used for activities, projects, or further study. The *Test Bank* includes approximately 700 questions in NCLEX, multiple-choice format, and there are approximately 30 *Transparency Masters* provided at the back of this ancillary.

✔ **Computerized test bank (Win/Mac CD-ROM).** This test bank is the same one found in the *Instructor's Manual and Test Bank* (i.e., approximately 700 questions in NCLEX, multiple-choice format) but is on a hybrid CD-ROM allowing exams to be customized and printed.

✔ **Transparency acetates.** A package of 58 transparencies (2- and 4-color) accompanies the text, as well as the other two Williams nutrition titles, *Nutrition and Diet Therapy* and *Essentials of Nutrition and Diet Therapy*.

✔ **Mosby's NutriTrac Nutrition Analysis CD-ROM.** A FREE nutrition analysis CD-ROM with a database of over 2,200 food items is included with every text. This software allows users to analyze nutrition and calculate food intake and energy expenditure for effective diet analysis.

✔ **MERLIN** *Merlin* **website.** This website was created specifically for this book: www.mosby.com/MERLIN/Williams/Basic/.
See the MERLIN page at the very beginning of the text for more information.

✔ **Nutrition resource center website.** This informative website is available at www.harcourthealth.com/Nutrition/ to provide you with all of the Harcourt Health Sciences nutrition texts in one convenient location.

A PERSONAL APPROACH

In the past, users of this text have responded very positively to the person-centered approach I have tried to develop. In this new edition, I have sought to maintain this approach in several ways.

Personal writing style. In this new edition, I have continued to use a writing style that reflects the very personal nature of human nutrition and health care and to speak directly to the reader. I wish to share my own self and feelings, which were born of many years of experience in clinical work and teaching. I want to create interest and involvement in our rapidly advancing knowledge of nutrition, the exciting process of learning, and sound humanistic practice. In this manner, I want to express my constant concern for students and their learning and for clients and patients and their needs.

Practical application. In almost all human endeavors, theory is only useful in its human application; so it is with nutritional care. Thus all of the chapters here supply expanded practical applications of current scientific knowledge in realistic terms. My goal is always to bring together science and human needs to make them "come alive" for students and, in turn, for their clients and patients. There often are no single, "pat" answers to health care problems, and individual situations require individual solutions. A basic understanding of the principles involved, however, makes for better person-centered care in any case.

ACKNOWLEDGEMENTS

A realistic and useful textbook is never the work of one person. It develops into the planned product through the committed hands and hearts of a number of persons. It would be impossible to name all the individuals involved here, but several groups deserve special recognition.

First, I am indebted to Mosby and the many persons there—new and old friends—who have had a part in this project. I especially thank my publisher and editorial staff—especially my editor of nutrition publications, Yvonne Alexopoulos, and my developmental editor, Melissa Boyle. I am also grateful for the help of my production editor, Jodi Everding. All of them helped to shape the manuscript and supported my efforts and goals. I also thank the marketing staff and the sales representatives scattered throughout the country and abroad for their encouragement and skills that help guide this result of my efforts to its ultimate users. You know who you are and how important each one of you is to this vital goal.

Second, I am grateful to the reviewers who gave their time and skills to help strengthen the manuscript.

Third, I am very grateful to all those persons who worked with me on my own staff during the various stages of preparing the manuscript, especially Mary Herbert, my chief research associate who gathered the comprehensive materials I requested and connected me to the university's vast network. I owe a special debt of gratitude to my editor, James C. Williams, for assisting in the research and writing of many of the learning aids articles, for expert copyediting throughout, and for producing the manuscript. To both of these key persons, I give special thanks for always being there when I needed them.

Fourth, many students, interns, colleagues, clients, and patients have enriched my life over the years; their contributions are revealed in all my work. Each one has taught me something about human experience, and I am grateful for those opportunities for personal growth.

And finally, most of all, I want to thank my family—my "home team." These beautiful people never cease to provide loving support for all my work, and to each one I am eternally grateful.

I hope that those who use this text will continue to give me feedback and suggestions. My purpose is to provide a useful and practical beginning text for students that can help them understand some of the elemental principles of nutritional science and apply them in personal patient care—and that they can enjoy.

Sue Rodwell Williams

Preface to the Student

Basic Nutrition and Diet Therapy is a market leader in nutrition textbooks for support personnel in health care. It provides careful explanations of the basic principles of scientific nutrition, and then presents their applications in person-centered care in health and disease.

The author, Sue Williams, provides this important information in an easy-to-read, user-friendly format by including helpful learning tools throughout the text. Check out the following features to familiarize yourself with the book and help you get the most value out of this text:

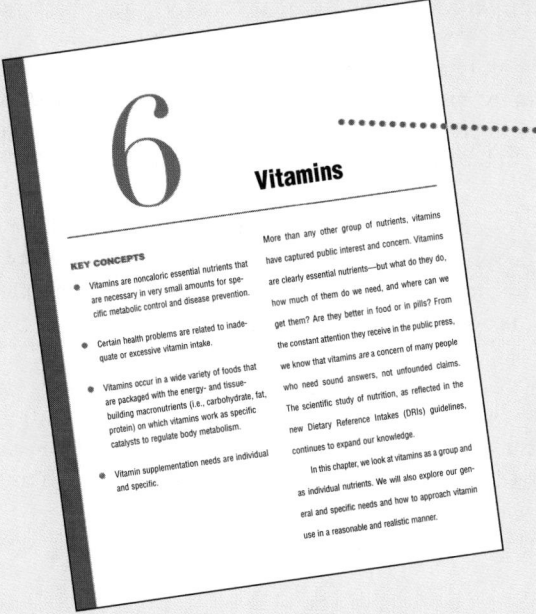

A short list of **Key Concepts** and a brief **chapter overview** begin each chapter to immediately draw you into the subject at hand.

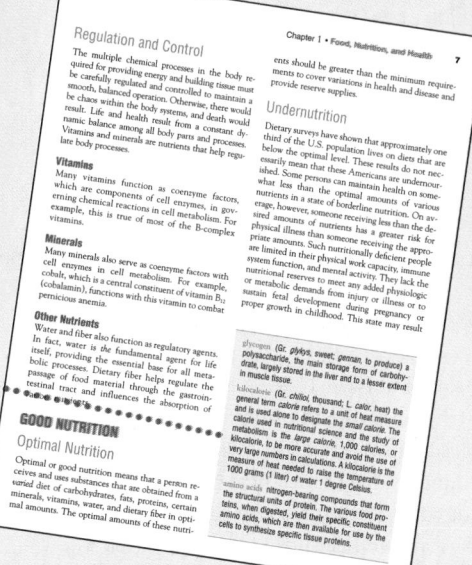

• **Definition boxes** throughout the text identify and define key terms important to your understanding and application of the material.

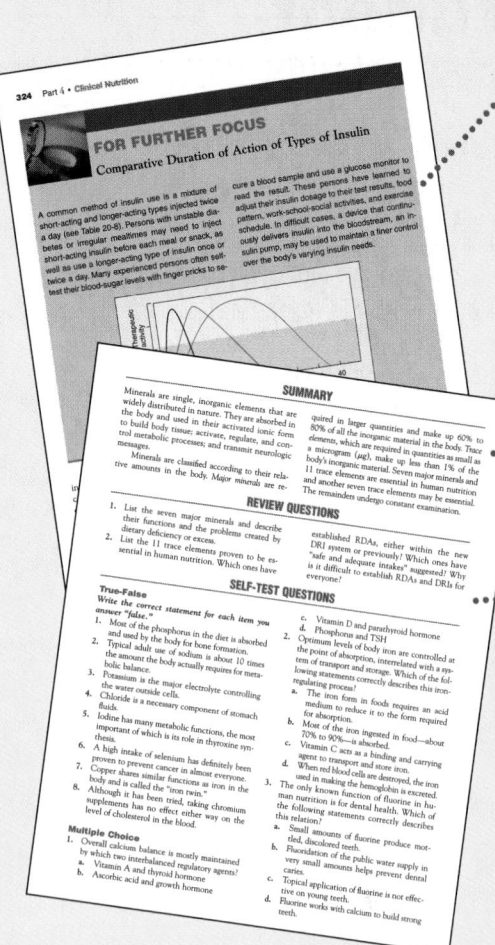

For Further Focus boxes and Clinical Applications boxes take you one step further in the discussion of a given topic, enhancing your understanding of concepts through further exploration or application.

A brief chapter Summary is included at the end of every chapter to review chapter highlights and help you see how particular chapters contribute to the book's overall focus.

Review Questions and Self-Test Questions are presented after each chapter summary for review and analysis and to allow you to apply key concepts to patient care problems.

Suggestions for Additional Study, References, and Further Reading are also provided after the self-test questions to complete the chapter.

Your free copy of the **NutriTrac Nutritional Analysis CD-ROM** is also included in the back of this text. NutriTrac provides the easiest way to analyze nutrition and calculate food intake and energy expenditure for effective diet analysis. Here's what you'll find: an updated food database with over 2,200 foods; 17 food categories; one of the most extensive lists of the latest reduced-fat and fat-free brands; an unlimited number of food-intake days, plus the ability to copy food from any meal from one day to another; NutriTrac Top 20 foods in nutrient density for any selected nutrient; and full print capabilities for all full-color graphics.

Be sure to visit our two new websites of interest. First, a brand new **MERLIN** website has been created specifically for this book at http://www.mosby.com/MERLIN/Williams/Basic/. See the Merlin page at the very beginning of this text for more information. Second, a **nutrition resource center** website is available at www.harcourthealth.com/Nutrition/ to provide you with all of the Harcourt Health Sciences nutrition texts in one convenient location.

We are pleased that you have included *Basic Nutrition and Diet Therapy* as part of your nutrition education. Be sure to check out our web site at www.mosby.com for all of your health science educational needs!

Contents

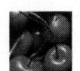

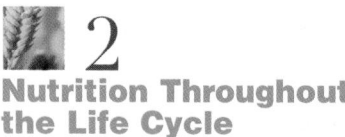

2
Nutrition Throughout
the Life Cycle

3
Community Nutrition
and Health Care

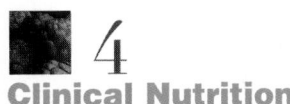

4
Clinical Nutrition

Appendixes

1

Introduction to Basic Principles of Nutritional Science

Food, Nutrition, and Health

KEY CONCEPTS

- Optimal personal and community nutrition is a major component of health promotion.

- Certain nutrients in food are essential to our health and well-being.

- Food and nutrient guides help us to plan a balanced diet according to individual needs and goals.

We live in a world with rapidly changing elements—our environment, food supply, population, and scientific knowledge. Within different environments, our bodies and our personalities change, and with them our personal needs and goals. These *constant changes* of life must be in some kind of *positive balance* to produce healthy living. To be realistic within these concepts of change and balance, our study of food, nutrition, and health care must therefore focus upon health promotion. Although we may view and define health and disease in different ways, a primary basis for promoting health and preventing disease must always be good food and the sound nutrition it provides. This basic study of nutrition, then, has primary importance in the following two ways: it is fundamental for our own health, and it is essential for the health and well-being of our patients and clients.

HEALTH PROMOTION

Basic Definitions

Nutrition and Dietetics

Nutrition concerns the food people eat and how their bodies use it. Nutritional science comprises the body of scientific knowledge governing humans' food requirements for maintenance, growth, activity, reproduction, and lactation. Dietetics is the health profession responsible for applying nutritional science to promote human health and treat disease. The registered dietitian (RD), especially the *clinical nutrition specialist* or the *public health nutritionist* in the community, is the nutrition authority on the health care team. These health care professionals carry the major responsibility of nutritional care of patients and clients.

Health and Wellness

Good nutrition is essential to good health throughout life, beginning with prenatal life and extending through old age. In its simplest terms, health is defined as the absence of disease; but this definition is too narrow. Life experience shows that the definition of health is much more. It must include broader attention to the roots of health in meeting basic human needs (i.e., physical, mental, psychologic, and social well-being). This approach recognizes the individual as a whole and relates health to both internal and external environments. The added positive concept of *wellness* carries this broader approach one step further. Wellness seeks for all persons full development of their potential, within whatever environment they may find themselves. It implies a balance between activities and goals: work vs. leisure, lifestyle choices vs. health risks, and personal needs vs. others' expectations. Wellness implies a positive dynamic state motivating a person to seek a higher level of function.

Wellness Movement and National Health Goals

The current wellness or fitness movement, which is rooted in the 1970s, continues to be a fundamental response to the medical care system's emphasis on illness and disease and the rising costs of medical care. Since the 1970s, "holistic" health and health promotion have focused on lifestyle and personal choice in helping persons and families develop plans for maintaining health and wellness. The U.S. national health goals continue to reflect this wellness philosophy. People are also becoming more comfortable with our rapidly developing modern biotechnology. The pivotal report, *Healthy People 2000*, published in 1990 by the U.S. Department of Health and Human Services, had wide influence.[1] The new report in this series, *Healthy People 2010*, continues to focus on the nation's main objective of positive health promotion and disease prevention. This report outlines specific objectives for meeting three broad, public health goals throughout the new century,[2] as follow:

1. An increase in the span of healthy life for Americans
2. Reduction of health disparities among Americans
3. Access to preventative health care services for all Americans

A major theme throughout the report is the encouragement of healthy choices in diet, weight control, and other risk factors for disease—especially in the report's specific nutrition objectives. Community health agencies continue to implement these goals and objectives in local and state public and private health programs, especially in areas where malnutrition and poverty exist. All of these efforts recognize personal nutrition as an integral component of health and health care for all persons.

Traditional and Preventive Approaches to Health

The *preventive* approach to health involves identifying risk factors that increase a person's chances of developing a particular health problem. By knowing these factors, persons can then choose behaviors that will prevent or minimize their risks for disease. On the other hand, the *traditional* approach to health only attempts change when symptoms of illness or disease already exist, at which point those who are ill seek out a physician to diagnose, treat, and "cure" the condition. The traditional approach has little value for lifelong positive health. Major chronic problems (e.g., heart disease or cancer) may be developing long before overt signs become apparent.

Importance of a Balanced Diet

Food and Health

Food has always been one of the necessities of life. Many people, however, are only concerned with food insofar as it relieves their hunger or satisfies their appetites—not with whether it supplies their bodies with all the components of good nutrition. The core practitioners of the health care team (i.e., physician, clinical dietitian, and nurse) are all aware of the important part that food plays in maintaining good health and recovering from illness. Chronic ill health in patients requires checking food habits as possible contributing factors. Therefore assessing a patient's nutritional status and identifying nutritional needs are primary activities in planning care.

Signs of Good Nutrition

A well-developed body, the ideal weight for body composition (i.e., ratio of muscle mass to fat) and height, and good muscle development and tone are all evidence of good nutrition. Additionally, skin is smooth and clear, hair is glossy, and eyes are clear and bright. Posture is good, and facial expression is alert. Appetite, digestion, and elimination are normal. Well-nourished persons are more likely to be mentally and physically alert and have a positive outlook on life. They are also more able to resist infectious diseases than undernourished persons. Within wide varieties of cultural food habits, a wise diet not only creates healthier persons but also extends their years of normal functioning.

FUNCTIONS OF NUTRIENTS IN FOOD

To sustain life, the nutrients in foods must perform three basic overall functions within the body, as follow:

1. Provide energy sources.
2. Build tissue.
3. Regulate metabolic processes.

Metabolism refers to the sum of all body processes that accomplish these three basic life-sustaining tasks.

---

health promotion (A.S. *hal*, hale, sound; L. *promovere*, to move forward) active involvement in behaviors or programs that advance positive well-being.

nutrition (L. *nutritic*, nourishment) the sum of the processes involved in taking in nutrients, assimilating and using them to maintain body tissue and provide energy; a foundation for life and health.

nutritional science the body of science, developed through controlled research, that relates to the processes involved in nutrition—international, community, and clinical.

dietetics management of diet and the use of food; the science concerned with the nutritional planning and preparation of foods.

registered dietitian (RD) a professional dietitian, accredited with an academic degree course from a university or graduate study program and having passed required registration examinations administered by the American Dietetic Association.

health a state of optimal well-being—physical, mental, and social; relative freedom from disease or disability.

metabolism (Gr. *metaballein*, to turn about, change, alter) the sum of all chemical changes that take place in the body by which it maintains itself and produces energy for its functioning. Products of the various reactions are called *metabolites*.

An important nutritional-metabolic fact emerges in the following outline of these three basic nutrient functions. This fact is the fundamental principle of *nutrient interaction*, which means two things: (1) individual nutrients have many specific metabolic functions, including primary and supporting roles; and (2) no nutrient ever works alone. The human body is a fascinating whole made up of many parts and processes. Intimate metabolic relationships exist among all the basic nutrients and their metabolic products. This key principle of nutrient interaction is demonstrated more clearly in the following chapters. Although the various nutrients may be separated for study purposes, remember that they do not exist that way in the human body. They always interact as a dynamic whole to produce and maintain the body.

Energy Sources

Carbohydrates

Dietary carbohydrates (e.g., starches and sugars) provide the body's primary source of fuel for heat and energy. They also maintain the body's back-up store of quick energy as glycogen, which is sometimes called "animal starch" (see Chapter 2). Human energy is measured in heat units called kilocalories (abbreviated kcalories or kcal [see Chapter 5]). Each gram of carbohydrate consumed yields 4 kcal of body energy. This number is called the "fuel factor" for carbohydrates. In a well-balanced diet, carbohydrates should provide about 55% to 60% of the total kcalories.

Fats

Dietary fats, from both animal and plant sources, provide the body's secondary—or storage—form of heat and energy. This form is more concentrated, yielding 9 kcal for each gram consumed and thus having a fuel factor of 9. In a well-balanced diet, fats should provide no more than 25% to 30% of the total kcalories, with most of this amount (approximately two thirds) being unsaturated fats from plant sources (see Chapter 3).

Proteins

The body may draw from dietary or tissue protein to obtain needed energy when the supply of fuel from carbohydrates and fats is insufficient. When this occurs, protein can yield 4 kcal/g, making its fuel factor 4. In a well-balanced diet, protein should provide about 15% of the total kcalories. Therefore although protein's primary function is tissue building, some of it may be available for energy as needed.

Tissue Building

Proteins

The primary function of protein is tissue building. Dietary protein provides amino acids, which are the building units necessary for constructing and repairing body tissues. Tissue building is a constant process that ensures growth and maintenance of a strong body structure and vital substances for its tissue functions.

Other Nutrients

Several other nutrients that contribute to building and maintaining tissues are described in the following paragraphs.

Minerals. For example, two major minerals—calcium and phosphorus—function in building and maintaining bone tissue. Another key mineral is iron, which contributes to building the oxygen carrier hemoglobin in red blood cells (RBCs).

Vitamins. An example of the use of a vitamin in tissue building is that of vitamin C in developing the cementing intercellular ground substance. This substance helps build strong tissue and prevents tissue bleeding.

Fatty acids. Fatty acids derived from fat metabolism help build the central fat substance of cell walls and promote the transport of fat-soluble materials across the cell wall.

Regulation and Control

The multiple chemical processes in the body required for providing energy and building tissue must be carefully regulated and controlled to maintain a smooth, balanced operation. Otherwise, there would be chaos within the body systems, and death would result. Life and health result from a constant dynamic balance among all body parts and processes. Vitamins and minerals are nutrients that help regulate body processes.

Vitamins

Many vitamins function as coenzyme factors, which are components of cell enzymes, in governing chemical reactions in cell metabolism. For example, this is true of most of the B-complex vitamins.

Minerals

Many minerals also serve as coenzyme factors with cell enzymes in cell metabolism. For example, cobalt, which is a central constituent of vitamin B_{12} (cobalamin), functions with this vitamin to combat pernicious anemia.

Other Nutrients

Water and fiber also function as regulatory agents. In fact, water is *the* fundamental agent for life itself, providing the essential base for all metabolic processes. Dietary fiber helps regulate the passage of food material through the gastrointestinal tract and influences the absorption of various nutrients.

GOOD NUTRITION

Optimal Nutrition

Optimal or good nutrition means that a person receives and uses substances that are obtained from a *varied* diet of carbohydrates, fats, proteins, certain minerals, vitamins, water, and dietary fiber in optimal amounts. The optimal amounts of these nutrients should be greater than the minimum requirements to cover variations in health and disease and provide reserve supplies.

Undernutrition

Dietary surveys have shown that approximately one third of the U.S. population lives on diets that are below the optimal level. These results do not necessarily mean that these Americans are undernourished. Some persons can maintain health on somewhat less than the optimal amounts of various nutrients in a state of borderline nutrition. On average, however, someone receiving less than the desired amounts of nutrients has a greater risk for physical illness than someone receiving the appropriate amounts. Such nutritionally deficient people are limited in their physical work capacity, immune system function, and mental activity. They lack the nutritional reserves to meet any added physiologic or metabolic demands from injury or illness or to sustain fetal development during pregnancy or proper growth in childhood. This state may result

---

glycogen (Gr. *glykys*, sweet; *gennan*, to produce) a polysaccharide, the main storage form of carbohydrate, largely stored in the liver and to a lesser extent in muscle tissue.

kilocalorie (Gr. *chilioi*, thousand; L. *calor*, heat) the general term *calorie* refers to a unit of heat measure and is used alone to designate the *small calorie*. The calorie used in nutritional science and the study of metabolism is the *large calorie*, 1,000 calories, or kilocalorie, to be more accurate and avoid the use of very large numbers in calculations. A kilocalorie is the measure of heat needed to raise the temperature of 1000 grams (1 liter) of water 1 degree Celsius.

amino acids nitrogen-bearing compounds that form the structural units of protein. The various food proteins, when digested, yield their specific constituent amino acids, which are then available for use by the cells to synthesize specific tissue proteins.

from poor eating habits or a continuously stressful environment with little or no income.

Malnutrition

Signs of more serious malnutrition appear when nutritional reserves are depleted and nutrient and energy intake is not sufficient to meet day-to-day needs or added metabolic stress. Many malnourished people live in conditions of poverty. Such conditions influence the health of all involved, but especially that of the most vulnerable persons (i.e., pregnant women, infants, children, and elderly adults). In the United States, one of the wealthiest countries on earth, many studies document widespread hunger and malnutrition among the poor, indicating that food-security problems involve urban development issues, economic policy, and more general poverty issues. In the United States alone, at least 20 million people suffer with hunger some days each month. Elderly persons, particularly those living alone or in rural areas, are vulnerable. Many studies document widespread hunger and malnutrition among the poor, especially among the growing number of homeless, including mothers with young children.[3,4] These children have stunted growth and episodes of infection and disease, which often have lasting effects on intellectual development.[5,6] Worldwide, about 40,000 to 50,000 people die *each day* from malnutrition, while an estimated 450 million to 1.3 billion people do not have enough to eat.[6]

Malnutrition also occurs sometimes in our hospitals. For example, extended illness—especially among older persons with chronic disease—places added stress on the body, and the daily nutrient and energy intake of these persons is insufficient to meet their needs.

Overnutrition

Some persons may be in a state of overnutrition that results from excess nutrient and energy intake over time. In a sense, overnutrition can be another form of malnutrition, especially when excess caloric intake produces harmful gross body weight (i.e., morbid obesity) (see Chapter 15). Harmful overnutrition can also occur in persons who use excessive (e.g., "megadose") amounts of nutrient supplements over time, producing damaging tissue effects (see Chapter 6).

NUTRIENT AND FOOD GUIDES FOR HEALTH PROMOTION

Nutrient Standards

Most of the developed countries of the world have established nutrition standards for major nutrients to serve as guidelines for maintaining healthy populations. These standards are not intended to indicate individual requirements or therapeutic needs but rather, on the basis of current scientific knowledge, to serve as a reference for intake levels of the essential nutrients to adequately meet the known nutritional needs of most healthy population groups. Although these standards are similar in different countries, they may vary somewhat according to the philosophy of the scientists and practitioners in a particular country on the purpose and use of such standards. In the United States, these standards have recently been updated and reorganized and are now called the Dietary Reference Intakes (DRIs).[7] With the growing population of elderly persons, the optimal allowances for older adults, due to poor diets or eating problems, are an increasing concern (see Chapter 12).

U.S. Standards: DRIs

The U.S. dietary standard has been enlarged and updated. The previous, simpler system used for calculating the standards for all age groups was called the Recommended Dietary Allowances (RDAs). At this writing, a new system is being developed to meet today's expanded needs. The system has been broadened to include several measures, the DRIs.[7,8] The new reference DRIs are a more comprehensive measure of a person's nutritional status and long-term health. The dietitian may use any or all of the following measures to determine a patient's or client's nutritional status:

- Redefined values for RDAs.
- Upper limits for safe intake values, guarding against excessive intakes with common usage of dietary vitamin/mineral supplements. This value is called the Tolerable Upper Intake Level (UL).
- Estimated Average Requirement (EAR).
- Adequate Intake (AI).

These new U.S. DRI nutrient standards for population groups are outlined by age and sex, with special attention to RDAs for older people[9] (see Appendix G). These standards are developed and maintained by a group of leading scientists and practitioners in the field of nutrition, working with the National Academy of Sciences in Washington, D.C. The Academy has numerous divisions of councils and is supported by the National Institutes of Health (Figure 1-1). The working group of nutrition scientists responsible for these nutrition standards comprises the Food and Nutrition Board

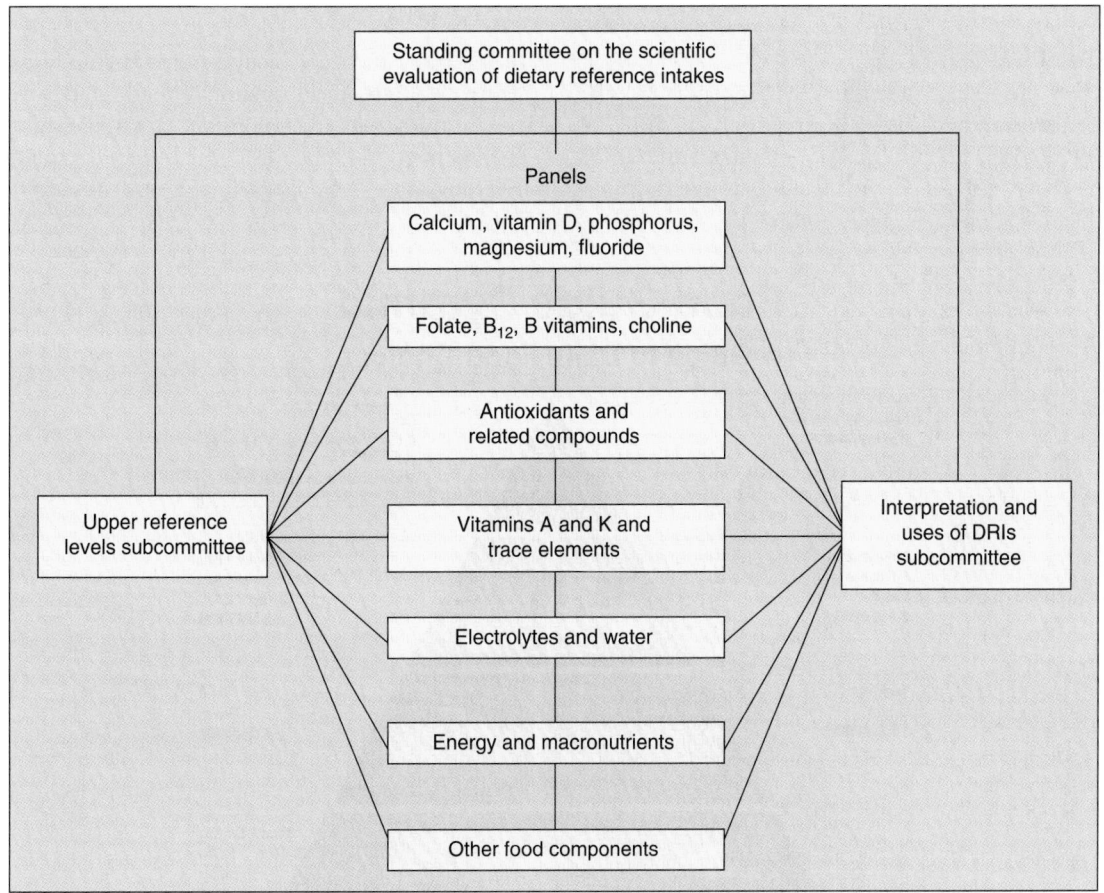

FIGURE 1-1 Dietary Reference Intakes (DRIs) panels of the Institute of Medicine of the National Academy of Sciences. (From Food and Nutrition Board, Institute of Medicine, National Academy of Sciences: *Dietary reference intakes for thiamin, riboflavin, niacin, vitamin B₆, folate, vitamin B₁₂, pantothenic acid, biotin, and choline,* Washington D.C., 1998, National Academy Press.)

of the National Research Council. Their working mandate is to determine the roles of the nutrients in maintaining optimum health and preventing disease.

The U.S. RDA standard was first published during World War II in 1943 as a guide for planning and obtaining food supplies for national defense and providing average population standards as a goal for good nutrition. Over the years, these standards have been revised and expanded about every 5 years to reflect increasing scientific knowledge and social concerns about nutrition and health.

Other Standards

Over the years, Canadian (see Appendix H) and British standards have been similar to the U.S. standards. The current U.S. standard, the DRIs, has been developed with Canadian nutrition sci-

ence associates and is similar to British standards. In less developed countries where factors such as the quality of the available protein foods must be considered, workers look to standards such as those set by the Food and Agriculture Organization (FAO) and the World Health Organization (WHO). Nonetheless, all of these standards provide a guideline to help health workers in a variety of population groups promote good health and prevent disease through sound nutrition.

Food Guides

To interpret and apply sound nutrient standards, health workers need practical food guides to use in nutrition education and food planning with persons and families. Such tools include the long-used U.S. Department of Agriculture

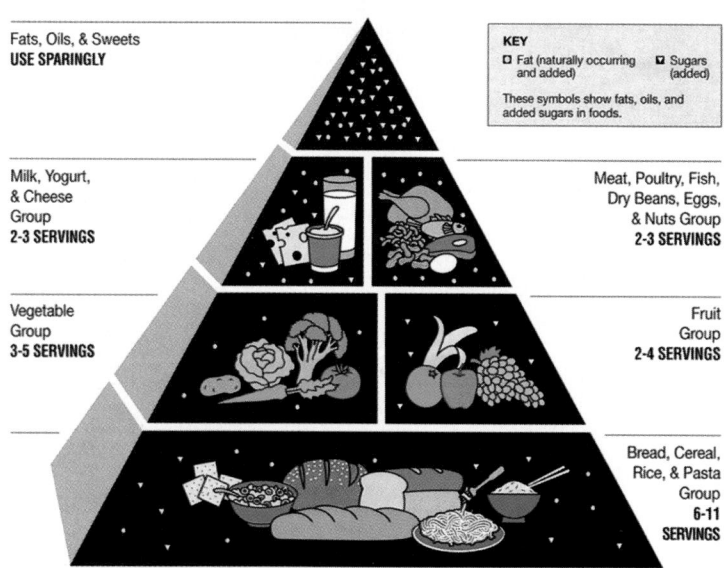

FIGURE 1-2   Food guide pyramid—a guide to daily food choices. (Adapted from the U.S. Department of Agriculture, 1992.)

(USDA) basic food groups guides and the more recent U.S. dietary guidelines.

Basic Food Groups Guide

The basic four food groups guide was developed by the USDA as a general food guide for planning a well-balanced diet. Previous editions of the USDA Basic Four Food Groups have had limitations in relation to rapid changes in food processing, marketing, or current public health concerns. The current edition, in five basic food groups, is especially striking; its visual proportional representation is the now well-known Food Guide Pyramid (Figure 1-2).

This visual has provided a simple practical nutrition education tool, even for young children in elementary schools. The pyramid also serves as a basis for general meal planning and evaluating a person's overall food-intake pattern. A summary outline of this food guide is given in Table 1-1. Major changes focus on a representative total diet emphasizing increased servings in the bread and cereal group (i.e., from 4/day to 6 to 11/day) and the vegetable and fruit groups (i.e., from 4/day to 5 to 9/day). The goal of these changes is to provide the bulk of dietary energy from carbohydrate, while limiting fat intake. Daily food-group choices may be spread over three or more meals, according to personal or family food patterns.

U.S. Dietary Guidelines

The U.S. dietary guidelines were issued as a result of growing public concerns beginning in the 1960s and the subsequent Senate investigations studying hunger and nutrition in the United States. These guidelines are based on our developing concern about chronic health problems in an aging population and a changing food environment. Controversy, centering mainly on the broad issue of the roles of government and science in maintaining health, surrounded the guidelines from the beginning. The USDA and the U.S. Department of Health and Human Services reissued this food guide in 1980 under the title, "The Dietary Guidelines for Americans." These guidelines relate current scientific thinking to America's leading health problems. A new updated statement is issued every 10 years.

Recent review by expert committees has only led to minimal changes over the past decade. The current set of guidelines, from 1995, is titled "Nutrition and Your Health: Dietary Guidelines for Americans."[10] This issue reflects a comprehensive evaluation of the scientific evidence of a relationship between diet and health, based on important findings in a current U.S. report issued jointly by the Departments of Agriculture and Health and Human Services: *Nutrition and Your Health: Dietary Guidelines for Americans* (see the Clinical Applications box, "Dietary Guidelines for Americans"). The seven statements in the current guidelines continue to serve as a useful general guide for a concerned public. Although no guidelines can guarantee health or well-being and

dietary reference intakes (DRIs) a system of reference values that can be used for assessing and planning diets for healthy populations and many other purposes. These values revise and enlarge the Recommended Dietary Allowances (RDAs), which have been published by the National Academy of Sciences since 1941.

recommended dietary allowances (RDAs) recommended daily allowances of nutrients and energy intake for population groups according to age and sex, with defined weight and height. Established and reviewed periodically by a representative group of nutritional scientists, in relation to current research. These standards vary little among the developed countries.

food guide pyramid a visual pattern of the current basic five food groups (bread-cereal, 6-11 servings; vegetable, 3-5 servings; fruit, 2-4 servings; milk-cheese, 2-3 servings; meat-dry beans-egg, 2-3 servings), arranged in a pyramid shape to indicate proportionate amounts of daily food choices. The largest food group, bread-cereal, forms the entire foundation. The next two narrowing tiers indicate relatively fewer daily portions of vegetables and fruits, and then of the milk-cheese and meat-egg groups. The small tip at the pyramid top indicates sparing use of fats, oils, and sweets.

TABLE 1-1   The Guide to Daily Food Choices—a Summary

Food group	Servings	Major contributions	Foods and serving sizes*
Bread, cereals, rice, pasta	6-11	Starch Thiamin Riboflavin† Iron Niacin Folate Magnesium‡ Fiber‡ Zinc	1 slice of bread 1 oz ready-to-eat cereal $1/2$-$3/4$ cup cooked cereal, rice, pasta
Vegetables	3-5	Vitamin A Vitamin C Folate Magnesium Fiber	$1/2$ cup raw or cooked vegetables 1 cup raw leafy vegetables
Fruits	2-4	Vitamin C Fiber	$1/4$ cup dried fruit $1/2$ cup cooked fruit $3/4$ cup juice 1 whole piece of fruit 1 melon wedge
Milk, yogurt, cheese	2 (adult§) 3 (children, teens, young adults, pregnant or lactating women)	Calcium Riboflavin Protein Potassium Zinc	1 cup milk $1^1/2$ oz cheese 2 oz processed cheese 1 cup yogurt 2 cups cottage cheese 1 cup custard/pudding $1^1/2$ cups ice cream
Meat, poultry, fish, dry beans, eggs, nuts	2-3	Protein Niacin Iron Vitamin B$_6$ Zinc Thiamin Vitamin B$_{12}$‖	2-3 oz cooked meat, poultry, fish 1-$1^1/2$ cups cooked dry beans 4 T peanut butter 2 eggs $1/2$-1 cup nuts
Fats, oils, sweets	Foods from this group should not replace any from the other groups. Amounts consumed should be determined by individual energy needs.		

Adapted from the U.S. Department of Agriculture, revised edition of former *Basic Four Food Groups Guide,* 1994. In Wardlaw GM, Insel PM, and Seyler MF: *Contemporary nutrition: issues and insights,* New York, 1992, McGraw-Hill. Used with permission of The McGraw-Hill Companies.

*May be reduced for child servings.
†If enriched.
‡Whole grains especially.
§≥25 years of age.
‖Only in animal food choices.

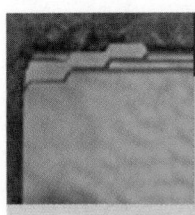

CLINICAL APPLICATIONS

Dietary Guidelines for Americans

Eat a Variety of Foods

About 40 different known nutrients—and probably other unknown factors—are needed to maintain health. No single food can supply all the essential nutrients in the amounts needed to maintain health. Therefore the greater the variety of foods used, the less likely a person is to develop either a deficiency or an excess of any single nutrient. One way to ensure variety, and with it a balanced diet, is to select foods each day from all the major food groups.

Maintain Healthy Weight

Excessive weight is associated with some chronic disorders (e.g., hypertension and diabetes) that also relate to heart disease. Healthy body weight, however, must be determined individually because many factors, such as body composition (i.e., muscle to fat ratio), body metabolism, genetics, and physical activity, are involved.

Choose a Diet Low in Fat, Saturated Fat, and Cholesterol

Americans have traditionally consumed diets high in fat. In some persons, excess fat leads to high levels of blood fats and cholesterol. Elevated levels of fats and cholesterol in blood are associated with a higher risk for coronary heart disease. Therefore it is wise to cut down on fats in general, using them only in moderation.

Choose a Diet with Plenty of Vegetables, Fruits, and Grain Products

Increasing the use of these foods will help supply more of the needed starches (i.e., complex carbohydrates) for energy, many essential nutrients, and necessary dietary fiber. Research indicates that certain types of dietary fiber may help control chronic bowel diseases, contribute to improved blood glucose management for persons with diabetes mellitus, and bind dietary cholesterol.

Use Sugars Only in Moderation

The major health hazard of eating too much sugar is tooth decay (i.e., dental caries). Contrary to popular opinion, however, too much sugar does not in itself cause diabetes but can contribute to poor control of diabetes in persons who have inherited the disease. Most Americans consume a relatively large amount of sugar, over 100 pounds per person per year, much of it in processed food products. Again, moderation is the key.

Use Salt and Sodium Only in Moderation

Our main source of dietary sodium is ordinary table salt. Excessive salt is not healthy for anyone and certainly not for persons who have high blood pressure. Many processed food products contain a considerable amount of salt and other sodium compounds, and many Americans use more salt than necessary in foods. Therefore it is wise to limit salt use in food preparation or at the table, as well as to reduce the use of "salty" food products. These reductions will lower individual salt tastes, which are learned habits and not biologic necessities. Enough sodium is present as a natural mineral in foods to meet usual needs.

If You Drink Alcoholic Beverages, Do So in Moderation

Alcoholic beverages tend to be high in kcalories and low in other nutrients. Limited food intake may accompany large alcohol intake. Also, heavy drinking contributes to chronic liver disease and some neurologic disorders, as well as some throat and neck cancers. Moreover, it is a major factor in highway deaths. Therefore if alcohol is used at all, moderation is the key, and *never* drink and drive.

From U.S. Department of Agriculture and U.S. Department of Health and Human Services: *Nutrition and your health: dietary guidelines for Americans,* ed 4, Home and Garden Bull No 232, Washington DC, 1995, U.S. Government Printing Office.

people differ widely in their food needs, these general statements can lead persons to evaluate their food habits and move toward general improvements. Good food habits based on moderation and variety can help to build sound healthy bodies.

Individual Needs

Person-Centered Care

Regardless of the type of food guide used, health workers must remember that food patterns vary with individual needs, tastes, habits, living situations, and energy demands. Persons who eat nutritionally balanced meals spread fairly evenly throughout the day, however, can usually work more efficiently and sustain a more even energy supply.

Changing Food Environment

In recent years, our food environment has been rapidly changing. There are more processed food items of variable or unknown nutrient quality. American food habits may have deteriorated in some ways. Despite a plentiful food supply, surveys give evidence of malnutrition, even among hospitalized patients. Nurses and other health workers have an important responsibility in observing patients' food intake carefully. In general, however, it is encouraging to note that Americans are gradually learning that what they eat does influence their health. Even fast food restaurants, where Americans often eat, are beginning to respond to their customers' desires for less fat, and some have also added self-help salad bars. Other chain, family, and university restaurants are developing and testing similar patterns in new menu items. More than ever, Americans are being selective about what they eat. Guided by the FDA nutrition labels on processed food items, shoppers' choices indicate an increased awareness of nutritional values. Details of these marketing regulations are given in Chapter 14.

SUMMARY

Good food and key nutrients are essential to life and health. In our changing world, an emphasis on health promotion and disease prevention through reducing health risks has become our primary health goal. The importance of a balanced diet in meeting this health goal through the functioning of its component nutrients is fundamental. Food guides that help persons plan such a healthy diet include the DRIs, the basic Food Guide Pyramid, and the U.S. dietary guidelines.

REVIEW QUESTIONS

1. What is the current U.S. national health goal? Define this goal in terms of health, wellness, and the differences between traditional and preventive approaches to health.
2. Why is a balanced diet important? List and describe some signs of good nutrition.
3. What are the three basic functions of foods and their nutrients? Describe the general roles of nutrients in relation to the following functions: (1) main nutrient(s) for that function, and (2) other contributing nutrients.
4. With regard to both purpose and use, compare a nutrient standard, such as the DRIs, with a food group guide, such as the Food Guide Pyramid.
5. Using the Food Guide Pyramid, plan a day's food pattern for a selected person with modifications according to the Dietary Guidelines for Americans.

SELF-TEST QUESTIONS

True-False

Write the correct statement for each item you answer "false."

1. The diet-planning tool Dietary Guidelines for Americans stresses the two basic concepts of variety and moderation in food habits.
2. Food processing has little influence on food taste, appearance, safety, or nutrient values.
3. Certain foods are called "complete foods" because they contain all the nutrients essential for full growth and health and are therefore essential in everyone's diet.

Multiple Choice

1. Nutrients are:
   a. Chemical elements or compounds in foods that have specific metabolic functions.
   b. Foods that are necessary for good health.
   c. Metabolic control substances, such as enzymes.
   d. Nourishing foods used to cure certain illnesses.
2. All nutrients needed by the body:
   a. Must be obtained by specific food combinations.
   b. Must be obtained by vitamin and/or mineral supplements.
   c. Have a variety of functions and uses in the body.
   d. Are supplied by a variety of foods in many different combinations.
3. All persons throughout life, as indicated by the DRIs, need:
   a. The same nutrients in varying amounts.
   b. The same amount of nutrients in any state of health.
   c. The same nutrients at any age in the same amounts.
   d. Different nutrients in varying amounts.

SUGGESTIONS FOR ADDITIONAL STUDY

1. Keep a notebook throughout the course. Cut out any articles on nutrition that you find; bring them to class for discussion and evaluation; then paste them in your notebook.
2. Make a list of your food intake for 3 days and analyze each day using the following: (1) the basic Food Guide Pyramid, and (2) the Dietary Guidelines for Americans. Compare the two results. Which of the two food guides do you think is more useful? Why?
3. At some time during the first half of the course, give a special report on the phase of nutrition that interests you most. Present your report to the class, then place it in your notebook.

REFERENCES

1. U.S. Department of Health and Human Services, Public Health Service: Healthy People 2000: National Health Promotion and Disease Prevention Objectives—Nutrition Priority Area, *Nutr Today* 25(6):29, 1990.
2. U.S. Department of Health and Human Services: *Healthy people 2010: understanding and improving health,* Washington, D.C., 2000, Government Printing Office.
3. Bassuk EL and others: Single mothers and welfare, *Sci Am* 275(4):60, 1996.
4. Bassuk EL and others: Homelessness in female-headed families: childhood and adult risk and protective factors, *Am J Pub Health* 87(2):241, 1997.
5. Brekey WR: It's time for the public health community to declare war on homelessness, *Am J Pub Health* 87(2):153, 1997.

6. Brown JL, Pollitt E: Malnutrition, poverty, and intellectual development, *Sci Am* 274(2):38, 1996.

7. Staff report, Public policy news: Translating the science behind the Dietary Reference Intakes, *J Am Diet Assoc* 98(7):756, 1998.

8. Yates AA, Schlicker SA, Suitor CW: Dietary Reference Intakes: the new basis for recommendation for calcium and related B vitamins, and choline, *J Am Diet Assoc* 98(6): 699, 1998.

9. Russell RM: New views on the RDAs for older adults, *J Am Diet Assoc* 97(5):515, 1997.

10. Kennedy E and others: The 1995 Dietary Guidelines for Americans, an overview, *J Am Diet Assoc* 96(3):234, 1996.

FURTHER READING

• Callaway CW: Dietary Guidelines for Americans: an historical perspective, *J Am Coll Nutr* 16(6):510, 1997.

This article describes the interesting history of the U.S. Dietary Guidelines since they were established in 1980. Each step along the way shows the insight and dedicated work of participating nutrition scientists and the increasing interest of the American public in the relationships between food habits and health.

• Raloff J: Why cutting fats may harm the heart, *Sci News* 155(12):181, 1999.

This interesting glimpse of new research in Berkeley, California helps us to understand that all fat in the diet is not bad but does require us to make distinctions between types of fat.

2

Carbohydrates

KEY CONCEPTS

- Carbohydrate foods provide practical body fuel sources because of their availability, relatively low cost, and storage capacity.

- Carbohydrate structure varies from simple to complex, so it can provide both quick and extended energy for the body.

- An indigestible carbohydrate, dietary fiber, serves separately as a body regulatory agent.

As discussed in Chapter 1, key nutrients in foods sustain life and promote health. These tremendous results are possible because the human body's unique use of these nutrients provides three essential life and health needs, as follow: (1) *energy* to do its work, (2) *building materials* to maintain its form and functions, and (3) *control agents* to regulate these processes efficiently.

These three basic life and health functions of nutrients are closely related—no nutrient ever works alone. For this study, as indicated in the previous chapter, we will look at each of the nutrients separately, remembering that in our bodies they do not exist or work that way. In this chapter, we consider the first of these life needs—*energy production*—and the body's primary fuel for its energy system—*carbohydrates*.

NATURE OF CARBOHYDRATES
Relation to Energy

Basic Fuel Source

Energy is a necessity for life. It is the power an organism requires to do its work. Any energy system must first have a basic fuel supply. In the human energy system, vast energy resources from the sun enable plants, through their internal system of photosynthesis, to transform solar energy into carbohydrates, the stored fuel form of plants.[1] Because the human body can rapidly break down these stores of quick and sustaining energy foods—sugars and starches, they provide our major source of energy.

Energy-Production System

To produce energy from a basic fuel supply, a successful energy system must be able to do the following three things: (1) change the basic fuel to a refined fuel that the machine is designed to use; (2) carry this refined fuel to the places that need it; and (3) burn this refined fuel in the special equipment set up at these places. Far more efficient than any man-made machine, the body easily does these three things. It digests its basic fuel, carbohydrate, changing it to glucose. The body then absorbs and, through blood circulation, carries this refined fuel to cells that need glucose. Glucose is burned in the specific and intricate equipment in these cells, and energy is released through the amazing process of cell metabolism. Because the human body can

TABLE 2-1 Summary of carbohydrate classes

Chemical class name	Class members	Sources
Polysaccharides	Starch	Grains and grain products
Multiple sugars, complex carbohydrates		Cereal, bread, crackers, and other baked goods
		Pasta
		Rice, corn, bulgur
		Legumes
		Potatoes and other vegetables
	Glycogen	Animal tissues, liver and muscle meats
	Dietary fiber	Whole grains
		Fruits
		Vegetables
		Seeds, nuts, skins
Disaccharides	Sucrose	"Table" sugar: sugar cane, sugar beets
Double sugars, simple carbohydrates		Molasses
	Lactose	Milk
	Maltose	Starch digestion, intermediate
		Sweetener in food products
		Starch digestion, final
Monosaccharides	Glucose (dextrose)	Corn syrup (large use in processed foods)
Single sugars, simple carbohydrates		
	Fructose	Fruits, honey
	Galactose	Lactose (milk)

rapidly break down the starches and sugars we eat to yield energy, carbohydrates are called "quick energy" foods and are our major source of energy.

Practical Dietary Importance

There are also practical reasons for the large quantities of carbohydrates in diets all over the world. First, carbohydrates are widely available, easily grown in grains, legumes, other vegetables, and fruits. In some countries, carbohydrate foods make up almost the entire diet of the people. In the typical American diet, about half of the total kcalories is in the form of carbohydrates. Second, carbohydrates are relatively low in cost when compared with many other food items. Third, carbohydrates may be easily stored. They can be kept in dry storage for relatively long periods without spoilage. Modern processing and packaging extend the shelf life of carbohydrate products almost indefinitely.

The U.S. Department of Agriculture (USDA) regularly surveys individual food intakes. These reports usually indicate that about half of the total kcalories in the American diet come from carbohydrates, with children consuming somewhat more than adults. Daily intake of sugars by Americans accounts for about 20% of total kcalories and may range as high as 40% in individuals consuming increased amounts of sweets and foods processed with high-fructose corn syrup. As a result, the typical American sugar consumption is always considerably higher than the FDA guidelines for a healthy diet. The remainder of the total carbohydrate kcalories comes from starches.

Classes of Carbohydrates

The name *carbohydrate* comes from its chemical nature. A carbohydrate is composed of carbon (C), hydrogen (H), and oxygen (O), with the hydrogen/oxygen ratio usually that of water: H_2O. Its abbreviated name, CHO, which is the combination of the chemical symbols of its three components, is often used in medical charts or various notations. The term *saccharide* used as a carbohydrate class name comes from the Latin word *saccharum*, meaning "sugar." Thus a saccharide unit is a single sugar

unit. Carbohydrates are classified according to the number of sugar, or saccharide, units making up their structure: *monosaccharides* have one sugar unit; *disaccharides* have two sugar units; and *polysaccharides* have many sugar units. Monosaccharides and disaccharides are small, simple structures of only one- and two-sugar units, so they are called simple carbohydrates. Polysaccharides, however, are large, complex compounds of many saccharide units in long chains, so they are called complex carbohydrates. For example, starch, the most significant polysaccharide in human nutrition, is made up of many coiled and branching chains in a tree-like structure. Each of the multiple branching chains is composed of 24 to 30 sugar units of glucose, which gradually split off in digestion to supply a steady source of energy over a period of time. Table 2-1 summarizes these classes of carbohydrates.

---

photosynthesis (Gr. *photos,* light; *synthesis,* putting together) process by which plants containing chlorophyll are able to manufacture carbohydrate by combining CO_2 from air and water from soil. Sunlight is used as energy; chlorophyll is a catalyst. $6\ CO_2 + 6\ H_2O + Energy \rightarrow Chlorophyll \rightarrow C_6H_{12}O_6 + 6\ O_2$

saccharide (L. *saccharum,* sugar) chemical name for sugar molecules. May occur as single molecules in monosaccharides (glucose, fructose, maltose), as two molecules in disaccharides (sucrose, lactose, maltose), or as multiple molecules in polysaccharides (starch, dietary fiber, glycogen).

simple carbohydrates sugars with a simple structure of one or two single sugar (saccharide) units. A monosaccharide is composed of one sugar unit; a disaccharide is composed of two sugar units.

complex carbohydrates larger, more complex molecules of carbohydrates composed of many sugar units (polysaccharides). Complex forms of dietary carbohydrates are starch, which is digestable and provides a major energy source, and dietary fiber, which is nondigestible (humans lack the necessary enzymes) and thus provides important bulk in the diet.

Monosaccharides

The three important simple single sugars in nutrition are glucose, fructose, and galactose.

Glucose. The basic single sugar in body metabolism is glucose, which is the form of sugar that circulates in the blood and is the primary fuel to the cells. It is not usually found as such in the diet, except for in corn syrup used alone or in processed food items. The body supply comes mainly from the digestion of starch. Glucose is a moderately sweet sugar. Glucose is also sometimes called *dextrose*.

Fructose. Fructose is found mainly in fruits, from which it gets its name, or in honey. Honey therefore is a form of sugar and cannot be used as a sugar substitute. The amount of fructose in fruits depends on the degree of ripeness. As a fruit ripens, some of its stored starch turns to sugar. High-fructose corn syrups are increasingly being used in processed food products and are a major factor of increased sugar intake. Fructose is the sweetest of the simple sugars.

Galactose. Galactose is also not usually found as such in the diet but comes mainly from the digestion of milk sugar, or lactose.

All of these monosaccharides, or simple single sugars, require no digestion. They are quickly absorbed from the intestine into the blood stream and carried to the liver. In the liver, they are converted by enzymes into glycogen for a constant back-up energy supply or used for immediate energy needs.

Disaccharides

Disaccharides are simple double sugars, comprised of two single-sugar units linked together. The three disaccharides important in nutrition are sucrose, lactose, and maltose.

Sucrose. Sucrose is common table sugar. Its two single-sugar units are glucose and fructose. Sucrose is used in the form of granulated, powdered, or brown sugar and is made from sugar cane or sugar beets. Molasses, a by-product of sugar production, is also a form of sucrose. When people speak of sugar in the diet, they usually mean sucrose.

Lactose. The sugar in milk is lactose. Its two single-sugar units are glucose and galactose. Lactose is the only common sugar not found in plants and is less soluble and sweet than sucrose. Lactose remains in the intestine longer than other sugars and encourages the growth of certain useful bacteria. It is formed in the mammary glands and composes about 40% of the milk solids. Cow's milk contains 4.8% lactose, and human milk contains 7% lactose. Because lactose aids in the absorption of calcium and phosphorus, the presence of all three nutrients in milk is a fortunate circumstance, as well as an example of why milk is one of nature's best "package" foods. About 75% of adults worldwide are lactose-intolerant but can tolerate such lactose-free milk products as cheese.[2,3]

Maltose. Maltose is not usually found as such in the diet. It is derived in the body from the intermediate digestive breakdown of starch. Because starch is made up entirely of many single glucose units, the two single sugar units that compose maltose are both glucose. Maltose is used as a sweetener in various processed foods.

The *sugar alcohols* are a group of sugar-related substances. Probably the most well-known of these compounds is sorbitol, which has been widely used as a sucrose substitute in various foods, candies, chewing gum, and beverages. Sugar alcohols such as sorbitol, however, share absorption with glucose in the small intestine, and then are digested by fermenting bacteria in the colon. Thus two negative results counteract the dietary use of sugar alcohols as a sugar substitute, as follow: (1) the kcalorie value of sugar alcohols is approximately that of glucose, so they contribute the same amount of energy and are not actually sugar-savers; and (2) their colonic fermentation causes diarrhea (see Chapter 18).

Polysaccharides

Polysaccharides are complex carbohydrates composed of many single sugar units. The important polysaccharides in nutrition include starch, glycogen, and dietary fiber.

Starch. Starches are by far the most significant polysaccharides in the diet. They are found in grains, in legumes and other vegetables, and in some fruits in minute amounts. Starches are more complex in structure than simple sugars. Thus they break down more slowly and supply energy over a longer period of time. For starch to be used more promptly by the body, the outer membrane can be broken down by grinding or cooking. Cooking of starch not only improves its flavor but also softens and ruptures the starch cells, making digestion easier. Starch mixtures thicken when cooked because the portion that encases the starch granules has a gel-like quality, thickening the starch mixture in the same way that pectin causes jelly to set.

Starch is the most important dietary carbohydrate worldwide. The value of starch in human nutrition and health has recently received a great deal of recognition. The U.S. dietary guidelines (see Chapter 1) recommend that about 50% to 55% of our total kcalories come from carbohydrates, with a greater portion of that intake coming from complex carbohydrate forms of starch. In many other countries where starch is a staple food, it makes up an even higher portion of the diet. The major food sources of starch (Figure 2-1) include grains in the form of cereals, pastas, crackers, breads, and other baked goods; legumes in the form of beans and peas; potatoes, rice, corn, and bulgur; and other vegetables, especially of the root variety.

The term *whole grain* is used for food products such as flours, breads, or cereals that are produced from unrefined grain, which is grain that still retains its outer bran layers and inner germ endosperm (Figure 2-2) and their nutrients (i.e., dietary fiber, minerals and vitamins). The term *enriched grains* refers to refined grain products to which key nutrients—usually minerals (e.g., iron and calcium) and vitamins (e.g., A, C, thiamin, riboflavin, and niacin)—have been added. Ready-to-eat breakfast cereals usually contain additional nutrients such as vitamins D, E, B_6, and folic acid, as well as the minerals phosphorus, magnesium, and zinc. These cereals, which are a favorite breakfast item for children, have become a major source of their vitamin and mineral intake.

Glycogen. Glycogen is similar in structure to starch, so it is sometimes called *animal starch*. The animal body contains little glycogen, however, and this small amount drains away when meat is prepared for sale. Glycogen is not a significant carbohydrate in diets. Rather, it is a carbohydrate formed within the body's tissues and is crucial to the body's metabolism and energy balance. Glycogen is found in the liver and muscles, where it is constantly recycled (i.e., broken down to form glucose for immediate energy needs and resynthesized for storage in the liver and muscles). These small stores of glycogen help sustain normal blood sugar during short-term fasting periods (e.g., during sleep) and provide immediate fuel for muscle action. These reserves also protect cells from depressed metabolic function and injury.

Dietary fiber. Several types of dietary fiber are polysaccharides. Because humans lack the necessary enzymes to digest dietary fiber, these substances do not have a direct energy value like other carbohydrates. Their inability to be digested, however, makes these materials important dietary assets. Increasing attention has focused on the relation of fiber to health promotion and disease prevention, especially to gastrointestinal problems

---

sorbitol a sugar alcohol formed in mammals from glucose and converted to fructose. Named for its initial discovery in nature, found in ripe berries of the tree *Sorbus acuparia;* also occurs in small quantities in various other berries, cherries, plums, and pears. Produced in food industry laboratories for use as a sweetener in candies, chewing gum, beverages, and other foodstuffs; side effect of diarrhea limits use.

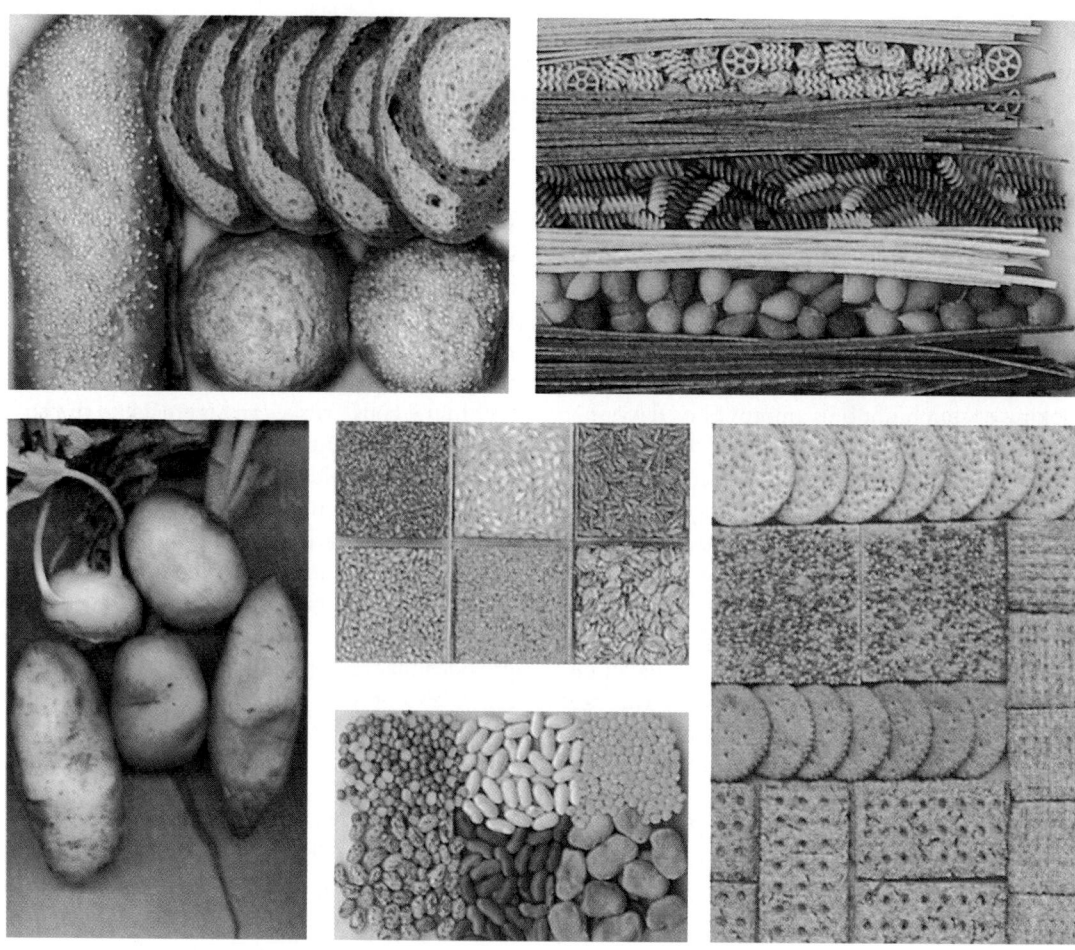

FIGURE 2-1 Complex carbohydrate foods. (Credit: Amy Buxton.)

and management of diabetes. The types of dietary fiber important in human nutrition are described in the following paragraphs.

Cellulose. Cellulose is the chief part of the framework of plants. It remains undigested in the gastrointestinal tract and provides important bulk to the diet. This bulk helps move the food mass along, stimulates normal muscle action in the intestine, and forms feces for elimination of waste products. The main sources of cellulose are the stems and leaves of vegetables and the coverings of seeds and grains.

Noncellulose polysaccharides. Hemicellulose, pectins, gums and mucilages, and algal substances are noncellulose polysaccharides. They absorb water and swell to a larger bulk, thus slowing the emptying of the food mass from the stomach, binding bile acids (including cholesterol) in the intestine, and preventing spastic colon pressure by providing bulk for normal muscle action. Noncellulose polysaccharides also provide fermentation material on which colon bacteria can work.

Lignin. Lignin, the only noncarbohydrate type of dietary fiber, is a large compound that forms the

TABLE 2-2   Summary of dietary fiber classes

	Source	Function
Cellulose	Main cell wall constituent of plants	Holds water; reduces elevated colonic intraluminal pressure; binds zinc
Noncellulose polysaccharides	Secretions of plants	Slow gastric emptying; provide fermentable material for colonic bacteria with production of gas and volatile fatty acids; bind bile acids and cholesterol
Gums	Plant secretions and seeds	
Mucilages		
Algal polysaccharides	Algae, seaweeds	
Pectin substances	Intercellular cement plant material	
Hemicellulose	Cell wall plant material	Holds water and increases stool bulk; reduces elevated colonic pressure; binds bile acids
Lignin	Woody part of plants	Antioxidant; binds bile acids, cholesterol, and metals

woody part of certain plants. It binds the cellulose fibers in plants, giving added strength and stiffness to plant cell walls. It also combines with bile acids and cholesterol in the human intestine, preventing their absorption.

Table 2-2 provides a summary of these dietary fiber classes, along with the sources and functions of each. As a means of simplification, dietary fiber is usually divided into two groups based on solubility. Cellulose, lignin, and most hemicelluloses are not soluble in water. The rest of the dietary fibers (e.g., most pectins and other polysaccharides such as gums and mucilages), however, are water-soluble. These two classes of dietary fiber based on solubility are summarized in Box 2-1. The looser physical structure and greater water-holding capacity of gums, mucilages, pectins, and algal polysaccharides (e.g., those derived from seaweed) partly account for their greater water-solubility. Note the ordered stacking of the structural chain segments in insoluble fibers such as cellulose.

In general, the food groups that provide needed dietary fiber include whole grains in their many food forms (i.e., legumes, vegetables, and fruits with as much of their skin remaining as possible). Whole grains provide a special natural "pack-

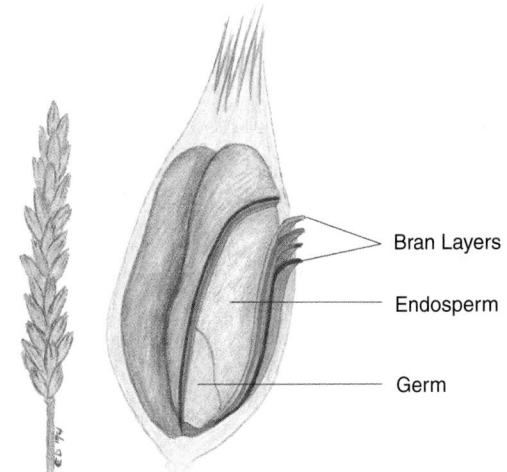

FIGURE 2-2   Kernel of wheat, showing bran layers, endosperm, and germ. (Credit: Eileen Draper.)

age" of both the complex carbohydrate starch and the fiber in its coating.[4,5] In addition, whole grains contain an abundance of vitamins and minerals.

Many health organizations have recommended increasing the intake of complex carbohydrates, in general, or dietary fiber, in particular, and a range of dietary intakes has been suggested by study groups. There is a growing discussion and consensus among scientists and the public to add complex carbohydrates to the nutrition label on foods.[6]

The Food and Nutrition Board has always indicated that a desirable fiber intake should not be achieved by adding concentrated fiber supplements to the diet, but by eating a higher fiber diet of whole grains, fruits, vegetables, and legumes, which also provide vitamins and minerals. A general daily increase to 25 g/1000 kcal to 40 g/1000 kcal of total dietary fiber appears to be a reasonable goal. This intake would require consistent use of whole grains, legumes, vegetables, fruits, seeds, and nuts. A table of the dietary fiber content of some commonly used foods is provided in Table 2-3 and Appendix C.

FUNCTIONS OF CARBOHYDRATES
Primary Energy Function

Basic Fuel Supply
The main function of carbohydrates is to provide the primary fuel for the body. To meet energy needs, carbohydrates burn in the body at the rate of 4 kcal/g. Thus the fuel factor for carbohydrates is 4. Carbohydrates furnish readily available energy that is needed not only for physical activities but also for all the work of the body cells. Fat is also a fuel, but the body only needs a small amount of dietary fat, mainly to supply the essential fatty acids (Chapter 3).

Reserve Fuel Supply
Glycogen reserves supply vital backup fuel. The total amount of carbohydrate in the body, including both glycogen and blood sugar, is relatively small. Without constant resupply, however, this total amount of available glucose only provides enough energy for about a half day of moderate activity. Therefore to maintain a normal blood glucose level and prevent a breakdown of fat and protein in tissue, individuals must eat carbohydrate foods regularly to meet energy demands.

BOX 2-1 Summary of soluble and insoluble fibers in total dietary fiber

Insoluble	Soluble
Cellulose	Gums
Most hemicelluloses	Mucilages
Lignin	Algal polysaccharides
	Most pectins

Special Tissue Functions

Carbohydrates also serve special functions in many body tissues as part of their basic function as the body's main energy source.

Liver
Glycogen reserves in the liver and muscles provide a constant exchange with the body's overall energy-balance system. These reserves, especially in the liver, protect cells from depressed metabolic function and resulting injury.

Protein and Fat
Carbohydrate helps regulate both protein and fat metabolism. If there is sufficient dietary carbohydrate to meet general body energy needs, protein will not have to be drained off to supply energy. Instead it will be used for its main purpose of tissue building. This *protein-sparing action* of carbohydrate thus protects protein, allowing it to be used for its major role in tissue growth and maintenance. Likewise, with sufficient carbohydrate for energy, fat will not be needed to supply large amounts of energy. Such a rapid breakdown of fat would produce excess materials called *ketones*, which result from incomplete fat oxidation in the cells. Ketones are strong acids, so this condition of acidosis, or *ketosis*, upsets the normal acid-base balance of the body and can become serious. This protective action of carbohydrate is called its *antiketogenic* effect.

Heart
The constant action of the heart muscle sustains life. Although fatty acids are the preferred regular fuel for the heart muscle, glycogen is vital emergency fuel. In

TABLE 2-3 Dietary fiber and kilocalorie values for selected foods

Foods	Serving	Dietary fiber (g)	Kcalories
Breads and cereals			
All Bran	1/3 cup	8.5	70
Bran (100%)	1/2 cup	8.4	75
Bran Buds	1/3 cup	7.9	75
Corn Bran	2/3 cup	5.4	100
Bran Chex	2/3 cup	4.6	90
Cracklin' Oat Bran	1/3 cup	4.3	110
Bran Flakes	3/4 cup	4.0	90
Air-popped popcorn	1 cup	2.5	25
Oatmeal	1 cup	2.2	144
Grapenuts	1/4 cup	1.4	100
Whole-wheat bread	1 slice	1.4	60
Legumes, cooked			
Kidney beans	1/2 cup	7.3	110
Lima beans	1/2 cup	4.5	130
Vegetables, cooked			
Green peas	1/2 cup	3.6	55
Corn	1/2 cup	2.9	70
Parsnip	1/2 cup	2.7	50
Potato, with skin	1 medium	2.5	95
Brussel sprouts	1/2 cup	2.3	30
Carrots	1/2 cup	2.3	25
Broccoli	1/2 cup	2.2	20
Beans, green	1/2 cup	1.6	15
Tomato, chopped	1/2 cup	1.5	17
Cabbage, red & white	1/2 cup	1.4	15
Kale	1/2 cup	1.4	20
Cauliflower	1/2 cup	1.1	15
Lettuce (fresh)	1 cup	0.8	7
Fruits			
Apple	1 medium	3.5	80
Raisins	1/4 cup	3.1	110
Prunes, dried	3	3.0	60
Strawberries	1 cup	3.0	45
Orange	1 medium	2.6	60
Banana	1 medium	2.4	105
Blueberries	1/2 cup	2.0	40
Dates, dried	3	1.9	70
Peach	1 medium	1.9	35

Continued

TABLE 2-3   Dietary fiber and kilocalorie values for selected foods—cont'd

Foods	Serving	Dietary fiber (g)	Kcalories
Fruits—cont'd			
Apricot, fresh	3 medium	1.8	50
Grapefruit	1/2 cup	1.6	40
Apricot, dried	5 halves	1.4	40
Cherries	10	1.2	50
Pineapple	1/2 cup	1.1	40

Adapted from Lanza E and Butrum RR: A critical review of food fiber analysis and data, *J Am Diet Assoc* 86:732, 1986.

a damaged heart, low glycogen stores or inadequate carbohydrate intake may cause symptoms of cardiac disorder and angina.

Central Nervous System

Constant carbohydrate intake and reserves are necessary for proper functioning of the central nervous system (CNS). The master center of the CNS, the brain, has no stored supply of glucose. Therefore it is especially dependent on a minute-to-minute supply of glucose from the blood. Sustained and profound shock from low blood sugar may cause brain damage and can result in death.

FOOD SOURCES OF CARBOHYDRATES

Starches

As indicated earlier, starches provide fundamental complex carbohydrate foods for slowly available glucose (SAG), thus sustaining the energy sources of primary rapidly available glucose (RAG).[1] Starches are the central type of food for a balanced diet. In unrefined forms, they also provide important sources of fiber and other nutrients.

Sugars

Sugar per se is not the villain in the story of health. The problem lies in the large quantities of sugar that many people consume, often to the exclusion of other important foods. High-sugar diets do carry health risks, such as dental caries and obesity. The average American consumes about one-third pound of sugar per day, which may lead to problems. So, as with many things, moderation is the key.

DIGESTION OF CARBOHYDRATES

Mouth

The digestion of carbohydrate foods, starches and sugars, begins in the mouth and progresses through the successive parts of the gastrointestinal tract, accomplished by two types of actions, as follow: (1) mechanical or muscle functions that break the food mass into smaller particles, and (2) chemical processes in which specific enzymes break down the food nutrients into still smaller usable metabolic products.[7] The chewing of the food, a process called *mastication*, breaks food into fine particles and mixes it with saliva. During this process, the salivary enzyme *ptyalin* is secreted by the *parotid* glands, which lie under each ear at the back of jaw. Ptyalin acts on starch to begin its breakdown into dextrins (i.e., intermediate starch breakdown products) and then maltose. Maltose is later changed into glucose.

Stomach

Wavelike contraction of the muscle fibers of the stomach wall continue the mechanical digestive

TABLE 2-4 Summary of carbohydrate digestion

Organ	Enzyme	Action
Mouth	Ptyalin	Starch → Dextrins → Maltose
Stomach	None	(Above action continued to minor degree)
Small intestine	Pancreatic amylopsin	Starch → Dextrins → Maltose
	Intestinal:	
	Sucrase	Sucrose → Glucose + Fructose
	Lactase	Lactose → Glucose + Galactose
	Maltase	Maltose → Glucose + Glucose

process. This action, which is called *peristalsis*, further mixes food particles with gastric secretions to facilitate chemical digestion. The gastric secretions contain no specific enzyme for the breakdown of carbohydrate. The hydrochloric acid in the stomach stops the action of the salivary ptyalin in the food mass. Before the food mixes completely with the acidic stomach secretions, however, up to 20% to 30% of the starch may have been changed to maltose. Muscle action continues to mix the food mass and move it to the lower part of the stomach. Here the food mass is a thick creamy *chyme*, ready for its controlled emptying through the *pyloric valve* into the *duodenum*, the first portion of the small intestine.

Small Intestine

Peristalsis continues to aid digestion in the small intestine by mixing and moving the chyme along the length of the tube. Chemical digestion of carbohydrate is completed in the small intestine by specific enzymes from both the pancreas and the intestine.

Pancreatic Secretions

Secretions from the *pancreas* enter the duodenum through the common bile duct. These secretions contain a starch enzyme, *pancreatic amylase*, which is commonly called *amylopsin*. This enzyme continues the breakdown of starch to maltose.

Intestinal Secretions

Secretions from small glands in the intestinal wall contain three disaccharidases: *sucrase, lactase,* and *maltase.* These specific enzymes act on their respective disaccharides to render the monosaccharides—glucose, galactose, and fructose—ready for absorption directly into the portal blood circulation.

A summary of the major aspects of carbohydrate digestion through the successive parts of the gastrointestinal tract is shown in Table 2-4. The

enzyme (Gr. *en,* in; *zyme,* leaven) specific proteins produced in cells that digest or change specific nutrients in specific chemical reactions without being changed themselves in the process. Their action is therefore that of a *catalyst.* Digestive enzymes in the gastrointestinal secretions act on food substances to break them down into simpler compounds. An enzyme is usually named according to the substance (substrate) on which it acts, with common word ending of *-ase;* for example, sucrase is the specific enzyme for sucrose, which it breaks down into glucose and fructose.

portal (L. *porta,* a portal or doorway) an entrance or gateway; for example, the portal blood circulation designates the entry of blood vessels from the intestines into the liver, carrying nutrients for major liver metabolism, then draining into the body's main systemic circulation to deliver metabolic products to body cells.

overall processes of absorption and metabolism of all of the energy-yielding nutrients together—carbohydrate, fat, and protein—are discussed in Chapter 9.

BODY NEEDS FOR CARBOHYDRATES

Dietary Reference Intakes (DRIs)

There is no single recommended dietary allowance for carbohydrate as such in the DRIs.[8] In the nutrient standards, energy needs are listed as total kcalories, which includes caloric intake from fat and protein, as well as carbohydrate. Additionally, there is no specific DRI standard for dietary fiber beyond the general recommendation that a desirable fiber intake be achieved by consumption of whole-grain cereals, legumes, vegetables, and fruits—which also provide minerals and vitamins, rather than by adding fiber concentrates as supplements.

U.S. Dietary Guidelines

The recommended amount of carbohydrate in the diet outlined in the U.S. dietary guidelines for health is given in percent of total kcalories. To achieve an optimal balance for health, these guidelines recommend that 55% to 60% of the total kcalories in the diet come from carbohydrates, with the large majority from *complex* carbohydrates, or starches. Achieving this balance would necessitate a reduction in the amount of sugar and sweets consumed, which would be an improvement in the health habits of many individuals.

SUMMARY

The primary source of energy for most of the world's population comes from carbohydrate foods. These foods are from widely distributed plant sources, such as grains, legumes, vegetables, and fruits. For the most part, these food products store easily and are relatively low in cost.

Two basic types of carbohydrates supply energy: complex and simple. Simple carbohydrates are made up of single and double sugar units (monosaccharides and disaccharides). Because simple carbohydrates are easy to digest and absorb, they provide quick energy. Complex carbohydrates, or polysaccharides, are made up of many sugar units. They break down more slowly and thus provide sustained energy over a longer period of time.

Dietary fiber in most of its forms is complex carbohydrate that is not digestible. It occurs mainly as the structural parts of plants and provides important bulk in the diet, affects nutrient absorption, and benefits health.

Carbohydrate digestion starts briefly in the mouth with the initial action of the salivary enzyme ptyalin to begin breaking down starch into maltose. There is no enzyme for starch breakdown in the stomach, but muscle action continues to mix the food mass and move it on to enter the small intestine. Final starch and disaccharide digestion occurs in the small intestine with the action of specific enzymes—sucrase, lactase, and maltase—to produce the single-sugar units glucose, fructose, and galactose, which then are absorbed directly into the portal blood circulation to the liver.

REVIEW QUESTIONS

1. Why is carbohydrate the predominant type of food in the world's diets? Give some basic examples of these carbohydrate foods.

2. What are the main classes of carbohydrates? Describe each in terms of general nature, functions, and main food sources.

3. Compare starches and sugars as a basic fuel. Why are complex carbohydrates a significant part of a healthy diet? What is the recommendation about the use of sugars in such a diet? Why?

4. Describe the types and functions of dietary fiber. What are the main food sources? What amount of fiber is generally recommended for a healthy diet.

5. What is glycogen? Why is it a vital tissue carbohydrate?

SELF-TEST QUESTIONS

True-False

Write the correct statement for each item you answer "false."

1. Carbohydrates are composed of carbon, hydrogen, oxygen, and nitrogen.
2. Starch is the main carbohydrate in our diet.
3. Lactose is a very sweet, simple, single sugar found in a number of foods.
4. Glucose is the form of sugar circulating in the blood.
5. Glycogen is an important long-term storage form of energy because relatively large amounts are stored in the liver and muscles.
6. Modern food processing and refinement have reduced dietary fiber.

Multiple Choice

1. Which of the following carbohydrate foods provides energy the *quickest*?
   a. Slice of bread
   b. Chocolate candy
   c. Milk
   d. Orange juice
2. A quickly available but limited form of energy is stored in the liver by conversion of glucose to:
   a. Glycerol.
   b. Glycogen.
   c. Protein.
   d. Fat.

SUGGESTIONS FOR ADDITIONAL STUDY

1. Cut pictures from magazines illustrating carbohydrate foods. Put them in your notebook under two headings, "Simple carbohydrates" and "Complex carbohydrates."

2. Compare the taste of a very ripe banana with that of a partially ripe one. Describe the difference in taste. Why are they different?

3. Check the carbohydrate and dietary fiber values on labels of six different food products.

REFERENCES

1. Nevins DJ: Sugars: their photosynthesis and subsequent biological interconversions, *Am J Clin Nutr* 6(suppl 55): 996S, 1995.
2. Levine B: ... About lactose intolerance, *Nutr Today* 31(2): 78, 1996.
3. Hertzler SR and others: How much lactose is low lactose?, *J Am Diet Assoc* 96(3):243, 1996.
4. Cummings JH, Englyst HN: Gastrointestinal effects of food carbohydrate, *Am J Clin Nutr* 61(suppl 55):938S, 1995.
5. Traber PG: Carbohydrate assimilation. In Yamada T, editor: *Textbook of gastroenterology*, vol 1, New York, 1995, Lippencott.
6. Special Workshop Report: Complex carbohydrates: the science and the label, *Nutr Rev* 53(7):186, 1995.
7. Marsh MN, Riley SA: Digestion and absorption of the nutrients and vitamins. In Feldman M, Scharschmidt BF, Sleisenger MH, editors: *Gastrointestinal and liver disease*, ed 6, vol 2, Philadelphia, 1998, Saunders.
8. Food and Nutrition Board, Institute of Medicine: *Dietary reference intakes*, Washington, D.C., 1998, National Academy Press.

FURTHER READING

- McNutt K, Senko A: Sugar replacers, *Nutr Today* 31(6):255, 1996.

  These consumer specialists describe their interesting experience with the growing group of sweeteners in the United States, which are collectively called sugar replacers. These intense sweeteners are extensively used in sugar-free food products.

- Filer LJ Jr, Reynolds WA: Lessons in comparative physiology: lactose intolerance, *Nutr Today* 32(2):79, 1997.

  These authors tell their fascinating experience with lactose intolerance in a pair of valuable juvenile Panda Bears on loan from China to the Los Angeles Zoo. The authors managed to diagnose the young bears' lactose intolerance and saved the bears' lives by substituting a special lactose-free enteral formula, which the young bears consumed with relish. The bears had no additional problems and, with a stopover rest at the San Francisco Zoo, arrived home in China in good health.

3

Fats

KEY CONCEPTS

- Fat in foods supplies essential diet and body tissue needs, both as an energy fuel and a structural material.

- Food from animal and plant sources supplies distinct forms of fat that affect health in different ways.

- Excess dietary fat, especially from animal food sources, is a health risk factor.

Americans and people in most other developed countries have traditionally eaten a diet relatively high in fat. In the United States, we have maintained a rich food pattern, with about 34% of our total caloric intake coming from fat. Now, however, we have well-established health concerns and are beginning to eat less fat, especially animal fats.

In this chapter, we consider fat as not only an essential nutrient, concentrated storage fuel, and tissue need but also—when in excess—a health hazard. We want to help keep attitudes and habits about fat and health realistic.

THE NATURE OF FATS

Fat as Fuel

Fats are a storage form of concentrated fuel for the human energy system. As such, they back up carbohydrates—the primary fuel—as an available energy source. In food, fats may be in the form of either solid fat or liquid oil. Fats are not soluble in water and are greasy.

Classes of Fats

Lipids

The overall name for the chemical group of fats and fat-related compounds is lipids, which comes from the Greek word *lipos*, meaning "fat." The word *lipid* appears in combination words used for fat-related health problems. For example, the condition of an elevated level of blood fats is called *hyperlipidemia.*

Triglycerides

Fats are made up of the same basic chemical elements that compose carbohydrates—carbon, hydrogen, and oxygen. As a group, fats are called glycerides because they are composed of *glycerol* with *fatty acids* attached. Whether in food or body tissue, fatty acids combine with glycerol to form glycerides. Most natural fats, whether in animal or plant sources, have three fatty acids attached to their glycerol base, so their chemical name is

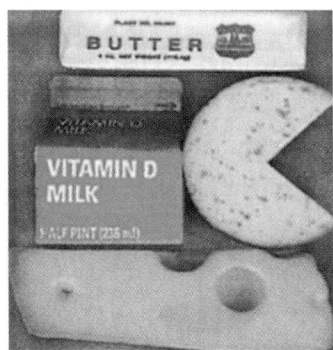
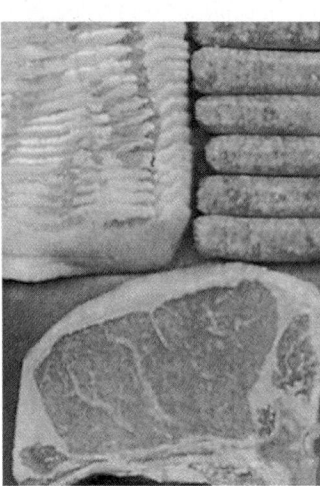
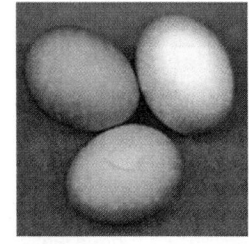
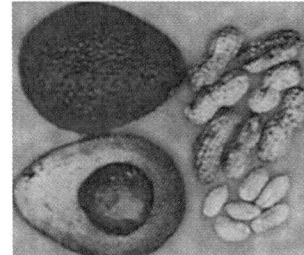
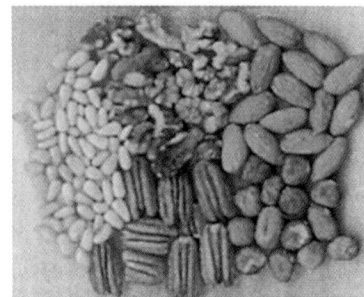
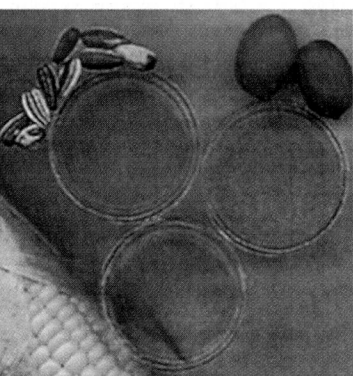
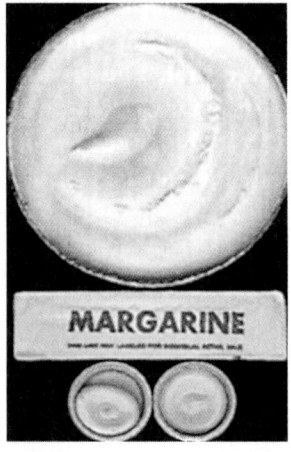

FIGURE 3-1 Food sources of fat. (Credit: Amy Buxton.)

triglyceride. When you encounter the word *triglycerides*, think of it as the chemical name for fat.

Fatty acids

The main building blocks of fats are fatty acids. Fatty acids have two significant characteristics, one of which relates to the concept of saturation and the other to essentiality.

Saturated fatty acid. When a substance is described as saturated, it contains all the material that it is capable of holding. For example, a sponge is saturated with water when it holds all the water that it can hold. Similarly, fatty acids are "saturated" or "unsaturated" according to whether or not they are filled with hydrogen. Thus a saturated fatty acid is one whose structure is filled with all of the hydrogen it can hold and as a result is heavier, denser, and more solid. If most of the fatty acids making up a fat are saturated, that fat is said to be a *saturated fat.* Such a fat would naturally be a more solid fat (e.g., meat fats). Most saturated fats are of animal origin (Figure 3-1).

Unsaturated fatty acid. A fatty acid that is not completely filled with all the hydrogen it can hold is unsaturated, and as a result is less heavy and less dense (e.g., a liquid oil). If most of the fatty acids making up a given fat are unsaturated, that fat is said to be an *unsaturated fat.* If the component fatty acids have *one* unfilled spot, the fat is called a *mono*unsaturated fat. For example, olives and olive oil, peanuts and peanut oil, canola oil (rapeseed), almonds, pecans, and avocados supply monounsaturated fats. If the component fatty acids have two or more unfilled spots, the fat is called a *poly*unsaturated fat. Examples of such fats, in order of their degree of unsaturation, are the vegetable oils: safflower, corn, cottonseed, and soybean. Fats from plant sources usually are unsaturated (Figure 3-2). Notable exceptions, however, are coconut and palm oils, which are saturated. Although world production of saturated tropical oils (e.g., palm, palm kernel, and coconut) increased rapidly since the 1970s, use of these oils in the United States has not followed this trend. These saturated oils have generally contributes less than 4% of Americans' total daily fat intake and only about 8% of their daily saturated fat intake.

Essential fatty acid. The term *essential* or *nonessential* is applied to a nutrient according to its relative necessity in the diet. A nutrient is essential if either of the following is true: (1) its absence will create a specific deficiency disease, or (2) the body cannot manufacture it and must obtain it from the diet. A diet with 10% or less of its total kcalories from fat cannot supply adequate amounts of essential fatty acids. The only fatty acids known to be essential for complete human nutrition are linoleic, linolenic, and arachidonic acids. Of these three, only linoleic acid is a true *dietary* essential fatty acid, because the body can synthesize the other two from it. All three of these fatty acids serve important functions related to tissue strength, cholesterol metabolism, muscle tone, blood clotting, and heart

---

lipids (Gr. *lipos,* fat) the chemical group name for organic substances of a fatty nature. The lipids include fats, oils, waxes, and other fat-related compounds such as cholesterol.

glycerides chemical group name for fats, from their base substance glycerol; formed from the glycerol base with one, two, or three fatty acids attached to make monoglycerides, diglycerides, and triglycerides. Glycerides are the principle constituents of adipose tissue and are found in animal and vegetable fats and oils.

triglycerides chemical name for fats in the body or in food; compound of three fatty acids attached to a glycerol base.

fatty acids the major structural components of fats.

saturated (L. *saturare,* to fill) state of being filled; state of fatty acid components of fats being filled in all their available carbon bonds with hydrogen, making the fat harder and more solid. Such solid food fats are from animal sources.

linoleic acid the ultimate essential fatty acid for humans.

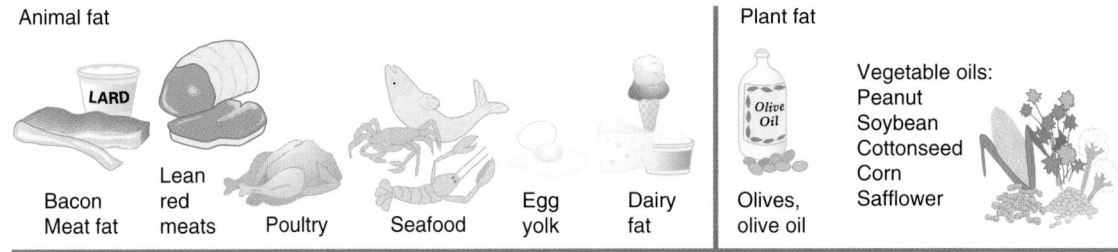

Animal fat

Plant fat

LARD

Olive Oil

Vegetable oils:
Peanut
Soybean
Cottonseed
Corn
Safflower

Bacon
Meat fat

Lean
red
meats

Poultry

Seafood

Egg
yolk

Dairy
fat

Olives,
olive oil

Saturated

Unsaturated

FIGURE 3-2   Spectrum of food fats according to degree of saturation of component fatty acid. (Credit: Eileen Draper.)

action. Linoleic acid is primarily found in polyunsaturated vegetable oils.

Lipoproteins

Lipoproteins are combinations of fat (lipids), protein (the protein part is called an *apoprotein*), and other fat-related substances, which are the major vehicle for the transport in the bloodstream. Because fat is insoluble in water and blood is mainly water, fat cannot travel freely in the bloodstream; it needs a water-soluble carrier. The body solves this problem by wrapping small particles of fat in a covering of protein, which is soluble in water. The blood then carries these little packages of fat to and from the cells to supply needed nutrients. Lipoproteins contain triglycerides, cholesterol, and other materials (e.g., fat-soluble vitamins). A lipoprotein's relative load of fat and protein determines its density. The higher the protein load, the higher the lipoprotein's density. The higher the fat load, the lower the lipoprotein's density. Groups of *low-density lipoproteins* (LDLs) carry fat and cholesterol to cells. Groups of *high-density lipoproteins* (HDLs) carry free cholesterol from body tissue to the liver for breakdown and excretion. All lipoproteins are closely associated with lipid disorders and the underlying blood vessel disease in heart attacks, *atherosclerosis*. These relationships are discussed in greater detail in Chapter 19.

Cholesterol

Although cholesterol is often discussed in connection with dietary fat, it is not a fat itself. Many people confuse it with saturated fats, but cholesterol belongs to a group of chemical substances called *sterols*. Its name comes from the body material where it was first identified—gallstones. Hence, "chole-" refers to the gallbladder or bile, and "-sterol" refers to the family group name. Cholesterol is a vital substance in human metabolism that occurs naturally in all animal foods. Because it is only synthesized in animal tissue, there is no cholesterol in plant foods. The main food sources of cholesterol are egg yolks and organ meats, such as liver and kidney, as well as other meats (see Appendix B). To ensure that it always has the relatively small amount of cholesterol required for sustaining life, the human body synthesizes the *endogenous* cholesterol in many body tissues—particularly in the liver, which is a major source, as well as small amounts in the adrenal cortex, skin, intestines, testes, and ovaries.

FUNCTIONS OF FAT

Fat in Foods

Energy

In addition to carbohydrate, fat is one of the body's fuels for energy production. Fat is also an important storage form of body fuel for energy reserves because carbohydrate is easily converted into it. Fat is a much more concentrated form of fuel, yielding 9 kcal/g when burned by the body, compared with carbohydrate's yield of 4 kcal/g.

Essential Nutrients

Food fats supply the essential fatty acids—especially linoleic acid—and cholesterol to supplement the amount synthesized by the body. Food fats also carry fat-soluble vitamins (see Chapter 6) and aid in their absorption.

Flavor and Satisfaction

Some fat in the diet adds flavor to foods and contributes to a feeling of *satiety* or satisfaction after a meal. These effects are partly caused by the slower rate of digestion of fats compared with that of carbohydrate. This satiety is also due to the fuller texture and body that fat gives to food mixtures and the slower emptying time of the stomach that it necessitates. The absence of this satiation and hunger delay experienced by some persons on low-fat diets may contribute to client dissatisfaction and problems with necessary changes in food habits.

Fat Substitutes

Several fat substitutes, compounds that are not absorbed and thus contribute little or no kcalories, are being marketed or tested to provide improved flavor and physical texture to low-fat foods and help reduce total dietary fat. Two examples of these fat substitutes are Simplesse (The Nutra-Sweet Company), which is made by reshaping the protein of milk whey or egg whites, and Olestra (Procter & Gamble), which is a nondigestible form of sucrose.

Fat in the Body

Adipose Tissue

Fat stored in various parts of the body is called adipose tissue, from the Latin word *adiposus* meaning "fatty." A weblike padding of this tissue supports and protects vital organs, and a layer of fat directly under the skin is important in regulating body temperature. A special fat covering protects nerve fibers and helps relay nerve impulses.

Cell Membrane Structure

Fat forms the fatty center of cell walls, helping to carry nutrient materials across cell membranes.

FOOD SOURCES OF FAT
Variety of Sources

Animal Fats

Animal sources supply saturated fats, as shown in Figure 3-2. Therefore food sources of saturated fats include meat fats (e.g., bacon and sausage), dairy fats and products (e.g., cream, ice cream, butter, cheese, and egg yolk). The American diet has traditionally featured meats and other foods of animal origin. Surveys have shown that animal products in particular (e.g., red meats [beef, veal, pork, lamb]; poultry, fish and shellfish; separate animal fats [lard], milk and milk products, and eggs) contribute more than half of the total fat to U.S. diets, three fourths of the saturated fat, and all of the cholesterol.

---

lipoproteins chemical complexes of fat with protein that serve as the major carriers of lipids in the plasma because most of the plasma fat is associated with them. They vary in density according to the size of the fat load being carried; the lower the density, the higher the fat load. The combination package with water-soluble protein makes possible the transport of nonwater-soluble fatty substances in the water-based blood circulation.

cholesterol (Gr. *chole,* bile; *steros,* solid) a fat-related compound, a sterol, synthesized only in animal tissues; a normal constituent of bile and a principal constituent of gallstones. In the body, cholesterol is synthesized mainly in the liver. In the diet, it is found only in animal food sources. In human body metabolism, cholesterol is important as a precursor of various steroid hormones such as sex hormones and adrenal corticoids. In disordered lipid metabolism, however, it is a major factor in atherosclerosis, the underlying disease process in coronary arteries that leads to heart attacks.

adipose (L. *adeps,* fat; *adiposus,* fatty) fat present in cells of adipose (fatty) tissue.

Red meats—especially beef, which is the major red meat consumed—that are more healthy with less fat, however, are being increasingly marketed. Pasture-fed lean beef with little tissue marbling of fat that is well-trimmed of external edge fat often contains less than 5% fat and has cholesterol-lowering effects. When regular, market beef cuts are used in the diet, however, there is little or no beneficial effect on serum cholesterol levels. These results indicate that the meat fat—not the moderate portions of very lean meat—increases cholesterol levels. Even greater cholesterol-lowering effects can be achieved from regular moderate use of polyunsaturated safflower oil or monounsaturated olive oil in the diet.[1]

Plant Fats

Plant sources supply unsaturated fats. Food sources for unsaturated fats include vegetable oils (e.g., safflower, corn, cottonseed, soybeans, peanuts, and olives) (see Figure 3-2), but, as indicated, coconut and palm oils are exceptions. These oils are saturated fats used mainly in commercially processed food items and identified on the labels.

Hydrogenated Fat

Margarine and shortenings are made from unsaturated vegetable oils when hydrogen is introduced into the fat molecule. This process is called *hydrogenation*, a word that frequently appears on the labels of such commercial fat products. To make margarine a substitute for butter, the hydrogenated product may also be churned with cultured milk, to give it a butter flavor, and fortified with vitamins A and D. Fortified margarine is the nutritional equivalent of butter and has the same caloric value. Margarine, which is economical, tasteful, and lower in saturated fat, is 80% fat and fortified with 15,000 International Units (IU) of vitamin A per pound.

Cis and trans fatty acid products. Health professionals have recently been concerned about the increasing number of hydrogenated (hardened) food products being made from the cis and trans

forms of unsaturated fatty acids.[2] These two chemical terms—cis and trans—refer to two different shapes that a fat molecule can have as its structure. The illustration here shows these two different structures in a molecule of oleic acid, which is a common monounsaturated fatty acid that has a chain of 18 carbon atoms:

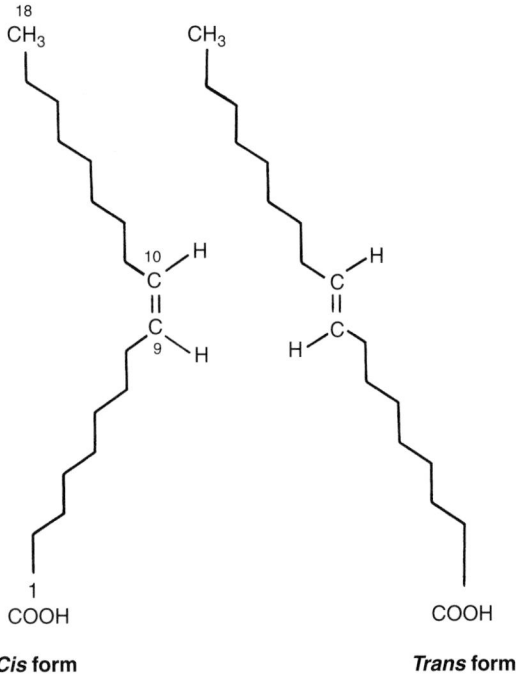

Cis form **Trans form**

All naturally occurring fatty acid molecules have a bend in the chain of atoms at the point of the chemical bond in the middle of the chain. This form is called *cis* (same side). When vegetable oils are partially hydrogenated to make food products, however, the normal bend is changed so that the chains of atoms are on opposite sides of the central bond. This form is called *trans* (opposite side).[2] Commercially hydrogenated fats in margarine and many other food products are in the *trans* form.[3] Increased use of these products, especially margarine, has stirred debate about accumulating trans fatty acids in the body.[4] Some of the observed effects include elevation of serum lipids, inhibited essential fatty acid metabolism, and modification of membrane properties. In response to these growing health concerns, the food industry has developed solid and soft tub *trans*-free fat products for concerned individuals.

Food Label Information

Nutrition labeling on food products, which is now mandated by U.S. law, provides particular information about fat. The nature and amount of dietary fat and cholesterol are special health concerns related to some cancers, coronary heart disease, diabetes, and obesity. U.S. Food and Drug Administration (FDA) food-labeling regulations provide the following mandatory and voluntary (italicized) information:

Nutrition panel content:

- Calories from fat
- *Calories from saturated fat*
- Total fat
- Saturated fat
- *Polyunsaturated fat*
- *Monounsaturated fat*
- Cholesterol

Fat-related health claims allowed:

- Fat and cancer
- Saturated fat and cholesterol and coronary heart disease

Characteristics of Food Fat Sources

For practical purposes, food fats can be classified as *visible* or *invisible* fats to help individuals become aware of all food sources of fat.

Visible Fat

The obvious fats are plain to see and include butter, margarine, separate cream, salad oils and dressings, lard, shortening, fat meat (e.g., bacon, sausage, and salt pork), and the visible fat of any meat. It is easier to control visible fats in the diet than those that are less apparent.

Invisible Fat

Some dietary fats are less visible, so individuals who want to control dietary fat must also be aware of these food sources. Invisible fats include cheese, the cream portion of homogenized milk, egg yolk, nuts, seeds, olives, avocados, and lean meat. Even when all of the visible fat has been removed from meat (e.g., the skin on poultry and the obvious fat on the lean portions), about 6% of the total fat surrounding the muscle fibers remains.

Digestibility and Market Availability of Food Fats

The digestibility of fats varies somewhat according to the food source and cooking method. Butter digests more completely than meat fat. Fried foods, especially those saturated with fat in the frying process, are digested more slowly than baked or broiled foods. When fried foods are cooked at too high of a temperature, they are more difficult to digest because substances in the fat break down into irritating materials. Fried foods should be consumed sparingly, and the temperature of the fat should be carefully controlled during frying. Although lower fat food products are now generally more available in our food markets, there are still many high-fat products available beckoning for the customer's attention. In any case, however, our overall health goal is to reduce the amount of excessive fat used in the diet.

BODY NEEDS FOR FAT

Dietary Fat and Health

American Diet

From reading world health reports and caring for malnourished patients, it is evident that fats make up an essential nutrient class.[4,5] The role of fat-modified foods in the American diet, however, has been increasing.[6,7] As is so often the case, the old maxim here holds true: you need what you need, but you don't need more than you need. The American diet has traditionally been high in fat. Fats in the diet supply flavor to the food we eat, as well as feel special in our mouths, providing a sense of satisfaction and enhancing our eating pleasure. We often eat more than we intended, however, or more than we need. The average amount of fat consumed per person, about 100 pounds per year, provides about 40% to 45% of the diet's total kcalories. This amount exceeds that needed by the average person. No more than 25% to 30% of the diet's total kcalories need to come from fat. Many individuals with health problems have adjusted to lower amounts of fat, with goals such as 10% to 15% of the total kcalories. This amount would easily provide an adequate amount of the essential fatty acids, especially linoleic acid, to meet the physiologic needs of the body.

Health Problems

If fat is vital to human health, what is the concern about fat in the diet? Research continues to validate results indicating that health problems from fat relate to too much dietary fat and too much of that fat from animal food sources.

Amount of fat. Too much fat in the diet supplies more kcalories than required for immediate energy needs. The excess is stored as increasing body fat. Increased body fat and weight have been associated with risk factors for health problems such as diabetes, hypertension, and heart disease. Look for more details about these relationships in the later section on clinical nutrition. How much fat is in your own diet? You might try figuring it out for a day (Box 3-1).

Type of fat. An excess of cholesterol and saturated fat in the diet, which comes from animal food sources, has been associated as a specific risk factor for atherosclerosis, the underlying blood vessel disease that contributes to heart attacks and strokes (see Chapter 19). A decrease in dietary saturated fats (i.e., using polyunsaturated and monounsaturated fats instead) has been shown to reduce serum total cholesterol in many individuals. When substituted for saturated fat in the diet, monounsaturated fats (e.g., olive oil) reduce the low-density lipoprotein (LDL) cholesterol, which is the main target for control.

Health Promotion

The ongoing movement in American health care is toward health promotion and disease prevention through reduction of risk factors related to chronic disease. Heart disease continues to be the leading

BOX 3-1 How Much Fat Are You Eating?

- Keep an accurate record of everything you eat or drink for 1 day. Be sure to estimate and add amounts of all fat or other nutrient seasonings used with your foods. (If you want a more representative picture and have a computer available with nutrient analysis programming, keep a 1-week record and calculate an average of the 7 days.)
- Calculate the total kilocalories (kcal) and grams of each of the energy nutrients (carbohydrate, fat, and protein) in everything you eat. Multiply the total grams of each energy nutrient by its respective fuel value:

$$\text{fat } \underline{\hspace{1cm}} \text{ g} \times 9 = \underline{\hspace{1cm}} \text{ kcal}$$
$$\text{protein } \underline{\hspace{1cm}} \text{ g} \times 4 = \underline{\hspace{1cm}} \text{ kcal}$$
$$\text{carbohydrate } \underline{\hspace{1cm}} \text{ g} \times 4 = \underline{\hspace{1cm}} \text{ kcal}$$

- Calculate the percentage of each energy nutrient in your total diet:

$$\frac{\text{Fat kcal}}{\text{Total kcal}} \times 100 = \% \text{ fat kcal in diet}$$

- Compare with fat in American diet (40% to 45%); compare with the U.S. dietary goals (25% to 30%).

cause of death in developed countries, and much attention is given to reducing the various risk factors leading to this disease. Excess dietary fat, particularly saturated fat and cholesterol, contributes to these risk factors, which include obesity, diabetes, elevated blood fats, and elevated blood pressure. Additional lifestyle risk factors include smoking, increased stress, and lack of exercise—especially in middle-aged and older individuals.[8] Thus a middle-aged or older adult who eats a high-fat diet, is overweight, and has a high level of blood cholesterol and blood pressure should reduce both weight and amount of dietary fat, especially animal fat. Today there is increasing emphasis—especially for persons at least 40 years of age—on the importance of keeping the body's total daily energy use in balance with the total daily caloric intake, especially of dietary fat.[9,10] Children are learning in grade school about healthier food habits with less fat. Healthier food habits are especially important for children in high-risk families (i.e., families having identified lipid disorders and heart disease at young adult ages) who should develop moderation in fat use, as well as other aspects of a healthy lifestyle, at an early age.

In addition, changes are gradually being made in the fast-food industry to reduce the traditional high-fat content of their menu items. For example, most of the fast food chains are shifting to leaner meat for hamburgers and more variety in food choices (e.g., grilled chicken and fish sandwiches; breakfast items such as fruit, waffles, pancakes, and hot and cold cereals; baked potatoes; chili; and fresh and packaged salads) and using vegetable oil for cooking french fries. Many fast food restaurants are experimenting and surveying customers about use of fat substitutes.

DIGESTION OF FATS

Mouth

The various animal and plant fats (triglycerides) that naturally occur in foods are taken into the body with the diet. The task is to change these basic fuel fats into a form of fat that is a refined fuel the cells can burn for energy. This key refined fuel form is the individual fatty acid. The body accomplishes this refinement through the process of fat digestion. When fat foods are eaten, some initial chemical fat breakdown may begin in the mouth by action of a *lingual lipase* that is secreted by Ebner's glands at the back of the tongue. The main action in this first portion of the gastrointestinal tract is mechanical, as fat foods are broken up into smaller particles through chewing and moistened for passage into the stomach with the total food mass.

Stomach

Little, if any, chemical fat digestion takes place in the stomach. General muscle action continues to mix the fat with the stomach contents. No significant amount of enzymes specific to fats is present in the gastric secretions except a *gastric lipase* (tributyrinase), which acts on emulsified butterfat. As the main gastric enzymes act on other specific nutrients in the food mix, fat is separated out from them and prepared for its major, chemical-specific breakdown in the small intestine.

Small Intestine

Fat digestion occurs primarily in the small intestine. The major enzymes necessary for the chemical changes are not present until fat reaches the small intestine. These specific digestive agents come from three major sources—a preparation agent from the gallbladder and specific enzymes from the pancreas and the small intestine itself.

Bile from the Gallbladder

The fat coming into the duodenum, the first section of the small intestine, stimulates the secretion of *cholecystokinin*, a local hormone from glands in the intestinal walls. In turn, cholecystokinin causes the gallbladder to contract, relax its opening muscle, and subsequently secrete bile into the intestine by way of the common bile duct. The bile is first produced in large dilute amounts in the liver, which then sends it to the gallbladder for concentration and storage so that it is ready for use with fat as needed. Bile is not an enzyme but functions as an emulsifier. Emulsification is not a chemical digestive process but is the important first preparation of fat for chemical digestion by its specific enzymes. This preparation process accomplishes two important tasks: (1) it breaks the fat into small particles, greatly enlarging the total surface area available for action of the enzyme; and (2) it lowers the surface tension of the finely dispersed and suspended fat particles, allowing the enzymes to penetrate more easily. This process is similar to the wetting action of detergents. The bile also provides an alkaline medium necessary for the action of the fat enzyme *enteric lipase*.

Enzymes from the Pancreas

Pancreatic juice flowing into the small intestine contains an enzyme for fat and another one for cholesterol. First, *pancreatic lipase*, a powerful fat enzyme, breaks off one fatty acid at a time from the glycerol base of fats (triglycerides). One fatty acid plus a diglyceride, then another fatty acid plus a monoglyceride, are produced in turn. Each succeeding step of this breakdown occurs with increasing difficulty. In fact, separation of the final fatty acid from the remaining monoglyceride is such a slow process that less than a third of the total fat present actually reaches complete breakdown. The final products of fat digestion to be absorbed are fatty acids, diglycerides, monoglycerides, and glycerol. Some remaining fat may pass into the large intestine for fecal elimination. Second, the enzyme *cholesterol enterase* acts on free cholesterol to form a combination of cholesterol and fatty acids in preparation for absorption into the lymph vessels and finally into the bloodstream (see Chapter 9).

Enzyme from the Small Intestine

The small intestine secretes an enzyme in the intestinal juice called *lecithinase*, which acts on leci-

thin, another lipid compound, breaking it down for absorption. Table 3-1 provides a summary of fat digestion in the successive parts of the gastrointestinal tract.

DIETARY FAT REQUIREMENTS

Dietary Reference Intakes/ Recommended Dietary Allowances

Healthy diet guidelines stress the health benefits of a diet low in fat, saturated fat, and cholesterol. All guidelines recommend that the fat content of the U.S. diet not exceed 30% of the total kcalories, less than 10% of the kcalories should be provided from saturated fats, and dietary cholesterol be limited to 300 mg/day (see Chapter 1). The current average consumption of fat is about 34% of the total kcalories. Both the current RDAs and the 1995 Dietary Guidelines for Americans include these recommendations. The forthcoming report by the Dietary Reference Intakes (DRIs) panel on energy and macronutrients will reemphasize these healthy guidelines.

U.S. Dietary Guidelines

In line with the current national health goal of health promotion through disease prevention by reducing identified risks of chronic disease, the U.S. dietary guidelines recommend general control of fat in the diet, especially saturated fat and cholesterol. Several practical ways of lowering fat in the diet are as follows:

- **Meat:** Use only lean cuts of all meats, and use more poultry and seafood. Remove skin from poultry and trim fat from all meats. Avoid added fat in cooking. Use smaller portions (e.g., 2 to 4 oz) of meat. For example, a boneless chicken breast is about 3 to 4 oz.
- **Eggs:** Limit intake of eggs to approximately two or three a week. Cook and serve without added fat. Use egg whites freely.

TABLE 3-1   Summary of fat digestion

Organ	Enzyme	Activity
Mouth	Small amount of lingual lipase	Some initial fat breakdown
		Mechanical, mastication
Stomach	No major enzyme	Mechanical separation of fats as protein and starch digested out
	Small amount of gastric lipase tributyrinase	Tributyrin (butterfat) to fatty acids and glycerol
Small intestine	Gallbladder bile salts (emulsifier)	Emulsifies fats
	Pancreatic lipase (steapsin)	Triglycerides to diglycerides and monoglycerides in turn, then fatty acids and glycerol

- **Milk and milk products:** Use low-fat or fat-free milk and milk products. Use cheeses with lower fat content.
- **Food preparation:** Avoid fat as much as possible in food preparation and cooking. Use alternative seasonings such as herbs, spices, lemon and lime juice, onion, garlic, fat-free broth, or wine. Use low-fat or fat-free salad dressings or herb-seasoned or wine vinegars.

bile (L. *bilis,* bile) a fluid secreted by the liver and transported to the gallbladder for concentration and storage; released into the duodenum with the entry of fat to facilitate enzymatic fat digestion by acting as an emulsifying agent.

emulsifier an agent that breaks down large fat globules into smaller, uniformly distributed particles; action accomplished in the intestine chiefly by bile acids, which lower the surface tension of the fat particles, breaking the fat into many smaller droplets, thus greatly increasing the surface area of fat and facilitating contact with the fat-digesting enzymes.

SUMMARY

Fat is an essential body nutrient, serving important body needs as a back-up storage fuel—secondary to carbohydrate—for energy. Fat also supplies important tissue needs as a structural material for cell walls, protective padding for vital organs, insulation to maintain body temperature, and covering for nerve fibers.

Food fats have different forms and body uses. Saturated fats come from animal food sources and carry health risks for the body. Unsaturated fats come from plant food sources and help reduce health risks. Cholesterol is a fat-related substance synthesized only by animals that in excess amounts also contributes to health risks.

Americans generally consume far more fat than they need or is healthy for them. For health promotion, reducing fats and saturated fat and maintaining a low-cholesterol diet are recommended. When various foods containing fat and cholesterol are eaten, specific digestive agents including bile and the major enzyme pancreatic lipase prepare and break down the fats (triglycerides) into fatty acids and glycerides for absorption via the lymphatic system into blood circulation.

REVIEW QUESTIONS

1. Compare fat with carbohydrate as a fuel source in the body's energy system. Name several other important functions of fat in human nutrition and health.
2. Define the terms *lipids, triglycerides, fatty acids, cholesterol,* and *lipoproteins.* Distinguish between saturated and unsaturated fats, giving food sources for each.
3. Why is a controlled amount of dietary fat recommended for health promotion? How much fat should a healthy diet contain?

SELF-TEST QUESTIONS

True-False

Write the correct statement for each item you answer "false."

1. Fat has the same energy value as carbohydrate.
2. Fat is composed of the same basic chemical elements as carbohydrate.
3. Corn oil is a saturated fat.
4. Polyunsaturated fats usually come from animal food sources.
5. Lipoproteins, produced mainly in the liver, carry fat in the blood.

Multiple Choice

1. The fuel form of fat found in food sources is:
   a. Triglyceride.
   b. Fatty acid.
   c. Glycerol.
   d. Lipoprotein.
2. Which of the following statements about the saturation of fats is correct?
   a. The degree of saturation does not depend on the relative amount of hydrogen in the fatty acids that make up the fat.
   b. The more unsaturated fats come from animal food sources.
   c. The more saturated the fat, the softer it tends to be.
   d. Fats composed of fatty acids with two or more "unfilled" spaces in their structure are called *polyunsaturated.*
3. If an individual implemented a low saturated fat diet to lower the risk for heart disease, which of the following foods would be used frequently?
   a. Whole milk
   b. Oil-vinegar salad dressing
   c. Butter
   d. Cheddar cheese

SUGGESTIONS FOR ADDITIONAL STUDY

1. Visit a community food market to survey fats and fat-related foods. Read the labels carefully. Look for the words *imitation, hydrogenated, polyunsaturated, saturated, P/S (polyunsaturated/saturated) ratio, fortified,* and *hardened,* as well as the P/S (polyunsaturated/saturated) ratio. Include foods such as margarines, shortenings, oils, frozen desserts, whipped toppings, cream substitutes, nondairy creamers, milks, egg and cheese foods, egg substitutes, and special low-fat cheeses in your survey. Make a list of the terms you find on labels of the fat-related food products and describe each product. What does each term mean? How has the product been processed? What nutrition information do you find on the label? Prepare a report of your survey for your notebook, as well as a class report.
2. Plan your meals for 1 day using as little fat as possible. Describe how you would prepare and serve food to avoid fat.

REFERENCES

1. Drewnoski A: Why do you like fat? *J Amer Diet Assoc* 27(suppl 7):S58, 1997.
2. Williams SR: *Essentials of nutrition and diet therapy,* ed 7, St Louis, 1999, Mosby.
3. Hernandez E, Lucas EW: Trends in transesterification of cottonseed oil, *Food Tech* 51(5):72, 1997.
4. Staff report, nutrition science and policy, WHO and FAO joint consultation: Fats and oils in human nutrition, *Nutr Rev* 53(7):202, 1995.
5. Klein S, Jeejeebhoy KN: The malnourished patient: nutrition assessment and management. In Feldman M, Scharschimedt BF, Sleisenger MH, eds: *Gastrointestinal and liver disease,* vol 1, ed 6, Philadelphia, 1998, W.B. Saunders.
6. Calloway CW: The role of fat-modified foods in the American diet, *Nutr Today* 33(4):156, 1998.
7. Sims LS: The politics of fat, *Nutr Today* 33(4):134, 1998.
8. Poelman ET: Effect of exercise on daily energy needs in older individuals, *Amer J Clin Nutr* 68(8):997, 1998 (editorial).
9. Carpenter WH and others: Total energy expenditure in free-living older African Americans and Caucasions, *Am J Physiol* 274:E96-101, 1998.
10. Bunyard LB and others: Energy requirements of middle-aged men are modifiable by physical activity, *Amer J Clin Nutr* 68(9):1136, 1998.

FURTHER READING

- Hahn NI: Replacing fat with food technology, *J Am Diet Assoc* 97(1):15, 1997.
- McNutt K: What's bothering Olestra opponents?, *Nutr Today* 32(1):41, 1997.

These interesting articles describe recently developed fat substitutes that are now available in the marketplace, with mixed responses from the public and professionals.

- Rolls BJ, Miller DL: Is the low-fat message giving people a license to eat more?, *J Am Coll Nutr* 16(6):535, 1997.
- Scarbrough FE: Some Food and Drug Administration perspectives of fat and fatty acids, *Am J Clin Nutr* 65(suppl): 1578S, 1997.

These authors provide interesting background about food labels and the need for better communication with consumers about fat in the American diet and health-related problems.

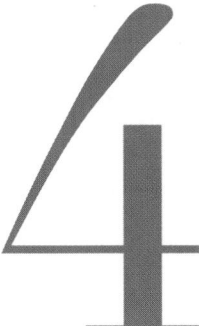

Proteins

KEY CONCEPTS

- Food proteins provide the amino acids necessary for building and maintaining body tissue.

- Protein balance, both within the body and in the diet, is essential to life and health.

- A food's value for meeting body protein needs is determined by its composition of essential amino acids.

Many different proteins in the body make human life possible. Each one of these thousands upon thousands of specific body proteins has a unique structure designed to do an assigned task. Amino acids are the essential units of our bodies and are the building blocks of all protein. We obtain amino acids from the variety of food proteins we eat every day. This chapter looks at the specific nature of proteins—both in our food and in our bodies. We will see why protein balance is essential to life and health and how we maintain that balance.

THE NATURE OF PROTEINS

Amino Acids: Basic Building Material

Role as Building Units

All protein, whether in our bodies or in the food we eat, is made up of building units or compounds known as amino acids. Amino acids are joined in unique, chain sequences to form specific proteins. When we eat protein foods, the protein (e.g., casein in milk and cheese, albumin in egg white, or gluten in wheat products) is broken down into amino acids in the digestive process. Amino acids are then reassembled in the body in the proper *specific* order to form *specific* tissue proteins (e.g., collagen in connective tissue; myosin in muscle tissue; hemoglobin in red blood cells [Figure 4-1], cell enzymes, or insulin) needed by the body. To maintain its solvency, each protein chain adopts a folded form, which can fold and unfold according to metabolic need.[1] Because proteins are relatively large structures and sometimes have difficulty making their way through the cell membrane, scientists are working on an efficient way for cells to make the needed protein themselves.[2] For example, protein-folding mistakes are involved in Alzheimer's disease, which robs many older adults of their mental capacity.[3]

Role as Nitrogen Supplier

Amino acids are named for their chemical nature. The word *amino* refers to compounds containing nitrogen. Like carbohydrates and fats, proteins have a basic structure of carbon, hydrogen, and oxygen. But unlike carbohydrates and fats, which contain no nitrogen, protein is about 16% nitrogen. In addition, some proteins contain small but valuable amounts of the minerals sulfur, phosphorus, iron, and iodine.

Classes of Amino Acids

There are 22 common amino acids, all of which are vital to human life and health. These amino acids are classified as essential or nonessential *in the diet*, however, according to whether the body can make them.

Essential Amino Acids

Ten amino acids are classified as essential amino acids because the body cannot manufacture them in sufficient quantity or at all. Thus, as the word *essential* implies, these amino acids are necessary in the diet (Box 4-1). During growth years, the amino acid arginine is especially essential to meet normal infancy and childhood growth demands. The remaining 12 nonessential amino acids are easily synthesized by the body to meet continuous needs throughout the life cycle.

Nonessential Amino Acids

In this instance, the word *nonessential* is misleading, because all amino acids have essential tissue-building and metabolic functions in the body. As used here, however, the term refers to the remaining 12 amino acids that the body can synthesize, so they are not essential in the diet.

Balance

The term *balance* refers to the relative intake and output of substances in the body to maintain the normal levels of these substances necessary for health in various circumstances during life. We can apply this concept of balance to life-sustaining protein and the nitrogen it supplies.

Protein Balance

The body's tissue proteins are constantly being broken down into amino acids, a process called *catabolism*, and then resynthesized into tissue proteins as needed, a process called *anabolism*. To

---

amino acids nitrogen-bearing compounds that form the structural units of protein. When digested, the various food proteins yield their constituent *amino acids*, which are then available for use by the cells to synthesize specific tissue proteins.

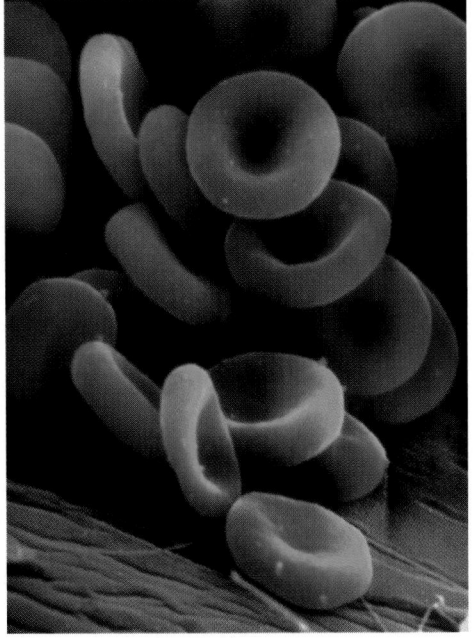

A Red blood cells

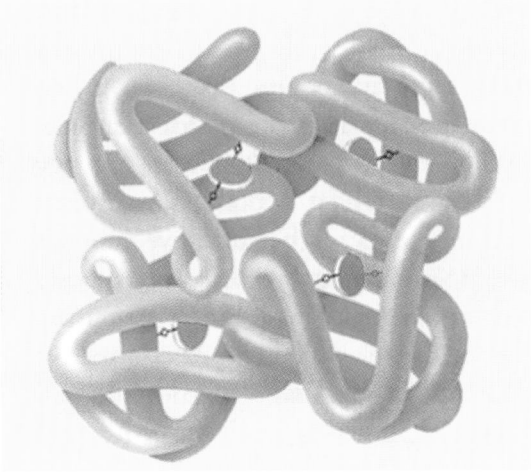

B

Hemoglobin molecule

FIGURE 4-1 Hemoglobin is an oxygen-carrying protein of red blood cells. (Credits: **A,** Copyright 1994 Dennis Kunkel, University of Hawaii. **B,** Christine Oleksyk Perchal, from Thibodeau GA, Patton KT: *Anatomy and physiology,* ed 4, St Louis, 1999, Mosby.)

BOX 4-1 Amino acids required in human nutrition, grouped according to nutritional (dietary) essentiality

Essential amino acids	Nonessential amino acids
Arginine	Alanine
Histidine	Aspargine
Isoleucine	Aspartic acid
Leucine	Cystine (cysteine)
Lysine	Glutamic acid
Methionine	Glutamine
Phenylalanine	Glycine
Threonine	Hydroxylysine
Tryptophan	Hydroxyproline
Valine	Proline
	Serine
	Tyrosine

maintain nitrogen balance, the part of the amino acids that contains nitrogen may be removed through a process called *deamination*, then converted to ammonia (NH_3), and excreted as urea in the urine. The remaining non-nitrogen residue can be used to make carbohydrate or fat or reattached to make another amino acid if necessary. The rate of this protein and nitrogen turnover varies in different tissues, according to their degree of metabolic activity.

This tissue turnover is a continuous process of reshaping, rebuilding, and adjusting as necessary to maintain overall protein balance within the body. The body also maintains a balance between tissue protein and plasma protein, which are then further balanced with dietary protein intake. With this finely balanced system, a "pool" of amino acids from both tissue protein and dietary protein is always available to meet construction needs (Figure 4-2).

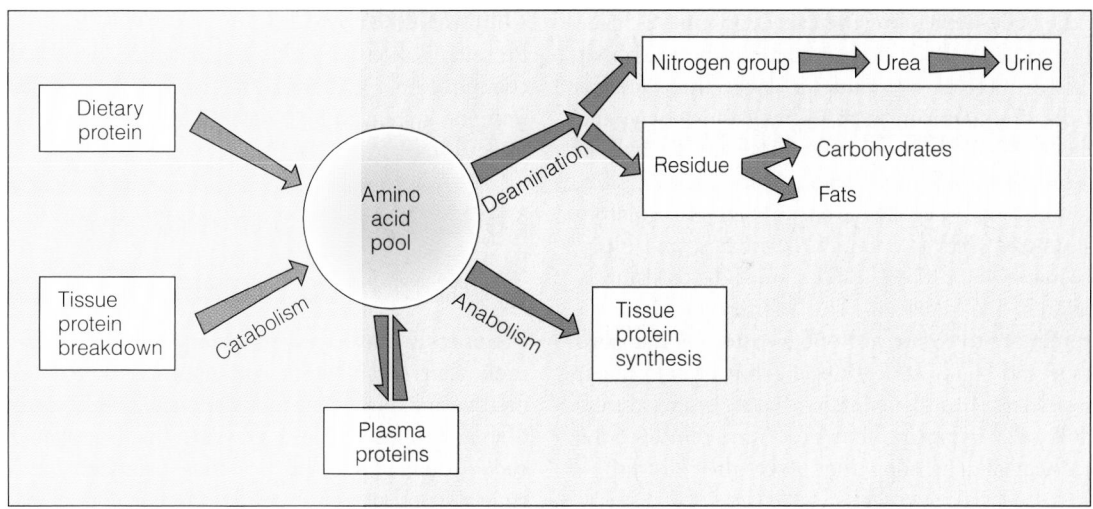

FIGURE 4-2   Balance between protein compartments and amino acid pool.

Nitrogen Balance

The body's nitrogen balance indicates how well its tissues are being maintained. The intake and use of dietary protein is measured by the amount of nitrogen intake in food protein and the amount of nitrogen excreted in the urine. For example, 1 g of urinary nitrogen results from the digestion and metabolism of 6.25 g of protein. Thus if 1 g of nitrogen is excreted in the urine for every 6.25 g of protein consumed, the body is said to be in nitrogen balance. This balance is the normal pattern in adult health, but at different times of life or in states of malnutrition or illness, the balance may be either positive or negative.

Positive nitrogen balance.   A positive nitrogen balance exists when the body takes in more nitrogen than it excretes, thus storing more nitrogen by building more tissue than it is losing nitrogen by breaking down tissue. This situation occurs normally during periods of rapid growth (e.g., infancy, childhood, adolescence) and during pregnancy and lactation. A positive nitrogen balance also occurs in individuals who have been ill or malnourished and are being "built back up" with increased nourishment. In such cases, protein is

stored to meet increased needs for tissue building and associated metabolic activity.

Negative nitrogen balance.   A negative nitrogen balance exists when the body takes in less nitrogen than it excretes. This means that the body has an inadequate protein intake and is losing nitrogen by breaking down more tissue than it is building up. This situation occurs in states of malnutrition and illness. For example, this nitrogen imbalance is seen in America when a specific protein deficiency—even when kcalories from carbohydrate and fat may be adequate—causes the classic protein deficiency disease kwashiorkor. Failure to maintain nitrogen balance may not become apparent for some time but will eventually cause loss of muscle tissue, impairment of body organs and functions, and increased susceptibility to infection. In children, negative nitrogen balance causes growth retardation.

FUNCTIONS OF PROTEIN
Primary Tissue Building

Protein is the fundamental structural material of every cell in the body. In fact, the largest portion of the body—excluding the water content—is made up of protein. Body protein, mainly the lean body mass of muscles, accounts for about three fourths of the dry matter in most tissues besides bone and adipose fat. Protein not only makes up the bulk of the muscles, internal organs, brain, nerves, skin, hair, and nails but also is a vital part of regulatory substances such as enzymes, hormones, and blood plasma. All of these tissues must be constantly repaired and replaced. The primary functions of protein are to repair worn-out, wasted, or damaged tissue and build up new tissue. Thus protein meets growth needs and maintains tissue health during adult years. In fact, proteins are always central to the biochemical machinery that makes the cells run.[4]

Additional Body Functions

In addition to its basic tissue-building function, protein has other body functions relating to energy, water balance, metabolism, and the body's defense system.

Energy System

As described in previous chapters, carbohydrate is the primary fuel source for the body's energy system, assisted by fat as a stored fuel. In times of need, protein may furnish additional body fuel to sustain body heat and energy, but this is a less-efficient, back-up source for use only when there is an insufficient supply of carbohydrate and fat. The available fuel factor of protein is 4 kcal/g.

Water Balance

Plasma protein, especially albumin, helps to control water balance throughout the body by exerting osmotic pressure to maintain normal circulation of tissue fluids and capillary blood flow.

Metabolism

Protein aids metabolic functions by the following: (1) combining with iron to form hemoglobin, the vital oxygen-carrier in the red blood cells (see Figure 4-1); and (2) manufacturing agents (e.g., digestive and cell enzymes) that control metabolic processes, as well as hormones.

Body Defense System

Protein is used to build special white blood cells (lymphocytes) and antibodies as part of the body's immune system to help defend against disease and infection.

FOOD SOURCES OF PROTEIN

Types of Food Proteins

Fortunately, most foods contain a mixture of proteins that complement one another. In a mixed diet, animal and plant foods provide a wide variety of many nutrients and proteins that supplement each other.[5] Thus the key to a balanced diet is *variety*. Food proteins are classified as complete or incomplete proteins, depending on their amino acid composition (Figure 4-3).

Complete Proteins

Protein foods that contain all of the 10 essential amino acids (see Box 4-1) in sufficient quantity and ratio to meet the body's needs are called *complete proteins*. These proteins are of animal origin (e.g., egg, milk, cheese, and meat), but gelatin is a notable exception. Although this protein food is an animal product, it is a relatively worthless protein because it lacks three essential amino acids—tryptophan, valine, and isoleucine—and has only small amounts of another—leucine.

Incomplete Proteins

Protein foods that are deficient in one or more of the 10 essential amino acids are called *incomplete proteins*. These proteins are of plant origin (e.g., grains, legumes, nuts, seeds, vegetables, and fruits) but are contained in foods that make valuable contributions to the total dietary protein.

Vegetarian Diets

Complementary Protein

The principle of complementary protein foods providing adequate amounts of essential amino acids forms the basis of planning vegetarian diets.[5] Current knowledge of protein metabolism

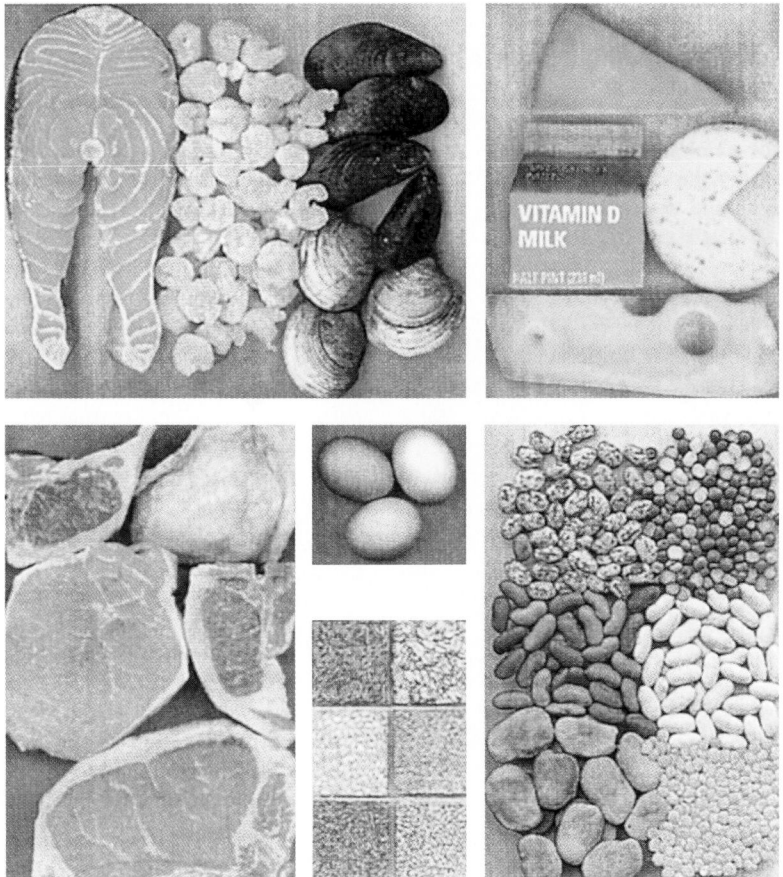

FIGURE 4-3 Complete and incomplete protein foods. (Credit: Amy Buxton.)

and the "pooling" of amino acid reserves (see Figure 4-2) indicates that even a mixture of plant proteins can provide adequate amounts of amino acids when our basic use of various grains is expanded to include soy protein and other dried legume (i.e., beans and peas) storage proteins.[6] A normal eating pattern through the day, together with the body's reserve supply of protein, usually ensures a complementary amino acid balance. The underlying requirement for vegetarians, as for all people, is to eat a sufficient amount of varied foods to meet normal nutrient and energy needs (see For Further Focus box, "Essential Amino Acids—10 or 12—and Their Complementary Food Proteins").

Types of Vegetarian Diets

Vegetarian diets differ according to the beliefs or needs of individuals following these food patterns. In general, there are three basic types, as follow:

Lacto-ovo vegetarians. Lacto-ovo vegetarians follow a food pattern that allows dairy products and eggs. Some may even accept fish and occasionally poultry. Their mixed diet of plant and animal food sources, excluding only meat—especially red meats, poses no nutritional problems.

Lacto-vegetarians. Lacto-vegetarians accept only dairy products from animal sources to complement their basic diet of plant foods. The use of milk and

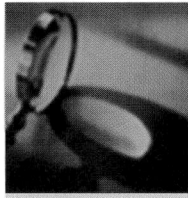

FOR FURTHER FOCUS

Essential Amino Acids—10 or 12—and Their Complementary Food Proteins

All of the 10 essential amino acids must be supplied by the diet. But two of them, phenylalanine and methionine, have helpers as interactive backup. The body makes the amino acids tyrosine, which can spare some of the phenylalanine, and cystine, which can interact with methionine. Therefore although there are only 10 essential amino acids because the body can't make them sufficiently or at all, sometimes—when the two helpers tyrosine and cystine are added—there are said to be 12 amino acids.

The real concern related to a vegetarian diet is in getting a balanced amount of the essential amino acids to complement each other and make complete food combinations. Only three of the 10 essential amino acids are critical, however, because if individuals eat foods to supply enough of these three in a combined pattern, sufficient amounts of the others are provided, as well. These three amino acids (i.e., lysine, methionine, and tryptophan) are thus called *limiting amino acids.* Of these three, lysine is the most limiting.

To make complementary food combinations to balance the needed amino acids, families of foods

(e.g., grains, legumes, and milk) must be mixed. For example, grains are low in lysine and high in methionine, while legumes are just the opposite—low in methionine and high in lysine. So basically, grains and legumes will always balance one another, and the addition of milk products and eggs will enhance their adequacy. Here are a few sample food combination dishes to illustrate:

- Rice + black-eyed peas—a Southern United States dish called "Hopping John"
- Whole wheat or bulgur + soybeans + sesame seeds—protein enhanced by the addition of yogurt
- Cornmeal + kidney beans—a combination in many Mexican dishes, protein enhanced by the addition of cheese
- Soybeans + peanuts + brown rice + bulgur wheat—an excellent sauce dish served over the rice and wheat

Prepared with a variety of herbs, spices, onions, and garlic to suit your taste, such dishes can supply needed nutrients and good eating.

milk products (e.g., cheese) with a varied mixed diet of whole or enriched grains, legumes, nuts, seeds, fruits, and vegetables in sufficient quantities to meet energy needs provides a balanced intake.

Vegans. Vegans follow a strict vegetarian diet and use no animal foods. Their food pattern is composed entirely of plant foods (e.g., whole or enriched grains, legumes, nuts, seeds, fruits, and vegetables). The use of soybeans, soy milk, soybean

curd (tofu), and processed soy protein products enhances the nutritional value of the diet, and these products are well-tolerated and accepted. Careful planning and sufficient food intake are necessary for adequate nutrition (Clinical Applications box, "Case Study: A Vegan Child and Her Family").

The American Dietetic Association's current position paper on vegetarian diets indicates that the former conscious combining of complementary plant proteins within every given meal is unnecessary.[6]

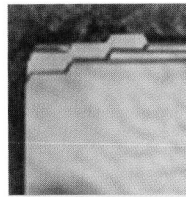

CLINICAL APPLICATIONS
CASE STUDY: A Vegan Child and Her Family

A vegan couple decided to raise their 2-year-old daughter on their strict vegetarian diet. Often the child did not finish her meals and ate snacks of fruits and biscuits. The parents eventually began to notice that she was not growing at the same rate as the other children and was becoming thin.

Questions for Analysis
1. What food patterns would you expect in this family? What dietary factor may have been involved in the child's poor growth?
2. What advice would you offer these parents to improve their child's nutritional status?
3. Plan 1 day's food for this family that would meet their nutritional needs within their vegetarian pattern. Indicate any added foods to meet the child's needs.
4. Would nutrient supplementation be indicated for this family, especially for the children? Why or why not? What would you suggest to them?

DIGESTION OF PROTEINS

Mouth

After the food protein is secured, it must be changed into the necessary, ready-to-use building units, amino acids. This work is done through the successive parts of the gastrointestinal tract by the mechanical and chemical processes of digestion. The mechanical breaking up of protein foods only occurs by chewing in the mouth. The food particles are mixed with saliva and passed on to the stomach as a semisolid mass.

Stomach

Because proteins are such large, complex structures, a series of enzymes is necessary to finally break them down and produce their structural units, amino acids. These chemical changes begin in the stomach. In fact, the stomach's chief digestive function overall is the partial first stage in the enzymatic breakdown of protein. The following three agents in the gastric secretions help with this task:

Pepsin

Pepsin is the main gastric enzyme, specific to proteins. It is first produced as an inactive proenzyme, *pepsinogen*, by a single layer of cells (i.e., the chief cells) in the stomach wall. The hydrochloric acid in the gastric juices then change pepsinogen to the enzyme pepsin. The active pepsin begins splitting the links between the protein's amino acids, which changes the large amino acid chains that make up the protein into smaller short chains called *peptides*. If the protein were held in the stomach longer,

---

proenzyme an inactive precursor (forerunner substance from which another substance is made) that is converted to the active enzyme by the action of an acid, another enzyme, or other means. Also called zymogen.

pepsin (Gr. *pepsis*, digestion) the main gastric enzyme specific for proteins. Pepsin begins breaking large protein molecules into shorter chain polypeptides; gastric hydrochloric acid necessary to activate.

pepsin could continue this breakdown until only the individual amino acids of the protein resulted. But with normal gastric emptying time, pepsin only completes the first stage of breakdown.

Hydrochloric Acid

Hydrochloric acid provides the acid medium necessary to convert pepsinogen to active pepsin.

Rennin

The gastric enzyme rennin is only present in infancy and childhood and is especially important in the infant's digestion of milk. Rennin and calcium act on the casein of milk to produce a curd. By coagulating milk into a more solid curd, rennin prevents the food from passing too rapidly from the infant's stomach to the small intestine.

Small Intestine

Protein digestion begins in the acidic medium of the stomach and is completed in the alkaline medium of the small intestine. Enzymes from secretions of both the pancreas and the intestine take part.

Pancreatic Secretions

The following three enzymes produced by the pancreas continue breaking down proteins into simpler and simpler substances:

1. Trypsin, secreted first as the inactive trypsinogen, is activated by a local hormone from glands in the wall of the duodenum, the first section of the small intestine. Then the active enzyme works on protein and large polypeptide fragments carried from the stomach. This enzymatic action produces small polypeptides and dipeptides.
2. Chymotrypsin, secreted first as the inactive chymotrypsinogen, is activated by the trypsin already present. The active enzyme then continues the same protein-splitting action of trypsin.

TABLE 4-1 Summary of protein digestion

| Organ | Enzyme | | | |
	Inactive precursor	Activator	Active enzyme	Digestive action
Mouth			None	Mechanical only
Stomach (acid)	Pepsinogen	Hydrochloric acid	Pepsin	Protein → polypeptides
			Rennin (infants) (calcium necessary for activity)	Casein → coagulated curd
Intestine (alkaline)				
Pancreas	Trypsinogen	Enterokinase	Trypsin	Protein, polypeptides → polypeptides, dipeptides
	Chymotrypsinogen	Active trypsin	Chymotrypsin	Protein, polypeptides → polypeptides, dipeptides
			Carboxypeptidase	Polypeptides → simpler peptides, dipeptides, amino acids
Intestine			Aminopeptidase	Polypeptides → peptides, dipeptides, amino acids
			Dipeptidase	Dipeptides → amino acids

3. Carboxypeptidase attacks the acid (carboxyl) end of the peptide chains, producing small peptides and some free amino acids.

Intestinal Secretions

Glands in the intestinal wall produce two more protein-splitting enzymes to complete the breakdown and free the remaining amino acids:

1. Aminopeptidase attacks the nitrogen-containing (amino) end of the peptide chains and releases amino acids one at a time, producing peptides and free amino acids.
2. Dipeptidase, the final enzyme in the protein-splitting system, completes the large task by breaking the remaining dipeptides into two free amino acids.

This finely coordinated system of protein-splitting enzymes breaks down the large, complex proteins into progressively smaller peptide chains and frees each individual amino acid—a tremendous overall task. The free amino acids are now ready to be absorbed directly into the portal blood circulation for use in building body tissues. A summary of this remarkable system of protein digestion is given in Table 4-1.

BODY NEEDS FOR PROTEIN

Protein Requirements: Influencing Factors

The following three factors influence our requirement for protein: (1) tissue growth needs, (2) quality of the dietary protein, and (3) additional needs from illness or disease.

Tissue Growth

During rapid growth periods of the human life cycle, more protein per unit of body size is required to build new tissue, as well as maintain present tissue. Human growth is most rapid during the following three periods: fetal growth during the mother's pregnancy, infant growth during the first year of life plus the lactation needs of a breastfeeding mother,

and adolescent growth and development into adulthood. Young childhood is a sustained time of continued growth but at a somewhat slower rate. For adults, protein requirements level off to meet tissue-maintenance needs, but individual needs may vary.

Dietary Protein Quality

The nature of the protein foods eaten and their pattern of amino acids significantly influence the quality of the dietary protein. Sufficient kcalories or energy intake—especially from nonprotein foods—is also necessary to conserve protein for tissue building. Finally, the digestion and absorption of the

rennin milk-curdling enzyme of the gastric juice of human infants and young animals such as calves. Do not confuse with *renin,* which is an important enzyme produced by the kidney that plays a vital role in producing angiotensin, a potent vasoconstrictor and stimulant for release of the hormone aldosterone from the adjacent adrenal glands.

trypsin a protein-splitting enzyme, secreted as the inactive proenzyme *trypsinogen* in the pancreas, that is activated and acts in the small intestine to reduce proteins to shorter chain polypeptides and dipeptides.

chymotrypsin a protein-splitting enzyme, secreted as the inactive proenzyme *chymotrypsinogen* in the pancreas, that is activated and acts in the small intestine to continue breaking down proteins into shorter chain polypeptides and dipeptides.

carboxypeptidase specific protein-splitting enzyme, secreted in inactive form in the pancreas, that is activated by trypsin in the small intestine to break off the acid (carboxyl, COOH) end of the peptide chain forming protein, producing smaller chained peptides and free amino acids.

aminopeptidase specific protein-splitting enzyme, secreted by small glands in the walls of the small intestine that breaks off the nitrogen-containing amino ($-NH_2$) end of the peptide chain forming protein, producing smaller chained peptides and free amino acids.

dipeptidase specific final enzyme in the protein-splitting system that produces the last two free amino acids.

protein consumed is affected by the comparative complexity of its structure, as well as its preparation and cooking. The comparative quality of protein foods has been determined by the four basic measures that follow:

1. *Chemical score (CS)* is a value derived from the amino acid pattern of the food. Using a high-quality protein food, such as egg, and giving it a value of 100, other foods are compared according to their amino acid ratios.
2. *Biologic value (BV)* is based on nitrogen balance.
3. *Net protein utilization (NPU)* is based on the biologic value and the degree of the food protein's digestibility.
4. *Protein efficiency ratio (PER)* is based on the weight gain of a growing test animal in relation to its protein intake.

Table 4-2 provides a comparison of various protein food scores based on these measures of protein quality. As seen in this table, egg and milk proteins lead all the lists. A sound diet is the best way for a healthy person to obtain quality protein. There is no need for amino acid supplements.

Illness or Disease

An illness or disease, especially when accompanied by fever and increased tissue breakdown (catabolism), increases the body's need for protein and kcalories for rebuilding tissue and to meet the demands of increased metabolic rate. Traumatic injury requires extensive tissue rebuilding. After surgery, extra protein is needed for wound healing and restoring losses. Extensive tissue destruction, as occurs with massive burns, requires a large protein increase for the healing and grafting processes.

Dietary Guides

Dietary Reference Intakes (DRIs) and Recommended Dietary Allowances (RDAs)

The RDAs continue to be the principal dietary guides for protein consumption and are part of

TABLE 4-2 Comparative protein quality of selected foods

Food	Chemical score*	BV†	NPU‡	PER§
Egg	100	100	94	3.92
Cow's milk	95	93	82	3.09
Fish	71	76	—	3.55
Beef	69	74	67	2.30
Unpolished rice	67	86	59	—
Peanuts	65	55	55	1.65
Oats	57	65	—	2.19
Polished rice	57	64	57	2.18
Whole wheat	53	65	49	1.53
Corn	49	72	36	—
Soybeans	47	73	61	2.32
Sesame seeds	42	62	53	1.77
Peas	37	64	55	1.57

Data adapted from Guthrie H: *Introductory nutrition,* ed 6, New York, 1986, McGraw-Hill; and from Food and Nutrition Board: *Recommended dietary allowances,* ed 10, Washington, DC, 1989, National Academy of Sciences.

*Amino acid   ‡Net protein utilization

†Biologic value   §Protein efficiency ratio

the new DRI standards. Guides for protein in the newer, more comprehensive DRI format are still being prepared and have not yet been published. The continuing RDA standards relate to the age and sex of the "average" person. For example, the reference man used for these determinations is aged 25 to 50 years and weighs 79 kg (174 lbs); the reference woman in this age group weighs 63 kg (138 lbs). Both are assumed to be in good health and doing moderate activity. The adult standards for protein are based on 0.8 g/kg desirable body weight per day. Thus the man described here would need about 63 g of protein per day; and his DRI for energy needs (kcalories) would be about 2900 kcal/day. The woman would need about 50 g protein/day; and her energy need is less—about 2200 kcal/day.

U.S. Dietary Guidelines

The dietary guidelines for Americans recommend that for adults, about 9% and no more than 13% of the diet's total kcalories come from protein, based on the latest guidelines from the National Academy of Sciences. There are no known benefits and

TABLE 4-3 Foods high in protein

Food	Approximate amount	Protein (g)
Beef, chuck roast	3 oz cooked	23.4
Beef, hamburger	3 oz cooked	20.5
Beef, round	3 oz cooked	24.7
Beef, cube steak	4 oz cooked	27.6
Lamb leg	3 oz cooked	21.6
Liver (beef, calf, or pork)	3 oz cooked	20.4
Pork loin	3 oz cooked	20.7
Ham	3 oz cooked	20.7
Veal, leg or shoulder	3 oz cooked	25.2
Chicken	¼ broiler	22.4
Chicken, fryer	½ breast (4 oz raw)	26.9
Chicken, hen, stewed	1 thigh or ½ breast	26.5
Duck, roasted	3 slices (3½ × 2¾ × ¼)	20.6
Goose, roasted	3 slices (3½ × 2¾ × ¼)	25.3
Turkey	3 slices (3½ × 2¾ × ¼)	27.8
Haddock	3 oz cooked	20.2
Halibut	3 oz cooked	21.0
Oysters	6 medium	15.1
Salmon	⅔ cup	20.5
Scallops	5-6 medium	23.8
Tuna	½ cup	15.9
Peanut butter	4 tbs	15.9
Milk	1 cup	8.5
Cottage cheese	5-6 tbs	19.5
American cheddar cheese	1 oz	7.0
Egg	1 medium	7.0

some potential health risks in the consumption of a diet with a high animal protein content, which also carries added fat. These risks relate to certain cancers, coronary heart disease associated with increased animal fat, urinary calcium loss and kidney stones, as well as chronic renal failure (see Chapter 21) associated with the increased protein. Therefore the National Research Council has recommended that adult protein intake be maintained at moderate levels, meeting the standard of 0.8 g/kg of desirable body weight per day, as described here (i.e., a moderate protein intake of 9% to 13% of the total day's kcalories). Americans generally eat more protein than necessary, especially in the form of meat, which carries considerable animal fat. Cutting down consumption of meat to leaner moderate portions would also bring the health benefits of reducing the intake of saturated animal fat. Table 4-3 provides a comparison of protein food portions.

SUMMARY

Proteins provide the human body with its primary tissue-building units, amino acids. Of the 22 known amino acids, 10 are essential in the diet because the body cannot manufacture them as it can the remaining ones. Foods that supply all the essential amino acids are called complete proteins. These foods are of animal origin (e.g., egg, milk, cheese, and meat). Plant protein foods (e.g., grains, legumes, nuts, seeds, vegetables, and fruits) are called incomplete because they lack one or more of the essential amino acids. Strict vegetarian diets use only plant proteins; but other vegetarian diets may use milk and egg, eliminating only meat.

Constant turnover of tissue protein occurs between tissue building (anabolism) and tissue breakdown (catabolism). Adequate dietary protein and a reserve "pool" of amino acids help to maintain this overall protein balance. Nitrogen balance is a measure of overall protein balance. A mixed diet of a variety of foods, together with sufficient nonprotein kcalories from the primary fuel foods, supplies a balance of protein and other nutrients. Only strict vegetarians—vegans—risk protein imbalance and other nutritional deficiencies in iron, zinc, calcium, and vitamin B_{12}.

After protein foods are eaten, a powerful digestive team of six protein-splitting enzymes frees individual unique amino acids for their vital tissue-building tasks.

Protein requirements are mainly influenced by growth needs and the nature of the diet in terms of protein quality and energy intake. Clinical influences on protein needs include fever, disease, surgery, or other trauma to body tissues.

REVIEW QUESTIONS

1. What is the difference between essential and nonessential amino acids? Why is this difference important?
2. Compare complete and incomplete protein foods. Give examples of each.
3. Describe the different types of vegetarian diets. Compare each in terms of protein quality and risk for nutrient deficiencies.
4. Describe the factors that influence protein requirements.

SELF-TEST QUESTIONS

True-False

Write the correct statement for each item you answer "false."

1. Complete proteins of high biologic value are found in whole grains, dried beans and peas, and nuts.
2. The primary function of dietary protein is to supply the necessary amino acids to build and repair body tissue.
3. Protein provides a main source of body heat and muscle energy.
4. The average American diet contains a relatively moderate amount of protein.
5. Because they are smaller, infants and young children need less protein per unit of body weight than adults.
6. In old age the protein requirement decreases because of decreased physical activity.
7. Healthy adults are in a state of nitrogen balance.
8. Positive nitrogen balance exists during periods of rapid growth (e.g., in infancy and adolescence).
9. When negative nitrogen balance exists, an individual is less able to resist infection and general health deteriorates.
10. Wheat and rice are complete protein foods of high biologic value.
11. Egg protein has a higher biologic value than meat protein.

Multiple Choice

1. Ten of the 22 amino acids are "essential," meaning that:
    a. The body cannot make them and must get them in the diet.
    b. They are essential in body processes and the rest are not.
    c. The body makes them because they are the life-essential ones.
    d. After making them, the body uses them for essential growth.
2. A complete protein food of high biologic value contains:
    a. All 22 of the amino acids in sufficient amounts to meet human requirements.
    b. The 10 essential amino acids in any proportion because the body can always fill in the necessary differences.
    c. All of the 22 amino acids from which the body can make additional amounts of the 10 essential ones, as necessary.
    d. All 10 of the essential amino acids in correct proportion to meet human requirements.
3. A state of negative nitrogen balance occurs during periods of:
    a. Pregnancy.
    b. Adolescence.
    c. Injury or surgery.
    d. Infancy.

SUGGESTIONS FOR ADDITIONAL STUDY

1. Collect illustrations of complete and incomplete protein foods for your notebook.
2. List the protein food combinations you usually have at daily meals.
3. Keep a record of everything you eat or drink for 1 day. Calculate your protein intake and compare it with your need according to the DRI guidelines. Identify your complete and incomplete protein food sources. How would you rate the protein quality of your diet?

REFERENCES

1. Cordes MHJ and others: Evolution of a protein fold in vitra, *Science* 284(5412), April 9, 325, 1999.
2. Strauss E: Introducing proteins into body cells, *Science* 285(5433):1466, 1999.
3. Peterson J: Simulations nab protein-folding mistakes, *Science News* 155(Mar 6):150, 1999.
4. Barinaga M: New clues to how proteins link up to run the cell, *Science* 283(Feb 26):1247, 1999.
5. Young VR, Pellett PL: Plant proteins in relation to human protein and amino acid nutrition, *Am J Clin Nutr* 5S:1203S, 1994.
6. Messina VK, Burke KI: Position of the American Dietetic Association: vegetarian diets, *J Am Diet Assoc* 97(11): 1317, 1997.

FURTHER READING

- Robertson L and others: *The new Laurel's kitchen*, ed 3, Berkeley, Calif., 1998, Ten Speed Press.

  This excellent book, revised and expanded in its third edition, combines sound nutrition with a wide variety of cooking suggestions and recipes for a vegetarian diet that are both healthy and delicious. Its pages are permeated by the warmth of its authors and their many practical guidelines and personal anecdotes. It remains one of the best vegetarian cookbooks.

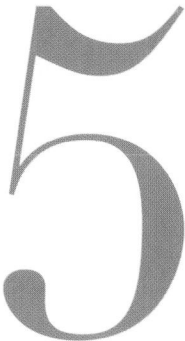

Energy Balance

KEY CONCEPTS

- Food energy is changed into body energy and cycled throughout the body to do its work.

- The body uses most of its energy intake for basal metabolic work needs.

- A balance between intake of food energy and output of body-work energy maintains life and health.

- States of being underweight and overweight reflect degrees of body energy imbalance.

Our efficient bodies constantly change the stored fuel energy in our food into the energy we use at work and play, as well as at rest. Overall energy metabolism deals with *change* and *balance*, the constant facts of life.

Many constant changes and balances in the nutrients that our food delivers to our body cells produce our needed energy. Fuel is "burned" and stored as necessary to provide a continuous flow of energy for our body's work.

In this chapter, we look at the "big picture" of energy balance among all the energy nutrients. We see how this energy intake is measured, cycled, and used to meet all our energy needs.

HUMAN ENERGY SYSTEM
Basic Energy Needs

The body needs constant energy to do the work required to maintain life and health. The actions involved are both voluntary and involuntary.

Voluntary Work and Exercise

Voluntary body work includes all the physical actions related to a person's usual activities, as well as any additional physical exercise. Although this visible, conscious action would seem to require most of our energy output, this is usually not true.

Involuntary Body Work

The greatest energy output is the result of involuntary body work, which includes all the activities in the body that are not consciously performed. These activities include such vital processes as circulation, respiration, digestion, and absorption, as well as many other internal activities that maintain life at all times.

Sources of Fuel

The energy needed for voluntary and involuntary body work requires fuel, which is provided in the form of nutrients. As presented in previous chapters, the only three "energy nutrients" are carbohydrate, fat, and protein. Carbohydrate is the body's primary fuel, with fat assisting as a storage fuel. Protein is occasionally a back-up fuel—and actually an inefficient one, at that—available as needed. The body must have a supply of the food fuels to provide energy for work and keep the body warm. If the sufficient primary fuel, carbohydrate, is not consumed to supply these body-energy needs, the body will burn more fat. To maintain health, the average daily food energy intake should equal the daily body energy needs.

Measurement of Energy

Unit of Measure: Kilocalorie

In common usage, the word *calorie* refers to the amount of energy in food or expended in physical actions. In human nutrition, however, the term *kilocalorie* (1000 calories) is used to designate the large calorie unit used in nutritional science to avoid dealing with such large numbers. A kilocalorie, abbreviated as *kcalorie* or *kcal*, is the amount of heat required to raise 1 kg of water 1° centigrade (C). Sometimes you may see the international unit of measure for energy, *joule* (J). The conversion factor for changing kilocalories (kcal) to kilojoules (kJ) is 4.184. Therefore 1 kcal equals 4.184 kJ.

Food Energy: Fuel Factors

As previously discussed, the three energy nutrients (i.e., carbohydrate and fat with protein as a back-up) have basic fuel factors. Beverage alcohol, from fermented grains and fruits, also adds fuel. These factors reflect their relative fuel densities, as follows: (1) carbohydrate: 4 kcal/g; (2) fat: 9 kcal/g; (3) protein: 4 kcal/g; and (4) alcohol: 7 kcal/g.

Caloric and Nutrient Density

The term *density* refers to the degree of concentration of material in a given substance. More material in a smaller amount of substance gives that substance a greater density. Thus the concept of *caloric density* refers to a higher concentration of energy (kcalories) in a smaller amount of food. Therefore, of the three energy nutrients, fat or foods high in fat have the highest caloric density. Similarly, foods may be evaluated in terms of their relative *nutrient density*. High nutrient density refers to a relatively high concentration of nutrients—from all nutrient groups—in smaller amounts of a given food. A number of food guides do not base their listed "food scores" on the concentration of nutrients in given foods but on the overall nutrient density in those foods as a general indicator of a food's contribution to health goals.

ENERGY BALANCE

Energy, like matter, cannot be "created." When we speak of energy as being "produced," we really mean that it is being transformed (i.e., changed in form and cycled throughout a system). Consider our human energy system as part of the total energy system on earth. In this sense, two energy systems support our lives: the one within us and the much larger one surrounding us, as follows:

1. **External energy cycle:** In our environment, the ultimate source of energy is the sun and its vast nuclear reactions. Using water and carbon dioxide as raw materials, plants transform the sun's radiation into stored chemical energy (i.e., mainly carbohydrate and some fat). The food chain continues as animals eat plants and transform plant energy into animal food energy.

2. **Internal energy cycle:** When we eat plant and animal foods, we change the stored energy into our own body fuels, glucose and fatty acids, and cycle them into various other energy forms to serve our body needs. These forms include the following: (1) chemical energy in the many new metabolic products made; (2) electric energy in brain and nerve tissue; (3) mechanical energy in muscle contraction; and (4) thermal energy in the heat to keep our bodies warm. As this internal energy cycle continues, we excrete water, exhale carbon dioxide, and radiate heat, returning these end-products to the external environment. The overall energy cycle repeats constantly, sustaining our lives.

Energy Intake

The total overall energy balance within the body depends on the energy intake in relation to the energy output. The main source of energy for all body work is food, backed up by stored energy in body tissues.

Sources of Food Energy

The three energy nutrients in food keep our bodies supplied with fuel. You can easily estimate your own energy intake by recording a day's actual food consumption, using a form such as the one in Table 5-1, and calculating its energy value (see Appendix A).

Sources of Stored Energy

When food is not available, as during sleep or longer periods of fasting or the extreme stress of starvation, the body draws from its stores of energy.

Glycogen. A 12- to 48-hour reserve of glycogen exists in liver and muscles and is quickly depleted if not replenished by daily food intake. For example, glycogen stores maintain normal blood glucose levels for body functions during sleep hours. Our first meal, breakfast—so named because it "breaks the fast," has a significant function for energy intake.

Adipose tissue. Although fat storage is larger than glycogen, the supply varies from person to person, and a balanced amount needs to be maintained as an added energy resource.

Muscle mass. Energy stored as protein exists in limited amounts in muscle mass, but this lean muscle mass must be maintained for health. Only during longer periods of fasting or starvation does the body turn to these tissues for energy.

Energy Output

The energy from our food and body reserves is spent in the necessary activities of various organs of the

---

calorie (L. *calor,* heat) a measure of heat. The *energy* required to do the work of the body is measured as the amount of *heat* produced by the body's work. The energy value of a food is expressed as the number of kilocalories a specified portion of the food will yield when oxidized in the body.

kilocalorie (Fr. *chilioi,* thousand; L. *calor,* heat) the general term *calorie* refers to a unit of heat measure and is used alone to designate the *small calorie* or as a general term in common language for the *large calorie,* the kilocalorie. The calorie used in nutritional science and the study of metabolism is the large calorie (1,000 calories) or kilocalorie, to be more accurate and avoid the use of very large numbers in calculations.

TABLE 5-1 Record of Food Energy Intake

List all meals and snacks for 1 day: Food (description and amount)	Carbohydrates (g)	Fat (g)	Protein (g)	Kcalories
Breakfast				
Lunch				
Snacks				
Dinner				
Snacks				
TOTAL				

body, such as body function work, regulation of body temperature, and the processes of tissue growth and repair. The total chemical changes that occur during all of these body activities are called *metabolism*. This exchange of energy in overall balance is usually expressed in kcalories. The energy output of the body is based on the following three demands for energy: (1) basal metabolism, (2) physical activity, and (3) eating.

Basal Metabolism

The term basal metabolism refers to the sum of all internal working activities of the body at rest. In general use, the terms *basal energy expenditure* (BEE), *resting energy expenditure* (REE), and *resting metabolic rate* (RMR) are interchangeable,[1,2] describing a vast amount of physiologic work. Most of the body's energy is spent maintaining these metabolic functions, although the majority of this amount is used by small but highly active tissues (e.g., liver, brain, heart, kidney, and gastrointestinal tract), which amount to less than 5% of the total body weight. These tissues, however, contribute about 60% of the total basal metabolism needs. Although resting muscle and adipose fat are far larger in mass, they contribute much less to the body's basal metabolic rate.

Measuring basal metabolic rate. Sometimes in clinical practice (e.g., on metabolic wards), a measure of the basal metabolic rate (BMR) is made by *indirect calorimetry.* This method indirectly measures the amount of energy a person uses while at rest. The test is done with a portable instrument on a cart at the bedside. The person breathes into an attached mouthpiece, and the normal exchange of oxygen and carbon dioxide in regular breathing is measured. The metabolic rate is calculated with a high degree of accuracy from the rate of oxygen utilization. In addition, *thyroid function tests* may be used as indirect measures of BMR because the thyroid hormone regulates BMR. These tests measure the activity of the thyroid gland and the blood levels of its hormone thyroxine. The tests also include measures of serum thyroxin levels and of serum–protein-bound iodine (PBI) and radioactive iodine uptake because iodine's basic function is in synthesizing thyroxine.

A general formula for calculating basal energy needs is to multiply 1 kcal/kg body weight (weight in pounds divided by 2.2) by the number of hours in a day. Thus the daily basal metabolic needs (in kcalories) are calculated as follows:

$$1 \text{ kcal} \times \text{kg body weight} \times 24 \text{ hrs}$$

The classic Harris-Benedict equations provide an alternate method of estimating the basal or resting energy expenditure for adult hospitalized patients, as follows:

Women: BEE = 655 + 9.56 × weight (kg) +
        1.85 × height (cm) − 4.68 × age

Men: BEE = 66.5 + 13.8 × weight (kg) +
        5 × height (cm) − 6.76 × age

Factors influencing BMR. Several factors that influence BMR should be kept in mind when related test results are read. The major factors affecting BMR relate to lean body mass, growth periods, and body temperature, as follow.[1,2]

- **Lean body mass:** The greatest factor affecting BMR is the relative amount of lean body mass in the body composition. This is due to the greater metabolic activity in lean tissues as compared with fat and bones. The BMR is higher in lean bodies, thus requiring more energy. It is lower in fat bodies, thus requiring less energy. Other factors such as surface area, sex, and age only influence BMR as they relate to the lean body mass.[2]

- **Growth periods:** During growth periods, the growth hormone stimulates cell metabolism and raises BMR 15% to 20%. Thus the BMR slowly rises during the first 5 years of life, levels off somewhat, rises again just before and during puberty, and then gradually declines into old age. During pregnancy, which is a rapid growth period, the BMR rises 20% to 25% due to the accelerated tissue growth and the increased work of the heart and lungs. During the following period of lactation, the breast-feeding mother's BMR increases further, and she needs extra kcalories to cover this added metabolic process.

- **Body temperature:** Fever increases BMR approximately 7% for each 0.83° C (1° F) rise in temperature. Diseases involving increased cell activity (e.g., cancer, cardiac failure) and respiratory problems (e.g., emphysema) usually increase the BMR. In the abnormal states of starvation and malnutrition, the BMR is lowered because the lean body mass is decreased. In cold weather—especially in freezing temperatures—the BMR rises somewhat to generate more body heat to maintain normal body temperature.

---

basal metabolism (Gr. *basis,* base; *metabole,* change) The amount of energy needed by the body for maintenance of life when a person is at digestive, physical, and emotional rest. This basal metabolic rate (BMR) is reported as the percent of variation in the person above or below the normal number of kilocalories required for a person of like height, weight, sex, and age.

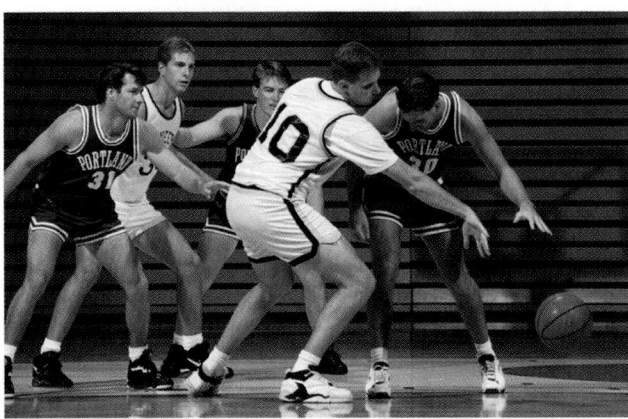

FIGURE 5-1   Energy output in exercise. (Credit: PhotoDisc.)

Physical Activity

Exercise involved in work or recreation (Figure 5-1) accounts for wide individual variations in energy output (see Chapter 16). Regular physical activity, balanced with adequate energy intake, is especially important for older persons to help offset the risk for heart disease and diabetes.[3-5] Physical activity has beneficial effects on both the body and mind throughout the adult years.[5] Some representative kcalorie expenditures in different types of work and recreation are given in Table 5-1. Mental work or study does not require additional kcalories; emotional states do not increase kcalorie needs but may require energy intake to compensate for muscle tension, restlessness, and agitated movements. The feeling of fatigue is caused by muscle tension or moving about.

Effect of Eating

After we eat, the food stimulates our metabolism and requires extra energy for digestion, absorption, and transport of the nutrients to the cells. This overall stimulating effect is called the *thermic effect of food* (TEF). About 5% to 10% of the body's total energy needs for metabolism relates to the handling of the food we eat.[2]

Total Energy Requirement

The basal energy requirement, individual physical activities, and the energy need involved with eating food (i.e., TEF) make up a person's overall total energy requirement. To maintain daily energy balance, food-energy intake must match body-energy output. An energy imbalance when food-energy intake exceeds body energy output causes obesity. Treatment should include a decrease in food kcalories and an increase in physical activity. Extreme weight loss (e.g., anorexia nervosa) results when food-energy intake does not meet body energy requirements. Treatment should include a gradual increase in food kcalories along with moderate activity and rest. A discussion of weight management is given in Chapter 15.

Where do you stand in your own energy balance? You can estimate your energy needs by using the steps in the Clinical Applications box, "Evaluate Your Own Daily Energy Requirements." You may instead wish to record your actual food and activities for a day and calculate your energy intake (kcalories) and output (kcalorie expenditure in light to heavy activities). Total your day's activity and compare it with the general type of similar activities given in Box 5-1. Estimate the total time you spent on a given activity by adding up the minutes you spent at any time on that activity, and then converting those minutes to hours (or decimal fractions of hours) for the day. For example, if you spent 10 minutes at one time and 5 minutes at another time doing the same thing, then your day's to-

BOX 5-1   Energy expenditure/hour during various activities*

Light activities: 120–150 kcal/hr	Light-moderate activities: 150–300 kcal/hr	Moderate activities: 300–420 kcal/hr	Heavy activities: 420–600 kcal/hr
Personal care	Housework	Yard work	Yard work
Dressing	Making beds	Digging	Chopping wood
Washing	Sweeping floors	Mowing lawn (not	Digging holes
Shaving	Ironing	motorized)	Shoveling snow
Sitting	Washing clothes	Pulling weeds	Walking
Rocking	Yard work	Walking	5 mph
Typing	Light gardening	3½-4 mph on level	Upstairs
Writing	Mowing lawn (power	surface	Up hills
Playing cards	mower)	Up and down small	Climbing
Peeling potatoes	Light work	hills	Recreation
Sewing	Auto repair	Recreation	Bicycling 11-12 mph
Playing piano	Painting	Badminton	or up and down
Standing or	Store clerk	Calisthenics	hills
slowly moving	Washing car	Ballet exercises	Cross-country skiing
around	Walking	Dancing (waltz,	Jogging 5 mph
Billiards	2-3 mph on level sur-	square)	Swimming
	face or down stairs	Golf (no cart)	Tennis (singles)
	Recreation	Ping-Pong	Water-skiing
	Bicycling 5½ mph on	Tennis (doubles)	
	level surface	Volleyball	
	Bowling		

*Energy expenditure depends on the physical fitness (i.e., amount of lean body mass) of the individual and continuity of exercise. Note that some of these activities can be used as aerobic activities to promote cardiovascular fitness. For more information, see Chapter 16.

tal for that activity is 15 min or 0.25 hr. Multiply this total time for a given type of activity by the average kcal/hr for that activity (see Box 5-1) and add them all up for the day's total kcalories. Use these basic steps to estimate your energy expenditure for a day's activities:

1. Total minutes of an activity ÷ 60 = hours of that activity
2. Total time (hr) × kcal/hr = total kcal/day for that activity
3. Total kcal/day of all activities = total kcal energy expenditure for day from activities

ENERGY REQUIREMENTS

General Life Cycle

Growth Periods

During periods of rapid growth, extra energy per unit of body weight is required to build new tissue. In childhood the most rapid growth occurs during infancy and adolescence, with continuous but slower growth in between (Table 5-2). The rapid growth of the fetus, placenta, and other maternal tissues makes increased energy intake during pregnancy and lactation a vital concern.

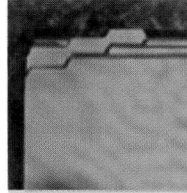

CLINICAL APPLICATIONS
Evaluate Your Own Daily Energy Requirements

Your total energy output (in kcal) per day is the sum of your body's three uses of energy:
1. Resting metabolic rate
2. Thermic effect of food
3. Physical activity

1. Basal metabolic rate (BMR):
Use general formula: Women: 0.9 kcal/kg/hr
                            Men: 1.0 kcal/kg/hr
Convert weight (lb) to kg: 1 kg = 2.2 lb
Multiply by formula:
    BMR (kcal) = 1 (or 0.9) × kg weight × 24 (hours in day)

2. Thermic effect of food intake (TEF):
The thermic effect of food is the energy the body uses in the processes of digestion and absorption. It averages 10% of the energy in the food.
    Record your food intake for one day (24 hours) and calculate approximate energy value (kcal), using either Table of Food Values in Appendix A or a simple computer program.
    Find energy cost of thermic effect of food (TEF):
    TEF (kcal) = 10% of total kcal in food consumed

3. Physical activity:
Estimate your general average level of physical activity.
    The energy used by physical activity can be approximated as a percentage of your **BMR** and varies with the degree of physical activity. Use this list to select your activity level:

Average Activity Level	Energy Cost: % of RMR
Sedentary	20%
Very light	30%
Moderate	40%
Heavy	50%

Find the energy cost of your activity level:
    Physical activity energy cost (kcal) = BMR × your activity %
For example, if you are sedentary (mostly sitting): BMR × 20%

4. Calculate your total energy output:
    Total energy output (kcal) = BMR + TEF + physical activity
Example 1:
A woman who weighs 130 lbs (59 kg), who eats an average of 1800 kcal per day, and who has started and maintains a regular physical exercise program.
    BMR   = 0.9 × 59 × 24 = 1274 kcal
    TEF   = 1800 × 10% = 180 kcal
    Activity = BMR × 40% = 510 kcal
    Total energy output   = 1964 kcal
Result: This woman will lose weight. Her energy output is around 150 kcal per day greater than her food intake. Because 1 lb of body weight equals approximately 3500 kcal, she will lose about 1 lb every 20 to 30 days with the above eating and exercise routine.
Example 2:
A man who weighs 180 lbs (82 kg), who eats an average of 2700 kcal per day, and who has a sedentary lifestyle.
    BMR   = 1 × 82 × 24 = 1968 kcal
    TEF   = 2700 × 10% = 270 kcal
    Activity = BMR × 20% = 394 kcal
    Total energy output   = 2632 kcal
Result: This man will tend to gain weight slowly over time. What would your clinical advice be to him?

TABLE 5-2 Approximate caloric allowances for ages 1 month to 19 years

Age	Kcalories per pound	Age	Kcalories per pound
Infants		Boys	
1-3 mo	54.3	13-15 yr	30.0
4-9 mo	49.5	16-19 yr	25.5
10-12 mo	45.5	Girls	
Children		13-15 yr	24.3
1-3 yr	45.0	16-19 yr	20.0
4-6 yr	40.0		
7-9 yr	40.0		
10-12 yr	32.0		

Adulthood

With full adult growth achieved, the energy needs of young adults level off, meeting requirements for tissue maintenance and usual physical activities. As the aging process continues, the gradual decline in BMR and physical activity decreases the energy requirement (Table 5-3). Therefore food choices should reflect a decline in caloric density and place greater emphasis on increased nutrient density.

U.S. Dietary Guidelines

The U.S. dietary guidelines for healthy Americans indicate energy needs by the following two recommendations: (1) maintain a healthy weight, and (2) choose a diet low in fat, saturated fat, and cholesterol. Fats, the most concentrated fuel source, have the highest caloric density; and most Americans eat too much fat. A healthier energy balance also comes from using sugars only in moderation and eating a diet with plenty of vegetables, fruits, and grain products (see Chapter 1).

TABLE 5-3 Gradual reduction of kcalorie needs during adulthood

Age	Kcalorie reduction (%) for maintenance of ideal weight*
30-40	3.0
40-50	3.0
50-60	7.5
60-70	7.5
70-80	10.0

*Added percent decreases for each decade past the age of 25.

SUMMARY

Energy is the force or power to do work. In the human energy system, energy intake is provided by food. This energy is measured in "large calories" (e.g., every 1000 calories), or *kilocalories* (*kcalorie, kcal*). Energy from food is cycled through our internal energy system in balance with the external environment's energy system, which is powered by the sun.

Metabolism is the sum of the body processes that change our food energy from the three energy nutrients (i.e., mainly carbohydrate, some fat, and protein as backup) into various forms of energy. These forms include *chemical* energy (in many metabolic products), *electrical* energy (in brain and nerve activities), *mechanical* energy (in muscle contraction), and *thermal* (heat) energy to keep us warm. Throughout this cycling of our body energy, metabolism is balanced by two types of metabolic actions, as follow: (1) *anabolism*, which builds tissue and stores energy; and (2) *catabolism*, which breaks down tissue and releases energy. When food is not available, the body draws on its stored energy: glycogen, fat, and tissue protein.

Total body energy requirements are based on the following: (1) basal (i.e., maintenance) metabolism needs, which are measured by the BMR and compose the largest portion of our energy needs; (2) energy for physical activities; and (3) the thermal effect of food (i.e., digesting food and absorbing and transporting nutrients).

REVIEW QUESTIONS

1. What are the fuel factors of the three energy nutrients? What are the fuel factors of alcohol? What do these figures mean? What is our primary energy nutrient? Why?

2. Define *basal metabolism*. What body tissues contribute most to our basal metabolic needs? Why? What factors influence basal energy needs (BMR)? Why?

3. What factors influence nonbasal energy needs?

SELF-TEST QUESTIONS

True-False
Write the correct statement for each item you answer "false."
1. Kilocalories are nutrients in foods.
2. Glycogen stores provide a long-lasting energy reserve to maintain blood-sugar levels.
3. Thyroid hormone controls the rate of overall body metabolism.
4. Because children are smaller, their energy requirements are less per kilogram (pound) of body weight than those of adults.
5. The process of catabolism builds new tissues.
6. Different persons doing the same amount of physical activity will require the same amount of energy in kcalories.

Multiple Choice
1. In human nutrition, the kilocalorie is used to:
   a. Provide nutrients.
   b. Measure body heat energy.
   c. Control energy reactions.
   d. Measure electrical energy.
2. In the following family of four, who has the highest energy needs per unit of body weight?
   a. 32-year-old mother
   b. 35-year-old father
   c. 2-month-old son
   d. 70-year-old grandmother
3. An overactive thyroid causes:
   a. Decreased energy need.
   b. No effect on energy need.
   c. Increased energy need.
   d. Obesity due to lower BMR.
4. Which of the following persons is using the most energy?
   a. Woman walking uphill
   b. Student studying for final examinations
   c. Teenager playing basketball
   d. Man driving a car
5. Which of these foods has the highest energy value per unit of weight?
   a. Bread
   b. Meat
   c. Potato
   d. Butter
6. A slice of bread contains 2 g of protein and 15 g of carbohydrate in the form of starch. What is its kcalorie value?
   a. 17 kcal
   b. 42 kcal
   c. 68 kcal
   d. 92 kcal

SUGGESTIONS FOR ADDITIONAL STUDY

1. Calculate your own energy balance for 1 day, based on your energy intake (i.e., food) and your energy output (i.e., basal metabolism, physical activities according to Table 5-1, and energy needed to handle your food after eating meals or snacks). Describe your energy balance in terms of your body weight.

2. Calculate the energy value (kcalories) of the following foods:
   - *1 cup milk:* carbohydrate, 12 g; fat, 10 g; protein, 8 g; kcalories, _____.
   - *½ cup ice cream:* carbohydrate, 15 g; fat, 9 g; protein, 3 g; kcalories, _____.
   - *½ cup cooked carrots:* carbohydrate, 7 g; fat, 0 g; protein, 2 g; kcalories, _____.
   - *½ grapefruit:* carbohydrate, 10 g; fat, 0 g; protein, 0 g; kcalories, _____.

3. List 10 of your favorite foods. Using Appendix A, check the kcalorie value of your usual portion of each one. Do any of these energy values surprise you?

REFERENCES

1. Guyton AC, Hall JE: *Textbook of medical physiology,* ed 9, Philadelphia,1996, W.B. Saunders.
2. Schutz Y, Jequier E: *Energy needs: assessment and requirements.* In Shils ME, Olson JA, Shike M, eds: *Modern nutrition in health and disease,* vol 1, ed 8, Philadelphia, 1994, Lea & Febiger.
3. Poehlman ET: Effect of exercise on daily energy needs in older individuals, *Am J Clin Nutr* 68:997, 1998.
4. Carpenter WH and others: Total energy needs of older African-Americans and Caucasians, *Am J Physiol* 274:E96-101, 1998.
5. Bunyard and others: Energy requirements of middle-aged men are modifiable by physical activity, *Am J Clin Nutr* 68:1136, 1998.

FURTHER READING

- The American Dietetic Association: *The healthy weight: a practical food guide,* Chicago, 1995, The Association.
- Position of the American Dietetic Association: weight management, *J Am Diet Assoc* 97(1):71, 1997.

These two important position papers from the American Dietetic Association discuss the importance of a healthy diet plan and physical activity that meet personal needs. The goal is to establish wise food habits and help persons develop and maintain a healthy lifestyle.

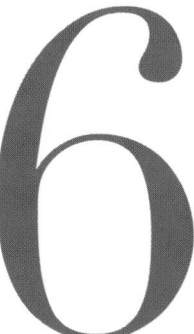

Vitamins

KEY CONCEPTS

- Vitamins are noncaloric essential nutrients that are necessary in very small amounts for specific metabolic control and disease prevention.

- Certain health problems are related to inadequate or excessive vitamin intake.

- Vitamins occur in a wide variety of foods that are packaged with the energy- and tissue-building macronutrients (i.e., carbohydrate, fat, protein) on which vitamins work as specific catalysts to regulate body metabolism.

- Vitamin supplementation needs are individual and specific.

More than any other group of nutrients, vitamins have captured public interest and concern. Vitamins are clearly essential nutrients—but what do they do, how much of them do we need, and where can we get them? Are they better in food or in pills? From the constant attention they receive in the public press, we know that vitamins *are* a concern of many people who need sound answers, not unfounded claims. The scientific study of nutrition, as reflected in the new Dietary Reference Intakes (DRIs) guidelines, continues to expand our knowledge.

In this chapter, we look at vitamins as a group and as individual nutrients. We will also explore our general and specific needs and how to approach vitamin use in a reasonable and realistic manner.

THE DIETARY REFERENCE INTAKES PROJECT

As we begin studying vitamins and minerals in nutrition, it is important to understand the system of national recommendations for their use and how these nutrient guidelines are expanding dramatically with the introduction of Dietary Reference Intakes (DRIs). Since 1941, the Recommended Dietary Allowances (RDAs), published by the National Academy of Sciences, has been the authoritative source setting standards for the minimum amounts of nutrients needed to protect almost all persons against the risk for nutrient deficiency. Since the last edition of the RDAs in 1989, both public awareness and research attention have shifted to reflect an increasing emphasis on nutrient requirements for maintaining optimum health for individuals and groups within the general population. This change of emphasis has resulted in the current DRIs project, which is also directed by the National Academy of Sciences. The creation of the new DRIs has involved hundreds of distinguished U.S. and Canadian scientists, divided into seven functional panels (see Figure 1-1), who have examined hundreds of nutritional studies on both the health benefits of nutrients and the hazards of taking too much of a nutrient. The new DRI recommendations are being published over several years in a series of seven volumes, the first three of which have been released as of publication of this text.[1-3]

The DRIs include recommendations for each gender and age group, as well as recommendations for pregnancy and lactation. For the first time, excessive amounts of nutrients are identified. The new DRIs incorporate and expand on the well-established RDAs. The DRIs encompass four interconnected categories of nutrient recommendations, as follow:

1. **Recommended Dietary Allowance (RDA)—** This is the daily intake of a nutrient that meets the needs of almost all healthy individuals of specific age and gender. Individuals should use the RDA as a guide to achieve adequate nutrient intake to decrease the risk of chronic disease. RDAs are only established when there is enough scientific evidence about a specific nutrient.

2. **Estimated Average Requirement (EAR)—** This is the intake level that meets the needs of half of the individuals in a specific group. This quantity is used as the basis for developing the RDA.

3. **Adequate Intake (AI)—**This is used as a guide when there is not enough scientific evidence available to establish the RDA figure. Both the RDA and the AI may be used as goals for individual intake.

4. **Tolerable Upper Intake Level (UL)—**This new indicator is not a recommended intake, but sets the maximum intake that is unlikely to pose adverse health risks in almost all healthy individuals. For most nutrients, the UL refers to the total daily intake from food, fortified food, and nutrient supplements.

In our study of vitamins in this chapter and minerals in the following chapter, we refer to the various DRI recommendations—especially the RDAs—whenever possible. The RDAs, now established for gender and age groups, continue to be the central guides on nutrient intake for most individuals.

THE NATURE OF VITAMINS
Discovery

Early Observations
Vitamins were largely discovered during the search for cures for classic diseases that were initially thought to be associated with dietary deficiencies. As early as 1753 a British naval surgeon, Dr. James Lind, observed that on long voyages when sailors were forced to live on very limited rations because no fresh foods were available, many of them became ill and died. When Lind gave some fresh lemons and limes (which are easily stored) to the sailors on a later voyage, no one became ill. This is also how

British sailors got the nickname "limeys." This vital clue then led to the discovery that *scurvy*, the curse of sailors, was caused by some dietary deficiency and was cured by adding certain fresh fruits to the diet.

Early Animal Experiments

In 1906, Dr. Frederich Hopkins of Cambridge University performed an experiment in which he fed a group of white rats a diet of a synthetic mixture of protein, fat, carbohydrate, mineral salts, and water. All of the animals became ill and died. When he added milk to the purified ration, however, all of the rats grew normally. This important discovery, that there are accessory food factors present in *natural* foods that are essential to life, reinforced the necessary foundation for the individual vitamin discoveries that followed.

Era of Vitamin Discovery

During the first half of the 1900s, the vitamins we now know of were discovered. The remarkable nature of these vital agents became more evident. A form of the name *vitamin* was first used in 1911 when Casimir Funk, a Polish chemist working at the Lister Institute in London, discovered a nitrogen-containing substance called an *amine*, which he thought was the chemical nature of these vital agents. So he called it *vitamine* ("vital-amine"). The final *e* was later dropped when other similarly vital substances turned out to be a variety of organic compounds. The name *vitamin* has been retained to designate compounds of this class of essential substances. At first, alphabet letter names were given to each vitamin discovered, but as the number quickly increased, this practice became confusing. In recent years, more specific names based on a vitamin's chemical structure or body function have been developed and the letter names largely dropped. Today these scientific names are preferred and commonly used, so they should be learned.

Definition

As each vitamin was discovered during the first half of the 1900s and the list grew, two character-istics clearly emerged to define a compound as a vitamin, as follow:

1. It must be a vital, organic, dietary substance that is not a carbohydrate, fat, protein, or mineral and is necessary in only very *small* amounts to perform a specific metabolic function or prevent an associated deficiency disease.
2. It cannot be manufactured by the body and therefore must be supplied by the diet.

On the basis of both of these characteristics, vitamins are essential to life and health. The amount of them that the body needs is very small (hence the designation "micronutrients"), unless some special state or condition creates an increased need in a particular person. The total volume of vitamins a healthy person normally requires per day would barely fill a teaspoon. Thus vitamins' units of measure (e.g., milligrams and micrograms) are exceedingly small and difficult to visualize (see For Further Focus box, "Small Measures for Small Needs"). All vitamins, however, are essential to existence.

Classes of Vitamins

Vitamins are usually classified as either *fat soluble* or *water soluble*. Although this is a somewhat arbitrary grouping with little real significance, it is the traditional grouping and is used here.[1] The fat-soluble vitamins, to use their to abbreviated letter group names, are A, D, E, and K. The water-soluble vitamins are C and all of the B vitamins.

Functions of Vitamins

Although each vitamin has its specific metabolic task, two general functions that have been ascribed to vitamins as a group are the following: (1) control agents in cell metabolism, and (2) components of body-tissue construction. A third function, preventing specific nutritional deficiency disease, may be considered a result of their primary role in cell metabolism.

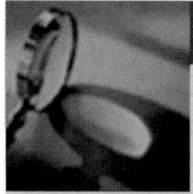

FOR FURTHER FOCUS
Small Measures for Small Needs

By definition, vitamins are essential nutrients required in small amounts for human health. But just how *very small* those amounts are is sometimes hard to imagine. Vitamins are measured in metric system terms such as *milligram* and *microgram*, but just how much is that? Perhaps comparing these amounts with commonly used household measures may help give you some idea.

Early in the age of scientific development, scientists realized that they needed a common language of measures that could be understood by all nations in order to fully exchange the rapidly developing scientific knowledge. Thus the metric system was born. Like our money, it is a simple decimal system, here applied to weights and measures. This system was developed in the mid-1800s by French scientists and named *Le Système International d'Unités*, which is abbreviated as SI units. Use of these more precise units is now widespread, especially because it is mandatory for all purposes in most countries besides the United States. The U.S. Congress passed the official Metric Conversion Act in 1975, but we have been slower to apply it to common use than other countries (see Appendix I). The use of this system in scientific work, however, is worldwide.

Compare the two metric measures used for vitamins in the United States. Following are the RDAs with common measures to see how small our need really is:

1. **Milligram** (mg) equals one-thousandth of a gram (28 grams = 1 oz; 1 g = about ¼ tsp). RDAs are measured in milligrams for vitamins E, C, thiamin, riboflavin, niacin, and B_6.
2. **Microgram** (mcg, or more often the Greek letter for "m"—μ) equals one-millionth of a gram. RDAs are measured in micrograms for vitamins A (retinol equivalents), D, K, folate, and B_{12}.

Small wonder that the total amount of vitamins we need in a day would scarcely fill a teaspoon—but that small amount makes the big difference between life and death.

Metabolic Control Agent: Coenzyme Partner

Specific enzymes and coenzymes control specific chemical reactions by acting as necessary *catalysts*. This term comes from the Greek word *katalysis*, meaning "to dissolve." In chemical usage, *catalyst* refers to substances such as enzymes that are necessary control agents for breaking down compounds but are not themselves consumed in the process.[4] In many cell reactions, a particular vitamin is required as a specific coenzyme partner with the regular cell enzyme to allow the reaction to proceed. Without the vitamin, the reaction cannot occur and the metabolic process involved cannot function. For example, several of the B vitamins (i.e., thiamin, niacin, and riboflavin) are essential components of the cell enzyme systems that metabolize glucose to produce energy.

Tissue Structure

Some of the vitamins act as tissue-building components. For example, vitamin C helps to deposit a cementlike substance in the spaces between cells to produce strong tissue. This material is called ground substance and is similar to collagen. In fact, the word *collagen* comes from a Greek word meaning "glue."

Prevention of Deficiency Diseases

If a vitamin deficiency becomes severe, a nutritional deficiency disease associated with the specific function of that vitamin becomes apparent. For example, the classic vitamin deficiency disease scurvy is caused by a lack of vitamin C. Scurvy is a hemorrhagic disease with bleeding into the joints and other internal tissues due to fragile capillaries breaking down under simple blood pressure. Without vitamin C to produce strong capillary walls, vital internal membranes finally disintegrate and death occurs, as with British sailors 200 years ago. The name given to the vitamin—*ascorbic acid*—comes from the Latin word *scorbutus*, meaning "scurvy," so the term *ascorbic* means "without scurvy." In developed countries today, we do not often see frank scurvy, but we *do* see it—even here in America—along with other forms and degrees of malnutrition among low-income and poverty-stricken population groups.

FAT-SOLUBLE VITAMINS

Retinol (Vitamin A)

Functions

Retinol performs the following functions in the body.

Vision. The chemical name *retinol* was given to vitamin A because of its major function in the retina of the eye. Retinol is an essential part of *rhodopsin*, which is a pigment in the eye commonly known as *visual purple*. This light-sensitive substance enables the eye to adjust to different amounts of available light. A mild deficiency of the vitamin causes night blindness, slow adaptation to darkness, or glare blindness.

Tissue strength. Retinol maintains healthy *epithelial* tissue, which is the vital protective tissue covering the body (i.e., the skin) and the inner mucous membranes in the nose, throat, eyes, gastrointestinal tract, and genitourinary tract. These tissues provide our primary barrier to infection.

Growth. Retinol is essential to the growth of skeletal and soft tissues and influences the stability of cell membranes and protein synthesis.

Deficiency Disease

Adequate intake of retinol prevents two eye conditions, as follow: (1) *xerosis*, which is itching and burning and red inflamed lids; and (2) *xerophthalmia*, which is blindness from severe deficiency.

Requirements

Retinol requirements are influenced by factors related to its two basic forms in food sources and its storage in the body. The DRI standards for retinol are currently under study; the established RDA standard for adults is 800 μg for women and 100 μg for men.

Food forms and units of measure. Retinol occurs in two forms, as follow: (1) retinol—the fully preformed vitamin A that is named as such because of its function in the retina of the eye, and (2) carotene—the "provitamin A," which is a pigment in yellow and green plants that the body converts to vitamin A. Because vitamin A comes in these two food forms and most of our intake is usually from *beta-carotene*, which becomes retinol in the body, vitamin A is currently measured in *retinol equivalents* (REs). Another measure sometimes used for vitamin A is that of International Units (IU). One IU of vitamin A equals 0.3 μg retinol or 0.6 μg beta-carotene (see the For Further Focus box, "Small Measures for Small Needs").

Body storage. The liver can store large amounts of retinol. In healthy individuals, the storage efficiency of retinol ingested in the liver is more than 50%, and the liver contains about 90% of the body's total store. Thus when persons take large supplements of retinol in addition to dietary sources, it is possible to take in a potentially toxic quantity.

Toxicity Symptoms

The condition created by excessive vitamin A intake is called *hypervitaminosis A*. Symptoms of this toxicity include joint pain, thickening of long bones, loss of hair, and jaundice. Excessive vitamin A may also cause liver injury with the following two results: (1) *portal hypertension*, which is elevated blood pressure in the blood circulation going directly to the liver from the gastrointestinal tract, carrying absorbed nutrient loads following meals; and (2) *ascites*, which is fluid accumulation in the abdominal cavity.

Food Sources

Fish-liver oils, liver, egg yolk, butter, and cream are sources of preformed, natural vitamin A. Fat-soluble vitamin A only occurs naturally in the fat part of milk. Low-fat and nonfat milks and the butter substitute margarine are good sources of vitamin A because they are fortified with added vitamin A. Some good sources of beta-carotene are green leafy vegetables such as Swiss chard, turnip greens, kale, and spinach; and yellow vegetables and fruits such as carrots, sweet potatoes or yams, yellow corn, yellow squash, apricots, and peaches. Both beta-carotene and preformed vitamin A require the presence of bile salts for proper absorption from the intestine. Bile acts as an antioxidant to protect and stabilize the easily oxidized vitamin, as well as transport it through the intestinal wall. Table 6-1 gives some comparative food sources of vitamin A.

Stability

Retinol is unstable in heat and in contact with air. Cooking vegetables in an uncovered pot destroys much of their vitamin content. Quicker cooking with little water helps to preserve the vitamins. If fats are rancid or vegetables are wilted, most of the vitamin A is destroyed.

Cholecalciferol (Vitamin D)

Vitamin D is not actually a true vitamin because it is made in our own bodies with the help of the sun's ultraviolet rays. It was mistakenly classed as a vitamin by its discoverers in 1922 because they were able to cure the childhood deficiency disease, rickets, with its only known natural form in fish liver oils. Today we know that the compound made in our skin by sunlight is actually a prohormone. This irradiated compound in the skin has been given the name cholecalciferol, often shortened to *calciferol*, because it is a fat-soluble *sterol* that controls calcium metabolism in bone-building. The initial compound in the skin is a *cholesterol* base. The irradiated cholesterol base in the skin, calciferol, is then activated by two successive enzymes—intermediate action in the liver and final action in the kidney—to become the active vitamin D hormone form called calcitriol that functions in the body.

---

retinol (L. *retina,* from *rēte,* net, eye vision; suffix *-ol,* an alcohol) the chemical name of vitamin A; derived from its vision function relating to the retina of the eye, which is the back inner lining of the eyeball that "catches" the lens light refractions to form images interpreted by the optic nerve and brain and makes the necessary light-dark adaptations.

carotene a group name of three red and yellow pigments (alpha-, beta-, and gamma-carotene) found in dark green and yellow vegetables and fruits. The one most important to human nutrition is beta-carotene because the body can convert it to vitamin A, thus making it a primary source of the vitamin.

prohormone a precursor substance that the body converts to a hormone. For example, a cholesterol compound in the skin is first irradiated by sunlight and then developed through successive enzyme actions in the liver and kidney into the vitamin D hormone, which then regulates calcium absorption and bone development. Only a few food sources of vitamin D are found in food fats (e.g., cream, butter, and egg yolks), but vitamin D occurs in other processed foods (e.g., breakfast cereals and milk) through enrichment.

cholecalciferol the chemical name for vitamin D in its inactive dietary form; often shortened to calciferol.

calcitriol the activated hormone form of vitamin D.

TABLE 6-1   Food sources of vitamin A

	Quantity	Vitamin A (μg RE)		Quantity	Vitamin A (μg RE)
Bread, cereal, rice, pasta			**Fruits, continued**		
This food group is not an important source of vitamin A.			Banana	1 med	69
			Canteloupe	¼ med	1386
Vegetables			Grapefruit (pink)	½ med	162
Asparagus	½ cup	196	Orange juice	½ cup	75
Beet greens	½ cup	1110	Papaya	1 cup (cubes)	735
Bok choy cabbage	½ cup	790	Peach	1 med	399
Broccoli (fresh)	1 med stalk	1350	Prunes (dried)	4 prunes	207
Broccoli (frozen)	½ cup (chopped)	721	Tangerine	1 med	108
Brussels sprouts	½ cup (4 sprouts)	121	Watermelon	1 wedge (4 × 8 in)	753
Carrots (raw)	½ cup (1 med)	2379	**Meat, poultry, fish, dry beans, eggs, nuts**		
Collard greens	½ cup	2223	Clams (canned)	3 oz	144
Corn	1 sm cob	93	Egg, whole	1 large	78
Dandelion greens	½ cup	1843	Liver, beef	3.5 oz	10,831
Green beans	½ cup	102	Liver, chicken	3.5 oz	4912
Green peas	½ cup	144	Salmon, pink (raw)	3 oz	30
Kale	½ cup	1369	**Milk, dairy products**		
Lima beans	½ cup	60	Cheddar cheese	1oz	90
Mustard greens	½ cup	1218	Milk, lowfat 2% (fortified)	8 fl oz	150
Pumpkin (canned)	½ cup	2352			
Romaine lettuce	½ cup (chopped)	157	Milk, skim (fortified)	8 fl oz	150
Spinach	½ cup	2187	Milk, whole (unfortified)	8 fl oz	101
Summer squash	½ cup	123			
Sweet potato (baked, in skin)	1 med	2769	Ricotta cheese, whole milk	½ cup	182
Tomato (cooked)	½ cup	325	Swiss cheese	1 oz	72
Winter squash	½ cup	1021	Yogurt, whole	8 fl oz	84
Fruits			**Fats, oils, sugar**		
Apricot (dried)	4 halves	490	Butter	1 tbsp	138
Apricot (fresh)	3 med	867	Margarine	1 tbsp	141
Avocado	1 med	189			

---

rickets (Gr. *rhachitis,* a spinal complaint) a disease of childhood characterized by softening of the bones from an inadequate intake of vitamin D and insufficient exposure to sunlight; also associated with impaired calcium and phosphorus metabolism.

Functions

Calcitriol performs the following functions in the body.

Absorption of calcium and phosphorus. The hormone form calcitriol acts physiologically with two other hormones, the *parathyroid hormone (PTH)* and the thyroid hormone *calcitonin.* In balance with these two hormones, the vitamin D hormone stimulates absorption of calcium and phosphorus in the small intestine.

Bone mineralization. Calcitriol, also works with calcium and phosphorus to form bone tissue by directly regulating the rate of deposit and resorption of these minerals in bone. This balancing process builds and maintains bone tissue. Thus calcitriol has been clinically used to treat *osteoporosis*, which is a type of bone loss in older women that leads to spontaneous fractures.

Deficiency Disease

A deficiency of calcitriol causes rickets, which is a condition characterized by malformation of skeletal tissue in growing children (Figure 6-1).

Requirements

A number of factors influence our requirements for vitamin D, and excessive intake is possible—especially in young infants. It is difficult to set requirements for this nutrient because of its unique hormonelike nature, its synthesis in the skin by the sun's irradiation of cholesterol there, and its limited food sources. The amount needed may vary between winter and summer, and with individual exposure to sunlight. People regularly exposed to sunlight (i.e., under appropriate conditions) have no requirement for vitamin D. A substantial proportion of the U.S. population, however, is exposed to very little sunlight—especially during certain seasons, so a dietary supply is needed. The new DRI research does not establish an RDA figure for vitamin D. Instead, AI levels are given as guidelines. For example, for both women and men from birth to age 50, the AI is 5 μg per day (200 IU). The DRIs also set the UL for vitamin D for persons over age 1 at 50 μg per day.

Toxicity Symptoms

Excess intake of vitamin D, especially in infants, can be toxic. Symptoms of toxicity, or *hypervitaminosis D*, include calcification of soft tissues such as kidneys and lungs, as well as fragile bones. Prolonged intake of cholecalciferol (i.e., above 50 μg/day [2000 IU], which is 10 times the new AI guideline) can pro-

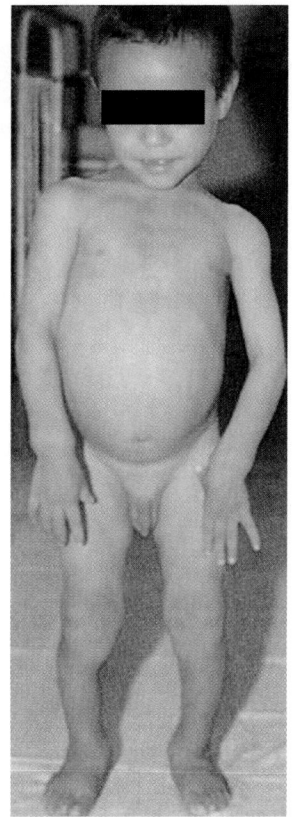

FIGURE 6-1 Child with rickets. Note his bowlegs. (From McLaren DS: *A colour atlas and text of diet-related disorders,* ed 2, London, 1992, Mosby Year Book Europe Limited. By permission of Mosby International Ltd.)

duce elevated levels of calcium in the blood in infants and calcium deposits in the kidney nephrons in both infants and adults, affecting overall kidney function. For example, infant feeding may provide an excess (i.e., as much as 100 μg [4000 IU] or more) of cholecalciferol when fortified milk and fortified cereal are used in addition to variable vitamin supplements. An infant (from birth to 1 year) only needs 5 μg (200 IU) of cholecalciferol daily.[1]

Food Sources

Only yeast and fish liver oils are natural sources of vitamin D. Therefore the only regular food

TABLE 6-2 Food sources of vitamin D

	Quantity	Vitamin D (μg)
Bread, cereal, rice, pasta		
Corn flakes	1 cup (1 oz)/28 g	1.00
Granola	¼ cup (1 oz)/28 g	1.23
Raisin bran	½ cup (1 oz)/28 g	1.23
Vegetables		
This food group is not an important source of vitamin D.		
Fruits		
This food group is not an important source of vitamin D.		
Meat, poultry, fish, dry beans, nuts		
This food group is not an important source of vitamin D.		
Eggs		
Egg, whole	1 large/50 g	0.68
Egg yolk	Yolk of 1 large egg/17 g	0.68
Milk, dairy products		
Cheddar cheese	1 oz/28 g	0.08
Cream cheese	1 oz/28 g	0.05
Evaporated milk (vitamin D fortified)	½ cup (4 fl oz)/126 g	2.50
Milk, whole or nonfat (vitamin D fortified)	1 qt/960 g	10.00
Milk, whole or nonfat (vitamin D fortified)	1 cup (8 fl oz)/240 g	2.50
Fats, oils, sugar		
Margarine	1 tbsp	1.50

sources of vitamin D are those that have been fortified with the vitamin (Table 6-2). Because it is a common food and also contains calcium and phosphorus, milk is the most practical carrier. The standard commercial practice is to add 10 μg (400 IU)/qt. But dairies and other producers must be closely regulated to ensure that this practice is consistently accurate (see the For Further Focus box "Vitamin D Toxicity: Too Much of a Good Thing"). Butter substitutes, such as margarines, are also fortified. Children on vitamin D-deficient diets (e.g., a rigid macrobiotic pattern with no milk products) are especially vulnerable to damaged bone development and rickets.

Stability

Vitamin D is stable to heat, aging, and storage.

Tocopherol (Vitamin E)

Early vitamin studies identified a substance necessary for animal reproduction that was chemically an alcohol. This substance was named tocopherol, from two Greek words: *tophos*, meaning "child-

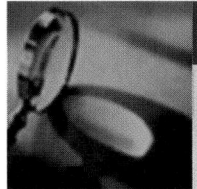

FOR FURTHER FOCUS
Vitamin D Toxicity: Too Much of a Good Thing

In the United States, milk has been fortified with vitamin D since the early 1930s. As a result, rickets has largely been eradicated. From the beginning, U.S. federal regulations have specified that each quart of milk contain 10 μg (400 IU) of vitamin D. The previous measure of International Units (IU) is passing from use in relation to vitamin needs because it is a less useful measure than the metric unit micrograms (μg), which can be measured and regulated directly.

Toxic amounts of vitamin D, however, can build up in the body easily because this vitamin is stored in fat tissue and released slowly. Even today, cases of toxicity occur, usually from excessively fortified

milk. For example, a U.S. outbreak was traced to a local dairy's sporadic addition—ranging from 20 μg to nearly 6000 μg/qt—of excessive vitamin D to milk during the fortification process, even though the regulation calls for only 10 μg. Young children who drank this dairy's milk for several years did not grow normally in height and developed kidney function problems due to excess calcium in their kidney tissues. Adults suffered progressive weakness, elevated blood levels of calcium, and bone pain.

For the most part, the American dairy industry is diligent about using correct procedures for fortifying milk, but this case demonstrated that too much of an essential vitamin can cause illness.

---

birth," and *phero*, meaning "to bring"—with the *-ol* ending for alcohol. Tocopherol soon became known as the antisterility vitamin, but it was soon demonstrated to have this effect only in rats and a few other animals, not in humans—all advertising claims for its contribution to sexual powers notwithstanding. A number of related compounds have since been discovered. Tocopherol (vitamin E) is actually the generic name for a group of similar fat-soluble nutrients. Three of these, designated alpha (α)-, beta (β)-, and gamma (γ)-tocopherol, display the most biologic activity. Of these three, α-tocopherol is the most significant in human nutrition and thus is used for measuring dietary needs.[3]

Functions
The single vital function of tocopherol relates to its action in many tissues as an antioxidant, which is an agent that prevents cellular structure from being broken down by oxygen (i.e., the process of oxidation).

Antioxidant function. Tocopherol acts as nature's most potent fat-soluble antioxidant. The polyunsaturated fatty acids (see Chapter 3) in lipid membranes of body tissues are particularly easy for oxygen to break down. Tocopherol can interrupt this oxidation process, protecting the fatty acids of the cell membrane from damage. For example, vitamin E can protect fragile red blood cell walls in premature infants from breaking down, causing anemia (see the Clinical Applications box, "Vitamin E and

---

tocopherol (Gr. *tokos*, childbirth; *pherein*, to carry) the chemical name for vitamin E, which was so named by early investigators because their initial work with rats indicated a reproductive function—which is not true with humans. In humans, vitamin E functions as a strong antioxidant that preserves structural membranes such as cell walls.

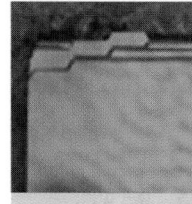

CLINICAL APPLICATIONS
Vitamin E and Premature Infants

A medical problem found in infants—especially premature ones—has responded positively to vitamin E therapy. This problem is *hemolytic anemia*.

Anemia is a blood condition characterized by loss of mature, functioning red blood cells. Different types of anemia are usually named according to cause or to the nature of an abnormal nonfunctioning cell produced instead of the normal cell. The name of this type of anemia comes from its cause. The word *hemolysis* comes from two roots, *hemo*-referring to blood, and *lysis* meaning dissolving or breaking. Therefore hemolysis means the bursting or dissolving of red blood cells, and the resulting condition is a hemolytic anemia. Vitamin E can help prevent this destruction of red blood cells and the loss of their vital oxygen-carrying hemoglobin because it is one of the body's foremost antioxidants.

An oxidant is a compound, or oxygen itself, that oxidizes other compounds, thereby breaking them down or changing them. Vitamin E is readily oxidized. When there is plenty of vitamin E among the other compounds exposed to an oxidant, vitamin E can, by its nature, take on the oxidative attack, thus protecting the others. Vitamin E is fat-soluble, so it is found among the polyunsaturated fatty acids that compose the core of the cell membranes in body tissues that are rich in fat. The cell membranes of red blood cells are particularly rich in these polyunsaturated lipids and are exposed to concentrated oxygen because they constantly circulate through the lungs. This situation would be destructive to the red blood cells if vitamin E was not present. Vitamin E takes the oxygen itself, protecting the polyunsaturated fatty acids and keeping the red blood cells intact to continue their life-sustaining journey throughout the body. Thus vitamin E acts as nature's most potent fat-soluble antioxidant. It interrupts the oxidative breakdown by free radicals (i.e., parts of compounds broken off by cell metabolism) in the cell, protecting the cell membrane fatty acids in cell membrane walls from the oxidative damage.

Infants fed formulas that are rich in polyunsaturated fatty acids and supplemented with iron (an oxidant) may develop hemolytic anemia as the fragile red blood cell membranes break down due to the high oxidative process of the cells and the induced deficiency of vitamin E. This protective need for increased vitamin E is especially great in small, premature infants fed formulas containing iron, which acts as an oxidant, and high concentrations of polyunsaturated fatty acids, which are vulnerable to oxidative breakdown. To avoid this problem and comply with American Academy of Pediatrics recommendations, manufacturers have increased the amount of vitamin E and lowered the iron in formulas for premature infants. The proportions of vitamin E, polyunsaturated fatty acids, and iron in today's improved formulas usually supply enough necessary nutrients, so in most cases supplements are no longer necessary to prevent hemolytic anemia in premature infants.

Premature Infants"). Vitamin E helps protect both red blood cells and muscle tissue cells.

Relation to selenium metabolism. Selenium is a trace mineral that works as a partner with tocopherol as an antioxidant. A selenium-containing enzyme is the second line of defense in preventing oxidative damage to cell membranes. Selenium spares tocopherol by reducing its requirement, just as tocopherol does for selenium.

Deficiency Disease

Young infants, especially premature infants who miss the final 1 to 2 months of gestation when tocopherol stores are normally built up, are particularly vulnerable to the tocopherol deficiency disease called hemolytic anemia. In this disease, the lipid membranes of red blood cells are easily oxidized by oxygen, and the continued loss of red blood cells leads to anemia. In older children and adults, a deficiency of tocopherol disrupts normal synthesis of *myelin*, the protective fat covering of nerve cells that helps them pass messages along to specific tissues. The main nerves involved are the following: (1) spinal cord fibers that affect physical activity (e.g., walking), and (2) the retina of the eye that affects vision.

Requirements

Tocopherol requirements are expressed in terms of *alpha-tocopherol* in mg/day. The new DRI recommendations state that the RDA standard for men and women age 14 and older is 15 mg/day, with lesser amounts required in childhood. Needs during the first year of infancy do not have an RDA figure, but an AI amount of 4 to 6 mg/day is used. The UL for all adults is set at 1,000 mg/day.

Toxicity Symptoms

Tocopherol is the only fat-soluble vitamin that has no toxic effect in humans. Its use as a supplement has not shown harmful effects.

Food Sources

The richest sources of tocopherol are vegetable oils. Note that vegetable oils are also the richest sources of polyunsaturated fatty acids, which vitamin E protects. Other food sources of tocopherol include milk, eggs, muscle meats, fish, cereals, and leafy vegetables. Table 6-3 provides a list of vitamin E food sources.

Stability

Tocopherol is stable to heat and acids but not to alkalis.

Vitamin K

In the early era of vitamin research, Henrik Dam, a biochemist at the University of Copenhagen, discovered a hemorrhagic disease in chicks that were fed a fat-free diet and determined that the factor responsible was the absence of a fat-soluble, blood-clotting vitamin. He called it "koagulationsvitamin," or vitamin K, and the letter name has stuck. Dam later succeeded in isolating and identifying the agent from alfalfa, for which he received the Nobel prize for physiology and medicine. As with a number of vitamins, not one but several forms of vitamin K compose a group of substances with similar biologic activity in blood-clotting. The major form found in plants and initially isolated from alfalfa by Dam is named phylloquinone because of its chemical structure. Phylloquinone is our dietary form of vitamin K. A second significant form, which is synthesized by intestinal bacteria and contributes about half of our daily supply, is *menaquinone*.

Functions

Vitamin K is known to have two metabolic functions in the body: blood clotting and bone development.

Blood-clotting. The basic function of vitamin K is in the blood-clotting process. Vitamin K is essential for maintaining normal levels of four of

---

phylloquinone a fat-soluble vitamin of the K group found in green plants or prepared synthetically.

TABLE 6-3   Food sources of vitamin E as alpha-tocopherol

	Quantity	Vitamin E (mg α-TE)
Bread, cereal, rice, pasta		
This food group is not an important source of vitamin E.		
Vegetables		
Asparagus (raw)	4 spears/58 g	1.15
Avocado (raw)	1 med/173 g	2.32
Brussels sprouts (boiled)	½ cup (4 sprouts)/78 g	0.66
Cabbage, green (raw)	½ cup shredded/35 g	0.58
Carrot (raw)	1 med/72 g	0.32
Lettuce, iceberg (raw)	¼ head/135 g	0.54
Spinach (raw)	½ cup chopped/28 g	0.53
Sweet potato (raw)	1 med/130 g	5.93
Fruits		
Apple (raw, with skin)	1 med/138 g	0.81
Apricot (canned)	4 halves/90 g	0.80
Banana (raw)	1 med/114 g	0.31
Mango (raw)	1 med/207 g	2.32
Pear (raw)	1 med/166 g	0.83
Meat, poultry, fish, dry beans, eggs		
This food group is not an important source of vitamin E.		
Nuts		
Almonds (dried)	1 oz (24 nuts)/28 g	6.72
Hazelnuts (dried)	1 oz/28 g	6.70
Peanut butter	1 tbsp/16 g	3.00
Peanuts (dried)	1 oz/28 g	2.56
Walnuts (dried)	1 oz (14 halves)/28 g	0.73
Milk, dairy products		
This food group is not an important source of vitamin E.		
Fats, oils, sugar		
Corn oil	1 tbsp/14 g	1.90
Cottonseed oil	1 tbsp/14 g	4.80
Olive oil	1 tbsp/14 g	1.60
Palm oil	1 tbsp/14 g	2.60
Peanut oil	1 tbsp/14 g	1.60
Safflower oil	1 tbsp/14 g	4.60
Soybean oil	1 tbsp/14 g	1.50

the 11 blood-clotting factors. The most familiar of these vitamin K-dependent blood factors is *prothrombin* (number II). Thus phylloquinone can serve as an antidote for the excess effects of anticoagulant drugs. Phylloquinone is often used in the control and prevention of certain types of hemorrhages. Because this fat-soluble vitamin is absorbed more completely if bile is present, conditions that hinder bile flow to the small intestine reduce blood-clotting ability. If bile salts are given with vitamin K concentrate, the blood-clotting time becomes normal.

Bone development. A more recently discovered function of vitamin K relates to bone development. Specific proteins found in bone and bone matrix are dependent on vitamin K for their synthesis and are involved with calcium in bone development. Like the blood-clotting proteins, these bone proteins bind calcium but function here to form bone crystals.

Deficiency Disease

Deficiency disease relating to vitamin K is not usually found in humans. A deficiency is unlikely except in clinical conditions related to blood-clotting, malabsorption, or lack of intestinal bacteria to synthesize the vitamin. For example, because the intestinal tract of a newborn is sterile, phylloquinone is routinely given to prevent hemorrhage when the cord is cut. Patients who are placed on poor diets after surgery and treated with antibiotics that kill intestinal bacteria are susceptible to vitamin K deficiency with resulting blood loss and poor wound healing.

Requirements

Because intestinal bacteria synthesize a form of vitamin K, a constant supply is normally available to support dietary sources. The DRI guidelines for vitamin K are not yet published. The RDA standard for men is 80 μg/day and for women is 65 μg. Because there is no specific information about the vitamin K requirements of children, values for them have been set at 1 μg/kg body weight. A recent study indicates that men and women in the 18- to 44-year-old age group reported dietary intakes below the current recommended intakes.[5]

Toxicity Symptoms

Toxicity from vitamin K—even when large amounts are taken over extended periods—has not been observed.

Food Sources

Green leafy vegetables, which provide 50 to 800 μg of phylloquinone per 100 g of food, are clearly the best dietary sources. Small but significant amounts of phylloquinone are contributed by milk and dairy products, meats, eggs, cereals, fruits and vegetables (Table 6-4).

Stability

Vitamin K as phylloquinone is fairly stable, although it is sensitive to light and irradiation. Therefore clinical preparations are kept in dark bottles. Table 6-5 provides a summary of the fat-soluble vitamins.

WATER-SOLUBLE VITAMINS
Ascorbic Acid (Vitamin C)

Functions

The basic function of ascorbic acid relates to tissue building. In this role, it serves body metabolism.

Cement substance between cells. Ascorbic acid is necessary to build and maintain strong tissues in general—but is especially important for connective tissues such as bone, cartilage, dentin, collagen, and capillary walls. Ascorbic acid acts like cement between cells, holding them together strongly. When ascorbic acid is absent, the ground substance that builds the cementing material does not develop into collagen. When ascorbic acid is adequate, this special connecting substance develops quickly. Blood vessel tissue particularly depends upon ascorbic acid to supply the cementing substance for strong capillary walls.

TABLE 6-4   Food sources of vitamin K

	Quantity	Vitamin K (μg)
Bread, cereal, rice, pasta		
Oats (dry)	100 g	63
Wheat bran	100 g	83
Whole wheat flour	100 g	30
Vegetables		
Broccoli (raw)	100 g	132
Cabbage (raw)	100 g	149
Cauliflower (raw)	100 g	191
Lentils (dry)	100 g	223
Lettuce, iceberg (raw)	100 g	112
Spinach (raw)	100 g	266
Turnip greens (raw)	100 g	650
Fruits		
This food group is not an important source of vitamin K.		
Meat, poultry, fish, dry beans, eggs, nuts		
Beef liver	100 g	104
Chicken liver	100 g	80
Pork liver	100 g	88
Milk, dairy products		
This food group is not an important source of vitamin K.		
Fats, oils, sugar		
Corn oil	100 g	60
Soybean oil	100 g	540

General body metabolism.   The more metabolically active body tissues (e.g., adrenal glands, brain, kidney, liver, pancreas, thymus, and spleen) have greater concentrations of ascorbic acid. The high concentration of ascorbic acid in the adrenal glands is depleted when the gland is stimulated. This depletion suggests an increased need for the vitamin during stress. There is also more ascorbic acid in a child's actively growing tissue than in adult tissue. Ascorbic acid is an essential partner of protein for tissue building. Furthermore, ascorbic acid also helps the body absorb iron and makes it available for hemoglobin production, thereby helping to prevent anemia. The general clinical needs of ascorbic acid relate to wound healing, fevers and infections, and growth periods.

Deficiency Disease

Ascorbic acid deficiency causes signs of tissue bleeding (e.g., easy bruising, pinpoint skin hemorrhages, bone and joint bleeding, easy bone fracture, poor wound healing, and soft bleeding gums with loosened teeth). Extreme deficiency produces the disease scurvy. Vitamin C was first called ascorbic acid (L. *a-*, prefix: without; *scorbutus*, scurvy) because of its ability to cure scurvy.

TABLE 6-5   A summary of fat-soluble vitamins

Vitamin	Functions	Results of deficiency	Food sources
A (retinol); provitamin A (carotene)	Vision cycle—adaption to light and dark; tissue growth, especially skin and mucous membranes; toxic in large amounts	Night blindness, xerophthalmia, susceptibility to epithelial infection, changes in skin and membranes	Retinol (animal foods): liver, egg yolk, cream, butter or fortified margarine, fortified milk; carotene (plant foods): green and yellow vegetables, fruits
D (cholecalciferol)	Absorption of calcium and phosphorous, calcification of bones; toxic in large amounts	Rickets, faulty bone growth	Fortified or irradiated milk, fish oils
E (tocopherol)	Antioxidant—protection of materials that oxidize easily; normal growth	Breakdown of red blood cells, anemia	Vegetable oils, vegetable greens, milk, eggs, meat, cereals
K (phylloquinone)	Normal blood clotting Bone development	Bleeding tendencies, hemorrhagic disease Poor bone growth	Green leafy vegetables, milk and dairy products, meats, eggs, cereals, fruits, vegetables

Requirements

Ascorbic acid provides antioxidant protection. To achieve this, the new DRI guidelines for adults over 18 establish an RDA of 75 mg/day for females and 90 mg/day for males, with increases for women during pregnancy and lactation. Because smokers suffer increased stress to their body tissues, the DRIs recommend that their intake be 35 mg/day higher. The UL for vitamin C in the DRI recommendations is 2,000 mg/day for adults.

Toxicity Symptoms

Ascorbic acid is not toxic to humans because any excess not used by the body for tissue maintenance is excreted in the urine.

Food Sources

The best food sources of ascorbic acid are citrus fruits. Additional sources include tomatoes, cabbage and other leafy vegetables, berries, melons, peppers, broccoli, potatoes (white and sweet), and other green and yellow vegetables in general (Table 6-6).

Stability

Ascorbic acid is easily oxidized upon exposure to air and heat. Therefore care must be taken in handling its food sources. Ascorbic acid is not stable to alkaline substances, so baking soda should not be added to food being cooked. Acidic fruits and vegetables retain their ascorbic acid content better than nonacid ones. The vitamin is also very soluble in water, so only small amounts of water should be used for cooking. Table 6-7 provides a summary of the uses and sources of ascorbic acid.

---

scurvy a vitamin-deficiency disease caused by a lack of vitamin C. It is a hemorrhagic disease with diffuse tissue bleeding, painful limbs and joints, thickened bones, and skin discoloration from tissue bleeding; bones fracture easily, wounds do not heal, gums are swollen and bleed, and teeth loosen.

ascorbic acid chemical name for vitamin C, from ability of the vitamin to cure scurvy.

TABLE 6-6 Food sources of vitamin C

	Quantity	Vitamin C (mg)
Bread, cereal, rice, pasta		
This food group is not an important source of vitamin C.		
Vegetables		
Asparagus (boiled)	½ cup (6 spears)	18
Avocado (raw)	1 med	14
Broccoli (raw)	½ cup	41
Brussels sprouts (boiled)	½ cup (4 sprouts)	48
Cauliflower (raw)	½ cup, pieces	36
Green pepper (raw)	½ cup, chopped	64
Kale (boiled)	½ cup	27
Potato (baked, with skin)	1 med	26
Sweet potato (baked)	1 med	28
Tomato (raw)	1 med	22
Fruits		
Cantaloupe (raw)	½ cup, pieces	34
Grapefruit, white	½ med	39
Kiwi (raw)	1 med	75
Lemon	1 med	31
Lemon juice (fresh)	8 fl oz	112
Orange juice (fresh)	8 fl oz	124
Orange, navel	1 med	80
Papaya (raw)	1 med	188
Pineapple (raw)	½ cup	12
Raspberries (raw)	½ cup	15
Strawberries (raw)	½ cup	44
Tangerine (raw)	1 med	26
Meat, poultry, fish, dry beans, eggs, nuts		
Beef liver (fried)	3.5 oz	23
Ham, lean (canned; vitamin C added)	3.5 oz	27
Lentils (boiled)	1 cup	3
Soybeans (boiled)	1 cup	3
Milk, dairy products		
Milk, skim	8 fl oz	2
Milk, whole	8 fl oz	4
Fats, oils, sugar		
This food group is not an important source of vitamin C.		

TABLE 6-7   A summary of vitamin C (ascorbic acid)

Functions	Clinical applications	Food sources
Intercellular cement substance; firm capillary walls and collagen formation Helps prepare iron for absorption and release to tissues for red blood cell formation	Scurvy (deficiency disease) Sore gums Hemorrhages, especially around bones and joints Tendency to bruise easily Stress reactions Growth periods Fevers and infections Wound healing, tissue formation Anemia	Citrus fruits, tomatoes, cabbage, leafy vegetables, potatoes, strawberries, melons, chili peppers, broccoli, chard, turnip greens, green peppers, other green and yellow vegetables

B-COMPLEX VITAMINS

All of the B-complex vitamins are water soluble. Each of the eight B vitamins is a separate vitamin in name, structure, and function. The earliest discoveries were related to classic diseases. The general role of B-complex vitamins is as coenzyme factor in various metabolic tasks. The B-complex vitamins can be grouped according to function, as follows: (1) classic deficiency disease factors: thiamin, riboflavin, and niacin; (2) more recently discovered coenzyme factors: B_6 (pyridoxine), pantothenic acid, and biotin; and (3) cell-growth and blood-forming factors: folate and B_{12} (cobalamin).

Thiamin

Functions

The vitamin name *thiamin* comes from its chemical-ringlike structure. The basic function of thiamin as a coenzyme factor relates to the production of energy from glucose and the storage of energy as fat, making energy available to support normal growth. Thiamin is especially necessary for maintaining good function of three body systems, as follow.

Gastrointestinal system.   Lack of thiamin causes poor appetite, indigestion, constipation and poor stomach action from lack of muscle tone, as well as deficient gastric hydrochloric acid secretion. The cells of smooth muscles and secretory glands must have energy to do their work; thiamin is a necessary agent for producing that energy.

Nervous system.   The central nervous system depends on glucose for energy to do its work. Without sufficient thiamin, this energy is not produced and the nerves cannot do their work. Alertness and reflex responses decrease; apathy, fatigue, and irritability

---

cobalamin the chemical name for the B-complex vitamin B_{12}; found mainly in animal protein food sources, so deficiencies are seen mostly among strict vegetarians (vegans). It is closely related to amino acid metabolism and formation of the heme portion of hemoglobin. Absence of its necessary absorbing agent in the gastric secretions, intrinsic factor, leads to pernicious anemia and degenerative effects on the nervous system, which requires continuing monthly cobalamin injections, bypassing the intestinal absorption defect, to control.

thiamin chemical name of a major B-complex vitamin; formerly called vitamin B_1, discovered in relation to the classic deficiency disease beriberi; important in body metabolism as a coenzyme factor in many cell reactions related to energy metabolism.

result. If the thiamin deficit continues, nerve tissue damage causes nerve irritation, pain, prickly or deadening sensations, and—finally—paralysis.

Cardiovascular system. Without constant energy, the heart muscle weakens and heart failure results. Blood circulation becomes involved when the muscles in vessel walls also weaken. This weakening causes the vessels to dilate, leading to fluid accumulation in the lower part of the legs.

Deficiency Disease

Thiamin was first discovered as the control agent relating to the classic deficiency disease beriberi, a paralyzing disease known since antiquity that was especially prevalent in Asian countries. The name describes the disease well; it is Singhalese for "I can't, I can't," because afflicted persons were always too ill to do anything. In industrialized societies, thiamin deficiency is largely associated with chronic alcoholism resulting in poor diet.

Requirements

Thiamin is directly related to the metabolic need for energy and carbohydrate. For healthy persons, the new DRI guidelines establish RDAs for adults over age 18 as 1.2 mg/day for men and 1.1 mg/day for women. Children require less. For infants up to 12 months, there is no RDA; the AI figure is 0.2 to 0.3 mg/day. Increased amounts are needed during

---

beriberi (Singhalese for "I can't, I can't") a disease of the peripheral nerves caused by a deficiency of thiamin (vitamin B_1); characterized by pain (neuritis) and paralysis of legs and arms, cardiovascular changes, and edema.

riboflavin chemical name of one of the early B vitamins, discovered in relation to an early vitamin-deficiency syndrome called "ariboflavinosis," that is mainly evidenced in breakdown of skin tissues and resulting infections; role as a coenzyme factor in many cell reactions related to energy and protein metabolism.

---

pregnancy and lactation, as well as in the treatment of infectious diseases and alcoholism. There is no UL for thiamin.

Toxicity Symptoms

Because excess thiamin is easily cleared by the kidneys, there is no evidence of toxicity from oral intake.

Food Sources

Although thiamin is widespread in almost all plant and animal tissues, its content is usually small. Thus thiamin deficiency is a distinct possibility when kcalories are markedly curtailed (e.g., in alcoholism or when a person is following a highly inadequate diet). Good food sources of thiamin include lean pork, beef, liver, whole or enriched grains (e.g., flour, bread, cereals), and legumes (Table 6-8). Eggs, fish, and a few vegetables are fair sources.

Stability

Thiamin is a fairly stable vitamin but is destroyed by alkalis and prolonged heat at high cooking temperatures. Because it is water-soluble, little cooking water should be used. When cooking water is retained in the dish being prepared, the vitamin is preserved.

Riboflavin

Functions

The name *riboflavin* comes from the chemical nature of the vitamin. It is a yellow-green fluorescent pigment—the Latin word *flavus* means "yellow"—containing a sugar named *ribose*, hence the name *riboflavin*. Riboflavin operates as a vital coenzyme factor in both energy production and tissue-protein building, so it is essential to tissue health and growth. Recent study has also related riboflavin to malaria and antioxidant activity.[6]

Deficiency Disease

Signs of riboflavin deficiency include cracked lips and mouth corners; a swollen red tongue; eyes burning, itching, and/or tearing from extra blood

TABLE 6-8 Food sources of thiamin

	Quantity	Thiamin (mg)
Bread, cereal, rice, pasta		
Bran flakes	1 cup	0.46
Bread, whole wheat	1 slice	0.10
Corn muffin	1 muffin	0.10
Egg noodles, enriched	1 cup	0.20
Pasta, enriched	1 cup	0.23
Rice, enriched	1 cup	0.23
Wheat flakes	1 cup	0.40
Vegetables		
Asparagus (boiled)	½ cup (6 spears)	0.09
Avocado (raw)	1 med	0.19
Brussels sprouts (boiled)	½ cup (4 sprouts)	0.08
Corn, yellow (boiled)	½ cup	0.18
Green peas (boiled)	½ cup	0.21
Potato (baked, with skin)	1 med	0.22
Fruits		
Figs (dried)	10 figs	0.13
Orange juice (fresh)	8 fl oz	0.22
Orange, navel (raw)	1 med	0.13
Raisins, seedless	⅔ cup	0.16
Meat, poultry, fish, dry beans, eggs, nuts		
Beef liver (fried)	3.5 oz	0.21
Black-eyed peas (boiled)	1 cup	0.35
Cashews (roasted)	1 oz	0.12
Chicken, light and dark (roasted, without skin)	3.5 oz	0.07
Chicken liver (simmered)	3.5 oz	0.15
Ham (canned)	3.5 oz	0.85
Kidney beans (boiled)	1 cup	0.28
Lentils (boiled)	1 cup	0.34
Lima beans (boiled)	1 cup	0.30
Navy beans (boiled)	1 cup	0.37
Peanuts (roasted)	1 oz	0.12
Pecans (dried)	1 oz	0.24
Pinto beans (boiled)	1 cup	0.32
Sirloin steak (broiled)	3.5 oz	0.13
Soybeans (boiled)	1 cup	0.27
Top round (broiled)	3.5 oz	0.12
Tuna (baked)	3 oz	0.24

Continued

TABLE 6-8   Food sources of thiamin—cont'd

	Quantity	Thiamin (mg)
Milk, dairy products		
Milk, skim	8 fl oz	0.09
Milk, whole	8 fl oz	0.09
Fats, oils, sugar		
This food group is not an important source of thiamin.		

vessels in the cornea; and a scaly greasy dermatitis in skin folds. Because nutritional deficiencies are usually multiple, riboflavin deficiencies seldom occur alone. They are most likely to occur with deficiencies of other B vitamins and protein. There is no specific deficiency disease comparable to beriberi. A rare deficiency condition of riboflavin has been given the general name ariboflavinosis. Its symptoms relate to tissue inflammation and breakdown and poor wound healing; even minor injuries easily become aggravated and do not heal well.

Requirements

Riboflavin needs are related to total energy requirements for age, level of exercise, body size, metabolic rate, and rate of growth. The DRI guidelines establish an RDA for daily riboflavin intake for adults age 18 and older of 1.3 mg/day and 1.1 mg/day for women. The RDA is higher for women during pregnancy (1.4 mg/day) and during lactation (1.6 mg/day). There is no RDA for infants up to 12 months old; the AI figure is 0.3 to 0.4 mg/day. There is no UL for riboflavin.

---

niacin chemical name for a B vitamin discovered in relation to the deficiency disease pellagra, largely a skin disorder; important as a co-enzyme factor in many cell reactions related to energy and protein metabolism.

Toxicity Symptoms

No adverse effects from riboflavin intake from food or supplements have been reported.

Food Sources

The most important food source of riboflavin is milk. Each serving of milk and milk products contains from 0.3 to 0.7 mg of riboflavin. Other good sources include animal protein sources, such as meats, poultry, and fish. Enriched grains are made to be good sources of riboflavin. Green vegetables such as broccoli, spinach, asparagus, and turnip greens are good natural sources. Table 6-9 gives a summary of riboflavin food sources.

Stability

Riboflavin is destroyed by light, so milk is now sold and stored in cartons instead of glass containers. Riboflavin is water-soluble.

Niacin

Functions

The coenzyme role of niacin is that of a partner with riboflavin and thiamin in the cell-metabolism system that produces energy. In addition, niacin has recently been shown to be a required part of important chemical reactions involved in DNA repair and calcium mobilization within the body.

Deficiency Disease

Symptoms of general niacin deficiency are weakness, poor appetite, indigestion, and various disorders of

TABLE 6-9 Food sources of riboflavin

	Quantity	Riboflavin (mg)
Bread, cereal, rice, pasta		
Bran flakes	1 cup	0.40
Bread, whole wheat	1 slice	0.05
English muffin, plain	1 muffin	0.18
Noodles, enriched	1 cup	0.19
Spaghetti, enriched	1 cup	0.11
Wheat flakes	1 cup	0.42
Vegetables		
Asparagus (boiled)	½ cup (6 spears)	0.11
Avocado (raw)	1 med	0.21
Mushrooms (boiled)	½ cup, pieces	0.23
Spinach (boiled)	½ cup	0.21
Sweet potato (baked)	1 med	0.15
Fruits		
Blueberries (raw)	1 cup	0.07
Figs (dried)	10 figs	0.17
Pear (raw)	1 med	0.07
Prunes (dried)	10 prunes	0.14
Raspberries (raw)	1 cup	0.11
Meat, poultry, fish, dry beans, eggs, nuts		
Almonds (oil roasted)	1 oz	0.28
Beef liver (fried)	3.5 oz	4.14
Chicken, dark (roasted, without skin)	3.5 oz	0.23
Chicken, light (roasted, without skin)	3.5 oz	0.12
Chicken liver (simmered)	3.5 oz	1.75
Clams (baked)	3 oz (9 small)	0.36
Egg, fresh	1 large	0.15
Ground beef, regular (broiled)	3.5 oz	0.19
Ham loin, lean (broiled)	3.5 oz	0.31
Kidney beans (boiled)	1 cup	0.10
Lentils (boiled)	1 cup	0.15
Lima beans (boiled)	1 cup	0.10
Mackerel (baked)	3 oz	0.35
Rainbow trout (baked)	3 oz	0.19
Sirloin steak (broiled)	3.5 oz	0.30
Soybeans (boiled)	1 cup	0.49
Top round (broiled)	3.5 oz	0.27

Continued

TABLE 6-9   Food sources of riboflavin—cont'd

	Quantity	Riboflavin (mg)
Milk, dairy products		
Brie cheese	1 oz	0.15
Buttermilk	8 fl oz	0.38
Cheddar cheese	1 oz	0.11
Cottage cheese, creamed	1 cup	0.34
Cottage cheese, 2% fat	1 cup	0.42
Milk, skim	8 fl oz	0.34
Milk, whole	8 fl oz	0.39
Ricotta cheese, whole milk	1 cup	0.48
Yogurt, whole	8 fl oz	0.32
Fats, oils, sugar		
This food group is not an important source of riboflavin.		

the skin and nervous system. Skin areas exposed to sunlight develop a dark scaly dermatitis. Continuing deficiency causes central nervous system damage with resulting confusion, apathy, disorientation, and neuritis. Such signs of nervous system damage are seen in chronic alcoholism. The deficiency disease associated with niacin is pellagra, which is characterized by dermatitis, diarrhea, dementia, weakness, vertigo, and anorexia. When therapeutic doses of niacin are given, pellagra symptoms cease. Pellagra was common in the United States and parts of Europe in the early twentieth century in regions where corn (which is low in niacin) was the primary staple food. Although pellagra has virtually disappeared in industrialized countries, it still occurs in India and parts of China and Africa.

Requirements

Factors such as age, growth, pregnancy and lactation, illness, tissue trauma, body size, and physical activity—all of which affect energy production—influence niacin requirements. Because the body can make some of its niacin from the essential amino acid *tryptophan*, the total niacin requirement is stated in terms of niacin equivalents to account for both sources. About 60 mg of tryptophan can pro-

duce 1 mg of niacin, so this amount is designated as a *niacin equivalent (NE)*. The DRI guidelines include an RDA standard for adults age 14 and over of 16 mg NE/day for men and 14 mg NE/day for women. The RDA is higher during pregnancy (18 mg NE/day) and lactation (17 mg NE/day). There is no RDA for infants up to 12 months old, but the AI amount is 2 to 3 mg NE/day. Niacin intake is generally adequate in the United States; the recently reported median intake of niacin from food is 28 mg NE/day for men and 18 mg NE/day for women, The DRIs establish a UL for adults of 35 mg NE/day, based on skin flushing as the primary adverse reaction.

Toxicity Symptoms

Excess intake of niacin can produce adverse physical effects, unlike thiamin and riboflavin, so a UL has been established. Although there is no evidence of adverse effects from niacin naturally occurring in foods, such effects have been observed as a result of excess niacin consumption from nonprescription vitamin supplements and fortified foods. The primary reaction is a reddened flush on the skin of the face, arms, and chest that is accompanied by burning, tingling, and itching. This reaction also occurs in many patients therapeutically treated with niacin.

Food Sources

Meat is a major source of niacin. The greatest intake of niacin in the United States comes from mixed dishes high in meat, poultry, or fish. In addition, niacin in ample in poultry as a main dish, enriched and whole grain breads and bread products, and fortified ready-to-eat cereals. Other good sources include legumes (e.g., peanuts, dried beans, and peas). Fruits and vegetables are relatively poor sources. Table 6-10 gives the food sources of niacin.

Stability

Niacin is stable to acid and heat but is lost when cooked with excess water, unless the cooking water is retained and consumed, as in soup.

Vitamin B_6

Functions

Vitamin B_6 is the collective name of a group of six related compounds (pyridoxine, pyridoxal, pyridoxamine, and their respective activated phosphate forms). The name pyridoxine comes from the vitamin's ringlike chemical structure, which is called a *pyridine ring*. Vitamin B_6 has an essential role in protein metabolism and function in many cell reactions involving amino acids. It aids neurotransmitter synthesis for brain activity and normal function of the central nervous system. Vitamin B_6 is stored in tissues throughout the body and participates in amino acid absorption, energy production, synthesis of the heme portion of hemoglobin, and niacin formation from typtophan. In its coenzyme role, vitamin B_6 is also active in carbohydrate and fat metabolism.

Deficiency Disease

A deficiency of vitamin B_6 is unlikely because the amounts in the general diet are large relative to the requirement. A deficiency of vitamin B_6 would cause abnormal central nervous system function with hyperirritability, neuritis, and possible convulsions. Certain types of anemia relate to a deficiency of the vitamin B_6 necessary to the formation of healthy hemoglobin.

Requirements

Because vitamin B_6 is involved in amino acid metabolism, its need varies directly with protein intake. The new DRI guidelines set the RDA standard for healthy adults up to age 50 at 1.3 mg/day for both men and women. For older adults, the RDA is slightly higher at 1.7 mg/day for men and 1.5 mg/day for women. The RDA is also higher during pregnancy (1.9 mg/day) and lactation (2.0 mg/day). The AI figure for infants up to 12 months is 0.1 to 0.3 mg/day. The UL for adults is 100 mg/day, based on nerve-damage studies.[2]

Toxicity Symptoms

High intake of vitamin B_6 from food sources has not been observed to lead to adverse effects, but when taken in large oral-supplement doses (e.g., in the treatment of carpal tunnel syndrome and premenstrual syndrome), vitamin B_6 can be associated with lack of muscular coordination and potential nerve damage. Symptoms disappear when use of large supplements is discontinued.

Food Sources

Vitamin B_6 is widespread in foods, but many sources provide only very small amounts. Good sources include grains, seeds, liver and kidney,

---

pellagra (L. *pelle,* skin; Gr. *agra,* seizure) deficiency disease caused by a lack of dietary niacin, and an inadequate amount of protein containing the amino acid tryptophan, a precursor of niacin. Pellagra is characterized by skin lesions that are aggravated by sunlight and by gastrointestinal, mucosal, neurologic, and mental symptoms. The four Ds often associated with pellagra are dermatitis, diarrhea, dementia, and death.

pyridoxine the chemical name of vitamin B_6. In its activated phosphate form, B_2-PO_4, pyridoxine functions as an important coenzyme factor in many reactions in cell metabolism related to amino acids, glucose, and fatty acids. Clinically, pyridoxine deficiency produces a specific anemia and disturbances of the central nervous system.

TABLE 6-10   Food sources of niacin

	Quantity	Niacin (mg NE)
Bread, cereal, rice, pasta		
Bread, whole wheat	1 slice	1.0
Corn meal, yellow, enriched	1 cup	4.8
Cream of wheat (regular, cooked)	¾ cup	1.1
Oatmeal (cooked)	¾ cup (⅓ cup dry)	0.2
Rice, white, enriched (cooked)	½ cup	1.1
Wheat flour, all-purpose, enriched	1 cup	4.8
Vegetables		
Asparagus (boiled)	½ cup (6 spears)	0.9
Avocado (raw)	1 med	3.3
Broccoli (raw)	½ cup, chopped	0.3
Carrot (raw)	1 med	0.7
Corn, yellow (boiled)	½ cup	1.3
Mushrooms (raw)	½ cup, pieces	1.4
Peas, green (boiled)	½ cup	1.6
Potato (baked, with skin)	1 med	3.3
Tomato (boiled)	½ cup	0.9
Tomato juice	6 fl oz	1.2
Fruits		
Banana (raw)	1 med	0.6
Figs (dried)	10 figs	1.3
Mango (raw)	1 med	1.2
Raspberries (raw)	1 cup	1.1
Meat, poultry, fish, dry beans, eggs, nuts		
Beef liver (fried)	3.5 oz	14.4
Chicken liver (simmered)	3.5 oz	4.5
Ground beef, regular (broiled)	3.5 oz	5.8
Ham cured, regular	3.5 oz	4.8
Peanut butter	1 tbsp	2.2
Peanuts (dry roasted)	1 oz	3.8
Salmon (baked)	3 oz	5.7
Sirloin steak (lean, broiled)	3.5 oz	4.3
Swordfish (baked)	3 oz	10.0
Top round, lean (broiled)	3.5 oz	6.0
Milk, dairy products		
Milk, skim	8 fl oz	0.2
Milk, whole	8 fl oz	0.2
Fats, oils, sugar		
This food group is not an important source of niacin.		

and other meats. There are limited amounts in milk, eggs, and vegetables. Table 6-11 gives food sources of vitamin B_6.

Stability

Vitamin B_6 is stable to heat but sensitive to light and alkalis.

Folate

Functions

The name folate comes from the Latin word *folium*, meaning "leaf," and was used because a major source of its original discovery was in dark green leafy vegetables. The term *folate* is now used as the common, generic name for this vitamin, which exists in many chemical forms. The most stable form of folate is folic acid, which is only rarely found in food but is the form usually used in vitamin supplements and fortified food products. In its basic coenzyme role, folate is essential to the formation of all body cells because it takes part in the creation of DNA, the important cell nucleus material that transmits genetic characteristics. Folate is also essential to the formation of hemoglobin.

Deficiency Disease

A direct deficiency of folate causes a special type of anemia—*megaloblastic anemia*, which is a particular risk during pregnancy due to increased fetal growth demands. Rapidly growing adolescents, especially ones following fad diets and who smoke, develop low levels of folate in the blood and risk anemia.

The role of adequate folate in reducing the serious public health problem of *neural tube defects* during pregnancy has received increasing study and public awareness in recent years. Neural tube defects, of which spina bifida is the one best known to the public, are the most common birth defects involving the brain and spinal cord, with incidence varying from 1 to 9 cases per 1000 births worldwide, with the highest rate occurring in Great Britain and Ireland. This defect occurs between 21 and 28 days after conception, before a woman may realize she is pregnant. Additional folic acid intake can significantly improve the folate status of women.[7] Therefore there is now a special requirement recommendation for increased folic acid intake for all women who are capable of becoming pregnant.

Requirements

The new DRI standards give a general RDA for folate for both men and women age 14 and older of 400 μg of dietary folate equivalent (DFE) per day. The DFE measure is used because food folate is about 50% less bioavailable to the body compared with synthetic folic acid. One μg of DFE equals 1 μg of food folate, 0.5 μg of folic acid taken on an empty stomach, or 0.6 μg of folic acid taken with food. In recognition of the role of folate in reducing the risk of neural tube defects, the DRIs include a new special RDA that all women who can become pregnant take an additional 400 μg daily of synthetic folic acid from fortified foods and/or supplements, in addition to natural folate from a varied diet. During pregnancy, the RDA is higher at 600 μg DFE/day to meet the increased requirements for fetal growth and is 500 μg DFE/day during lactation. For infants, the observed AI is 65 μg DFE/day during the first 6 months, and 80 μg DFE/day from 7 to 12 months. The UL for adults has been set at 1,000 μg/day of folic acid—not of DFE, not counting food folate. The DRI recommendations are aimed at providing adequate safety allowances that include specific population groups at risk, such as pregnant women, adolescents, and older adults—especially those with the added burden of low socioeconomic circumstances.[8,9]

Toxicity Symptoms

No negative effects have been observed from the excess consumption of folate from foods. There is some evidence, however, that excess intake of folic acid from supplements or fortified food products may have toxic effects—especially in persons deficient in vitamin B_{12}, which is reflected in the new UL figure.

Food Sources

Folate is widely distributed in foods. Rich sources include green leafy vegetables, liver, yeast, and

TABLE 6-11   Food sources of vitamin B_6 (pyridoxine)

	Quantity	Pyridoxine (mg)
Bread, cereal, rice, pasta		
Wheat germ (toasted)	¼ cup (1 oz)	0.28
Vegetables		
Avocado (raw)	1 med	0.48
Asparagus (boiled)	1 med	0.13
Broccoli (boiled)	½ cup	0.15
Carrot (raw)	1 med	0.11
Potato (baked, with skin)	1 med	0.70
Fruits		
Apple (raw, with skin)	1 med	0.07
Banana (raw)	1 med	0.66
Figs (dried)	10 figs	0.42
Grape juice (bottled)	8 fl oz	0.16
Meat, poultry, fish, dry beans, eggs, nuts		
Beef liver (fried)	3.5 oz	0.27
Cashews (roasted)	1 oz	0.07
Chicken, light meat (roasted, without skin)	3.5 oz	0.60
Chicken liver (simmered)	3.5 oz	0.58
Ground beef, regular (broiled)	3.5 oz	0.27
Ham (canned)	3.5 oz	0.48
Kidney beans (boiled)	1 cup	0.21
Lentils (boiled)	1 cup	0.35
Lima beans (boiled)	1 cup	0.30
Navy beans (boiled)	1 cup	0.30
Peanut butter (chunk style)	1 tbsp	0.14
Peanut butter (creamy)	1 tbsp	0.06
Peanuts (roasted)	1 oz	0.07
Pinto beans (boiled)	1 cup	0.27
Sirloin steak (broiled)	3.5 oz	0.45
Soybeans (boiled)	1 cup	0.40
Swordfish (baked)	3 oz	0.32
Top round (broiled)	3.5 oz	0.56
Walnuts (dried)	1 oz	0.16
Milk, dairy products		
Milk, skim	8 fl oz	0.10
Milk, whole	8 fl oz	0.10
Fats, oils, sugar		
This food group is not an important source of vitamin B_6.		

TABLE 6-12 Food sources of folate

	Quantity	Folate (μg)
Bread, cereal, rice, pasta		
Bread, whole wheat	1 slice	14
Wheat germ (toasted)	¼ cup (1 oz)	100
Vegetables		
Asparagus (boiled)	½ cup (6 spears)	88
Avocado (raw)	1 med	113
Peas, green (boiled)	1 cup	51
Spinach (boiled)	1 cup	262
Fruits		
Banana (raw)	1 med	22
Figs (dried)	10 figs	14
Orange (raw)	1 med	47
Strawberries (raw)	1 cup	26
Meat, poultry, fish, dry beans, eggs, nuts		
Beef liver (fried)	3.5 oz	220
Black beans (boiled)	1 cup	256
Black-eyed peas (boiled)	1 cup	356
Chicken liver (simmered)	3.5 oz	770
Chick-peas (boiled)	1 cup	282
Egg, whole	1 large	32
Green beans (boiled)	1 cup	42
Kidney beans (boiled)	1 cup	229
Lima beans, baby (boiled)	1 cup	273
Navy beans (boiled)	1 cup	255
Peanut butter	1 tbsp	13
Peanuts (dry roasted)	1 oz	41
Pinto beans (boiled)	1 cup	294
Milk, dairy products		
Milk, whole	8 fl oz	12
Yogurt, whole	8 fl oz	17
Fats, oils, sugar		
This food group is not an important source of folate.		

legumes (Table 6-12). Natural folate from food sources is important in a varied healthy diet.[10] As part of efforts to reduce the public health problem of neural tube defects in babies, the United States Food and Drug Administration (USFDA) has re-quired all manufacturers to add folic acid to certain grain products (e.g., enriched white flour, white rice, corn grits, cornmeal, noodles, fortified break-fast cereals, bread, rolls, and buns) since January 1998. The special new DRI recommendation that women capable of becoming pregnant consume folic acid from supplements or from fortified foods (e.g., enriched grains) is one of only two current RDAs that specifically recommend vitamin sources besides those readily available in a varied diet of natural foods. (The other such recommendation concerns vitamin B_{12} and older persons.)

Stability

Folate is a relatively stable vitamin, but storage and cooking losses can be high, especially when cooked in excess water. As much as 50% of food folate may be destroyed during household preparation, food processing, and storage.

Cobalamin (Vitamin B₁₂)

Functions

Vitamin B_{12} refers to cobalamin, the general term for a group of biologically active compounds whose name derives from its unique structure with a single red atom of the trace element cobalt at its center. In its coenzyme role, vitamin B_{12} is essential for normal blood formation due to its role in the synthesis of the nonprotein *heme* portion of hemoglobin. Vitamin B_{12} is also essential for proper nervous system function.

Deficiency Disease

The search for the controlling agent responsible for a special anemia—*pernicious anemia*—led to the discovery of vitamin B_{12}. A component of the digestive gastric secretions called *intrinsic factor* is necessary for absorption of vitamin B_{12} into the bloodstream. When this factor is missing, the vitamin cannot be absorbed to do its job in making hemoglobin, and pernicious anemia results. In such cases, vitamin B_{12} must be given by injection to bypass the absorption defect.

Requirements

Although it is essential, the amount of dietary vitamin B_{12} needed for normal human metabolism is very small, consisting of only a few micrograms. The usual mixed diet easily provides this much and more. The new DRI guidelines establish an RDA

for men and women ages 19 to 50 of 2.4 μg/day. The RDA during pregnancy is 2.6 μg/day; during lactation, the figure is 2.8 μg/day. There is no RDA for infants up to 12 months old. An observed AI during the first year is 0.4 to 0.5 μg/day. There is evidence that from 10% to 30% of people over age 50 may poorly absorb vitamin B_{12} from food sources. Therefore the DRIs include a special recommendation that both men and women over 50 should meet their RDA primarily from foods fortified by vitamin B_{12} or from supplements.

Toxicity Symptoms

Vitamin B_{12} does not produce adverse effects in healthy individuals when its intake from food or supplements exceeds body needs. Therefore no UL has been established.

Food Sources

Because vitamin B_{12} occurs as a protein complex in foods, its food sources are mostly from animals. The initial source, however, is synthesizing bacteria in the gastrointestinal tract of herbivorous animals. Some synthesis is done by human intestinal bacteria, but our major source is animal foods. The richest sources are liver and kidney, lean meat, milk, eggs, and cheese (Table 6-13). Natural dietary deficiency in a mixed diet is unknown. The only reported cases have been in some vegans (see Chapter 4), for whom cobalamin supplements are recommended to prevent such deficiency. The general symptoms of such a deficiency include nervous disorders, sore mouth and tongue, amenorrhea, and neuritis.

Stability

Vitamin B_{12} is stable in ordinary cooking processes.

Pantothenic Acid

Functions

The name *pantothenic acid* refers to the vitamin's widespread functions in the body and sources in food. It is based on the Greek word *pantothen*, which means "from every side." Pantothenic acid is present in all forms of living things and is essen-

TABLE 6-13   Food sources of vitamin B$_{12}$ (cobalamin)

	Quantity	Vitamin B$_{12}$ (μg)
Bread, cereal, rice, pasta		
This food group is not an important source of vitamin B$_{12}$.		
Vegetables		
This food group is not an important source of vitamin B$_{12}$.		
Fruits		
This food group is not an important source of vitamin B$_{12}$.		
Meat, poultry, fish, dry beans, eggs, nuts		
Beef liver (fried)	3.5 oz	111.80
Chicken liver (simmered)	3.5 oz	19.39
Chicken, white meat (roasted)	3.5 oz	0.34
Clams (steamed)	3 oz (9 small)	84.06
Egg, fresh	1 large	0.77
Ground beef, regular (broiled)	3.5 oz	2.93
Ham, cured, regular	3.5 oz	0.80
Mackerel (baked)	3 oz	16.15
Oysters (steamed)	3 oz (12 med)	32.53
Salmon (baked)	3 oz	4.93
Sirloin steak (lean, broiled	3.5 oz	2.85
Swordfish (baked)	3 oz	1.72
Top round, lean (broiled)	3.5 oz	2.48
Milk, dairy products		
Cheddar cheese	3.5 oz	0.83
Milk, skim	8 fl oz	0.93
Milk, whole	8 fl oz	0.87
Swiss cheese	3.5 oz	1.68
Yogurt, whole	8 fl oz	0.84
Fats, oils, sugar		
This food group is not an important source of vitamin B$_{12}$.		

tial to all forms of life. In its coenzyme role, it is essential to the synthesis and functioning of the body's key activating agent, *coenzyme* A, which controls many cell metabolic reactions involving fat and cholesterol, heme formation, and amino acid activation.

Deficiency Disease

Given its widespread natural occurrence, deficiencies of pantothenic acid are unlikely. The only cases

pantothenic acid (Gr. *pantothen,* from all sides, in every corner) a B-complex vitamin found widely distributed in nature and occurring throughout the body tissues. Its one role—which is a major one—is as an essential constituent of the body's main activating agent, coenzyme A. This special compound has extensive metabolic responsibility in activating a number of compounds in many tissues; it is a key energy metabolism substance in every cell.

of deficiency were in individuals fed synthetic diets with virtually no pantothenic acid.

Requirements

No specific RDA for pantothenic acid is given in the new DRI guidelines. The usual intake range of the American diet is 4 to 7 mg/day. The DRIs set an AI amount for persons age 14 and older of 5 mg/day. The AI is slightly higher during pregnancy (6 mg/day) and lactation (7 mg/day). For infants during the first year, the observed AI is 1.7 to 1.8 mg/day.

Toxicity Symptoms

There have been no observed adverse effects associated with pantothenic acid in humans or animals. Therefore the DRI guidelines have not established a UL for this vitamin.

Food Sources

Pantothenic acid occurs as widely in foods as in body tissues. It is found in all animal and plant cells and is especially abundant in animal tissues, whole grain cereals, and legumes (Table 6-14). Smaller amounts are found in milk, vegetables, and fruits.

Stability

Pantothenic acid is stable to acid and heat but is sensitive to alkalis and water-soluble.

Biotin

Functions

The minute traces of biotin in the body perform multiple metabolic tasks. In its coenzyme role, biotin serves as a partner with coenzyme A, of which pantothenic acid is an essential part. Biotin is also involved in the synthesis of both fatty acids and amino acids.

Deficiency Disease

Because the potency of biotin is great—even in its tiny microgram amounts in the body, there is no known natural deficiency. The only induced deficiencies have occurred in patients on long-term total parenteral nutrition (TPN) without biotin sup-

plementation. Occasional cases of inborn errors of biotin metabolism have been observed.

Requirements

The amount of biotin needed for metabolism is extremely small, measured in micrograms. The DRI guidelines do not establish an RDA for biotin. An AI figure has been set based on intakes of healthy individuals. The AI for adults age 18 and older is 30 μg/day. For infants during the first 12 months, the observed AI is 5 to 6 μg/day. The AI during pregnancy is also 30 μg/day; during lactation, it is 35 μg/day. The body also receives a supply of biotin synthesized by intestinal bacteria.

Toxicity Symptoms

There is no known biotin toxicity or adverse effects from its consumption in humans or animals. No data currently support setting a UL for biotin.

Food Sources

Biotin is widely distributed in natural foods but is not equally available to the body from various foods. For example, the biotin of corn and soy meals is completely bioavailable (i.e., able to be digested and absorbed by the body). The biotin in wheat, however, is almost completely unavailable to the body. The best food sources of biotin are liver, egg yolk, soy flour, cereals (except bound forms in wheat), other meats, tomatoes, and yeast. Fruits are poor sources.

Stability

Biotin is a stable vitamin, but it is water-soluble.

A summary of these B vitamins is given in Table 6-15.

Choline

Functions

Choline is a water-soluble nutrient associated with the B-complex vitamins. Choline has been insufficiently studied thus far. The new DRI guidelines include choline but state that there is insufficient human data to determine if choline is essential in the human diet.[2] The human body may be able

TABLE 6-14 Food sources of pantothenic acid

	Quantity	Pantothenic acid (mg)
Bread, cereal, rice, pasta		
All-bran	1/3 cup (1 oz)	0.49
Bagel	1 bagel	0.20
Bread, whole wheat	1 slice	0.18
English muffin, plain	1 muffin	0.29
Oatmeal, regular (quick)	3/4 cup (1 oz)	0.35
Shredded wheat	1 oz	0.24
Soybean flour (defatted)	1/2 cup	1.00
Wheat germ (toasted)	1/4 cup (1 oz)	0.39
Vegetables		
Avocado (raw)	1 med	1.68
Broccoli (raw)	1/2 cup, chopped	0.24
Corn, yellow (boiled)	1/2 cup	0.72
Potato (baked, with skin)	1 med	1.12
Squash, winter, all varieties (baked)	1/2 cup	0.36
Sweet potato (boiled)	1/2 cup, mashed	0.87
Tomato (boiled)	1/2 cup	0.35
Fruits		
Apricots (raw)	3 med	0.25
Banana (raw)	1 med	0.30
Figs (dried)	10 figs	0.81
Orange juice (fresh)	8 fl oz	0.47
Orange, navel (raw)	1 med	0.35
Papaya (raw)	1 med	0.66
Pomegranate (raw)	1 med	0.92
Meat, poultry, fish, dry beans, eggs, nuts		
Almonds (dried)	1 oz (24 nuts)	0.13
Beef liver (fried)	3.5 oz	5.92
Black beans (boiled)	1/2 cup	0.24
Black-eyed peas (boiled)	1/2 cup	0.35
Cashews (roasted)	1 oz (18 med nuts)	0.34
Chicken, dark meat (roasted, without skin)	3.5 oz	1.21
Chicken, light meat (roasted, without skin)	3.5 oz	0.97
Chicken liver (simmered)	3.5 oz	5.41
Egg, fresh	1 large	0.86
Egg yolk, fresh	Yolk of 1 large egg	0.75

Continued

TABLE 6-14 Food sources of pantothenic acid—cont'd

	Quantity	Pantothenic acid (mg)
Meat, poultry, fish, dry beans, eggs, nuts—cont'd		
Garbanzo beans (boiled)	½ cup	0.24
Ground beef, regular (broiled)	3.5 oz	0.33
Ham, cured, regular	3.5 oz	0.50
Lentils (boiled)	½ cup	0.63
Lima beans (boiled)	½ cup	0.35
Peanut butter (chunky style)	2 tbsp	0.31
Peanuts (roasted)	1 oz	0.39
Pinto beans (boiled)	½ cup	0.25
Salmon (smoked)	3 oz	0.74
Sirloin steak (broiled)	3.5 oz	0.35
Top round (broiled)	3.5 oz	0.48
Turkey, light meat (roasted, without skin)	3.5 oz	0.68
Milk, dairy products		
American cheese, processed	1 oz	0.14
Blue cheese	1 oz	0.49
Cheddar cheese	1 oz	0.12
Milk, skim	8 fl oz	0.81
Milk, whole	8 fl oz	0.76
Yogurt, whole	8 fl oz	0.88
Fats, oils, sugar		

This food group is not an important source of pantothenic acid.

to synthesize internally adequate choline at some stages of life. As a nutrient, choline is important in maintaining the structural integrity of cell membranes. Choline is also active in the synthesis of *acetylcholine*, which is a neurotransmitter involved in memory storage, muscle control, and other functions.

Deficiency Disease
A deficiency of choline from food sources appears to be associated with liver damage. In clinical settings, patients fed with TPN solutions that did not include choline also developed liver damage, which was resolved with choline supplementation.

Requirements
There is insufficient data on which to establish an RDA for choline. Therefore the DRI guidelines have no RDA for choline but give an AI level for adults of 550 mg/day for men over age 14 and 425 mg/day for women over age 18. During pregnancy, the AI is 450 mg/day; during lactation, it is 550 mg/day because an ample amount of choline is secreted into human milk. For infants, the observed AI figure is 125 to 150 mg/day during the first year.

Toxicity Symptoms
Choline has a low level of toxicity. Adverse effects have only been observed in cases where the choline

TABLE 6-15   A summary of B-complex vitamins

Vitamin	Functions	Results of deficiency*	Food sources
Thiamin	Normal growth; coenzyme in carbohydrate metabolism; normal function of heart, nerves, and muscle	Beriberi; GI: loss of appetite, gastric distress, indigestion, deficient hydrochloric acid; CNS: fatigue, nerve damage, paralysis; CV: heart failure, edema of legs especially	Pork, beef, liver, whole or enriched grains, legumes
Riboflavin	Normal growth and vigor; coenzyme in protein and energy metabolism	Ariboflavinosis; wound aggravation, cracks at corners of mouth, swollen red tongue, eye irritation, skin eruptions	Milk, meats, enriched cereals, green vegetables
Niacin (precursor: tryptophan)	Coenzyme in energy production; normal growth, health of skin, normal activity of stomach, intestines, and nervous system	Pellagra; weakness, lack of energy, and loss of appetite; skin: scaly dermatitis; CNS: neuritis, confusion	Meat, peanuts, legumes, enriched grains
Pyridoxine (B_6)	Coenzyme in amino acid metabolism: protein synthesis, heme formation, brain activity; carrier for amino acid absorption	Anemia; CNS: hyper-irritability, convulsions, neuritis	Grains, seeds, liver and kidney, meats; milk, eggs, vegetables
Pantothenic acid	Coenzyme in formation of coenzyme A: fat, cholesterol, and heme formation and amino acid activation	Unlikely because of widespread occurrence	Meats, cereals, legumes; milk, vegetables, fruits
Biotin	Coenzyme A partner; synthesis of fatty acids, amino acids, purines	Natural deficiency unknown	Liver, egg yolk, soy flour, cereals (except bound form in wheat), tomatoes, yeast
Folate	Part of DNA, growth and development of red blood cells	Certain type of anemia: megaloblastic (large, immature red blood cells); neural tube defects	Liver, green leafy vegetables, legumes, yeast
Cobalamin (B_{12})	Coenzyme in synthesis of heme for hemoglobin, normal red blood cell formation	Pernicious anemia (B_{12} is necessary extrinsic factor that combines with intrinsic factor of gastric secretions for absorption)	Liver, kidney, lean meats, milk, eggs, cheese

*Key: *GI,* gastrointestinal; *CNS,* central nervous system; *CV,* cardiovascular.

intake was several times greater than normal intake from food. Very high doses of choline have been associated with lowered blood pressure, fishy body odor, sweating, salivation, and reduced growth rate.

Food Sources

Choline is found naturally in a wide variety of foods. Milk, eggs, liver, and peanuts are especially rich sources of choline. A normal, varied diet can deliver 1 gram of choline per day, and typical dietary intake for adults in the United States has been estimated to be 700 to 1000 mg/day.

Stability

Choline is a stable vitamin and is water-soluble like all of the B-complex vitamins.

THE ISSUE OF VITAMIN SUPPLEMENTATION

Ongoing Debate

The debate between users and producers of vitamin supplements and those who think they have no place in health maintenance continues, fueled by extremists on both sides. On one hand, conservative health workers may dismiss anyone who suggests a need for vitamin supplements. On the other hand, self-proclaimed and noncredentialed nutrition "experts" may push megadoses of everything from A to Z to cure anything. Who is right? Probably someone with sound knowledge in addition to *wisdom*, who suggests a course between these two extremes. Some people think that all persons should meet the precise RDA standards for all essential nutrients, but as the new DRI guidelines emphasize, the RDA amounts have been designed to meet the average needs of healthy population groups—not individual needs, which can vary widely in different circumstances. For individual needs, wise practitioners take an individual approach based on personal assessment of need. Not all of the ideas expressed in the ongoing debate over vitamins are equal or have scientific basis.

Concept of Biochemical Individuality

The term *biochemical individuality* is important. It means that the body's chemical composition is not the same for every individual, and that this pattern changes within a given person at different times under various circumstances, during the normal life cycle and in disease. The concept of biochemical individuality cannot be overlooked when individual nutritional needs are assessed, because it is influenced by things such as age, sex, personal habits, work, living situation, and health status. Consider some of the following factors:

Life Cycle Needs

At different ages and situations through the life cycle, additional vitamins are needed.

Pregnancy and lactation. The new DRI guidelines explicitly establish separate recommendations for women during pregnancy and lactation that take into account the increased nutrient requirements at these times. To prevent possible birth defect damage early in pregnancy, the DRIs recommend that women capable of becoming pregnant take additional folic acid (folate) from supplements. Women may find it difficult to meet the increased nutrient needs of pregnancy by diet alone due to food availability, tolerances, food preferences, or other factors that can lead to a marginal diet. Supplements may then become a necessary way of ensuring adequate intake to meet the increased nutrient demands.

Infancy. Specific supplements for breast-feeding infants are recommended by the American Academy of Pediatrics to prevent certain clinical problems. These supplements include vitamins K and D and the trace minerals iron and fluoride (see Chapter 11). These nutrients are included in the composition of commercial formulas for bottle-fed babies.

Aging. The aging process may increase the need for some nutrients because of decreased food intake and impaired nutrient absorption, storage, and usage (see Chapter 12). Marginal deficiencies of ascorbic acid, thiamin, riboflavin, pyridoxine, and cobalamin have occurred in elderly persons, even in some individuals using supplements.

Lifestyle

Personal lifestyle choices and habits may also influence individual needs for nutrient supplementation.

Oral contraceptive use. Women using oral contraceptive agents (i.e., "the pill") as a means of family planning find that this practice lowers serum levels of several B vitamins, including pyridoxine and niacin, as well as of vitamin C. If general nutrient-intake levels are marginal, some supplements may be needed. Of course, poor diets need improvement.

Restricted diets. Persons who are always "dieting" may find it difficult to meet many of the nutrient standards, particularly if their meals provide less than 1200 kcal/day. Very strict diets are not recommended anyway. A wise weight-reduction program should meet all nutrient needs. Persons on strict vegetarian diets will need supplements of vitamin B_{12} (cobalamin) because its food source is animal proteins.

Exercise programs. Women on extensive exercise programs may increase their requirement for riboflavin. The combination of reducing diet and increasing exercise increases this need even more. This combination may indicate the need for a B-complex supplement, especially in women who do not tolerate milk—the major food source of riboflavin.

Smoking. This unhealthy habit, especially among women during their childbearing years, affects health and can reduce vitamin C levels by as much as 30%. If dietary intake is marginal and the smoker cannot stop the habit, a small supplement of vitamin C (e.g., 100 mg/day) may help compensate.

Alcohol. Chronic or abusive use of alcohol can interfere with absorption of B-complex vitamins—especially thiamin—and even destroy folate. Again, multivitamin supplements rich in B vitamins will help. A change in alcohol use must accompany this nutritional therapy, however, to prevent deficiency effects from recurring.

Caffeine. In large quantities (e.g., the amount in four to six cups of coffee a day), caffeine flushes water-soluble vitamins out of the body faster than usual. Small supplements of B vitamins and ascorbic acid may help, but reduced caffeine intake is recommended.

Disease

In states of disease, malnutrition, debilitation, or hypermetabolic demand, each patient requires careful nutrition assessment. In cases of need, nutritional support—including therapeutic supplementation as indicated—becomes part of the total medical therapy. Diet and supplementation needs for nutrition therapy are planned to meet individual clinical requirements. Increased nutrient needs are particularly evident in cases of long-term illness.

Megadoses

Persons taking megadoses of vitamins are using them as drugs. At such high pharmacologic levels, vitamins no longer operate as nutritional agents. The body uses both nutrients and drugs in specific amounts to do the following: (1) control or improve a physiologic condition or illness; (2) prevent a disease; or (3) relieve symptoms. The similarity of nutrients and drugs, however, ends there for many people. Most people generally realize that too much of any drug can be harmful—or even fatal, and so take care to avoid overdosing, but too many people do not apply this same logic to nutrients and learn the dangers of vitamin megadosing the hard way.

Toxic Effects

Fat-soluble vitamins—especially vitamin A, can be stored in large amounts in the liver. Therefore the potential toxicity of megadoses, including liver and brain damage in extreme cases, is well known.

Many people take physician- or self-prescribed megadoses of water-soluble vitamins, believing them to be safe because they are not stored in the body. The toxic effects of at least two such megadoses, however, are known. For example, megadoses of vitamin B$_6$ prescribed by gynecologists at up to 5 g/day for long periods of time as therapy for premenstrual syndrome (PMS) caused lack of muscular coordination and in some cases severe nerve damage. Megadoses of ascorbic acid (i.e., over 2 g/day) have caused gastrointestinal pain, raised the risk for kidney stone formation, and reduced the action of leukocytes (special white blood cells) against bacteria. Meanwhile, scientific research has failed to confirm that such megadoses cure colds or lower cholesterol or lower cancer risk—which are the reasons why these large amounts were used in the first place.

"Artificially Induced" Deficiencies

When blood levels of one nutrient taken in megadoses rise above normal, the increased need for the other nutrients with which it works in the body create deficiency symptoms. Deficiencies also occur when a person suddenly stops taking the large amounts and a "rebound effect" results. For example, infants born to mothers who took megadoses of ascorbic acid during pregnancy have developed scurvy when their high nutrient supply was cut off at birth.

Supplementation Principles

To summarize, the following basic principles may help guide nutrient supplementation decisions:

- **Read the new labels carefully.** As labels on dietary supplements come more in line with the Nutrition Labeling and Education Act of 1990, which reformed current labels on food products, consumers can have access to safe products without unfounded health claims. Professional health associations support such improved labeling on food supplements, as well as on foods. Consumers want to know a product's ingredients, toxicity levels, and any potential side effects, as well as that any health claims made are based on significant scientific agreement.

- **Vitamins, like drugs, can be harmful in large amounts.** The only time larger doses may be helpful is when the body already has a severe deficiency or is unable to absorb or metabolize the nutrient efficiently.

- **Identified individual needs govern specific supplement use.** Each person's need should be the basis for determining which nutrients and amounts are used. This helps prevent problems of excess, which may increase with a cumulative effect over time. The "blanket insurance" approach may well put more money in the multi-package manufacturer's pocket—not desired health in the buyer's body.

- **All nutrients work together to promote good health.** Adding large amounts of one vitamin only makes the body think it is not getting enough of the others and increases the risk for developing deficiency symptoms.

- **Food remains the best source of nutrients.** Most foods are the best "package deals" in nutrition. They provide a wide variety of nutrients in every bite, as compared with the dozen or so found in a vitamin bottle. And, *by itself*, a vitamin can do nothing. Its action is catalytic, so it must have substrate material (i.e., carbohydrate, protein, fat, and their metabolites) on which to work. With careful selection of a wide variety of foods and storage techniques and meal planning and preparation, most people can secure an ample amount of essential nutrients. Then specific supplements for certain individuals in specific circumstances will have far more effect.

PHYTOCHEMICALS

Certain plant compounds called *phytochemicals* have been identified in relation to health benefits. These newly discovered compounds are similar to vitamins in functions and importance. The term *phytochemical* comes from the Greek word *phyton*, meaning "plant," which indicates the chemical nature of the compound. This term describes a wide variety of chemical compounds produced by plants that act as either antioxidants or hormones in the originating plant or the person eating the plants.[11-13] The message is loud and clear: "Eat more fruits and vegetables!"

SUMMARY

Vitamins are organic, noncaloric food substances that are required in very small amounts for certain metabolic tasks. Vitamins cannot be made by the body, but a balanced diet usually supplies sufficient vitamin intake. In individually identified situations, however, a designated supplement amount may be needed. Megadoses carry significant risk and are on the level of drug abuse.

The fat-soluble vitamins are A, D, E, and K. Their metabolic tasks are mainly structural. The water-soluble vitamins are vitamin C (ascorbic acid), the eight B-complex vitamins (i.e., thiamin, riboflavin, niacin, vitamin B_6, folate, vitamin B_{12}, pantothenic acid, and biotin), and choline. Their major metabolic tasks relate to their roles as coenzyme factors—except for vitamin C, which helps protein build strong tissue. Little toxicity has been associated with these vitamins because they are water-soluble and excess is excreted in the urine. Megadose habits with two water-soluble vitamins have brought the following results on the level of drug abuse: (1) large amounts of pyridoxine (B_6) have caused severe nerve damage; and (2) large amounts of vitamin C have been associated with gastrointestinal problems and kidney stones. The possibility of toxicity is increased for fat-soluble vitamins because the body can store them. Such toxicity is no longer so rare because of the current popularity of large vitamin A (retinol) supplements.

All water-soluble vitamins—especially vitamin C—are easily oxidized, so care must be taken in food storage and preparation.

REVIEW QUESTIONS

1. What is a vitamin? Describe three general functions of vitamins and give examples of each.
2. How would you advise a friend who was taking self-prescribed vitamin supplements? Give reasons and examples to support your answer.
3. Describe the effects of three vitamins that some persons take in large amounts. What are the risks involved in such megadoses?
4. Describe four situations in which vitamin supplements should be used. Give reasons and examples in each case.
5. List four principles to guide a person's decisions about vitamin supplements, and explain the basis for each one.

SELF-TEST QUESTIONS

True-False
Write the correct statement for each item you answer "false."
1. A coenzyme acts alone to control a number of different types of reactions.
2. Carotene is preformed vitamin A found in animal food sources.
3. Exposure to sunlight produces vitamin D from cholesterol in the skin.

4. Extra vitamin C is stored in the liver to meet tissue-infection demands.
5. Vitamin D and sufficient calcium and phosphorus can prevent rickets.
6. Vitamin K is found in meat, especially liver, and in leafy vegetables.

Multiple Choice

1. Vitamin A is fat-soluble and produced by humans from carotene in plant foods or consumed as the fully formed vitamin in animal foods. Therefore which of the following supplies the greatest amount of this vitamin?
   a. Oranges
   b. Green leafy vegetables
   c. Carrots
   d. Tomatoes
2. If you wanted to increase the vitamin C content of your diet, which of the following foods would you choose in larger amounts?
   a. Liver, other organ meats, and seafood
   b. Potatoes, enriched cereals, and fortified margarine
   c. Green peppers, tomatoes, and oranges
   d. Milk, cheese, and eggs
3. Which of the following statements is true about the sources of vitamin K?
   a. Vitamin K is found in a wide variety of foods, so no deficiency can occur.
   b. Vitamin K is easily absorbed without assistance so we can get all we absorb into our systems.
   c. Vitamin K is rarely found in foods, so a natural deficiency can occur.
   d. Most of our vitamin K for metabolic needs is produced by internal bacteria.

SUGGESTIONS FOR ADDITIONAL STUDY

1. Use the following activities to survey the marketing and use of vitamins:
   a. Interview six persons to determine how many are buying and using vitamin pills and which vitamins they are using, in what amounts, and for what reasons.
   b. Interview several clerks in pharmacies concerning any increase in sales of vitamin pills, and if so, the possible reasons why.
   c. Visit a health food store, posing as a potential customer. Ask about taking vitamin pills, which ones to take, and the possible benefits of each. Look over the stock carefully, reading labels and advertisements. Ask for any literature (e.g., booklets, leaflets, ads) to take with you to help you decide which ones to buy.
   d. Survey and evaluate vitamin advertisements in magazines, newspapers, and television.

   Evaluate all of your survey information and prepare a report of your results for class discussion.

2. Analyze your dietary intake of retinol and ascorbic acid by recording all of your food intake for 1 day and checking the total amount of each vitamin. Compare your totals to the RDA standards contained in the new DRI guidelines. Where do you stand? What foods could you add to your diet to increase your intake of each vitamin?

REFERENCES

1. Food and Nutrition Board, Institute of Medicine: *Dietary reference intakes for calcium, phosphorous, magnesium, vitamin D, and fluoride*, Washington, DC, 1998, National Academy Press.

2. Food and Nutrition Board, Institute of Medicine: *Dietary reference intakes for thiamin, riboflavin, niacin, vitamin B₆, folate. vitamin B₁₂, pantothenic acid, biotin, and choline*, Washington, DC, 1999, National Academy Press.

3. Food and Nutrition Board, Institute of Medicine: *Dietary reference intakes for vitamin C, vitamin E, selenium, and carotenoids,* Washington, DC, 2000, National Academy Press.

4. Marsh MN, Riley SA: *Digestion and absorption of nutrients and vitamins.* In Feldman M, Scharschmidt BF, Sleisenger MH, eds: *Gastrointestinal and liver disease,* ed 6, vol 2, Philadelphia, 1998, Saunders.

5. Booth SL and others: Food sources and dietary intakes of vitamin K_1 (phylloquinone) in the American diet, *J Am Diet Assoc* 96(2):149, 1996.

6. Rivlin RS, Dutta P: Vitamin B_2 (riboflavin): relevance to malaria and antioxidant activity, *Nutr Today* 30(2):62, 1995.

7. Cuskelly GJ and others: Fortification with low amounts of folic acid makes a significant difference in folate status in young women: implications for the prevention of neural tube defects, *Am J Clin Nutr* 70(2):234, 1999.

8. Staff report—Nutrition science and policy: folic acid fortification, *Nutr Rev* 54(3):94, 1996.

9. Koehler KM and others: Folate nutrition and older adults: challenges and opportunities, *J Am Diet Assoc* 97(2):167, 1997.

10. Brouwer IA and others: Dietary folate from vegetables and citrus fruits decrease plasma homocysteine concentration in humans in a dietary controlled trial, *J Nutr* 129(4):1135, 1999.

11. Craig WJ: Phytochemicals: guardians of our health, *J Am Diet Assoc* 97(suppl 2):S199, 1997.

12. Polsinelli ML and others: Plasma carotenoids as biomarkers of fruit and vegetable servings in women, *J Am Diet Assoc* 98(2):194, 1998.

13. Bertram JS: Carotenoids and gene regulation, *Nutr Rev* 56(6): 182, 1999.

FURTHER READING

- American Academy of Pediatrics, Committee on Genetics: Folic acid for the prevention of neural tube defects, *Pediatrics* 104(2):325, 1999.
- Kloeblen AS: Folate knowledge, intake from fortified grain products, and periconceptional supplementation patterns of a sample of low-income pregnant women according to the Health Belief Model, *J Am Diet Assoc* 99(1):33, 1999.

Here the six physicians forming the Committee on Genetics of the American Academy of Pediatrics, with the full support of all AAP members, endorse the U.S. Public Health Service recommendation that all women capable of becoming pregnant consume 400 μg of folate acid daily to prevent having a baby born with neural tube defects. This vital need is illustrated in a follow-up study in a high-risk population that included teaching the subjects how they may easily attain this daily goal of folate intake through the use of fortified grain products.

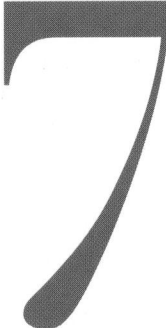

Minerals

KEY CONCEPTS

- The human body requires a variety of minerals in different amounts to do numerous metabolic tasks.

- A mixed diet of varied foods and adequate energy value is our best source of the minerals necessary for health, with individual supplements used according to specific age and growth needs or clinical requirements.

- Of the total amount of minerals a person consumes, only a relatively limited amount is available to the body.

When the earth was forming, shifting oceans and mountains deposited a large number of minerals into earth materials. Over time, these minerals moved from rocks to soil to plants to animals and then to humans. As a result, the mineral content of the human body is quite similar to that of the earth.

Minerals, which are single, inert elements, may seem simple when compared with vitamins, which are large, complex, organic compounds. Mineral micronutrients, however, perform a fascinating variety of metabolic tasks essential to our lives.

In this chapter, we look at this array of minerals to see how they differ from vitamins in the variety of their tasks and in the amounts, ranging from relatively large to exceedingly small, necessary to do these jobs.

THE DIETARY REFERENCE INTAKES PROJECT

The study of minerals and their many functions in human nutrition continues to be a subject of intense scientific investigation and public interest. As discussed fully in the previous chapter on vitamins, the Dietary Reference Intakes (DRIs) are a new system of recommendations for the use of these nutrients in healthy populations. The publication of DRI reference information, under the direction of the National Academy of Sciences, will take place over several years and involve numerous scientists from the United States and Canada. The first three of a projected series of seven reference volumes have been published. The new DRIs, which include recommendations for each gender and age group, incorporate and expand on the well-known system of RDAs.

Within the DRI system, there are four interconnected categories of recommendations, as follow: (1) the *Recommended Dietary Allowance (RDA)*, which is the daily intake that meets the needs of almost all healthy individuals in a specified group; (2) the *Estimated Average Requirement (EAR)*, which is used as the basis for developing the RDA and is the intake that meets the needs of half of the individuals in the group; (3) the *Adequate Intake (AI)*, which is a guideline used when there is not enough scientific evidence available to establish an RDA; and (4) the *Tolerable Upper Intake Level (UL)*, which is a new guideline that sets the maximum intake of a nutrient that is unlikely to pose a health risk in healthy individuals. In this chapter, we will refer to the DRI recommendations—especially the new RDAs—for minerals whenever possible because the RDAs remain the central guide to nutrient intake for most persons. The Dietary Reference Intake recommendations have currently been published for the following minerals: calcium, phosphorus, magnesium, fluoride, and selenium.[1,2]

THE NATURE OF BODY MINERALS

Most living matter is made up of five fundamental elements: hydrogen, carbon, nitrogen, oxygen, and sulfur, which are the building blocks of life. The minerals that are necessary in human nutrition are single, inorganic elements that are widely distributed in nature. Of the 54 known earth elements in the periodic table, 25 are essential to human life and function. These 25 elements—in varying amounts—perform a variety of metabolic functions in the body.

Variety of Functions

These seemingly simple, single elements, in comparison with the much larger complex organic structure of vitamins, perform an impressive variety of metabolic jobs for the body. They build, activate, regulate, transmit, and control. For example, sodium and potassium control water balance. Calcium and phosphorus build the body framework. Iron helps build the vital oxygen carrier hemoglobin. Cobalt is the central core of vitamin B_{12}. Iodine builds thyroid hormone, which in turn regulates the overall rate of all body metabolism. Thus, far from being static and inert, minerals are active essential participants, helping to control many of the body's overall metabolic processes.

Variety in Amount Needed

As described in the previous chapter, all vitamins are required in very small amounts to do their jobs. Minerals, however, occur in varying amounts in the body. For example, calcium forms a relatively large amount (i.e., about 2%) of the body weight, with most of this amount being bone tissue. An adult who weighs 150 pounds has about 3 lbs of calcium in the body. On the other hand, iron occurs in very small amounts. The same adult has only about 3 g (about one tenth of an ounce) of iron in the body. In both cases, the amount of each mineral is essential for its specific task.

Classes of Body Minerals

This varying amount of individual minerals in the body provides the basis for classifying them into two main groups.

Major Minerals

Elements are not called major minerals because they are more important but because they occur in larger amounts in the body. The major minerals are defined as those requiring an intake of more than 100 mg/day. The seven major minerals are calcium, phosphorus, sodium, potassium, magnesium, chlorine, and sulfur.

Trace Elements

The remaining 18 elements make up the group of trace elements. These minerals are not less important but occur in very small amounts in the body. Trace elements are generally defined as those having a required intake of less than 100 mg/day. Trace elements are equally essential for their specific vital tasks. Table 7-1 provides a helpful study guide.

Control of Amount and Distribution

The correct amount of minerals for body needs is usually controlled at either the point of absorption or the points of tissue uptake.

Absorption

Minerals are absorbed and used in the body in their activated *ionic* (i.e., carrying an electric charge [+ or −]) form. The following general factors influence how much of a mineral is actually absorbed into the body system from the gastrointestinal tract: (1) *food form*—minerals in animal foods are usually more readily absorbed than those in plant foods; (2) *body need*—if the body is deficient, more is absorbed than if the body has enough; and (3) *tissue health*—if the absorbing tissue surface is affected by disease, its absorptive capacity is greatly diminished.

Tissue Uptake

Some minerals are controlled by regulating hormones at the point of their "target" tissue uptake, with the excess being excreted in the urine. For example, the thyroid-stimulating hormone (TSH) controls the uptake of iodine from the blood according to the amount needed to make the thyroid hormone *thyroxine*. When more thyroxine is needed, more iodine is taken up by the thyroid gland under TSH stimulation and less is excreted. At other times when blood levels of thyroxine are normal, less iodine is taken up by the thyroid gland and more is excreted.

TABLE 7-1   Major minerals and trace elements in human nutrition

| | Trace elements | |
Major minerals (required intake over 100 mg/day)	Essential (required intake under 100 mg/day)	Essentiality unclear
Calcium (Ca)	Iron (Fe)	Silicon (Si)
Phosphorus (P)	Iodine (I)	Vanadium (V)
Sodium (Na)	Zinc (Zn)	Nickel (Ni)
Potassium (K)	Selenium (Se)	Tin (Sn)
Magnesium (Mg)	Fluoride (Fl)	Cadmium (Cd)
Chlorine (Cl)	Copper (Cu)	Arsenic (As)
Sulfur (S)	Manganese (Mn)	Aluminum (Al)
	Chromium (Cr)	
	Molybdenum (Mo)	
	Cobalt (Co)	
	Boron (B)	

Occurrence in the Body

Body minerals are found in several forms in places related to their functions. The two basic forms in which minerals occur in the body are as follows: (1) *free*—mineral atoms or molecules may be free as *ions* (meaning that they carry an electric charge) in body fluids (e.g., sodium in tissue fluids, which helps to control water balance); and (2) *combined*—minerals may be combined with other minerals (e.g., calcium with phosphorus to form bone) or with organic substances (e.g., iron with heme and globin to form the organic compound hemoglobin).

ISSUE OF MINERAL SUPPLEMENTATION

The same principles in the previous chapter relating to vitamin supplements also guide the use of mineral supplements. Special needs during growth periods and in clinical situations may require individual supplements of specific major minerals or trace elements.

Life Cycle Needs

Added minerals may be needed during rapid growth periods in the life cycle.

Pregnancy and Lactation

Women require added calcium, phosphorus, and iron to meet the demands of rapid fetal growth and milk production, and breast-fed infants may need additional fluoride.[3]

Adolescence

The rapid growth during adolescence requires increased calcium and phosphorous for growth of long bones. If an adolescent's diet provides insufficient calcium, additional amounts may be indicated to increase bone density and decrease the risk for bone density problems (e.g., osteoporosis) in later adult years (see Chapter 12). Supplements combining iron with folate may be indicated for adolescent girls who may soon enter the childbearing years.[4,5]

Adulthood

Healthy adults do not need mineral supplementation, but questions have been raised in media and advertising about the need for calcium to prevent and treat osteoporosis. Although currently marketed to prevent osteoporosis, calcium supplements alone have little effect—especially when the diet is poor. A well-rounded, varied diet combined with adequate physical exercise will maintain optimal bone health in most adults. In addition, an idiopathic (i.e., cause unknown) form of osteoporosis that occurs in young adults does not respond to calcium supplements. At any adult age, calcium supplements alone neither prevent nor successfully treat osteoporosis, the cause of which is not clear and involves multiple factors. Calcium may be used as part of a treatment program together with vitamin D hormone, estrogen, and increased physical activity.

Clinical Needs

Persons with certain clinical problems or those at high risk for developing such problems require mineral supplements.

---

major minerals the group of minerals, also called macronutrients, that are required by the body in amounts of more than 100 mg/day. The seven major minerals in the body are calcium, phosphorus, sodium, potassium, magnesium, chlorine, and sulfur.

trace elements the group of elements, also called micronutrients, that are required by the body in smaller amounts of less than 100 mg/day. The 11 essential elements in the body are iron, iodine, zinc, copper, manganese, chromium, cobalt, selenium, molybdenum, fluoride, and boron.

osteoporosis (Gr. *osteon,* bone; *poros,* passage, pore) abnormal thinning of the bone, producing a porous, fragile, lattice-like bone tissue of enlarged spaces that is prone to fracture or deformity.

Iron-Deficiency Anemia

One of the most prevalent health problems encountered in population surveys is iron-deficiency anemia. The need for increased iron has long been established for pregnant and breast-feeding women.[3] The following high-risk groups may also need to supplement their diets: adolescent girls on poor diets, low-income adolescent boys, athletes, vegetarians, and elderly persons on poor diets.

Weight-Loss Programs

The Women's Healthy Lifestyle Project was a recent study of the association between body weight and bone mineral density (BMD); 236 healthy women aged 44 to 50 participated with a goal of modest weight loss or preventing weight gain.[6] All of these women were randomly assigned to a control group or to a lifestyle-intervention group of behavior modification designed to reduce dietary fat and caloric intake. The women in the weight loss group who modified their lifestyles to lose weight, however, lost more BMD than those in the weight-stable control group. Therefore programs for weight loss must consider the possible results of BMD loss and iron status, and should be planned accordingly.[7]

Zinc Deficiency

Increased use of processed foods and vegetarian diets have increased concern about possible zinc deficiency, especially in pregnant and lactating women, children, and elderly persons. Signs of deficiency are slow growth, impaired taste and smell, poor wound healing, and skin problems, but it takes 3 to 24 weeks for symptoms to appear. Others at risk include alcoholics, persons on long-term low-calorie diets, and elderly persons in long-term institutional care.

Potassium-Losing Drugs

Persons requiring long-term use of potassium-losing diuretic drugs for treatment of hypertension may need potassium-replacement supplements. Increased intake of foods high in potassium is also necessary.

MAJOR MINERALS

Calcium

Functions

Most of the U.S. food and nutrition surveys, such as those conducted regularly by the U.S. Department of Agriculture (USDA) and the National Center for Health Statistics, indicate that calcium is one of the minerals most likely to be deficient, as measured by national surveys. Men and boys typically consume about 25% more calcium than women and girls, simply because men and boys usually eat larger amounts of food. The absorption of dietary calcium depends on the following: (1) the food form (i.e., plant forms are usually bound with other substances and not readily available); and (2) the interaction of three hormones (i.e., vitamin D hormone, parathyroid hormone [PTH], and calcitonin [from the thyroid gland]) that directly control absorption, along with indirect metabolic stimuli from the estrogen hormones (i.e., sex hormones produced in the ovaries and testes). Once absorbed, calcium has four basic functions in the body.

Bone and tooth formation. Most of the body calcium—over 99%—is found in bones and teeth. About 1% to 2% of normal adult body weight is calcium. When calcium phosphate is removed from bone, the remaining tissue is flexible cartilage. If dietary calcium is insufficient during childhood growth, especially during initial formation of the fetal skeleton and rapid growth of long bones during adolescence, the production of healthy bone tissue is hindered. Teeth are calcified before they erupt from the gums, so later dietary calcium does not affect tooth structure as it does the continuing balance of calcium in bone tissue.

Blood clotting. Calcium is essential for the formation of fibrin to compose the blood clot.

Muscle and nerve action. Calcium ions stimulate muscle contraction and transmit impulses along nerve fibers.

Metabolic reactions. Calcium is required for many general metabolic functions in the body. Such functions include absorption of vitamin B_{12}, activation of the fat-splitting enzyme pancreatic lipase, and secretion of insulin from special cells in the pancreas where it is synthesized. Calcium also occurs in cell membranes, where it governs how permeable the membrane is to nutrients.

Requirements

As part of the Dietary Reference Intakes (DRIs) project, the scientific panel on calcium reviewed all current research and concluded that there is not enough scientific knowledge of this nutrient's requirements through life to establish new specific RDAs for calcium. Although calcium is an area of active research, the DRI panel reports that the following are still areas of concern: uncertainties about the nutritional significance of some research data; a lack of firm agreement between observed survey information and experimental laboratory data; and a lack of long-term longitudinal data connecting calcium intake with long-term bone density loss. Therefore the DRIs set AI levels for calcium instead of a new RDA. The AI amounts should provide sufficient calcium nourishment for the body, while recognizing that a lower intake may be adequate for many individuals. Although there is currently no RDA for calcium, the UL has been established, based on the maximum calcium intake above which there is a risk of adverse effects—primarily kidney stone formation (which affects 12% of the United States population), kidney failure, and metabolic action inhibiting the body's absorption of other minerals (e.g., iron, zinc, magnesium, and phosphorus).[1]

The DRI guidelines give AI levels by age group. For all infants up to 6 months old, the AI level is 210 mg/day; for infants 7 through 12 months, the AI is 270 mg/day. The need increases during the growth years of childhood and adolescence, during which the AIs are as follows: 1 to 3 years, 500 mg/day; 4 to 8 years, 800 mg/day; and 9 to 18 years, 1300 mg/day. For both men and women aged 19 to 50 years, the AI for desirable calcium retention is 1000 mg/day, with a rise to 1200 mg/day for those over 50 years old. During pregnancy and lactation, the AI amount is currently set equal to the level for the general age group, as follows: 1300 mg/day for up to age 18, and 1000 mg/day for ages 19 years and older. Excess calcium intake is usually associated with excessive use of high-dose supplements. The new UL is set at 2500 mg/day for individuals aged 1 year and older.

Food Sources

Milk and milk products are the most important sources of readily available calcium (Figure 7-1). The calcium in these dairy products is well absorbed, whereas the calcium in most leafy plant sources is not readily available. Not all of the milk in the diet must be consumed as a beverage. Milk may be used in cooking (e.g., in soups, sauces, puddings) or in milk products such as yogurt, cheese,

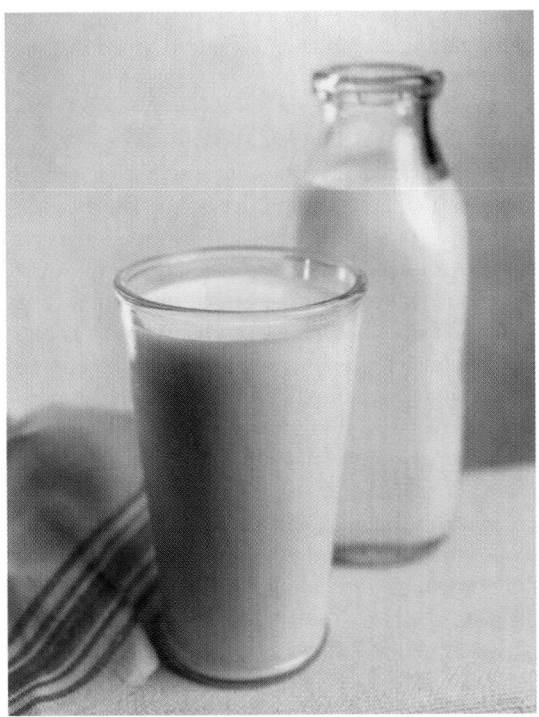

FIGURE 7-1 Milk is the major food source of calcium. (Credit: PhotoDisc.)

and ice cream. Secondary sources of calcium include grains, egg yolks, legumes, and nuts. In Swiss chard and beet greens, the calcium is bound with oxalic acid and not available. Oxalic acid is a compound found in plants such as spinach, rhubarb, and certain other vegetables and nuts, that forms insoluble salts—oxalates—with calcium, interfering with calcium absorption. Other green vegetables such as broccoli, kale, and mustard and turnip greens, however, are better calcium sources because they do not contain oxalic acid. Phytate, another plant compound in grains such as wheat, can bind calcium and interfere with its absorption. Excessive dietary fiber can decrease calcium absorption. Table 7-2 lists calcium food sources.

In addition to food sources, calcium intake from supplements is widespread. Surveys show that almost 25% of women in the United States take supplements containing calcium.[1] The bioavailability of calcium from supplements depends on the dose and whether it is taken in the preferred manner with a meal. Calcium is best absorbed in doses of 500 mg or less.

Deficiency States

If available calcium is insufficient during growth years, various bone deformities occur. The gross deficiency disease *rickets* is related to not enough vitamin D to support adequate calcium absorption. A decrease of calcium in the blood, in relation to its serum partner phosphorus, results in *tetany*, a condition characterized by abnormal muscle spasms. The major calcium-related clinical condition today is osteoporosis, which is an abnormal thinning of the bones—especially in postmenopausal women that is characterized by reduced bone mass, increased bone fragility, and a greater risk for fracture. Each year in the United States, over 1.5 million bone fractures—including 300,000 hip fractures—are associated with osteoporosis. Among postmenopausal American women, the incidence of osteoporosis is 21% for Caucasians and Asians, 16% for Hispanics, and 10% for African Americans.[1] The reasons for these observed differences by race are unclear.

Osteoporosis is not a primary calcium deficiency disease as such but results from a combination of factors that create chronic calcium deficiency. These factors include inadequate intake, poor intestinal absorption connected with hormones controlling calcium absorption and metabolism, and physical exercise that stimulates muscle insertion action on bones and determines the strength, shape, and mass of bone. Lack of physical exercise contributes to the development of osteoporosis; and immobility following injury or disease can cause serious loss of bone tissue. Bone is a dynamic tissue, with both new bone formation and resorption constantly occurring. A portion of the skeleton is reabsorbed and replaced by new bone each year; this bone remodeling can affect up to 50% of the total amount of bone per year in young children and about 5% in adults. Bone resorption exceeds formation, however, after menopause and with aging in general for both men and women. The precise cause of the imbalance in bone calcium deposit and resorption in osteoporosis—a balance that most adults normally maintain—is unknown. Thus increased calcium *alone*—in diet or supplements—will neither prevent osteoporosis in susceptible adults nor successfully treat diagnosed cases. Therapies that reduce bone loss in osteoporosis include combinations of the various factors involved: calcium, the active hormonal form of vitamin D, and estrogens.

Phosphorus

Functions

The phosphorus atom in nature is most commonly found combined with four oxygen atoms to form the phosphate molecule. Phosphorus serves as a partner with calcium in the major task of bone formation but also functions in the following other metabolic processes:

Bone and tooth formation. The calcification of bones and teeth depends on the fixing of phosphorus as calcium phosphate in the bone-forming tissue. The ratio of calcium to phosphorus in typical bone tissue is about 1.5:1.

TABLE 7-2 Food sources of calcium

	Quantity	Calcium (mg)
Bread, cereal, rice, pasta		
Bran muffin, homemade	1 muffin	54
Bread, whole wheat	1 slice	18
Corn muffin, from mix	1 muffin	96
Cream of wheat (cooked)	¾ cup	38
Pasta, enriched (cooked)	1 cup	16
Rice, enriched	1 cup	21
Wheat flakes	1 cup	43
Vegetables		
Artichoke (boiled)	1 med	47
Asparagus (boiled)	½ cup (6 spears)	22
Avocado (raw)	1 med	19
Broccoli (raw)	½ cup	21
Brussels sprouts (boiled)	½ cup (4 sprouts)	28
Carrots (raw)	1 med	19
Collards (boiled)	1 cup	148
Corn, yellow (boiled)	½ cup	2
Kale (chopped)	½ cup	47
Peas, green (boiled)	½ cup	19
Potato (baked, with skin)	1 med	115
Tomato (raw)	1 med	8
Fruits		
Apricots (raw)	3 med	15
Banana (raw)	1 med	7
Cantaloupe (raw)	½ cup	8
Figs (dried)	10 figs	269
Orange juice (fresh)	8 fl oz	27
Orange, navel (raw)	1 med	56
Papaya (raw)	1 med	72
Raspberries (raw)	½ cup	14
Strawberries (raw)	½ cup	11
Tangerine (raw)	1 med	12
Meat, poultry, fish, dry beans, eggs, nuts		
Almonds (roasted)	1 oz	148
Beef liver (fried)	3.5 oz	11
Cashews (roasted)	1 oz	13
Chicken, dark (roasted, without skin)	3.5 oz	179
Chicken light (roasted, without skin)	3.5 oz	216
Egg, whole	1 large	90

Continued

TABLE 7-2 Food sources of calcium—cont'd

	Quantity	Calcium (mg)
Meat, poultry, fish, dry beans, eggs, nuts—cont'd		
Ham (canned)	3.5 oz	6
Kidney beans (boiled)	1 cup	50
Lentils (boiled)	1 cup	37
Lima beans (boiled)	1 cup	32
Peanuts (roasted)	1 oz	15
Soybeans (boiled)	1 cup	175
Milk, dairy products		
Milk, skim	8 fl oz	302
Milk, whole	8 fl oz	290
Yogurt, whole	8 fl oz	355
Fats, oils		
This food group is not an important source of calcium.		
Sugar		
Brown sugar	1 cup	123
Molasses, barbados	1 tbsp	49

Energy metabolism. Phosphorus—in the form of phosphate—is necessary for the controlled oxidation of carbohydrate, fat, and protein in producing and storing available energy for the body. Phosphate contributes to energy and protein metabolism, and to cell function and genetic inheritance as an essential component of cell enzymes, thiamin, and the critical cell compounds DNA and RNA, which control cell reproduction.

Acid-base balance. Phosphate is an important buffer material to prevent changes in the acidity of body fluids.

Requirements

The typical American diet contains enough phosphorus. Surveys indicate that for those over aged 9, the mean daily phosphorus intake is around 1500 mg/day for men and 1000 mg/day for women. The DRI guidelines have established new Recommended Dietary Allowances (RDAs) for phosphorus for both men and women aged 19 and older of 700 mg/day. For children, the RDA varies with the stage of growth. For ages 1 to 3 years, the RDA is 460 mg/day; for ages 4 to 8 years, it is 500 mg/day. For ages 9 to 18 years—which is a period of very rapid bone growth, the RDA is 1250 mg/day. Healthy infants fed human milk receive adequate phosphorus. The AI level during the first 6 months is 100 mg/day, and from 7 to 12 months is 275 mg/day. For women during pregnancy and lactation, there is no additional phosphorus intake recommended above the RDA for the age group. Thus the RDA during pregnancy and lactation is 1250 mg/day for women aged 18 and younger, and 700 mg/day for those aged 19 and older. The DRI guidelines also establish the UL for phosphorus of 4000 mg/day for persons aged 9 to 70 years.

Food Sources

Phosphorus is an essential part of all living tissue and is found in all animal and plant cells. Therefore sufficient phosphorus is found in the natural food supply, whether animal or plant, of virtually all animals. High-protein foods are rich in phosphorus, so milk and milk products, meat, fish, and eggs are the primary sources of phosphorus in the average diet. For humans, the bioavailability of phosphorus from plant seeds (e.g., cereal grains, beans, peas, other legumes, and nuts) is much lower because they contain *phytic acid*, which is a storage form of phosphorus that humans can-not digest directly. However, the digestive enzymes found in other foods and in intestinal bacteria can help the body receive up to 50% of its phosphorus from these seed sources. Table 7-3 gives some main food sources of phosphorus.

Deficiency States

Because phosphorus is widely distributed in foods, a deficiency is rare. A state of nearly total starvation would be needed to create a dietary phosphorus deficiency. The only evidence of deficiency has been among persons who for weeks or months habitually consume large amounts of antacids containing aluminum hydroxide. Aluminum hydroxide binds phosphorus, making it unavailable for absorption. Phosphorus deficiency results in bone loss and is characterized by weakness, loss of appetite, fatigue, and pain.

Sodium

Functions

Sodium is one of the most plentiful minerals in the body. About 120 mg (4 oz) is present in an adult body. The main function of sodium is body-water balance, as discussed in Chapter 8. Sodium also has important tasks in acid-base balance and in muscle action.

Water balance. Ionized sodium is the major guardian of the body's water *outside* the cells, which helps to prevent dehydration. Variation in sodium concentration largely controls the movement of water from one body part to another via *osmosis*. Sodium is also an integral part of the digestive juices secreted into the gastrointestinal tract, most of which are then reabsorbed.

Acid-base balance. Sodium accounts for about 90% of the alkalinity of fluids outside of cells and helps to balance acid-forming elements. Excess alkalinity, a condition called *alkalosis*, may result from the continued use of antacid drugs containing sodium.

Muscle action. Sodium ions, in partnership with potassium, are necessary for the normal response of stimulated nerves, the transmission of nerve impulses to muscles, and the contraction of muscle fibers.

Glucose absorption. Sodium, an essential part of the cell membrane system, transports glucose across membranes in the small intestine.

Requirements

The body is able to function on various amounts of dietary sodium through mechanisms designed to conserve or excrete the mineral. As a result, there is not a specific RDA for sodium within the new DRI guidelines. Individual sodium needs vary greatly depending on growth stages, sweat loss, and medical conditions (e.g., diarrhea). The classic RDA standards include an estimated minimum requirement of the three major electrolytes needed for body fluid balance: sodium, chloride, and potassium. This standard sets a minimum sodium intake of 500 mg/day for healthy persons over age 10. The sodium content of the average American diet, which contains a high amount of processed foods, usually far exceeds this RDA minimum. Americans consume an average of 10 g of table salt daily, or 4000 mg of sodium.

Food Sources

Common table salt, as used in cooking, seasoning, and processing foods, is the main dietary source of sodium. Sodium occurs naturally in foods and is, in general, most prevalent in foods of animal origin. There is enough sodium in natural food sources to meet the body's needs. When food manufacturers add salt and other sodium compounds to processed foods, sodium intake levels increase dramatically.

TABLE 7-3 Food sources of phosphorus

	Quantity	Phosphorus (mg)
Bread, cereal, rice, pasta		
Bran flakes	¾ cup	158
Bran muffin, homemade	1 muffin	111
Bread, whole wheat	1 slice	65
Cream of wheat (cooked)	¾ cup	31
English muffin, plain	1 muffin	64
Oatmeal (cooked)	¾ cup	133
Pasta, enriched (cooked)	1 cup	70
Rice, enriched (cooked)	1 cup	57
Wheat flakes	1 cup	98
Vegetables		
Artichoke (boiled)	1 med	72
Avocado (raw)	1 med	73
Brussels sprouts (boiled)	½ cup (4 sprouts)	44
Carrots (raw)	1 med	32
Corn, yellow (boiled)	½ cup	84
Peas, green (boiled)	½ cup	94
Potato (baked, with skin)	1 med	115
Spinach (boiled)	½ cup	50
Sweet potato (baked)	1 med	62
Fruits		
Figs (dried)	10 figs	128
Kiwi fruit (raw)	1 med	31
Orange juice (fresh)	8 fl oz	42
Orange, navel (raw)	1 med	27
Raisins, seedless	⅔ cup	97
Meat, poultry, fish, dry beans, eggs, nuts		
Almonds (roasted)	1 oz (22 nuts)	156
Bacon (fried)	3 med	64
Beef liver (fried)	3.5 oz	461
Beef top round, lean (broiled)	3.5 oz	246
Black-eyed peas (boiled)	1 cup	266
Chicken, dark (roasted, without skin)	3.5 oz	179
Chicken light (roasted, without skin)	3.5 oz	216
Chick-peas (boiled)	1 cup	275
Clams, canned	3 oz	287
Cod (baked)	3 oz	117
Crab, Alaska king (steamed)	3 oz	238
Egg, whole	1 large	90

TABLE 7-3   Food sources of phosphorus—cont'd

	Quantity	Phosphorus (mg)
Meat, poultry, fish, dry beans, eggs, nuts—cont'd		
Ground beef, regular (broiled)	3.5 oz	170
Halibut (baked)	3 oz	242
Ham, canned (lean)	3.5 oz	224
Lentils (boiled)	1 cup	356
Lobster (steamed)	3 oz	157
Oysters (steamed)	3 oz (12 med)	236
Peanut butter, creamy	1 tbsp	60
Peanuts (roasted)	1 oz	100
Pinto beans (boiled)	1 cup	273
Sirloin steak, lean (broiled)	3.5 oz	244
Sole (baked)	3.5 oz	344
Soybeans (boiled)	1 cup	421
Trout, rainbow (baked)	3 oz	272
Tuna, light, canned in water	3 oz	158
Walnuts, dried	1 oz	132
Milk, dairy products		
Cheddar cheese	1 cup	145
Cottage cheese, creamed	1 cup	277
Milk, skim	8 fl oz	247
Milk, whole	8 fl oz	227
Swiss cheese	1 oz	171
Yogurt, whole	8 fl oz	215
Fats, oils, sugar		
This food group is not an important source of phosphorus.		

For example, cured ham has about 20 times more sodium as raw pork. Natural food sources include animal products like milk, meat, and eggs, and vegetables like carrots, beets, leafy greens, and celery. (See Appendix D for sodium and potassium content of foods and Appendix E for salt-free seasoning guides.)

Deficiency States

Because the body's need for sodium is low, a deficiency state rarely occurs. Exceptions occur during heavy body sweating, as may be the case with those engaged in heavy labor or athletes doing strenuous physical exercise in a hot environment. Such persons may need additional salt to replace these heavy sodium losses. Commercial sports drinks, which replace sodium, glucose, and fluid, may be useful for athletes in endurance events. Most persons will not require these beverages for nonendurance activities.

Potassium

Functions

The adult body contains about 270 mg (9 oz) of potassium, nearly twice the amount of sodium.

Potassium is not only a partner with sodium in the body's water balance, it also has many metabolic functions, as follow:

Water balance.   Potassium is the major electrolyte controlling the water *inside* cells. It balances with the sodium concentration in the water outside cells.

Metabolic reactions.   Potassium plays a role in the conversion of blood glucose to stored glycogen, the storage of nitrogen in muscle protein, and the production of energy.

Muscle action.   Potassium ions also contribute to nerve-impulse transmission to stimulate muscle action. Along with magnesium and sodium, potassium acts as a muscle relaxant in balance with calcium, which causes muscle contraction. The heart muscle is very sensitive to potassium levels; therefore proper concentration of potassium in the blood is particularly important.

Insulin release.   Potassium is involved when a rise in blood-glucose level triggers a release of insulin from the pancreas.

Blood pressure.   Sodium is one of the main dietary factors linked to elevated blood pressure; however, elevated blood pressure may be more related to the sodium/potassium ratio than to the actual amount of dietary sodium. A potassium intake equal to that of sodium may be the preventative factor.

Requirements

As with sodium, the present DRI guidelines do not establish an RDA for potassium, although potassium is a dietary essential. A future DRI reference volume will include the electrolytes such as sodium, potassium, and chloride. The minimum potassium need appears to be approximately 2000 mg/day. The National Research Council recommends an increase in potassium intake through increased consumption of fruits and vegetables. This would raise the adult potassium intake to about 3500 mg/day, which is ample for average needs.[3] A healthy varied diet contains 2000 to 4000 mg/day of potassium. Table 7-4 lists food sources of potassium.

Food Sources

Because potassium is an essential part of all living cells, it is abundant in natural foods. The richest dietary sources of potassium are unprocessed foods, fruits such as oranges and bananas, vegetables such as broccoli and leafy green vegetables, fresh meats, whole grains, and milk products. Those who eat large amounts of fruits and vegetables have a high potassium intake. The plant form of potassium is very soluble; therefore much of the potassium content may be lost when cooked with excessive water (unless the water is retained). Box 7-1 lists the comparative potassium content of some selected foods.

Deficiency States

Symptoms of potassium deficiency are well-defined but are seldom related to inadequate dietary intake. Potassium deficiency is more likely to develop during such clinical situations as prolonged vomiting or diarrhea, use of diuretic drugs, severe malnutrition, and surgery. Deficiency is also a concern during the use of hypertension drugs, because the diuretic causes a reduction in potassium. Those who couple diuretics with the excessive use of drugs that replace potassium may also experience a potassium imbalance. Characteristic symptoms of imbalance include heart muscle problems with possible cardiac arrest, weakness of respiratory muscles with breathing difficulties, poor intestinal muscle tone with resulting bloating, and overall muscle weakness. This is especially true in cases of elderly persons who have impaired kidney function and thus difficulty excreting potassium.

Magnesium

Functions

Magnesium has widespread metabolic functions and is present in all body cells. An adult body contains about 25 g of magnesium (a little less than an ounce). About 60% of this magnesium is present in the bones.

TABLE 7-4   Food sources of potassium

	Quantity	Potassium (mg)
Bread, cereal, rice, pasta		
Bran flakes	¾ cup	184
Bran muffin, homemade	1 muffin	99
Bread, whole wheat	1 slice	44
Oatmeal (cooked)	¾ cup	99
Pasta, enriched (cooked)	1 cup	85
Rice, white, enriched	1 cup	57
Wheat flakes	1 cup	110
Wheat germ, toasted	¼ cup (1 oz)	268
Vegetables		
Artichoke (boiled)	1 med	316
Asparagus (boiled)	½ cup (6 spears)	279
Avocado (raw)	1 med	1,097
Broccoli (raw)	½ cup, chopped	143
Brussels sprouts (boiled)	½ cup (4 sprouts)	247
Carrots (raw)	1 med	233
Corn, yellow (boiled)	½ cup	204
Mushrooms (boiled)	½ cup, pieces	277
Potato (baked, with skin)	1 med	844
Spinach (boiled)	½ cup	419
Sweet potato (baked)	1 med	397
Tomato (raw)	1 med	254
Fruits		
Apple (raw, with skin)	1 med	159
Banana	1 med	451
Cantaloupe	1 cup, pieces	494
Dates (dried)	10 dates	541
Figs (dried)	10 figs	1,332
Orange juice (fresh)	8 fl oz	486
Orange, navel	1 med	250
Prunes (dried)	10 prunes	626
Prune juice (canned)	8 fl oz	706
Raisins, seedless	⅔ cup	751
Meat, poultry, fish, dry beans, eggs, nuts		
Almonds (dry roasted)	1 oz (22 nuts)	219
Beef liver (fried)	3.5 oz	364
Beef top round, lean (broiled)	3.5 oz	442
Black-eyed peas (boiled)	1 cup	476

Continued

TABLE 7-4 Food sources of potassium—cont'd

	Quantity	Potassium (mg)
Meat, poultry, fish, dry beans, eggs, nuts—cont'd		
Chicken, dark (roasted, without skin)	3.5 oz	240
Chicken light (roasted, without skin)	3.5 oz	247
Clams (steamed)	3 oz (9 small)	534
Crab, blue (steamed)	3 oz	275
Egg, whole	1 large	65
Ground beef, regular (broiled)	3.5 oz	292
Halibut (baked)	3 oz	490
Ham, canned (lean)	3.5 oz	364
Lentils (boiled)	1 cup	731
Lima beans (boiled)	1 cup	955
Lobster (steamed)	3 oz	299
Mackerel (baked)	3 oz	341
Oysters (steamed)	3 oz (12 med)	389
Peanut butter, creamy	1 tbsp	110
Peanuts (dry roasted)	1 oz	184
Pinto beans (boiled)	1 cup	800
Salmon (baked)	3 oz	319
Sirloin steak, lean (broiled)	3.5 oz	403
Soybeans (boiled)	1 cup	886
Trout, rainbow (baked)	3 oz	539
Tuna, light, canned in water (with salt)	3 oz	267
Milk, dairy products		
Cottage cheese, creamed	1 cup	177
Milk, skim	8 fl oz	406
Milk, whole	8 fl oz	368
Yogurt, whole	8 fl oz	351
Fats, oils		
This food group is not an important source of potassium.		
Sugar		
Molasses, black	1 tbsp	585
Sugar, brown	1 cup	499

BOX 7-1 Potassium content per average serving of some selected foods

Group A (600 mg)	Group B (400 mg)	Group C (300 mg)	Group D (200 mg)
Dried apricots	Bananas	Avocados	Fruit cocktail
Dried peaches	Grapefruit	Cantaloupe	Grapes
Lima beans	Orange juice	Cherries	Peaches
Parsnips	Artichokes	Green beans	Pineapple
Spinach, fresh	Broccoli	Fresh tomatoes	Plums
Tomato juice	Brussels sprouts	Milk	Prunes, dried
Sweet potatoes	Carrots		Strawberries
	Cauliflower		Asparagus
	Corn		Cabbage
	Winter squash		Green peas
	Turnip greens		
	White potatoes		
	Liver		
	Pork		
	Beef		
	Chicken		
	Fish		
	Peanut butter		
	Cashew nuts		

General metabolism. Magnesium is a required catalyst for over 300 reactions in cells that produce energy, synthesize body compounds, or absorb and transport nutrients.

Protein synthesis. Magnesium activates amino acids for protein synthesis and facilitates the synthesis and maintenance of the cell genetic material, DNA. When cells replicate, they must produce new protein. This replication process requires a precise amount of magnesium to function correctly.

Muscle action. Magnesium ions help conduct the nerve impulses that stimulate muscle contraction. Magnesium, in balance with calcium, acts as a relaxant during muscle activity, which stimulates contraction.

Basal metabolic rate. Magnesium influences the secretion of the thyroid hormone thyroxine, thus helping the body maintain a normal metabolic rate and adapt to cold temperatures.

Requirements

The new DRI guidelines establish RDA amounts by age group and gender. For the age group of 14 to 18 years, the RDA is 410 mg/day for men and 360 mg/day for women. For those aged 19 to 30 years, the RDA is 400 mg/day for men and 310 mg/day for women. For persons 31 years of age and older, the RDA is 420 mg/day for men and 320 mg/day for women. The RDA is the same for both boys and girls during childhood and early adolescence: 80 mg/day for ages 1 to 3 years; 130 mg/day for ages 4 to 8 years; 240 mg/day for ages 9 to 13 years. For infants, the AI level is 30 mg/day during the first 6 months and 75 mg/day from 7 to 12 months. The RDA is somewhat higher during pregnancy: 400 mg/day for women aged 18 and younger; 350 to 360 mg/day for women 19 and older. There is not an increased magnesium recommendation during lactation. Magnesium consumed as a natural component of food has not been observed to have any adverse effects at high intake levels. Therefore the DRI standards establish the UL only for magnesium intake from supplements and pharmaceutic preparations. The UL from such sources is 350 mg/day for persons aged 9 and older, with lesser amounts for children.[1]

Food Sources

Although magnesium is relatively common in foods, the content level is variable. Unprocessed foods have the highest concentrations of magnesium. Major food sources include nuts, soybeans, cocoa, seafood, whole grains, dried beans and peas, and green vegetables. Relatively poor sources include most fruits other than bananas, milk, meat, and fish. More than 80% of the magnesium content in cereal grains is lost with the removal of the germ and outer layers. Significant amounts of magnesium may also be present in drinking water in regions that have hard water with a fairly high mineral content.

Deficiency States

A magnesium deficiency that is purely dietary is very rare in persons consuming natural diets. Symptoms of magnesium deficiency have been observed in clinical situations such as starvation, persistent vomiting or diarrhea with loss of magnesium-rich gastrointestinal fluids, and surgical trauma. Magnesium depletion is also found in various diseases involving cardiovascular and neuromuscular function, in diabetes mellitus, in kidney disease, and in alcoholism. Deficiency symptoms include muscle weakness and cramps, hypertension, and blood vessel constriction in the heart and brain.

Chloride

Functions

Chloride is the chemical form of chlorine as it appears in the human body. Chloride accounts for about 3% of the body's total mineral content and is widely distributed throughout body tissues. Predominantly, chloride is found in the fluid outside cells where it helps control the water and acid-base balances. Its two significant functions involve digestion and respiration.

Digestion. Chloride is a key element in the hydrochloric acid secreted in gastric juices. The action of gastric enzymes requires the proper acidity level of the stomach fluids. This acid secretion also helps maintain the acid-base balance in body fluids.

Respiration. Chloride ions help red blood cells transport large amounts of carbon dioxide to the lungs for release in breathing. The chloride ions move easily in and out of red blood cells in balance with the carbon dioxide to counteract any potential changes in the acid-base balance. This movement of chloride in and out of red blood cells is called the *chloride shift*.

Requirements

As noted for sodium and potassium, new DRI standards for chloride do not presently exist. The classic RDA standards estimated the minimum requirements of the major electrolytes in body fluid balance: sodium, chloride, and potassium. This standard sets a minimum intake of chloride for healthy persons over age 10 as 750 mg/day, and recommends lesser amounts for infants and children. The intake level of chloride from food and the normal loss of chloride levels from the body parallel sodium.[3]

Food Sources

Dietary chloride is provided almost entirely by sodium chloride, which is the chemical name for ordinary table salt. The kidneys are very efficient in reabsorbing chloride when the dietary intake is low.

Deficiency States

Dietary deficiency of chloride does not occur under normal circumstances. Chloride loss parallels sodium loss in clinical cases of diarrhea, vomiting, or heavy sweating.

Sulfur

Functions

An essential part of protein structure, sulfur is present in all body cells and participates in widespread metabolic and structural functions.

Hair, skin, and nails. Sulfur is involved in the structure of hair, skin, and nails through its presence in two amino acids—methionine and cystine—that are concentrated in the tissue protein keratin.

General metabolic functions. Combined with hydrogen, sulfur is important as a high-energy bond in building many tissue compounds. Sulfur helps transfer energy as needed in various tissues.

Vitamin structure. Sulfur is a part of several vitamins (e.g., thiamin, pantothenic acid, and biotin) that in turn act as coenzymes in cell metabolism.

Collagen structure. Sulfur is necessary for collagen synthesis and thus is important in building connective tissue.

Requirements

Dietary requirements for sulfur are not stated as such because sulfur is supplied by protein foods containing the amino acids methionine and cystine.

Food Sources

A diet with adequate protein contains adequate sulfur. Sulfur is primarily available to the body as part of the organic sulfur compounds in its two amino acid carriers, methionine and cystine. Thus animal protein foods are the main dietary sources of sulfur. Sulfur is widely available in meat, eggs, milk, cheese, legumes, and nuts.

Deficiency States

Deficiency states have not been reported. Such conditions would only relate to general protein malnutrition and the absence of the sulfur-carrying amino acids methionine and cystine. Table 7-5 provides a summary of the major minerals.

TRACE ELEMENTS

Iron

Functions

Iron has the longest and best described history of all the micronutrients. Iron is essential for life but toxic in excess. Thus the body has developed exquisite systems for balancing iron intake and excretion and for efficiently transporting iron in and out of cells to maintain health.[7-9] Iron functions both in the synthesis of hemoglobin and in the body's general metabolism. The human body contains only about 45 mg iron/kg body weight.

Hemoglobin synthesis. Most of the body's iron, about 70%, occurs in red blood cells. Iron is an essential component of heme, the nonprotein part of the hemoglobin structure. Hemoglobin in red blood cells carries oxygen to the cells for cell oxidation and metabolism. Iron is also a necessary part of myoglobin, which is a similar compound in muscle tissue.

General metabolism. Iron is required for proper glucose metabolism in the cell, antibody production, drug detoxification in the liver, collagen and purine synthesis and carotene conversion to vitamin A. To accomplish these vital functions, precise mechanisms regulate the amount of iron in the body according to the body's need.

Requirements

Presently, the DRI project has not published the new DRI guidelines for iron or the remaining trace elements. The requirements for iron, however, have been studied for a long time. Adult require-

TABLE 7-5 A summary of major minerals

Mineral	Metabolism	Physiologic functions	Clinical application	Requirements	Food sources
Calcium (Ca)	Absorption according to body need, aided by vitamin D; hindered by binding agents (oxalates), or excessive fiber. Parathyroid hormone controls absorption and mobilization	Bone formation Teeth Blood clotting Muscle contraction and relaxation Heart action Nerve transmission	Tetany—decrease in ionized serum calcium Rickets Osteoporosis	Adults: 1000-1200 mg* Pregnancy and lactation: 1000-1300 mg* Infants: 2100-2700 mg* Children: 500-1300 mg*	Milk Cheese Whole grains Egg yolk Legumes, nuts Green leafy vegetables
Phosphorus (P)	Absorption with calcium aided by vitamin D; hindered by excess binding agents (aluminum)	Bone and tooth formation Overall metabolism Energy metabolism (enzymes) Acid-base balance	Bone loss Poor growth	Adults: 700 mg Pregnancy and lactation: 700-1250 mg Infants: 100-275 mg* Children: 460-1250 mg	Milk Cheese Meat Egg yolk Whole grains Legumes, nuts
Sodium (Na)	Readily absorbed	Major extracellular fluid control Water balance Acid-base balance Muscle action; transmission of nerve impulse and resulting contraction	Fluid shifts and control Buffer system Losses in gastrointestinal disorders Dehydration	Limit to 2.4 g or less	Table salt (NaCl) Milk Meat Egg Baking soda Baking powder Carrots, beets, spinach, celery

*Adequate intake (AI) levels.

Mineral	Metabolism	Physiologic Functions	Clinical Applications	Requirement	Food Sources
Potassium (K)	Secreted and reabsorbed in digestive juices	Major intracellular fluid control Acid-base balance Regulates nerve impulse and muscle contraction Glycogen formation Protein synthesis Energy metabolism	Fluid shifts Heart action—low serum potassium (cardiac arrest) Insulin release Blood pressure factor	About 2000-3500 mg Diet adequate in protein, calcium, and iron contains adequate potassium	Fruits Vegetables Meats Whole grains Legumes
Magnesium (Mg)	Absorption increased by parathyroid hormone	Aids thyroid hormone secretion, normal BMR Activator and coenzyme in carbohydrate and protein metabolism Muscle, nerve action	Tremor, spasm; low serum level following gastrointestinal losses or renal losses from alcoholism, convulsions	Adults: 310-420 mg Pregnancy and lactation: 350-400 mg Deficiency in humans unlikely	Whole grains Nuts Legumes Green vegetables (chlorophyll)
Chlorine (Cl)	Absorbed readily	Acid-base balance—chloride shift Gastric hydrochloric acid—digestion	Hypochloremic alkalosis in prolonged vomiting, diarrhea, tube drainage	About 750 mg	Table salt
Sulfur (S)	Absorbed as such and as constituent of sulfur-containing amino acids methionine and cystine	Essential constituent of cell protein Hair, skin, nails Vitamin structure Collagen structure High-energy sulfur bonds in energy metabolism	General protein malnutrition	Diet adequate in protein contains adequate sulfur	Meat Egg Cheese Milk Nuts, legumes

TABLE 7-6   Characteristics of heme and nonheme portions of dietary iron

Heme (smallest portion)	Nonheme (largest portion)
Food sources	
None in plant sources; 40 % of iron in animal sources	All iron in plant sources; 60 % of iron in animal sources
Absorption rate	
Rapid; transported and absorbed intact	Slow; tightly bound in organic molecules

ments for iron differ between men and women. The classic RDAs establish standards of 10 mg/day for men 19 years of age and older and 15 mg/day for women 11 to 50 years of age. The RDA is 6 mg/day for infants during the first 6 months; 10 mg/day for all children aged 6 months to 10 years; 12 mg/day for boys 11 to 18 years of age; 10 mg/day for women aged 50 and older.[3] Women require more iron to cover the loss during menstruation and the demand during pregnancy. During pregnancy, a woman's RDA for iron doubles to 30 mg/day. This increase usually requires an iron supplement because neither the usual American diet nor the iron stores of many women can meet the increased iron demands.

Food Sources

The typical Western diet provides an average of 6 mg of iron per 1000 kcalories of energy intake. Iron is widely distributed in the U.S. food supply mainly in meat, eggs, vegetables and cereals. Iron is especially present in liver and fortified cereal products. Although fruits, vegetables, and juices contain varying amounts of iron, as a group, they are another major source of dietary iron. The body absorbs iron more easily in conjunction with vitamin C. Iron occurs in food in two forms, *heme* and *nonheme*, a factor that affects its absorption and hence its availability to the body. Heme iron is the most easily absorbed form of dietary iron, but it contributes the smallest amount of the total dietary iron, because it comes from none of the plant food sources and only 40% of the animal food sources (Table 7-6). Nonheme iron is less easily absorbed because it occurs in a more tightly bound form in foods, yet the majority of our food sources—60% of the animal food sources and all of the plant food sources—contain this form. To help enhance the absorption and availability of this larger amount of dietary nonheme iron, food sources of vitamin C, moderate amounts of lean meats, and enriched cereal products must be included in the diet. Table 7-7 lists food sources of iron.

Deficiency States

The major condition indicating a deficiency of iron is anemia, which is characterized by a decrease in the number of red blood cells, a drop in the amount of cell hemoglobin, or both. Iron deficiency anemia is the most prevalent nutritional problem in the world today. More than 2 billion people worldwide are iron deficient; women and children are affected more than others. This lack of iron and the inability to use it may result from several causes, as follow: (1) inadequate supply of dietary iron; (2) excessive blood loss; (3) inability to form hemoglobin in the absence of other necessary factors such as vitamin

---

anemia (Gr. *an-*, negative prefix; *haima*, blood) blood condition characterized by a decreased number of circulating red blood cells or hemoglobin or both.

TABLE 7-7 Food sources of iron

	Quantity	Iron (mg)
Bread, cereal, rice, pasta		
Bran flakes	¾ cup	4.50
Bran muffin, homemade	1 muffin	1.26
Bread, whole wheat	1 slice	0.86
Cream of wheat, regular (cooked)	¾ cup	7.70
Oatmeal (cooked)	¾ cup	1.19
Pasta, enriched (cooked)	1 cup	2.40
Rice, white, enriched (cooked)	1 cup	1.80
Wheat flakes	1 cup	4.45
Vegetables		
Artichoke (boiled)	1 med	1.62
Avocado (raw)	1 med	2.04
Broccoli (boiled)	½ cup	0.89
Brussels sprouts (boiled)	½ cup	0.94
Peas, green (boiled)	½ cup	1.24
Potato (baked, with skin)	1 med	2.75
Spinach (boiled)	½ cup	3.21
Fruits		
Dates (dried)	10 dates	0.96
Figs (dried)	10 figs	4.18
Prune juice (canned)	8 fl oz	3.03
Prunes (dried)	10 prunes	2.08
Raisins, seedless	⅔ cup	2.08
Meat, poultry, fish, dry beans, eggs, nuts		
Almonds (roasted)	1 oz (22 nuts)	1.08
Beef liver (fried)	3.5 oz	6.28
Beef top round, lean (broiled)	3.5 oz	2.88
Black-eyed peas (boiled)	1 cup	4.29
Cashews (roasted)	1 oz	1.70
Chicken, dark (roasted, without skin)	3.5 oz	1.33
Chicken light (roasted, without skin)	3.5 oz	1.06
Chick-peas (boiled)	1 cup	4.74
Clams (steamed)	3 oz (9 small)	23.76
Crab, blue (steamed)	3 oz	0.77
Egg, whole	1 large	1.04
Ground beef, regular (broiled)	3.5 oz	2.44
Halibut (baked)	3 oz	0.91
Ham, canned (lean)	3.5 oz	0.94

Continued

TABLE 7-7 Food sources of iron—cont'd

	Quantity	Iron (mg)
Meat, poultry, fish, dry beans, eggs, nuts—cont'd		
Lentils (boiled)	1 cup	6.59
Lima beans (boiled)	1 cup	4.50
Mackerel (baked)	3 oz	1.33
Oysters (steamed)	3 oz (12 med)	11.39
Pinto beans (boiled)	1 cup	4.47
Shrimp (steamed)	3 oz (15 large)	2.62
Sirloin steak, lean (broiled)	3.5 oz	3.36
Sole (baked)	3.5 oz	1.40
Soybeans (boiled)	1 cup	8.84
Trout, rainbow (baked)	3 oz	2.07
Tuna, light, canned in water	3 oz	2.72
Milk, dairy products		
Cheddar cheese	1 oz	0.19
Cottage cheese, creamed	1 cup	0.29
Milk, skim	8 fl oz	0.10
Milk, whole	8 fl oz	0.12
Yogurt, whole	8 fl oz	0.11
Fats, oils		
This food group is not an important source of iron.		
Sugar		
Molasses, black	1 tbsp	3.20
Sugar, brown	1 cup	4.90

B_{12} (e.g., pernicious anemia); (4) lack of gastric hydrochloric acid necessary to help liberate iron for absorption; (5) presence of various inhibitors of iron absorption (e.g., phosphate or phytate); or (6) mucosal lesions affecting the absorbent surface area.

Iodine

Functions

Iodine, like iron, has a long history of study. The average adult body contains only 20 to 50 mg of iodine. In human nutrition, iodine's basic function is to participate in the thyroid gland's synthesis of the hormone thyroxine. The pituitary gland releases the thyroid stimulating hormone (TSH), which controls the thyroid gland's uptake of iodine, in direct response to the level of thyroxine circulating in the blood. When the blood level of thyroxine decreases below normal, the pituitary gland releases more TSH, thus stimulating the thyroid gland to take up more iodine to make more thyroxine. The transport form of iodine in the blood is called serum *protein-bound iodine* (PBI). After thyroxine (i.e., in its two forms having hormonal activity—T3 and T4) is used to stimulate metabolic processes in cells, it is broken down in the liver and the iodine portion is excreted in bile as inorganic iodine. Therefore the basic overall function of iodine relates to the control of the body's BMR by its role in synthesizing the controlling hormone thyroxine.

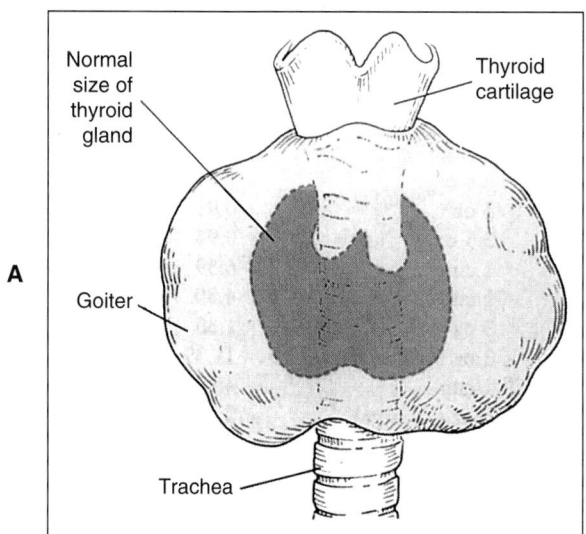
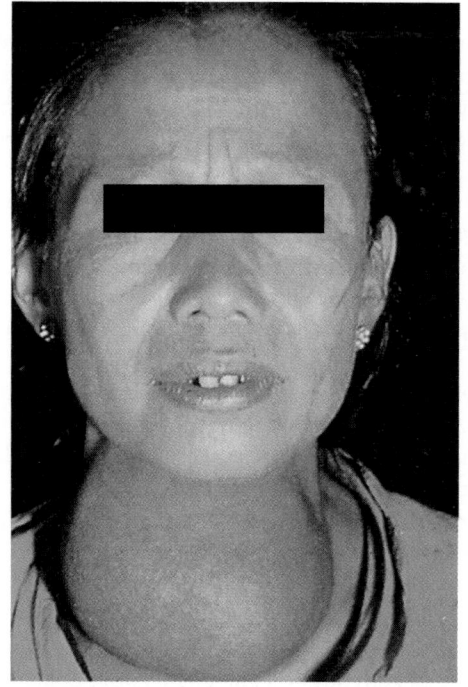

A

B

FIGURE 7-2 Goiter; the extreme enlargement shown here is a result of extended duration of iodine deficiency. (Photo credit: Lester V. Bergman/The Bergman Collection, Project Masters, Inc, Princeton, NJ.)

Requirements

At this time the new DRI reference volume for trace elements such as iodine is unpublished. The body's need for iodine has undergone extensive study. To maintain desirable tissue levels of iodine, the adult body's minimum requirement is 50 to 75 µg/day; therefore to provide an extra margin of safety, the classic RDAs recommend an intake of 150 µg/day for all persons aged 11 and older. Lesser amounts are indicated for infants and children. During pregnancy, the need increases to 175 µg/day and during lactation it increases to 200 µg/day.[3]

Food Sources

The amount of iodine in natural food sources varies considerably depending on the iodine content of the soil. Seafood provides a good amount of iodine. The major reliable source, however, is iodized table salt, with each gram containing 76 µg

of iodine. The presence of salt in processed foods supplies iodine even for those persons who do not use table salt.

Deficiency States

A lack of iodine in the diet contributes to several deficiency diseases, as follow:

Goiter. A lack of iodine in the diet causes the classic condition of goiter, which often occurs in areas where the water and soil contain little iodine (Figure 7-2). Some 800 million people live in these iodine deficient areas of underdeveloped countries

---

goiter (L. *gutter,* throat) an enlarged thyroid gland caused by lack of enough available iodine to produce the thyroid hormone thyroxine.

where goiter is a large health problem. Goiter is characterized by an enlargement of the thyroid gland, sometimes to tremendous size. When the thyroid gland is starved for iodine, it cannot produce a normal amount of thyroxine. With this low level of thyroxine in the blood, the pituitary gland continues to put out more and more TSH. These large amounts of TSH continually stimulate the nonproductive thyroid gland, causing it to increase greatly in size. Such an iodine-starved thyroid gland may weigh 0.45 to 0.67 kg (1 to 1.5 lbs) or more.

Cretinism. The condition of cretinism is characterized by physical deformity, dwarfism, and mental retardation. This serious condition occurs in children born to mothers who had limited iodine intake during adolescence and pregnancy. During pregnancy, the mother's iodine need takes precedence over that of the developing child. Thus the fetus suffers from iodine deficiency, and the lack continues following birth. These children are retarded in both physical and mental development. If the condition is discovered at birth and treatment is started immediately, however, many of the symptoms are reversible. If the condition continues beyond early childhood, the physical and mental retardation becomes permanent.

Hypothyroidism. An adult form of hypothyroidism called *myxedema* occurs when a poorly functioning thyroid gland cannot make enough thyroxine and the BMR is greatly reduced. The symptoms of this condition are thin, coarse hair, dry skin, poor cold tolerance, weight gain, and a low, husky voice.

Hyperthyroidism. An opposite condition, hyperthyroidism, in which the accelerated thyroid produces excessive thyroxine and the BMR is greatly increased, may also occur in adults. Hyperthyroidism is known as Graves' disease, or *exophthalmic goiter,* from the general symptom of protruding eyeballs. Other symptoms include weight loss, hand tremors and general nervousness, increased appetite, and intolerance of heat.

Iodine Overload

Occasionally, dairy farming methods may cause an excessive intake of iodine. These dairy farm methods include the use of iodized salt licks for the animals and the application of disinfectants that contain iodine on cow udders, milking machines, and milk storage tanks. Other compounds containing iodine are used as additives to animal feed. Compounds containing iodine also act as dough oxidizers in the continuous bread-making process, adding about 500 μg/100 g of bread. Increased incidental intake of iodine may cause an overload for some persons. Excess iodine may result in acnelike skin lesions or may worsen the preexisting acne of adolescents or young adults. Excessive amounts may also cause "iodine goiter," which could be misdiagnosed as goiter caused by insufficient iodine. Continued use of iodized salt, however, is still a wise practice for several reasons, as follow: (1) moderately excessive iodine is relatively harmless; (2) persons living in certain regions may be at greater risk of goiter; and (3) individual iodine intake is highly variable and may be insufficient (e.g., depending on geographic location and food supply). Also, persons with disorders affecting the thyroid gland may have adverse effects from excessive iodine.

Zinc

Functions

Zinc is an essential trace element with wide clinical significance. Zinc is especially important during growth periods such as pregnancy, lactation, infancy, childhood, and adolescence. The amount of zinc in the adult body is about 1.5 g in women and 2.5 g in men. Zinc is present in minute quantities in all body organs, tissues, fluids, and secretions. In these tissues, zinc participates in three different types of metabolic functions, as follow:

Enzyme constituent. Zinc's wide tissue distribution reflects its broad metabolic activity as an essential part of cell enzyme systems. Over 70 such zinc enzymes have been identified. In its role in protein metabolism, zinc is associated with wound healing and healthy skin. It has great influence on any rapidly growing tissues, so its effect on reproduction is highly significant.

Insulin storage. Zinc combines readily with insulin in the pancreas, serving as a storage form of the hormone. The pancreas of a person with diabetes contains only about half of the normal amount of zinc.

Immune system. A considerable amount of zinc bound to protein is present in the leukocytes (i.e., white blood cells), which are a major component of the body's immune system. Zinc affects the immune system through its essential role in the synthesis of nucleic acids (i.e., DNA and RNA) and protein. Zinc is also needed for lymphocyte transformation. Lymphoid tissue, which gives rise to lymphocytes (i.e., the major white cell populations involved in the body's immune system), contains a large amount of zinc. The leukocytes of patients with leukemia, for example, contain about 10% less zinc than normal.

Requirements
The forthcoming reference volume on trace elements will include the requirements for zinc within the new DRI standards. The classic RDA standard for zinc is 15 mg/day for men aged 11 and older and 12 mg/day for women aged 11 and older. The RDA for infants is 5 mg/day during the first year and 10 mg/day for children 1 to 10 years of age. Pregnant women require 15 mg/day to meet fetal growth needs and 19 mg/day for lactation. The zinc content of the typical mixed diet of adults in the United States has been reported to furnish from 10 to 15 mg/day.

Food Sources
The greatest source of dietary zinc in the United States is meat, which supplies about 70% of the zinc consumed. Seafood, particularly oysters, is another excellent source of zinc. Eggs are also a good source. Legumes and whole grains are additional sources, but they are less available to the body. A balanced diet usually meets adult needs for zinc, but considerable evidence shows that diets high in processed foods may be low in zinc. Animal food sources supply a major portion of dietary zinc. Pure vegetarians, especially women, may be at risk for developing marginal zinc deficiency. Table 7-8 gives food sources of zinc.

Deficiency States
Zinc is imperative during periods of rapid tissue growth such as childhood and adolescence. Retarded physical growth (i.e., dwarfism) and retarded sexual maturation, especially in males, have been observed in some populations where dietary intake of zinc is low. Impaired taste and smell (i.e., hypogeusia and hyposmia) are improved with increased zinc intake. Zinc deficiency commonly causes poor wound healing in hospital patients. Surgical patients and older patients may need supplements. Patients with poor appetites—subsisting on marginal diets in the face of chronic wounds and illnesses and tissue breakdown—may be particularly vulnerable to developing a zinc deficiency (see the Clinical Applications box, "Zinc Barriers").

Selenium

Functions
Selenium is present in all body tissues except fat. The highest concentrations of selenium appear in the liver, kidney, heart, and spleen. Selenium functions with specific proteins as an essential part of an antioxidant enzyme that protects cells and their lipid membranes from oxidative damage. In this role, selenium balances vitamin E; each element spares the other. Selenium functions as a part of the protein center of teeth and participates in the regulation of thyroid hormone action and the regulation of vitamin C activity. Recently, the focus on selenium has been on its role as an antioxidant and as an element that may function to protect cells against cancer. In some animal model studies, high selenium intakes reduced the frequency of cancer. Several recent human studies suggest that selenium may have a protective role regarding certain cancers. The DRI panel on antioxidants reviewed the current scientific research on selenium. The panel concluded that although selenium intakes higher

TABLE 7-8   Food sources of zinc

	Quantity	Zinc (mg)
Bread, cereal, rice, pasta		
Bran muffin, homemade	1 muffin	1.08
Bread, whole wheat	1 slice	0.42
Cream of wheat (cooked)	¾ cup	0.24
English muffin, plain	1 muffin	0.41
Oatmeal (cooked)	¾ cup	0.86
Pasta, enriched (cooked)	1 cup	0.70
Wheat flakes	1 cup	0.63
Vegetables		
Artichoke (boiled)	1 med	0.43
Asparagus (boiled)	½ cup (6 spears)	0.43
Avocado (raw)	1 med	0.73
Broccoli (raw)	½ cup	0.18
Brussels sprouts (boiled)	½ cup (4 sprouts)	0.25
Carrots (raw)	1 med	0.14
Collards (boiled)	½ cup	0.23
Kale (boiled, chopped)	½ cup	0.15
Peas, green (boiled)	½ cup	0.95
Potato (baked, with skin)	1 med	0.65
Tomato (raw)	1 med	0.13
Fruits		
Apricots (raw)	3 med	0.28
Banana (raw)	1 med	0.19
Cantaloupe (raw)	½ cup	0.25
Figs (dried)	10 figs	0.94
Orange juice (fresh)	8 fl oz	0.13
Orange, naval (raw)	1 med	0.08
Meat, poultry, fish, dry beans, eggs, nuts		
Almonds (roasted)	1 oz (22 nuts)	1.39
Beef liver (fried)	3.5 oz	6.07
Cashews (roasted)	1 oz	1.59
Chicken, dark (roasted, without skin)	3.5 oz	2.80
Chicken light (roasted, without skin)	3.5 oz	1.23
Chick-peas (boiled)	1 cup	2.51
Clams, canned	3 oz	2.32
Crab, Alaska king (steamed)	3 oz	6.48
Egg, whole	1 large	0.72
Ham, canned (lean)	3.5 oz	1.93

TABLE 7-8 Food sources of zinc—cont'd

	Quantity	Zinc (mg)
Meat, poultry, fish, dry beans, eggs, nuts—cont'd		
Kidney beans (boiled)	1 cup	1.89
Lentils (boiled)	1 cup	2.50
Lima beans (boiled)	1 cup	1.79
Lobster (steamed)	3 oz	2.48
Oysters (steamed)	3 oz (12 med)	154.62
Peanuts (roasted)	1 oz	0.93
Soybeans (boiled)	1 cup	1.98
Milk, dairy products		
Milk, skim	8 fl oz	0.98
Milk, whole	8 fl oz	0.93
Yogurt, whole	8 fl oz	1.34
Fats, oils, sugar		
This food group is not an important source of zinc.		

than the RDA level may have an anticancer effect in humans, more large-scale research is necessary to establish such an effect.[2]

Requirements

The new DRI reference volume on antioxidants includes the revised RDAs for selenium. The recommendations are by age group, without a gender difference. For both men and women aged 14 and older, the RDA amount is 55 µg/day. The RDA is progressively reduced for children: 40 µg/day for 9 to 13 years of age; 30 µg/day for 4 to 8 years of age; and 20 µg/day for 1 to 3 years of age. The DRI does not establish a RDA for infants. Based on mean intakes of human milk, an infant's observed AI level is 15 µg/day for the first 6 months and 20 µg/day for 7 to 12 months. The recommended intake during pregnancy is 60 µg/day and 70 µg/day during lactation.[2] Recent studies have found that the selenium compounds in breast milk are more biologically available to infants than the selenium in formulas.[10] The DRIs establish the UL for selenium at 400 mg/day for persons aged 14 and older.

Food Sources

Most selenium in food is highly available to the body. The amount of selenium in food is dependent upon the quantity of selenium in the soil used to graze animals and grow plants. Unlike plants, animals require selenium. Seafood, kidney and liver are consistently good sources of selenium. To a lesser extent, other meats also provide selenium. Grains and other seeds are more variable, depending on the selenium content of the soil in which they are grown. Fruits and vegetables generally contain little selenium. In the United States and Canada, the dietary intake of selenium varies by geographic region, but these local differences are reduced by the national food distribution system.

Deficiency States

Selenium deficiency results in two significant conditions. The first is Keshan disease, named after the area in China where it was discovered. This heart muscle disease affects young children and women of child bearing age and can lead to heart failure resulting from cardiomyopathy (i.e., degeneration of

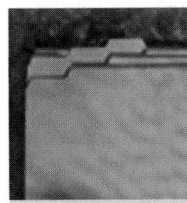

CLINICAL APPLICATIONS

Zinc Barriers

Are people eating more zinc but absorbing it less? Current trends toward a "heart-healthy" diet may be the reason why. Some Americans may be at risk for developing a zinc deficiency—not because they are avoiding zinc-rich foods, but because they are choosing foods and supplements that reduce its availability for absorption. For example:

- Animal foods, rich in readily available zinc, are consumed less by an increasingly cholesterol-conscious public.
- Dietary fiber, which is being promoted by some persons as a cardiovascular panacea, may hinder absorption and create a negative zinc balance.
- Food processing may make zinc less available.
- Vitamin-mineral supplements may contain iron/zinc ratios greater than 3:1 and provide enough iron to inhibit zinc absorption.

The risk for zinc deficiency is greatest among pregnant and breast-feeding women. Low levels of zinc can reduce the amount of protein available to carry iron and vitamin A to the target tissues and can reduce the mother's appetite and taste for foods. As a result, the fetus is at even greater risk for inadequate growth and development.

All of these conditions, plus milling processes that remove excessive amounts of zinc from grains, have resulted in an average adult intake of 12.5 mg/day, with elderly adults sometimes consuming only 7 to 10 mg zinc daily. This is less than the 15 mg/day recommended for all adult men and the 12 mg/day recommended for all adult women. The recommended intake for pregnant women is 15 mg/day and for lactating women it is 19 mg/day.

The following will help persons put more zinc in their diets:

- Include some form of animal food (e.g., meat, milk, eggs) in the diet each day to ensure a minimal intake of zinc.
- Avoid extensive use of alcohol.
- Avoid "crash" diets.

Signs of zinc deficiency are fairly rare in the United States but are becoming more apparent among at risk persons (e.g., older adults hospitalized with long-term chronic illness). There is no need, however, for the general public to try to overprotect themselves with massive supplement doses. These large doses may compete with other elements such as iron and create other deficiency problems. Excess zinc can lead to nausea, abdominal pain, anemia, and immune system impairment. As with all other nutrients, too much of a good thing can sometimes be as bad as—or even worse than—too little.

---

the heart muscle). A selenium deficiency clearly predisposes people to Keshan disease, because it may make them more vulnerable to a cardiotoxic virus. Research indicates that an adequate intake of selenium plays a role in preventing this disease. The other selenium deficiency that requires clinical intervention involves patients on total parenteral nutrition (TPN). These patients may experience muscular discomfort or weakness, low blood levels of the antioxidant enzyme that contains selenium (i.e., glutathione peroxide) and low levels of selenium in plasma and red cells.

Other Essential Trace Elements

The remaining seven essential trace elements—fluoride, copper, manganese, chromium, molybdenum, cobalt, and boron—do not have established recommended intake levels because it is difficult to quantify their human requirements. Presently, DRI guidelines only include fluoride from this group and only establish the AI amounts. For copper, manganese, chromium, and molybdenum, the classic RDAs recommend only "safe and adequate" ranges of intake. Cobalt does not have a recommended intake because it is supplied in vitamin B_{12}. Studies on boron are not sufficient enough to establish a recommended intake. Following is a brief review of the seven remaining essential trace elements.

Fluoride

Fluoride forms a strong bond with calcium, which means that fluoride accumulates in calcified body tissues, such as bones and teeth. Fluoride's main function in human nutrition is to prevent dental caries. Fluoride strengthens the ability of the tooth structure to withstand the erosive effect of bacterial acids. The continuous intake of fluoride throughout life maximizes the protective effect of fluoride on teeth and maintains an adequate level of fluoride in tooth enamel. To a great extent, the fluoridation of the public water supply—for which the optimal level is 1.0 mg/liter—is responsible for the remarkable decline in dental caries in recent decades. The use of fluoridated toothpaste (0.1%) and improved dental hygiene habits also produces dental benefits. Because fluoride stimulates new bone formation, it became an experimental drug in the treatment of osteoporosis. Presently, no evidence supports fluoride's ability to prevent osteoporosis. According to the new DRI guidelines, there is an insufficient amount of knowledge regarding fluoride; therefore specific RDAs are currently unattainable. Alternatively, the DRI lists observed AI amounts by age group. For adults aged 19 and older, the AI is 4 mg/day for men and 3 mg/day for women, with smaller amounts for children. There is not a recommended increase in fluoride intake during pregnancy and lactation. The DRI guidelines set the UL for fluoride at 10 mg/day for persons aged 9 and older. Fish, fish products, and tea contain the highest concentrations of fluoride in foods. Cooking in fluoridated water raises the fluoride levels in many foods.

Copper

This trace element has frequently been called the "iron twin" because the two are metabolized in much the same way and share functions as components of cell enzymes. Both are also related to energy production and hemoglobin synthesis. Severe copper deficiency is rare, attributable to individual adaptation to somewhat lower intakes, but copper depletion sufficient enough to cause low blood levels has been observed during TPN and in cases of anemia. For adults, the classic RDAs estimate a safe and adequate range of dietary copper intake at 1.5 to 3.0 mg/day, which regular United States diets supply. Natural foods contain a wide distribution of copper. Its richest food sources are organ meats—especially liver, followed by seafood, nuts, and seeds, including legumes and grains.

Manganese

The adult body contains about 20 mg of manganese, found mainly in the liver, pancreas, pituitary gland, and bone. Although it is considered a dietary essential, manganese is toxic at high levels.[11] Manganese functions like other trace elements as an essential part of cell enzymes that catalyze many important metabolic reactions. Absorption and retention of manganese are associated with serum ferritin concentration.[12] Manganese deficiency is rare, but it has been reported in cases of diabetes and pancreatic insufficiency and in protein-energy malnutrition states such as *kwashiorkor*. Manganese toxicity occurs as an industrial disease, *inhalation toxicity*, in miners and other workers with prolonged exposure to manganese dust. The excess manganese accumulates in the liver and central nervous system, producing severe neuromuscular symptoms similar to those of Parkinson's disease. The classic RDAs estimate a safe and adequate range of 2.5 to

5.0 mg/day for adults and 1.0 to 2.0 mg/day for children. The best food sources of manganese are of plant origin. Whole grains, cereal products, and teas are the richest food sources, and fruits and vegetables are somewhat less rich. Dairy products, meat, fish, and poultry are poor sources of manganese.

Chromium

The precise amount of chromium present in body tissues is uncertain because analysis is difficult. Although large geographic variations occur, the total body content is less than 6 mg. Chromium functions as an essential component of the organic complex *glucose tolerance factor* (GTF), which stimulates the action of insulin. Insulin resistance shown by impaired glucose tolerance has responded positively to chromium supplements, restoring normal blood glucose levels. Chromium supplements are also effective in the treatment of elevated serum cholesterol, lowering LDL cholesterol and increasing HDL cholesterol. For adults, the classic RDAs give a safe and adequate range of chromium intake of 50 to 200 μg/day. Brewer's yeast is a rich source of chromium, and most grains and cereal products contain significant amounts.

Molybdenum

Absorption studies indicate that molybdenum is better absorbed than many minerals, and inadequate dietary intake is unlikely.[13] The amount of molybdenum in the body is exceedingly small; it ranges from 0.1 to 1 μg per gram of body tissue. Molybdenum functions as a catalyst component in several cell enzyme systems and is essential for a number of metabolic reactions. For adults, the classic RDAs give a safe and adequate range of 75 to 250 μg/day. The amounts of molybdenum in foods vary considerably, depending on the growth environment. Food sources include legumes, whole grains, milk, leafy vegetables, and organ meats.

Cobalt

Cobalt occurs in trace amounts in body tissues and stores itself mainly in the liver. As an essential part of vitamin B_{12} (cobalamin), cobalt's only known function is associated with the formation of red blood cells. Vitamin B_{12} is the only provider of cobalt in the human diet. The human requirement is unknown, but is evidently minute. For example, as little as 0.045 to 0.09 μg/day maintains bone marrow function in persons with pernicious anemia. Cobalt is widely distributed in nature, but for our needs, the essential part of vitamin B_{12} is obtained only in the preformed vitamin. The cobalt is synthesized in animals by intestinal bacteria.

Boron

Boron has long been known as an essential micronutrient for plant growth, but now there is increasing evidence that it is essential for the growth of animals and humans, as well. For example, the understanding of boron's role with calcium in bone building is becoming much clearer. As an essential element in the diet, boron is available in widely used foods.[14] Because of the volume used, coffee and milk are two top contributors of boron in the diet; other sources include peanuts and peanut butter, other nuts, raisins, and wine.

Probably Essential Trace Elements

The seven remaining trace elements found in human tissue are silicon, vanadium, nickel, tin, cadmium, arsenic, and aluminum. These elements are being studied to determine their precise functions in the body. Most of them have already been found to be essential to the nutrition of specific animals and are probably essential in human nutrition, as well, although how they are metabolized in humans is not yet fully defined. Because these elements occur in such small amounts, they are more difficult to study and primary dietary deficiency is highly unlikely. With increased use of long-term TPN therapy, however, these elements may be of increasing clinical concern. Table 7-9 provides a summary of selected trace elements.

TABLE 7-9 A summary of selected trace elements

Element	Metabolism	Physiologic functions	Clinical application	Requirements	Food sources
Iron (Fe)	Absorption according to body need; aided by vitamin C Heme and nonheme forms Excretion from tissue in minute quantities; body conserves then reuses	Hemoglobin formation Cellular oxidation of glucose Myoglobin in muscle Antibody production Drug detoxification Carotene conversion to vitamin A Collagen synthesis	Growth Pregnancy demands Deficiency—anemia	Men: 10 mg Women: 15 mg Pregnancy: 30 mg Lactation: 15 mg Children: 10-15 mg	Liver Meats Egg yolk Whole grains Enriched bread and cereal Dark green vegetables Legumes, nuts
Iodine (I)	Absorbed as iodides, taken up by thyroid gland under control of thyroid-stimulating hormone (TSH) Excretion by kidney	Synthesis of thyroxine, the thyroid hormone, which regulates cell oxidation BMR regulation	Deficiency—endemic colloid goiter; creatinism Hypothyroidism Hyperthyroidism	Men 150 μg Women 150 μg Infants: 35-45 μg Children: 70-150 μg	Iodized salt Seafood
Zinc (Zn)	Transported with plasma proteins Excretion largely intestinal Stored in liver, muscle, bone, and organs	Essential enzyme constituent Combined with insulin for storage of the hormone Immune system leukocytes	Wound healing Taste and smell acuity Retarded sexual and physical development	Men: 15 mg Women: 12 mg Children: 10-15 mg Infants: 5 mg	Meat Seafood, especially oysters Eggs Milk Whole grains Legumes
Copper (Cu)	Stored in muscle, bone, liver, heart, kidney, and central nervous system Iron twin	Associated with iron in energy production Hemoglobin synthesis Absorption and transport of iron	TPN deficiency Anemia	Adults: 1.5-3.0 mg Children 1.0-2.5 mg (estimated)	Liver Seafood Whole grains Legumes, nuts

Continued

TABLE 7-9 A summary of selected trace elements—cont'd

Element	Metabolism	Physiologic functions	Clinical application	Requirements	Food sources
Manganese (Mn)	Absorption limited Excretion mainly by intestine	Activates reactions in: Urea formation Protein metabolism Glucose oxidation Lipoprotein clearance and synthesis of fatty acids	Clinical deficiency in protein-energy malnutrition Inhalation toxicity in miners	Adults: 2-5 mg (estimated) Children: 1-2 mg	Cereals, whole grain Soybeans Legumes, nuts Tea Vegetables Fruits
Chromium (Cr)	Improves faulty uptake of glucose by body tissues as part of glucose tolerance factor	Associated with glucose metabolism; raises abnormally low fasting blood sugar levels	Possible link with cardiovascular disorders and diabetes	Adults: 50-200 μg Children: 20-200 μg (estimated)	Whole grains Cereal products
Cobalt (Co)	Absorbed chiefly as constituent of vitamin B_{12}	Constituent of vitamin B_{12}; essential factor in red blood cell formation	Deficiency associated with deficiency of vitamin B_{12}—pernicious anemia	Unknown	Supplied by preformed vitamin B_{12}
Selenium (Se)	Active as cofactor in cell oxidation enzyme systems	Associated with vitamin E as antioxidant; protects lipid in cell membrane	Keshan disease, heart muscle failure TPN deficiency	Men: 55 μg Women: 55 μg Children: 20-40 μg	Seafoods Kidney Liver Meats Whole grains
Molybdenum (Mo)	Minute traces in the body	Constituent of specific enzymes involved in purine conversion to uric acid Aldehyde oxidation		Adults: 75-250 μg (estimated)	Organ meats Milk Whole grains Leafy vegetables Legumes
Fluorine (Fl)	Deposited in bones and teeth	Associated with dental health	Small amount prevents dental caries Excess causes endemic dental fluorosis	Adults: 3-4 mg (estimated) Children: 0.5-2.5 mg	Fluoridated water (1 ppm Fl)

SUMMARY

Minerals are single, inorganic elements that are widely distributed in nature. They are absorbed in the body and used in their activated ionic form to build body tissue; activate, regulate, and control metabolic processes; and transmit neurologic messages.

Minerals are classified according to their relative amounts in the body. *Major minerals* are required in larger quantities and make up 60% to 80% of all the inorganic material in the body. *Trace elements*, which are required in quantities as small as a microgram (μg), make up less than 1% of the body's inorganic material. Seven major minerals and 11 trace elements are essential in human nutrition and another seven trace elements may be essential. The remainders undergo constant examination.

REVIEW QUESTIONS

1. List the seven major minerals and describe their functions and the problems created by dietary deficiency or excess.
2. List the 11 trace elements proven to be essential in human nutrition. Which ones have established RDAs, either within the new DRI system or previously? Which ones have "safe and adequate intakes" suggested? Why is it difficult to establish RDAs and DRIs for everyone?

SELF-TEST QUESTIONS

True-False

Write the correct statement for each item you answer "false."

1. Most of the phosphorus in the diet is absorbed and used by the body for bone formation.
2. Typical adult use of sodium is about 10 times the amount the body actually requires for metabolic balance.
3. Potassium is the major electrolyte controlling the water outside cells.
4. Chloride is a necessary component of stomach fluids.
5. Iodine has many metabolic functions, the most important of which is its role in thyroxine synthesis.
6. A high intake of selenium has definitely been proven to prevent cancer in almost everyone.
7. Copper shares similar functions as iron in the body and is called the "iron twin."
8. Although it has been tried, taking chromium supplements has no effect either way on the level of cholesterol in the blood.

Multiple Choice

1. Overall calcium balance is mostly maintained by which two interbalanced regulatory agents?
   a. Vitamin A and thyroid hormone
   b. Ascorbic acid and growth hormone
   c. Vitamin D and parathyroid hormone
   d. Phosphorus and TSH
2. Optimum levels of body iron are controlled at the point of absorption, interrelated with a system of transport and storage. Which of the following statements correctly describes this iron-regulating process?
   a. The iron form in foods requires an acid medium to reduce it to the form required for absorption.
   b. Most of the iron ingested in food—about 70% to 90%—is absorbed.
   c. Vitamin C acts as a binding and carrying agent to transport and store iron.
   d. When red blood cells are destroyed, the iron used in making the hemoglobin is excreted.
3. The only known function of fluorine in human nutrition is for dental health. Which of the following statements correctly describes this relation?
   a. Small amounts of fluorine produce mottled, discolored teeth.
   b. Fluoridation of the public water supply in very small amounts helps prevent dental caries.
   c. Topical application of fluorine is not effective on young teeth.
   d. Fluorine works with calcium to build strong teeth.

SUGGESTIONS FOR ADDITIONAL STUDY

1. Survey food products in a community supermarket to identify items that are fortified with minerals. Read the labels carefully to determine the mineral form added and the quantity used. Do you think each mineral addition is good for the consumer? If so, why?

2. Visit a health food store, using the same procedure you followed in your vitamin study, this time to survey various mineral supplements. Discuss your findings and evaluations with your class.

3. Using Table 7-7 and the food value table in Appendix A, compute the amount of iron in each of the following foods and compare your results: (1) 3 oz beef liver, (2) 3 oz beef round steak, (3) 1 tablespoon molasses, (4) 1 tablespoon raisins, (5) 1 cup cooked kale, and (6) 6 dried prunes (plain or cooked).

4. Prepare a chart comparing the calcium values of several of the main food sources of calcium with those of some less rich sources. List some ways you can incorporate more dairy products into your diet besides drinking milk.

REFERENCES

1. Food and Nutrition Board, Institute of Medicine: *Dietary reference intakes for calcium, phosphorous, magnesium, vitamin D, and fluoride*, Washington, DC, 1998, National Academy Press.

2. Food and Nutrition Board, Institute of Medicine: *Dietary reference intakes for vitamin C, vitamin E, selenium, and carotenoids*, Washington, DC, 2000, National Academy Press.

3. Food and Nutrition Board, National Research Council, *Recommended dietary allowances*, ed 10, Washington, DC, 1989, National Academy Press.

4. Tee E-S and others: School administered weekly iron-folate supplements improve hemoglobin and ferritin concentrations in Malaysian adolescent females, *Am J Clin Nutr* 69(6):1249, 1999.

5. Picciano MF: Iron and folate supplementation in adolescent females, *Am J Clin Nutr* 69(6):1069, 1999.

6. Salamone LM and others: Effect of a lifestyle intervention on bone mineral density (BMD) in premenopausal women: a randomized trial, *Am J Clin Nutr* 70(1):97, 1999.

7. Monsen ER: The ironies of iron, *Am J Clin Nutr* 69(2):831, 1999.

8. Hunt JR, Roughead ZK: Nonheme-iron absorption, fecal ferritin excretion, and blood indexes of iron status in women consuming controlled lactoovovegetarian diets for 8 weeks, *Am J Clin Nutr* 69(3):944, 1999.

9. Andrews and others: Iron transport across biologic membranes, *Nutr Rev* 57(4):114, 1999.

10. Alaejos MS, Romero SD: Selenium in human lactation, *Nutr Rev* 53(6):159, 1995.

11. Greger JL, Malecki EA: Manganese: How do we know our limits?, *Nutr Today* 32(3):116, 1997.

12. Finley JW: Manganese absorption and retention by young women is associated with serum ferritin concentration, *Am J Clin Nutr* 70(1):37, 1999.

13. Turnlund JR and others: Molybdenum absorption and utilization in humans from soy and kale intrinsically labeled with stable isotopes of molybdenum, *Am J Clin Nutr* 69(8):1217, 1999.

14. Naghii MR and others: The boron content of selected foods and the estimation of its daily intake among free-living subjects, *Am Coll Nutr* 15(6):614 1996.

FURTHER READING

• Rainey CJ and others: Daily boron intake from the American diet, *J Am Diet Assoc* 99(3):335, 1999.

  This article reviews the increasing amount of information emerging on the role of the trace element boron and its sources in our diet. The authors provide a useful list of 50 major food sources ranked by item quantity and frequency of use in the typical American diet.

8

Water Balance

KEY CONCEPTS

- Throughout the body, water exists as a unified whole with constant ebb and flow among its interfacing parts.

- Collective water compartments, inside and outside of cells, maintain a balanced distribution of total body water.

- The concentration of various solute particles in the body's water solution determines internal shifts and balances of water.

- A state of dynamic equilibrium (i.e., homeostasis) among all parts of the body's water-balance system sustains life.

Water is the most vital nutrient to human existence. In fact, the majority of the earth's surface is covered by water. Our lives, and those of all other life forms sharing this planet, depend on a constant supply of water from the earth's ever-moving cycle. We can survive far longer without food than we can without water. Only our constant need for air is more demanding.

One of our most basic nutritional tasks is meeting this need for a continuous supply of water. Ensuring a balanced distribution of this precious water to all our body cells is a primary physiologic function.

In this chapter, we look briefly at the finely developed water-balance system in the body. We see how this system works and the various parts and processes that sustain it, thereby sustaining life itself.

BODY WATER FUNCTIONS AND REQUIREMENTS

Water: The Fundamental Nutrient

Basic principles

Three basic principles are essential to an understanding of the balance and uses of water in the human body.

A unified whole. The human body forms one continuous body of water. The "sea within" is contained by a protective envelope of skin. Enclosed within the skin, body water moves freely to all parts, controlled only by water's chemical nature.[1] Virtually every space inside and outside of cells is filled with water-based body fluids. Therefore in this warm, watery, chemical environment, all the processes necessary to life are sustained. Water is indeed an essential nutrient required for life.

Body water compartments. Water does not simply slosh around in the body. The key word *compartment* is generally used in human physiology to refer to the dynamic systems within the body's water-based environment of storage and transport of materials (e.g., water or blood) that are vital for life. The body's water compartment can be treated as a whole, encompassing all the water in the body, as well as in separate individual locations throughout the body (e.g., in cells and blood vessels) where the body stores and uses water. At the cellular level, compartments of water are separated by *membranes*. The body's dynamic mechanisms are constantly shifting water to places of the greatest need and maintaining an equilibrium among all parts.

Particles in the water solution. The concentration and distribution of *particles* in the water solution in various places throughout the body determine all of the internal shifts and balances in the total body water.

Homeostasis

Thus you can picture body water as a unified whole, sustained in critical balance to protect life. The body's state of dynamic balance is called homeostasis. Many years ago a thoughtful physiologist, W.B. Cannon, viewed these balance principles as "body wisdom."[2] He applied the term *homeostasis* to the capacity built into the body to maintain its life systems, despite what enters the system from the outside. The first part of the word, *homeo-*, is from a Greek word meaning "similar." The second half of the word, *-stasis*, is from another Greek root, meaning "balance." The body has a great capacity to employ numerous, finely balanced, *homeostatic mechanisms* to protect its vital water supply.

Body Water Functions

To serve life-sustaining functions, our body water supply acts as a solvent; serves as a means of transport; and provides form and structure, temperature control, and lubrication for the body.

- **Solvent:** Water provides the basic liquid solvent for all of the body's chemical processes. The word *hydrolysis* is used to describe this water-based chemical activity in the body. The first part of the word, *hydro-*, means "water," and the second part, *-lysis*, means "to break apart." Thus with water as the basic solvent, multiple water solutions may be formed as needed throughout the body to allow all of its life-sustaining metabolic activities (e.g., energy production and tissue building) to proceed.
- **Transport:** Water circulates throughout the body in the form of blood and various other body secretions and tissue fluids. In this circulating fluid, the many nutrients, secretions, metabolites (i.e., products formed in body metabolism), and other materials can be carried freely about to meet the needs of all the body cells. The body cell is the functional unit of life. Its fundamental needs for oxygen and nourishment, as well as needs for all its chemical activities, must be met at all times.
- **Body form and structure:** Water also helps to give structure and form to the body by filling in spaces within body tissues. For example, striated (from the Latin for "furrow" or "line")

muscle contains more water than any other body tissue except blood.

- **Body temperature:** Water is necessary to help maintain a stable body temperature. As the temperature rises, sweat increases and evaporates, thus cooling the body.
- **Body lubricant:** Water also has a lubricating effect on moving parts of the body. For example, fluid within the body joints (i.e., *synovial* fluid) helps to provide smooth movement of the many joint parts.

Body Water Requirements

The body's requirement for water varies according to several factors: temperature, activity level, functional losses, metabolic needs, and age.

- **Surrounding Temperature:** As the temperature rises in the surrounding environment, body water is lost to help maintain the body temperature, and thus more water intake is required to offset it. This increasing temperature may be caused by the natural climate or the heat of a work environment.
- **Activity level:** Heavy work or extensive physical activity, such as in sports, increases the water requirement for two reasons: (1) more water is lost as sweat, and (2) more water is required for the increased metabolic work involved in the physical activity.
- **Functional losses:** When any disease process interferes with the normal functioning of the body, water requirements are affected. For example, in gastrointestinal problems such as prolonged diarrhea, large amounts of water may be lost. In such cases, replacement of this lost water is vital to prevent dehydration.
- **Metabolic needs:** The work of body metabolism requires water. A general rule is that about 1000 ml of water—as water and other water-based beverages—is required for every 1000 kcalories in the diet. On average, beverages supply about two thirds of the body's water intake. Solid foods supply the remaining one third.

- **Age:** Age plays an important role in determining body needs, especially in the case of an infant. An infant needs about 1500 ml of water per day. Water intake is critical for an infant because of the following: (1) an infant's body content of water is large (i.e., about 70% to 75% of the total body weight), and (2) a relatively large amount of this total body water is outside of the cells, and thus more easily lost.

In order to meet adult fluid needs, and thus be well-hydrated, the average sedentary woman should consume about 2200 ml (9 cups) of liquids per day. A sedentary man should consume about 2900 ml (12 cups) of fluid per day.[1] Very active persons, however, require more fluid. Elderly adults especially need to avoid becoming dehydrated.[3]

THE HUMAN WATER BALANCE SYSTEM
Body Water: The Solvent

Amount and Distribution

In a man's body, 55% to 65% of the total body weight is water; in a woman's body, 45% to 55% is water.[1] The higher water content of men generally results from their greater muscle mass, because muscle contains a relatively large amount of water. This total body water is divided into two major categories or *compartments*, depending on its placement in the body.

Total water outside cells. The total body water outside of the cells is called the *extracellular fluid* (ECF). This water collectively makes up about 20% of the total body weight. About one fourth of this

---

homeostasis (Gr. *homoios*, like, unchanging; *stasis*, standing, stable) the state of relative dynamic equilibrium within the body's internal environment; a balance achieved through the operation of various interrelated physiologic mechanisms.

water (i.e., 5% of the body weight) is contained in the blood plasma. The remaining three fourths (i.e., 15% of the body weight) is composed of the following: (1) water surrounding the cells and bathing the tissues; (2) water in dense tissue such as bone; and (3) water moving through the body in various tissue secretions. The water in the blood plasma includes the total fluid in the heart and all the blood vessels. The fluid surrounding the cells in the tissues is called *interstitial fluid*. This tissue circulation helps to move materials in and out of body cells to sustain life. Fluid in transit includes all the water in various body fluids and secretions, such as those of the salivary glands, thyroid gland, liver, pancreas, gallbladder, gastrointestinal tract, gonads, various mucous membranes, skin, kidneys, and eye spaces.

Total water inside cells. Total body water inside the cells is called the *intracellular fluid* (ICF). This water collectively amounts to about twice of that outside the cells, making up about 45% to 55% of the total body weight. This is not surprising, however, because the cell is the basic unit of life and all life-sustaining work (i.e., metabolism) is done within the cells.

The relative amounts of water in the different body water compartments are compared in Table 8-1.

Overall water balance. Water enters and leaves the body by various routes, controlled by basic mechanisms such as thirst and hormones. Special attention must be given to the water needs of the elderly, whose thirst sensation may be decreased.[3,4] The average adult metabolizes 2.5 to 3 L of water per day in a balance between intake and output.

Water intake. Water enters the body in three main forms, as follow: (1) as preformed water in liquids that are drunk; (2) as preformed water in foods that are eaten; and (3) as a product of cell oxidation when nutrients are burned in the body for energy (e.g., meta-

TABLE 8-1 Volumes of body fluid compartments*

Body fluid	Infant	Adult male	Adult female	
Extracellular fluid				
Plasma	4	4	4	
Interstitial fluid	26	15	10	
Intracellular fluid	45	38	33	
TOTAL	75	57	47	

*Percentage of body weight

(From Thibodeau GA, Patton KT: *Anatomy and physiology,* ed 3, St. Louis, 1996, Mosby. Art credit: Rolin Graphics.)

bolic water or "water of oxidation"). The approximate water intake of an average adult is 2600 ml/day.

The vital need for water in older adults, however, is too often overlooked. The normal thirst mechanism usually diminishes with age, so dehydration can easily occur. Many older persons suffer from dry mouth caused by severe reduction in the flow of saliva, which in turn affects their food intake. This condition may be associated with the use of certain medications, disease, or radiation therapy to the head and neck. Conscious attention to adequate fluid intake (i.e., not less than the recommended minimum of 1500 to 2000 ml daily and not dependent on normal thirst) is an important part of health maintenance and care.[4]

Water output. Water leaves the body through the kidneys, skin, lungs, and feces. Of these output routes, the largest amount of water exits through the kidneys. A certain amount of water must be excreted as urine to carry out the various products of metabolism that the body does not need. This is called *obligatory* water loss because it is compulsory for survival and must occur daily for health. An additional amount of water may also be put out by the kidneys each day, depending on body activities and needs. This additional, or *optional*, water loss varies according to the climate and physical activity. For example, athletes require a large increase in water intake, especially in hot weather. In any event, the American College of Sports Medicine recommends drinking 500 ml of water 2 hours before the start of competition.[5] Some athletes hyperhydrate with glycerol because of its osmotic properties, but more research is required before this action can be recommended.[6] On average, the daily water output from the body totals about 2600 ml, which balances the average intake of water.

Table 8-2 summarizes the comparative intake and output of body water balance.

Solute Particles in Solution

The solutes in body water are a variety of particles in varying concentrations. Two main types of particles control water balance in the body: electrolytes and plasma protein.

Electrolytes

Electrolytes are small, inorganic substances (i.e., either single-mineral elements or small compounds) that can dissociate or break apart in a solution and carry an electrical charge.[7] These charged particles are called *ions*, from the Greek word meaning "wanderer." Thus these particles are free to wander throughout a solution to maintain its chemical

TABLE 8-2 Approximate daily adult intake and output of water

	Intake (replacement) ml/day		Output (loss)	
			Obligatory (insensible) ml/day	Optional (according to need) ml/day
Preformed		Lungs	350	
Liquids	1200-1500	Skin		
In foods	700-1000	Diffusion	350	
Metabolism	200-300	Sweat	100	±250
(oxidation		Kidneys	900	±500
of food)		Feces	150	
TOTAL	2100-2800	TOTAL	1850	750
(approx. 2600 ml/day)		(approx. 2600 ml/day)		

balance. In any chemical solution, the separate particles are constantly in balance between cations and anions.

Cations. These are ions carrying a positive charge (e.g., sodium [Na$^+$], potassium [K$^+$], calcium [Ca^{++}], and magnesium [Mg^{++}]).

Anions. These are ions carrying a negative charge (e.g., chloride [Cl$^-$], carbonate [HCO$_3^-$], phosphate [HPO$_4^{--}$], and sulfate [SO$_4^{--}$]). The constant balance between the two major electrolytes—sodium [Na$^+$] outside the cell and potassium [K$^+$] inside the cell—maintains water balance between these two water compartments. Because of their small size, these electrolytes can diffuse freely across most membranes of the body, thereby maintaining a constant balance between the water outside the cell and that inside the cell.

The balance between cation and anion concentrations in the body fluids maintains a state of chemical neutrality in these fluids that is necessary to life. Electrolyte concentration in body fluids is measured in terms of *milliequivalents* (mEq). The number of electrolytes per unit of fluid in a solution is expressed as mEq/L. Table 8-3 outlines the balance between cations and anions in the two body-fluid compartments. The number of particles in each compartment are exactly balanced.

Plasma Proteins

Plasma proteins, mainly in the form of albumin and globulin, are organic compounds of large molecular size. They do not move as freely across membranes as electrolytes, which are much smaller. Thus plasma protein molecules are retained in blood vessels and make up a major substance in circulating blood, controlling water movement in the body and guarding blood volume by influencing the shift of water in and out of capillaries in balance with the surrounding water. In this function, these plasma proteins are called *colloids*, from the

TABLE 8-3 Balance of cation and anion concentrations in extracellular fluid (ECF) and intracellular fluid (ICF), which maintains electroneutrality within each compartment

	ECF (mEq/L)	ICF (mEq/L)
Cation		
Sodium (Na$^+$)	142	35
Potassium (K$^+$)	5	123
Calcium (Ca^{++})	5	15
Magnesium (Mg^{++})	3	2
TOTAL	155	175
Anion		
Chloride (Cl$^-$)	104	5
Phosphate (HPO$_4^-$)	2	80
Sulfate (SO$_4^-$)	1	10
Protein	16	70
Carbonate (HCO$_3^-$)	27	10
Organic acids	5	
TOTAL	155	175

Greek word *kolla*, meaning "glue," and form *colloidal* solutions. Because of their large size, these particles or molecules normally remain in the blood vessels, where they exert colloidal osmotic pressure (COP) to maintain the integrity of the blood volume. Cell protein helps to guard cell water in a similar manner.

Small Organic Compounds

In addition to electrolytes and plasma protein, other small organic compounds are dissolved in body water. Their concentration is too small, however, to ordinarily influence shifts of water. Although in some instances, they are found in abnormally large concentrations and do influence water movement. For example, glucose is one of these small particles in body fluids, and it only influences water loss from the body when it is in abnormal concentrations (e.g., in uncontrolled diabetes).

Separating Membranes

Two quite different types of membranes separate and contain body water throughout the body. These membranes are the capillary membrane and the cell membrane.

Capillary Membrane

The walls of the capillaries are fairly free membranes because they are thin and porous. Therefore water molecules and small particles can move freely across these membranes. Such small particles having free passage across capillary walls include electrolytes and various nutrient materials. As indicated, however, larger particles such as plasma protein molecules cannot pass through the small pores in the capillary membrane. These larger molecules remain in the capillary vessel and exert an important pressure control (i.e., COP) to keep the water circulating from capillaries and surrounding tissue cells.

Cell Membrane

The cell walls are thicker membranes that are specially constructed to protect and nourish the cell contents. To accomplish these tasks, cell membranes are structured almost in sandwich fashion, with outer layers and penetrating channels of protein and an inner structure of fat material. Special transport mechanisms are necessary to carry substances across cell membranes.

Forces Moving Water and Solutes Across Membranes

As a result of the presence of these separating membranes (i.e., the capillary membrane and the cell membrane), certain physical and chemical forces are created to control the movement of body water and particles in solution across these membranes.

Osmosis

The term osmosis comes from the Greek word *osmos*, which means "a driving or pushing force, an impulse." Osmosis describes nature's fundamental impulse to balance or equalize opposing forces. In human physiology, the term *osmosis* is used to describe the process or force (e.g., "osmotic pressure") that impels water molecules to move throughout the body. When solutions of different concentrations exist on either side of semipermeable body membranes, the pressure of the crowded water molecules moves them across the membrane to help equalize the solutions on both sides. Therefore

---

colloidal osmotic pressure (COP) **fluid pressure produced by the protein molecules in the plasma and in the cell. Because proteins are large molecules, they do not pass through the separating membranes of the capillary walls. Thus they remain in their respective compartments, exerting a constant osmotic pull that protects vital plasma and cell fluid volumes in these areas.**

osmosis (Gr. *osmos,* a thrusting) passage of a solvent such as water through a membrane that separates solutions of different concentrations, tending to equalize the concentration pressures of the solutions on both sides of the membrane.

osmosis can be defined as the force that moves water molecules from an area of greater concentration of water molecules (i.e., with fewer particles in solution) to an area of lesser concentration of water molecules (i.e., with more particles in solution). Therefore osmosis distributes water molecules more evenly throughout the body (i.e., water balance) and thus provides a solvent base for materials the water must carry.

Diffusion

The force of diffusion operates similarly to osmosis but instead applies to the particles in solution in the water. Diffusion is the force by which these particles move outward in all directions from an area of greater concentration of particles to an area of lesser concentration of particles. The relative movements of water molecules and solute particles by osmosis and diffusion effectively balance solution concentrations—and hence pressures—on both sides of the separating membrane. The two balancing forces of osmosis and diffusion are shown in Figure 8-1.

Filtration

Water is forced or filtered through the pores of membranes when the pressure on both sides of the membrane is different. This difference in pressure results from the differences in the particle concentrations of the two solutions, causing water and small particles to move back and forth between capillaries and cells according to shifting pressures.

Active Transport

Particles in solution that are vital to body processes must move across membranes throughout the body at all times, even when the pressures are against their flow. Thus some type of energy-driven *active transport* is necessary to carry these particles "upstream" across separating membranes. Such active transport mechanisms usually require some sort of carrier partner to help "ferry" the particles across the membrane. For example, glucose enters absorbing cells through an active transport mechanism involving sodium (Na^+) as a "ferrying" partner.

Pinocytosis

Sometimes larger particles, such as proteins and fats, enter absorbing cells by the process of *pinocytosis* (Figure 8-2), which means "cell drinking." In this process, larger molecules attach themselves to the thicker cell membrane and are then engulfed by

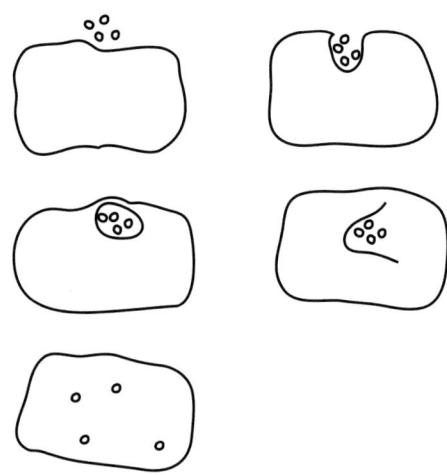

FIGURE 8-2   Pinocytosis—engulfing of large molecules by the cell. (Redrawn from Williams SR: *Essentials of nutrition and diet therapy,* ed 7, St Louis, 1999, Mosby.)

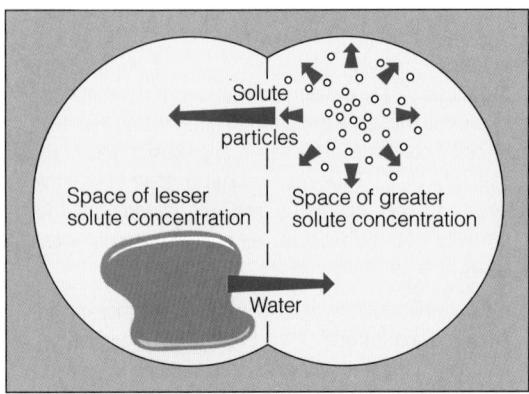

FIGURE 8-1   Movement of molecules, water, and solutes by osmosis and diffusion

the cell. In this way, they are encased in a *vacuole* (L. *vacuus*, meaning "empty"; plus ending *-ole*, meaning "small"), which is a small space or cavity formed in the protoplasm of the cell. In this small cavity the nutrient particles are carried across the cell membrane and into the cell. Once inside the cell, the vacuole opens and the particles are metabolized by the cell enzymes. For example, pinocytosis is one of the basic mechanisms by which fat is absorbed from the small intestine.

Tissue Water Circulation: The Capillary Fluid Shift Mechanism

One of the body's most important controls to maintain overall water balance is the *capillary fluid shift mechanism*. This control operates a balancing act between opposing fluid pressures to nourish the life of the cell.

Purpose

Water and other nutrients are constantly circulated through the body tissues by the blood vessels. To nourish cells, however, the water and nutrients must get out of the tissue blood vessels—the capillaries—and into the cells. Then water and the cell's metabolites, products of cell metabolism leaving the cell, must get back into the capillaries to circulate all over the body. In other words, essential water, nutrients, and oxygen must be pushed out of blood circulation into tissue circulation; then water, cell metabolites, and carbon dioxide must be pulled back into blood circulation to distribute their goods throughout the body and dispose of metabolic wastes through the kidneys. The body maintains this constant flow of water through the tissues—carrying materials to and from the cells—by means of a balance of opposing fluid pressures, as follows: (1) *hydrostatic pressure*, an intracapillary blood pressure from the contracting muscle of the heart pushing blood into circulation; and (2) *colloidal osmotic pressure* from the plasma proteins drawing tissue fluids back into ongoing circulation. A *filtration* process operates according to the differences in osmotic pressure on either side of the capillary membrane.

Process

When blood first enters the capillary system from the larger vessels coming from the heart—the arterioles, the greater blood pressure from the pumping heart muscle forces water and small particles (e.g., glucose) into the tissues to bathe and nourish the cells. This force of blood pressure is an example of *hydrostatic* pressure (*hydro-* meaning "water" and *-static* meaning "balance"). Plasma protein particles, however, are too large to go through the pores of capillary membranes. When the circulating tissue fluids are ready to reenter the blood capillaries, the initial blood pressure has diminished. The COP of the concentrated protein particles remaining in the capillary vessel is now the greater influence, drawing the water and its metabolites back into the ending capillary circulation after they have served the cells and carrying them on to the receptive larger vessels—the venules—for blood circulation back to the heart. A small amount of normal turgor pressure of the resisting tissue of the capillary membrane remains the same and operates throughout the system. This fundamental fluid shift mechanism constantly controls water balance through its capillary-tissue circulation to nourish cells all over the body. This vital fluid flow through tissue is maintained by the balance between blood pressure and the osmotic pressure of the plasma protein particles. This key tissue circulation balance is illustrated in Figure 8-3.

Organ Systems Involved

In addition to the blood circulation, the human water-balance system uses the circulations of two other major organ systems to control the overall water balance of the body. The other systems involved are the gastrointestinal circulation, which supports digestion and absorption of nutrients, and the renal circulation, which maintains normal blood levels of various nutrients and metabolites.

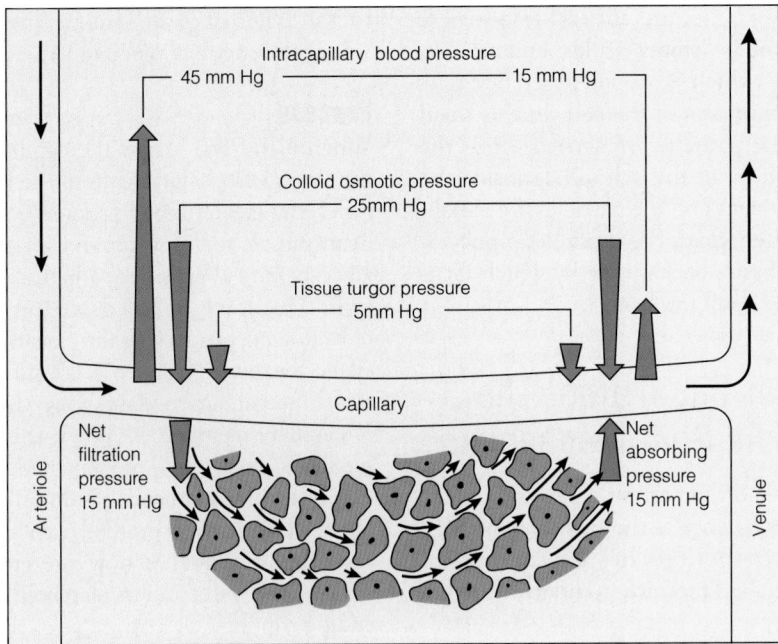

FIGURE 8-3   The fluid shift mechanism. Note the balance of pressures that controls the flow of fluid.

Gastrointestinal Circulation

Water from the blood plasma, containing vital electrolytes, is constantly secreted into the gastrointestinal tract to aid the processes of food digestion and nutrient absorption. This large circulation of water and electrolytes constantly moves among the blood plasma, the secreting cells, and the gastrointestinal tract. In the latter portion of the intestine, most of the water and electrolytes are then reabsorbed into the blood to circulate over and over again. This constant movement of a large volume of water and its electrolytes among the blood, the secreting cells, and the gastrointestinal tract is called *gastrointestinal circulation*. The sheer magnitude of this vital gastrointestinal circulation, as shown in Table 8-4, indicates the seriousness of fluid loss from the upper or lower portion of the gastrointestinal tract. This circulation is maintained in *isotonicity* with the surrounding water outside of cells (i.e., including the blood) and carries risk for clinical imbalances, as follow:

Law of isotonicity. The gastrointestinal fluids are part of the water compartment outside of cells, which includes the blood circulation. All of these fluids are held in isotonicity, meaning a state of equal osmotic pressure resulting from equal concentrations of electrolytes and other solute particles. For example, when a person drinks water (i.e., plain water without any solutes or accompanying food), electrolytes and salts enter the intestine from the surrounding blood plasma fluid to equalize pressures. If a concentrated solution of food mix is ingested, additional water is then drawn into the intestine from the surrounding blood plasma to dilute the intestinal contents. In each instance, water and electrolytes move among the parts of the extracellular fluid compartment to maintain solutions that

TABLE 8-4 Approximate total volume of digestive secretions produced in 24 hours by an adult of average size

Secretion	Volume (ml)
Saliva	1500
Gastric	2500
Bile	500
Pancreatic	700
Intestinal	3000
TOTAL	8200

TABLE 8-5 Approximate concentration of certain electrolytes in digestive fluids (mEq/L)

Secretion	Na$^+$	K$^+$	Cl$^-$	HCO
Saliva	10	25	10	15
Gastric	40	10	145	0
Pancreatic	140	5	40	110
Jejunal	135	5	110	30
Bile	140	10	110	40

are *isotonic* (i.e., have an equal concentration of particles) in the gastrointestinal tract with the surrounding fluid. If an imbalance of the pressures involved goes unchecked, it will eventually draw on the intracellular fluid compartment in an effort to restore balances, creating a risk for critical cell dehydration.

Clinical applications. The law of isotonicity has many clinical implications. For example, what would happen if a patient undergoing gastric suctioning drank water? Or if a patient being fed by tube were given the formula too rapidly at too concentrated a dilution? In the first case, the water would cause the stomach to produce more secretions containing electrolytes. Then the electrolytes would be lost in the suctioning. In turn the plasma, from which the electrolytes were supplied, would be gradually depleted of these electrolytes and unable to supply them to tissue cells. In the second case, the concentrated (i.e., *hypertonic*) solution given by tube would cause water to shift into the intestine to dilute the solution, thus rapidly shrinking the surrounding blood volume. This condition would then produce symptoms of shock, reflecting the body's effort to restore blood volume.

Because of the large amounts of water and electrolytes involved, upper and lower gastrointestinal losses are the most common cause of clinical fluid and electrolyte problems. Such problems exist, for example, in cases of persistent vomiting or prolonged diarrhea, in which large amounts of precious water and electrolytes are lost (see Clinical Applications box, "Principles of Oral Rehydration Therapy"). The large numbers of electrolytes involved in gastrointestinal circulation are shown in Table 8-5.

Renal Circulation

The kidneys maintain the appropriate levels of all constituents of blood by filtering the blood and then selectively reabsorbing water and needed materials to be carried throughout the body. Through this continual "laundering" of the blood by the millions of nephrons in the kidneys, water balance and the proper solution of blood are maintained. When disease occurs in the kidneys and this filtration process does not operate normally, water imbalances occur.

Hormonal Controls

Two basic hormonal controls operate in the kidneys to help maintain constant body water balance, as follows:

ADH mechanism. Antidiuretic hormone (ADH), also called *vasopressin*, is produced by the pituitary gland. ADH is a water-conserving mechanism, operating on the kidneys' nephrons to cause reabsorption of water. In any stress situation with threatened

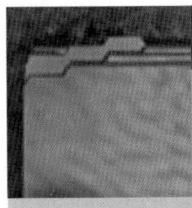

CLINICAL APPLICATIONS
Principles of Oral Rehydration Therapy

The principles of electrolyte absorption are the basis for development of a method to rehydrate children suffering from diarrhea. Although diarrhea is usually considered a trivial problem in developed countries, it is responsible for the deaths of one fourth to one half of all children under 4 years of age worldwide. Although 90% of the mortality of diarrhea is associated with fluid loss, the mere provision of water alone can be dangerous.

Intravenous (IV) therapy, developed by Darrow in the 1940s, provided sodium chloride—a base—and potassium in water and proved very successful. Unfortunately, however, IV therapy is not readily available to those who need it most. A large number of isolated, poor rural families—in both developed and developing countries—do not have access to health care facilities because of their lack of transportation and money. Fortunately, though, the World Health Organization (WHO) has developed an oral rehydration therapy (ORT) that is much less expensive and is being used in the United States, as well as in undeveloped countries. If safe drinking water is made available, the ORT solution can easily be mixed at home under the guidance of a public health worker and administered by a family member. The ingredients are 1 L of safe water, 3.5 g table salt (i.e., sodium chloride), 2.5 g baking soda (i.e., sodium bicarbonate), 1.5 g potassium chloride, and 20 g glucose. This ORT is based upon principles of sodium absorption in the small intestine.

Transport of metabolic compounds
A number of metabolic compounds—principally glucose but also certain amino acids, dipeptides, and disaccharides—depend on sodium to cross the intestinal wall.

Additive effects
The more substances present, the better the absorption of sodium. The rate at which sodium is absorbed depends on the presence of substances such as glucose or other protein metabolic products.

Water absorption
The rate of water absorption is enhanced as sodium absorption improves. Thus a solution of sodium and potassium salts plus glucose is an IV solution that can be given orally.

In addition to the ORT, infants and older children with acute diarrhea should also be fed so that the added burden of malnutrition from fasting is avoided. Such fasting practices were based on the former belief that recovery was more effective if the bowel was allowed to rest and heal. To the contrary, children should be fed their regular age diets (i.e., breast feeding, formula, or solid foods), allowed to determine the amount of food they need, and given extra food as the diarrhea subsides to recover nutritional deficits. Food choices should be guided by individual tolerances. Use of the old so-called BRAT diet (i.e., bananas, rice, applesauce, and tea or toast) is not recommended because it does not include typical foods consumed by infants and small children and only compounds the energy-nutrient decline.

or real loss of body water, this hormone is triggered to conserve vital body water.

Aldosterone mechanism. The hormone *aldosterone* is produced by the adrenal glands, which are located on top of each kidney, in response to a reduced renal filtration rate or decreased sodium level. Aldosterone operates on the kidneys' nephrons to cause reabsorption of sodium. Therefore it is primarily a sodium-conserving mechanism but also exerts a secondary control over water reabsorption. Both ADH and aldosterone may be activated by stress situations, such as body injury or surgery.

HUMAN ACID-BASE BALANCE SYSTEM

The optimal degree of acidity or alkalinity must be maintained in various body water solutions and secretions to support human life. This vital balance is achieved by solutions of both acids and bases with the correct proportions of each controlled by a buffer system.

Acids and Bases

The concept of acids and bases relates to *hydrogen* ions both in its measurement symbol—pH—and in its defining of the terms *acid* and *base*.

Measurement
A substance is *more or less* acid, according to the degree of its concentration of hydrogen ions. Its degree of acidity is therefore expressed in terms of **pH.** The abbreviation *pH* is derived from a mathematical term, which refers to the power of the Hydrogen ion concentration. A pH of 7 is the neutral point between an acid and a base. Because pH is in effect a negative mathematical factor, the higher the hydrogen ion concentration (i.e., more acid), the lower the pH number. Similarly, the lower the hydrogen ion concentration (i.e., less acid), the higher the pH number. Because a pH of 7 is the neutral

point, substances with a pH *below* 7 are *acid*. Substances with a pH *above* 7 are *alkaline*. More precise definitions of acids and bases are based on the hydrogen ion concentration.

Acids. An acid is defined as a compound that has more hydrogen ions, enough to give some away. When in solution, it releases extra hydrogen ions.

Bases. A base is a compound that has fewer hydrogen ions. Thus in solution it takes up extra hydrogen ions, effectively reducing the solution's acidity.

Acid-Base Buffer System

The body deals with degrees of acidity by maintaining buffer systems to handle excess acid. A buffer system is a mixture of acidic and alkaline components—an acid and a base partner—that together protect a solution from wide variations in its pH, even when strong bases or acids are added to it. For example, if a strong acid is added to a buffered solution, the base partner reacts with the acid to form a weaker acid. If a strong base is added to the solution, the acid partner combines with the intruder to form a weaker base. In both cases, the pH is restored to its starting balance point.

Main Buffer System
The human body contains many buffer systems because only a relatively narrow range of pH is compatible with life. The carbonic acid [H_2CO_3]/base bicarbonate [$NaHCO_3$] buffer system, however, is the body's main buffer system for the following three reasons.

Available materials. The raw materials for producing the acid partner carbonic acid (H_2CO_3) are readily available. Water (H_2O) and carbon dioxide (CO_2) are always accessible.

Ease of adjustment. The lungs and the kidneys can easily adjust to changes in the acid and base partners, quickly returning body fluids to normal pH level. The normal pH of the fluids outside of cells is 7.4, with a range of 7.35 to 7.45. pH must be maintained within this narrow range to sustain the life of the cells.

Base-to-acid ratio.   The carbonic acid/base bicarbonate buffer system is able to maintain this essential degree of acidity in the body fluids because the base bicarbonate partner in this buffer system is about 20 times as abundant as the carbonic acid partner. This *20:1 ratio* is maintained even though the absolute amounts of the two partners may fluctuate during adjustment periods. Whether or not added base or acid enters the system, as long as the 20:1 ratio is maintained, the extracellular fluid (ECF) acid-base balance is held constant. This way, the life of the cells is protected.

SUMMARY

The human body is approximately 50% to 60% water. The primary functions of body water are to give form and structure to the body tissue, provide the water environment necessary for cell work, and control body temperature. Body water is distributed in two collective body water compartments: intracellular and extracellular. The water inside cells is the larger portion, accounting for about 40% of the total body weight. The water outside cells consists of the fluid in spaces between cells (i.e., interstitial and lymph fluid), the blood plasma, the secretions in transit (e.g., the gastrointestinal circulation) and the smaller amount of fluid in cartilage and bone.

The overall water balance of the body is maintained by fluid intake and output. The distribution of body water is controlled by two types of solute particles, as follow: (1) electrolytes, mainly charged mineral elements; and (2) plasma protein, mainly albumin. These solute particles influence the movement of water across cell or capillary membranes, allowing tissue circulation to nourish cells.

The acid-base buffer system, which is mainly controlled by the lungs and the kidneys, uses electrolytes and hydrogen ions to maintain a normal ECF pH of about 7.4. This pH level is necessary to sustain cell life.

REVIEW QUESTIONS

1. Why is the total body water considered a unified whole? What does the term *body compartment* mean? How does this term apply to body water balance?
2. Define the term *homeostasis*. Give examples of how this state is maintained in the body.
3. List and describe five functions of body water. Describe five factors that influence water requirements to supply these body water functions.
4. Apply your knowledge of the capillary fluid shift mechanism to account for the gross body edema seen in starving children.

SELF-TEST QUESTIONS

Matching
Match the terms provided below with the corresponding items listed here:

____ 1. Chief electrolyte guarding the water outside of cells

____ 2. An ion carrying a negative electrical charge

____ 3. Sodium-conserving mechanism or control agent

_____ **4.** Simple passage of water molecules through a membrane separating solutions of different concentrations from the side of lower concentration of solute particles to that of higher concentration of particles, thus tending to equalize the solutions

_____ **5.** A substance (element or compound) that, in solution, conducts an electrical current and is dissociated into cations and anions

_____ **6.** Particles in solution, such as electrolytes and protein

_____ **7.** State of dynamic equilibrium maintained by an organism among all its parts and controlled by many finely balanced mechanisms

_____ **8.** Chief electrolyte guarding the water inside of cells

_____ **9.** Major plasma protein that guards and maintains the blood volume

_____ **10.** Abnormal increase in water held in body tissues

_____ **11.** An ion carrying a positive electrical charge

_____ **12.** The body's means of maintaining tissue water circulation by means of opposing fluid pressures

_____ **13.** Force exerted by a contained fluid (e.g., blood pressure)

_____ **14.** Movement of particles throughout a solution and across membranes outward from the area of denser concentration of particles to all surrounding spaces

_____ **15.** A type of fluid outside of cells

_____ **16.** Movement of particles in solution across cell membranes and against normal osmotic pressures, involving a carrier and energy for the work

a. osmosis
b. solutes
c. diffusion
d. cation
e. interstitial fluid
f. homeostasis
g. anion
h. K^+
i. albumin
j. hydrostatic pressure
k. Na^+
l. electrolyte
m. active transport
n. aldosterone
o. capillary fluid shift mechanism
p. edema

SUGGESTIONS FOR ADDITIONAL STUDY

1. Keep a 3-day record of your total fluid intake from all sources, including water. Note the circumstances under which you took in these fluids. How did thirst influence your intake? Evaluate your intake in terms of the total amount of fluid consumed and the nutrients contributed by each source.

2. Observe some type of athletic competition. What provisions do the participants to cover water loss? Do these provisions appear to be adequate? Why would athletes require increased water intake? Record your observations and discuss them in class.

REFERENCES

1. Kleiner SM: Water: an essential but overlooked nutrient, _J Am Diet Assoc_ 99(2):200, 1999.

2. Cannon WB: _The wisdom of the body_, New York, 1932, W.W. Norton and Co., Inc.

3. Sansevero AC: Dehydration in the elderly: strategies for prevention and management, _Nurse Pract_ 22(2):41, 1997.

4. Chidester JC: Spangler AA: Fluid intake in the institutionalized elderly, _J Am Diet Assoc_ 97(1):23, 1997.

5. American College of Sports Medicine Position stand: exercise and fluid replacement, _Med Sci Sports Exer_ 28:iv-vii, 1996.

6. Wagner DR: Hyperhydrating with glycerol: implications for athletic performance, _J Am Diet Assoc_ 99(2):207, 1999.

7. Oh MS: _Water, electrolyte, and acid-base balance_. In Shils ME, Olson JA, Shike M, eds: _Modern nutrition in health and disease_, vol 1, ed 8, Philadelphia, 1994, Lea & Febiger.

FURTHER READING

• McCleary K: The fitness report: when water works and when it doesn't, *Am Health* 5(5):26, 1986.

This classic article is a practical guide describing the need for more water for activities in the summer's heat, especially highlighting the dangers of dehydration and water intoxication.

• Robinson JR: Water, the indispensable nutrient, *Nutr Today* 5(1):16, 1970.

This classic but still current article by a New Zealand physician who is a world authority clearly describes the processes involved in body water balance. This article is filled with excellent charts and diagrams to illustrate key principles.

• Wagner DR: Hyperhydrating with glycerol: implications for athletic performance, *J Am Diet Assoc* 99(2):207, 1999.

The author, who is a professor of exercise and sports science at a California university, alerts us to the pros and cons of using the sport supplement glycerol, a natural body sugar, as an extra energy source with water or sports drinks.

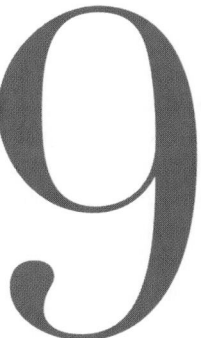

Digestion and Absorption

KEY CONCEPTS

● Through a balanced system of mechanical and chemical change, our food is broken down into simpler substances and the food's nutrients are released and reformed for the body's use.

● Special organ structures and functions conduct these changes through the successive parts of the overall system.

As described previously in this text, the nutrients our bodies require do not come to us ready to use but come packaged as foods in a variety of forms. Our body cells cannot use nutrients in these forms, so our foods must be changed to simpler substances. In this process, we must also free the food nutrients and reform and reroute them to meet our special life needs.

In this chapter, we see how this marvelous process of change takes place. We view the overall process of food digestion and nutrient absorption as one continuous *whole* made up of a series of successive events. Throughout this chapter, we review the unique body structures and functions that make this process—and our lives—possible.

DIGESTION

Basic Principles

Principle of Change

Our body cells cannot use foods as we eat them. They must be changed into simpler substances and then into other—even simpler—substances that our cells can use to sustain our lives. Preparing food for our body's use involves many changes that make up the overall process of digestion, absorption, and metabolism.

Digestion is the process in which food is broken up in the gastrointestinal tract, releasing many nutrients in forms the body can use.

Absorption is the process in which these nutrients are carried into the body's circulation system and delivered to the cells.

Cell metabolism is the sum of the vast number of chemical changes in the cell—the functional unit of life—that finally produces the es-

sential materials we need for energy, tissue building, and metabolic controls.

Principle of Wholeness

The parts of this overall process of change do not exist separately but make up one continuous *whole*. The different parts of the gastrointestinal tract and their relative positions within the whole gastrointestinal tract are shown in Figure 9-1. Food components travel *together* through this system for delivery to the cells.

Mechanical and Chemical Changes

In order for nutrients to be delivered to cells, the food we eat must go through a series of mechanical and chemical changes. Together, these two types of actions make up the overall process of digestion.

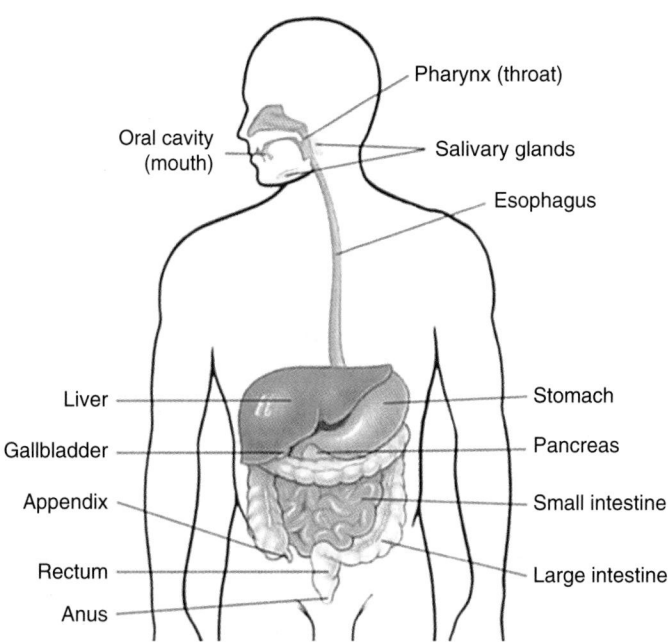

FIGURE 9-1   The gastrointestinal system. Through the successive parts of the system, multiple activities of digestion liberate and reform food nutrients for our use. (Credit: Joan Beck, from Seeley RR, Stephens TD, Tate P: *Anatomy and physiology,* ed 3, New York, 1995, McGraw-Hill.)

Mechanical Digestion: Gastrointestinal Motility

Beginning in the mouth, muscles and nerves in the walls of the gastrointestinal tract coordinate their actions to provide the necessary motility for digestion to proceed. The word *motility* means the ability to move spontaneously. This automatic response to the presence of food enables the system to break up the food mass and move it along the digestive pathway at the best rate. Muscles and nerves work together to produce this smoothly running motility.

Muscles.   The layers of smooth muscle composing the gastrointestinal wall interact to provide two general types of movement, as follows: (1) *muscle tone* or tonic contraction, which ensures continuous passage of the food mass and valve control along the way; and (2) *periodic muscle contraction and relaxation*, which are rhythmical waves that mix the food mass and move it forward. These alternating muscular contractions and relaxations that force the contents forward are known as *peristalsis*, a term from two Greek words: *peri-* meaning "around" and *-stalsis* meaning "contraction."

Nerves.   Specific nerves regulate these muscle actions. A complex network of nerves in the gastrointestinal wall extends from the esophagus to the anus. This network is called the intramural nerve plexus. These nerves do three things, as follow: (1) control muscle tone in the wall; (2) regulate the rate and intensity of the alternating muscle contractions; and (3) coordinate all of the various movements. When all is well, these many, finely tuned movements flow together like those of a great symphony, and you are unaware of them. But when all is not well, you feel the discord as pain.

Chemical Digestion: Gastrointestinal Secretions

A number of secretions work together to make chemical digestion possible. There are generally five types of substances involved: the basic enzymes that break down the food materials, and four other substances that help these enzymes do their specific jobs.

Enzymes.   Digestive enzymes are proteins, specific in kind and quantity for breaking down specific nutrients.

Hydrochloric acid and buffer ions.   Hydrochloric acid and buffer ions are needed to produce the correct pH (i.e., degree of acidity or alkalinity) required for enzyme activity.

Mucus.   Secretions of mucus lubricate and protect the mucosal tissues lining the gastrointestinal tract, as well as help to mix the food mass.

Water and electrolytes.   The products of digestion are carried and circulated through the tract and into the tissues by water and electrolytes.

Bile.   Made in the liver and stored in the gallbladder, bile divides fat into smaller pieces to expose more surface area for the actions of fat enzymes.

Special secretory cells in the intestinal tract and nearby accessory organs (i.e., pancreas and liver) produce these enzymes for their specific jobs in chemical digestion. The secretory action of these special cells or glands is stimulated by the following: (1) the presence of food, (2) nerve impulse, or (3) hormones specific for certain nutrients.

Digestion in the Mouth and Esophagus

Mechanical Digestion

In the mouth, the process of *mastication* (i.e., biting and chewing) begins to break up the food into smaller particles. The teeth and oral structure are particularly suited for this work. After the food is chewed, the mixed mass of food particles is swallowed and passes down the esophagus largely by peristaltic waves controlled by nerve reflexes. Muscles at the base of the tongue facilitate the swallowing process. Then, if the body is in the usual upright position, gravity aids the movement of food down the esophagus. At the entrance to the stomach, the gastroesophageal sphincter muscle that controls food passage relaxes to allow the food to enter, then constricts again to retain the food. If this muscle does not work properly or a part of the stomach protrudes upward into the chest (thorax) causing the fairly common *hiatal hernia*, "heartburn" from the bit of acid-mixed food being pushed back up into the lower esophagus is felt after eating. Heartburn has nothing to do with the heart but has been called this because sensations are perceived as originating in the region of the heart.

Chemical Digestion

The salivary glands secrete material containing a salivary amylase called *ptyalin*. *Amylase* is the general name for any starch-splitting enzyme. Small glands at the back of the tongue secrete a *lingual lipase*. *Lipase* is the general name for any fat-splitting enzyme, but in this case the food does not remain in the mouth long enough for much chemical action to occur. The salivary glands also secrete a mucous

material that lubricates and binds food particles to facilitate the swallowing of each food *bolus*, or lump of food material. Mucous glands also line the esophagus, and their secretions help move the food mass toward the stomach.

Digestion in the Stomach

Mechanical Digestion

The major parts of the stomach are shown in Figure 9-2. Under sphincter muscle control from the esophagus, which joins the stomach at the cardiac notch, the food enters the *fundus*—the upper portion of the stomach—in individual bolus lumps as swallowed. In the body of the stomach, muscles in the stomach wall gradually knead, store, mix, and propel the food mass forward in slow, controlled movements. By the time the food mass reaches the *antrum*—the lower portion of the stomach, it is now a semiliquid, acid-food mix called chyme. A

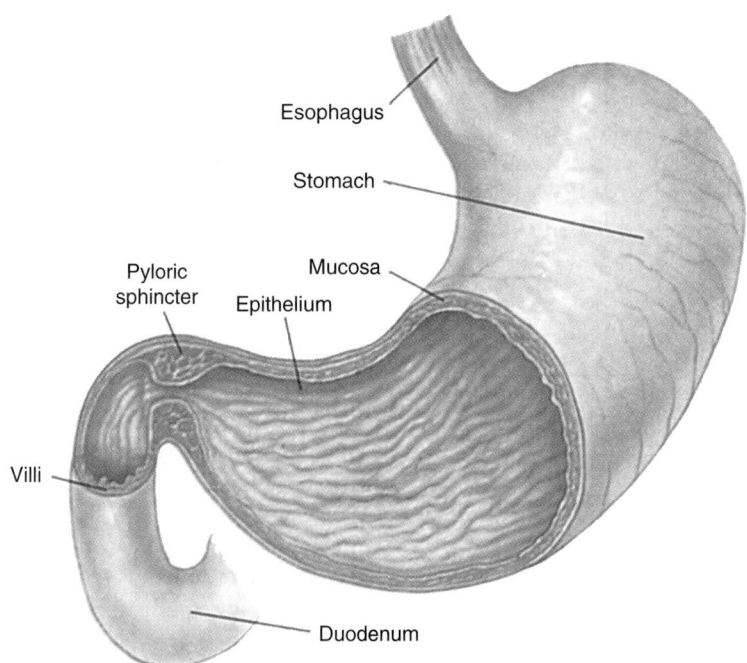

Esophagus

Stomach

Pyloric
sphincter

Mucosa

Epithelium

Villi

Duodenum

FIGURE 9-2 Stomach. (Credit: Bill Ober, from Raven PH, Johnson GB: *Biology,* ed 3, NewYork, 1992, McGraw-Hill.)

constricting sphincter muscle at the end of the stomach, the *pyloric valve*, controls the flow at this point. This valve releases the acidic chyme slowly so that it can be quickly buffered by the alkaline intestinal secretions and not irritate the mucosal lining of the *duodenum*, which is the first section of the small intestine. The caloric density of a meal, which is mainly due to its fat component—not just its volume or particular composition, influences the rate of stomach emptying at the pyloric valve.[1]

Chemical Digestion

The gastric secretions contain three types of materials that aid chemical digestion in the stomach.

Acid. Special cells produce hydrochloric acid to create the necessary degree of acidity for gastric enzymes to work.

Mucus. Special mucous secretions protect the stomach lining from the erosive effect of the acid. Secretions also bind and mix the food mass and help move it along.

Enzymes. The inactive enzyme form *pepsinogen* is secreted by special cells and is activated by the acid to become the major protein-splitting enzyme pepsin. Other cells produce small amounts of a specific gastric lipase called *tributyrinase* because it works on tributyrin (butterfat), but this is a relatively minor activity in the stomach.

Various sensations, emotions, and foods stimulate nerve impulses that trigger these secretions. It is not without reason that the stomach is said to "mirror the person within." For example, anger and hostility increase secretions. Fear and depression decrease secretions, as well as inhibit blood flow and motility. Additional hormonal stimulus comes when food enters the stomach.

Digestion in the Small Intestine

Up to this point, digestion of food has been largely mechanical, delivering a semifluid mixture of fine food particles and watery secretions to the small intestine. Chemical digestion has been minimal. Thus the major task of digestion and the absorption that follows occurs in the small intestine. The structural parts, synchronized movements, and array of specific enzymes of the small intestine are highly developed for the all-important, final task of mechanical and chemical digestion.

Mechanical Digestion

Under the control of nerve impulses, walls stretch from the food mass or hormonal stimuli, and the intestinal muscles produce several types of movement that aid digestion, as follow[2]:

- *Peristaltic waves* slowly push the food mass forward, sometimes with long, sweeping waves over the entire length of the intestine.
- *Pendular movements* from small, local muscles sweep back and forth, stirring the chyme at the mucosal surface.
- *Segmentation rings* from the alternating contraction and relaxation of circular muscles progressively chop the food mass into successive soft lumps and mix them with secretions.
- *Longitudinal rotation* by long muscles running the length of the intestine rolls the slowly moving food mass in a spiral motion, mixing it and exposing new surfaces for absorption.
- *Surface villi motions* stir and mix the chyme at the intestinal wall, exposing additional nutrients for absorption.

---

salivary amylase (Gr. *amylon,* starch) a starch-splitting enzyme in the mouth, sometimes called *ptyalin* (Gr. *ptyalon,* spittle) that is secreted by the salivary glands.

chyme (Gr. *chymos,* juice) semifluid flood mass in the gstrointestinal tract following gastric digestion.

pepsin (Gr. *pepsis,* digestion) the main gastric enzyme specific for proteins. Pepsin begins breaking large protein molecules into shorter chain polypeptides; gastric hydrochloric acid is necessary to activate.

Chemical Digestion

To meet the major burden of chemical digestion, this portion of the gastrointestinal system, together with its accessory organs—pancreas, liver, and gallbladder—supplies many secretory materials.

Pancreatic enzymes

1. *Carbohydrate*: Pancreatic amylase converts starch to the disaccharides maltose and sucrose.
2. *Protein*: Trypsin and chymotrypsin split large protein molecules into smaller and smaller peptide fragments, and finally into single amino acids. Carboxypeptidase removes end amino acids from peptide chains.
3. *Fat*: Pancreatic lipase converts fat to glycerides and fatty acids.

Intestinal enzymes

1. *Carbohydrate*: Disaccharidases (e.g., maltase, lactase, sucrase) convert their respective disaccharides (e.g., maltose, lactose, sucrose) to monosaccharides (e.g., glucose, fructose, galactose). Most of the world's population does not actually produce enough lactase to digest lactose (milk sugar). As a result, these individuals cannot tolerate milk and milk products well, unless they are in some "predigested" form (e.g., yogurt, buttermilk, or cheese, or lactase-treated milk).
2. *Protein*: The intestinal enzyme enterokinase activates trypsinogen (from the pancreas) to become the protein-splitting enzyme trypsin. Amino peptidase removes end amino acids

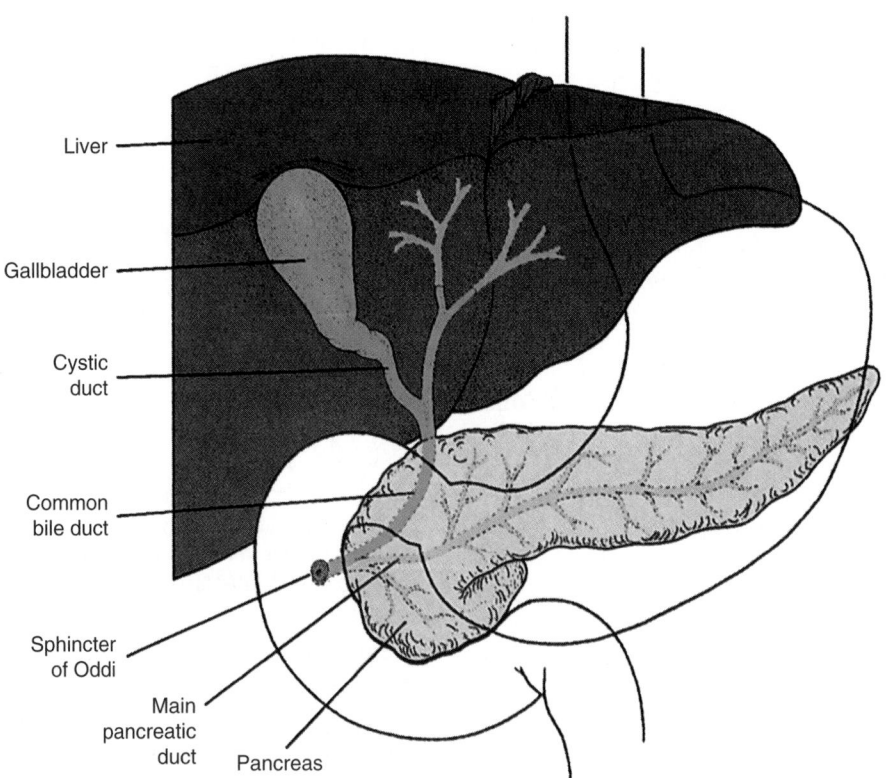

Liver

Gallbladder

Cystic duct

Common bile duct

Sphincter of Oddi

Main pancreatic duct

Pancreas

FIGURE 9-3 Organs of the biliary system and the pancreatic ducts.

from polypeptides. Dipeptidase splits dipeptides into their two remaining amino acids.

3. *Fat*: Intestinal lipase splits fat into glycerides and fatty acids.

Mucus.   Large quantities of mucus, secreted by intestinal glands, protect the mucosal lining from irritation and erosion caused by the highly acidic gastric contents entering the duodenum.

Bile.   The emulsifying agent bile is an important aid to fat digestion and absorption. Bile is produced by the liver and stored in the adjacent gallbladder, ready for use when fat enters the intestine.

Hormones.   The hormone *secretin*, which is produced by the mucosal glands in the first part of the intestine, controls the secretion and acidity of enzymes from the pancreas. The resulting alkaline environment in the small intestine—pH 8—is necessary for the activity of the pancreatic enzymes. The hormone *cholecystokinin*, which is secreted by intestinal mucosal glands when fat enters, triggers release of bile from the gallbladder to emulsify the fat.

The arrangement of the accessory organs to the duodenum, the first section of the small intestine, is shown in Figure 9-3. These organs compose the biliary system and have vital roles in digestion and metabolism. The liver is sometimes called the "metabolic capital" of the body because it has numerous functions in the metabolism of all the converging nutrients. The portal blood circulation drains the small intestine directly to the liver for immediate cell enzyme work in energy production, protein metabolism, and rapid conversion of fat into lipoproteins for transport to body cells. A metabolic "pool" of nutrients and metabolites is maintained for a constant supply of cells and to provide for metabolic waste removal (e.g., ultimate removal of nitrogen and maintenance of nitrogen balance). The liver's many metabolic functions are reviewed in greater detail in Chapter 18.

The various nerve and hormone controls of digestion are illustrated in Figure 9-4. Although

small individual summaries of digestion are given in each of the major nutrient chapters, a general summary of the entire digestive processes is given in Table 9-1 so that the overall process can be viewed as it is—one continuous, integrated *whole*.

ABSORPTION

When digestion is complete, our original food has been changed into simple end products that are the nutrients ready for the cells to use. Carbohydrate foods are reduced to the *simple sugars* glucose, fructose, and galactose. Fats are transformed into *fatty acids* and *glycerides*. Protein foods are changed to single *amino acids*. Vitamins and minerals are also liberated. With a water base for solution and transport, in addition to the necessary electrolytes, the whole fluid food-derived mass is now prepared for absorption as part of the large "gastrointestinal circulation." The large, 10-L volume of this daily circulating absorption is shown in Table 9-2. For many nutrients—especially certain vitamins and

pancreatic amylase major starch-splitting enzyme that is secreted by the pancreas and acts in the small intestine.

trypsin (Gr. *trypein*, to rub; *pepsis*, digestion) a protein-splitting enzyme formed in the small intestine by action of enterokinase on the inactive precursor trypsinogen.

chymotrypsin (Gr. *chymos*, semifluid food mass from digestion; *trypein*, enzyme trypsin) one of the protein-splitting and milk-curdling pancreatic enzymes activated in the small intestine from the precursor chymotrypsinogen; breaks specific amino acid peptide links of protein.

carboxypeptidase (L. *carbo-*, carbon; *oxy*, oxygen) a protein enzyme that splits off the chemical group *carboxyl* (-COOH) at the end of peptide chains.

pancreatic lipase (Gr. *lipos*, fat) a major fat-splitting enzyme produced by the pancreas and secreted into the small intestine to digest fat.

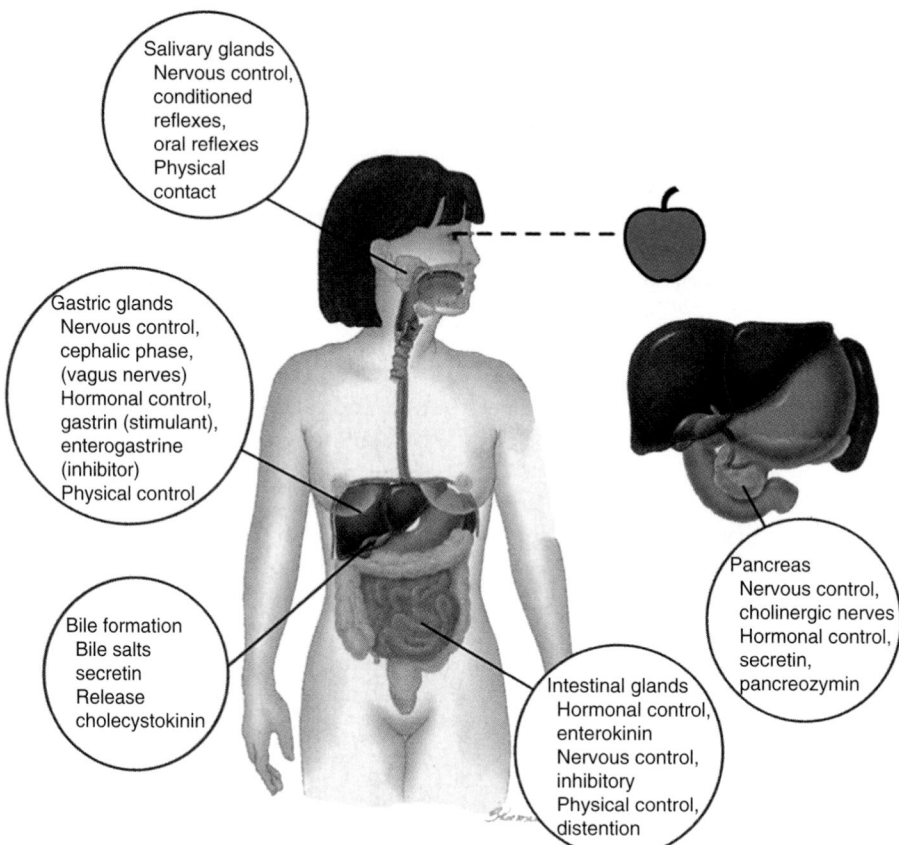

FIGURE 9-4 Summary of the factors influencing secretions of the gastrointestinal tract. (Credit: Modified from Lisa Shoemaker; apple by Eileen Draper, from Thibodeau GA, Patton KT: *Anatomy and physiology,* ed 4, St. Louis, 1999, Mosby.)

minerals, the point of absorption becomes the vital "gatekeeper" that determines how much of a given nutrient is kept for body use. This degree of *bioavailability* is a factor in setting dietary intake standards.[3,4]

Absorption in the Small Intestine

Special Absorbing Structures

Three important structures of the surface of the intestinal wall are particularly adapted to ensure maximum absorption of essential nutrients freed from food in the digestive process (Figure 9-5).

1. *Mucosal folds:* Like the hills and valleys of a mountain range, the surface of the small intestine piles into many folds. Mucosal folds can easily be seen when such tissue is examined.

2. *Villi:* Closer examination under a regular light microscope reveals small, fingerlike projections—the villi—covering the piled-up folds of mucosal lining. These little villi further increase the area of exposed surface. Each villus has an ample supply of blood vessels to receive protein and carbohydrate materials, as well as a special lymph vessel to receive fat materials. This lymph vessel is

TABLE 9-1 Summary of digestive processes

Carbohydrate	Protein	Fat
Mouth		
Starch $\xrightarrow{\text{Ptyalin}}$ Dextrins		Fat $\xrightarrow{\text{Lipase}}$ Glycerides
Stomach		
	Protein $\xrightarrow{\text{Hydrochloric acid}}$ Polypeptides (Pepsin)	Tributyrin (butterfat) $\xrightarrow{\text{Tributyrinase}}$ Glycerol Fatty acids
Small intestine		
Pancreas	*Pancreas*	*Pancreas*
(Disaccharides)	Protein, Polypeptides $\xrightarrow{\text{Trypsin}}$ Dipeptides	Fat $\xrightarrow{\text{Lipase}}$ Glycerol
Starch $\xrightarrow{\text{Amylase}}$ Maltose and sucrose	Protein, Polypeptides $\xrightarrow{\text{Chymotrypsin}}$ Dipeptides	Glycerides](di-, mono-) Fatty acids]
	Polypeptides, Dipeptides $\xrightarrow{\text{Carboxypeptidase}}$ Amino acids	
Intestine	*Intestine*	*Intestine*
(Monosaccharides)	Polypeptides, Dipeptides $\xrightarrow{\text{Aminopeptidase}}$ Amino acids	Fat $\xrightarrow{\text{Lipase}}$ Glycerol
Lactose $\xrightarrow{\text{Lactase}}$ Glucose and galactose	Dipeptides $\xrightarrow{\text{Dipeptidase}}$ Amino acids	Glycerides](di-, mono-) Fatty acids]
Sucrose $\xrightarrow{\text{Sucrase}}$ Glucose and fructose		*Liver and gallbladder*
Maltose $\xrightarrow{\text{Maltase}}$ Glucose and glucose		Fat $\xrightarrow{\text{Bile}}$ Emulsified fat

TABLE 9-2   Daily absorption volume in human gastrointestinal system

	Intake (L)	Intestinal absorption (L)	Elimination (L)
Food ingested	1.5		
Gastrointestinal secretions	8.5		
TOTAL	10.0		
Fluid absorbed in small intestine		9.5	
Fluid absorbed in large intestine		0.4	
TOTAL		9.9	
Feces			0.1

called a *lacteal* because the fatty chyme is creamy at this point and looks like milk.

3. *Microvilli:* Even closer examination with an electron microscope reveals a multiple covering of smaller projections on the surface of each tiny villus. The covering of microvilli on each villus is called a *brush border* because it looks like bristles on a brush.

These three unique structures of the inner intestinal wall—folds, villi, and microvilli—combine to make the inner surface some 600 times the area of the outer surface of the intestine. The length of the small intestine is about 660 cm (22 feet). This remarkable organ is well-adapted to deliver its precious nutrients into circulation to the body cells. In fact, the small intestine can scarcely be equaled in its feat of providing such an absorbing surface area in so compact a space. It has been estimated that if its entire surface were spread out on a flat plane, the total surface area would be as large or larger than half a basketball court. Far from being the lowly "gut," the small intestine is actually one of the most highly developed, exquisitely fashioned, specialized tissues in the human body.[5]

Absorption Processes

A number of absorbing processes complete the task of moving vital nutrients across the inner intestinal wall and into body circulation. These processes include diffusion—both passive or simple for small materials and carrier-assisted for larger items, energy-driven active transport with the help of a "ferrying" substance, and penetration of larger materials through engulfing pinocytosis (see Chapter 8).

Routes of Absorption

Most of the products of digestion are water-soluble nutrients, which can therefore be absorbed directly

---

mucosal folds (L. *mucus,* mucosa) large visible folds of the mucus lining of the small intestine that increase the absorbing surface area.

villi (L. *villus,* tuft of hair) small protrusions from the surface of a membrane; fingerlike projections covering mucosal surfaces of the small intestine that further increases the absorbing surface area; visible through a regular microscope.

microvilli (Gr. *mikros,* small; L. *villus,* tuft of hair) exceedingly small hairlike projections covering all villi on the surface of the small intestine and greatly extending the total absorbing surface area; visible through electron microscope.

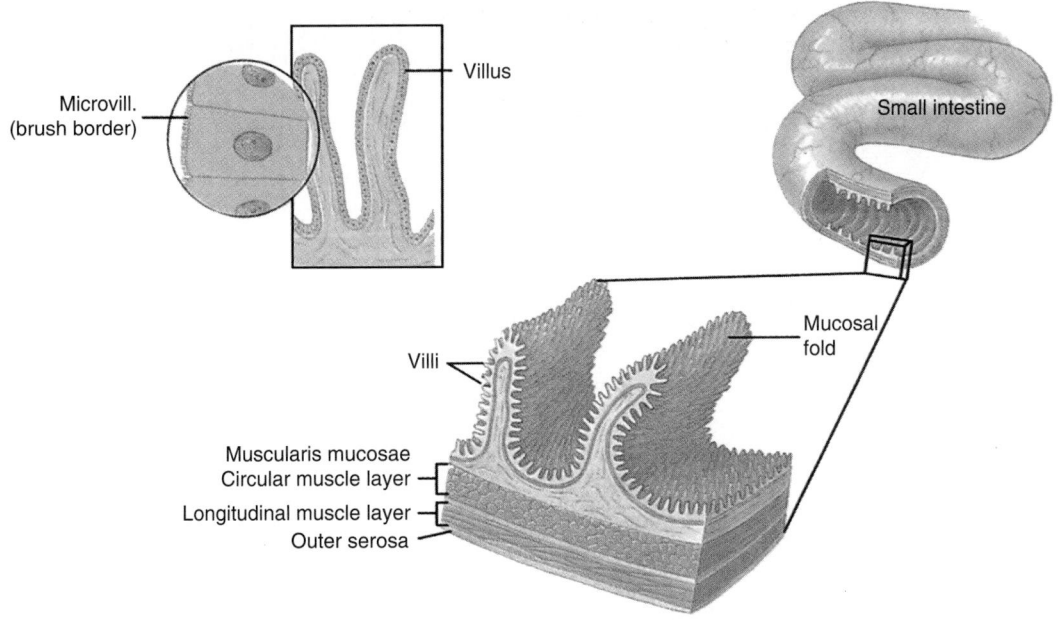

FIGURE 9-5 Intestinal wall. Note the arrangement of muscle layers and the structures of the mucosa that increase the surface area for absorption—mucosal folds, villi, and microvilli. (Credit: Medical and Scientific Illustration.)

into the bloodstream. Because fatty materials are not water-soluble, another route must be provided. These fat molecules pass into the lymph vessels in the villi (i.e., the lacteals), flow into the larger lymph vessels of the body, and eventually enter the blood.

Absorption in the Large Intestine

Water

The main absorptive task remaining for the large intestine is to take up needed body water. Most of the water in the chyme entering the large intestine is absorbed in the first half of the colon. Only a

small amount (about 100 ml) remains to form and eliminate the feces.

Dietary Fiber

Food fiber is not digested because humans lack the specific enzymes required. Dietary fiber, however, contributes important bulk to the food mass throughout the process of digestion-absorption and helps to form the feces. The formation and passage of intestinal gas is a normal process but is embarrassing to some individuals (see Clinical Applications box, "The Sometimes Embarrassing Effects of Digestion-Absorption"). Table 9-3 summarizes major features of intestinal nutrient absorption.

SUMMARY

Necessary nutrients as they occur in food are not available to us but must be changed, released, regrouped, and rerouted in forms our body cells can use. Two closely related activities—digestion and absorption—ensure that key food nutrients

are delivered to the cells so that the multiple metabolic tasks that sustain our lives can be completed.

Mechanical digestion consists of spontaneous muscular activity that is responsible for the

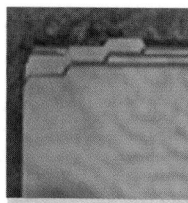

CLINICAL APPLICATIONS

The Sometimes Embarrassing Effects of Digestion-Absorption

After eating a meal or certain foods, some persons complain of the discomfort and/or embarrassment of gas. This gas is a normal byproduct of digestion, but when it becomes painful or apparent to others it may become a physical and social problem.

The gastrointestinal tract normally holds about 3 oz of gas that move along with the food mass and are silently absorbed into the bloodstream. Sometimes extra gas collects in the stomach or intestine, creating an embarrassing—though usually harmless—situation.

Stomach gas

Gas in the stomach results from air bubbles trapped there and occurs when a person eats too fast, drinks through a straw, or otherwise takes in extra air while eating. Burping relieves this gas, but these tips may help to avoid a social slip:

- Avoid carbonated beverages.
- Don't gulp.
- Chew with your mouth closed.
- Don't drink from a can or through a straw.
- Don't eat when you're nervous.

Intestinal gas

The passing of gas from the intestine is usually a social embarrassment. This gas forms in the colon, where bacteria attack undigested items, causing them to decompose and produce gas. Carbohydrates release hydrogen, carbon dioxide, and—in some people with certain types of bacteria in the gut—*methane*. All three of these products are odorless (though noisy) gases. Protein produces *hydrogen sulfide* and such volatile compounds as *indole* and *skatole*, which add a distinctive aroma to the expelled air. The following suggestions may help to control the problem:

- Cut down on simple carbohydrates (i.e., sugars). Especially observe milk's effect because *lactose intolerance* may be the real culprit. Substitute cultured forms such as yogurt or milk treated with a lactase product such as LactAid.
- Use a prior leaching process before cooking dry beans, to remove indigestible saccharides such as *raffinose* and *stachyose*. Although humans cannot digest these substances, they provide a feast for bacteria in the intestines. This simple procedure eliminates a major portion of these gas-forming saccharides. First, put washed beans into a large pot, add 4 cups of water for each pound (about 2 cups) of beans, and boil beans uncovered for 2 minutes. Then remove pot from heat, cover, and let stand for 1 hour. Finally, drain and rinse the beans, add 8 cups fresh water, bring to a boil, reduce heat, and simmer in covered pot for 1 to 2 hours, until beans are tender. Season as desired.
- Eliminate known food offenders. These vary among individuals but some of the most common offenders are beans (if not prepared for cooking as described above), onions, cabbage, and high-fiber wheat products.

Once relief is achieved, *slowly* add more complex carbohydrates and high fiber foods back to the diet. Once small amounts are tolerated, try moderate increases. If there is still no relief, medical help may be needed to rule out or treat an overactive gastrointestinal tract.

TABLE 9-3 Intestinal absorption of some major nutrients

Nutrient	Form	Means of absorption	Control agent or required cofactor	Route
Carbohydrate	Monosaccharides (glucose and galactose)	Competitive	—	Blood
		Selective	—	
		Active transport via sodium pump	Sodium	
Protein	Amino acids	Selective	—	Blood
	Some dipeptides	Carrier transport systems	Pyridoxine (pyridoxal phosphate)	Blood
	Whole protein (rare)	Pinocytosis	—	Blood
Fat	Fatty acids	Fatty acid-bile complex (micelles)	Bile	Lymph
	Glycerides (mono-, di-)		—	Lymph
	Few triglycerides (neutral fat)	Pinocytosis	—	Lymph
Vitamins	B_{12}	Carrier transport	Intrinsic factor (IF)	Blood
	A	Bile complex	Bile	Blood
	K	Bile complex	Bile	From large intestine to blood
Minerals	Sodium	Active transport via sodium pump	—	Blood
	Calcium	Active transport	Vitamin D	Blood
	Iron	Active transport	Ferritin mechanism	Blood (as transferritin)
Water	Water	Osmosis	—	Blood, lymph, interstitial fluid

following: (1) initial mechanical breakdown by means such as mastication, and (2) movement of the food mass along the gastrointestinal tract by motions such as peristalsis. Chemical digestion involves enzymatic action that breaks food down into smaller and smaller components and releases its nutrients for absorption.

Absorption involves the passage of food nutrients from the intestines to the bloodstream across the intestinal wall. It occurs mainly in the small intestine by means of highly efficient intestinal wall structures that, together with a number of effective absorbing mechanisms, increase the absorbent surface area.

REVIEW QUESTIONS

1. Describe the types of muscle movement involved in mechanical digestion. What does the word *motility* mean? How are the nerves involved?

2. Identify digestive enzymes and any related substances secreted by the following glands: salivary and mucosal glands, pancreas, and liver. What activities they perform on carbohydrates,

proteins, and fats? What stimulates the release of these enzymes? What inhibits their activity?

3. Describe four mechanisms of nutrient absorption from the small intestine. Describe the routes taken by the breakdown products of carbohydrates, proteins, and fats after absorption. Why must an alternate route to the bloodstream be provided?

4. What functions does the large intestine perform?

SELF-TEST QUESTIONS

True-False

Write the correct statement for each item you answer "false."

1. The digestive products of a large meal are difficult to absorb because the overall area of the absorbant surface of the intestines is relatively small.

2. Before they can work, some enzymes must be activated by hydrochloric acid or other enzymes.

3. Bile is an enzyme specifically used for fat breakdown.

4. The "gastrointestinal circulation" provides a constant supply of water and electrolytes to carry digestive secretions and substances being produced.

5. Secretions from the gastrointestinal accessory organs—the gallbladder and the pancreas—mix with gastric secretions to aid digestion.

6. An enzyme may work on more than one nutrient.

7. Bile is released from the gallbladder in response to a hormonal stimulus.

Multiple Choice

1. During digestion, the major muscle action that moves the food mass forward in regular rhythmic waves is called:
   a. Valve contraction.
   b. Segmentation ring motion.
   c. Muscle tone.
   d. Peristalsis.

2. Gastrointestinal secretory action is affected by:
   a. Blood pressure.
   b. Peristalsis.
   c. Speed of eating.
   d. Emotions such as anger and fear.

3. Mucus is an important gastrointestinal secretion because it:
   a. Causes chemical changes in substances to prepare for enzyme action.
   b. Helps create proper degree of acidity for enzymes to act.
   c. Lubricates and protects the gastrointestinal lining.
   d. Helps to emulsify fats for enzyme action.

4. Pepsin is:
   a. Produced in the small intestine to act on protein.
   b. A gastric enzyme that acts on protein.
   c. Produced in the pancreas to act on fat.
   d. Produced in the small intestine to act on fat.

5. Bile is an important secretion that is:
   a. Produced by the gallbladder.
   b. Stored in the liver.
   c. An aid to protein digestion.
   d. A fat-emulsifying agent.

6. The route of fat absorption is:
   a. The lymphatic system via the villi lacteals.
   b. Directly into the portal blood circulation.
   c. With the aid of bile directly into the villi blood capillaries.
   d. With the aid of protein directly into the portal blood circulation.

SUGGESTIONS FOR ADDITIONAL STUDY

1. On 3 successive days eat the following breakfasts:

    Day 1: All fruit breakfast—eat several fruits and fruit juices only.

    Day 2: Eat only fruit juice, 1-2 slices of white toast with jelly, and hot tea or coffee with sugar.

    Day 3: Eat only 1-2 slices of toast with a generous amount of butter or margarine, 2-4 slices of bacon, 2 eggs scrambled in the bacon fat, and tea or coffee with cream.

    On each day, record the time that you first felt hungry. Compare each breakfast's food combination. Which food combination satisfied you for the longest? How do you account for this difference?

REFERENCES

1. Green HL, Moran JR: *The gastrointestinal tract: regulator of nutrient absorption*. In Shils ME, Olson JA, Shike M, eds: *Modern nutrition in health and disease*, ed 8, Philadelphia, 1994, Lea & Febiger.
2. Guyton AC, Hall JE: *Textbook of medical physiology*, ed 9, Philadelphia, 1996, Saunders.
3. National Research Council, Food and Nutrition Board: *Recommended dietary allowances*, ed 10, Washington, D.C., 1989, National Academy Press.
4. National Research Council, Food and Nutrition Board, Committee on diet and health: *Diet and health, implications for reducing chronic disease risks*, Washington, D.C., 1989, National Academy Press.
5. Marsh MN, Riley SA: *Digestion and absorption of nutrients and vitamins*. In Feldman M, Scharschmidt BF, Sleisenger MH eds: *Gastrointestinal and liver disease*, ed 6, vol 2, Philadelphia, 1998, Saunders.

FURTHER READING

• Hertzler SR and others: How much lactose is low lactose?, *J Am Diet Assoc* 96(3):243, 1996.
• Strocchi A, Levitt MD: *Intestinal gas*. In Feldman M, Scharschmidt BF, Sleisenger MH, eds: *Gastrointestinal and liver disease*, vol 1, ed 6, Philadelphia, 1998, Saunders.

These interesting references will provide clear answers to your questions about why persons worldwide who are allergic to milk have lactose intolerance and thus cannot drink milk or eat foods made with the milk sugar lactose.

• Mattes RD: Physiologic responses to sensory stimulation by food: nutritional implications, *J Am Diet Assoc* 97(4):406, 1997.

This author explains the various physical responses we may have experienced while eating particular foods.

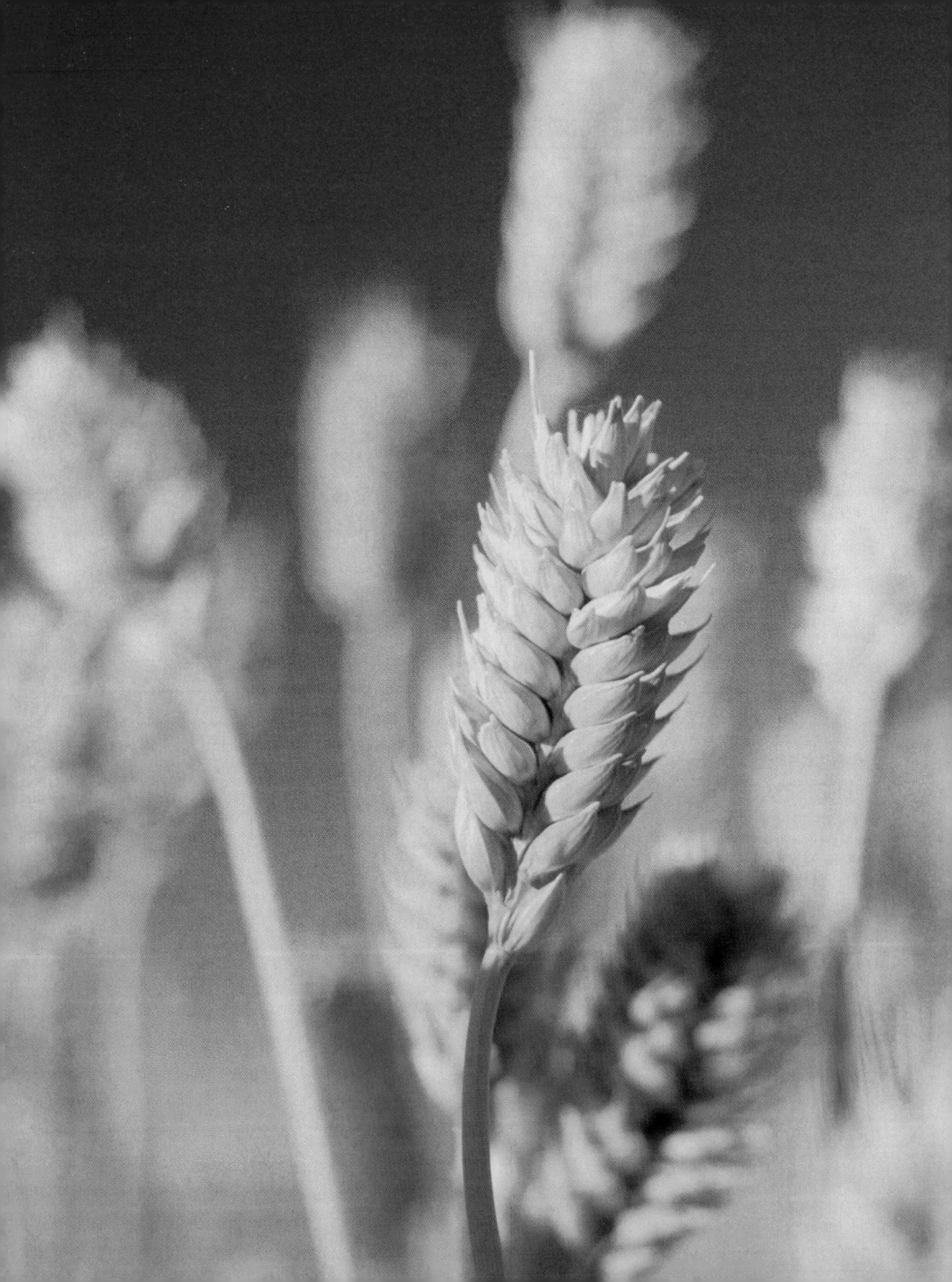

Nutrition Throughout the Life Cycle

2

10

Nutrition during Pregnancy and Lactation

KEY CONCEPTS

● The mother's food habits and nutritional status before conception, as well as during pregnancy, influence the outcome of the pregnancy.

● Pregnancy is a prime example of physiologic synergism in which the mother, fetus, and placenta collaborate to sustain and nurture new life.

● Through the food a pregnant woman eats, she gives her unborn child the nourishment required to begin and sustain fetal growth and development.

● Through her diet, a breast-feeding mother continues to provide all of her nursing baby's nutritional needs.

Healthy body tissues depend directly on certain essential nutrients in food. This is especially true during pregnancy because a whole new body is being formed. The tremendous growth of a baby from the moment of conception to the time of birth depends entirely on nourishment from the mother's food. The complex processes of rapid, specialized human growth demand increased amounts of nutrients from the mother.

In this chapter we look at the beginnings of life and see that the infant's fetal development and the mother's supporting tissues directly relate to the mother's diet. We explore the nutritional needs of pregnancy and the lactation period that follows and recognize the vital role each plays in producing a healthy infant.

MATERNAL NUTRITION AND THE OUTCOME OF PREGNANCY

Not many years ago, traditional practices and diet during pregnancy were highly restrictive in nature, built upon assumptions and folklore of the past and having little or no basis in scientific fact. Early obstetricians even developed the notion that semi-starvation of the mother during pregnancy was a blessing in disguise because it produced a small, lightweight baby who was easy to deliver. To this end, they used a diet restricted in kcalories, protein, water, and salt for pregnant women.

Developments in both nutritional and medical science have refuted these ideas and laid a sound base for positive nutrition in current maternal care. Old dogma, however, dies hard. Shreds of old beliefs are sometimes still evidenced, but we now know that it is very important to both the mother's and child's health that a pregnant woman eat a well-balanced diet with increased amounts of all the essential nutrients. In fact, women who have always eaten a well-balanced diet are in a good state of nutrition at conception—even before they know they are pregnant. Such women have a better chance of having a healthy baby and remaining in good health than women who have been undernourished.

POSITIVE NUTRITIONAL DEMANDS OF PREGNANCY

The 9 months between the time of conception and the birth of a fully formed baby is a marvelous period of rapid growth and intricate functional development. All of these tremendous activities require increased energy and nutrient support to produce a positive, healthy outcome. General guidelines for these increases are provided in both the classic RDA and the new comprehensive DRI standards[1-5] (see Appendix G).

The RDA and DRI guidelines are based on general needs for healthy populations. Some women (e.g., those who are poorly nourished when becoming pregnant or those carrying additional risks) demand more

nutritional support. First, we review the basic nutritional needs for positive support of a normal pregnancy, with emphasis on critical energy and protein requirements and key mineral and vitamin needs. In each case, there are reasons for the increased demand, the general amount of increase, and the food sources to supply it. In the following section, we underscore the importance of sufficient weight gain and the problems facing high-risk mothers and infants.

Energy Needs

Reasons for Increased Need

Energy intake during pregnancy is measured in terms of the kcalorie value of the food the mother eats. The mother needs more kcalories for two important reasons, as follow: (1) to supply the increased fuel demanded by the enlarged metabolic workload, and (2) to spare protein for the added tissue-building requirements. At least 36 kcal/kg are required for efficient use of protein during pregnancy. For these reasons, the mother must have more food—especially more nutrient-dense food.[6]

Amount of Energy Increase

The national standard recommends an increase of about 300 kcal per day (i.e., for a total of about 2200 to 2500 kcals) during pregnancy, which is about a 15% to 20% increase over the energy need of nonpregnant women. Even more energy is needed by active, large, or nutritionally deficient women, who may require as much as 2700 to 3000 kcals per day. The emphasis should always be on ample kcalories to secure nutrient and energy needs. Sufficient weight gain is vital to a successful pregnancy and indicates if sufficient kcalories are provided. Increased carbohydrate in the diet is the preferred source of these increased energy demands, especially during late pregnancy and lactation.

Protein Needs

Reasons for Increased Need

Protein is a primary need during pregnancy because it is the growth element for body tissues. Reasons for this increased need reflect the tremendous growth involved in pregnancy.

Rapid growth of the baby. The mere increase in size of the infant from one cell to millions of cells in a 3.2-kg (7-lb) child in only 9 months indicates the relatively large amount of protein required for such rapid growth.

Development of the placenta. The placenta is the fetus's lifeline to the mother. The mature placenta requires sufficient protein for its complete development as a vital and unique organ to sustain, support, and nourish the fetus during growth.

Growth of maternal tissues. To support the pregnancy, increased development of breast and uterine tissue is required.

Increased maternal blood volume. The mother's blood volume increases 20% to 50% during pregnancy. More circulating blood is necessary to nourish the child and support most of the increased metabolic workload. With extra blood volume, however, comes a need for more synthesis of blood components—especially hemoglobin and plasma protein, which are proteins vital to the pregnancy. The hemoglobin increase supplies oxygen to the growing number of cells, and the plasma protein (albumin) increase helps the greater blood volume circulate enough tissue fluids between the capillaries and the cells. Albumin in the blood provides the osmotic force constantly needed to pull the tissue fluids back into circulation after they have bathed and nourished the cells, thus preventing an abnormal accumulation of water in the tissues beyond the normal physiologic edema of pregnancy.

Amniotic fluid. Amniotic fluid surrounds the fetus during growth and guards it against shock or injury. Amniotic fluid contains proteins, so its formation requires still more protein.

Storage reserves. Increased storage reserves of tissue—especially fuel stores as adipose fat tissues—are needed in the mother's body to prepare for the large amount of energy required during labor, delivery, the immediate postpartum period, and lactation.

Amount of Increase

Protein intake should increase to 10 g per day during pregnancy, making the total protein need 60 g/day. This increase is about a 20% increase over the average adult requirement. A large number of high-risk or active pregnant women, however, need even more protein.

Food Sources

The only *complete* protein foods of high biologic value are milk, egg, cheese, and meat. Certain other *incomplete* proteins from plant sources such as legumes and grains contribute additional secondary amounts. Protein-rich foods also contribute other nutrients, such as calcium, iron, and B vitamins. The amounts of these foods that supply the needed protein are indicated in the daily core food plan given in Table 10-1.

Key Mineral and Vitamin Needs

Increases in all minerals and vitamins are needed during pregnancy to meet the greater structural and metabolic requirements. These increases are

---

hemoglobin (Gr. *haima*, blood; L. *globus*, globe) a conjugated protein in red blood cells that is composed of a compact, rounded mass of polypeptide chains forming *globin,* the protein portion, and attached to an iron-containing red pigment called *heme*. Carries oxygen in the blood to cells.

plasma protein any of a number of protein substances carried in the circulating blood. A major one is *albumin,* which maintains the fluid volume of the blood through its colloidal osmotic pressure.

albumin (L. *albus,* white) a major protein in many animal and plant tissues; specialized plasma protein maintaining normal blood pressure.

TABLE 10-1 Daily food guide for women

Food group	One serving equals	Recommended minimum servings		
		Nonpregnant		Pregnant/ lactating
		11–24 yr	25+ yr	
Protein foods	**ANIMAL PROTEIN:**	5	5	7
Provide protein, iron, zinc, and B vitamins for growth of muscles, bone, blood, and nerves. Vegetable protein provides fiber to prevent constipation.	1 oz cooked chicken or turkey			
	1 oz cooked lean beef, lamb, or pork			
	1 oz or ¼ cup fish or other seafood			
	1 egg			
	2 fish sticks or hot dogs			
	2 slices luncheon meat			
	VEGETABLE PROTEIN:	A half serving of vegetable protein daily		One serving of vegetable protein daily
	½ cup cooked dry beans, lentils, or split peas			
	3 oz tofu			
	1 oz or ¼ cup peanuts, pumpkin, or sunflower seeds			
	1½ oz or ⅓ cup other nuts			
	2 tbsp peanut butter			
Milk products	8 oz milk	3	2	3
Provide protein and calcium to build strong bones, teeth, and healthy nerves and muscles and to promote normal blood clotting.	8 oz yogurt			
	1 cup milk shake			
	1½ cups cream soup (made with milk)			
	1½ oz or ⅓ cup grated cheese (like cheddar, Monterey, mozzarella, or Swiss)			
	1½-2 slices presliced American cheese			
	4 tbsp Parmesan cheese			
	2 cups cottage cheese			
	1 cup pudding			
	1 cup custard or flan			
	1½ cups ice milk, ice cream, or frozen yogurt			
Breads, cereals, grains	1 slice bread	7	6	7
Provide carbohydrates and B vitamins for energy and healthy nerves. Also provide iron for healthy blood. Whole grains provide fiber to prevent constipation.	1 dinner roll	Four servings of whole grain products daily		Four servings of whole grain products daily
	½ bun or bagel			
	½ English muffin or pita			
	1 small tortilla			
	¾ cup dry cereal			
	½ cup granola			
	½ cup cooked cereal			
	½ cup rice			
	½ cup noodles or spaghetti			
	¼ cup wheat germ			
	1 4-inch pancake or waffle			
	1 small muffin			
	8 medium crackers			
	4 graham cracker squares			
	3 cups popcorn			

Vitamin C-rich fruits and vegetables

Provide vitamin C to prevent infection and promote healing and iron absorption. Also provide fiber to prevent constipation.

6 oz orange, grapefruit, or fruit juice enriched with vitamin C	
6 oz tomato juice or vegetable juice cocktail	
1 orange, kiwi, or mango	
½ grapefruit or cantaloupe	
½ cup papaya	
2 tangerines	
½ cup strawberries	
½ cup cooked or 1 cup raw cabbage	
½ cup broccoli, brussels sprouts, or cauliflower	
½ cup snow peas, sweet peppers, or tomato puree	
2 tomatoes	1 1

Vitamin A-rich fruits and vegetables

Provide beta-carotene and vitamin A to prevent infection and promote wound healing and night vision. Also provide fiber to prevent constipation.

6 oz apricot nectar or vegetable juice cocktail	
3 raw or ¼ cup dried apricots, ¼ cantaloupe or mango	
1 small or ½ cup sliced carrots	
2 tomatoes	
½ cup cooked or 1 cup raw spinach	
½ cup cooked greens (beet, chard, collards, dandelion, kale, mustard)	
½ cup pumpkin, sweet potato, winter squash, or yams	1 1 1

Other fruits and vegetables

Provide carbohydrates for energy and fiber to prevent constipation.

6 oz fruit juice (if not listed above)	
1 medium or ½ cup sliced fruit (apple, banana, peach, pear)	
½ cup berries (other than strawberries)	
½ cup cherries or grapes	
½ cup pineapple	
½ cup watermelon	
¼ cup dried fruit	
½ cup sliced vegetable (asparagus, beets, green beans, celery, corn, eggplant, mushrooms, onion, peas, potato, summer squash, zucchini)	
½ artichoke	
1 cup lettuce	3 3 3

Unsaturated fats

Provide vitamin E to protect tissue.

⅛ med. avocado	
1 tsp margarine	
1 tsp mayonnaise	
1 tsp vegetable oil	
2 tsp salad dressing (mayonnaise-based)	
1 tbsp salad dressing (oil-based)	3 3 3

NOTE: The Daily Food Guide for Women may not provide all the kcalories you require. The best way to increase your intake is to include more than the minimum servings recommended.

Adapted from California Department of Health Services, Maternal and Child Health: *Nutrition during pregnancy and postpartum period: a manual for health care professionals,* Sacramento, 1990, CDHS.

indicated in the RDA and DRI tables in Appendix G. Several of these essential substances have key roles in pregnancy, however, and require special attention.

Calcium

A good supply of calcium, along with phosphorus and vitamin D, is essential for fetal development of bones and teeth, as well as the mother's own body needs. Calcium is also necessary for proper clotting of blood. A diet that includes 3 to 4 cups of fortified milk daily plus generous amounts of green vegetables, enriched whole grains, and eggs usually supplies enough calcium. In cases of poor maternal stores or pregnancies involving more than one fetus, calcium supplements are needed. Because food sources of the major minerals calcium and phosphorus are almost the same, a diet sufficient in calcium also provides enough phosphorus.

Iron and Iodine

Particular attention is given to iron and iodine intake during pregnancy. Iron is essential for the increased hemoglobin synthesis required for the greater maternal blood volume, as well as for the baby's necessary prenatal storage of iron. Because iron occurs in small amounts in food sources, and much of this intake is not in a readily absorbable form, the maternal diet alone can rarely meet needs. Thus the current standard recommends a daily iron intake of 30 g, which is twice a woman's normal need. Because the increased pregnancy requirement cannot be met by the iron content of typical U.S. diets or the iron stores of some women, however, daily iron supplements are usually recommended.[5] Adequate iodine intake is essential for producing more thyroxine, which is the thyroid hormone needed in greater amounts to control the increased basal metabolic rate during pregnancy. This increased iodine need is easily ensured by the use of iodized salt.

Vitamins

Increased attention to all vitamins is needed to support a healthy pregnancy. Vitamins A and C are needed in increased amounts during pregnancy because they are both important elements in tissue growth. The B vitamins are needed in increased amounts because of their vital roles as coenzyme factors in energy production and protein metabolism. Folate is especially needed to build mature red blood cells.

Folate is also particularly needed during the early periconceptional period (i.e., from about 2 months before conception to week 6 of gestation) to ensure healthy embryonic tissue development and prevent malformation of the *neural tube*.[7] This tissue forms during the critical period from 17 to 30 days gestation and grows into the mature infant's spinal column and its network of nerves. A neural tube defect results in a malformed spinal cord and the severely disabling condition spina bifida, which affects about 3000 newborns in the United States each year. The DRI standard recommends a daily folate intake of 600 μg, which is more than a nonpregnant woman's need of 400 μg/day. Women who do not eat well or have less than optimal food habits may need a folate supplement during pregnancy.

The increased vitamin D need to ensure absorption and utilization of calcium and phosphorus for fetal bone growth is met by the mother's intake of 3 to 4 cups of fortified milk in her daily food plan. Fortified milk contains 10 μg (400 IU) of cholecalciferol (vitamin D) per quart, which is twice the AI amount. The mother's general exposure to sunlight will produce more.

Daily Food Plan

General Basic Plan

Some form of a food plan must be developed for pregnant women on an individual basis to meet their increased nutritional needs. Such a core plan (see Table 10-1) can serve as a guideline, with additional amounts of foods used as needed for sufficient kcalories. This core food plan is built upon basic foods available in American markets and designed to supply necessary nutrient increases. The standards for individual nutrients apply throughout the pregnancy, so such a core food guide with additional foods as needed should provide the required nutrients. Energy needs increase as the pregnancy progresses, and the recommended increment of 300 kcal/day applies to the second and third trimesters. Adolescent, underweight, or malnourished women, however, need special attention to increased energy needs from the outset of the pregnancy.

Alternate Food Patterns

The core food plan provided here may be only a starting point for women with alternate food patterns. Such food patterns exist among women from different ethnic backgrounds, belief systems, and lifestyles, making individual diet counseling essential. *Specific nutrients*—not necessarily specific foods—are required for successful pregnancies and may be found in a variety of foods. Wise health workers encourage pregnant women to use foods that serve both their personal and nutritional needs, whatever such foods may be. Many resources have been developed to serve as guides for a variety of alternative food patterns (e.g., ethnic and vegetarian) (see the further reading list and the Clinical Applications box, "Case Study: A Vegan Child and Her Family," in Chapter 4). If the mother's vegetarian pattern includes dairy products and eggs (lacto-ovo), there is no problem in achieving a sound diet to meet pregnancy needs by increasing the use of animal proteins. Strict vegans who are pregnant are at greater risk.[2] Vitamin B$_{12}$ supplements are mandatory at DRI levels of 2.6 μg/day during pregnancy and 2.8 μg/day during lactation.[2]

Specific counseling on avoidance of alcohol, caffeine, tobacco, and drugs during pregnancy is essential. Information about the direct effects of poor nutrition on the fetus—especially as related to brain development and later learning problems and developmental delays—helps to motivate many pregnant women to choose a well-selected diet of optimal nutritional value. Given the American obsession with thinness—especially among teenage girls, pregnancy is no time to diet.

Basic Principles

Whatever the food pattern, two important principles govern the prenatal diet, as follow: (1) pregnant women should eat a sufficient *quantity* of food, and (2) pregnant women should eat *regular meals and snacks*, avoiding any habit of fasting or skipping meals—especially breakfast.

GENERAL CONCERNS

Functional Gastrointestinal Problems

Nausea and Vomiting

The so-called morning sickness of early pregnancy is usually mild, only occurring briefly during the first trimester. It is caused by hormonal adaptations in the first weeks and may be increased by stress or anxieties about the pregnancy itself. The following simple treatment usually helps relieve symptoms: small frequent meals and snacks that are fairly dry and consist mostly of easily digested energy foods (e.g., carbohydrates) with liquids between—not with—meals. If this sickness becomes severe and prolonged, a condition called *hyperemesis*, medical treatment is required.

Constipation

Although usually a minor complaint, constipation may occur in the latter part of pregnancy as a result of the increasing pressure of the enlarging uterus and the muscle-relaxing effect of placental hormones on the gastrointestinal tract, reducing normal peristalsis. Helpful remedies include adequate exercise, increased fluid intake, and naturally laxative foods such as whole grains, dried

---

spina bifida (L. *spina,* spine; *bifidus,* cleft into two parts or branches) congenital defect in the embryonic-fetal closing of the neural tube to form a portion of the lower spine, leaving the spine unclosed and the spinal cord open in various degrees of exposure and damage.

fruits (especially prunes and figs), and other fruits and juices. Pregnant women should avoid artificial laxatives.

Hemorrhoids

Hemorrhoids (i.e., enlarged veins in the anus, often protruding through the anal sphincter) are a fairly common complaint during the latter part of pregnancy. This vein enlargement is usually caused by the increased weight of the baby and the downward pressure it produces. Hemorrhoids may cause considerable discomfort, burning, and itching and may even rupture and bleed under the pressure of a bowel movement, causing the mother more anxiety. Hemorrhoids are usually controlled by the dietary suggestions given for constipation. Sufficient rest during the latter part of the day may also help relieve some of the downward pressure of the uterus on the lower intestine.

Heartburn

The related complaints of heartburn or a "full feeling" are sometimes voiced by pregnant women. These discomforts occur especially after meals and are caused by the pressure of the enlarging uterus crowding the stomach. Gastric reflux of some of the food (i.e., now a liquid food mass mixed with stomach acid) in the stomach may occur in the lower esophagus, causing irritation and a burning sensation. This common complaint has nothing to do with heart action but is called heartburn because of the close position of the lower esophagus to the heart. The full feeling comes from general gastric pressure, lack of normal space in the area, a large meal, or gas formation. These complaints are usually relieved by dividing the day's food intake into a series of small meals and avoiding large meals at any time. Comfort is also improved by wearing loose-fitting clothing.

Effects of Iron Supplements

An iron supplement is usually given during pregnancy to meet the increased need for iron. The effects of added iron include gray or black stools and sometimes nausea, constipation, or diarrhea. To help avoid food-related effects, iron supplements should be taken an hour before or 2 hours after a meal with a liquid such as water or orange juice—not milk or tea. The effect of the iron in the body is increased with orange juice and decreased with milk, other dairy foods, eggs, whole grain bread and cereal, and tea.

Weight Gain During Pregnancy

Amount and Quality

The mother's optimal weight gain during pregnancy, sufficient to support and nurture her and the fetus, is essential. Weight gain should not be viewed negatively because it is a positive reflection of good nutritional status and contributes to a successful course and outcome of pregnancy and should be assessed individually. The average weight gained is about 11 to 13 kg (25 to 30 lbs) as indicated in Table 10-2. A report of the National Academy of Sciences, *Nutrition During Pregnancy*, recommends setting weight gain goals together with the pregnant woman according to her normal nutritional status and weight-for-height, as follows:[5]

- Normal weight women—25 to 35 lb
- Underweight women—28 to 40 lb

TABLE 10-2 Approximate weight of products of a normal pregnancy

Products	Weight
Fetus	3400 g (7.5 lb)
Placenta	450 g (1 lb)
Amniotic fluid	900 g (2 lb)
Uterus (weight increase)	1100 g (2.5 lb)
Breast tissue (weight increase)	1400 g (3 lb)
Blood volume (weight increase)	1800 g (4 lb) (1500 ml)
Maternal stores	1800-3600 g (4-8 lb)
TOTAL	11000-13000 g (11-13 kg; 24-28 lb)

- Overweight women—15 to 25 lb
- Teenagers—35 to 40 lb (upper end of the recommended range)
- Twin pregnancy—35 to 45 lb (total target)

The important consideration in each case is not only the quantity of the weight gain but also the *quality* of the gain and the foods consumed to bring it about. There is a definite connection between high-risk, low–birth-weight babies and inadequate maternal weight gain during the pregnancy. Severe caloric restriction during pregnancy is not normal and potentially harmful to the developing fetus and to the mother. Such a restricted diet cannot supply all the energy and nutrients essential to the growth process during pregnancy. Thus weight reduction should *never* be undertaken during pregnancy. To the contrary, adequate weight gain—which is more for underweight women—should be supported with the use of a nourishing, well-balanced diet.

Rate of Weight Gain

About 1 to 2 kg (2 to 4 lbs) is the average amount of weight gain during the first trimester (i.e., first 3 months) of pregnancy. Thereafter about 0.5 kg (1 lb) a week during the remainder of the pregnancy is usual, although some women need to gain more. Only unusual patterns of gain (e.g., a sudden sharp increase in weight after the 20th week of pregnancy, possibly indicating excessive and abnormal water retention) must be watched. On the other hand, an insufficient or low maternal weight gain in the second or third trimester increases the risk for intrauterine growth retardation.[6,14] Increased energy demand is normal during late pregnancy and prepares for full infant growth needs and the mother's approaching delivery and lactation. Carbohydrate becomes the preferred energy source.

Role of Sodium

Just as with restriction of kcalories, routine restriction of sodium during pregnancy is physiologically unsound and unfounded. A regular, moderate amount (e.g., about 2 to 3 g/day) of dietary sodium is needed and can be achieved through the general use of salt in cooking and seasoning with limitations of extra use (e.g., a "heavy hand with the shaker") at the table, as well as of obviously salty processed foods. Maintenance of the increased volume of maternal blood, which is normal during pregnancy to support the increased metabolic work, requires adequate amounts of sodium and protein. The National Research Council and the professional nutrition and obstetrics guidelines have labeled routine use of salt-free diets and diuretics as potentially dangerous.

High-Risk Mothers and Infants

Identify Risk Factors Involved

To avoid the results of poor nutrition during pregnancy, mothers at risk should be identified as soon as possible. Pregnancy among teenage girls continues to be a problem in the United States (see Clinical Applications box, "Pregnant Teenagers"). Risk factors that identify the age extremes—teenagers and older women, who have special needs during pregnancy—are given in the Clinical Applications box, "Nutritional Risk Factors in Pregnancy." These nutrition-related factors are based on clinical evidence of inadequate nutrition. Do not wait for clinical symptoms of poor nutrition to appear. The best approach is to identify poor food patterns and prevent nutritional problems from developing. Three types of dietary patterns that will not support optimal maternal and fetal nutrition are as follows: (1) insufficient food intake, (2) poor food selection, and (3) poor food distribution throughout the day.

Plan Personal Care

Every pregnant woman needs personalized care and support during pregnancy. Women with risk factors such as those listed here, however, have special counseling needs. In each case, we must work with the mother in a sensitive and supportive manner to help her develop a healthy food plan that is both practical and nourishing. Dangerous practices, such as diet fads, extreme macrobiotic diets, or *pica*, need to be identified.[10] Pica is the name given to a perverted

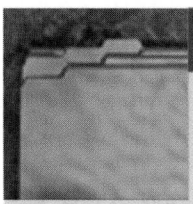

CLINICAL APPLICATIONS
Pregnant Teenagers

Teenage pregnancy continues to be a major public health problem in the United States. Few situations are as life-changing for a single teenage girl and her family as an unintended pregnancy. Depending on how she and her family—as well as her partner—resolve the crisis, there may be lifelong consequences not only for them but also for the broader community.

Pregnant teenagers are at high risk for pregnancy complications and poor outcome with increased rates of low birth weight and infant mortality. The following two problems contribute to these complications: (1) the physiologic demands of the pregnancy compromise the teenager's needs for her own unfinished growth and development; and (2) the psychosocial influences of low income; inadequate diet; the teenage peer culture's experimentation with alcohol, smoking and other drugs; and often little or no access to appropriate prenatal care significantly contribute to a lack of nutritional support for the pregnancy. Early nutrition intervention is essential and can change the course of events and the pregnancy outcome but is not an easy task. Changes from the inconsistent, often poor food pattern of teenagers are difficult to achieve, and their care is challenging. Experienced, sensitive health workers in teen clinics emphasize the need for supportive individual and group nutrition counseling. Nutrition-management programs recommend the following additional suggestions:

- **Know each client personally.** All nutrition services must be tailored to the unique needs and characteristics of each pregnant teenager. Many have lower educational levels and even limited reading skills to which educational material must be adapted. Low-income teens lack the financial resources to maintain an adequate diet, and those living at home may have little control over the food available to them. Personal stress over the pregnancy is paramount and nutrition concerns are often not a priority. Skipping meals and snacking are common; even dieting is frequent.

- **Seek ways to motivate clients.** Schedule appointments on days that clients are coming in to pick up their WIC food packages. Invite the teen's mother and friends to accompany her to group counseling sessions so they can support any recommendations made. Make each recommendation concrete and reasonable. Avoid scare tactics.

- **Make appropriate assessments.** Use simple, concrete forms for evaluating dietary intake (e.g., the basic five food groups of the well-known Food Guide Pyramid [see Chapter 1]). This traditional model can be used, with increased amounts indicated for pregnancy, for both education and assessment at a level teenagers can understand.

- **Make practical interventions.** Plan short, enjoyable, active learning sessions. Use positive reinforcement liberally. Provide specific suggestions for carrying out changes at home. Review progress in follow-up sessions. Always maintain a positive, supportive atmosphere.

- **Support the teenager's responsibility.** Help the teenager learn to be responsible. In the final analysis, pregnant teenagers must take on responsibility—often for the first time—for their own nourishment and for the nourishment of others. Helping them in a supportive manner to understand and carry out this responsibility, which ultimately only they can do, is a main objective of nutrition counseling. Nutrition consultants must be skillful in establishing the kind of rapport and relationship where these responsibilities can develop and grow.

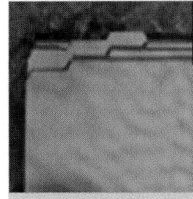

CLINICAL APPLICATIONS
Nutritional Risk Factors in Pregnancy

Risk factors presented at the onset of pregnancy:
- Age: ≤15 years or ≥35 years
- Frequent pregnancies: three or more during a 2-year period
- Poor obstetric history or poor fetal performance
- Poverty
- Bizarre or trendy food habits
- Abuse of nicotine, alcohol, or drugs
- Therapeutic diet required for a chronic disorder
- Weight: <85% or >120% of standard weight

Risk factors occurring during pregnancy:
- Low hemoglobin and/or hematocrit: Hgb <12.0 g; Hct <35.0 mg/dl
- Inadequate weight gain: Any weight loss *or* weight gain of <1 kg (2 lb) per month after the first trimester
- Excessive weight gain: >1 kg (2 lb) per week after the first trimester

appetite or craving for unnatural foods (e.g., chalk, laundry starch, or clay), a practice sometimes seen in pregnancy or in malnourished children.

Recognize Special Counseling Needs
In addition to avoiding dangerous practices such as those stated here, several special needs—including those related to age and *parity* (i.e., number of pregnancies and time in between), detrimental lifestyle habits, and socioeconomic problems—require sensitive counseling.

Age and parity. Pregnancies at either age extreme of the reproductive cycle carry special problems. The adolescent pregnancy adds many social and nutritional risks as its social upheaval and physical demands are imposed on an immature, teenage girl. Sensitive counseling must involve both information and emotional support with good prenatal care throughout. On the other hand, pregnant women who are over 35 years of age and having their first child also require special attention. These women may be more at risk for high blood pressure (i.e., either preexisting or pregnancy-induced) and

need guidance about the rate of weight gain and excessive use of sodium. In addition, women with a high parity rate (i.e., who have had several pregnancies within a limited number of years) may wish to have family-planning guidance because they enter each successive pregnancy at a higher risk, drained of nutritional resources and usually facing the increasing physical and economic pressures of child care. Such counseling may include discussions of acceptable means of contraception and nutrition information and support.

Social habits: alcohol, cigarettes, and drugs. These three personal lifestyle habits cause fetal damage and are contraindicated during pregnancy. Extensive, habitual alcohol use leads to the well-documented *fetal alcohol syndrome* (FAS), which has become a leading cause of mental retardation and other birth defects.[11] Cigarette smoking during pregnancy causes placental abnormalities and fetal damage, including prematurity and low–birth-weight (see Clinical Application box, "Who Will Have the Low–Birth-Weight Baby"), largely due to impaired oxygen transport.[12]

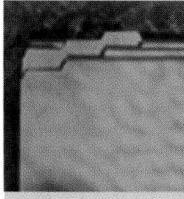

CLINICAL APPLICATIONS
Who Will Have the Low–Birth-Weight Baby?

The number of babies weighing less than 2500 g (5 lb) at birth is still a problem. Perinatal nutritionists are aware of the dietary factors—especially poor weight gain during pregnancy—that influence this increase. The prevalence of the turn-of-the-century adage to "grow the baby to fit the pelvis" continues to influence some physicians, nurses, and expectant mothers to limit prenatal weight gain to 9 kg (20 lb) or less to avoid obstetric problems at delivery. This practice is harmful and is refuted by current evidence that a weight gain of 25 to 35 lb for average-weight women and 28 to 40 lb for underweight women correlates with a birth weight of over 2500 g (5 lb).

The obsession with weight control during pregnancy can lead to harmful restrictions of vital energy and nutrients. Weight reduction should *never* be attempted during pregnancy. Such diets are extremely dangerous to the fetus. Even the common habit of skipping breakfast—especially late in pregnancy, may impair intellectual development by quickly producing a state of pseudostarvation. Increased ketoacidosis from fat breakdown can cause neurologic damage to the fetus.

Nondietary factors influencing the trend toward more low–birth-weight (LBW) babies include the following:

- Rise in number of older first-time mothers (i.e., over 35 years of age)
- Rise in number of teenage pregnancies
- Previous induced abortions
- Technologic advances in neonatal care, which keeps premature infants alive longer
- Race: nonwhites have higher rates of LBW infants than whites

To reduce the risk of LBW infants in mothers you may be counseling, you may want to do the following:

- Explain the reasons for gaining sufficient weight as recommended
- Help mothers who smoke or drink to stop using cigarettes or alcohol
- Monitor excessive weight gain and sodium intake in older first-time mothers, who are at risk for prenatal essential hypertension and obesity
- Explore the eating habits of teenagers, working with the girl and the baby's father, if possible, to include nutrient-dense foods in her meals and snacks
- Stay informed of federal, state, and local supplemental food programs (e.g., the WIC program [see Chapter 14]) that ensure an adequate intake of nutrients in low-income women
- Encourage regular eating patterns throughout pregnancy

Drug use, both medicinal and recreational, poses many problems. Self-medication with over-the-counter drugs carries potential adverse effects. The use of illegal drugs is especially dangerous to the developing fetus, causing the baby to be born addicted or with AIDS from the mother's use of contaminated needles. Dangers come not only from the drug itself or contaminated needles but also from the impurities that street drugs contain. Vitamin abuse from megadosing with basic nutrients such as vitamin A during pregnancy may also bring fetal damage. Drugs made from vitamin A compounds (e.g., retinoids such as *etretinoin* [Accutane], which is prescribed for severe acne) have caused spontaneous abortion of malformed fetuses by women who conceived during such acne treatment. Thus the use of these drugs without contraception is definitely contraindicated.

Caffeine. Depending on extent of its use, the effect of caffeine during pregnancy is much milder than the effects of the agents discussed previously. Caffeine, however, is still a widely used drug that can cross the placenta and enter fetal circulation. Its use at pharmacologic levels has been associated with low–birth-weight babies.[13] A pharmacologic dose of caffeine (i.e., 250 mg) is contained in 2 cups of coffee, 3.5 cups of tea, or 5 12-oz colas, so such use is not recommended. Responsible health agencies recommend that pregnant women avoid caffeine-containing beverages and that products containing caffeine are plainly labeled to inform consumers.

Socioeconomic problems. Special counseling is required for women and young girls living in low-income situations. Poverty especially puts pregnant women in grave difficulty because they need resources for financial assistance and food supplements. Nutritionists and social workers on the health care team can provide special counseling and referrals. Community resources include programs such as the special Supplemental Food Program for Women, Infants, and Children (WIC), which has helped many low-income mothers have healthy babies (Figure 10-1).

Complications of Pregnancy

Anemia
Anemia is common during pregnancy. About 10% of the women in large U.S. prenatal clinics have low hemoglobin and hematocrit levels. Anemia is more prevalent among poor women, many of whom live on marginal diets barely adequate for subsistence but is by no means restricted to lower economic groups. A deficiency of iron or folate in the

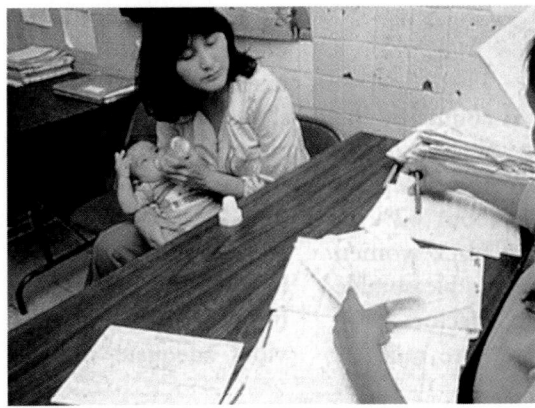

FIGURE 10-1 This mother is a participant in the WIC program. (Credit: U.S. Department of Agriculture.)

mother's diet can cause nutritional anemia, so dietary intake must be determined and supplements used as indicated.[2] During the second and third trimesters of pregnancy, a low-dose iron supplement of 30 mg of ferrous iron daily can provide the amount of extra iron needed.

Neural Tube Defect
The DRI recommendation of 400 μg/day for women who are capable of becoming pregnant is increased to 600 μg/day during pregnancy.[2] This is especially important when individual dietary adequacy is doubtful or there is a genetic high risk for neural tube defect in the family. Women who do not frequently eat fruit, juices, whole-grain or fortified cereals, and green leafy vegetables are likely to have low folate intake.

Intrauterine Growth Failure
Many studies have shown what good sense and experience clearly indicate: children born with intrauterine growth retardation (IUGR) have multiple survival and growth problems.[14] Many factors may contribute to IUGR, but low prepregnancy weight gain—primarily inadequate weight gain during pregnancy—and continuing to smoke are strong factors. In adolescents, low weight gain by

20 weeks into the pregnancy has been shown to carry a twofold risk.[14]

Pregnancy-Induced Hypertension (PIH)

Formerly called *toxemia*, pregnancy-induced hypertension (PIH) is primarily a disease of malnutrition that is especially related to diets low in protein, kcalories, calcium, and salt. Such malnutrition affects the liver and its metabolic activities. PIH has classically been associated with poverty and most often found in women subsisting on inadequate diets with little or no prenatal care. Symptoms of PIH, which occur in late pregnancy near term, are elevated blood pressure, abnormal and excessive water retention, albumin in the urine, and—in severe cases—convulsions, a condition called *eclampsia*. Specific treatment varies according to individual symptoms and needs, but in any case optimal nutrition is basic. Emphasis is given to adequate dietary protein, kcalories, salt, minerals, and vitamins.

Gestational Diabetes

During pregnancy, sugar in the urine (i.e., *glycosuria*) is not uncommon. In susceptible women, it results from the increased metabolic workload during pregnancy and the increased volume of blood with its load of metabolites including glucose. Some of this extra glucose then "spills over" into the urine. For this reason, prenatal clinics routinely screen each pregnant woman and provide careful follow-up for those who show glycosuria or have blood glucose levels above 110 mg (6.1 mmol/L) within 2 hours after a meal. Particular attention is given to women at higher risk for developing pregnancy-induced (i.e., *gestational*) diabetes, including those age 30 and over who are overweight and unfit and have a history of any of the following predisposing factors:

- Family diabetes
- Previously unexplained stillbirths
- Large babies weighing 4 kg (9 lb) or more
- Habitual abortions
- Birth of babies with multiple congenital defects
- Excessive obesity

Gestational diabetes occurs in about 2% to 13% of pregnant women. Although only 20% to 30% of these women subsequently develop diabetes, it is nevertheless important to identify them and provide close follow-up testing and treatment with special diet and insulin as needed. These women are at higher risk for fetal damage, prematurity, or delivery of a very large baby—a complicating condition called *macrosomia* that is associated with survival dangers. Current studies of pregnant women have also shown elevated blood lipid levels where there had been no previous history.[15]

Pre-Existing Disease

Pre-existing clinical conditions, such as hypertension, diabetes, phenylketonuria (PKU), or other diseases, complicate pregnancy. In each case, a woman's pregnancy is managed—usually by a team of specialists—according to the principles of care related to pregnancy and the particular disease involved.

LACTATION

Trends

In America and other developed countries, the number of mothers choosing to breast-feed their babies has been increasing but has leveled off somewhat at present, with about 62% of white women and 25% of black women nursing their babies and finding it a pleasurable experience (Figure 10-2). The following factors have contributed to this choice: (1) more mothers are informed about the benefits of breast feeding; (2) practitioners recognize that human milk can meet unique infant needs, as shown in Table 10-3; (3) maternity wards and alternative birth centers are being modified to support successful lactation; and (4) community support is more available, even in some workplaces.[16-18] Almost all women who choose to breast feed their infants can do so.[19] Well-nourished mothers who breast feed exclusively provide adequate nutrition from 2 to 15 months, with solid foods usually added to the baby's diet at about 6 months of age.

Nutritional Needs

The basic diet followed during pregnancy, as well as the prenatal nutrient supplement used, can be continued through the lactation period. In general, attention to three lactation supports is needed.

Diet

Milk production requires energy (i.e., about 800 kcal/day) for both the process and the product. Thus more food is needed for more kcalories. Because some of this energy need may be partially met by extra fat stored during pregnancy, the national standard is 500 kcal/day throughout lactation more than a woman's normal need of about 2200 kcal, for a total of 2700 kcal/day. The need for protein during lactation is 15 g/day more than a woman's normal need of 50 g, for a total of 65 g/day. These lactation energy and nutrient increases are shown in the RDA standards (see Appendix G). The core food plan for meeting these lactation needs (see Table 10-1) includes 4 to 5 cups of milk; 6 to 8 oz lean meat; 1 to 2 eggs; 1 to 2 servings of dark green or yellow vegetables; 2 servings of vitamin C-rich fruits and vegetables; 4 to 6 servings of other vegetables, fruits, and juices; 10 servings of whole-grain or enriched breads and cereals; and moderate amounts of butter or fortified margarine. Notice the increases in the amount of each food group needed during pregnancy.

Fluids

Because milk is a fluid tissue, breast feeding mothers need fluids for adequate milk production. Water and other beverages such as juices and milk add to the fluid necessary to produce milk. Beverages containing alcohol and caffeine should be limited or avoided because they are secreted to some extent in the mother's milk.

Rest and Relaxation

In addition to the increased diet and adequate fluids, breast feeding mothers require rest, moderate exercise, and relaxation. The nurse and dietitian often help by counseling mothers about their new family situations and may help them to develop plans to meet their personal needs.

Advantages of Breast Feeding

There are many physiologic and practical advantages to breast feeding, including the following: (1) *fewer infections*, because the mother transfers certain antibodies or immune properties in human

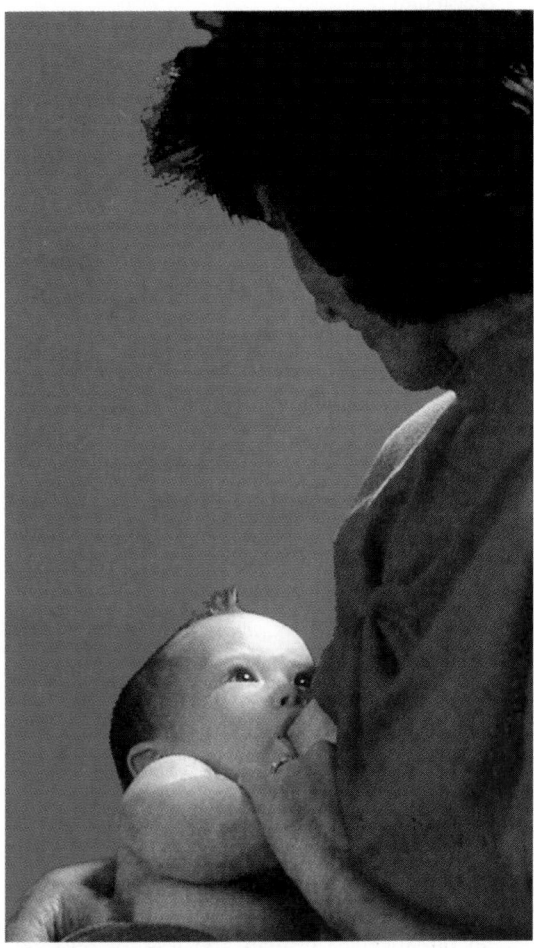

FIGURE 10-2 Breast-feeding infant and mother. (Credit: La Leche League.)

TABLE 10-3 Nutritional components of human milk (per 100 ml)

Milk component	Colostrum*	Transitional†	Mature‡	Cow's milk
Kilocalories	57.0	63.0	65.0	65.0
Vitamins, fat-soluble:				
A (μg)	151.0	88.0	75.0	41.0
D (IU)	—	—	5.0	2.5
E (mg)	1.5	0.9	0.25	0.07
K (μg)	—	—	1.5	6.0
Vitamins, water-soluble:				
Thiamin (μg)	1.9	5.9	14.0	43.0
Riboflavin (μg)	30.0	37.0	40.0	145.0
Niacin (μg)	75.0	175.0	160.0	82.0
Panthothenic acid (μg)	183.0	288.0	246.0	340.0
Biotin (μg)	0.06	0.35	0.6	2.8
Vitamin B_{12} (μg)	0.05	0.04	0.1	0.6
Vitamin C (mg)	5.9	7.1	5.0	1.1

*On delivery.

†Delivery to approximately 4 weeks.

‡Human milk after approximately 4 weeks.

milk to her nursing infant; (2) *fewer allergies and intolerances*, especially in allergy-prone infants, because cow's milk contains a number of potentially allergy-causing proteins that human milk does not have; (3) *ease of digestion*, because human milk forms a softer curd in the gastrointestinal tract that is easier for the infant to digest; and (4) *convenience and economy*, because the mother is freed from the time and expense involved in buying and preparing formula, and her breast milk is always ready and sterile. In a recent position paper, the American Dietetic Association encourages breast feeding for all able mothers.[19]

SUMMARY

Pregnancy involves the fundamental interaction of the following three distinct—yet unified—biologic entities: the fetus, the placenta, and the mother. Maternal needs also reflect the increasing nutritional needs of the fetus and the placenta. Optimal weight gain varies with the normal nutritional status and weight of the woman, with a goal of about 25 to 35 lb for a woman of average weight but more for an underweight woman and less for an overweight woman. Sufficient weight gain is important during pregnancy to support the rapid growth taking place. The nutritional quality of the diet, however, is as significant as the actual weight gain.

Common problems during pregnancy include first-trimester nausea and vomiting associated with hormonal adaptations and later constipation, hemorrhoids, or heartburn resulting from the pressure of the enlarging uterus. These problems are usually relieved without medication by simple, often temporary, changes in the diet. Unusual or irregular eating habits, age, parity, prepartum weight status, and low income are among the many related conditions that put pregnant women at risk for complications.

The ultimate goal of prenatal care is a healthy infant and a healthy mother who can breast feed her child, if she chooses to do so. Human milk provides essential nutrients in quantities that are uniquely suited for optimal infant growth and development.

REVIEW QUESTIONS

1. List six nutrients that are required in larger amounts during pregnancy. Describe their special roles, and identify four food sources of each.
2. Identify two common gastrointestinal problems associated with pregnancy and describe the diet management of each.
3. List and describe five major nutritional factors to support lactation. What additional, nonnutritional needs does the breast feeding mother have, and what suggestions can you give to help her meet them?

SELF-TEST QUESTIONS

True-False

Write the correct statement for each item you answer "false."

1. The development of the fetus is directly related to the diet of the mother.
2. Strict weight control during pregnancy is necessary to avoid complications.
3. Salt should be removed from the pregnant woman's diet to prevent edema.
4. A higher risk for pregnancy complications occurs in teenage and older women.
5. A woman's diet prior to pregnancy has little effect on the outcome of her pregnancy.
6. No woman should ever gain more than 15 to 20 lbs during pregnancy.
7. Rapid growth of the fetal skeleton requires increased calcium in the mother's diet.
8. Inadequate vitamin D during pregnancy contributes to faulty skeletal development in the fetus.
9. Anemia is common during pregnancy because iron requirements are increased.
10. Additional kcalories and fluids are needed during lactation.

Multiple Choice

1. Blood volume _____ during pregnancy.
   a. Increases
   b. Decreases
   c. Remains unchanged
   d. Fluctuates widely
2. Which of the following foods are complete proteins of high biologic value and hence should be increased during pregnancy?
   a. Enriched whole grains and breads
   b. Milk, eggs, and cheese
   c. Beans, peas, and lentils
   d. Nuts and seeds
3. Which of the following foods has the highest iron content to help meet the need for increased iron during pregnancy?
   a. Lean beef
   b. Liver
   c. Orange juice
   d. Milk
4. The increased need for vitamin A during pregnancy may be met by increased use of foods such as:
   a. Nonfat milk.
   b. Extra egg whites.
   c. Citrus fruits.
   d. Carrots.

SUGGESTIONS FOR ADDITIONAL STUDY

1. Nutritional Analysis of a Pregnant Woman's Diet:

A. Using the general guides in this book, interview a pregnant woman to learn about her food habits and environment.

B. From your account of her typical daily food intake pattern, calculate her intake of the following key nutrients: kcalories, protein, calcium, iron, vitamin A, and vitamin C.

C. Using the information from your interview about her living and family situation and her food habits, plan with her a suitable daily food plan to meet her increased nutritional needs during pregnancy.

2. Cultural Food Pattern in Pregnancy

A. Select any one of the various cultural food patterns. Plan a prenatal diet within this pattern to meet the increased nutritional demands of pregnancy.

B. If possible, interview a pregnant woman of this cultural group and analyze her diet.

3. Diet for Lactation

A. Interview a breast feeding mother of a newborn baby to determine her food habits and questions about a diet during lactation.

B. Discuss with her the lactation process and help her with successful breast feeding techniques.

REFERENCES

1. Food and Nutrition Board, Institute of Medicine: *Dietary reference intakes for calcium, phosphorous, magnesium, vitamin D, and fluoride*, Washington, DC, 1998, National Academy Press.
2. Food and Nutrition Board, Institute of Medicine: *Dietary reference intakes for thiamin, riboflavin, niacin, vitamin B6, folate, vitamin B12, pantothenic acid, biotin, and choline*, National Academy Press, Washington, DC, 1999.
3. Food and Nutrition Board, Institute of Medicine: *Dietary reference intakes for vitamin C, vitamin E, selenium, and carotenoids*, Washington, DC, 2000, National Academy Press.
4. National Research Council, Food and Nutrition Board: *Recommended dietary allowances*, ed 10, Washington, DC, 1989, National Academy Press.
5. National Academy of Sciences, Committee on Nutritional Status During Pregnancy and Lactation, Food and Nutrition Board: *Nutrition during pregnancy*, Washington, DC, 1990, National Academy Press.
6. Butte, NF and others: Adjustments in energy expenditure and substrate utilization during late pregnancy and lactation, *Am J Clin Nutr* 69(1):299, 1999.
7. Slattery ML, Janerich DT: The epidemiology of neural tube defects: a review of dietary intake and the related factors as etiologic agents, *Am J Epidemiol* 33(6):526, 1991.
8. Kloeben AS: Folate knowledge, intake from fortified grain products, and periconceptional supplementation patterns of a sample of low-income pregnant women according to the Health Belief Model, *J Am Diet Assoc* 99(1):33, 1999.
9. Mackey AD, Picciano MF: Maternal folate status during extended lactation and the effect of supplemental folic acid, *Am J Clin Nutr* 69(1):285, 1999.
10. Rainville AJ: Pica practices of pregnant women are associated with lower maternal hemoglobin level at delivery, *J Am Diet Assoc* 98(3):293, 1998.
11. Larroque B and others: Moderate prenatal alcohol exposure and psychomotor development at preschool age, *Am J Public Health* 85(12):1654, 1995.
12. Hellerstadt WL and others: The effects of cigarette smoking and normal weight women, *Am J Public Health* 87(4): 591, 1997.
13. Hinds TS and others: The effect of caffeine on pregnancy outcome variables, *Nutr Rev* (7):203, 1996.
14. Strauss RS, Dietz WH: Low maternal weight gain in the second or third trimester increases the risk for intrauterine growth retardation, *J Nutr* 129(5):988, 1999.
15. Jovanovic L: Time to reassess the optimal dietary prescription for women with gestational diabetes, *Am J Clin Nutr* 70 (1):3, 1999.
16. Beshgetor D and others: Attitudes toward breast-feeding among WIC employees in San Diego County, *J Am Diet Assoc* 99(1):86, 1999.
17. Chezem J, Friesen C: Attendance at breast-feeding support meetings: relationship to demographic characteristics and duration of lactation in women planning postpartum employment, *J Am Diet Assoc* 99(1):83, 1999.
18. Kannan S and others: Cultural influences on infant feeding beliefs of mothers, *J Am Diet Assoc* 99(1):88, 1999.
19. Position of The American Dietetic Association: promotion of breast-feeding, *J Am Diet Assoc*, 1997: 97(6):662, 1997.

FURTHER READING

- Gord C: Nutrition for a healthy pregnancy: national guidelines for the childbearing years, *Can J Diet Pract Res* 60(2): Summer 1999.

  This excellent resource provides helpful guidance for healthy pregnancies, as well as important information for identifying women at nutritional risk.

- Vozenilek GP: What they don't know could hurt them: increasing public awareness of folic acid and neural tube defects, *J Am Diet Assoc* 99(1):20, 1999.

  This brief article draws a clear picture of the cloud of ignorance that still hangs over the general population about the devastating results of neural tube defects in an affected child from birth, due to the mother's folic acid deficiency early in pregnancy.

11

Nutrition in Infancy, Childhood, and Adolescence

KEY CONCEPTS

- Normal growth of individual children varies within a relatively wide range of measures.

- Human growth and development require both nutritional and psychosocial support.

- A variety of food patterns and habits supply the energy and nutrient requirements of normal growth and development, although basic nutritional needs change with each growth period.

In any culture, food nurtures both the physical and the personal "growing up" process for each infant, child, or adolescent. Food, feeding, and eating during these significant years of childhood do not and cannot exist apart from the broader overall process of growth and development. The *whole* process produces the *whole* person.

In this chapter, we consider food and feeding in an individual and unique manner, as a basic part of "growing up" for each person. We then relate the various age-group nutritional needs and food patterns to individual psychosocial development, as well as physical growth.

NUTRITION FOR GROWTH AND DEVELOPMENT

Life Cycle Growth Pattern

The normal human life cycle follows four general stages of overall growth, with individual variances along the way.

Infancy

Growth is rapid during the first year of life, with the rate tapering off somewhat in the latter half of the year. Most infants double their birth weight by the time they are 6 months of age and triple it by 1 year of age.

Childhood

Between infancy and adolescence, the childhood growth rate slows and becomes irregular. Growth occurs in small spurts, during which children have increased appetites and eat accordingly. Plateaus occur in between, during which children have little or no appetite and eat less. Parents who recognize this as a normal growth pattern in the "latent period of childhood" will relax, enjoy their child, and not make eating a battle issue.

Adolescence

The onset of puberty begins the second stage of rapid growth, which continues until adult maturity. The flooding sex hormones and increased growth hormone bring multiple and often bewildering body changes to young adolescents. During this period, long bones grow rapidly, sex characteristics develop, and fat and muscle mass increase.

Adulthood

With physical maturity comes the final phase of a normal life cycle. Physical growth levels off during adulthood and then gradually declines during old age. Mental and psychosocial development, however, lasts a lifetime.

Measuring Childhood Growth

Individual Growth Rates

Children grow normally at widely varying rates. Therefore the best counsel for parents is that children are *individuals*. One child should not be compared with another. Growth is not inadequate because its rate does not equal that of another child. General measures of growth in children relate not only to physical development but also to mental, emotional, social, and cultural growth.

Physical Growth

Growth charts such as those developed by the National Center for Health Statistics (NCHS) provide a broad base for growth in children today. These charts are based on large numbers of children representing our national population. They are used as guides to see an individual child's pattern of physical growth in relation to the general percentile growth curves on the charts. Individual measures of physical growth in a child include weight and height, body measurements, general signs of health, laboratory tests, and nutritional study of general eating habits.

Psychosocial Development

Tests are used to measure mental, emotional, social, and cultural growth and development. Food is intimately related to these aspects of psychosocial development, as well as to physical growth. The growing child does not learn food attitudes and habits in a vacuum but in close personal and social relationships.

NUTRITIONAL REQUIREMENTS FOR GROWTH

Energy Needs

Kilocalories

The demand for energy, as measured in kcalories from food, is relatively large during childhood. The general recommendations for energy and nutrient needs at different ages are given in the RDA and DRI tables in Appendix G. Individual need, however, varies with age and condition. For example, the total daily caloric intake of a 5-year-old child is spent in the following way:

Basal metabolism—50%
Physical activities—25%
Tissue growth—12%
Fecal loss—8%
Metabolic effect of food—5%

Energy Nutrients

Of the total kcalories, carbohydrate is the main energy source. It also acts as a protein-sparer so that the protein vital for building tissue during childhood growth is not diverted for energy needs. Fat is a back-up energy source and also supplies *linoleic acid*, which is the essential fatty acid necessary for growth.

Protein Needs

Protein is the fundamental *tissue-building* substance of the body. It supplies the essential, specific building materials—amino acids—for tissue growth and maintenance. As a child grows, the protein requirements per unit of body weight gradually decrease. For example, for the first 6 months of life, the protein requirements of an infant are 2.2 g/kg of body weight; but the protein needs of a fully grown adult are only 0.8 g/kg. A healthy, active, growing child usually eats enough of a variety of foods to supply the necessary protein and kcalories for overall growth.

TABLE 11-1 Approximate daily fluid needs during growth years

Age	ml/kg	Age	ml/kg
0-3 months	120	4-7 years	95
3-6 months	115	7-11 years	90
6-12 months	110	11-19 years	50
1-4 years	100	>19 years	30

Water Requirements

Water is an essential nutrient, second only to oxygen for life itself. Metabolic needs—especially during periods of rapid growth—demand adequate fluid intake. For example, compare infant and adult water needs. Infants require more water per unit of body weight than adults for two important reasons, as follow: (1) a greater percentage of the infant's total body weight is made up of water, and (2) a larger proportion of the infant's total body water is outside the cells and hence more easily available for loss, resulting in serious dehydration. In 1 day, an infant generally consumes an amount of water equivalent to 10% to 15% of body weight, whereas an adult consumes a daily amount equivalent to 2% to 4% of body weight. Table 11-1 provides a summary of the approximate daily fluid needs during growth years.

Mineral and Vitamin Needs

Though yielding no energy themselves, the macronutrient minerals and vitamins have important roles in tissue growth and maintenance, as well as in overall energy metabolism. Positive childhood growth depends on adequate amounts of all of these essential substances (as indicated in the RDA and DRI tables in Appendix G), but several of these essential materials are of special concern during rapid growth years.

Calcium

Calcium is needed throughout the growth years—especially during the most rapid growth periods of infancy and adolescence. In infancy, mineralization of the skeleton is completed, bones grow larger, and teeth are formed from initial buds. In adolescence, the skeleton grows most rapidly to its adult size. Bone density, particularly in long bones and vertebrae, demands adequate calcium, along with phosphorus and vitamin D. In fact, as a preventive measure to reduce the risk for osteoporosis in older adults, both research and clinical experience indicate that calcium must be emphasized during adolescence. Calcium intake during rapid adolescent bone growth (i.e., both in size and density) is far more effective than the use of more poorly absorbed calcium supplements in older adult years.[1]

Iron

Iron is essential for hemoglobin formation. The infant's fetal store is depleted 4 to 6 months after birth and the first infant food, milk, provides little iron. Iron in human milk, however, is more easily absorbed, and commercial formulas are usually iron-fortified. The addition of solid foods (e.g., enriched cereal, egg yolk, and meat) at 4 to 6 months of age help supply the need for iron.

Hypervitaminosis

Excess amounts of two vitamins, A and D, are of concern in feeding children (see Chapter 6). Excess intake may occur over prolonged periods as a result of ignorance, carelessness, or misunderstanding. Parents should only provide the amount directed and no more.

AGE GROUP NEEDS

Infancy

At birth, we begin our development in our particular "world" as unique human beings. As we grow older, this process continues throughout our lives. Food is intimately related at each stage because our physical growth and personal psychosocial development go hand in hand.[1]

Immature Infants

Special care is crucial for tiny, immature babies. There are two main types of immature babies, defined by weight and gestational age.

Weight.   Defined by birth weight, low–birth-weight (LBW) babies weigh less than 2500 g (5 lb); very low–birth-weight (VLBW) babies weigh less than 1500 g (3 lb); extremely low–birth-weight (ELBW) babies weigh less than 990 g (2 lb).

Gestational age.   Defined by gestational age, premature babies are born preterm (i.e., at under 270

days of gestation) and weigh less than 2500 g (5 lb). Small-for-gestational-age (SGA) babies are born at full term but have suffered some degree of intrauterine growth failure before birth and have general growth retardation and low weight.

All of these infants have problems catching up with growth and nutrition. Because their bodies are not fully formed, they differ from full-term infants of normal weight. Immature infants have the following: (1) more body water, less protein, and fewer minerals; (2) little subcutaneous fat, so they must be kept warm; (3) poorly calcified bones; (4) incomplete nerve and muscle development, making their sucking reflexes weak; (5) limited ability for digestion-absorption and renal function; and (6) an immature liver lacking developed metabolic enzyme systems or adequate iron stores. To survive, these "tiniest babies" require special feeding.

Type of milk.   Immature babies have grown well on both breast milk and special formulas. Most preterm and immature babies are fed special commercial formulas, however, for a number of reasons. Table 11-2 compares these special formulas with standard, full-term infant formulas and human milk.

Methods of feeding.   Tube feeding and peripheral vein feeding are used in special cases, but both carry hazards and are avoided if possible. For most immature infants, bottle feeding—using one of the newer special formulas—can be successful with much care and support.

Full-Term Infants

Mature newborns have more finely developed body systems and grow rapidly, gaining about 168 g (6 ounces) per week during the first 6 months. The feeding process is an important component of the bonding relationship between parent and child. The mother may choose to breast feed her baby or use a formula and add solid foods later (i.e., at about 4 to 6 months of age) when the baby can handle them.

TABLE 11-2 Nutritional value of special formulas and human milk for the preterm infant

Nutritional component	Advisable intake by birth weight		Human milk		Standard formulas	Special premature formulas		
	1.0 kg (2.2 lb)	1.5 kg (3.3 lb)	Preterm	Mature	Enfamil* Similac† SMA‡	Enfamil Premature with Whey*	Similac Special Care†	"Preemie" SMA‡
Kilocalories/deciliter			73	73	67	81	81	81
Protein (g/100 kcal)	3.1	2.7	2.3§	1.5	2.2	3.0	2.7	2.5
Vitamins, fat-soluble								
D (IU/120 kcal/kg/day)	600	600	—	4.0	70-75	75	180	76
E (IU/120 kcal/kg/day)	30	30	—	0.3	2-3	2	4	2
Vitamins, water-soluble								
Folic acid (µg/120 kcal/kg/day)	60	60	—	8.0	9-19	36	45	14
Vitamin C (mg/120 kcal/kg/day)	60	60	—	7.0	10	10	45	10
Minerals								
Calcium (mg/100 kcal)	160	140	40	43.0	66-78	117	178	92
Phosphorus (mg/100 kcal)	108	95	18.0	20.0	49-66	58	89	49
Sodium (mEq/100 kcal)	2.7	2.3	1.5‖	0.8	1.0-1.8	1.7	1.9	1.7

*Mead Johnson Nutritonal Division, Evansville, Ind.
†Ross Laboratories, Columbus, Ohio.
‡Wyeth Laboratories, Philadelphia.
§Range: 1.9-2.8 g/100 kcal.
‖Range: 0.9-2.3 mEq/100 kcal.

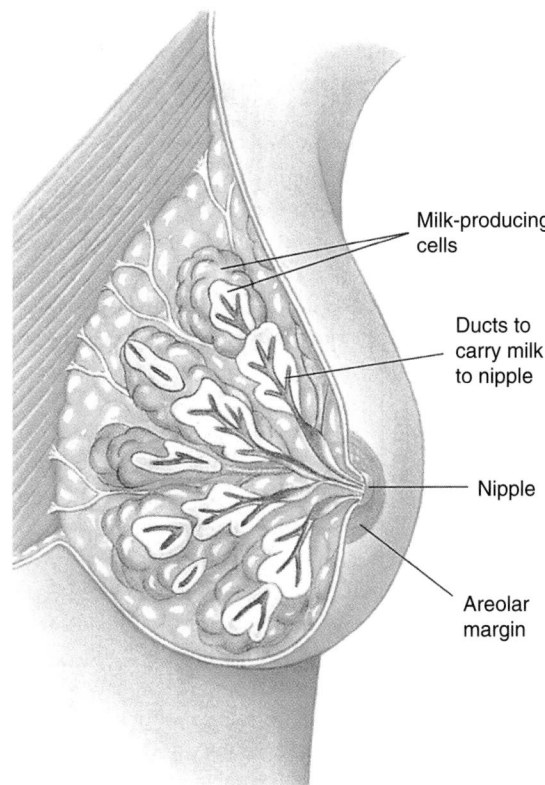

FIGURE 11-1 The anatomy of the breast. (From Wardlaw GM, Insel PM: *Perspectives in nutrition,* ed 3, New York, 1996, McGraw-Hill.)

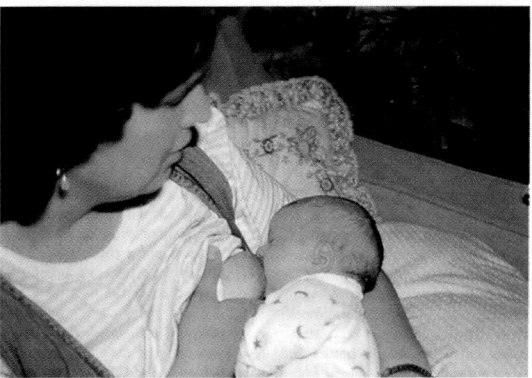

FIGURE 11-2 Breast-feeding the newborn infant. Note that the mother avoids touching the infant's outer cheek so as not to counteract the infant's natural rooting reflex at the touch of the breast. (Courtesy Marjorie Pyle, RNC, Lifecircle, Costa Mesa, CA. From Dickason EJ, Silverman BL, Schult MO: *Maternal-infant nursing care,* ed 2, St Louis, 1994, Mosby.)

Breast Feeding

Human milk is the ideal first food for infants and is the primary recommendation of pediatricians and nutritionists. The nutrients in human milk are uniquely adapted to meet the growth needs of the infant, in forms more easily digested, absorbed, and used. Breast feeding supports early immunity for the baby, helps the mother's uterus quickly return to normal size, and facilitates the important mother-child bonding process. Breast feeding can be successfully started and maintained by most women who try, have support, and use an increased diet for lactation (see Chapter 10). The female breasts or mammary glands are highly specialized secretory organs (Figure 11-1). During pregnancy the breasts prepare for lactation and, toward term, produce a thin, fluid premilk called colostrum. As the infant grows, the breast milk develops and adapts in composition to match the needs of the developing child. The newborn rooting reflex, oral needs for sucking, and basic hunger drive usually make breast feeding simple for the healthy, relaxed mothers (Figure 11-2). Working mothers who want to breast feed their babies can do so by using manual expression and a breast pump while at work, as well as freezing and storing 1- or 2-oz amounts of milk in sealed plastic baby bottle liners for later use. Child care facilities provided in some business and industry settings support breast feeding by employed mothers.

colostrum (L. *colostrum,* pre-milk) a thin, yellow fluid first secreted by the mammary gland a few days before and after childbirth, preceding the mature breast milk. It contains up to 20% protein including a large amount of lactalbumin, more minerals, and less lactose and fat than milk, as well as immunoglobulins that represent the antibodies found in maternal blood.

Breast feeding mothers can find support and guidance through local groups of the national La Leche League or professional certified lactation counselors who are registered dietitians or nurses.

Bottle Feeding

If a mother chooses not to breast feed or some condition in either the mother or baby prevents it, bottle feeding of an appropriate formula is an acceptable alternative. Sterile procedures in formula preparation, the amount of formula consumed, and weaning from the bottle are some of the concerns mothers have voiced.

Cleaning bottles and nipples.   Rinse bottles and nipples after each feeding, using special bottle and nipple brushes and forcing water through nipple holes to prevent milk from crusting in them.

Preparing the formula.   Whether preparing a single bottle for each feeding or a day's batch, scrub, rinse, and sterilize all equipment by the *terminal sterilization* method. Most mothers who bottle feed their infants use a standard commercial formula (see Table 11-2). In some cases of potential milk allergy or intolerance, a soy-based formula (not soy milk) is sometimes used. For infants who are allergic to both cow's milk and soy-based formulas, a special predigested formula such as Pregestimil or Nutramigen (both from Mead-Johnson) or Alimentum (Ross) may be medically advised. With any commercial formula, manufacturer's instructions for mixing concentrated or powdered formula with water should be precisely and consistently followed; and the formula should be refrigerated until use. Throughout the process, scrupulous cleanliness and accurate dilution are essential to prevent infection and illness. Most babies who are hospitalized for vomiting and diarrhea are bottle-fed. A ready-to-feed formula only requires a sterile nipple and bypasses many problems but is more expensive.

Feeding the formula.   Babies drink formula either cold or warm—they just like it to be consistent. Tilt the bottle to keep the nipple full of milk to prevent air-swallowing and hold the baby's head somewhat elevated during feeding to facilitate the passage of milk into the stomach. Never prop the bottle and leave the baby alone to feed—especially as a pacifier at sleep time. This practice deprives the infant of the cuddling that is a vital part of nuturing and also allows milk to pool in the mouth, causing choking, earache, or *bottle mouth* with early tooth decay. Never put a child to sleep with a bottle of milk or fruit juice or other caloric liquid pooling in the mouth.

Weaning

Throughout the feeding process, wise parents learn early to recognize their baby's signs of hunger and satiety and follow the baby's leads. Babies are individuals and set their own particular needs according to age, activity level, growth rate, and metabolic efficiency. A newborn has a very small stomach and can hold only an ounce or two but gradually takes more as the stomach capacity enlarges relative to overall body growth. The amounts of increasing intake during the first 6 months vary and reflect individual growth patterns, but the following quantities are average:

- *1 month:* 2-3 oz, 6-8 feedings, 20 oz total
- *2 months:* 4-5 oz, 6-7 feedings, 28 oz total
- *3 months:* 6-7 oz, 5-6 feedings, 30 oz total
- *4 months:* 6-8 oz, 4-5 feedings, 30 oz total
- *5 months:* 7-8 oz, 4-5 feedings, 34 oz total
- *6 months:* 7-8 oz, 4-5 feedings, 38 oz total

By 6 to 8 months of age as increasing amounts of other foods are used, weaning from bottle feeding takes place naturally as the primitive need for suckling fades. Most older babies with growing physical capacities and desires for independence wean themselves as they learn to drink from a cup.

Cow's Milk

An infant should never be fed regular, whole cow's milk during the first year of life. Unmodified cow's milk is not suitable for infants; its concentration may cause gastrointestinal bleeding and provides too heavy a load of solutes for the infant's renal system. Infants and young children should also not be fed cow's milks of reduced fat content (e.g., skim or low-fat milk) for the following reasons: (1) *insufficient energy* is provided, and (2) *linoleic acid*, the essential fatty acid for growth in the fat portion, is not available. To meet infant needs during the first year of life, the American Academy of Pediatrics recommends breast milk supplemented by vitamin D and fluoride from birth and iron supplement after 4 months of age, with the gradual addition of suitable foods beginning at about 6 months.[2] An alternative appropriate formula may be the mother's choice in place of breast milk.

Solid Food Additions

In some groups, such as urban African-Americans, there is a traditional pattern of starting solid foods early.[3] The usual practice, however, is to introduce solid foods at about 6 months of age. There is no nutritional need for solid foods to be added to an infant's diet before 6 months of age. Because the infant's system cannot use solid foods well before 6 months, they are not yet needed. When solid foods are started, there is no one specific sequence of food additions that must be followed. A general guide is given in Table 11-3, but individual needs and responses vary and suggestions of individual practitioners are the guide. Foods are usually introduced one at a time in small amounts so that if there is an adverse reaction, the offending is food identified. Over time, the child is introduced to a variety of foods and comes to enjoy many of them (Figure 11-3).[4-6] A variety of commercial baby foods are available and are now prepared without added sugar, salt, or monosodium glutamate. Some mothers prefer to prepare their own baby food. Baby food can be easily prepared at home by cooking and straining vegetables and fruits, freezing a batch at a time in ice cube trays, and storing the cubes in plastic bags in the freezer. A single cube can later be conveniently reheated for feed-

ing. Throughout the early feeding period–whatever plan is followed, the following basic principles should guide the feeding process: (1) *necessary nutrients*–not any specific food or sequence–are needed, (2) food is a basis of *learning*, and (3) *normal physical development* guides the feeding behavior (see the For Further Focus box, "How Infants Learn to Eat"). Good food habits begin early in life and continue as the child grows. By 8 or 9 months of age, infants should be able to eat so-called table foods (i.e., cooked, chopped, simply seasoned foods) without needing special infant foods.

Summary Guidelines

The Nutrition Committee of the American Academy of Pediatrics (AAP) has provided the following recommendations to guide infant feeding:

- **Breast feeding** provides the ideal first food for the infant, continued for the first full year of life supplemented with vitamin D and fluoride from birth and iron supplements after 4 months of age.
- **Commercial formulas** provide an alternative to breast feeding during the first year of life; fluoride supplements may be need to be mixed in if the local water supply is not fluoridated.
- **Solid foods** may be introduced at approximately 4 to 6 months of age, after the extrusion reflex of early infancy disappears and the ability to swallow solid food is established. Current studies indicate, however, that baby food is sometimes introduced earlier than recommended.[3]
- **Whole cow's milk** may be introduced at the end of the first year if breast feeding has been completely discontinued and infants are

---

wean (Middle English, 1000 AD, *wenen*, to accustom) to gradually accustom a young child to food other than the mother's milk or a bottle-fed substitute formula as the child's natural need to suckle wanes.

TABLE 11-3 Guideline for adding solid foods to infant's diet during the first year

Foods added*	Feeding
6 to 7 months	
Cereal and strained cooked fruit	10 AM and 6 PM
Egg yolk (at first, hard boiled and sieved, soft boiled or poached later)	
Strained cooked vegetable and strained meat	2 PM
Zweiback or hard toast	At any feeding
7 to 9 months	
Meat: beef, lamb, or liver (broiled or baked and finely chopped)	10 AM and 6 PM
Potato: baked or boiled and mashed or sieved	
9 months to 1 year or older—suggested meal plan	
Milk	7 AM
240 ml (8 oz)	
Cereal	
2-3 tbsp	
Strained fruit	
2-3 tbsp	
Zweiback or dry toast	
Milk	12 NOON
240 ml (8 oz)	
Vegetables	
2-3 tbsp	
Chopped meat or one whole egg	
Puddings or cooked fruit	
2-3 tbsp	
Milk	3 PM
120 ml (4 oz)	
Toast, zweiback, or crackers	
Milk	6 PM
240 ml (8 oz)	
Whole egg or chopped meat	
2 tbsp	
Potato: baked or mashed	
2-3 tbsp	
Pudding or cooked fruit	
Zweiback or toast	

*Semisolid foods should be given immediately before milk feeding. One or two teaspoons should be given at first. If food is accepted and tolerated well, the amount should be increased 1 to 2 tbsp per feeding.

NOTE: Banana or cottage cheese may be used as substitution for any meal.

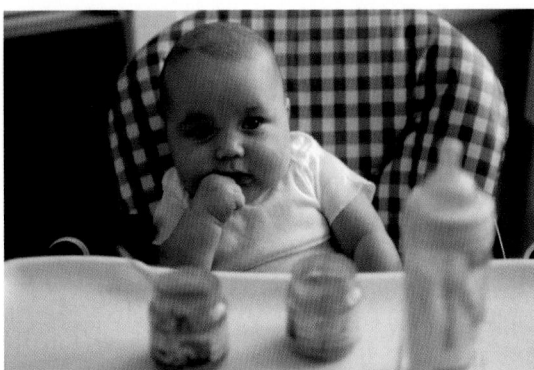

FIGURE 11-3 This child is taking a variety of solid food additions and developing wide tastes. Here, feeding serves as a source not only of physical growth but also of psychosocial development. Optimal physical development and security are evident, the result of sound nutrition and loving care. (Credit: PhotoDisc.)

consuming one third of their kcalories as a balanced mixture of solid foods including cereals, vegetables, fruits, and other foods to supply adequate sources of vitamin C and iron. Reduced fat cow's milk is not recommended.

- **Iron-fortified formula** should be used for older infants (e.g., above 6 months of age) who do not consume a significant portion of their kcalories from added solid foods.
- **Allergens** such as wheat, egg white, citrus juice, nut butters, and chocolate should not be introduced as early solid foods but added later after tolerance has been established through their gradual use.
- **Honey** should not be given to infants under 1 year of age because botulism spores have been reported in honey and the immune system capacity of young infants cannot resist this infection.
- **Physically irritating foods** such as hot dogs, nuts, grapes, carrots, and round candy may cause choking and aspiration, so they are best delayed for careful use only with older children and not given to infants.

Throughout the first year of life, the requirements for physical growth and psychosocial development are met by human milk or formula, a variety of solid food additions, and a loving, trusting relationship between parents and child.

Childhood

Toddlers (1 to 3 years)

Once children learn to walk at about 1 year of age, these toddlers are off and away, into everything and learning new skills. This dawning sense of self, which is a fundamental foundation for ultimate maturity, carries over into many areas—including food. After parents are accustomed to the rapid growth and resulting appetite of the first year of life, they may be concerned when they see their toddler eating less food and at times having little appetite, while being easily distracted from food to another activity (see Clinical Applications box, "Toddler and Preschooler Feeding Made Simple"). Increasing the variety of foods helps children develop good food habits. The food preferences of young children grow directly from the frequency of a food's use in pleasant surroundings and the increased opportunity to become familiar with a number of foods. Sweets should be reserved for special occasions—and not used habitually or as bribes to get a child to eat.

Infant Failure to Thrive

The term *failure to thrive* has been used in pediatrics to describe a child who does not measure up to usual growth and development standards. Sometimes pediatricians use a brief hospital stay to classify infants who fail to thrive. Careful nutrition assessment is essential to identifying underlying causes of feeding problems. The following factors may be involved:

- **Clinical disease**—Central nervous system disorders, endocrine disease, congenital defects, or partial intestinal obstruction.
- **Neuromotor problems**—Poor sucking or abnormal muscle tone from the retention of

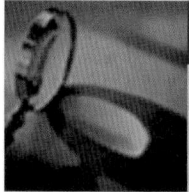

FOR FURTHER FOCUS

How Infants Learn To Eat

Guided by reflexes and gradually developing muscle controls during their first year of life, infants learn many things about living in their particular environment. A most basic need is food, which infants obtain through a normal developmental sequence of feeding behaviors in the process of learning to eat.

Age 1 to 3 months
Rooting, sucking, and swallowing reflexes are present at birth, along with the tonic neck reflex. Therefore infants secure their first food, milk, with a suckling pattern in which the tongue is projected during a swallow. In the beginning, head control is poor but develops by the third month of life.

Age 4 to 6 months
The early rooting and biting reflexes fade, and the tonic neck reflex has faded by 16 weeks. Infants now change from a suckling pattern with a protruded tongue to a mature, stronger suck with liquids, and a munching pattern begins. Infants are now able to grasp objects with a fistlike palmar grip, bringing them to the mouth and biting them.

Age 7 to 9 months
The gag reflex weakens as infants begin chewing solid foods and develop a normal controlled gag along with control of the choking reflex. Munching movements now develop as older infants increase their intake of solid foods and chew with a rotary motion. These infants can sit alone, secure items and release them and resecure them, and hold a bottle alone. They begin to develop a pincer grasp to pick up very small items between the thumb and forefinger and put them in the mouth.

Age 10 to 12 months
Older infants can now reach for a spoon. They bite nipples, spoons, and crunchy foods; can grasp a bottle and foods and bring them to the mouth; and, with assistance, can drink from a cup that is held. These infants have tongue control to lick food morsels off the lower lip and can finger-feed themselves with a refined pincer grasp. These normal developmental behaviors are the basis for the following progressive pattern of introducing semisolid and table foods to older infants:

> *4 to 6 months*—Add iron-fortified infant cereals, starting with less allergenic rice and progressing to wheat and mixed grains.

> *6 to 8 months*—Add strained fruits and vegetables, progressing to strained or finely chopped table meats. Add finger foods (e.g., arrowroot biscuits or over-dried toast) that can be secured with a palmar grasp.

> *9 to 12 months*—Gradually delete strained foods and introduce various table foods (e.g., chopped, well-cooked vegetables and meats and chopped, well-cooked or canned fruits). Use smaller finger foods as the pincer grasp develops. Add other well-cooked mashed or chopped table foods, all prepared without added salt or sugar, and help the child to drink moderate amounts of juice by cup.

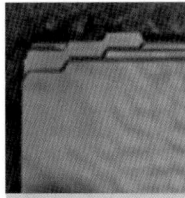

CLINICAL APPLICATIONS

Toddler and Preschooler Feeding Made Simple

Parents waste a lot of time coaxing, arguing, begging, and even threatening their 2- to 5-year-olds to eat more than one and a half peas at dinner time. You can help save parents time, tears, and energy by developing child-feeding strategies based on the normal developmental needs of their little ones.

First, remind parents that:

- **Their children are not growing as fast as they did during the first year of life.** Consequently, they need less food.
- **Children's energy needs are irregular.** Just watch their activity level. Provide food as needed to help their bodies keep up with the many activities "planned" for each day.

Second, offer a few suggestions that make child-feeding easier:

- **Offer a variety of foods.** After a taste, put new food aside if not taken; then try again later to help develop broad tastes.
- **Serve small portions.** Let children ask for seconds if they're still hungry.
- **Guide children in serving themselves small portions.** Like adults, children's eyes tend to be bigger than their stomachs. Constant, gentle reminders help them learn when to stop.
- **Avoid overseasoning.** Let tastes develop gradually. If a food is too spicy, no amount of screaming or cajoling will make them eat it.
- **Don't force foods that the child dislikes.** Individual food dislikes usually don't last very long. If the child shuns one food, offer a similar one if it's available at that meal (e.g., offer a fruit if the child rejects a vegetable) so that

there's little chance of deficiency signs cropping up soon.

- **Don't put away the main meal before serving dessert.** If there is a dessert, hold on to the main meal food. Amazing but true: if they're still hungry, some children will ask for more food from the main meal after finishing dessert.
- **Keep "quick-fix" nutritious foods around for "off-hour" meals.** The word "snack" isn't appropriate for the amount of food some youngsters eat between regular meals. To keep parents from turning into permanent short-order chefs, keep foods such as fruit, cheese, peanut butter, bread, and crackers to serve between meals and to provide essential nutrients.
- **Enroll the child in a nursery school or preschool program.** Because food is not always available in the classroom, little students learn to eat at regular times. They also tend to try foods they rejected at home, probably because of peer pressure or a desire to impress a new authority figure—the teacher.
- **Be patient.** Remember that while adults may be discussing world events over broccoli, toddlers are just now learning how to pick it up with their fork.

Toddlers may take longer. They may not even eat at all. But with flexibility, time, patience, and a sense of humor, most parents find that they can get enough nutrients into their children to keep them alive and happy throughout the preschool years. Happily, when presented with nutritious food choices, preschoolers tend to self-regulate their intake to meet energy needs without adult intervention.

primitive reflexes that should have already faded; eating, chewing, and swallowing problems.

- **Dietary practices**—Parental misconceptions and beliefs about what constitutes a "normal" diet for infants; inappropriate formula feeding or improper dilutions in mixing formula.
- **Unusual nutrient needs or losses**—Adequate diet for growth but inadequate nutrient absorption and thus excessive fecal loss; hypermetabolic state requiring increased dietary intake.
- **Psychosocial problems**—Family environment and relationships resulting in emotional deprivation of the child, requiring medical-nutritional intervention; similar problems may also occur later (e.g., between 2 and 4 years of age) when parents and children have conflicts about normal changes caused by slowed childhood growth and energy needs that result in changing food patterns, food jags (i.e., brief sprees or binges of eating one particular food), erratic appetites, reduced milk intake, and disinterest in eating.

Failure to thrive is often caused by a complex of factors; and there are no easy solutions. Careful history taking, supportive nutritional guidance, and warm personal care are required to influence growth patterns in these infants and young children and are a big help to these families. Careful and sensitive correction of the social and environmental issues surrounding the problem is essential.

Preschool Children (3 to 5 years)

Physical growth and appetite continue in spurts. Mental capacities develop and the expanding environment is gradually explored. Children continue to form life patterns in attitudes and basic eating habits as a result of social and emotional experiences. These varying experiences frequently lead to food jags that last a few days but are usually short-lived and of no major concern. Again, the key is food variety and relatively small portions. Group eating becomes a significant means of socialization (see Clinical Applications box, "Toddler and Preschooler Feeding Made Simple") For example, during preschool food preferences grow according to what the group is eating. Children in kindergarten also have early learning about healthy eating. In one school, they participated in food preparation and then ate what they had prepared as part of their "Five a Day, Let's Eat and Play" program.[7] Children in another kindergarten planted and tended gardens of various vegetables as part of their "Growing Healthy project."[8] In such situations a child learns a variety of different food habits and forms new social relationships.

School-Age Children (5 to 12 years)

The generally slow and irregular growth rate continues in the early school years, and body changes occur gradually. In the year or two before adolescence—in particular, reserves are being laid for the rapid growth period ahead. This is the last lull before the storm. By this time, body types are established and growth rates vary widely. Girls' development usually outdistances boys' in the latter part of this period. With the stimulus of school and a variety of learning activities, children experience increasing mental and social development, the ability to work out problems, and competitive activities. They begin moving from dependence on parental patterns to the standards of peers, in preparation for coming maturity.

Food preferences are the products of earlier years, but school-age children are increasingly exposed to new stimuli—including television—that influence food habits. Table 11-4 lists some favorite foods of American children. The relation of sound nutrition to learning has long been established, and breakfast is particularly important for school-age children. The school lunch program provides a nourishing noon meal for many children who would otherwise lack one. The classroom also provides positive learning opportunities, particularly when parents provide support at home. An interested and motivated teacher can integrate nutrition into many other learning activities. School breakfast and lunch programs, which have a large effect on a child's health, are described in Chapter 13.

BOX 11-1 Favorite food choices of American children (listed in order of priority)

Breakfast	Lunch or dinner	Vegetables	Fruit	Beverage	Desserts	Sandwiches
Cereal	Steak or roast beef	Corn	Apple	Cola or soda	Ice cream	Peanut butter and jelly
Pancakes or waffles	Pizza	Carrots	Orange	Milk	Cake	Meat or cold cuts
Eggs	Spaghetti	Beans	Peach	Fruit punch	Pie	
French toast	Chicken	Tomatoes	Grape	Root beer	Pudding	Ham
Toast	Hamburger	Peas	Banana	Juices (other than orange)	Gelatin dessert	Tuna fish
Sweet rolls	Fish	Greens, collards, or spinach	Watermelon	Orange juice	Banana split	Cheese
Doughnuts	Macaroni and cheese	Potatoes	Pear	Lemonade	Brownie	Bacon, lettuce, and tomato
						Roast beef

American School Health Association, Kent, Ohio. Modified from survey data of Lamme AJ and Lamme LL: Children's food preferences, *J Sch Health* 50(7):397, September 1980. Reprinted with permission.

Adolescence (12 to 18 years)

Physical Growth

The final growth spurt of childhood occurs with the onset of puberty. This rapid growth is evident in increasing body size and development of sex characteristics in response to hormonal influences. The rate of these changes varies widely among individual boys and girls, but particularly distinct growth patterns emerge.[9] Girls develop an increasing amount of fat deposit, especially in the abdominal area. As the bony pelvis widens in preparation for future childbearing and subcutaneous fat increases, the size of the hips also increases, causing much anxiety to many figure-conscious young girls. In boys, physical growth is seen more in increased muscle mass and long-bone growth. At first a boy's growth spurt is slower than that of a girl, but he soon passes her in weight and height.

Eating Patterns

Teenagers' eating habits are greatly influenced by their rapid growth—and hence their need for energy, as well as by their self-conscious peer pressure—and hence their acceptance of popular food fads. Teenagers tend to skip lunch more often than breakfast, derive a great deal of their energy from snacks, eat at fast food restaurants because these are frequent "hangouts," and are likely to eat any kind of food at any time of day. Unfortunately, some teenagers begin to get a significant portion of their total caloric intake in the form of alcohol. Even a mild form of alcohol abuse, when combined with the elevated nutritional demands of adolescence, can easily affect their nutritional status. In general overall nutrition, boys usually fare better than girls. Their larger appetite and sheer volume of food consumed usually ensure an adequate intake of nutrients. On the other hand, under a greater social pressure for thinness, girls may tend to restrict their food and have inadequate nutrient intake.

Eating Disorders

Social, family, and personal pressures concerning figure control strongly influence many young girls. As a result, they sometimes follow unwise, self-imposed "crash" diets for weight loss. In some cases, self-starvation occurs. Complex and far-reaching eating disorders such as *anorexia nervosa* and *bulimia nervosa* may develop.[10] Psychologists have traditionally identified mothers as the main source of family pressure to remain thin. Fathers also have a role if they are emotionally distant and do not provide important feedback to build self-worth and self-esteem in their young daughters. Fathers must help their daughters see themselves as loved no matter what they weigh, so they are not as vulnerable to social influences that equate extreme thinness with beauty. Eating disorders can have severe effects and involve a distorted body image and a morbid, irrational pursuit of thinness. Such disordered eating often begins in the early adolescent years, when many girls see themselves as "fat" even though their average weight is often below the normal weight for their height. Malnutrition may exist. These eating disorders are discussed further in Chapter 15 on weight management.

Teenage Pregnancy

The number of teenage pregnancies continues to be a problem. With a background of inadequate diet, many of these girls are poorly prepared for the demands of pregnancy (see Chapter 10, Clinical Applications box "Pregnant Teenagers"). They must complete their own growth and development while supplying the extra needs of the baby. A teenage girl who is not very nutritionally prepared for pregnancy is at risk for complications such as abortion, premature labor, pregnancy-induced hypertension (PIH), and delivery of an immature, low birth weight baby. A girl who has maintained good nutrition has a better chance to deliver a healthy baby. These young mothers need much personal support and health care counseling to help reduce their infant mortality rate.

SUMMARY

Positive growth and development of healthy children depend on optimal nutritional support. In turn, this good nutrition depends on many social, psychologic, cultural, and environmental influences that affect individual growth potential throughout the life cycle.

From birth, the nutritional needs of children change with each unique growth period. *Infants* experience rapid growth. Human milk is preferred as their first food, with solid foods delayed until about 6 months of age when their metabolic processes have matured. *Toddlers, preschoolers,* and *school-age children* experience slowed and irregular growth. During this period, their energy demands are less,

but they require a well-balanced diet for continued growth and health. Social and cultural factors influence their developing food habits.

Adolescents experience a large growth spurt before adulthood. This rapid growth involves both physical and sexual maturing. Boys usually obtain their increased caloric and nutrient demands because they eat larger amounts of food. Girls more often feel social and peer pressure to restrict their food to control their weight, causing some to develop severe eating disorders. This pressure may also prevent them from forming the nutritional reserves necessary for future childbearing.

REVIEW QUESTIONS

1. Describe the major factors responsible for the differences in the nutritional and feeding needs of pre- and full-term infants.
2. Why is breast feeding the preferred method of feeding infants? Compare breast feeding with the commercial formulas available for bottle-fed babies.
3. Outline a general schedule for a new mother to use as a guide for adding solid foods to her baby's diet during the first year of life.

4. Compare the changes in growth and development of toddlers, preschoolers, and school-age children. What factors influence their nutritional needs and eating habits?
5. Describe factors that influence the changing nutritional needs and eating habits of adolescents. Who is usually at greater nutritional risk during this period—boys or girls? Why? What suggestions do you have for reducing the nutritional risk at this vulnerable age?

SELF-TEST QUESTIONS

True-False
Write the correct statement for each item you answer "false."
1. A good way to keep infants and toddlers from being overweight is to use nonfat milk in their diets.
2. A variety of carbohydrate foods in a child's diet helps provide all the essential amino acids for growth.

3. Hypervitaminosis C is possible during the growth period when an excess of the vitamin is given to infants.
4. The rooting and sucking reflexes must be learned before a newborn infant can obtain milk from the breast.
5. A toddler needs at least a quart of milk a day to meet increased growth needs.

Multiple Choice

1. Fat is needed in the child's diet to supply:
   a. Fat-soluble vitamins.
   b. Water-soluble vitamins.
   c. Essential amino acids.
   d. Essential fatty acids.
2. An iron deficiency in childhood is associated with the following disease:
   a. Scurvy
   b. Rickets
   c. Anemia
   d. Pellagra

3. Growth and development of a school-age child are characterized by:
   a. A rapid increase in physical growth with increased food requirements.
   b. More rapid growth of girls in the latter part of the period.
   c. Body changes associated with sexual maturity.
   d. Increased dependence on parental standards or habits.

SUGGESTIONS FOR ADDITIONAL STUDY

1. Nutrition for Growth

Select a child in one of the stages of growth from infancy through adolescence. Using the guidelines in this text, interview the mother and child (depending on age) about the food and feeding and/or eating practices. Analyze your findings, using the general guides in this text for each age group, as well as the RDA and DRI standards and food value table.

According to your findings, plan with the mother and child (depending on age) a satisfying food plan to provide both nutritional and psychosocial support for the child's growth and development.

2. Snack Foods for Growing Children

Prepare a discussion for a group of parents of toddlers and preschool children. Develop snack ideas with recipes and suggestions for use. Demonstrate the preparation of some of these snacks and have the parents form a taste-testing panel. If the children are present, have them taste and respond to the products. Write a brief report of your project and discuss it with your class.

REFERENCES

1. Glinsman WH and others: Dietary guidelines for infants: a timely reminder, *Nutr Rev* 54(2):50, 1996.
2. American Academy of Pediatrics Work Group on Breast-Feeding: Policy statement on breast-feeding, *Pediatrics* 100(Dec):1035, 1997.
3. Browner YL and others: Early introduction of solid foods among urban African-American participants in WIC, *J Am Diet Assoc* 99(4):457, 1999.
4. Skinner JD and others: Transitions in infant feeding during the first year of life, *J Am Coll Nutr* 16(3):209, 1997.
5. Reed DB: Focus groups identify desirable features of nutrition programs for low-income mothers of preschool children, *J Am Diet Assoc* 96(5):501, 1996.
6. Birch LL: Children's food acceptance patterns, *Nutr Today* 31(6):234, 1996.
7. Levy PM, Cooper J: Five a day, let's eat and play: a nutrition education program for preschool children, *J Nutr Ed* 31:235B, 1999.
8. Casen KL: Children are "growing healthy" in South Carolina, *J Nutr Educ* 31:235A, 1999.
9. Cameron JL: Nutritional determinants of puberty, *Nutr Rev* 54(2):S17, 1996.
10. Nash M: Conferences, symposia, and reports: conference on adolescent nutritional disorders: prevention and treatment, *Nutr Today* 31(2):68, 1996.

FURTHER READING

- Johnson RK, Nicklas TA: Position of The American Dietetic Association: Dietary guidance for healthy children aged 2 to 11 years, *J Am Diet Assoc* 99(1):93, 1999.

  This new position paper from The American Dietetic Association states the association's current position on the nutritional guidance for young children up to age 11. This paper also indicates the need for regular exercise.
- Bronner YL: Nutritional status outcomes for children: ethnic, cultural, and environmental contexts, *J Am Diet Assoc* 96(9):891, 1996.

  This excellent literature review explores relationships between nutritional status outcomes among ethnically diverse children and their cultural environments.

- Kenedy E, Goldberg J: What are American children eating? Implications for public policy, *Nutr Rev* 53(5):111,1995.

  These authors review the changing health and demographic profile of the United States population with resulting changes in children's food patterns, and the impact of these changes on children's health.

12

Nutrition for Adults: The Early, Middle, and Later Years

KEY CONCEPTS

- Gradual aging throughout the adult years is an *individual* process based on genetic heritage and life experience.

- Aging is a total life process—with biologic, nutritional, social, economic, psychologic, and spiritual aspects.

The rapid growth and development of the adolescent years bring us to physical maturity as adults. Physical growth in size levels off but continues in the constant cell growth and reproduction necessary to maintain our bodies. Other aspects of growth and development (e.g., mental, social, psychologic, and spiritual) continue for a lifetime.

Food and nutrition continue to provide essential support during the adult aging process. Life expectancy is lengthening, so health promotion and disease prevention are even more important as we seek to ensure quality of life throughout our extended years.

In this chapter, we explore the ways that positive nutrition and good food can help adults lead healthier and happier lives.

ADULTHOOD: CONTINUING HUMAN GROWTH AND DEVELOPMENT

Coming of Age in America

As the pace of modern life becomes faster in the twenty-first century, adults in America are experiencing tremendous change in the composition of the population and in the impact of technology on the economy.[1] The new report of the U.S. Department of Health and Human Services, *Healthy People 2010: Understanding and Improving Health*, presents national goals of helping all people make informed decisions about their health.[2] The work of the U.S. Census Bureau and the President's Council of Economic Advisors also report on important changes in the population and the economy.[3,4]

Population and Age Distribution

By the year 2010, according to the U.S. Census Bureau, the U.S. population will have grown to 300 million people—up 9% from the year 2000 total of 275 million. The average size of American households will continue to decline, from 2.59 to 2.53 persons. The U.S. population will continue to become older for the next several decades, with its median age increasing from 36 years in 2000 to 37 years in 2010. The older segments of the population will grow significantly during this period; people over age 65 will increase from 35 to 40 million, and those over 85 will increase from 4.3 to 5.8 million.

Life Expectancy and Quality of Life

Life expectancy has increased dramatically over the past century, from only 47 years in 1900 to 77 years in 2000. By 2010, the average life expectancy will rise to 78 years. By gender, life expectancy in 2010 it will be 74 for males and 81 for females. There are, however, substantial differences among different population groups nationally, and household income, along with gender and race, are major factors. Women outlive men by an average of 6 years. Americans consistently value the health-related quality of life—our personal sense of physical and mental health and our ability to act within our environment—to be extremely important and the quality of life is a major focus of the Healthy People initiative.[2]

Racial and Ethnic Composition

By the year 2010, a shifting racial and ethnic pattern will continue to reshape the American population. The U.S. Census Bureau projects that the proportion of whites in the population, not including Hispanic Americans, will decline from 72% in 2000 to 68% in 2010. Hispanic Americans, the fastest growing group in the country, will grow to 43 million people (14%), becoming the second largest segment of the population. By 2010, African Americans will number 37 million (12%).

Economic Expansion

During the second half of the 1990s, the United States economy experienced dramatic sustained growth.[4] By the year 2010, over 50% of all jobs will be in information industries or require technical skills. The largest group of new entrants into the labor force will continue to be women, who will make up 50% of the total work force by 2005—up from 46% in 2000.

Shaping Influences on Adult Growth and Development

Today's adults are growing and developing within this broader, rapidly changing world. The overall process of human aging begins at birth and lasts a lifetime. Each stage has unique potential for growth and fulfillment. The periods of adulthood—young, middle, and older years—are no exception. Many individual and group events mark our course; but at each stage, four basic areas of adult life—physical, psychosocial, socioeconomic, and nutritional—shape its general growth and development.

Physical Growth

Because physical maturity is reached in the late teen years, overall physical growth of the human body, governed by its genetic potential, levels off in the early adult years. Physical growth is no longer a process of increasing numbers of cells and body size but is the vital growth of new cells to replace old ones. This process maintains vigor and wholeness of body structure and function, increases learning, and strengthens mental capacities. Then at older ages, physical growth gradually declines and individual vigor reflects the health status of preceding years.

Psychosocial Development

Human personality development continues through the adult years. Three unique stages of personal psychosocial growth progress through the young, middle, and older years.

Young adults (18 to 40 years). With physical maturity, young adults are increasingly independent. They form many new relationships, adopt new roles, and make many choices concerning continued education, career, jobs, marriage, and family. Young adults experience considerable stress but also significant personal growth. These are years of career beginnings, establishing one's own home, and starting young children on their way through the same life stages—all part of early personal strug- gles to make one's way in the world. Sometimes health problems relate to these early stress periods.

Middle adults (40 to 60 years). The middle years often present an opportunity to expand personal growth. In most cases, children have grown and gone to make their own lives, and parents may have a sense of "it's my turn now." This is also a time of coming to terms with what life has offered, a "regrouping" of ideas, life directions, and activities. There is also a sort of regeneration of one's own life in the lives of young people following along a similar path. Early evidence of chronic disease appears in some middle adults. Wellness, health promotion,

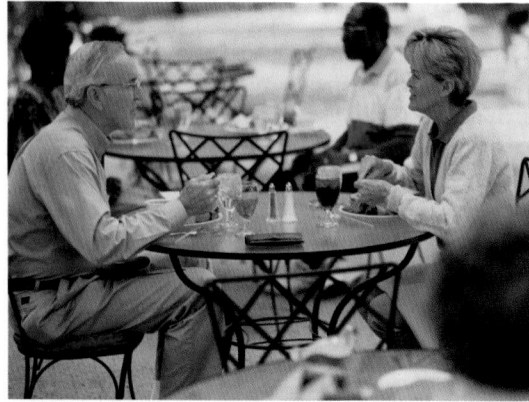

FIGURE 12-1 Retired couple enjoying a good meal. (Credit: PhotoDisc.)

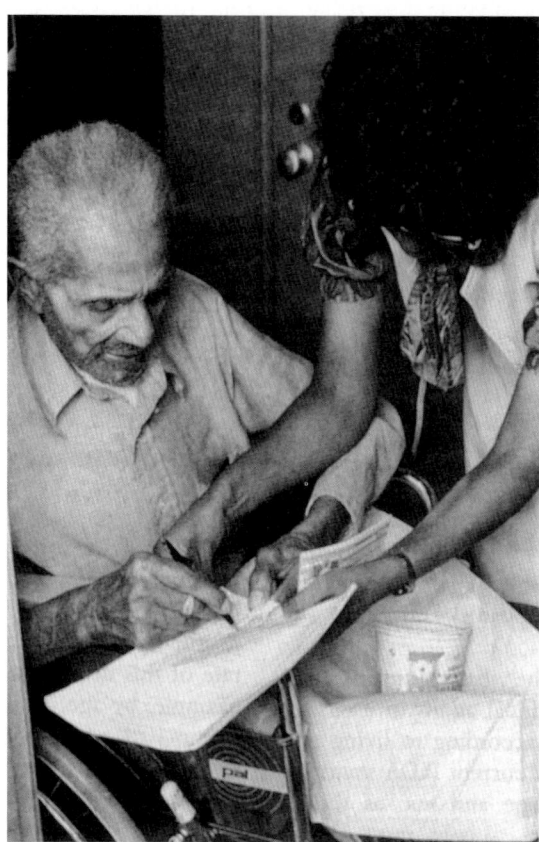

FIGURE 12-2 Elderly disabled man assisted by the Food Stamp Program to obtain needed food. (Credit: U.S. Department of Agriculture.)

and reduction of disease risks are becoming the focus of health care.

Older adults (60 years and older). Adults vary widely in their personal and physical resources to deal with older age. They may have a sense of wholeness and completeness, or they may increasingly withdraw from life. If the outcome of their life experiences is positive, they arrive at older ages as rich persons—rich in wisdom of their years—and enjoy life and health (Figure 12-1), enriching the lives of those around them. But some elderly people arrive at these years poorly equipped to deal with adjustments of aging and health problems that may arise.

Socioeconomic Status

We all grow up and live our lives in a social and cultural context. Now our rapidly changing world is experiencing major social and economic shifts. Most adults and their families are feeling the strain in some way. These pressures directly influence food security and health. As they grow older, many older persons find themselves under increasing financial pressure. Economic insecurity creates added stress and often leads to the need for food assistance (Figure 12-2). Sometimes social and financial pressures, along with a decreasing sense of acceptance and productivity, cause many elderly persons to feel unwanted and unworthy. All people need a sense of belonging, achievement, and self-esteem. Instead many elderly people are often lonely, restless, unhappy, and uncertain. In medical charts and clinical conferences, their medical diagnosis is increasingly given as "the dwindles."[5,6] Basic needs common to older persons are economic security, personal effectiveness, suitable housing, constructive and enjoyable activities, satisfying social relationships, and spiritual values.

Nutritional Needs

The basic energy and nutrient needs of individual adults in each age group vary according to living and working situations. The RDAs and the other DRI standards for healthy adults by age and sex, as shown in Appendix G, supply most needs, but the aging process influences individual nutritional needs.

THE AGING PROCESS AND NUTRITIONAL NEEDS

General Physiologic Changes

Biologic Changes

Human biologic growth, and then decline, extends over the entire life span. Throughout life, all experiences make their imprint on individual genetic heritage. Everyone ages in different ways, depending on individual make-up and resources. During middle and older adulthood, however, there is generally a gradual loss of functioning cells with reduced cell metabolism. As a result, body organ systems gradually lose some capacity to do their jobs and maintain their reserves. The rate of this decline accelerates in later life. For example, by age 70 the kidneys and lungs lose about 10% of their former weight, the liver loses 18% of its weight, and skeletal muscle is reduced by 40%.

Effect on Food Patterns

Some of the physical changes of aging affect food patterns. For example, secretion of digestive juices and motility of gastrointestinal muscles gradually decrease, causing decreased absorption and use of nutrients. Decreased taste, smell, and vision also affect appetite and persons eat less. Older persons often experience increased concern about body functions, more social stress, personal losses, and fewer social opportunities to maintain self-esteem. All of these concerns affect food intake. Much of what we consider "just aging" in older people is really the result of poor nutrition. Lack of sufficient nourishment is the primary nutrition problem of older adults.

Individuality of The Aging Process

The general process of senescence affects all older adults, although the biologic changes in aging are

---

senescence (L. *senescere*, to grow old) the process or condition of growing old.

general, each person is unique, and older persons show a wide variety of individual responses. Individuals get old at different rates and in different ways, depending on their genetic heritage and their health and nutrition resources of past years. Each older adult has specific needs.

Nutritional Needs

Kilocalories—Energy

Because of gradual loss of functioning body cells and reduced physical activity, adults generally require less energy intake as they grow older. The current national standard is based on estimates of 5% decreased metabolic activity in middle and older years.[7] The recommended allowance for energy need is 1900 kcal/day for women over age 51 and 2300 kcal/day for men of the same age, but these are only estimates. Individual physical and health status, as well as living situations, vary among older adults. Our knowledge of the energy and nutrient needs of elderly persons also has many gaps. For example, there is doubt about traditional standards of "ideal" weight based on weight-for-height tables. Ongoing review of these tables indicates that the weight ranges associated with longer lives are not necessarily the "desirable" weights given but weights 10% to 25% greater. Thus thin older adults, rather than those of moderate weight, have a reduced life expectancy. The basic fuels required to supply these energy needs are primarily carbohydrate with moderate fat.

Carbohydrate.   About 50% to 60% of the total diet kcalories should come from carbohydrate foods, with the majority being mostly complex carbohydrates (e.g., starches). Easily absorbed sugars may also be used for energy. Carbohydrate metabolism is usually undisturbed in older age. The fasting blood glucose level is essentially unchanged in the aged. They can choose freely among carbohydrate foods according to individual needs, desires, and physical responses.

Fat.   Fats usually contribute about 30% of total kcalories and provide a back-up energy source, important fat-soluble vitamins, and essential fatty acids. A reasonable goal is to avoid large quantities of fat and emphasize the quality of the fat used. Fat digestion and absorption may be delayed in elderly persons, but these functions are not greatly disturbed. Sufficient fat for helping food taste better aids appetite and in some cases provides needed kcalories to prevent excessive weight loss.

Protein.   The current national standard recommends an adult protein intake of 0.8 g/kg of body weight, making the total protein need 63 g/day for an average-weight man and 50 g/day for an average-weight woman. This amount of protein provides about 13% to 15% of the total kcalories (see Chapter 3). There may be an increased need for protein during illness, convalescence, or a wasting disease. In any case, protein needs are related to two basic factors, as follow: (1) the protein quality—the quantity and ratio of its amino acids, and (2) adequate total kcalories in the diet. Healthy adults do not need supplemental amino acid preparations, which are an expensive and inefficient source of available nitrogen.

Vitamins and Minerals

A diet with a variety of foods should supply vitamins and minerals in the amounts needed for healthy adults. Normal aging does not usually require increased amounts. Individual problems may arise from inadequate intake rather than increased need. Several of these essential nutrients, however, may need special attention in relation to two possible health problems in aging.

Osteoporosis.   Vitamin D and calcium are essential nutrients for growth and maintenance of healthy bone tissue. Older adults, especially white and Asian women, carry a risk as high as 50% for developing the bone disease *osteoporosis*.[8] Contributing factors include the following: (1) less use of calcium-rich food such as milk and other dairy products; (2) loss of appetite and lack adequate body fat; (3) less outdoor physical exercise; and (4) decreased capacity of the skin to produce vitamin D with exposure to sunlight.[9,10] The new DRI standards give an Adequate Intake (AI) level for vitamin D of 5 μg/day (200 IU) for both men and women from birth to age 50 (see Chapter 6).[11] The usual dietary intake in the United States as measured by a previous USDA survey is 1.25 to 1.75 μg/day (50 to 70 IU), so apparently vitamin D stores are enriched in most people by regular exposure to sunlight.

Anemia.   The poor diet of many older adults lacks sufficient iron to prevent iron-deficiency *anemia*. These individuals need attention and encouragement to help them eat more iron-rich foods.

The Question of Nutrient Supplementation
There is no evidence that *healthy* adults in their middle and older years require additional nutrient supplements, but use of supplements is widespread. Surveys indicate that about 40% of adult Americans take vitamin supplements regularly, with much higher use in Western states. The use of nutritional supplements by elderly adults, usually on a self-prescribed basis, is common. Although such routine use may not be necessary, supplements are often required for persons in debilitated states. This is especially true for the malnutrition often seen in homebound elderly persons, for example, as is clearly shown in a recent comprehensive study in Texas of a rural Hispanic population who were at serious nutritional risk.[12] Such persons need a nourishing diet to help restore tissue strength and health. These are the same concerns of many other middle-aged women who are more interested in health and nutrition than in weight and appearance.[13]

CLINICAL NEEDS
Health Promotion and Disease Prevention

Reduction of Risk for Chronic Disease
The emphasis of adult health care is on reducing individual risks for developing chronic disease as persons grow older. This approach has always been used in development of the U.S. dietary guidelines and the national health objectives. These guidelines outline lifestyle changes that we can make to live healthier lives, as follow: (1) eat a variety of foods; (2) maintain a healthy weight; (3) choose a diet low in fat, saturated fat, and cholesterol; (4) choose a diet with plenty of vegetables, fruits, and grain products; (5) only use sugars in moderation; (6) only use salt and sodium in moderation; and (7) if you drink alcoholic beverages, do so in moderation (see Clinical Applications box, "Dietary Guidelines for Americans," in Chapter 1). The guidelines emphasize individual needs and good eating habits based on moderation and variety.

Nutritional Status
Many of the health problems of older adults are not only due to general aging but also to states of malnutrition (see Clinical Applications box, "Feeding Older Adults with Sensitivity"). This undernourishment may develop for several reasons, as follow: (1) poor food habits, often from lack of appetite or loneliness and not wanting to eat alone, as well as lack of sufficient money to buy needed food; (2) oral problems, such as poor teeth or poorly fitting dentures; (3) general gastrointestinal problems, such as declining salivary secretions and dry mouth with diminished thirst and taste sensations, less hydrochloric acid secretion in the stomach, decreased enzyme and mucus secretion in the intestines, and general decline in gastrointestinal motility. Older adults may voice concerns about adequate dietary fiber. Individual medical complaints range from vague indigestion or "irritable colon" to specific diseases such as *peptic ulcer* or *diverticulitis* (see Chapter 18).

Weight Management
Both excessive weight loss and excessive weight gain can be signs of malnutrition. Many of the same depressed living situations and emotional factors described here may also lead to excessive weight gain. Overeating or undereating become a compensation for the conditions encountered in older age. Poor food choices result, and physical activity is usually decreased.

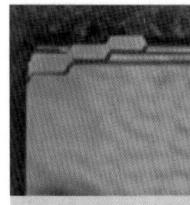

CLINICAL APPLICATIONS
Feeding Older Adults with Sensitivity

Many older adults have eating problems and may easily become malnourished. Each is a unique individual with particular needs and requires sensitive support to meet both nutritional and personal requirements. A personal approach, providing assistance for eating when needed, can help meet these needs.

Basic Guidelines

- *Analyze food habits carefully.* Learn about the attitudes, situations, and desires of the older person. Nutritional needs can be met with a variety of foods, so make suggestions in a practical, realistic, and supportive manner.
- *Never moralize.* Never say, "Eat this because it's good for you." This approach has little value for anyone, especially for those struggling to maintain their personal integrity and self-esteem in a youth-oriented, age-fearing culture that largely alienates its aged.
- *Encourage food variety.* Mix new foods with familiar "comfort foods." New tastes and seasonings often encourage appetite and increase interest in eating. Many people think that a bland

diet is best for all elderly persons—*it is not.* The decreased taste sensitivity of aging necessitates added attention to variety and seasoning. Smaller amounts of food and more frequent meals may also encourage better nutrition.

Assisted Feeding Suggestions

- Make no negative remarks about the food served.
- Identify the food being served.
- Allow the person at least three bites of the same food before going on to another food to allow time for the taste buds to become accustomed to the food.
- Give sufficient time for the person to chew and swallow
- If using a syringe to feed, never feed more than 30 cc (1 oz) at a time to allow enough time for the person to swallow and always remove the syringe from the mouth during swallowing.
- Give liquids throughout the meal, not just at the beginning and end.

Individual Approach

In all cases, personal and realistic planning with every person is essential. Individual personalities and problems are unique, and individual needs vary widely. A malnourished older person needs much personal, sensitive support to build improved eating habits (see the two Clinical Applications boxes, "Feeding Older Adults with Sensitivity" and "Case Study: Situational Problem of an Elderly Woman").

Chronic Diseases of Aging

Diet Modifications

Chronic diseases of aging (e.g., heart disease, cancer, diabetes, and renal disease) may occur in adult years or at a younger age when family history for them exists. Diet modifications and nutritional support are an important part of therapy. Details of these modified diets are given in Chapter 17 and following

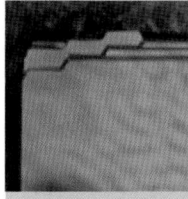

CLINICAL APPLICATIONS

Case Study: Situational Problem of an Elderly Woman

Mrs. Johnson, a 78-year-old widow, lives alone in a three-bedroom house in a large city. A year ago a fall resulted in a broken hip, and now she depends on a walker for limited mobility. Her husband died suddenly 6 months ago, and almost all of her friends have died or are disabled. Her only child, a daughter, lives in a distant city and does not care to bear the burden of responsibility for her mother. Mrs. Johnson's only income is a monthly Social Security check for $160. Her monthly property taxes, insurance payments, and utility bills amount to $130.

A recent medical examination revealed that Mrs. Johnson is severely anemic and has lost 20 pounds in the past 3 months. Her current weight is 82 pounds; she is 5 feet, 4 inches tall. Mrs. Johnson states that she has not been hungry, and her daily diet is repetitious: broth, a little cottage cheese and canned fruit, saltine crackers, and hot tea. She lacks energy, rarely leaves

the house, and appears emaciated and generally distraught.

Questions for Analysis

1. Identify Mrs. Johnson's personal problems and describe how they might have influenced her eating habits. How has her physical problem influenced her food intake?

2. What nutritional improvements could she make in her diet (include food suggestions), and how are these related to her physical needs at this stage of her life?

3. What practical suggestions do you have for helping Mrs. Johnson cope with her physical and social environment? What resources, income sources, food, and companionship can you suggest? How do you think these suggestions would benefit her nutritional status and overall health?

chapters. In any situation, individual needs and food plans are essential for successful therapy.

Drugs

Because people are living longer, many with chronic diseases, older adults may be taking as many as 8 to 12 different prescription drugs for multiple health problems, in addition to over-the-counter drugs. Many drug-nutrient-food interactions can occur (see Chapter 17). Each person needs careful evaluation of all drugs used and instruction on how to take these medications in relation to food intake. Many drugs affect ap-

petite or absorption and use of nutrients, possibly contributing to malnutrition.

COMMUNITY RESOURCES

Government Programs for Older Americans

Older Americans Act

The Administration on Aging of the U.S. Department of Health and Human Services administers programs for older adults under the Older Americans

Act Amendments of 1987. Nutrition programs are promoted through Title III—Grants for State and Community Programs on Aging, Part C—Nutrition Services. These services include both congregate and home-delivered meals, with related nutrition education and food-service components.

Congregate meals. This program provides older Americans—particularly those with low incomes—with low-cost, nutritionally sound meals in senior centers and other public or private community facilities. In these settings, older adults can gather for a hot noon meal and have access to both good food and social support.

Home-delivered meals. For those who are ill or disabled and cannot attend the congregate meals, meals are delivered by couriers to their homes. This service meets nutritional needs and provides human contact and support. The couriers are usually volunteers concerned about the people and their needs. A courier is often the only person a homebound individual may contact during the day.

U.S. Department of Agriculture

The U.S. Department of Agriculture (USDA) provides both research and services for older adults.

Research centers. Research centers for studies on aging are being established in various areas of the United States. For example, a Human Nutrition Research Center on Aging has been built at Tufts University in Boston and is the largest research facility in the U.S. specifically authorized by Congress to study the role of nutrition in aging. Studies there involve research on topics such as the protein needs of the aged, the nutritional status of elderly men and women, and the prevention and slowing of osteoporosis through nutritional support. Much more knowledge about the nutritional requirements of older adults is needed in order to provide better care.

Extension services. The USDA operates agricultural extension services in state "land grant" universities, including food- and nutrition-education services. County home advisors help communities with practical materials and counsel for elderly persons and community workers.

Public Health Service (PHS)

The Public Health Service (PHS) is a major division of the U.S. Department of Health and Human Services. Skilled health professionals work in the community through local and state public health departments. Public health nutritionists are important members of this health care team, providing nutrition counseling and education and helping with various food-assistance programs.

Professional Organizations and Resources

National Groups

The American Geriatric Society and the Gerontological Society are national professional organizations of physicians, nurses, nutritionists, and other interested health workers. These societies publish journals and promote community and government efforts to meet needs of aging persons.

Community Groups

Local medical societies, nursing organizations, and dietetic associations sponsor various programs to help meet the needs of elderly people. An increasing number of qualified nutritionists, who are registered dietitians, are also in private practice in most communities and can supply a variety of individual and group services. Senior centers in local communities are also resources.

Volunteer Organizations

Many activities of volunteer health organizations (e.g., the American Heart Association and the American Diabetes Association) relate to the needs of older persons.

SUMMARY

Meeting the nutritional needs of adults—especially older adults—is a challenge for several reasons. We have lacked sufficient research on which to base the determination of energy and nutrient needs as persons grow older. Current and past social, economic, and psychologic factors influence needs, and the biologic process of aging differs widely in individuals. Moreover, standards for older adults are mainly based on data available for younger adult populations or requirements to counteract the disease processes of aging (e.g., heart disease).

Much of the illness in older adults results from malnutrition—not from the effects of aging. Thus in working with older people, food habits must be carefully analyzed and approached with encouragement to make any positive changes. Individual supportive guidance and patience are required, using available nutrition resources as needed.

REVIEW QUESTIONS

1. Identify three major biologic changes that occur with aging and give an example of each.
2. Identify and describe three major factors contributing to malnutrition in older adults.

How do these factors influence the nutrition-counseling process?

3. List and describe the resources of several agencies providing nutrition-related services for elderly persons.

SELF-TEST QUESTIONS

True-False

Write the correct statement for each item you answer "false."

1. Old persons in American society are generally given much value and made to feel needed and productive.
2. In American health care, much progress has been made in the control of chronic disease in old age and related medical and social care practices in meeting the needs of the aged.
3. Beginning at about the age of 30, a gradual increase occurs in the performance capacity of most organ systems that lasts throughout adulthood.
4. We have an extensive research base of knowledge about the nutritional needs of elderly persons and can state their specific energy and nutrient requirements.
5. The simplest basis for judging the adequacy of kcalorie intake is the maintenance of normal weight.

6. The protein requirement increases with age.
7. Most elderly persons require additional supplements of vitamins and minerals.

Multiple Choice

1. The basic biologic changes of old age include:
   a. An increase in the number of cells.
   b. A decreasing sense of self-worth.
   c. An increased basal metabolic rate.
   d. A gradual loss of functioning cells and reduced cell metabolism.
2. Protein needs in adulthood are influenced by (circle all that apply):
   a. The biologic value of the dietary protein being used.
   b. The adequacy of the diet's energy value (kcalories).
   c. The individual's state of health.
   d. The nature of the dietary fats (i.e., the saturated to unsaturated ratio).

3. Which of the following responses is an example of a physiologic change in aging? (Circle all that apply.)
   a. Increased cell metabolism to meet increased aging needs
   b. Decreased gastrointestinal motility
   c. A gradual increase in the body's reserve capacity
   d. Decreased digestive secretions

4. Which of the following actions would help elderly persons in finding solutions to health problems? (Circle all that apply.)
   a. Analyze the individual living situation and food habits carefully.
   b. Reinforce good habits, leave harmless ones alone, and suggest needed changes that are practical within the living situation.
   c. Encourage variety in foods and seasonings.
   d. Explore and use available community resources for assistance.

SUGGESTIONS FOR ADDITIONAL STUDY

1. Nutritional Analysis of an Older Adult's Diet
Select an older adult and plan a home visit, individually or in a small group of two to three students. In the home, interview this person and observe food use and habits. For example, go with the person into the kitchen and show your interest in facilities for cooking and food storage. Note the food products in the refrigerator and on the shelves.

Analyze your findings in terms of kcalories (energy value) and the following four nutrients: protein, vitamin D, calcium, and iron. Also note the nature of the carbohydrates (i.e., complex, simple, fiber) and fats (i.e., animal or plant sources) used. Plan with the person a suitable diet with suggestions to meet the following priorities: (1) variety in foods and seasonings, (2) personal desires, (3) practical living situation, and (4) nutritional needs.

If possible, go with the person to a nearby market and suggest some tips for wise buying of food products. Return to the home and help prepare a meal or snack, discussing the values of various food items. Follow up with a later visit, if possible, to provide additional support and encouragement to continue any needed improvements in food habits.

2. Community Senior Citizens Center
Arrange for an informal interview with the center director to learn about the center's activities and programs. Plan with the director a follow-up visit for one of the center activities. Informally discuss some of the center's programs and activities with persons there. Bring your findings to class.

REFERENCES

1. Chernoff R: Baby boomers come of age: nutrition in the 21st century, *J Am Diet Assoc* 95(6):650, 1995.
2. U.S. Department of Health and Human Services: *Healthy people 2010: understanding and improving health*, Washington, DC, 2000, U.S. Department of Health and Human Services, Government Printing Office.
3. U.S. Census Bureau, U.S. Department of Commerce: *Statistical abstract of the United States 1999*, ed 119, Washington, DC, 1999, U.S. Department of Commerce, Government Printing Office.
4. Council of Economic Advisors: *Economic report of the President*, Washington, DC, 2000, Council of Economic Advisors, Government Printing Office.
5. Egbert AM: The dwindles: failure to thrive in older patients, *Nutr Rev* 54(1):S25, 1996.
6. Cass R, Shea ME: Recognizing depression in older adults: the role of the dietitian, *JAMA* 96(10):1042, 1996.
7. National Research Council, Food and Nutrition Board: *Recommended dietary allowances*, ed 10, Washington, DC, 1989, National Academy Press.

8. Marriot BM: Editorial: vitamin D supplement—a word of caution, *Ann Intern Med* 127(3):231, 1997.

9. Packard PT, Heaney RP: Medical nutrition therapy for patients with osteoporosis, *J Am Diet Assoc* 97(414), 1997.

10. Ullom-Minnich P: Prevention of osteoporosis and fractures, *Am Fam Phys* 60(1):7, 1999.

11. Food and Nutrition Board, Institute of Medicine: *Dietary reference intakes for calcium, phosphorus, magnesium, vitamin D, and fluoride*, Washington, DC, 1997, National Academy Press.

12. Marshall JA and others: Indicators of nutritional risk in a rural elderly Hispanic and non-Hispanic white population: the San Luis Valley health and aging study, *J Am Diet Assoc* 99(3):315, 1999.

13. Lahmann PH, Kumanyika SK: Attitudes about health and nutrition are more indicative of dietary quality in 50- to 75-year old women than weight and appearance concerns, *J Am Diet Assoc* 99(4):475, 1999.

FURTHER READING

• Bernard MA and others: Common health problems among minority elders, *J Am Diet Assoc* 97(7):771, 1997.

This article reviews the primary health problems of elderly people in four of our most prominent minority population groups: African Americans, Hispanic Americans, Asian/Pacific Islander Americans, and Native Americans. This highly useful information will assist health workers in decision-making in dietary counseling.

• Pennington JAT and others: Update: diet-related observational studies supported by the National Institutes of Health, *Nutr Today* 34(1):29, 1999.

This report describes current and recent NIH studies, including a unique study of 700 extremely frail, homebound elderly patients aged 60 to 101 years.

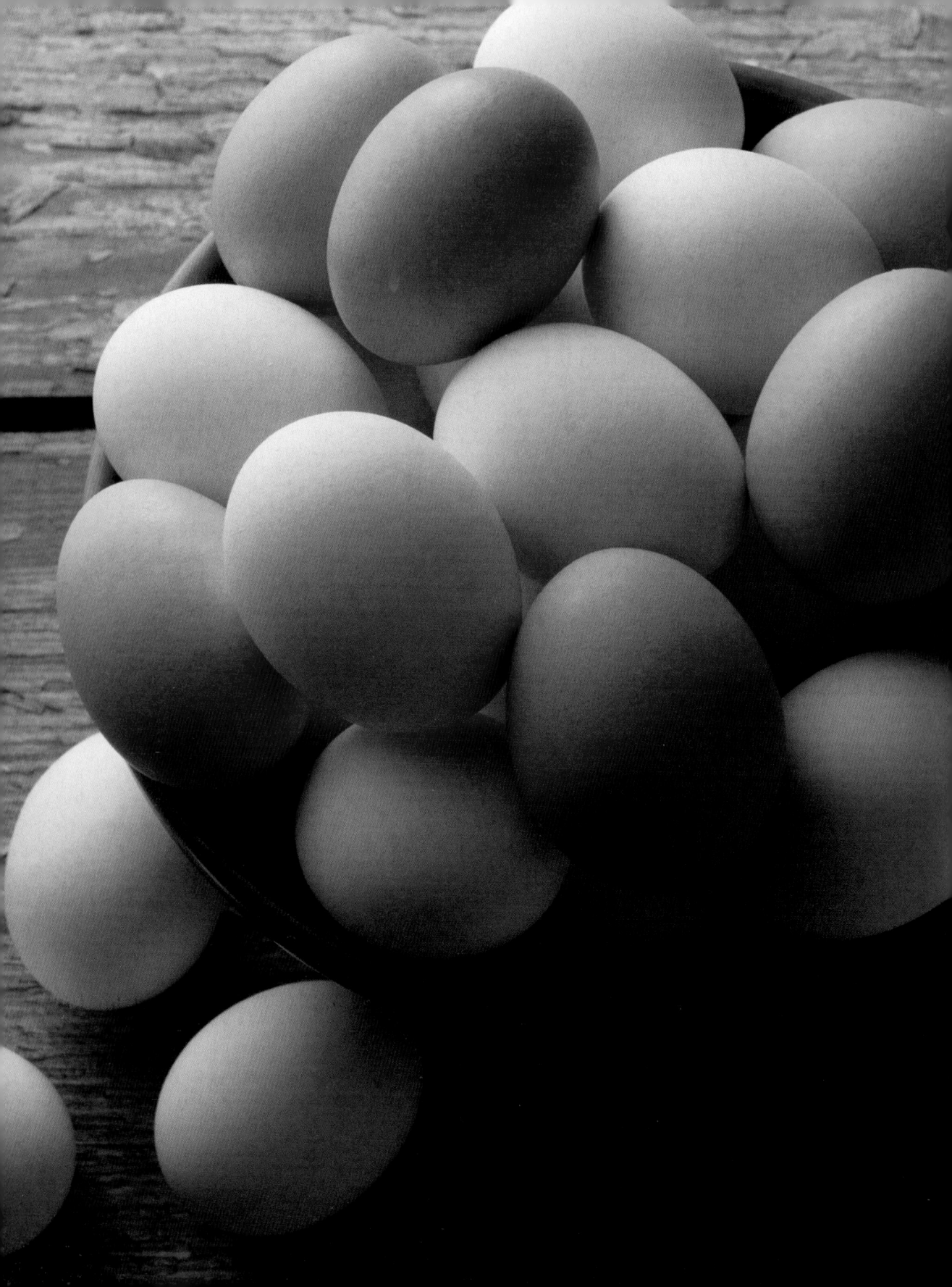

Community
Nutrition and
Health Care

3

13

Community Food Supply and Health

KEY CONCEPTS

- Modern food production, processing, and marketing have both positive and negative influences on food safety.

- Many organisms in contaminated food transmit disease.

- Poverty effectively prevents individuals and families from having adequate access to their surrounding community food supply.

The health of a community largely depends on the safety of its available food and water supply. Our system of government control agencies and regulations, along with local and state public health officials, works diligently at maintaining a safe food supply and is generally—but not always—successful. There are problems because our technologic advances are quickly changing our total environment, and such progress brings new problems.

In this chapter, we explore factors that influence the safety of the food we eat. Our bountiful food supply is accompanied by certain hazards. Potential health problems related to our food supply can also arise from two other sources—food-borne disease and poverty.

FOOD SAFETY

The character of America's food supply has radically changed over the years. These changes, which have swept the food-marketing system, are rooted in widespread social change and in scientific advance. The agricultural and food processing industries have developed various chemicals to increase and preserve our food supply. Critics, however, voice concerns about how these changes have affected food safety and the overall environment. Their concerns center on pesticides and food additives.

Agricultural Pesticides

Reasons for Use

Large American agricultural corporations, as well as individual farmers, use a number of chemicals to promote their crop yields. These materials have made the advances in food production required to feed a growing population possible. For example, farmers use certain chemicals to control a wide variety of destructive insects, kill weeds, control plant diseases, stop fruit from dropping prematurely, and cause leaves to fall. Thus these substances facilitate harvesting, make seeds sprout, keep seeds from rotting before they sprout, increase yield, and generally improve marketing quality.

Problems

Concerns and confusion continue about the use and effects of these chemicals. Problems have developed in four main areas, as follow: (1) the pesticide residues on foods; (2) the gradual leaching of the chemicals into ground water and surrounding wells; (3) the increased exposure of farm workers to these strong chemicals; and (4) the increased amount of chemicals required as insects develop a tolerance. Over time, use of these chemicals has created our pesticide dilemma—what do we do in the face of conflicting interests? Thousands of pesticides are in use, and testing them fully and consistently is a difficult task.

Scientists are constantly at work to improve technology for day-to-day testing of difficult-to-detect food residues.[1]

A basic problem focuses on the difficulty of assessing the risks of specific pesticides in use. Such assessment is important for children, who are more vulnerable to larger amounts, as well as for adults, who are eating an increasing amount of fresh vegetables and fruits in their daily diets.

Alternative Agriculture

An increasing number of concerned farmers, with help from soil scientists, are turning to alternative agricultural methods instead of heavy reliance on pesticide use. They are developing systems of sustainable agriculture that produce large amounts of high-quality food, protect the land and its resources, preserve the environment, and are profitable.[1] An increasing number of farmers, especially in California—the major supplier of U.S. fruits and vegetables, are introducing organic farming. They are entirely using this system of nonchemical control practices or combining it with limited pesticide use in a farming system known as Integrated Pest Management. These agricultural systems combine traditional conservation practices and modern technology. The science of agrogenetics is also being developed as part of this technology. Through these studies, plant physiologists are developing strains of genetically modified foods that reduce the need for toxic pesticides and herbicides.[2]

Food Additives

Over the past few decades, *food additives* (i.e., chemicals intentionally added to foods) have become part of our food supply. Our current variety of food market items would be impossible without them. Additives have helped turn corner grocery stores into our giant supermarket chains. Scientific advances have created these processed food products, and our changing society has created the market for them. Our expanding population, greater work force, and more complex family life have increased our desire for more variety and convenience in foods, as well as for better safety and quality.[3,4] Food additives help achieve these needs and serve many purposes. For example, additives do the following:

(1) enrich foods with added nutrients; (2) produce uniform qualities (e.g., color, flavor, aroma, texture, and general appearance); (3) standardize many functional factors (e.g., thickening or stabilization [keeping parts from separating]); (4) preserve foods by preventing oxidation; and (5) control acidity or alkalinity to improve flavor, texture, and the cooked product. Table 13-1 lists some examples of food additives. A number of micronutrients and antioxidants are used as additives in processed foods, not for their ability to increase nutrient content but for their technical effects either during processing or in the final product.

Government Control Agencies

Several government agencies now help control the safety and quality of our food. Concerned sections in the U.S. Department of Health and Human Services are the Food and Drug Administration (FDA) and the Public Health Service (PHS). The U.S. Department of Agriculture (USDA) controls the use of pesticides in farming; related work is assigned to the Agricultural Research Service and the Consumer Marketing Service. The Federal Trade Commission and the National Bureau of Standards also protect the consumer. Of these various agencies, the FDA primarily controls food safety.

Food and Drug Administration

Enforcement of federal food-safety regulations. The FDA is a law enforcement agency charged by Congress to ensure, among other things, that our food supply is safe, pure, and wholesome. With able commissioners, the agency has cleared its backlog of assessment work and strengthened itself through tough enforcement of regulations. The agency enforces federal food-safety regulations through various activities, including the following: (1) enforcing food sanitation and quality control; (2) controlling chemical contaminants and pesticides; (3) controlling food additives; (4) regulating the movement of foods across state lines; (5) maintaining the nutrition labeling of foods; (6) ensuring the safety of public food service; and (7) ensuring the safety of meat

and milk. The agency's methods of enforcement are recall, seizure, injunction, and prosecution. The use of recalls is the most common method, followed by seizures of contaminated food.

Consumer education. The FDA's division of consumer education conducts an active program of protection through consumer education and general public information. Special attention is given to nutrition misinformation. Materials are prepared and distributed to individuals, students, and community groups. Consumer specialists work through all FDA district offices.

Research. Along with the USDA's Agricultural Research Service, FDA scientists continually evaluate foods and food components through their own

---

sustainable agriculture a system of agriculture that combines traditional conservation-minded farming techniques with modern technologies. Sustainable systems use modern equipment, certified seed, and soil- and water-conservation practices with emphasis on rotating crops, building up the soil, diversifying crops and livestock, and controlling pests naturally. Major goals are safe soil preservation and avoidance of a heavy dependence on pesticides and chemical fertilizers.

organic farming farming methods that use natural means of pest control by choosing hardy plant varieties that resist diseases and introduce beneficial insects to thrive and help control entrenched populations of destructive ones, thus avoiding dependence on stronger and stronger pesticides as resistant insects multiply. These methods also use time-tested natural means of enriching soil (e.g., crop rotation and cycling plant mulch and manure) for healthier soil and pesticide-free foods.

agrogenetics application of the science of genetic engineering to agriculture to produce hardier plant species that are more resistant to pests and disease.

TABLE 13-1 Examples of food additives

Function	Chemical compound	Common food uses
Acid, alkalis, buffers	Sodium bicarbonate	Baking powder
	Tartaric acid	Fruit sherbets
		Cheese spread
Antibiotics	Chlortetracycline	Dip for dressed poultry
Anticaking agents	Aluminum calcium silicate	Table salt
Antimycotics	Calcium propionate	Bread
	Sodium propionate	Bread
	Sorbic acid	Cheese
Antioxidants	Butylated hydroxyanisole (BHA)	Fats
	Butylated hydroxytoluene (BHT)	Fats
Bleaching agents	Benzoyl peroxide	Wheat flour
	Chlorine dioxide	
	Oxides of nitrogen	
Color preservative	Sodium benzoate	Green peas
		Maraschino cherries
Coloring agents	Annatto	Butter, margarine
	Carotene	
Emulsifiers	Lecithin	Bakery goods
	Monoglycerides and diglycerides	Dairy products
		Confections
	Propylene glycol alginate	
Flavoring agents	Amyl acetate	Soft drinks
	Benzaldehyde	Bakery goods
	Methyl salicylate	Candy; ice cream
	Essential oils; natural extractives	Canned meats
	Monosodium glutamate	
Nonnutritive sweeteners	Saccharin	Diet canned fruit
	Aspartame	Low-calorie soft drinks
Nutrient supplements	Potassium iodide	Iodized salt
	Vitamin C	Fruit juices
	Vitamin D	Milk
	Vitamin A	Margarine
	B vitamins, iron	Bread and cereal
Sequestrants	Sodium citrate	Dairy products
	Calcium pyrophosphoric acid	
Stabilizers and thickeners	Pectin	Jellies
	Vegetable gums (carob bean, carrageenan, guar)	Dairy desserts and chocolate milk
	Gelatin	Confections
	Agar-agar	"Low-calorie" salad dressings
Yeast foods and dough conditioners	Ammonium chloride	Bread, rolls
	Calcium sulfate	
	Calcium phosphate	

research (Figure 13-1). In the more distant past, FDA views and policies have varied with administrators and sometimes left much to be desired. Nevertheless, in the more recent past and today, broader views more in tune with today's needs prevail. Today people want to know more than just that a given food will not kill them; they want to know if it has any positive nutritional value. For a more health-conscious public and a changed marketplace, the FDA is developing nutrition guidelines for a variety of food products, including main dishes, meat substitutes, groups of foods having high malnutrition risks, fruit juices and fruit drinks, and snack foods. The development of these guidelines is a broad jump from the attitudes of more distant administrators involving a purely regulatory function. Such guidelines are rapidly progressing to meet our changing needs in these changing times.

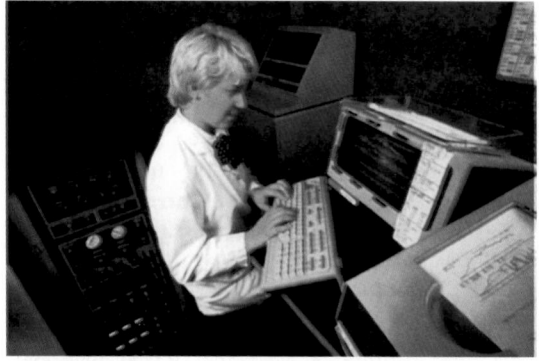

FIGURE 13-1   Research in food chemistry. A chemist in the U.S. Department of Agriculture's Grand Forks Nutrition Research Center analyzes the amount of copper absorbed from food eaten by volunteers. (Credit: Agricultural Research Service, USDA.)

Development of Food Labels

Early Development of Label Regulations
In the mid-1960s, the FDA established "truth in packaging" regulations that dealt mainly with food standards. As food processing developed and the number of items grew, the labels also needed to have more nutritional information added. Both types of label information are important to consumers.

Food standards. The basic *standard of identity* requires that labels on foods not having an established reference standard must list all the ingredients in the order of amount found in the product. Other food standard information on labels relates to food quality, fill of container, and enrichment.

Nutritional information. Under regulations adopted in 1973, the FDA began developing a labeling system that describes a food item's nutritional value to meet the increasing nutritional interest and concern of consumers. Some producers began to add limited information on their own to meet this increasing market demand. Many persons became concerned that nutrition labeling was inadequate, but the real problem was

what, how much, and in what format. Information about nutrients and food constituents that consumer groups believed should be listed on labels included the amount of macronutrients (i.e., carbohydrate, protein, fat) and their total energy value (i.e., calories), key micronutrients (i.e., vitamins, minerals), sodium, cholesterol, and saturated fat. Concerned public and professional groups also wanted nutrients to be identified in terms of percentages of the current DRI or RDA standard per defined portion.[5,6]

Development of Current FDA Nutrition Labeling Regulations

Background of Present FDA Label Regulations
Over the immediate past few years, two factors fueled rapid progress toward better food labels. These factors were the following: (1) the increase in the variety of food products entering the U.S. marketplace, and (2) the changing patterns of American food habits. Both of these realities led many health-conscious consumers and professionals alike to increasingly rely on nutrition labeling on foods to help meet health goals.[5,6] A number of labeling problems—including

lack of uniformity, misleading health claims, and indefinite terms such as "natural" and "light"—persisted. These problems indicated a need to reorganize and coordinate the entire food labeling system. This need had been reinforced by three previous landmark reports relating nutrition and diet to national health goals: *The Surgeon General's Report on Nutrition and Health*, the National Research Council's *Diet and Health*, and the Public Health Service's national health goals and objectives to be reached by the year 2000, *Healthy People 2000*. Based on these reports, the Institute of Medicine of the National Academy of Sciences established a Committee on the Nutrition Components of Food Labeling to study and report on the scientific issues and practical needs involved in food-labeling reform. The report of this committee provided basic guidelines for the rule-making process conducted by FDA and the U.S. Departments of Agriculture and Health and Human Services, for submission to the U.S. Congress to achieve the needed reforms (see the For Further Focus box, "Nutrition Labeling: Recommendations for a New Century"). Three areas of concern formed the basis of recommendations from the Institute of Medicine, National Research Council, as follow: (1) foods for mandatory regulations; (2) the format of label information; and (3) education of consumers. This report became the basic guideline for the final law and regulations enacted by Congress in 1994.

Current Food Label Format

The food label format that is so familiar to us now is very different from the one used in the 1970s and 1980s. The title *Nutrition Facts* is printed in bold eye-catching lettering. Because the classic vitamin B deficiency diseases are no longer a public health problem in the United States, these micronutrients are now deleted, giving room for the current focus on macronutrients that have a greater effect on chronic diseases.

An example of the revised food label format is given in Figure 13-2. Manufacturers of processed foods may choose to include additional nutrients, such as calories from saturated fat, polyunsaturated fat, monounsaturated fat, potassium, soluble and in-

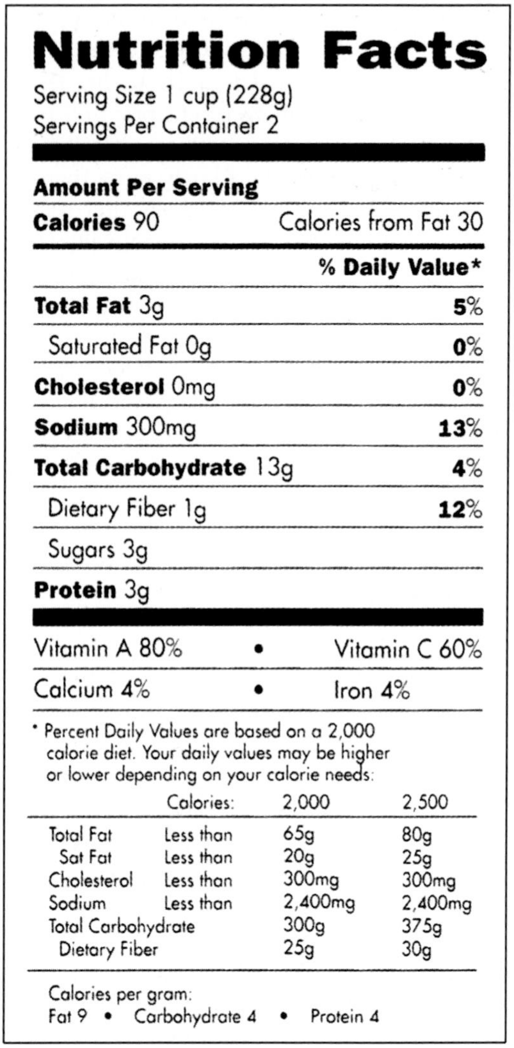

FIGURE 13-2 Example of a food product label showing the detailed Nutrition Facts box of nutrition information mandated by FDA under the Nutrition Labeling and Education Act. (From the Food and Drug Administration, Washington, DC.)

soluble fiber, sugar alcohol (e.g., sorbitol), other carbohydrates, and/or other vitamins and minerals.

Another key term is *daily value*, which refers to two separate label nutrient reference values, based on current RDAs, as follow: (1) the Reference

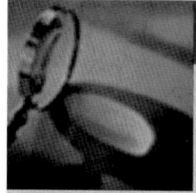

FOR FURTHER FOCUS

Nutrition Labeling: Recommendations for a New Century

There is no longer any doubt. The U.S. government is now committed by law to the food labeling reform mandated by a health-conscious public, a proliferation of new health-related food products marketplace, and concerned health professionals. It is apparent that nutrition "sells" in today's consumer market.

As part of the rule-making process and final regulations to administer the Nutrition Labeling and Education Act (NLEA) at the FDA and USDA, the initial report and recommendations of the Institute of Medicine's Committee on the Nutrition Components of Food Labeling, National Academy of Sciences, formed the foundation for final implementation of the law. This baseline focus resulted from a 1-year study requested by the U.S. Departments of Health and Human Services (DHHS) and Agriculture (USDA). The study committee made the following recommendations, which are embodied in NLEA law:

Foods Covered by Nutrition Labeling:

- Nutrition labeling should be mandatory on most packaged foods.
- Nutrition labeling should be provided at the point of purchase for produce, seafood, meats, and poultry.
- Restaurants should make the nutrient content of menu items available to customers on request.

Label Presentation

- The FDA and USDA should set standardized serving sizes.
- More complete ingredient listings should be provided on all foods.
- A modified regulatory scheme should be established for the development and approval of lower-fat alternative foods that currently have standards of identity.

Educating Consumers

- A well-designed nutrition labeling program should be fashioned as one part of a comprehensive education program, concurrent with the adoption of new regulations on the labeling of nutrition content and format, to help consumers make wise dietary choices.

From the beginning of the process, Congress wanted to develop legislative proposals to clarify the legal basis for reforms. The food industry, health professionals, and consumer groups wanted to promote changes in nutrition labeling that reflect the actual current dietary guidelines (RDAs) and related product development. These recommendations of the committee have provided a helpful foundation for all concerned.

Daily Intakes (RDIs), referring to current DRI and RDA standards for vitamins and minerals, and (2) the Daily Reference Values (DRVs), referring to current RDAs for macronutrients (see the For Further Focus Box, "A Glossary of Terms for Current Labels"). In addition, the serving size (i.e., the amount of the food customarily consumed) must be given and expressed in household measures, followed by the metric weight in parentheses and the total number of servings per container.

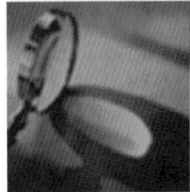

FOR FURTHER FOCUS

A Glossary of Terms for Current Labels

To improve communication between producers and consumers, we must all use the same "dictionary" supplied by the FDA. Whether these terms are used in the common format of nutrition information in the box titled "Nutrition Facts" or elsewhere as part of the manufacturer's product description, everyone must work from the same FDA "dictionary." The following is a sampling:

Nutrition Facts Box

Daily values (DV)

DVs are reference values that relates the nutrition information to a total daily diet of 2,000 kcalories, which is appropriate for most women and teenage girls, and some sedentary men. The footnote indicates the daily values for a 2,500-kcalorie diet, which meets the needs of most men, teenage boys, and active women. To help consumers determine how a food fits into a healthy diet, the following nutrients, in the order given, must be listed as percent of the daily value (DV%):

- Total fat
- Saturated fat
- Cholesterol
- Sodium
- Total carbohydrate
- Dietary fiber
- Vitamins A and C
- Calcium and iron

Daily Reference Value (DRV)

As part of the DVs listed here, the DRVs are a set of dietary standards for the following eight nutrients: total fat, saturated fat, cholesterol, total carbohydrate, dietary fiber, protein, potassium, and sodium. DRVs do not appear on the label because they are part of a food's DV.

Reference Daily Intake (RDI)

As part of the DVs listed here, the RDIs are a set of dietary standards for essential vitamins and minerals, and—in some cases—protein. RDIs are based on the actual Recommended Dietary Allowances (RDAs), which are now part of the new Dietary Reference Intakes (DRI) standards. This replaced the old confusing term "US RDA," which was developed by food manufacturers as an estimate based on old RDAs. RDIs do not appear on the label because they are part of a food's DV.

Descriptive Terms on Products

The FDA has specifically defined many terms that manufacturers must follow if they wish to use the term on their product. The following are some examples:

- **Fat free:** Less than 0.5 g of fat per serving.
- **Low cholesterol:** 20 mg of cholesterol or less per serving and per 100 g; 2 g saturated fat or less per serving. Any label claim about low cholesterol is prohibited for all foods that contain more than 2 g of saturated fat per serving.
- **Light** or **Lite:** At least a one-third reduction in kcalories (i.e., 40 kcal with minimum fat reduction of 3 g; if fat contributes 50% or more of total kcalories, fat content must be reduced by 50% compared with the reference food).
- **Less sodium:** At least a 25% reduction; 140 mg or less per reference amount per serving.
- **High:** 20% or more of the DV per serving.
- **Reduced saturated fat:** At least 25% less saturated fat per reference amount than an appropriate reference food.
- **Lean:** Applied to meat, poultry, and seafood; less than 10 g of fat, 4 g of saturated fat, and 95 mg of cholesterol per reference amount, and 100 g for individual foods.

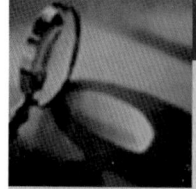

FOR FURTHER FOCUS

A Glossary of Terms for Current Labels—cont'd

- **Extra Lean:** Applied to meat, poultry, and seafood; less than 5 g of fat, 2 g of saturated fat, and 95 mg of cholesterol per reference amounts and 100 g for individual foods.

Health Claims

The FDA guidelines indicate that any health claim on a label must be supported by substantial scientific evidence and has found that the following claims meet this test and can be used:
- Sodium and hypertension
- Calcium and osteoporosis

- Dietary fat and cancer
- Dietary cholesterol and saturated fat and coronary heart disease
- Fiber-containing grain products, fruits, and vegetables and cancer
- Grain products and fruits and vegetables that contain fiber—especially soluble fiber and coronary heart disease
- Fruits and vegetables rich in vitamins A or C and cancer

FOOD-BORNE DISEASE

Costs of Food-Borne Disease

Many disease-bearing organisms inhabit our environment and can contaminate our food and water. We have learned much about them in past years and have taken many steps to control their spread. Lapses in our control still occur, however, resulting in high incidences of illness and death, as well as greater economic cost. This effect is probably greatest in developing countries of the world because few facts are known about real costs, although great costs also occur in developed countries. Recent reports for the United States and Canada included accounts of real economic costs that effect government public health facilities, private health care centers, nursing care centers, as well as patients' personal earnings from inability to work. For example, preliminary U.S. estimates of food-borne disease have been previously reported as 12.6 million cases per year with costs for medical care and personal salary losses totaling approximately $8.4 billion.[7] Microbiologic diseases (bacterial and viral) represented 84% of these U.S.

costs, compared with 88% in Canada. The important U.S. diseases reported with less economic impact were *Salmonellosis* and staphylococcal poisoning, costing annually $4.0 billion and $1.5 billion respectively. Other costly types of food-borne disease include *listeriosis, trichinosis, C. perfringens* enteritis, and botulism. The reported cost per case of botulism annually in the United States was estimated to be $322,200, but its total comparative effect was much lower (i.e., only $87 million) because relatively few cases (270), occurred.[7]

Examples of common infections in home and community breakouts have included *Listeria, Salmonella,* and *E. coli.*[8] Recent sources of these infections include water from public drinking water at a county fair, ice cream from a widespread distributor, and raw milk or soft cheeses.[9,10]

Food Sanitation

Food and Its Environment

Control of food-borne disease obviously focuses on strict sanitation measures and rigid personal hygiene. First, the food itself should be of good quality and not defective or diseased. Second, its dry or cold storage should protect it from deterioration or decay, which is especially important for such recently developed products as refrigerated convenience foods, the fastest-growing segment of the convenience food market and potentially the most dangerous because they are not sterile. These vacuum-packaged or modified-atmosphere chilled food products are only minimally processed—not sterilized—and risk temperature abuse. Home refrigerator temperatures should be held at 40° F or lower. At temperatures above 45° F, any precooked or leftover foods are potential reservoirs that survive the cooking and can recontaminate the cooked food. For food safety, it pays to be careful at all critical points, as follow[11,12]:

- Cook thoroughly when you first cook a food.
- If you cook ahead, cool food rapidly in small, shallow containers; and freeze it for longer keeping.
- When you cook in a microwave oven, cover food, heat or cook thoroughly, and allow standing time to finish cooking.
- Any time you are unsure of a food's safety, THROW IT OUT!

All food preparation areas must be scrupulously clean, and foods must be washed or cleaned well. Cooking procedures and temperatures must be followed as directed. All utensils, dishes, and anything else coming in contact with food must be clean. Leftover food must be stored and reused appropriately or discarded. Garbage must be contained and disposed of in a sanitary manner. We know about all of these measures but do not always practice them.

Food Handlers

All persons handling food, especially those working with public food services, should follow strict rules of personal hygiene. For example, simple hand washing, along with clean clothing and aprons, is imperative. Basic rules of hygiene should apply to all persons handling food, whether they work in food processing and packaging plants, process and package foods in markets, or prepare and serve food in restaurants. In addition, persons with infectious disease obviously should not work around food, although this sometimes occurs.

Food Contamination

Bacterial Food Infections

Bacterial food infections result from eating food contaminated by large colonies of different types of bacteria. Specific diseases result from specific bacteria (e.g., *salmonellosis*, *shigellosis*, and *listeriosis*).

Salmonellosis is caused by *Salmonella*, a bacteria named for the American veterinarian-pathologist Daniel Salmon (1850-1914), who first isolated and identified the species commonly causing human food-borne infections—*S. typhi* and *S. paratyphi*. These organisms grow readily in common foods such as milk, custard, egg dishes, salad dressing, and sandwich fillings. Seafood, especially shellfish such as oysters and clams, from polluted waters may also be a source of infection. Unsanitary handling of foods and utensils can spread the bacteria. Resulting cases of gastroenteritis may vary from mild diarrhea to severe attacks. Practices of immunization, pasteurization, and sanitary regulations involving community water and food supplies, as well as food handlers, help to control such outbreaks. Because incubation and multiplication of the bacteria take time (after the food is eaten), symptoms of food infection develop relatively slowly (i.e., usually at least 12 to 24 hours later).

Shigellosis is caused by the bacteria *Shigella*, named for the Japanese physician Kiyoshi Shiga (1870-1957), who first discovered a main species of the organism—*S. dysenteriae*—during a dysentery epidemic in Japan in 1898. Shigellosis is usually confined to the large intestine and may vary from a mild transient intestinal disturbance in adults to fatal dysentery in young children. The bacteria grow easily in foods—especially in milk, which is a common vehicle of transmission to infants and children. The boiling of water or pasteurization of milk kills the organisms, but the food or milk may easily be reinfected through unsanitary handling by a carrier. The disease is spread similarly to how salmonella is transmitted (i.e., by feces, fingers, flies, milk, and food and articles handled by unsanitary carriers).

Listeriosis is caused by the bacteria *Listeria*, which was named for the English surgeon Baron Joseph Lister (1827-1912), who first applied knowledge of bacterial infection to the principles of antiseptic surgery in a benchmark 1867 publication that lead to "clean" operations and the development of modern surgery. Only within the past 20 years, however, has knowledge of bacteria's role in directly causing food-borne disease in humans (i.e., both occasional illness and disease epidemics) increased and the major species causing human illness—*L. monocytogenes*—been identified.[8] Before 1981, *Listeria* was thought to be only an organism of animal disease transmitted to humans by direct contact with infected animals. Now it is clear, however, that this organism widely occurs in the environment and in high-risk individuals such as elderly persons, pregnant women, infants, or patients with suppressed immune systems and can produce rare but often fatal illness, with severe symptoms such as diarrhea, flulike fever and headache, pneumonia, sepsis, meningitis, and endocarditis. Food-borne disease has been traced to a variety of foods including soft cheese, poultry, seafood, raw milk, commercially broken and refrigerated raw liquid whole eggs, and meat products (e.g., pate).[13] A recent case of Listeria in a young pregnant woman was traced to hot dogs and ham in a public restaurant.[14]

Bacterial Food Poisoning

Food poisoning is caused by the ingestion of bacterial toxins that have been produced in the food by the growth of specific kinds of bacteria before the food is eaten. The powerful toxin is ingested directly, so symptoms of the food poisoning develop rapidly (i.e., usually 1 to 6 hours after the food is eaten). Two types of bacterial food poisoning are most commonly responsible, *staphylococcal* and *clostridial*.

Staphyloccal food poisoning was named for the shape of the causative organism, which is mainly *Staphylococcus aureus*—round bacteria forming masses of cells (Gr. *staphyl*—bunch of grapes;

kokkus—berry), is the most common form of bacterial food poisoning in the United States. Powerful preformed toxins in the contaminated food produce illness rapidly (i.e., 1 to 6 hours after ingestion). The symptoms appear suddenly and include severe cramping and abdominal pain with nausea, vomiting, and diarrhea, usually accompanied by sweating, headache, fever, and sometimes prostration and shock. Recovery is fairly rapid, however, and symptoms subside within 24 hours (see the Clinical Applications Box, "Case Study: A Community Food Poisoning Incident"). The amount of toxin ingested and the susceptibility of the individual eating it determine the degree of severity. The source of the contamination is usually a staphylococcal infection on the hand of a worker preparing the food. This infection is often minor and considered harmless or even unnoticed by the food handler. Foods that are particularly effective culture beds for staphylococci and their toxins include custard or cream-filled bakery goods, processed meats, ham, tongue, cheese, ice cream, potato salad, sauces, chicken and ham salads, and combination dishes such as spaghetti and casseroles. The toxin causes no change in the normal appearance, odor, or taste of the food, so the victim has no warning. A careful food history helps determine the source of the poisoning, and portions of the food are obtained for bacterial examination, if possible. Few bacteria may be found because heating kills the organisms but does not destroy toxin produced.

Clostridial food poisoning was named for the spore-forming rod-shaped bacteria (Gr. *kloster*, spindle), mainly *Clostridium perfringes* and *Clostridium botulinum*, that can also form powerful toxins in infected foods. *C. perfringes* spores are widespread in the environment (e.g., in soil, water, dust, refuse, and everywhere else). This organism multiplies in cooked meat and meat dishes and develops its toxin in foods held at warm or room temperatures for an extended time. A number of outbreaks from food eaten in restaurants, college dining rooms, and school cafeterias have been reported. In each case, cooked meat was improperly prepared and/or refrigerated. Control rests principally on

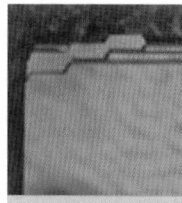

CLINICAL APPLICATIONS

Case Study: A Community Food Poisoning Incident

John and Eva Wesson, a middle-aged couple, agreed that their lodge dinner had been the best they had ever had, especially the dessert—custard-filled cream puffs, John's favorite. He had eaten two of them, despite Eva's protests. Maybe that was why he began to feel ill shortly after they arrived home. Eva's stomach felt a little upset too, so they both took some antacid pills, thinking their "stomachaches" were from eating more rich food than they were accustomed to having. They went to bed early.

By 11:00 PM, however, Eva woke up alarmed. John was vomiting and having diarrhea and increasingly severe stomach cramps. He complained of a headache, and his pajamas were wet with sweat. He had a fever and appeared to be in shock. Eva began to have similar pains and symptoms, although they were not as severe as John's.

The phone rang. It was one of their friends who had been at the lodge dinner. She and her husband were also experiencing the same reactions.

Now Eva was really frightened. John had recently begun to have some heart trouble and she thought this attack was related. By now he was prostrate, unable to move. Eva immediately called their physician, who arranged for John to be taken to the hospital. After treatment in the emergency room for shock, followed by observational care and rest the following day, John's symptoms had subsided and he was allowed to go home. The doctor advised them to eat lightly for a few days and get more rest and said that he would investigate the cause in the meantime. During the next few days, John and Eva learned that almost all of their friends who had been at the lodge dinner had had an experience similar to theirs.

The doctor contacted the public health department to report the incident. His was one of several similar calls, a public health officer said, and the department was already investigating.

The following week, the officer returned the doctor's call to report his findings. The cream puffs that the lodge restaurant served that evening had been purchased from a local bakery. At the bakery, health officials had located a worker with an infected cut on his little finger: "a small thing," the worker said. He couldn't understand what all the fuss was about.

The health officials also located the delivery truck driver, who had started out at midmorning to make his rounds and take the cream puffs to the restaurant. On questioning the driver, however, they learned that the truck had broken down during the afternoon deliveries before he reached the restaurant. The driver said that he had been irritated by a 3-hour wait at the garage while the truck was being fixed. But he still got the order to the restaurant in time for the dinner, he said, so what was the problem?

At the restaurant, the chef said that everyone was so busy with the dinner that when the cream puffs finally arrived, no one had time to give much notice to them. They had decided that there was no point in putting the cream puffs in the refrigerator at the time because they were to be served in a short while.

When John and Eva's doctor called them afterward to report the story, John and Eva decided they would not eat at that restaurant again. Besides, by then John had lost his taste for cream puffs.

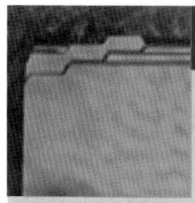

CLINICAL APPLICATIONS
Case Study: A Community Food Poisoning Incident—cont'd

Questions for analysis

1. Why is control of the community's food supply an important responsibility of the health department?
2. What disease agents may be carried by food or water?
3. What was the agent causing John and Eva's illness? Was this a food infection or a food poisoning? How do you know? While the investigation was going on and before John and Eva learned the real cause of their illness, John thought it must have been caused by "those things farmers and food processors put into food these days. I've been reading about those tings in the paper. It's a wonder we're not sick all the time."
4. What substances did John mean? Can you give some examples?
5. Why are these materials used for growing and processing food?
6. What controls do we have for their use?
7. What are some ways in which food is protected from its point of production to our tables? How can food be preserved for later use?
8. What agency controls food safety and quality? How does it do so?

careful preparation and adequate cooking of meats, prompt service, and immediate refrigeration at sufficiently low temperatures. The bacteria *C. botulinum* causes far more serious, often fatal food poisoning—*botulism*—from ingestion of food containing its powerful toxin. Depending on the dose of toxin taken and the individual response, the illness may vary from mild discomfort to death within 24 hours. Mortality rates are high. Nausea, vomiting, weakness, and dizziness are initial complaints. The toxin progressively irritates motor nerve cells and blocks transmission of neural impulses at the nerve terminals, causing gradual paralysis. Sudden respiratory paralysis with airway obstruction is the major cause of death. *C. botulinum* spores are widespread in soil throughout the world and may be carried on harvested food to the canning process. Like all *clostridia*, this species is anaerobic or nearly so. The relatively air-free can and the canning temperatures (above 27° C [80° F]) provide good conditions for toxin production. The development of

high standards in the commercial canning industry has eliminated this source of botulism, but cases still result each year, mainly from ingestion of carelessly home-canned foods. Because boiling for 10 minutes destroys the toxin (not the spore), all home-canned food, no matter how well preserved it is considered to be, should be boiled for at least 10 minutes before it is eaten. In the United States, the states of Alaska and Washington have the highest incidence of botulism, with Alaska having by far the greater number of cases because of native habits of eating uncooked or partially cooked meat that has been fermented, dried, or frozen. Table 13-2 summarizes these examples of bacterial sources of food contamination.

> **anaerobic** (Gr. *an-*, without; *aēr*, air; *bios*, life) a microorganism that can live and grow in an oxygen-free environment.

TABLE 13-2   Selected examples of bacterial food-borne disease

Food-borne disease	Causative organisms Genus Species	Food source	Symptoms and course
Bacterial food infections			
Salmonellosis	Salmonella _S. typhi_ _S. paratyphi_	Milk, custards, egg dishes, salad dressings, sandwich fillings, polluted shellfish	Mild to severe diarrhea, cramps, vomiting. Appears 12-24 hours or more after eating; lasts 1-7 days.
Shigellosis	Shigella _S. dysenteriae_	Milk and milk products, seafood, and salads	Mild diarrhea to fatal dysentery (especially in young children). Appears 7-36 hours after eating; lasts 3-14 days.
Listeriosis	Listeria _L. monocytogenes_	Soft cheese, poultry, seafood, raw milk, meat products (paté)	Severe diarrhea, fever, headache, pneumonia, meningitis, endocarditis. Symptoms begin after 3-21 days.
Bacterial food poisoning			
(Enterotoxins) Staphylococcal	Staphylococcus _S. aureus_	Custards, cream fillings, processed meats, ham, cheese, ice cream, potato salad, sauces, casseroles	Severe abdominal pain, cramps, vomiting, diarrhea, sweating, headache, fever, pros tration. Appears suddenly 1-6 hours after eating; symptoms generally subside within 24 hours.
Clostridial Perfringes enteritis	Clostridium _C. perfringes_	Cooked meat, meat dishes held at warm temperature	Mild diarrhea, vomiting. Appears 8-24 hours after eating; lasts a day or less.
Botulism	_C. botulinum_	Improperly home canned foods; smoked and salted fish, ham, sausage, shellfish	Symptoms range from mild discomfort to death within 24 hours; initial nausea, vomiting, weakness, dizziness, progressing to motor and sometimes fatal breathing paralysis.

Viruses

Illnesses produced by viral contamination of food are few when compared with those produced by bacterial sources. These include upper respiratory infections (e.g., colds and influenza) and viral infectious hepatitis. Explosive epidemics of infectious hepatitis have occurred in schools, towns, and other communities after fecal contamination of water, milk, or food. Contaminated shellfish from polluted waters have also caused several outbreaks. Again, stringent control of community water and food supplies, as well as personal hygiene and sanitary practices of food handlers, is essential for prevention of disease.

Parasites

The following two types of worms are of serious concern in relation to food: (1) roundworms, such as the *trichina* (*Trichinella spiralis*) worm found in pork, and (2) flatworms, such as the common tapeworms of beef and pork. The following control measures are essential: (1) laws controlling hog and cattle food sources and pastures to prevent transmission of the parasites to the meat produced for market; and (2) avoidance of rare beef or underdone pork as an added personal precaution.

Environmental Food Contaminants

Heavy metals such as lead and mercury may also contaminate food and water, as well as the air and environmental objects. Children are especially vulnerable to lead poisoning, particularly children of poor families sheltered in urban hotels or other impoverished areas with peeling lead paint. Of all sources of lead—even in the overall population, paint is the most important source. It is estimated that 30 million homes in the United States have leaden paint surfaces, and young children live in 3 million homes that have peeling, deteriorated lead surfaces.[15] These children face lead exposure by eating paint chips or breathing airborne particles of paint dust from abrasive paint removal before remodeling, which is a situation that may last for a while within the house after remodeling is complete. Drinking water is a major source of lead in high-risk households whose water comes through leaden service pipes or plumbing joints that have been sealed with lead solder.[16] Current U.S. Environmental Protection Agency (EPA) rules for public drinking water, however, have lowered the controlled lead exposure levels even further (see For Further Focus Box, "Lead in Children's Diets"). Lead pigment has also been found in foods wrapped in labeled, soft plastic (e.g., bread)—not only when the wrapping is turned inside out and reused to store food but also when it is thrown away and the lead becomes part of the environmental waste.[17] Children suffering these elevated lead exposures develop brain damage with subsequent learning deficits from what has been called a "silent, relentless destroyer of brain cells."[15]

Mercury poisoning was first reported in 1953 after the massive exposure of a local population in Japan from seafood from water contaminated by the waste discharge of a local plastics factory. Over a third of the affected individuals died, with many suffering neurologic problems (e.g., mental confusion, convulsions, and coma) and many infants and children suffering permanent brain damage. A similar incident occurred again in Japan in 1964. During the winter of 1971-1972 another mercury poisoning disaster occurred in Iraq when barley and wheat grain treated with methylmercury as a fungicide had been purchased from Mexico. The grain sacks carried a written warning, but only in Spanish. The USFDA limits possible mercury contamination by closely inspecting the seafood and pesticide residues on crops.

FOOD NEEDS AND COSTS
Hunger and Malnutrition

World Malnutrition

The daily news makes us increasingly aware that malnutrition—even famine and death—exists in many countries of the world, as well as that hunger and disease go hand in hand. Many environmental problems influence malnutrition. It is not only a problem of agriculture and soil erosion and drought but also of sanitation, culture, social problems, and economic and political structure. For example, close to U.S. borders, peoples of Mexico and Central and South America are plagued by social conditions such as economic depression, revolution, inequity, and desperate poverty. Figure 13-3 shows the interaction of some of the factors that lead to malnutrition.

American Malnutrition

Hunger, however, does not stop at the U.S. border. In the United States—one of the wealthiest countries on earth, many studies document hunger and malnutrition among the poor. At both the governmental and personal levels of any society, food availability and use involves both money and politics. Various factors are involved, such as land-management practices, water distribution, long-term use of questionable pesticides, food production and

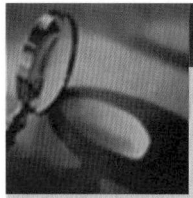

FOR FURTHER FOCUS
Lead in Children's Diets

Lead poisoning has been a major public health problem for centuries. New studies show that lead not only poisons our air and soil but also contaminates the food we eat, the dust in our homes, and the water that we drink. The most disturbing of all, however, is its danger to our children, especially during the first 6 years of life.

More than 250,000 children in the United States, most between the ages of 2 and 3 years, are found to have absorbed excessive amounts of lead each year. Most health workers have assumed that these children obtained most of the excess lead from lead-based paint chips or contaminated dirt or dust, but researchers have found that 55% to 85% of this daily lead intake is contributed by food and water. About 25% of the lead in food comes from canned vegetables, fruits, and juices—especially acidic foods that extract any lead from the cans. The lead pigment used to print labels on soft plastic food packaging can also be a source, especially if families reuse the bag for food storage.

Increased research has shown that even low levels of lead can have damaging effects on chil-dren, as well as adults, leading the Environmental Protection Agency (EPA) to issue new rules to reduce the levels of lead in U.S. drinking water. These new rules, phased in from 1992 to 1993, established a monitoring system in which the lead values of tap water must not exceed 15 parts per billion (ppb), lowering the previous standards of 50 ppb for drinking water.

The brain-damaging effects of lead poisoning in young children are associated with anemia, fatigue, poor attention span, and learning ability. The new federal definition of lead toxicity is now 10 μg/dl, putting at least 17% of all children—and 50% of children in poverty—with blood levels above this newly defined level at neurotoxic risk. Recognizing the increasing danger of childhood lead poisoning, the Department of Health and Human Services has started a plan of prevention, reduced exposure, and national surveillance to eradicate this serious problem. These measures are not new, but this degree of federal commitment is—and none too soon to meet this increasing threat to the living environment and health of every child.

distribution policies, and food assistance programs for individuals and families in need. A "culture of poverty" often develops among the poor and is reinforced by society's values and attitudes.

Food Assistance Programs

In situations of economic stress and natural disasters, individuals and families need financial help. There are currently persons in the United States who experience hunger each day. You may need to discuss available food assistance programs and make appropriate referrals.

Commodity Distribution Program

Under this Act, the federal government purchases market surpluses of food items to support the prices of agricultural products. These items include both perishable goods and price-supported basic and nonperishable commodities. This accumulation of

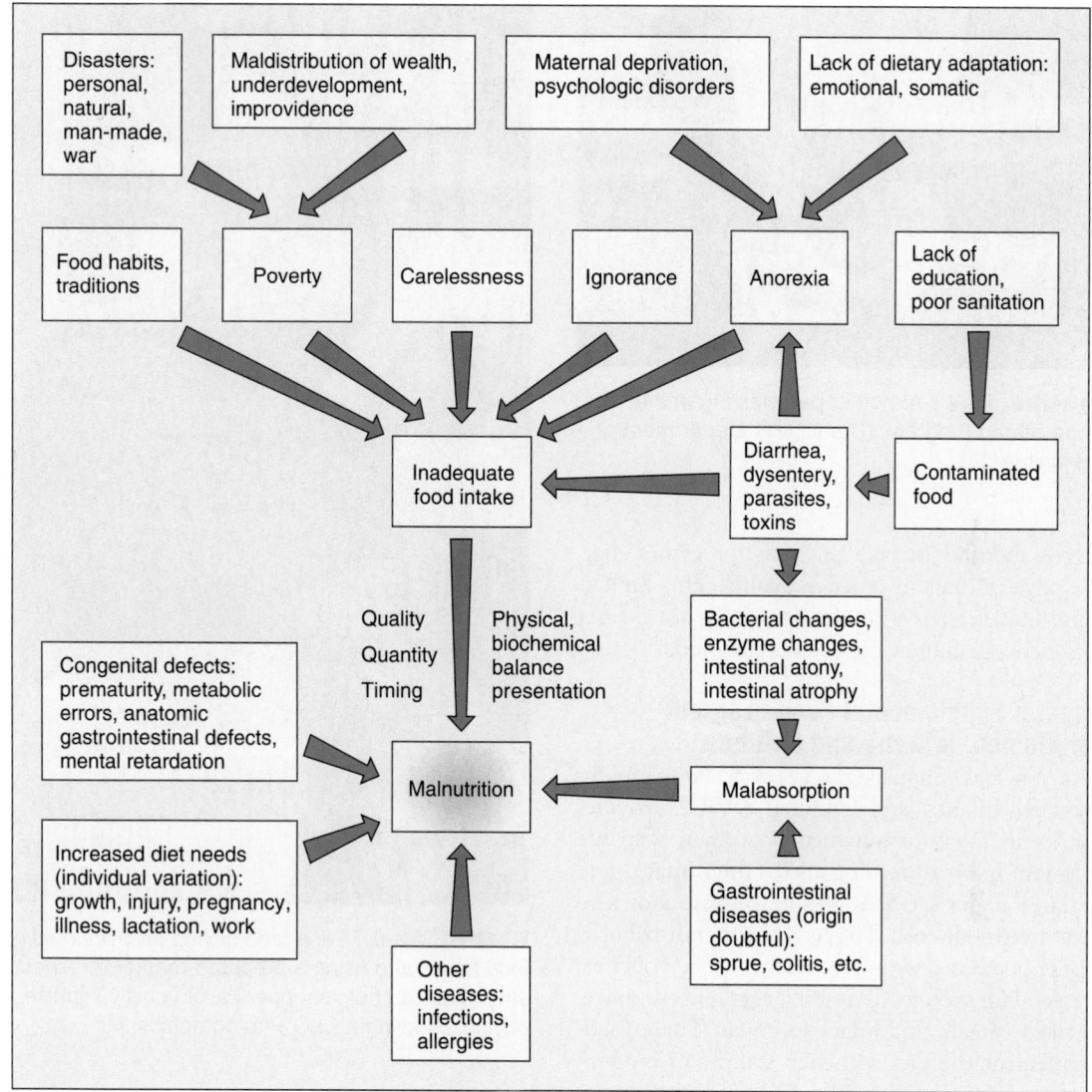

FIGURE 13-3 Multiple etiology of malnutrition. (Modified from Williams, CD: *Lancet* 2:342, 1962. © by the Lancet Ltd.)

food stocks led to the creation of the present program as a means of distributing the stored products to persons in need (Figure 13-4).

Food Stamp Program

The Food Stamp Program began in the late depression years of the 1930s and was further developed in the 1960s and 1970s. This program has helped many poor persons purchase needed food, although federal cuts in the 1980s curtailed its help to many persons in need. Under this program, the person or "household" is issued coupons, or "food stamps," which are supposed to sufficiently cover the household's food needs for 1 month. Households must

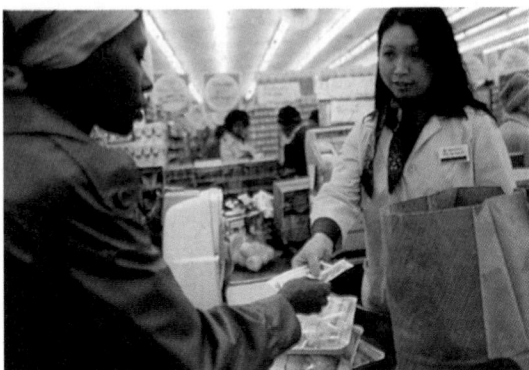

FIGURE 13-4 A mother participating in the Food Stamp Program. (Credit: U.S. Department of Agriculture.)

have a monthly income below the program's eligible poverty limit in order to qualify. This limit is quite low. Persons who qualify usually just do not make enough money to buy necessary food.

Special Supplemental Food Program for Women, Infants, and Children

The Special Supplemental Food Program for Women, Infants, and Children (WIC) provides nutritious foods to low-income women who are pregnant or breast feeding and to their infants and children under age 5, as well as to those shown to be at nutritional risk. The food is either distributed free or purchased with free vouchers. The vouchers are good for such foods as milk, eggs, cheese, juice, fortified cereals, and infant formulas. These foods supplement the diet with rich sources of protein, iron, and certain vitamins to help reduce risk factors such as poor growth patterns, low birth weight or prematurity, toxemia, miscarriage, and anemia.

National School Lunch and Breakfast Programs

These programs enable schools to provide nutritious lunches and breakfasts to students. Poor children eat free or at reduced-rates, and this is often their main food intake of the day. Other students pay somewhat less than the full cost of the meal. The lunches

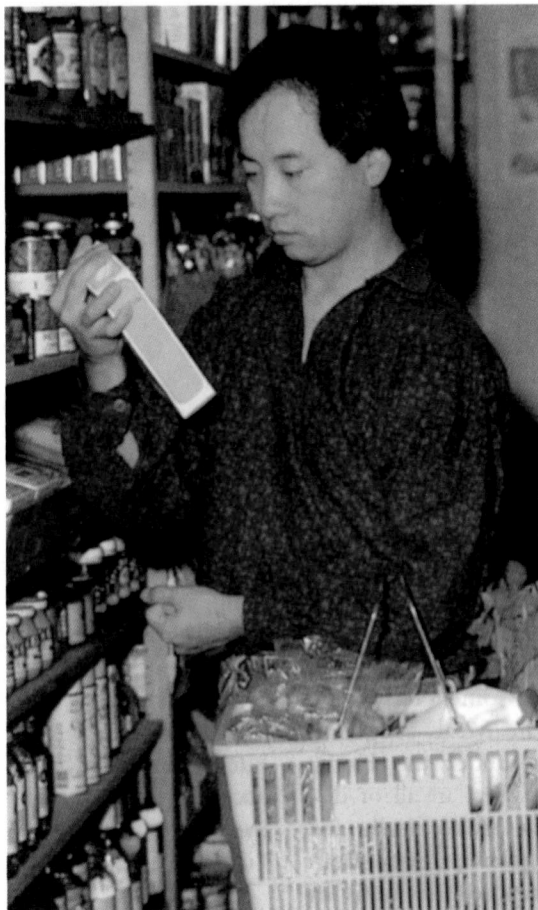

FIGURE 13-5 Wise food buying involves reading food labels and using a prepared market list. These strategies can help shoppers avoid costly impulse buying. (Copyright CLG Photographics, Inc.)

are required to fulfill approximately one third of a child's RDA standard for energy and nutrients.

Older Americans Program

Under this act, two types of food programs benefit the growing number of elderly citizens in the United States. Regardless of their income, all persons over 60 can eat hot lunches at some community center under the Congregate Meals Program or, if they are ill or disabled, receive meals at home under the Home-Delivered Meals Program. The act specifies that economically and socially needy persons are given priority. Both programs accept voluntary contributions for meals.

Food Buying and Handling Practices

For many American families, the problem is spending their limited food dollars wisely. Shopping for food often is no easy task, especially when each marketed item in a supermarket's overabundant supply shouts, "Buy me!" Food marketing is big business, and producers compete for prize placement and shelf space. A large supermarket may stock 8000 or more different food items, with more added daily. A single food item may be marketed a dozen different ways at as many different prices. In diet counseling, clients and families typically express their greatest need as help with buying food. The following wise shopping and handling practices will help provide healthy foods, as well as control food costs.

Plan Ahead

Use market guides in newspapers, plan general menus, and keep a checklist of kitchen supplies. Make out a list ahead of time according to the location of items in a regularly used market (Figure 13-5). Such planning controls "impulse buying" and extra trips.

Buy Wisely

Know the market, market items, packaging, labels, grades, brands, portion yields, measures, and food values in various market units. Read labels carefully. Watch for sale items. Only buy in quantity if it results in real savings and the food can be adequately stored or used. Be cautious in selecting so-called convenience foods. The time saved may not be worth the added cost. For fresh foods and good buys, also try alternative food sources such as farmers' markets, consumer co-ops, and gardens.

Store Food Safely

Control food waste and prevent illness from food spoilage or contamination. Conserve food by storing items according to the nature and use of each. Use dry storage, covered containers, and correct temperature refrigeration as needed. Keep opened and partly used food items at the front of the shelf for early use. Avoid plate waste by preparing only the amount needed. Use leftovers in creative ways.

Cook Food Well

Use cooking processes that retain maximum food value and maintain food safety. Prepare food with imagination and good sense. Give zest and appeal to dishes with a variety of seasonings, combinations, and serving arrangements. No matter how much they know about nutrition and health, people usually eat because they are hungry and the food looks and tastes good—not necessarily because it is healthy.

SUMMARY

Common public concerns about the safety of the community food supply center on the use of chemicals as pesticides and food additives. These substances have produced an abundant food supply but have also brought dangers and require control. The FDA is the main government agency established to maintain this control and conducts activities related to areas such as food safety, food labeling, food standards, consumer education, and research.

Food-borne disease may be caused by numerous organisms such as bacteria, viruses, and parasites that can contaminate food. Rigorous public health measures control sanitation of food areas and personal hygiene of food handlers. The same standards should apply to home food preparation and storage.

Families under economic stress need counseling about financial assistance. Various U.S. food assistance programs help families in need, and referrals can be made to appropriate agencies. Families may also need assistance buying and handling food.

REVIEW QUESTIONS

1. What is the basis of concern about food additives and pesticide residues?
2. What are some ways agriculture is changing to reduce the use of pesticides and their danger to workers, as well as to protect the land?
3. Describe ways that various organisms may contaminate food. What standards of food preparation and handling should be used to keep food safe?

4. Describe the development of food label reform and the nature of the new food labels.
5. List and describe food assistance programs available to help low income families. What other local resources are available in your community?
6. List and discuss the wise food buying and handling practices described in this chapter. How many of these practices do you follow in selecting, storing, and preparing foods?

SELF-TEST QUESTIONS

True-False

Write the correct statement for each item you answer "false."

1. U.S. surveys reveal little or no real malnutrition.
2. The politics of a region or country is not involved in the nutritional status of the people.
3. The number of new processed food items using food additives has declined in recent years because of public pressure and concern.
4. The use of pesticides on farm crops and food additives in processed foods is controlled by the USDA and FDA.
5. Food poisoning is caused by viral contamination of food.
6. The Commodity Distribution Program buys agricultural food surpluses to support market prices of food and distributes these goods to needy persons.
7. The number of poor persons assisted by the Food Stamp Program has been increasing due to expanded federal support.

8. The Older Americans Program provides group meals for all persons over 60 years of age, regardless of their income.

Multiple Choice

1. Food additives are used in processed food items to (circle all that apply):
   a. Preserve food and lengthen its market life.
   b. Enrich food with added nutrients.
   c. Improve flavor, texture, and appearance.
   d. Enhance or improve some physical property of the food.
2. The use of food additives in food products is controlled by the:
   a. U.S. Public Health Service.
   b. U.S. Department of Agriculture.
   c. Food and Drug Administration.
   d. Federal Trade Commission.

SUGGESTIONS FOR ADDITIONAL STUDY

1. Food Market Survey: Food Labeling

Visit a local community food market and survey the variety of food products. Find at least 10 new, processed food items. Read the labels carefully, and study the nature and use of each item.

a. List the food items you located. Describe each in terms of its nature, packaging, and use.
b. What does the label on each item tell you about the product's relative nutritional

value? Are any food additives used? If so, determine the purpose of as many as you can. Call your nearest FDA district office for information or write to the federal FDA office in Washington, DC for information on food additives.

c. What specific nutrition information did you find on each label?

d. How would you evaluate these processed food items?

2. Market Survey of Comparative Food Costs

Visit a community food market and compare the different forms (e.g., fresh, canned, frozen, processed) of 10 food items. List the different forms you found for each food item with the unit price for each form.

a. What form was the least expensive in each case?

b. In view of your findings, what suggestions can you give for economical food buying?

c. What factors influence the cost of food items?

REFERENCES

1. Hahn NI: Growing a healthy food system, *J Am Diet Assoc* 97(9):950, 1997.
2. McMahon KE, Cameron MA: Consumers and key nutrition trends for 1998, *Nutr Today* 33(1):19, 1998.
3. Tippett KS and others: Food consumption surveys in the U.S. Department of Agriculture, *Nutr Today* 34(1):33, 1999.
4. Glanz K and others: Why Americans eat what they do: taste, nutrition, cost, convenience, and weight concerns as influences on food consumption, *J Am Diet Assoc* 98(10):1118, 1998.
5. Neuhouser ML and others: Use of food nutrition labels is associated with lower fat intake, *J Am Diet Assoc* 99(1): 45, 1999.
6. Staff: Practice points: translating research into practice: food labels benefit consumers and dietetic professionals, *J Am Diet Assoc* 99(1):53, 1999.
7. U.S. Department of Agriculture, Food Safety and Inspection Service (FSIS): *Listeria* awareness, *J Am Diet Assoc* 99(6):660, 1999.
8. Bildstein C: About food safety and spoilage, *Nutr Today* 34(1):27, 1999

9. Spake A: Death came with the water, *E. coli* breaks out at county fair, *U.S. News & World Report*, 127(11):56, Sept 20, 1999.
10. Mahon BE and others: Consequences in Georgia of a nationwide outbreak of salmonella infections: what you don't know might hurt you, *Am J Public Health* 89(1):31, 1999.
11. Henneman A: Don't mess with food safety myths, *Nutr Today* 34(1):23, 1999.
12. U.S. Department of Agriculture, Food Safety Inspection Services: *A quick consumer guide to food safety* HG248, Washington, DC, 1990, U.S. Government Printing Office.
13. Duggan J, Phillips CA: Listeria in the domestic environment, *Nutr Food Sci* 98(2):73, 1998.
14. Spake A: Deadly hot dogs and ham, *U.S. News & World Report* 126(7):62, 1999.
15. Needleman HL: Childhood lead poisoning: a disease for the history texts, *Am J Public Health* 81(6):685, 1991.
16. Report: New lead rules for water, *Sci News* 139(20):308, 1991.
17. Weisel C and others: Soft plastic bread wrapping lead content and reuse by families, *Amer J Public Health* 81(6): 756, 1991.

FURTHER READING

• Henneman A: Don't mess with food safety myths!, *Nutr Today* 34(1):23, 1999.

This short and to-the-point article is aptly titled. The author is a food safety educator who blasts the myths and presents the warnings about food preparation and storage in simple language. Her final words are to the point: "When in doubt, throw it out!"

• McMahon KE, Cameron MA: Consumers and key nutrition trends, *Nutr Today* 33(1):19, 1998.

As we stand at the beginning of a new century, it blows one's mind to think about the tremendous changes that are occurring rapidly in family lifestyles and food preparation. With working parents, the trend is more convenience and efficiency, with a key message of balance, variety, and moderation. These authors provide a comprehensive, current view and look ahead to things to come.

14

Food Habits and Cultural Patterns

KEY CONCEPTS

- Personal food habits develop as part of one's social and cultural heritage, as well as changing lifestyles and life situations.

- Short-term food patterns, or fads, stem from food misinformation that appeals to some human need.

- The force of social change brings changes in food patterns.

Why do people eat what they eat? We know that food is necessary to sustain life and health. We also know that people eat certain foods for many other reasons— least of all perhaps for good health and nutrition, although these are increasing concerns. As stated in Chapter 13, the broader food environment from which persons have to choose is often influenced by factors such as politics and poverty, which limit personal control and choice.

We attach many meanings to food. All of our food habits are intimately related to our whole way of life: our values, beliefs, and situation. Sometimes, however, these food beliefs come from food misinformation and fads rather than sound nutrition knowledge. Here we examine some of these influences.

CULTURAL DEVELOPMENT OF FOOD HABITS

Food habits, like any other form of human behavior, do not develop in a vacuum. They grow from many personal, cultural, social, economic, and psychologic influences. For each of us, these factors are interwoven.

Strength of Personal Culture

Culture involves much more than the major and historic aspects of a person's communal life (e.g., language, religion, politics, technology) but also develops from all the habits of everyday living and family relationships, such as preparing and serving food, caring for children, feeding them, and lulling them to sleep. We learn these things as we grow up. In a gradual process of conscious and unconscious learning, our culture's values, attitudes, habits, and practices become a deep part of our lives. Although we may revise or reject parts of this heritage as adults, it remains within us to influence our lives and pass on to following generations. Americans have a broad heritage of food habits; indeed, it is our respect for this wonderful cultural diversity that "helps us to eat right."[1]

Food in a Culture

Food habits are among the oldest and most deeply rooted aspects of many cultures. Cultural background largely determines what is eaten as well as when and how it is eaten, but much variation exists, of course. All types of customs—whether rational or irrational, beneficial or injurious—are found in every part of the world. Whatever the situation, however, food habits are primarily based on food availability, economics, and personal food meanings and beliefs. Many foods in any culture take on symbolic meanings related to major life experiences from birth, to death, to religion, to politics, and to general social organization. From ancient times, ceremonies and religious rites involving food have surrounded certain events and seasons. Food gathering, preparing, and serving have followed specific customs, many of which remain today.

Some Traditional Cultural Food Patterns

The United States has been called a "melting pot" of ethnic and racial groups. In more recent years, however, this image is no longer appropriate. We have come to recognize and even celebrate our diversity as a basis for national strength. This recognition is especially strong in the diversity of our cultural food patterns.

Many different cultural food patterns are part of American family and community life. These patterns have contributed special dishes or modes of cooking to American eating habits. In turn, many of these cultural food habits have been Americanized. Traditional foods are used more regularly by older members of the family, with younger members of the family using them mainly on special occasions or holidays. Nevertheless, traditional foods have strong meanings and bind families and cultural communities in close fellowship.[2] A few representative cultural food patterns are briefly reviewed here. Individual tastes and geographic patterns may vary somewhat, but these food patterns connected with culture have a strong influence on how we eat.[3]

Religious Dietary Laws

Jewish

All Jewish festivals are religious in nature and have historical significance,[4] but the observance of Jewish food laws differs among the three basic groups within Judaism: (1) Orthodox, strict observance; (2) Conservative, less strict; and (3) Reform, less ceremonial emphasis and minimum general use. The basic body of dietary laws is called the *Rules of Kashruth*. Foods selected and prepared according to these rules are called *kosher*, from the Hebrew word meaning "fit, proper." These laws originally had special ritual significance. Current Jewish dietary laws apply this significance to laws governing the slaughter, preparation, and serving of meat; the combining of meat and milk; and the use of fish and eggs. Various food restrictions exist.

- **Meat**—No pork is used. Forequarters of other meats are allowed, as well as all commonly used forms of poultry. All forms of meat are rigidly cleansed of all blood.
- **Meat and milk**—The combining of meat and milk is not allowed. Orthodox homes maintain two sets of dishes, one for serving meat and the other for meals using dairy products.
- **Fish**—Only fish with fins and scales are allowed. These may be eaten with either meat or dairy meals. No shellfish or eels may be used.
- **Eggs**—No egg with a blood spot may be eaten. Eggs may be used with either meat or dairy meals.

Influence of festivals. Many traditional Jewish foods relate to festivals of the Jewish calendar that commemorate significant events in Jewish history. Often, special Sabbath foods are used. A few representative foods include the following:

- **Bagels**—Doughnut-shaped, hard yeast rolls.
- **Blintzes**—Thin, filled, rolled pancakes.
- **Borscht (borsch)**—Soup of meat stock, beaten egg or sour cream, beets, cabbage, or spinach; served hot or cold.
- **Challah**—Sabbath loaf of white bread, shaped as a twist or coil, used at the beginning of the meal after the kiddush, the blessing over wine.
- **Gefullte (gefilte) fish**—From a German word meaning "stuffed fish"; usually the first course of Sabbath evening meal; made of chopped and seasoned fish filet, stuffed back into the skin or rolled into balls.
- **Kasha**—Buckwheat groats (hulled kernels), used as a cooked cereal or as a potato substitute with gravy.
- **Knishes**—Pastry filled with ground meat or cheese.

- **Lox**—Smoked, salted salmon.
- **Matzo**—Flat, unleavened bread.
- **Strudel**—Thin pastry filled with fruit and nuts, rolled, and baked.

Moslem

Moslem dietary laws are based on the restriction or prohibition of some foods and the promotion of others, derived from Islamic teachings in the Koran. The laws are binding and must be followed at all times—even during pregnancy, hospitalization, or travel. These laws are also binding to visitors in the host Moslem country. The general rule is that "all foods are permitted" unless specifically conditioned or prohibited.[5]

- **Milk products**—Permitted at all times.
- **Fruits and vegetables**—Permitted except if fermented or poisonous.
- **Breads and cereals**—Permitted unless contaminated or harmful.
- **Meats**—Seafood (including fish, shellfish, eels, and sea animals) and land animals (except swine) are permitted; pork is strictly prohibited.
- **Alcohol**—Strictly prohibited.

Any food combinations are used as long as no prohibited items are included. Milk and meat may be eaten together, in contrast to Jewish kosher laws. The Koran mentions certain foods as being of special value, such as figs, olives, dates, honey, milk, and buttermilk. Prohibited foods by the Moslem dietary laws may be eaten when no other sources of food are available.

Representative foods. A number of favorite foods and dishes are used as appetizers, main dishes, snacks, or salads. The following are some of these foods:

- **Bulgur (or burghel)**—Partially cooked and dried cracked wheat, available in coarse grind as a base for pilaf or fine grind for use in tabouli and kibbeh.

- **Falafel**—A "fast food" made from a seasoned paste of ground soaked beans formed into shapes and fried.
- **Fatayeh**—Snack or appetizer similar to a small pizza with toppings of cheese, meat, or spinach.
- **Kibbeh**—Meat dish made of cracked wheat shell filled with small pieces of lamb and fried in oil.
- **Pilaf**—Sautéed, seasoned bulgur or rice steamed in a bouillon, sometimes with poultry, meat, or shellfish.
- **Pita**—Flat circular bread, torn or cut into pieces, stuffed with sandwich fillings or used as scoops for a dip such as *hummus* made from garbanzo beans.
- **Tabouli**—Salad made from soaked bulghur combined with chopped tomatoes, parsley, mint, green onion, mixed with olive oil and lemon juice.

Influence of festivals. Among the Moslem people, a 30-day period of daylight fasting is required during Ramadan, the ninth month of the Islamic lunar calendar, thus this period rotates through all seasons.[5] The fourth pillar of Islam commanded by the Koran is fasting. Ramadan was chosen for the sacred fast because it was when Mohammed received the first of the revelations that were subsequently compiled to form the Koran, and it is also the month when his followers first drove their enemies from Mecca in 624 AD. During the month of Ramadan, Moslems all over the world observe daily fasting, taking no food or drink from dawn to sunset. Nights, however, are often spent in special feasts. First, an appetizer is taken, such as dates or a fruit drink, followed by the family's "evening breakfast," the *iftar*. At the end of Ramadan, a traditional feast lasting up to 3 days climaxes the observance. Special dishes, with delicacies such as thin pancakes dipped in powdered sugar, savory buns, and dried fruits, mark this occasion (see For Further Focus Box, "Id al-Fitr, The Post-Ramadan Festival").

Spanish and Native American Influences

Mexican

The food habits of the early Spanish settlers and Indian nations form the basis of the current food patterns of persons of Mexican heritage who now live in the United States, chiefly in the Southwest.[6] The following three foods are basic to this pattern: dried beans, chili peppers, and corn. Variations and additions may be found in different places or among those of different income levels. Relatively small amounts of meat are used, and eggs are occasionally eaten. Some fruit (e.g., oranges, apples, and bananas) is used, depending on availability. For centuries, corn has been the basic grain used for bread in the form of tortillas, which are flat cakes baked on a hot surface or griddle. Some wheat is now being used in making tortillas; and rice and oat are added cereals. Coffee is a main beverage. Major seasonings are chili peppers, onions, and garlic; the basic fat is lard.

Puerto Rican

The Puerto Rican people share a common heritage with the Mexicans, so much of their food pattern is similar.[6] Puerto Ricans, however, add tropical fruits and vegetables, many of which are available in their neighborhood markets in the United States. *Viandas*, which are starchy vegetables and fruits such as plantain and green bananas, are a main type of food. Two other basic foods are rice and beans. Milk, meat, yellow and green vegetables, and other fruits are used in limited quantities; but dried codfish is a staple. Coffee is a main beverage. The main cooking fat is usually lard.

Ramadan (*Ar. ramādan,* the host month) the ninth month of the Muslim year, a period of daily fasting from sunrise to sunset.

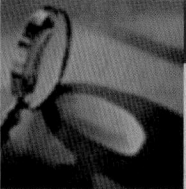

FOR FURTHER FOCUS
Id al-Fitr, The Post-Ramadan Festival

In Moslem countries at the conclusion of Ramadan—Islam's holy month of prayer and fasting, wealthy merchants and princes traditionally hold public feasts for the needy. This is the festival of Id al-Fitr.

Over the years, many delicacies have been served to symbolize the joy of returning from fasting and the heightened sense of unity, brotherhood, and charity that the fasting experience has brought to the people. Among the foods served are chicken or veal sauteed with eggplant and onions, then simmered slowly in pomegranate juice and spiced with turmeric and cardamom seeds. The highlight of the meal is usually kharuf mahshi, which is a whole lamb (symbol of sacrifice) stuffed with a rich dressing made of dried fruits, cracked wheat, pine nuts, almonds, and onions and seasoned with ginger and coriander. The stuffed lamb is baked in hot ashes for many hours, so that it is tender enough to be pulled apart and eaten with the fingers.

At the conclusion of the meal, rich pastries and candies are served. These may be flavored with spices or flower petals. Some of the sweets are taken home and savored as long as possible as a reminder of the festival.

Native American

The Native American population—Indian and Alaska Natives—is mainly composed of more than 500 federally recognized diverse groups living on reservations, in small rural communities, or in metropolitan cities.[3] Despite their individual diversity, the various groups share a spiritual attachment to the land and a determination to retain their culture. Food has great religious and social significance and is an integral part not only of celebrations and ceremonies but also of everyday hospitality, which includes a serious obligation for serving food. Foods may be prepared and used in different ways from region to region and vary according to what can be grown locally, harvested or hunted on the land or fished from its rivers, or is available in food markets. Among the Native American groups of the Southwest United States, the food pattern of the Navajo people, whose reservation extends over a 25,000-square mile area at the junction of three states—New Mexico, Arizona, and Utah, is an example.[3]

The Navajos learned farming from the early Pueblo people, establishing corn and other crops as staples. They later learned herding from the Spaniards, making sheep and goats available for food and wool. Some families also raised chickens, pigs, and cattle. Today, Navajo food habits combine traditional dietary staples with modern food products from available supermarkets and fast-food restaurants. Meat (e.g., fresh mutton, beef, pork, chicken, or smoked or processed meat) is eaten daily. Other staples include bread—tortillas or fry bread, blue corn bread and cornmeal mush; beverages—coffee, soft drinks and other fruit-flavored sweet ades; eggs; vegetables—corn, potatoes, green beans, tomatoes; and some fresh or canned fruit. Frying is a common method of food preparation; lard and shortening are main cooking fats. Some health concerns are growing, however, about an increased use of modern convenience or snack foods that are high in fat, sugar, calories, and sodium, especially among children and teenagers.

Influences of the Southern United States

African-Americans

The black populations, especially in the Southern states, have contributed a rich heritage to American food patterns, particularly to Southern cooking as a whole. Similar to their moving music styles (e.g., spirituals, blues, gospel, and jazz), the food patterns of Southern blacks were born of hard times and developed through a creative ability to turn any basic staples at hand into memorable food. Although regional differences occur, as with any basic food pattern, the representative use of foods from basic food groups is evident, as follows:

- **Breads and cereals**—Traditional breads include hot breads such as biscuits, spoonbread (i.e., a souffle-like dish of cornmeal mush with beaten eggs), cornmeal muffins, and skillet cornbread. Cooked cereals such as cornmeal mush, hominy grits (ground corn), and oatmeal are commonly used. Cooked cereal is generally used more than ready-to-eat dry cereal.
- **Eggs and dairy products**—Eggs and some cheese are used; but little milk is used, probably due to the greater prevalence of lactose intolerance among African-Americans.
- **Vegetables**—Leafy greens, such as turnip greens, collards, mustard greens, and spinach, are frequently used and usually cooked with bacon or salt pork. Cabbage is boiled or chopped raw with a salad dressing (e.g., coleslaw). Other vegetables used include okra (coated with cornmeal and fried), sweet potatoes (baked whole or sliced and "candied" with added sugar), green beans, tomatoes, potatoes, corn, butter beans (i.e., lima beans), and dried beans such as black-eyed peas or red or pinto beans cooked with smoked ham hocks and served over rice. Black-eyed peas over rice is a dish called Hopping John that is traditionally served on New Year's Day to bring good luck for the new year.

- **Fruits**—Commonly used fruits include apples, peaches, berries, oranges, bananas, and juices.
- **Meat**—Pork is a common meat, including fresh cuts and ribs, sausage, and smoked ham. Some beef is used, mainly ground for meat loaf or hamburgers. Poultry is frequently used, mainly as fried chicken and baked holiday turkey. Organ meats, such as liver, heart, intestines (chitterlings), or poultry giblets (gizzard and heart), are used. When available, fish includes catfish, some flounder, and shellfish (e.g., crab and shrimp). Frying is a common method of cooking; lard, shortening, or vegetable oils are fats used.
- **Desserts**—Favorites include pies (e.g., pecan, sweet potato, pumpkin) and deep-dish peach or berry cobblers; cakes (e.g., coconut and chocolate); and bread pudding to use up leftover bread.
- **Beverages**—Coffee, apple cider, fruit juices, lemonade, iced tea, carbonated soft drinks, and buttermilk, which is a more-tolerated, cultured form of milk, are used.

French Americans

The Cajun people of the southwestern coastal waterways in southern Louisiana have contributed a unique cuisine and food pattern to America's rich and varied fare. This pattern continues to provide a unique model for rapidly expanding forms of American ethnic food.[7] The Cajuns are descendents of the early French colonists of Acadia, a peninsula on the eastern coast of Canada now known as Nova Scotia. In the prerevolutionary

Cajun (Derivative, *Acadian*) a group of people with an enduring tradition whose French Catholic ancestors established permanent communities in the southern Louisiana coastal waterways after being expelled from Acadia (now Nova Scotia, Canada) by the reigning English in the late eighteenth century; developed unique food pattern from blend of native French influence and mix of Creole cooking found in the new land.

wars between France and Britain, both countries contended for the area of Acadia; but after Britain finally won control of all Canada, fear of an Acadian revolt led to a forcible deportation of the French colonists in 1755. After a long and difficult journey down the Atlantic coast, then westward along the Gulf of Mexico, a group of the impoverished Acadians finally settled along the bayou country of what is now Louisiana. To support themselves, they developed their unique food pattern from the seafood at hand and what they could grow and harvest. Over time, they blended their own French culinary background with the Creole cooking they found in their new homeland around New Orleans, which had combined classical French cuisine with other European, American Indian, and African styles of cooking.

Thus the unique Cajun food pattern of the Southern United States represents an ethnic blending of cultures using basic foods available in the area. Cajun foods are strong-flavored and spicy, with the abundant seafood as a base, and usually cooked as a stew and served over rice. The well-known hot chili sauce, made of crushed and fermented red chili peppers blended with spices and vinegar and sold all over the world under the trade name Tabasco Sauce, is still made by generations of a Cajun family on Avery Island on the coastal waterway of southern Louisiana. The most popular shellfish native to the region is the crawfish, which is now grown commercially in the fertile rice paddies of the bayou areas. Catfish, red snapper, shrimp, blue crab, and oysters are some of the other seafood used. Cajun dishes usually start with a *roux* made from heated oil and flour mixed with liquid to form a sauce base. Vegetables, then meat or seafood and seasonings, are added to form a stew. Vegetables used include onions, bell peppers, parsley, shallots, and tomatoes; seasonings are Cayenne (red) pepper, hot pepper sauce (Tabasco), crushed black pepper, white pepper, bay leaves, thyme, and filé powder. Filé powder is made from ground sassafras leaves and serves both to season and thicken the dish being made. Some typical Cajun dishes include

seafood or chicken gumbo, jambalaya (a dish of Creole origin, combining rice, chicken, ham, pork, sausage, broth, vegetables, and seasonings), red beans and rice, blackened catfish or red snapper (i.e., blackened with pepper and seasonings and seared in a hot pan), barbecued shrimp, breaded catfish with Creole sauce, and boiled crawfish. Breads and starches include French bread, hush puppies (fried cornbread-mixture balls, originally named because they were thrown to hungry hunting dogs around a hunting party's campfire to keep them from barking), cornbread muffins, cush-cush (cornmeal mush cooked with milk), grits (gruel made of ground white corn), rice, and yams. Vegetables include okra, squash, onions, bell peppers, and tomatoes. Desserts include ambrosia (fresh peeled orange segments and juice with sliced bananas and freshly grated coconut), sweet potato pie, pecan pie, berry pie, bread pudding, or pecan pralines.

Asian Food Patterns

Chinese

Chinese cooks believe that refrigeration diminishes natural flavors, so they select the freshest foods possible, hold them the shortest time possible, and cook them quickly at a high temperature in a *wok* (i.e., a basic round-bottom pan) with small amounts of fat and liquid. The wok allows heat to be controlled in a quick stir-frying method that preserves natural flavor, color, and texture. Vegetables cooked just before serving are still crisp and flavorful when served. Meat is used more in small amounts in combined dishes than as a single main entree. Little milk is used, but eggs and soybean products (e.g., tofu) add other sources of protein. Foods that have been dried, salted, pickled, spiced, candied, or canned may be added as garnishes or relishes to mask some flavors or textures or enhance others. Fruits are usually eaten fresh. Rice is the staple grain used at most meals. The traditional beverage is unsweetened green tea. Seasonings include soy sauce, ginger, almonds, and sesame seed. Peanut oil is a main cooking fat.[8]

Japanese

In some ways, Japanese food patterns are similar to those of the Chinese. Rice is a basic grain at meals, soy sauce is used for seasoning, and tea is the main beverage. The Japanese diet contains more seafood, especially raw fish items called *sushi*. Many varieties of fish and shellfish are used. Vegetables are usually steamed; pickled vegetables are also used. Fresh fruit is eaten in season; a tray of fruit is a regular course at main meals.

Southeast Asian

Since 1971, in the wake of the war in Vietnam, more than 340,000 Southeast Asians have come to the United States as refugees. The largest group of refugees are Vietnamese, but others have come from the adjacent war-torn countries of Laos and Cambodia. They have settled mainly in California, with other groups in Florida, Texas, Illinois, and Pennsylvania. As a whole, their food patterns are similar. They are having an effect on American diet and agriculture, and Asian grocery stores are stocking many traditional Asian food items. Rice, both long grain and glutinous, forms the basis of the Indonesian food pattern and is eaten at most meals. The Vietnamese usually eat their rice plain in a separate rice bowl—not mixed with other foods, whereas other Southeast Asians may eat rice in mixed dishes.

Soups are also commonly used at meals. Many fresh fruits and vegetables are used along with fresh herbs and other seasonings such as chives, spring onions, chili peppers, ginger root, coriander, turmeric, and fish sauce. Many kinds of seafood—fish and shellfish—are used, as well as chicken, duck, pork, and beef. Stir-frying in a wok type of pan with a small amount of lard or peanut oil is a common method of cooking. A variety of vegetables and seasonings are used, with small amounts of seafood or meat added.

Since coming to the United States, Vietnamese have made some diet changes that reflect American influence. These changes include the use of more eggs, beef, and pork but less seafood, more candy and other sweet snacks, bread, fast foods, soft drinks, butter and margarine, and coffee.

Mediterranean Influences

Italian

The sharing of food is an important part of Italian life. Meals are associated with warmth and fellowship, and special occasions are shared with families and friends. Bread and pasta are basic foods. Milk, seldom used alone, is typically mixed with coffee in equal portions. Cheese is a favorite food, with many popular varieties. Meats, poultry, and fish are used in many ways, and the varied Italian sausages and cold cuts are famous. Vegetables are used alone, in mixed main dishes or soups, in sauces, and in salads. Seasonings include herbs and spices, garlic, wine, olive oil, tomato puree, and salt pork. Main dishes are prepared by initially browning vegetables and seasonings in olive oil; adding meat or fish for browning, as well; covering with such liquids as wine, broth, or tomato sauce; and simmering slowly on low heat for several hours. Fresh fruit is often dessert or a snack.[9]

Greek

Everyday meals are simple, but Greek holiday meals are occasions for serving many delicacies. Bread is always the center of every meal, with other foods considered accompaniments. Milk is seldom used as a beverage but rather as the cultured form of yogurt. Cheese is a favorite food, especially *feta*, a special white cheese made from sheep's milk and preserved in brine. Lamb is a favorite meat, but others—especially fish—are also used. Eggs are sometimes a main dish but never a breakfast food. Many vegetables are used, often as a main entree, cooked with broth, tomato sauce, onions, olive oil, and parsley. A typical salad of thinly sliced raw vegetables and feta cheese, dressed with olive oil and vinegar, is often served with meals. Rice is a main grain in many dishes. Fruit is an everyday dessert, but rich pastries, such as *baklava*, are served on special occasions.[9]

SOCIAL, PSYCHOLOGIC, AND ECONOMIC INFLUENCES ON FOOD HABITS

Social Influences

Social Structure

Human group behavior reveals many activities, processes, and structures that make up social life. In any society, social groups are formed largely by factors such as economic status, education, residence, occupation, or family. Values and habits vary in different groups. Subgroups also develop on the basis of region, religion, age, sex, social class, health concerns, special interests, ethnic backgrounds, politics, or other common concerns. All of our various group affiliations influence our basic habit patterns, including our food attitudes and habits.

Food and Social Factors

In our social relationships, food is a symbol of acceptance, warmth, and friendliness. People tend to accept food or food advice more readily from friends or acquaintances or from persons they view as trusted authorities. These influences are especially strong in our family relationships. Food habits that are closely associated with family sentiments stay with us throughout life. Throughout adulthood, certain foods trigger a flood of childhood memories and are valued for reasons apart from any nutritional value.

Psychologic Influences

Understanding Diet Patterns

We begin to understand diet patterns better when we also see the psychologic influences involved. Food has many personal meanings and relationships to personal needs. Our social relationships, in turn, affect our individual behavior. Many of these psychologic factors are rooted in childhood experiences with food in the family. For example, when a child is hurt or disappointed, parents may offer a sweet food to help the child feel better. Then when

we feel hurt as adults, we turn to those sweets to help us feel good again. Now we are learning that this food behavior may actually have some physiologic components, as well. Certain foods, especially sweets and other pleasurable tastes, apparently stimulate "feel good" body chemicals in the brain called *endorphins* that give us a mild "high" or help relieve pain.

Food and Psychosocial Development

Because food is so fundamental to our physical survival, it also relates closely to our psychosocial development as individuals. From infancy to old age, our emotional maturity grows along with our physical development. At each stage of human growth, food habits are part of both physical and psychosocial development. For example, when 2-year-old toddlers are struggling with their first steps toward eventual independence from their parents, they learn that they can control their parents through food and often become picky eaters, refusing to eat any new foods. Psychologists now believe that another normal developmental factor is involved, which they call *food neophobia*, or fear of unfamiliar foods. This universal trait may be an instinct from our evolutionary past that protected children from eating harmful foods when they were just becoming independent from their mothers.

Economic Influences

Family Income and Food Habits

Except perhaps for the relatively small group of very wealthy individuals, most American families live under socioeconomic pressures, especially in periods of recession and inflation. The problems of middle-income families differ in relative terms, but it is the low-income families—especially those in poverty situations—that suffer extreme needs. These families often lack adequate housing and may have little or no access to educational opportunities. As a result, they are poorly prepared for jobs and often only make a day-to-day living at low-paying work or are unemployed. Nearly one in every eight Americans lives in a family with an income below the federal poverty level, and about one in every four children younger than 6 years are members of such families.[10] It is no wonder that people with low incomes bear the greater burden of unnecessary illness and malnutrition.

Food Assistance Programs

Many low-income families are helped to better health by developing better food habits through community projects conducted by the U.S. Federal Extension Service working at the county level. These county Extension agents—home economists and their aides from the community—help families to use better food-buying practices, acquire skills in food preparation, and improve eating habits. Meals are more balanced, better use is made of government-donated commodity foods, and federal food stamps are spent more wisely. Some of the economical ways of handling food and available food-assistance programs are discussed in Chapter 13.

FOOD MISINFORMATION AND FADS

The word *fad* is a shortened form of an old word *faddle* (retained today in the phrase "fiddle-faddle"), meaning "to play with." A fad is something one "plays with" for a while. A fad is any popular fashion or pursuit, without substantial basis, that is embraced with fervor. Food fads are scientifically unsubstantiated beliefs about certain foods that may persist for a time in a given community or society. The word *fallacy* (L. *fallacia*, a trick to deceive) means "a deceptive, misleading, or false notion or belief." Therefore food fallacies are false or misleading beliefs that underlie food fads. The word *quack*, as used in this sense, is a shortened form of *quicksalver*, a term invented centuries ago by the Dutch to describe the pseudophysician or pseudoprofessor who sold worthless salves, "magic" elixirs, and cure-all tonics. He proclaimed his wares in a patter that skeptical people compared to the quacking of a duck. In medicine, nutrition, and allied health fields, a

quack is a fraudulent pretender who claims to have skill, knowledge, or qualifications that he or she does not possess. The motive for such quackery is usually money, and the quack uses some cruel hoax to feed on the physical and emotional needs of his or her victims. The food quack exists because food faddists exist.

Unscientific statements about food often mislead consumers and contribute to poor food habits. False information may come from folklore or fraud. We need to make wise food choices and recognize misinformation as such, based on sound scientific knowledge from responsible authorities.

Food Fads

Types of Claims

Food faddists make exaggerated claims for certain types of food. These claims fall into four basic groups, as follow:

1. **Food cures**—Certain foods will cure specific conditions.
2. **Harmful foods**—Certain foods are harmful and should be omitted from the diet.
3. **Food combinations**—Special food combinations restore health and are effective in reducing weight.
4. **"Natural" foods**—Only so-called "natural" foods can meet body needs and prevent disease. The term *natural food* is generally used by persons who consider all processed foods (including those that are enriched or fortified) as unhealthy. On the other hand, growing foods by organic farming is not a fad. It is an environmentally sound, positive practice now being developed by soil scientists that uses sustainable agriculture methods to avoid pesticides and restore the land (see Chapter 13).

Basic Error

Look at these claims carefully. On the surface they seem to be simple statements about food and health. Further observation, however, reveals that each one focuses on foods per se, not on the specific chemical components in food, the *nutrients*, which are the actual physiologic agents of life and health. Certain individuals may be allergic to specific foods and obviously should avoid them. Also, certain foods may supply relatively large amounts of certain nutrients and are therefore good sources of those nutrients. The *nutrients*, however—not the specific foods, have specific functions in the body. Each of these nutrients is found in a wide variety of different foods. Remember, persons require specific nutrients, never specific foods.

Dangers

Why should health workers be concerned about food fads and their effect on food habits? What harm do food fads cause? Food fads generally involve four possible dangers, as follow.

Dangers to health. Responsibility for care of one's health is fundamental. Self-diagnosis and self-treatment can be dangerous, however, especially when such action follows questionable sources. By following such a course, persons with real illness may fail to seek appropriate medical care. Many ill and anxious people have been misled by fraudulent claims of cures and have postponed effective therapy.

Cost. Some foods and supplements used by faddists are harmless, but many are expensive. Money spent for useless items is wasted. When dollars are scarce, a family may neglect to buy foods that will fill its basic needs and instead purchase a "guaranteed cure."

Lack of sound knowledge. Misinformation hinders the development of individuals, and society and ignores lines opened up by scientific progress. Certain superstitions that are perpetuated can counteract sound teaching about health.

Distrust of the food market. Our food environment is changing. We need to be watchful, but a blanket rejection of *all* modern food production is unwarranted. We must develop intelligent concerns and rational approaches to meet our nutritional needs. A wise course is to select a variety of primary foods "closer to the source" or that have minimal processing, and then add a few carefully selected processed items for specific uses. We can evaluate each food product on its own merits in terms of individual needs (i.e., nutrient contribution, personal values, safety, and cost).

Vulnerable Groups

Food fads appeal especially to certain groups of people with particular needs and concerns.

Elderly Persons

Fear of the changes of aging leads many middle-aged and older adults to grasp at exaggerated claims that some product will restore vigor. Persons in pain living with chronic illness reach out for the "special supplement" that promises a sure cure. Desperately ill and lonely persons are easy prey for a cruel hoax.

Young Persons

Figure-conscious girls and muscle-minded boys may respond to crash programs and claims offering the "perfect body." Many who are lonely or have exaggerated ideas of glamour hope to achieve peer group acceptance by these means.

Obese Persons

Obesity is one of the most disturbing personal concerns and frustrating health problems in America today (see Chapter 15). Obese persons face a constant barrage of propaganda pushing diets, pills, candies, wafers, formulas, and devices. Many of these persons are likely to follow fads.

Athletes and Coaches

This group is a prime target for those who push miracle supplements (see Chapter 16). Always looking for the added something to give them the "competitive edge," athletes tend to fall prey to nutrition myths and hoaxes. Two such examples of substances being used by well-known athletes who influence many young players are the amino acid, creatine, and anabolic steroids.[11,12] Such misuse of drugs is harmful in the long run and dishonest behavior in young athletes in competition but also—at the dangerous rate taken by some aspiring young athletes—can be deadly.

Entertainers

Persons in the public eye are often taken in by false claims that certain foods, drugs, or dietary combinations will maintain the physical appearance and strength on which their careers depend.

Others

The vulnerability of the groups listed previously is obvious, but many other people in the general population follow the appeal of various food fads. Misinformation hinders the efforts of health professionals and concerned consumers to raise community nutrition standards.

What Is the Answer?

What can be done to counter food habits associated with food fads, misinformation, or even outright deception? What can—and *should*—health workers do? An attitude of "do as I say, not as I do" achieves nothing. Health workers cannot counsel or teach others until they have first examined their own habits. Helpful instruction is based on personal conviction, practice, and enthusiasm. Then the following approaches to positive teaching can be used.

Use Reliable Sources

Sound background knowledge is essential, as follows: (1) know the product being pushed and the persons behind it, (2) know how human physiology really works, and (3) know the scientific method of problem-solving (i.e., collect the facts, identify the real problem, determine a reasonable solution or action, carry it out, and evaluate the results). Sound community resources include the following:

- Extension Service home economists working in the community through state and county

Extension Service offices and directing highly successful community nutrition activities, such as their Expanded Food and Nutrition Education Program (EFNEP). These specialists develop many food and nutrition guides—especially for those with limited education or little skill with English as a second language. The Food and Drug Administration (FDA) and U.S. Department of Agriculture (USDA) produce many educational materials related to food and nutrition (see Chapter 13). Requests for these mostly free materials can be directed to FDA and USDA agency offices.
- Public Health nutritionists located in county and state public health offices and special programs, such as WIC.
- Registered dietitians in local medical care centers, serving hospitalized patients, outpatient clinics, and others in private practice.

Recognize Human Needs

Consider the emotional needs that food and food rituals help fulfill. Everyone has such needs; they are part of life. Use these needs in a positive way in your nutrition teaching. Even if a person is using food as an emotional "crutch," the emotional need is very real. We must never "break crutches" without offering a better and wiser way of support.

Be Alert to Teaching Opportunities

Use any opportunity that arises to present sound nutrition and health information, formally or informally. Learn about the available resources described previously (e.g., local or state university agricultural extension services, volunteer health agencies, clinic and hospital facilities, public health departments, and professional health organizations). Develop communication skills, avoid monotony, and use a well-disciplined imagination. Otherwise, your message will not convince consumers of the falsehoods behind the attractive skills of the food faddist or bogus "nutritionist" credentialed by a "mail-order school" or best-selling "diet book."

BOX 14-1 Factors determining food choices

Physical Factors
Food supply available
Food technology
Geography, agriculture, distribution
Personal economics, income
Sanitation, housing
Season, climate
Storage and cooking facilities

Social Factors
Advertising
Culture
Education, nutrition and general

Social Factors—cont'd
Political and economic policies
Religion and social class, role
Social problems, poverty, or alcoholism

Physiologic Factors
Allergy
Disability
Health-disease status
Heredity
Personal food acceptance
Needs, energy, or nutrients
Therapeutic diets

Think Scientifically

You can teach even very young children to use the problem-solving approach to everyday situations. Children are naturally curious. With their eternal "Why?", they often seek evidence to support statements they hear. You must teach them and others the value of three basic questions, as follow: (1) "What do you mean?"; (2) "How do you know?"; and (3) "What is your evidence?"

Know Responsible Authorities

The FDA has the legal responsibility of controlling the quality and safety of the food and drug products marketed in the United States. This is a tremendous task, however, and requires public help. Other governmental, professional, and private organizations can provide additional resources.

CHANGES IN AMERICAN FOOD HABITS
Personal Food Choices

Basic Determinants

As we have seen, universal factors determining personal food choices clearly arise from physical, social, and physiologic needs. Box 14-1 summarizes some of these factors. Changing our own eating patterns is difficult enough; helping our clients and patients to make needed changes for positive health reasons is even more difficult. Such teaching requires a sensitive and flexible understanding of the complex factors involved.

Factors Influencing Change

Ethnic patterns and regional cultural habits are strong influences in our lives. They establish our early food habits and make changing those habits difficult. On the other hand, our changing society puts the old in conflict with the new. Some newer factors influence changes in our food habits.[13]

- **Income**—The generally improved economic situation of society provides sufficient income in most cases to give us more choice and time.
- **Technology**—Expansion in the fields of science and technology increases the number and variety of food items available.
- **Environment**—Our rapidly changing environment results in concerns about our food and health.
- **Vision**—Our expanding mass media, especially television, stimulates many options for

new items and changes our expectations and desires. The current market target for television advertisements is younger children, who then influence the family's buying habits.

Changing American Food Patterns

The stereotype of the all-American family of parents and two children eating three meals a day with no snacks in between is no longer the norm. We have made far-reaching changes in our way of living and, subsequently, in our food habits.

Households

American households are increasing in number and changing in nature. Most new households are groups of unrelated persons or persons living alone. U.S. Census Bureau projections are that from 2000 to 2010 the number of non-family households will increase 17%, while family households will increase 9%.[14] The average size of American households is projected to decline from 2.59 persons in 2000 to 2.53 persons by 2010. Married couple households from 2000 to 2010 will decline from 54% to 52% of all households.[14] These changes reflect our rapidly changing society.

Working Women

The number of women in the workforce continues to increase rapidly and is not likely to reverse. This trend is not restricted to any social, economic, or ethnic group. Women of all racial and ethnic groups will be the major entrants into the U.S. labor market. The U.S. Department of Labor reports that women were 46% of the total national workforce in 1999.[14] This is a widespread change in society. Working parents increasingly rely on food items and cooking methods that save time, space, and labor.

Family Meals

Family meals as we have known them have changed. Breakfasts and lunches are seldom eaten in a family setting. Half of Americans between the ages of 22 and 40, as well as many children, skip breakfast regularly, and 25% skip lunch. About 25% of American households do not have a sit-down dinner as often as 5 nights a week.

Meals and Snacks

Our habits have changed dramatically as to when we eat and whether we eat with our families. Midmorning and midafternoon breaks at work usually involve food or beverage. Evening television snacks plus a midnight refrigerator raid are common. Nutrition hardliners of the old school may denounce this snacking behavior, but they are out of step. Americans are moving toward a concept of *balanced days* instead of *balanced meals*. They are increasing the number of times a day they eat to as many as 11 "eating occasions," a pattern recently termed *grazing*. This shift is not necessarily bad, depending on the nature of the periodic snacking or more constant "grazing." In fact, studies indicate that frequent small meals are better for the body than three larger meals per day, especially when healthy snacking and grazing contribute to needed nutrient and energy intake (see For Further Focus box, "Snacking: An All-American Food Habit").

Health and Fitness

Americans' interest in health and fitness is increasing, which has affected food buying in several ways, with more nutrition awareness, weight concern, and interest in gourmet or specialty foods. New lines of so-called light foods are popular.

Economical Buying

More Americans are making diet changes to save money. They are seeking bargains and cutting back on expensive "convenience foods." They are buying in larger packages and in bulk and doing less "store-hopping," staying with a store that maintains fairer overall prices. Americans are less loyal to brand names and buy more generic products; they are also using food labels both for unit pricing and "calorie-counting."

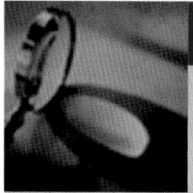

FOR FURTHER FOCUS
Snacking: An All-American Food Habit

The snack market in the United States continues to grow. Consumer spending for all foods has increased, with a greater portion of the increase being spent for snacks—mainly salty snacks, cookies, and crackers. Other popular snacks include soft drinks, candies, gum, fresh fruit, bakery items, milk, and chips.

Snacking is said to "ruin your appetite," and we certainly consume too many soft drinks, but is snacking all bad? Not necessarily. Surveys have shown a direct association between more complete nutrition and an increase in snacking.

Those who snack more show higher nutrient percentages in the "adequate" range of the DRI and RDA standards. Many people snack on foods that are not "empty extras" but essential contributions to total nutritional adequacy (e.g., fruit, cheese, eggs, bread, and crackers).

Snacking, or "grazing" as some persons do with more frequent nibbling, is clearly a significant component of food behavior. Rather than rule against the practice, we need to promote snack foods that enhance nutritional well-being.

Fast Foods

At least once, most Americans have eaten in a fast-food restaurant, averaging about one in 12 meals a year per person. From McDonald's modest beginning in 1955 in Des Plaines, Illinois, the fast-food business has grown into a multibillion-dollar enterprise that now captures almost half of the money spent on meals away from home. As family income rises, so does the consumption of fast foods, especially among the middle class.

All of the social changes listed here have radically changed the food marketplace in America. Our food habits reflect this changing market and society.

SUMMARY

We all grow up and live our lives in a social setting. We each inherit a culture and live in our particular social structure, complete with its food habits and attitudes about eating. We need to understand the effects on health that are associated with major social and economic shifts. We must also understand current social forces to best help persons make dietary changes to benefit their health. We must meet concerns about food misinformation.

The food patterns of Americans are changing. We increasingly rely on new forms of food in our fast, complex lives. More women are working; households are getting smaller; more people are living alone; and our meal patterns are different. We search for less fancy, lower-cost food items, and also cook creatively. We are generally more nutrition- and health-conscious. Fast food outlets and snacking are social habits here to stay.

REVIEW QUESTIONS

1. What is the meaning of culture? How does it affect our food patterns?
2. What social and psychologic factors influence our food habits? Give examples of personal meanings related to food.
3. Why does the public tend to accept nutrition misinformation and fads so easily? What groups of people are more susceptible? Select one such group and give some effective approaches you might use to reach them.
4. What are current trends in American food habits? Discuss their implications for nutrition and health.

SELF-TEST QUESTIONS

True-False

Write the correct statement for each item you answer "false."

1. Food habits result from instinctive behavioral responses throughout life.
2. The structure of American social classes is largely determined by occupation, income and education, and residence.
3. Lifestyles change as society's values change.
4. From the time of birth, eating is a social act that is built on social relationships.
5. Food fads are usually long-lasting and seldom change.
6. Special food combinations are effective as weight-reducing diets and have special therapeutic effects.

Multiple Choice

1. A healthy body requires:
   a. Specific foods to control specific functions.
   b. Certain food combinations to achieve specific physiologic effects.
   c. Natural foods to prevent disease.
   d. Specific nutrients in various foods to perform specific body functions.
2. Food habits in a given culture are largely based on (circle all that apply):
   a. Food availability.
   b. Genetic differences in food tastes.
   c. Food economics, market practices, and food distribution.
   d. Symbolic meanings attached to certain foods.
3. In the Jewish food pattern, the word *kosher* refers to food prepared by (circle all that apply):
   a. Ritual slaughter of allowed animals for maximum blood drainage.
   b. Avoiding the combination of meat and milk in the same meal.
   c. Special seasoning to avoid use of salt.
   d. Special cooking of food combinations to ensure purity and digestibility.
4. The basic grain used in the Mexican food pattern is:
   a. Rice.
   b. Corn.
   c. Wheat.
   d. Oat.
5. Stir-frying is a basic cooking method used in the food pattern of:
   a. Mexicans.
   b. Jews.
   c. Chinese.
   d. Greeks.

SUGGESTIONS FOR ADDITIONAL STUDY

1. Cultural Food Pattern Survey

Select a person of a cultural background that is different from your own. Interview this person about food habits. Inquire about food items most commonly used and general methods of preparing them. Then ask about the basic meal pattern for a day. If possible, visit a market that carries these foods and seasonings and survey the items there. Also arrange to have a home or restaurant meal of this cultural food pattern. Compare your findings with the discussion in your textbook and other resources, as well as with other cultural patterns in your class discussion.

2. Food Fad Survey

Select a person (or persons) in one of the vulnerable groups discussed in relation to food misinformation and fads. Interview them about any food or supplement practices or misinformation they may have encountered. Ask them how they feel about these practices or if they can offer any suggestions about these practices. Summarize your findings and list any approaches you think can help correct these beliefs or practices. Review your report with those of others presented in your follow-up class discussion.

REFERENCES

1. Kittler PG, Sucher KP: *Food and culture in America*, ed 2, New York, 1998, The West Group.
2. Counihan C, Van Esterik P, editors: *Food and culture: a reader*, New York, 1997, Routledge.
3. Barer-Stein T: *You eat what you are: people, culture, and food traditions*, ed 2, New York, 1999, Culture Concepts.
4. Kittler PG, Sucher KP: *Cultural foods: traditions and trends*, New York, 1999, Wadsworth Publishing Co.
5. Zubila S, Tapper R: *Culinary cultures of the Middle East*, New York, 1995, IB Tauris.
6. Sanjur D: *Hispanic foodways, nutrition, and health*, Boston, 1995, Allyn & Bacon.
7. Gabacia DR: *We are what we eat: ethnic food and the making of Americans*, Cambridge, Mass, 1998, Harvard University Press.
8. Davidson A: *The Oxford companion to food*, New York, 1999, Oxford University Press.
9. Fieldhouse P: *Food and nutrition: customs and culture*, ed 2, New York, 1995, Chapman and Hall USA.
10. U.S. Department of Health and Human Services: *Healthy People 2010: understanding and improving health*, Washington, DC, 2000, U.S. Department of Health and Human Services, Government Printing Office.
11. Juhn MS, O'Kane JW, Vincent DM: Oral creatine supplement in male collegiate athletics: a survey of dosing habits and side effects, *J Am Diet Assoc* 99(5):593, 1999.
12. Nmakwe N: Anabolic steroids and cardiovascular risk in athletes, *Nutr Today* 31(5):206, 1996.
13. Southgate DAT: Dietary change: changing patterns of eating; in Meiselman HL and MacFie HJH, editors: *Food choices, acceptance, and consumption*, London, 1999, Chapman & Hall.
14. U.S. Census Bureau, U.S. Department of Commerce: *Statistical abstract of the United States 1999*, ed 119, Washington, DC, 1999, U.S. Department of Commerce, Government Printing Office.

FURTHER READING

- Juhn MS, O'Kane JW, Vinci DM: Oral creatine supplementation in male collegiate athletes: a survey of dosing habits and side effects, *J Am Diet Assoc* 99(5):593, 1999.
- Wagner DR: Hyperhydrating with glycerol: implications for athletic performance, *J Am Diet Assoc* 99(2):207, 1999.

These two articles provide sound scientific background to help athletes—especially younger, still growing athletes—who are straining to win, sometimes at whatever the cost to their bodies, and who thus are vulnerable to nutrition myths. In this effort, they may push to the limit—exceeding cautions—and suffer harmful side effects. The potential misuse of two substances (creatine and glycerol) is clearly described, with the basis for caution presented in each case.

- Bell D, Valentine G: *Consuming geographies: we are what we eat*, New York, 1997, Routledge.
- Griffiths S, Wallace J, editors: *Consuming passions: food in an age of anxiety*, New York, 1998, Manchester University Press.

These two fascinating little books hold a wealth of information about why we eat what we do.

15

Weight Management

KEY CONCEPTS

- America's obsession with thinness carries social and physiologic costs.

- Underlying causes of obesity are a complex of psychosocial, physiologic, and genetic factors.

- Realistic weight management focuses on the individual and health promotion.

At least one out of every four Americans is on a weight-reduction diet. Use of these "diets" seems to increase daily, with a new "diet book" constantly appearing in the public press. Despite this obsession and the fact that weight loss is big business, Americans are actually getting heavier. The average American has gained about 2.25 kg (5 lb) over the past decade or so. Why has this occurred?

Much of the answer lies in our changing lifestyle. Our technology is producing a more sedentary society, and all of these popular "diets" do not work. Only about 5% of dieters maintain their weight at the new lower level after such a diet. In this chapter, we examine the problem of weight management and seek a more positive and realistic health model that recognizes personal needs and sound weight goals.

THE PROBLEM OF OBESITY AND WEIGHT CONTROL

Body Weight and Body Fat

Definitions

Obesity is not "simple," though we have often called it that in general practice. Obesity develops from many interwoven factors—including personal, physical, and genetic factors—and is difficult to define. As used in the traditional medical sense, *obesity* is a clinical term for excess body weight generally applied to persons who are at least 20% above a desired weight for height. Over the past 4 decades the percentage of overweight and obese adults age 20 years or older has increased to about 55%.[1] We must always remember, however, that every person is different, and *normal* values in healthy persons vary. Until recently, we had also overlooked the important factor of *age* in setting a reasonable body weight for adults. With advancing age, body weight usually increases until about age 50 for men and age 70 for women, then declines. Extreme thinness carries more overall health risk than being moderately overweight as persons grow older.

The terms *overweight* and *obesity* are often used interchangeably, but they actually have different meanings. The word *overweight* simply means a body weight that is above a population weight-for-height standard. The word *obesity*, however, is a more specific term that comes from a Latin root (*obedere*, to devour) and means "very fat." Thus it refers to the *degree of fatness* (i.e., the relative excess amount of fat in the total body composition), which is the real health problem. For example, a football player in peak condition can be extremely "overweight" according to standard weight-height charts. That is, he can weigh considerably more than the average man of the same height, but much more of his weight is lean muscle mass—not excess fat (Figure 15-1).

Body Composition

Therefore it is more correct to talk in terms of *fatness* and *leanness*—or body composition—than use the term *overweight*. Health professionals (i.e., usually the registered dietitian on the health care team) measure body fatness in working with overweight or obese persons. They use calipers to measure the widths of skin folds at specific body sites, because most of the body fat is deposited in layers just under the skin. These measures are then used in special formulas to calculate an approximate body fat composition. A more precise method, underwater weighing, is used in athletic programs or

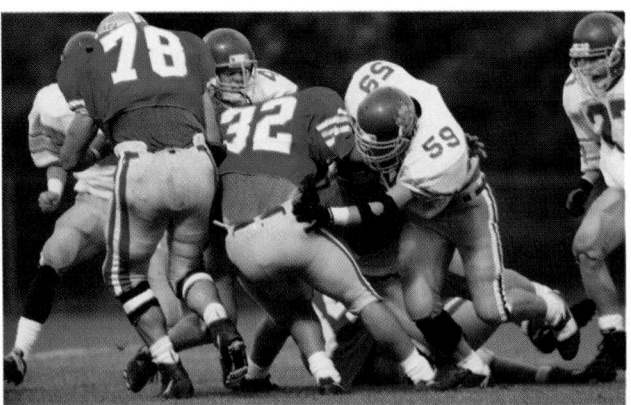

FIGURE 15-1 According to standard weight-height charts, some football players would be considered overweight. These charts should be used with discretion. (Credit: PhotoDisc.)

research studies and ensures that obesity can be better defined in terms of body fat content. The standard body fat content for healthy men, estimated from underwater body weighing, ranges from about 14% to 28% of total body weight. For women it is somewhat larger: 15% to 30%. Obesity occurs when the percentage of body fat exceeds these estimates.

Measures of Weight Maintenance Goals

Former General Guide

In prior years, a general rule of thumb was passed along to determine weight goals, as follows:

- *Males*—106 pounds for the first 5 feet, then add 6 pounds/inch, plus or minus 10 pounds.
- *Females*—100 pounds for the first 5 feet, then add 5 pounds/inch, plus or minus 10 pounds.

This guide is no longer used because it produces unrealistically low weights, especially for women, and does not account for age differences.

Standard Weight-Height Tables

These tables are tools or general population guides and should be regarded only as such. Individual needs as a whole must be considered. One of the standard tables in use in the United States is the Metropolitan Life Insurance Company's "ideal" weight-for-height charts, which are based on life expectancy information gathered since the 1930s from its population of life insurance policy holders (mostly white adult males in its beginnings). Many people have questioned how well these tables represent our total current population, even with the relatively minor changes made in a 1983 revision.

Studies also show that health risks are as great—if not greater—for very thin low-weight persons as for extremely obese ones. Within each age group, both extremely thin and extremely fat persons have higher mortality rates. Therefore it seems that we should try to be neither excessively over-weight nor excessively underweight, and that the multitude of health problems attributed to *moderate* amounts of overweight are unfounded.

More recent height-weight tables have been developed based on the National Research Council data on weight and health, the current U.S. dietary guidelines, and recent medical studies.[1,2] These more realistic guides, shown in Table 15-1, relate height and adult age ranges to good ranges of body weight.

Ideal Weight

The term *ideal weight* is not very useful. It may give you a "ballpark" figure but not much more. You should be wary of this term for two important reasons.

Individual variation. The basic problem with "ideal weight" is that it varies with different people at different times under different circumstances. Any person's ideal weight depends on many factors including age, body shape, metabolic rate, genetic makeup, sex, and physical activity. Persons need varying amounts of weight and can carry different amounts in good health. Specific individual situations govern needs.

Necessity of body fat. In our zeal to lose weight, we may forget that some body fat is essential to survival, as is evidenced in cases of starvation. Victims of starvation die of fat loss—not protein depletion. For mere survival, males require 3% body fat, and females require 12%. Menstruation begins when the female body reaches a certain size or, more precisely, when a young girl's body fat reaches a critical point of body weight (i.e., about 20%). This is the amount needed for ovulation, and thus any eventual pregnancy.

---

body composition the relative sizes of the four basic body compartments that make up the total body: lean body mass (muscle mass), fat, water, and bone.

TABLE 15-1 Good body weights-for-height for adults, expressed in pounds (for height, in feet-inches) and kilograms (for height, in centimeters)*

Height (ft-in)†	19-34 years		35 years +		cm	19-34 years		35 years +	
	Average weight (lb)	Range (lb)	Average weight (lb)	Range (lb)		Average weight (kg)	Range (kg)	Average weight (kg)	Range (kg)
5'0"	112	97-128	123	108-138	152	51	44-58	55	49-62
5'1"	116	101-132	127	111-143	155	53	46-60	58	40-65
5'2"	120	104-137	131	115-148	157	54	47-62	59	52-67
5'3"	124	107-141	135	119-152	160	56	49-64	61	54-69
5'4"	128	111-146	140	122-157	163	58	51-66	64	56-72
5'5"	132	114-150	144	126-162	165	60	52-68	65	57-74
5'6"	136	118-155	148	130-167	168	62	54-71	68	59-76
5'7"	140	121-160	153	134-172	170	64	55-72	69	61-78
5'8"	144	125-164	158	138-178	173	66	57-75	72	63-81
5'9"	149	129-169	162	142-183	175	67	58-77	74	64-83
5'10"	153	132-174	167	146-188	178	70	60-79	76	67-86
5'11"	157	136-179	172	151-194	180	71	62-81	78	68-88
6'0"	162	140-184	177	155-199	183	74	64-84	80	70-90
6'1"	166	144-189	182	159-205	185	75	65-86	82	72-92
6'2"	171	148-195	187	164-210	188	78	67-88	85	74-95
6'3"	176	152-200	192	168-216	191	80	69-91	88	77-99
6'4"	180	156-205	197	173-222	193	82	71-93	89	78-101
6'5"	185	160-211	202	177-228	196	85	73-96	92	81-104
6'6"	190	164-216	208	182-234	198	86	75-98	94	82-106

Data adapted from U.S. Department of Agriculture, U.S. Department of Health and Human Services: *Nutrition and your health: dietary guidelines for Americans,* ed 4, Washington, D.C., 1995, U.S. Government Printing Office; and from Bray GA: Pathophysiology of obesity. *Am J Clin Nutr* 55:448S, 1992.

*Without clothes.

†Without shoes.

Obesity and Health

Weight Extremes

Clearly massive, or *morbid*, obesity is a health hazard in itself and is a medical problem because it places severe strain on all body systems. Both extremes of weight—fatness and thinness—pose medical problems.

Overweight and Health Problems

The most recent National Health and Examination Survey (NHANES III) data indicated a marked increase in the prevalence of overweight in the United States.[2] Experts have estimated that 97 million American adults are overweight or obese, which increases their risk of related conditions such as hypertension, type 2 diabetes, and breast, prostate, and colon cancers.[3] The major problem affecting most Americans is the degree of general overweight that is a risk to positive health. Current studies indicate that direct relationships between overweight and disease have been demonstrated in the following two conditions: adult type 2 non–insulin-dependent diabetes mellitus (NIDDM) and hypertension, which may contribute to cardiovascular disease. Health risks exist in *extreme* obesity, but unless a person is at least 30% over the normal weight-for-height ratio, the relation of weight to mortality is questionable.

Indirect Relationship to Disease

As studies show, general obesity *is* directly related to type 2 diabetes mellitus and hypertension. These two conditions are also risk factors in coronary heart disease, which is a much larger health problem. Thus general obesity is an indirect factor in heart disease. Losing excessive weight is associated with improvement of hypertension and diabetes. Weight loss can bring significant reductions in elevated blood glucose or blood pressure in obese persons with type 2 diabetes mellitus or hypertension. In turn, these improvements reduce risks related to heart disease.

Causes of Obesity

Basic Energy Balance

How does a person become overweight? Although some persons suffer from congenital obesity, a major cause of obesity in sedentary Americans is *lack of exercise*. In fact, a simple, well-defined walking program can help reduce the amount of body fat in overweight persons, even without any noticeable changes in dietary intake. Thus regular exercise by itself has a significant effect on reducing fat and increasing lean body content.[3]

The overall underlying energy imbalance (i.e., more energy intake as food than energy output as physical activity and basal metabolic needs) is the ultimate basis of excess weight. The excess intake is stored in the body. About 3,500 kcal is the equivalent of 1 lb (.45 kg) of body fat (Box 15-1). This is part of the answer. We also know from experience, however, that some overweight persons only eat moderate amounts of food, and that some persons of average weight eat much more but never seem to gain. Because many individual differences exist, more factors must be involved.

Genetic Base

The discovery of the obesity gene is a tale of 8 years of tedious work. A research group at Rockefeller Uni-

versity first reported their finding in test animals, an overweight strain of laboratory mice. Soon thereafter these researchers located the human equivalent of this gene.[4] In 1995, this team and two other research groups also reported similar findings of a hormonelike protein product of the gene that apparently acts on the satiety centers in the brain, for one place, to control appropriate eating behavior and fat storage.[5,6] The researchers named the hormone *leptin*, from the Greek word *leptos*, meaning thin or slender. In late 1995, after continued study, other groups working on the same problem reported a major breakthrough with the finding of a leptin receptor in the human brain. This discovery helped scientists to understand how leptin works to control body weight, ultimately enabling them to develop antiobesity drugs.[7]

Follow-up studies of leptin use have reported disappointing results overall, although the drug did prove effective in a small percentage of the test participants.[8-10] Ongoing research seeks to learn what made the few who had positive experience with leptin respond as they did.

Additional studies are focusing on population groups such as the Pima Indians, whose naturally low leptin concentration and low resting metabolic rate may possibly be an expression of a "thrifty genotype."[11] Such research seeks to find answers to questions about a possible genetic influence.

Genetic and Family Factors

Genetic inheritance probably influences a person's chance of becoming fat more than any other factor. Family food patterns reinforce this genetic base.

Genetic control. A genetic base regulates differences in body fat and sex in weight. In some types of obesity, genetic-metabolic controls regulate the amount of body fat an individual carries.[12] A person then eats to regain or lose whatever amount of fat the body is naturally set or programmed for, according to the weight below or above this internally regulated point. Thus persons who have unnaturally lost body fat below their programmed level—either by strenuous "dieting" or lack of food, will eat to regain to their genetic fat point when food is available again. Similarly, persons with lower programmed fat

BOX 15-1   Kilocalorie adjustment required for weight loss

To lose 454 g (1 lb) a week—500 fewer kcal daily
        Basis of estimation
        1 lb body fat   = 454 g
        1 g pure fat   = 9 kcal
        1 g body fat   = 7.7 kcal (some water in fat cells)
        454 g × 9 kcal/g   = 4086 kcal/454 g fat (pure fat)
        454 g × 7.7 kcal/g = 3496 kcal/454 g body fat (or 3500 kcal)
        500 kcal × 7 days = 3500 kcal = 454 g body fat

levels who have gained excess body fat above their genetic level by eating more, although their body metabolism remains unchanged by pushing food, will lose this excess fat when they resume their regular food intake. It seems that the only way to help lower a higher genetic setting for body fat is through an increase in regular exercise.

Family reinforcement.   In the long run, however, excess body weight may have its start not so much in individual gene control as in the family food patterns learned in early years. An individual's genetic predisposition for increased body fat is then reinforced by family food patterns. If one parent is obese, a child's chance of becoming obese is modest. This chance is greater if both parents are obese. It is rare that a child will become obese if neither parent is obese. In addition to genetic influence, families also exert social pressure and teach children habits and attitudes toward food. Thus it is wise to begin developing healthy eating habits, with fat-controlled cooking and the family enjoying meals together, during childhood and teenage years.

Physiologic factors.   The amount of body fat a person carries, whether through inheritance or eating habits, is related to the number and size of fat cells in the body. Critical periods for developing obesity occur during early growth periods when cells are multiplying rapidly in childhood and adolescence. Once the body has added extra fat calls for more fuel storage, these cells remain and can store varying amounts of fat. Middle-aged and older adults may store more fat when they get less exercise.[15] Women store more fat during pregnancy and after menopause because hormones are involved.[16]

Psychosocial factors.   Many persons respond to emotional stress by eating—especially foods they regard as "comfort" foods. Social pressures—especially on women—to maintain our cultural "ideal" thin body type also contribute to eating disorders and social discrimination against obese persons.

Individual Differences and Extreme Practices

Individual Energy-Balance Levels

As we have seen, several factors influence a person's individual point of energy balance. Some persons do have more genetic-based metabolic efficiency (i.e., they just "burn" food more readily than others do). Also, when you calculate a person's energy balance, which is a worthwhile general exercise, your figures indicate only an *approximate* value. Reported food values represent averages of many samples of that food tested. Many factors (e.g., including basal metabolic rate [BMR], body size, lean body mass, age, sex, and physical activity) also influence how much energy a person "burns up." These calculations, however, provide useful general information and indicate areas of individual needs and goals.

Extreme Practices

Individual differences in energy needs, along with social pressures, lead many overweight persons to use extreme measures to lose weight—often at risk to their health.

Fad diets. A constant array of "diet books" floods the American market. These books usually sell briefly and then fade away, largely because their "quick fixes" do not work. There are no magic, simple answers to a far more complex problem. Most of the fad diets fail on the following two counts:

1. **Scientific inaccuracies and misinformation.** As a result of scientific inaccuracies and misinformation, these fad diets are often nutritionally inadequate.
2. **Failure to address the necessity of changing long-term habits.** Persons are often set up for failure to maintain a healthy individual weight once it is achieved. The basic behavioral problem involved in changing food and exercise habits for life—actually a new lifestyle—is unrecognized.

For some persons the degree of kilocaloric restriction required places impossible demands, so they find themselves caught in a vicious cycle of chronic dieting syndrome and its harmful physical and psychologic effects. These people often become caught up in the big business of the U.S. diet industry, where a large amount of money may be spent each year on a wide range of weight loss diets, products, and services.

Fasting. This drastic approach takes many forms, from literal fasting to use of very–low-calorie diets of special formulas, possibly causing the effects of semistarvation: acidosis, low blood pressure, electrolyte loss, tissue protein loss, and decreased basal metabolic rate (BMR). Sometimes loss of sufficient heart muscle causes death. At best, some programs have failed to help persons maintain the new weight after weight loss when refeeding begins.

Clothing and body wraps. Special "sauna suits" or body wrapping is claimed to help weight loss in special spots of the body or clear up so-called *cellulite* tissue, which simply does not exist. The word *cellulite* was coined by a European beauty operator years ago and has no basis in scientific fact. Any spot reducing is only achieved by special exercises designed to use the particular muscles in that area in repeated workouts; the fat is certainly not sweated or pressed out as claimed. Some persons endure such mummylike body wrapping in an attempt to reduce body size. The resulting small weight loss, however, is only caused by temporary water loss. The only way to lose weight is to burn up more kcalories than are consumed.

Drugs. Various amphetamine compounds, commonly called "speed," were once popular in the medical treatment of obesity but are no longer used because of their danger to health. Typical over-the-counter drugs have included *phenylpropylamine (PPA)* (Dexatrim), which is a stimulant similar to amphetamine. Dexatrim has been linked to increased blood pressure and damage to blood vessels in the brain, which can lead to central nervous system disorders such as confusion, stroke, hallucination, and psychotic behavior. No diuretics or hormones (e.g., as thyroid hormone or steroids) should ever be used to affect body weight or leanness without strict medical indication and supervision.

A new pair of related weight loss drugs, fenfluramine and phentermine, were recently produced and prescribed to be used together in the popular

chronic dieting syndrome the cyclic pattern of weight loss by dieting to achieve an unnatural but culturally ideal body thinness, then regaining weight by compulsive food binges in response to stress, anxiety, and hunger. This abnormal psychophysiologic food pattern becomes chronic, changing a person's natural body metabolism and relative body composition to the abnormal state of a "metabolically obese" person of normal weight.

fen-phen combination for weight reduction. Shortly, however, physicians found that a number of persons using these drugs were developing pulmonary hypertension and heart-valve problems—sometimes fatally.[17] Thus the U.S. Food and Drug Administration, with the support of the medical community, quickly removed these drugs from the market. Physicians are now debating the use of drugs in the treatment of obesity.[18,19]

Surgery. Surgical techniques are usually reserved for the medical treatment of extreme, morbid obesity. A former surgical procedure, the *ileal bypass,* is no longer done because it caused many malabsorption and malnutrition problems but is of historical interest and caution. Problems have also followed other procedures previously used to treat obesity, such as wiring the jaws shut to prevent normal eating or inserting a free-floating "gastric bubble" to give a feeling of fullness and reduce food intake. Current surgical procedures focus on gastric bypass and include several forms of *gastroplasty* (Figure 15-2). These types of surgical intervention are designed to reduce the space for food in the stomach, thus limiting appetite and eating but are not without problems and require a skilled team of specialists, including nutritional care. These surgeries also require careful patient selection and preparation, as well as contin-

uous follow-ups in partnership with the patient and family. A more limited type of cosmetic surgery that was developed in the 1980s and is still occasionally used is a form of local fat removal, lipectomy, which is commonly called liposuction. Lipectomy is used to remove fat deposits under the skin in places of cosmetic or figure concern, such as the hips or thighs. A thin tube is inserted through a small incision in the skin, and the desired amount of fat is suctioned away. This procedure is quite painful, however, and carries risks such as infection, large disfiguring skin depressions, or blood clots that can lead to dangerous circulatory problems or even kidney failure. Any surgical procedure carries some risk and may cause other problems and side effects.

SOUND WEIGHT-MANAGEMENT PROGRAM

Essential Characteristics

There are no short-cuts to successful weight control; it requires hard work and strong individual motivation. Weight management must be a personalized program that focuses on changed food and exercise behaviors and stress-relaxation habits. This program must build a healthy lifestyle and

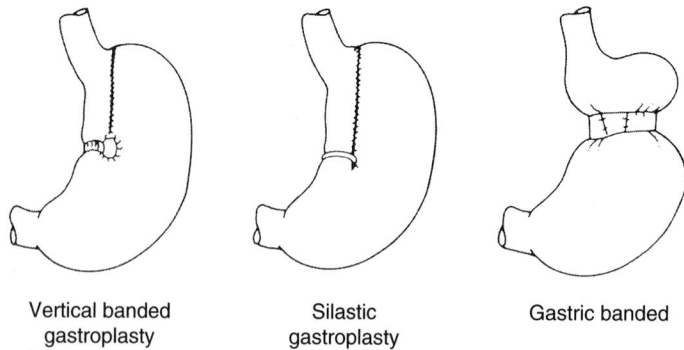

| Vertical banded | Silastic | Gastric banded |
| gastroplasty | gastroplasty | |

FIGURE 15-2 Gastroplasty is a type of restrictive gastric surgical procedure used for treatment of severe obesity. (Adapted from Grace DM: Gastric restriction procedures for treating severe obesity, *Am J Clin Nutr* 55:556S, 1992, and Mason EE and others: Perioperative risks and safety of surgery for severe obesity, *Am J Clin Nutr* 55:573S, 1992.)

have support from the individual, family, or group with follow-ups.

Behavior Modification

Basic Principles

Food behavior is rooted in many human experiences and associations, as well as environmental situations. Addictive forms of eating responses and conditioning are often produced. Behavior-oriented therapies are designed to help obese persons change patterns that contribute to excessive weight, such as excess food and eating, as well as lack of exercise. By understanding behaviors and changing associations with undesirable habits—reconditioning them into new desirable behavior patterns, overweight individuals can plan constructive actions to meet their personal health goals. This behavioral approach must begin with a detailed examination of each undesirable eating behavior with regard to the following three basic aspects: (1) *cues or antecedents*—What stimulates the behavior?; (2) *response*—What happens during the eating or not exercising behavior after the cue?; (3) *consequences*—What happens after the response to the eating or not exercising behavior that serves to reinforce it?

Basic Strategies and Actions

A program of personal behavior modification for weight management is directed toward the following: (1) control of eating behavior (i.e., the when, why, where, how, and how much); and (2) promotion of physical activity to increase energy output. Three progressive actions follow in planning individual strategies:

Define problem behavior. *Specifically* define the problem behavior and the desired behavior outcome. This process clearly establishes specific goals and contributing objectives.

Record and analyze baseline behavior. Record eating and exercise behavior and analyze it carefully in terms of setting and persons involved. What types of habit patterns emerge? How often do these

patterns occur? What conditions seem to "trigger" the behavior? What consequent events seem to maintain the habits (e.g., time and pace, places, persons, social responses, hunger before and after, emotional mood, other factors)?

Plan behavior-management strategy. Set up controls of the external environment involving the situational forces related to each of the three behavior areas involved: what goes before, the response, and the results. Then break these identified links to old undesirable behaviors and recondition them to the desired new eating and exercise behaviors. Think of as many creative ways as possible for reconditioning some of your own food and exercise behaviors that you may wish to change. The Clinical Applications box, "Breaking Old Links: Strategies for Changing Food Behavior," provides a few examples.

Dietary Principles

The central dietary approach in a weight-management program that could achieve a degree of *lasting* success must be based on five characteristics, as follow:

1. **Realistic goals**—Goals must be realistic in terms of overall loss and rate of loss (i.e., no more than 1 to 2 pounds/week).
2. **Kilocalories reduced according to need**—The diet must have sufficient kcalories in relation to individual output of energy to produce a gradual weight loss of 1 to 2 pounds/week.
3. **Nutritional adequacy**—The diet must be nutritionally adequate. Lower caloric levels may

---

lipectomy (Gr. *lipos,* fat; *ektomē,* excision) surgical removal of subcutaneous fat by suction through a tube inserted into a surface incision, or by removing larger amounts of subcutaneous fat by major surgical incision.

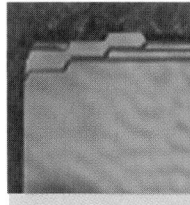

CLINICAL APPLICATIONS

Breaking Old Links: Strategies for Changing Food Behavior

Old habits die hard. They are never easy to change but, in the case of undesirable eating behaviors that contribute to excess body fat and are harmful to health, are worth the effort. Here are some behavioral suggestions.

First Deal with Behavioral Cues

Eliminate as many cues for the problem behavior as possible. Avoid situations and contacts associated with problem foods, put temptation out of reach, and make the problem behavior as difficult as possible. Freeze leftovers, remove problem food items from the kitchen or store them in hard-to-get places, and take a route other than by the familiar bakery or candy shop home.

Suppress the cues that can't be entirely eliminated. Control social situations that maintain the behavior, reward the alternate desired behavior, have a trusted person monitor eating patterns, minimize contact with excessive food, use smaller plates to make smaller food portions appear larger, control "poor me" moods with positive non-food "treat" activities or physical activity.

Strengthen cues for desirable behaviors. Collect information and guides for a wide array of appropriate food choices and amounts. Use food behavior aids (e.g., records, a diary, or a journal). Distribute appropriate foods in desirable food meal/snack patterns. Make desirable food behavior as attractive and good-tasting as possible.

Next Deal with Actual Food Behavior in Response to Cues

Slow the pace of eating—Take one bite at a time and place utensil on the plate between bites. Chew each bite slowly. Sip a beverage. Consciously plan bits of conversation with meal companions for between bites. Delay starting the meal when first seated. Visualize eating in slow motion. Enhance the social aspect of eating.

Savor the food—Eat slowly, sensing the taste, smell, and texture of the food. Develop and practice these sensory feelings to the extent that they can be described and brought to mind afterward. Look for food seasonings and combinations that will enhance this process and bring to mind positive feelings about the food experience.

Finally Deal with the Follow-Up Behavior that Results

Decelerate the problem behavior. Slow down its frequency, and respond neutrally when it occurs rather than with negative talk or thoughts. Give social reinforcement to the decreasing number of times the problem behavior is occurring. Focus on the ultimate consequences of the undesirable behavior in health problems.

Accelerate the desired behavior. Update the progress records or personal journal daily. Respond positively to all desired behavior; provide some sort of material reinforcement for positive behavior. Provide social reinforcement for all constructive efforts to modify behavior.

Such a program requires effort and motivation and work. Continuously evaluate progress toward desired behavior goals. Then plan individual or group maintenance and support activities during an extended follow-up period.

need supplementation. The ratio of energy nutrients (i.e., carbohydrate, fat, and protein) should have an appropriate balance based on a wide variety of food sources.

4. **Culturally desirable**—The food plan must be similar enough to an individual's cultural eating pattern to form the basis for *permanent* alteration of eating habits. It must be a good, personal lifetime plan.

5. **Kcalorie readjustment to maintain weight**—When the desired weight level is reached, the kcalorie level is adjusted according to maintenance needs. The changed basic habits of eating provide the continuing means of weight control.

Basic Energy-Balance Components

The two sides of energy balance are *energy intake* in the form of food and *energy output* in the form of metabolic work and physical activity. For successful weight reduction, both of these basic components must be changed.

Energy Input: Food Behaviors

The energy value of the food intake must be reduced. To accomplish this, the usual amount of food served and eaten should be noted. Then smaller portions, attractively served, should be used. The food should be eaten *slowly*, and its taste and texture savored. Seasonings such as fat, sugar, and salt should be reduced; and the fiber content increased. A variety of foods should be chosen from a basic food guide, such as the food exchange lists (see Appendix F), in the amounts suggested in Table 15-2. These guides can serve as a focus for sound nutrition education. Whole primary foods should be emphasized, and few processed foods used. Food should be fairly evenly distributed throughout the day. Some practical suggestions are given in the Clinical Applications box, "Practical Suggestions for Changing Food Behaviors."

Energy Output: Exercise Behaviors

Energy output in physical activity must be increased. Plan a regular daily exercise schedule, starting with simple walking for about a half hour each day and building to a brisk pace. Some form of aerobic exercise (e.g., swimming or running) should be added, or a set of body exercises should be developed (see the For Further Focus box, "Benefits of Aerobic Exercise in Weight Management,"). An exercise class may be helpful (Figure 15-3).

Principles of a Sound Food Plan

On the basis of a careful diet history (see Chapter 17), a sound personalized food plan can be developed with the client and should involve each of the following principles of nutritional balance.

Energy Balance

In general, a decrease of 1000 kcalories daily is needed to lose about 2 pounds/week; a decrease of 500 kcalories is needed to lose 1 pound/week (see Table 15-1). An average sound diet for women is about 1200 kcal/day; but for larger women and men, it is about 1500 to 1800 kcal/day. Some persons may wish to determine their general total energy needs as a basis for diet-planning (Table 15-3).

Nutrient Balance

Basic energy nutrients are outlined in the diet to achieve the following nutrient balance:

- *Carbohydrate*—about 55% of the total kcalories, with emphasis on complex forms such as starch with fiber, and a limit on simple sugars
- *Protein*—about 15% of the total kcalories, with emphasis on lean food and small portions
- *Fat*—about 30% of the total kcalories, with emphasis on low animal fats, scant total use, and alternate nonfat seasonings

This nutrient balance approximates the recommendations of the U.S. dietary guidelines for healthy Americans (see Chapter 1). This can serve as a good general guide for long-term habits.

TABLE 15-2   Weight-reduction food plans using the exchange system of dietary control*
(total kilocalorie distribution: 50% carbohydrate, 20% protein, 30% fat)

Food exchange groups	1000 kcal	1200 kcal	1500 kcal	1800 kcal
Total number exchanges/day				
Milk (nonfat)	2	2	2	2
Vegetable	3	3	4	4
Fruit	3	3	4	4
Starch/bread	4	5	7	9
Meat (lean or medium fat)	3	4	5	7
Fat	4	4	5	5
Meal pattern of food exchanges				
Breakfast				
Fruit	1	1	1	1
Meat			1	1
Starch/bread	1	1	2	2
Fat	1	1	1	1
Milk	½	½	½	½
Lunch/supper				
Meat	1	1	1	2
Vegetables	1	1	2	2
Starch/bread	1	2	2	3
Fat	1	1	2	2
Fruit	1	1	1	1
Milk	½	½	½	½
Dinner				
Meat	2	2	2	3
Vegetables	2	2	2	2
Starch/bread	1	1	2	3
Fat	2	2	2	2
Fruit			1	1
Milk	½	½	½	½
Snack (afternoon or evening)				
Milk	½	½	½	½
Meat		1	1	1
Starch/bread	1	1	1	1
Fruit	1	1	1	1

*See food exchange lists in Appendix F.

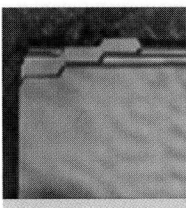

CLINICAL APPLICATIONS

Practical Suggestions for Changing Food Behaviors

Goals

Be realistic. Don't set your goals too high. Adapt your rate of loss to 450 to 900 g (1 to 2 lbs). If visible tools are helpful motivation techniques, use them.

Kilocalories

Don't be an obsessive "calorie counter." Simply become familiar with food exchanges in your diet list and learn the general values of some of your home dishes, then modify recipes or make occasional substitutes.

Plateaus

Anticipate plateaus; they happen to everyone. Plateaus are related to water accumulation as fat is lost. Increase exercise during these periods to help get started again.

Binges

Don't be discouraged when you break down and have a binge—this happens to most persons. Simply keep them infrequent and, when possible, plan ahead for special occasions. Adjust the following day's diet or the remainder of the same day accordingly.

Special Diet Foods

There is no need to purchase special "low-calorie" foods. Learn to read labels carefully. Most special diet foods are expensive foods that are not much lower in kilocalories than regular foods.

Home Meals

Try to avoid making a separate menu for yourself. Adapt your needs to the family meal, adjusting the seasoning or method of preparation to lower kilocalories—especially by reducing or omitting fat.

Eating Away from Home

Watch portions. When you are a guest, limit extras such as sauces and dressings and trim meat well. In restaurants, select singly prepared items rather than combination dishes. Avoid items with heavy sauces or fat seasonings and fried foods. Select fruit or sherbet for dessert rather than pastries.

Appetite Control

Avoid dependence on appetite-depressant medications, which are usually only crutches. Try nibbling on food items from the free food list or save other meal items, such as fruit or bread exchanges, for use between meals.

Meal Pattern

Eat three or more meals a day. If you are used to three meals, then leave it at that. If snacks between meals help you, then plan part of your day's allowance to account for them. The main thing is that you don't take all of your kilocalories at one time. Avoid the all-too-common pattern of no breakfast, little or no lunch, and a huge dinner.

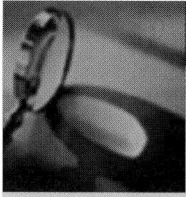

FOR FURTHER FOCUS

Benefits of Aerobic Exercise in Weight Management

The goal of weight management is to reduce excess body fat and, in most cases, to build *lean body mass (LBM)*. Both tissues are lost, however, when a person tries to reach a weight goal merely by reducing food intake.

Optimal body composition can be achieved by combining food restriction with aerobic exercise. Aerobic exercise consists of activities that are sustained long enough to draw on the body's fat reserve for fuel while oxygen intake is increased (thus the name *aerobic*). Lean body tissue burns fats in the presence of oxygen. Therefore aerobic activity is best suited for achieving the ideal balance of high LBM and low fatty tissue in the body.

The benefits of aerobic exercise to an overweight person in a weight-management program include the following:

- Lowered genetic setting for body fat
- Suppressed appetite
- Reduced total body fat
- Higher basal metabolic rate
- Increased circulatory and respiratory function
- Increased energy expenditure
- Retention of tissue protein and building of LBM levels

Sometimes persons complain about the slow rate of weight loss, the difficulty in controlling appetite, and the consistent "flabbiness" despite continuing diet management. These persons may welcome the suggestion of aerobic activity to help meet these needs. A brisk daily walk, jumping rope, swimming, bicycling, jogging, running, or some other activity may be sustained long enough for it to have an aerobic effect. Carefully note the physical stress this activity may place on individuals who have not exercised for some time or have medical problems related to exertion. These persons should have a medical checkup before beginning such a program on their own or joining a local gymnasium or other community fitness center.

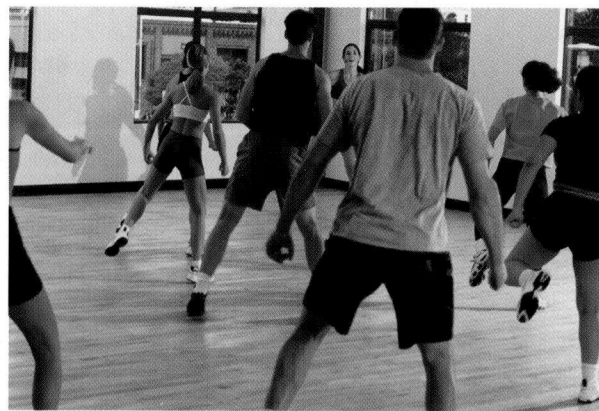

FIGURE 15-3 An exercise class provides regular support for an effective weight-management plan. (Credit: PhotoDisc.)

TABLE 15-3   General approximations for daily adult basal and activity energy needs

Daily energy needs (basis for calculations)		Male (70 kg) kcal	Female (58 kg) kcal
Basal energy needs			
1 kcal/kg/hr		70 kg × 24 hr = 1680	58 kg × 24 hr = 1392
Activity energy needs			
Sedentary	+20% basal	1680 + 336 = 2016	1392 + 278 = 1670
Very light	+30% basal	1680 + 504 = 2484	1392 + 418 = 1810
Moderate	+40% basal	1680 + 672 = 2352	1392 + 557 = 1949
Heavy	+50% basal	1680 + 840 = 2520	1392 + 696 = 2088

Distribution Balance

Spread the food fairly evenly through the day to meet energy needs. If you have certain "problem times" of the day, plan simple snacks for those periods.

Food Guide

The revised food exchange lists (Appendix F) follow the general U.S. dietary guidelines for healthy Americans. Table 15-2 provides some examples of basic food plans for weight reduction. This basic food exchange system is a good general reference guide for comparative food values and portions, variety in food choices, and basic meal planning. Alternatively, a simpler plan can be outlined using the basic food groups of the Food Guide Pyramid (see Chapter 1). With either plan, food items can be combined into desired dishes. Alternate nonfat seasonings (e.g., herbs, spices, onion, garlic, lemon and lime juice, vinegar, wine, broth, mustard, and other condiments) can be used.

Preventive Approach

The most positive work with weight management seems aimed at *prevention*. Current studies indicate that the U.S. population of children and adolescents are getting fatter, and the fatter members are becoming more obese, with a major culprit being lack of exercise—mainly from hours of television viewing. Support for young parents and children before an obese condition develops will help prevent many problems later in adulthood. This support and guidance should include early nutrition counseling and education, helping to build positive health habits—especially in positive eating behaviors and increased exercise behaviors of active play and physical activities.

THE PROBLEM OF UNDERWEIGHT

General Causes and Treatment

Extremes in underweight, just as in overweight, can bring serious health problems. Although general underweight is a less common problem in the U.S. population than overweight, it does occur and is usually associated with poor living conditions or long-term disease. A person who is more than 10% below the average weight for height and age is considered underweight; and being at least 20% below the average is cause for concern. Serious results may occur in these persons, especially young children. Their resistance to infection is lowered, general health is poor, and strength is reduced.

Causes

Underweight is associated with conditions that cause general malnutrition, including the following:

- **Wasting disease**—Long-term wasting disease with chronic infection and fever that raise the basal metabolic rate (BMR).

- **Poor food intake**—Diminished food intake resulting from (1) psychologic factors that cause a person to refuse to eat, (2) loss of appetite, or (3) personal poverty and limited available food supply.
- **Malabsorption**—Poor nutrient absorption resulting from (1) long-lasting diarrhea, (2) a diseased gastrointestinal tract, or (3) excessive use of laxatives.
- **Hormonal imbalance**—Hyperthyroidism or any other abnormalities may increase the caloric needs of the body.
- **Energy imbalance**—This can result from greatly increased physical activity without a corresponding increase in food.
- **Poor living situation**—An unhealthy home environment can result in irregular and inadequate meals, where eating is considered unimportant and an indifferent attitude toward food exists.

Dietary Treatment

Underweight persons require special nutritional care to rebuild their body tissues and regain their health. Any food plan needs to be adapted to each person's unique situation—whether it involves personal needs, living situation, economic needs, and/or any underlying disease. The dietary goal, according to each person's tolerance, is to increase both

energy and nutrient intake, with adherence to the following needs:

- **High-caloric diet,** at least 50% above the standard requirement.
- **High protein,** to rebuild tissues.
- **High carbohydrate,** to provide the primary energy source in an easily digested form.
- **Moderate fat,** to add kcalories without exceeding tolerance limits.
- **Good sources of vitamins and minerals,** including supplements when individual deficiencies require them.

A variety of food attractively served helps to revive the appetite and increase the desire to eat more. Nourishing meals and snacks should be spread through the day and often include favorite foods. A basic aim is to help build good food habits, so that improved nutritional status and weight can be maintained once they are regained. Residents in long-term care facilities are especially vulnerable to weight-loss problems and have special needs (see Clinical Applications box, "Problems of Weight Loss Among Older Adults in Long-Term Care Facilities"). This rehabilitation process requires creative counseling of each individual and family, along with practical guides and support. In some cases, tube feeding or vein feeding (i.e., total parenteral nutrition [TPN]) may be necessary (see Chapters 22 and 23).

anorexia nervosa (Gr. *an-*, negative prefix; *orexis*, appetite) extreme psychophysiologic aversion to food resulting in life-threatening weight loss. A psychiatric eating disorder resulting from a morbid fear of fatness in which a person's distorted body image is reflected as fat when the body is actually malnourished and extremely thin from self-starvation.

bulimia nervosa (L. *bous*, ox; *limos*, hunger) a psychiatric eating disorder related to a person's fear of fatness, in which cycles of gorging on large quantities of food are followed by self-induced vomiting and use of diuretics and laxatives to maintain a "normal" body weight

Extreme, Self-Imposed Eating Disorders

Sometimes family and personal tensions, as well as social pressures, for thinness cause adolescent girls—some even starting in grade school—and young women to develop serious body image and eating problems that may become psychiatric disorders. No matter what they weigh, these women always see themselves as fat and develop a deep-seated fear of food and fatness. Two forms of these extreme eating disorders are anorexia nervosa and bulimia nervosa. A third less extreme disorder, *compulsive overeating,* is fueled by our cultural drive for thinness and the

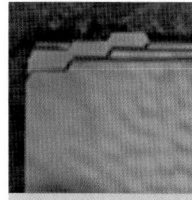

CLINICAL APPLICATIONS

Problems of Weight Loss Among Older Adults in Long-Term Care Facilities

The American population of older adults age 65 and above is rapidly increasing. In the year 2000, this older population numbers over 36 million. The most rapid population increase over the next decade will be among those over 85 years of age. Many of these elderly persons will require long-term care in nursing homes.

One of the problems encountered with these elderly residents is low body weight and rapid unintentional weight loss. These can become serious health problems and are a sensitive indicator of malnutrition, contributing to illness and death. Because weight loss is such a strong predictor of morbidity and mortality in clinical settings, early and continuing observation to assess needs is important—especially in relation to factors that contribute to weight loss.

In general, the weight loss can be caused by physical effects related to the metabolic changes of aging or disease or by factors that alter the amount and type of food eaten. Physical disease such as cancer can cause extreme weight loss from metabolic abnormalities, taste changes and loss of appetite, and nausea and vomiting. Other diseases underlying weight loss may be gastrointestinal problems, uncontrolled diabetes, and cardiovascular disorders such as congestive heart failure, pulmonary disease, infection, or alcoholism. Psychologic factors or psychiatric disorders may also contribute to malnutrition and weight loss through depression, memory loss, disorientation, apathy, or appetite disturbance. Some altered mental states may be caused by nutritional deficiencies, such as low levels of folate and B-complex vitamins, as well

as by protein-calorie malnutrition. These conditions can be corrected with specific nutritional support.

The following additional physiologic, psychologic, and social factors may influence food intake and body weight and contribute to malnutrition in elderly persons:

Body composition changes—Height and body weight gradually decline. Body weight peaks between the ages of 34 and 54 in men and 55 and 65 in women, decreasing thereafter. Body fat losses are generally not significant. The greatest cause of weight loss is a decline in body water, due in part to weakening of the normal thirst mechanism. Therefore a feeling of thirst cannot be depended on to secure adequate water intake, so water must frequently be offered and encouraged. More constant attention to fluid intake also helps with the common problem of *xerostomia* (dry mouth) in older adults, which is due to inadequate salivary secretions to help with eating, thus contributing to malnutrition. Lean body mass also declines with age, resulting in a lower basal metabolic rate, and decreased physical activity and energy requirements. Thus any possible increase in physical activity and use of nutrient-dense foods is encouraged.

Taste changes—Regeneration of taste cells slows with age, but the extent and effect on food intake varies widely. The sense of smell also declines with age and may affect taste. Increased use of appropriate seasoning and flavoring in food preparation is needed.

Dentition—About 50% of all Americans have lost their teeth by the age of 65. Many have

Continued

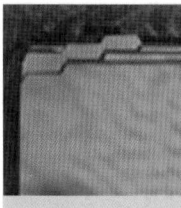

CLINICAL APPLICATIONS
Problems of Weight Loss Among Older Adults in Long-Term Care Facilities—cont'd

dentures, but chewing problems are often present. About half of the nursing home populations studied report chewing, biting, and swallowing problems that interfere with eating and adequate food intake. Assessment of specific need and dental care solutions help correct eating problems.

Gastrointestinal problems—Delayed gastric emptying may contribute to distention and lack of appetite. A decrease in gastric secretions, including hydrochloric acid, may hinder absorption of vitamin B_{12}, folate, and iron, thus contributing to anemia and loss of appetite. Constipation is a common complaint, often leading to laxative abuse and resulting in interference with nutrient absorption from chronic diarrhea. Increase in dietary fiber and liquids can help provide a more natural approach to establishing normal bowel action.

Drug/nutrient interactions—Elderly persons often take a number of prescribed and over-the-counter drugs, some of which are a direct cause of anorexia, nausea, and vomiting. Other drugs are indirect causes by inducing nutrient malabsorption, leading to deficiencies that in turn bring anorexia and weight loss. Drug therapy for elderly patients should have constant medical, nutritional, and nursing monitoring to provide for appropriate use.

Functional disabilities—Eating problems can prevent or alter the capacity of elderly persons to take in sufficient food. These problems may vary from more difficult functional disabilities that interfere with putting food into the mouth and swallowing (i.e., problems that often require a trained therapist) to dependence on feeding assistance that can be provided by sensitive nursing care.

Social problems—Socioeconomic problems are often involved with care of the elderly. For example, a specially trained geriatric social worker can help work out possible sources of financial assistance. A sense of social isolation can also lead to decreased food intake. Family support is necessary, as well as sensitive contacts with nursing home staff and residents and as much involvement as possible in group activities.

Health workers in geriatric settings need continuing education and sensitization to the potential dangers of low body weight and weight loss. Aged persons with acute and chronic illnesses and functional disabilities are at the greatest risk for nutrition-related problems. These persons need continuing nutrition assessment and monitoring of body weight. Some of the restrictions of "special diets" should be relaxed or discontinued when risk of malnutrition is evident, with the goal of increasing nutrient intake and making eating as enjoyable as possible.

resulting chronic dieting syndrome and may sow the seeds of more dangerous extreme disorders.

Anorexia Nervosa
This complex psychologic problem results in self-imposed starvation. A young girl who is usually a high achiever constantly pushing herself toward perfection sees food and her body as things that she can control. Her distorted body image—she sees herself as fat even when she is really emaciated (Figure 15-4)—keeps her in a state of near panic. She plans her days around ways of avoiding food, which becomes a full-time obsession and she grows more depressed, irritable, and anxious.

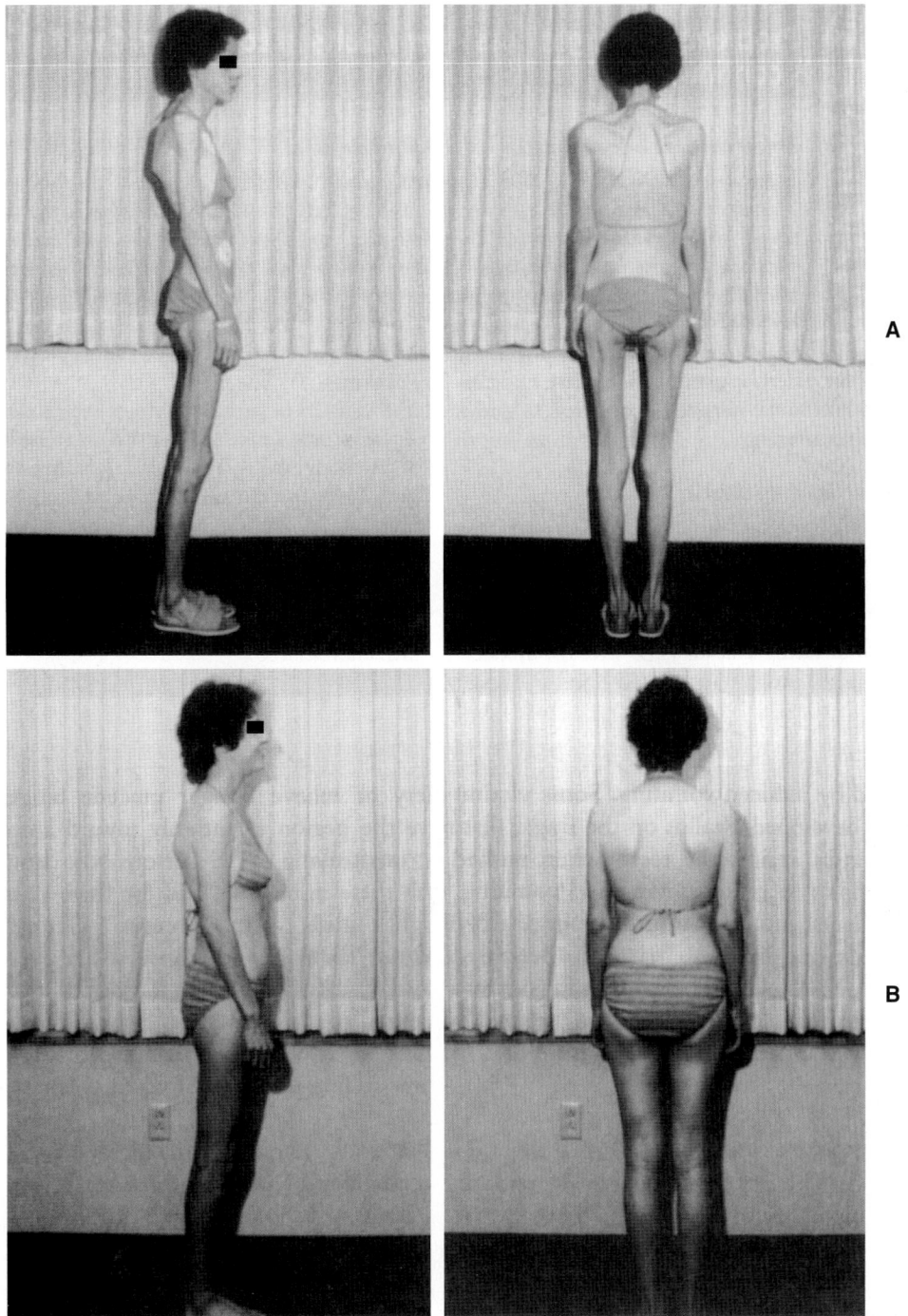

FIGURE 15-4   **A,** Anorectic woman before treatment. **B,** Same patient after gradual refeeding, nutritional management, and psychologic therapy. (Courtesy Sycamore Hospital, a division of Kettering Medical Center, Dayton, Ohio.)

Bulimia Nervosa

In a sense, a bulimic is a "failed anorexic." The young woman with bulimia nervosa also suffers from similar obsessions about her body and food. She also learns, however, that she can control her food and weight by *binge-purge* cycles. Compulsive binging on huge amounts of food is followed by induced vomiting. Some victims have even developed a callus on the finger that regularly rubs against the teeth when pushed into the throat to cause gagging and vomiting. Oral and dental problems from the purging behavior include oral mucosal irritation, decreased salivary secretions and dry mouth (xerostomia), and irreversible enamel erosion. Many bulimics also use laxatives and diuretics to "purge" their bodies further.

Compulsive Overeating

This eating disorder includes binging episodes without the purging behavior of bulimics. This reactive type of eating follows some stress or anxiety as an emotional eating pattern to soothe or relieve painful feelings. The binges may be triggered by psychologic factors involving self and body image, with unrealistic weight goals. Dietary restriction and failure to achieve satiety or relieve hunger precede binges and relentlessly drive individuals toward a continuous, unsatisfying cycle. Persons who attempt to reach these unrealistic—and (for them) unnatural—weight goals are "forever dieting" (i.e., chronic dieting syndrome). After each weight loss, rebound eating occurs, followed by more attempts to lose weight. Thus the weight cycling—with its physiologic effects compounding the psychologic problem—begins.

Treatment

These psychologic disorders require therapy from a team of skilled professionals, including physicians, psychologists, and nutritionists. Even with the best of care, recovery is slow—a day at a time—and the word *cure* is not often used. Continuing support groups are important, and national organizations provide resources.

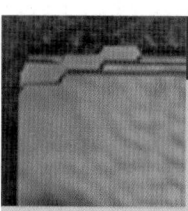

CLINICAL APPLICATIONS

CASE STUDY: John's Energy-Balance and Weight-Management Plan

John is a college student leading a more or less sedentary life because of classes and study. He is interested in wrestling, however, and wants very much to make the team. To do so, he must lose some excess weight.

John begins to look carefully at his energy-balance picture. His weight is 180 pounds, and his average food intake each day is approximately 3000 kcal. Next he plans a means of losing weight by reversing his energy balance.

Questions for Analysis

1. What does John decide his present daily total energy (kcalories) must be?
2. How does this total energy need compare with his food-energy intake?
3. To lose about 2 pounds/week, how much should he reduce the caloric value of his daily diet?
4. Besides reducing his diet kcalories, what else could John do to help reverse his energy balance and improve his body condition?

SUMMARY

In the traditional medical model, obesity has been viewed as an illness and a health hazard—which is true in cases of extreme or morbid obesity. Newer approaches view moderate overweight differently, however, in terms of the important aspect of fatness and leanness or body composition and propose a more person-centered positive health model (see Clinical Applications box, "Case Study: John's Energy-Balance and Weight-Management Plan").

The American obsession with thinness has created new weight-management problems: eating disorders that result in self-starvation. These psychologic disorders require professional team therapy, including medical, psychologic, and nutritional care.

Planning a weight-management program, either for an overweight or underweight person, must involve the metabolic and energy needs of the individual. Personal food choices and habits, as well as fatty tissue needs during different stages of the life cycle, must be considered. Important aspects of such a weight-reduction program include changing food behaviors and increasing physical activity. A sound program is based on reduced kcalories for gradual weight loss and nutrient balance to meet the health standards of the U.S. dietary goals, with meals distributed throughout the day for energy needs. The ideal plan begins with prevention, stressing the formation of positive food habits in early childhood to prevent major problems later in life.

REVIEW QUESTIONS

1. Why is the term *ideal weight* difficult to define? Explain some of the problems in determining this measure. What role does it play in weight management?
2. What does *set-point* mean in relation to individual weight? How does it relate to diet and exercise in a personal weight-management program?
3. Describe the components of a positive health model for weight management. What are the basic principles of a sound food plan for such a program?
4. Describe factors influencing the development of an underweight malnourished condition. Explain the dietary treatment required.
5. Describe the two major eating disorders associated with a growing obsession with thinness. What are the contributing social and psychologic factors? What is the treatment? How does the chronic dieting syndrome relate?

SELF-TEST QUESTIONS

True-False
Write the correct statement for each item you answer "false."

1. Development of childhood obesity results from genetics and family food practices that produce a decreased ratio of fat cells to lean cells.
2. Decreasing the energy expended in physical activity is a means of weight control.
3. During adolescence, boys usually have a higher deposit of subcutaneous fat tissue than girls.

4. A reasonable weight-reduction diet for an adult has an energy value of about 1200 to 1500 kcal, depending on individual size and need.

5. A weight-reduction diet should not use between-meal snacks.

Multiple Choice

1. Overweight is a direct risk factor in which of the following conditions (circle all that apply)?
   a. Surgery
   b. Type 2 diabetes mellitus
   c. Liver disease
   d. Hypertension

2. A reduction of 1000 kcal in the daily diet of an obese person would enable him or her to lose weight at which of the following rates?
   a. 1 lb/wk
   b. 2 lb/wk
   c. 3 lb/wk
   d. 4 lb/wk

3. Which two of the following portions of food have the lowest caloric value and may be used as necessary in a weight-control diet (circle all that apply)?
   a. Lean meat, 4 oz dinner portion
   b. Medium-sized baked potato
   c. 1 slice of bread
   d. 1 glass (8 oz) of whole milk

SUGGESTIONS FOR ADDITIONAL STUDY

1. Individual Project: Personal Energy Balance
Determine your own personal energy balance by making the following comparison between your energy output or requirements and your energy intake in food.

Energy output
- Record your weight in pounds and convert it to kilograms.
- Calculate your approximate basal energy needs.
- Estimate your general activity level (see Table 15-3) and calculate your approximate activity energy needs.
- What is your approximate total energy-output need in kcalories?
- Do you need more energy for physical activity or basal metabolism? Does this answer surprise you?

Energy intake
- Record your usual food intake for 1 day. Be sure to list portion sizes and method of seasoning and preparation.
- Use the food value tables in Appendix A to calculate the total approximate caloric value of your day's food.

- Compare your total energy input (food) with your total energy output (energy needs).

What is your present state of energy balance? Compare your present body weight with the standard weight-height tables inside the front cover of the book and with the tables given in Table 15-1. By your calculated state of energy balance, where do you stand? What plan do you suggest to maintain or change your present energy balance?

2. Weight-Control Products and Programs
Organize project groups in your class. Assign several group members to visit various pharmacies, markets, and health food stores to survey products advertised for weight control. Read the labels carefully. Evaluate the claims made by each product. Check the costs. Talk with the clerk about each product's value. Ask questions such as "Do you think this would help me lose weight?", "How does it work?", and "Do you sell many of these items?" Note any customers' reactions. Check any diet books displayed and, if possible, purchase a few for class evaluation.

Assign other group members to investigate various community weight-control programs. If possible, interview someone working for the program and someone participating in it. Compare individual responses and attitudes. How do the programs operate and what do they cost? Have a follow-up discussion of all your findings in class. Compare the products and programs investigated and evaluate them in terms of the principles of sound weight reduction you have learned.

REFERENCES

1. Expert Panel on the Identification, Evaluation, and Treatment of Overweight in Adults: Clinical guidelines on the Identification, Evaluation, and Treatment of Overweight and Obesity in Adults, *Am J Clin Nutr* 68(5):899, 1998.
2. Flegal KM: Trends in body weight in the U.S. population, *Nutr Rev* 54(4):S97, 1996.
3. Expert Panel on the Identification, Evaluation, and Treatment of Overweight and Obesity in Adults: Clinical Guidelines on the identification, evaluation, and treatment of overweight and obesity in adults: executive summary, *Am J Clin Nutr* 98(6):8, 1998.
4. Zhang Y and others: Positional cloning of the mouse *obese* gene and the human homologue, *Nature* 372(6505):425, 1994.
5. Halaas JL and others: Weight-reducing effects of the plasma protein encoded by the *obese* gene, *Science* 269(5223):540, 1995.
6. Barinaga M: Obesity: leptin receptor weighs in, *Science* 271(5245):29, 1996.
7. Wolf G: The weight-reducing plasma protein encoded by the obese gene, *Nutr Rev* 54(3):91, 1996.
8. Couzin J: Hormone research: leptin's uncertain promise, *U.S. News & World Report* 127(18):84, 8 Nov 1999.
9. Schultz S: Health: news you can use, why we're fat: gender and age matter more than you may realize, *U.S. News & World Report* 127(18):82, 8 Nov 1999.
10. Gura T: Obesity research: leptin not impressive in clinical trial, *Science* 286(5441):881, 29 Oct 1999.
11. Fox CS and others: Is a low leptin concentration, a low resting metabolic rate, or both the expression of the "thrifty genotype"? Results from the Pima Indians, *Am J Clin Nutr* 68(10):1053, 1998.
12. Montague CT and others: Congenital leptin deficiency is associated with severe early onset obesity in humans, *Nature* 387(5):903, 1997.
13. Hill JO, Peters JC: Environmental contributions to the obesity epidemic, *Science* 280(11):1371, 1998.
14. Fischman J: Cutting kids' weight: family meals, not TV dinners, *U.S. News & World Report* 236(5441):881, 1999.
15. Evans WJ, Cyr-Campbell D: Nutrition, exercise, and healthy aging, *J Am Diet Assoc* 97(5):632, 1997.
16. Jensen W, Rogers J: Obesity in older persons, *J Am Diet Assoc* 98(11):1308, 1998.
17. Schwartz MW, Seeley RJ: The new biology of body weight regulation, *J Am Diet Assoc* 97(1):54, 1997.
18. Mulrine A: Beyond fen-phen: the scramble to develop a miracle drug, *U.S. News & World Report*, 15 Feb 1999.
19. Editor, Controversies: Should drugs be used in the treatment of obesity?, *Am J Clin Nutr* 67(1):1, 1998.

FURTHER READING

- Nonas CA: A model for chronic care of obesity through dietary treatment, *J Am Diet Assoc* 98(10, suppl 2):S16, 1998.
- Aronne LJ: Modern medical management of obesity: the role of pharmaceutical intervention, *J Am Diet Assoc* 98(10, suppl 2):S23, 1998.
- Foreyt JP: The role of the behavioral counselor in obesity treatment, *J Am Diet Assoc* 98(10, suppl 2):S27, 1998.
- Rippe JM, Hess S: The role of physical activity in the prevention and management of obesity, *J Am Diet Assoc* 98(10, suppl 2):S31, 1998.
- Frank A: The multidisciplinary approach to obesity management: the physician's role and team care alternatives, *J Am Diet Assoc* 98(10, suppl 2):S44, 1998.
- Rippe JM and others: Panel discussion: the obesity epidemic—a mandate for a multidisciplinary approach, *J Am Diet Assoc* 98(10, suppl 2):S55. 1998.

This series of articles from a recent meeting of physicians, dietitians, behaviorists, and pharmacists provides a wealth of information about the team roles in helping people maintain a healthy weight. Nurses relate to each of these specialists in being closest to the person in need of help to reach and maintain a healthy weight.

First, read and discuss the first and final reports in the series—the dietitian's overall fundamental dietary treatment and summary panel—to get a basic overview. Then as interest and time permit, review the related roles of medical management, behavioral counselor, physical activity, and role of the pharmacist as needed. The final report of the full panel discussions and interactions sums up the importance of weight management in relation to other chronic diseases such as diabetes, cardiovascular disease, and hypertension and the team approach to the difficult problem of personal weight management.

16

Nutrition and Physical Fitness

KEY CONCEPTS

- Healthy muscle structure and function depend on appropriate energy fuels and tissue-building material, as well as oxygen and water.

- Different levels of physical activity and athletic performance draw on different body fuel sources.

- A sedentary lifestyle contributes to health problems.

- A healthy personal exercise program combines both general and aerobic activities.

Public interest in physical fitness has been growing recently, sparked by the modern approach of preventive medicine and positive health promotion. This approach has been stimulated by the effort to prevent or control various chronic diseases in our aging population.

In this chapter, we see that nutrition and physical fitness are essential interrelated parts of positive health promotion. Both reduce risks associated with chronic diseases, and both are important therapies in dealing with already developed chronic conditions. We need to provide our clients and patients with sound guidelines for physical fitness for use with both recreational desires and health demands. We must also practice these sound guidelines ourselves.

PHYSICAL ACTIVITY AND ENERGY SOURCES

The Growing Physical Fitness Movement

Americans are generally active people. In 1997, 60% of American adults engaged in some form of leisure-time physical activity, and 64% of adolescents engaged in vigorous physical activity three or more times per week. In the same year, however, only 15% of adults followed the national recommendation of 30 minutes of moderate physical activity five or more times per week.[1] Physical fitness is no longer just a fad or a trend, but increased participation in regular physical activity remains a national health goal. In its new report, *Healthy People 2010: Understanding and Improving Health,* the U.S. Department of Health and Human Services has set health-related goals for Americans in nutrition and physical fitness to be reached by the year 2010. The 2010 target for participation in regular moderate-to-vigorous physical activity is for 30% of adults and 85% of adolescents.[1]

The health benefits of physical activity are not reserved just for athletes.[2,3] In a personally planned program to meet individual needs, any person can develop a healthy lifestyle. The longer people follow some form of regular exercise, the more committed they become.[4,5] The new fashion for walking and "soft" workouts has enabled more people to participate (e.g., those who cannot enter marathons or do "go-for-the-burn" aerobics). Many of these persons are older adults who have health problems that moderate exercise helps control.[3] They find that regular exercise not only helps their health problem but also helps them feel more in control of their lives.

Muscle Action and Body Fuels

Muscle Structure and Function

Millions of special cells and fibers make up our skeletal muscle mass. These coordinated structures make all of our physical activity possible. They are stimulated and controlled by nerve end-ings to produce smooth muscle contraction and relaxation.

Fuel Sources

All of this action requires fuel to burn for energy. These fuel sources are our basic energy nutrients (i.e., primarily carbohydrate and some fat). Their metabolic products—glucose, glycogen, and fatty acids—provide ready fuels for immediate, short-term, and long-term energy needs. A good diet to meet these needs is essential, whatever the level of physical activity.

Fluids and Oxygen

Fluids

More water is necessary—but often overlooked—for increased activity and exercise.[6] With continued exercise, the body temperature rises due to the release of heat as part of the energy produced. To control this temperature rise, the body sends as much heat as possible to the skin, where it is released in sweat. Over time, and especially in hot weather, this excessive sweating can lead to *dehydration,* which is a serious complication. To prevent dehydration, water must be replaced more frequently.[5,6] Athletes who are engaged in longer and more demanding endurance events—especially in a warm environment, however, may use one of the newer, mild saline and glucose (6% solution) sports drinks that have rapid gastric emptying and intestinal absorption times.[7]

Oxygen

The constant supply of oxygen necessary for life becomes all the more important during exercise. A person's ability to deliver this vital oxygen to the tissues for energy production determines how much exercise can be done. This aerobic capacity depends on two basic factors, as follow: (1) the fitness of the lungs, heart, and blood vessels; and (2) the body composition.

Body fitness. Physical fitness may be defined in terms of aerobic capacity, which is the body's ability to deliver and use oxygen in sufficient quantities to meet the demands of increasing levels of exercise. Aerobic capacity varies with body size, so it is measured by amount of oxygen consumed per kilogram of body weight per minute. The lungs, heart, and blood vessels deliver this necessary oxygen to the cells, so their fitness is essential.

Body composition.   Body tissues that use more oxygen make up the *lean body mass*, which is mainly muscle mass. These tissues are the active metabolic tissues of the body. A person's aerobic capacity depends on the percentage of body fat and lean body mass. Body composition is determined by the relative amounts of these two components of body weight.

DIET AND EXERCISE
General Nutrient Needs

Nutrient Stores
For athletes, as well as for active persons, proper diet choices are essential for the winning performance, daily energy needs, and nutrient reserves.[6] When nutrient reserves become depleted during continuous exercise, the body burns its fuel stores to meet increasing energy demands and requires replenishing. With prolonged exercise, nutrient levels fall too low to sustain the body's continued demands. Fatigue follows, and exhaustion may result. Carbohydrate and fat are basic fuels to maintain these energy reserves; very little energy is drawn from protein. These general needs apply to all individuals, although children have special growth needs.[8]

Carbohydrate
The major nutrient for energy support in exercise is carbohydrate. The carbohydrate body-energy reserve comes from the following two sources: (1) circulating *blood glucose*, and (2) *glycogen* stored in muscle cells and the liver. Thus for active persons, carbohydrate should contribute about 60% to 65% of the daily diet's kcalories. Athletes competing in prolonged endurance events will need more (i.e., 65% to 70%) energy from carbohydrate.[7] Complex carbohydrates, or starches, are preferred to simple sugars. On the whole, more complex starches break down more slowly and help maintain blood sugar levels more evenly, avoiding low blood sugar drops. Starches are also more readily converted to glycogen to maintain this store of constant primary fuel.

Simple sugars, on the other hand, are less efficient at maintaining the body's glycogen stores and are mainly converted to fat and stored as such. Simple sugars also trigger a sharper insulin response, contributing to the dangers of follow-up hypoglycemia. Many studies have shown that low-carbohydrate diets hinder exercise performance. Athletes especially experience fatigue, dehydration, and hypoglycemia. Well-conditioned athletes sometimes use a glycogen-loading procedure to build up glycogen stores for endurance events of 1 hour or more. In addition, complex carbohydrates supply needed fiber, vitamins, and minerals.

Fat
In the presence of oxygen, *fatty acids* serve as a fuel source from stored fat tissue. Note that fat as a fuel source is not drawn from the diet directly but from body fat stores. There is no basis for increased levels of fat in the diet. There is a need for some dietary fat, however, to supply *linoleic acid*, the body's essential fatty acid. Although some fat is necessary in the diet of an active person, a moderate amount is sufficient. The total fat should not exceed about 25% to 30% of the diet's total daily kcalories.

---

aerobic capacity (Gr. *aer,* air or gas) requiring oxygen to proceed. Milliliters of oxygen consumed per kilogram of body weight per minute, as influenced by body composition.

hypoglycemia (Gr. *hypo,* under; *glykys,* sweet; *haima,* blood) an abnormally low blood sugar level that may lead to muscle tremors, cold sweat, headache, and confusion.

Protein

Some amino acid breakdown may occur during exercise, but protein is usually discounted as a fuel source because it makes an insignificant contribution to energy. No more than the usual adult requirement is needed to meet general needs during exercise, which amount to about 10% to 15% of the total day's kcalories from protein. Most Americans actually eat about twice this amount and put a taxing load on the kidneys, which can contribute to dehydration because the excess nitrogen must be excreted. High-protein diets can also lead to increased calcium loss in the urine.

Vitamins and Minerals

Vitamins and minerals cannot be used as fuel. They are not oxidized or used up in the energy production process. They are essential in this process but only as co-enzyme partners (see Chapter 6). Increased exercise does not require increased vita-

TABLE 16-1 Approximate energy expenditure per hour for an adult weighing 70 kg (154 pounds) and performing different activities

Activity	Kcalories per hour
Sleeping	65
Lying still, awake	75
Sitting at rest	100
Standing relaxed	105
Dressing and undressing	120
Rapid typing	140
Light exercise	170
Walking slowly (2.5 mph)	200
Active exercise	290
Intensive exercise	450
Swimming	500
Running (5.5 mph)	580
Very intense exercise	600
Walking very fast (5.2 mph)	640
Walking up stairs	1110

mins or minerals. Exercise generally increases the body's efficient use of vitamins and minerals. Because athletes require more energy, their larger intake of good food also increases their dietary intake of vitamins and minerals. Female and adolescent athletes, however, need to focus special attention on iron and may require therapeutic iron supplements if the levels of iron in their blood are consistently low.

Exercise and Energy

Kilocalories

Physical activity requires kcalories. Table 16-1 gives some examples of the amount of kcalories expended in general activities. (See also Table 15-3 for a comparison of the energy expenditure of a very active person with that of an inactive person.) Exercise raises the kcalorie need and helps regulate appetite to meet these needs. Persons at moderate exercise levels have actually been shown to eat less than inactive persons. Exercise is the only way to regulate an individual's internal genetic *set-point*, regulating how much body fat the person will carry naturally (see Chapter 15). This body-fat point is raised (i.e., more body fat is stored) when the susceptible individual becomes inactive. This point is lowered when the person exercises regularly.

Nutrient Ratios

Active persons, even athletes, require no more protein or fat than inactive persons. Carbohydrate is the preferred fuel and is the critical food for the active person—not only prior to an exercise period but also during the recovery period afterward. The complex carbohydrate forms (i.e., starches) not only sustain energy needs but also supply added fiber, vitamins, and minerals. Thus the recommended ratio of energy nutrients to support physical activity may be summarized as follows:

- *Carbohydrate*: 55% to 60% of total kcalories
- *Fat*: 25% to 30% of total kcalories
- *Protein*: 10% to 15% of total kcalories

Athletic Performance

Misinformation

Athletes and their coaches are particularly susceptible to magic claims and myths about foods and dietary supplements. All athletes, particularly those involved in very competitive sports, constantly search for the competitive edge. Knowing this, manufacturers sometimes make distorted or false claims for products. In addition, the world of athletics holds numerous superstitions and myths about food and nutrients, as follow:

- Athletes need protein for extra energy.
- Extra protein builds bigger and stronger muscles.
- Muscle tissue breaks down during exercise, and protein supplements are needed to replace it.
- Vitamin supplements enable athletes to use more energy.
- Vitamins and minerals are burned up in workouts and training sessions.
- Electrolyte solutions are important during exercise to replace sweat loss.
- A pregame meal of steak and eggs ensures maximum performance.
- Sugar is needed before and during performance to maintain energy levels.
- Drinking water during exercise will produce cramps.

General Training Diet

Anyone who exercises regularly, especially athletes in training, needs to apply the general principles of exercise and energy described in the previous discussion.

Carbohydrate.   Moderate to high amounts, about 55% to 70% of total kcalories, are needed. Endurance athletes need the higher value, with 500 to 600 g/day of carbohydrate.[6,8] Compare these values with the typical American diet of 46% of the total kcalories from carbohydrate.

Fat.   Moderate to low amounts, about 15% to 30% of the total kcalories are needed. Compare these values with the typical American diet of 38% to 40% of the total kcalories from fat.

Protein.   Potein should comprise the remainder of the diet, in moderate amounts (e.g., about 15% to 30%).

Total energy.   Athletes need varying amounts of energy, depending on body size and the type of training or competition involved. A small person may need only about 1800 kcal/day to sustain body weight and normal daily activities, whereas a larger, muscular man may need about 3000. Consider these different basic needs and add the additional energy needed for a given sport training. For example, endurance bicycle races in mountain areas may require an additional 4000 kcal/day. Thus some athletes in training may require as many as 7000 kcal/day just to maintain weight. Others may only need 1800 kcal/day at most.[3,6] A well-planned individual program is necessary.

Athletes should consume a variety of foods. The food groups of the Food Guide Pyramid (see Chapter 1) may serve as a simple guide, with relative increases in amounts as needed. Many choices and portions from the starch and fruit groups will replace glycogen losses from the previous day's workouts and provide adequate glycogen stores in the muscles. Box 16-1 gives carbohydrate values for selected foods to use in planning an athlete's low-fat, moderate-protein, high-carbohydrate diet to include 500 to 600 g carbohydrate each day.

Competition: Glycogen Loading

To prepare for an athletic event, especially an endurance event, athletes usually follow a dietary process called *glycogen loading* (see For Further Focus box, "Carbohydrate Loading for Endurance"). The current practice, which has been modified from earlier more stressful plans and takes place the week before the event, is a moderate, gradual

BOX 16-1 Grams of Carbohydrate in One Serving of Common Foods

Carbohydrate Group

STARCHES

Bread; Cereals and Grains; Starchy Vegetables; Crackers and Snacks; Beans, Peas, and Lentils; Starchy Foods Prepared With Fat

One serving contains **15 grams of carbohydrate.**

One serving is:

½ cup bran cereals

¼ cup Grape-Nuts

1½ cups puffed cereal

½ cup grits

⅓ cup rice, white or brown

½ cup bulgur

½ cup pasta

⅓ cup baked beans

½ cup corn

½ cup beans and peas (garbanzo, pinto, kidney, white, split, black-eyed)

½ cup lentils

⅔ cup lima beans

½ cup geen peas

1 cup winter squash (acorn, butternut, pumpkin)

½ cup yam, sweet potato, plain

1 small (3 oz) potato, baked or boiled

16-25 (3 oz) French-fried potatoes

½ (1 oz) bagel

1 (1½ oz) small muffin

½ English muffin

1 slice (1 oz) bread, white, whole-wheat, pumpernickel, rye

½ (1 oz) hot dog or hamburger bun

¾ oz pretzels

6 Saltine-type crackers

1 waffle, 4½-in square

2 pancakes, 4-in across

2 taco shells, 6-in across

1 tortilla, corn, 6-in across

1 tortilla, flour, 6-in across

1 biscuit, 2½-in across

½ pita, 6-in across

FRUIT

One serving contains **15 grams of carbohydrate.**

One serving is:

1 (4 oz) apple, unpeeled, small

4 whole (5½ oz) apricots, fresh

1 (4 oz) banana, small

½ (4 oz) pear, large, fresh

1¼ cup whole strawberries

12 (3 oz) cherries, sweet, fresh

17 (3 oz) grapes, small

½ (11 oz) grapefruit, large

1 (5 oz) nectarine, small

1 (6½ oz) orange, small

1 (6 oz) peach, medium, fresh

1 slice (13½ oz) of 1¼ cup cubes of watermelon

2 (5 oz) plums, small

½ cup apple juice/cider

⅓ cup fruit juice blends, 100% juice

½ cup orange juice

½ cup grapefruit juice

MILK

One serving contains **12 grams of carbohydrate.**

One serving is:

1 cup fat-free milk

1 cup ½% milk

1 cup 1% milk

¾ cup plain low-fat yogurt

BOX 16-1 Grams of Carbohydrate in One Serving of Common Foods—cont'd

Other Carbohydrates

One serving contains **15 grams of carbohydrate.**
One serving is:

Cake, frosted, 2-in square
Cake, unfrosted, 2-in square
3 gingersnaps
5 vanilla wafers
2 small cookies or sandwich cookies
with creme filling

½ cup ice cream
½ cup sherbert, sorbet
⅓ cup yogurt, frozen, low-fat,
fat-free
1 granola bar

Vegetable

One serving contains **5 grams of carbohydrate.**
One serving is:

½ cup cooked vegetables
1 cup raw vegetables
½ cup vegetable juice
Examples include: carrots, asparagus, beans (green, wax, Italian), beets, broccoli, cauliflower, onions, spinach, summer squash, greens (collard, kale, mustard, turnip), cucumbers, turnips, tomatoes.

Adapted from American Diabetes Association, Inc., The American Dietetic Association: *Exchange lists for meal planning,* 1995, ADA/ADA.

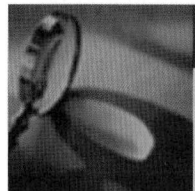

FOR FURTHER FOCUS

Carbohydrate Loading for Endurance

Glycogen is the body storage form of carbohydrate, designed to provide an immediate source of backup fuel and protect blood glucose levels during the fasting hours of sleep. Glycogen is restored with each day's food intake, but during heavy exercise, normal glycogen stores are quickly used up and the person reaches the point of exhaustion. In athletics, this is a no-win situation.

During the 1960s, trainers and coaches began to explore ways of avoiding this state of exhaustion in their players during endurance events. The trainers and coaches reasoned that if the athletes exercised heavily and ate a low-carbohydrate diet for 3 days to use up the stored glycogen, then only exercised lightly and ate a high-carbohydrate diet for the next 3 days, their glycogen stores would become supersaturated, enabling them to perform at a higher level. When this practice was tested, tests proved the increase in the glycogen stores in muscle and the athletes' performance was nearly twice their former workload.

This practice in athletics has become known as *glycogen loading* and is specifically designed for endurance sports. Today a less stressful, modified process of tapered depletion is used to prevent possible injury to muscle tissue and can thus be used more often than the previously used schedule and is more productive in the long run.

TABLE 16-2   Modified depletion-taper precompetition program for glycogen loading

Day	Exercise	Diet
1	90-minute period at 70% to 75% Vo_2 max*	Mixed diet, 50% carbohydrate (350 g)
2-3	Gradual tapering of time and intensity	Diet above continued
4-5	Tapering of exercise time and intensity continues	Mixed diet, 70% carbohydrate (550 g)
6	Complete rest	Diet above continued
7	Day of completion	High-carbohydrate pre-event diet

Adapted from Wright ED: Carbohydrate nutrition and exercise, *Clin Nutr* 7(1):18, 1988.
*Maximum uptake volume of oxygen.

BOX 16-2   Sample pregame meal

1 cup spaghetti, tomato sauce 1 slice French bread 1 cup apple juice	This sample pregame meal includes approximately 300 kcal; high complex carbohydrate; and low protein, fat, and fiber.

tapering of exercise while the diet is increased in carbohydrate (Table 16-2).

Pregame Meal

The ideal pregame meal is a light one (e.g., approximately 300 kcal) that is eaten about 2 to 4 hours before the event. This meal should be high in complex carbohydrates and relatively low in protein, with little fat or fiber.[3] This schedule for the meal gives the body time to digest, absorb, and transform it into stored glycogen. Good food choices include pasta, bread, bagels, muffins, and cereal with nonfat milk. Box 16-2 provides a sample pregame meal.

Hydration

Dehydration can be a serious problem for athletes. The extent of dehydration depends on the follow-

ing: (1) the intensity and duration of the exercise; (2) the surrounding temperature; (3) the level of fitness; and (4) the pregame or preexercise state of hydration. The thirst mechanism cannot keep up with the exercise, so to prevent dehydration athletes are advised to drink more water than they think they need frequently (Figure 16-1). Cold water absorbs more quickly, so athletes should drink small cups of it every 15 minutes during long athletic events. A number of sports drinks with added sugar, electrolytes, and flavorings have been marketed, but questions have been raised about their use or misuse (see For Further Focus box, "Sorting Out the Sports Drink Story"). Adding electrolytes and sugar to water delays its emptying from the stomach. Except for endurance events, plain cold water is usually the rehydration fluid of choice. Electrolytes will be replaced with the athlete's next meal.

Ergogenic Aids

Athletes always want to win. Since ancient times, they have been seeking and experimenting with some "magic" substance or treatment to gain the competitive edge. Today these substances are known as ergogenic aids. Most are worthless fads, but one current practice—the use of steroids—is of great concern because it is dan-

---

ergogenic (Gr. *ergon,* work; *gennan,* to produce) the tendency to increase work output; various substances that increase work or exercise capacity and output.

steroids (Gr. *stereos,* solid; L. *-ol, oleum,* oil) the group name for lipid-based sterols, including hormones, bile acids, and cholesterol.

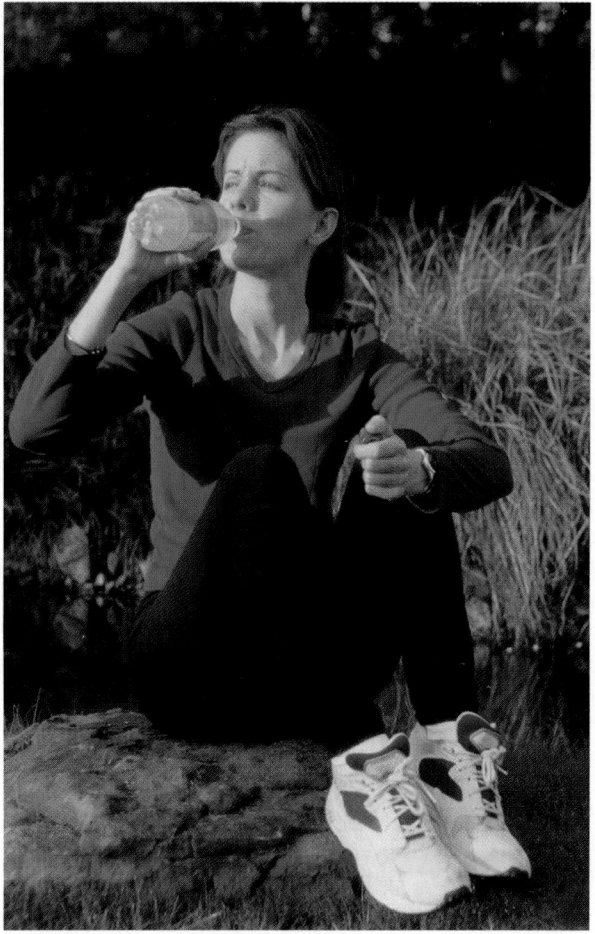

FIGURE 16-1 Frequent small drinks of cold water during extended exercise prevent dehydration. (Credit: PhotoDisc.)

gerous and, in athletics, illegal. Though seldom, an athlete in the Olympic Games is occasionally disqualified for using steroids. The use of steroids is widespread among athletes and body builders, sometimes starting as early as high school or even junior high school. These steroids are synthetic sex hormones that have two actions, as follow: (1) *anabolic* (tissue growth), and (2) *androgenic* (masculinization). Athletes often take these drugs in megadoses 10 to 30 times their normal body hormonal output to increase muscle size, strength, and performance. The physiologic side effects, however, can be devastating, varying from premature closure of bone growth, thus stunting normal skeletal development, and liver injury to accelerated heart disease, high blood pressure, sterility and many other physical effects.[9,10] Psychologic effects vary from increasing aggressiveness, drug dependence, and mood swings to depression, decreased sex drive, and violent rage. Many serious athletes face the hard choice of not using these dangerous drugs and facing a large field of opponents who are using them—and reaping the competitive edge, or of using the drugs and risking the side effects and potential official discovery and disqualification.

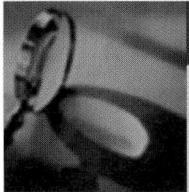

FOR FURTHER FOCUS
Sorting Out the Sports Drink Story

The current story of the so-called sports drinks developed from the belief that water alone does not meet hydration needs during exercise. We now know that the ideal fluid to prevent dehydration depends on how demanding the exercise is and how long it lasts.

For nonendurance exercise, physically fit athletes do perfectly well on plain water. Long-term endurance athletes, especially in hot weather, however, need both water and fuel (e.g., carbohydrate). For example, without carbohydrate replacement, a long-distance marathon runner would soon run out of muscle glycogen and slow down. Also, in such a demanding run when the body can sweat as much as 6% of its weight, it cannot keep cool enough and the overall system overheats, leading to heatstroke and collapse. Simply adding sugar to water causes the water to be held in the stomach longer, however, where it does nothing for the immediate needs of the body tissues.

The first group of sports drinks began with a solution called Gatorade, named by its developers for their university's football team. They reasoned that if they analyzed their players' sweat they could replace lost minerals and water, then add some flavoring, coloring, and sugars to make it more acceptable, and it would do a better job than plain water. Although Gatorade was highly profitable for the university and the manufacturer, subsequent studies showed that regular nonendurance athletes did not need it. Plain water served their needs very well, and they obtained minerals in their diet.

A second category of sports drinks has been developed to meet both the water and energy needs of athletes in longer-lasting endurance events. More dilute 10% sugar solutions, using glucose or *glucose polymers* (i.e., short chains of about five glucose molecules) that are not sweet, are being used. In the more dilute solutions, both energy-sustaining sugars quickly leave the stomach and provide a continuing fuel and water source for the endurance athlete.

Other products entering the sports drink market have been "Gatorade clones" that claim to add no sugar but supply ample amounts of fructose and glucose in their fruit juice base. Fructose does not leave the stomach rapidly and is absorbed more slowly from the intestine than glucose, often causing bloating or diarrhea. Still other products add multiple vitamins (i.e., yielding 137% of the RDA in a single 10-ounce bottle) to their fruit juice base but contain no minerals. All of these vitamins won't help performance at all, and on a hot day a sweating athlete could easily down a megadose in four or five bottles.

So sort out the claims of sports drinks; they are not for everyone. In the long run, special sports drinks meet needs of athletes in endurance events. For nonendurance activities, however, most persons don't need them. After all, water is the best solution for regular needs—and costs far less.

PLANNING A PERSONAL EXERCISE PROGRAM

Health Benefits

Exercise benefits overall health in general. The sense of fitness it brings helps one to "feel good." In addition to this general sense of well-being, however, exercise—especially when mixed with aerobic forms—has special benefits for persons with certain health problems.

Coronary Heart Disease

Exercise reduces risks for heart disease in several ways related to heart function, blood cholesterol levels, and oxygen transport.

Heart muscle function. The heart is a four-chambered organ of muscle that is about the size of a fist in adults. Its ability to pump blood depends on its development. As with any muscle, this development depends on how much the heart is used. Exercise, especially aerobic conditioning, strengthens and enlarges this muscular organ, enabling it to pump more blood per beat, a capacity called *stroke volume*. One effect of training and a physical exercise program is increased stroke volume of the strengthened heart, which enables the heart to pump more blood per minute without an undue increase in the heart rate. The heart's ability to pump enough blood during exercise determines the degree of aerobic capacity in healthy persons.

Blood cholesterol levels. Exercise raises blood levels of high-density lipoprotein (HDL), which is called "good cholesterol" because it carries surplus cholesterol from the tissues to the liver for breakdown and removal from the body (see Chapter 19). Exercise also lowers blood levels of low-density lipoprotein (LDL), which is called "bad cholesterol" because it carries at least two-thirds of the total blood cholesterol to body tissues, raising the potential of cholesterol deposits in major arteries of

the heart. Both of these exercise effects lower the risks for diseased arteries.

Oxygen-carrying capacity. Exercise also enhances the circulatory system by increasing the oxygen-carrying capacity of the blood. The strengthened heart muscle can pump out more blood per beat, thus resulting in a healthy circulating blood volume without an increased heart rate (i.e., the number of beats per minute).

Hypertension

The risk for cardiovascular complications increases continuously with increasing levels of blood pressure.[11,12] When blood pressure is measured, persons with mild essential hypertension show a systolic blood pressure (i.e., the upper notation) of 140 to 159 mm Hg or a diastolic blood pressure (i.e., the lower notation) of 90 to 104 mm Hg (see Chapter 19) or both. Persons with mild hypertension represent the overwhelming majority of hypertensive individuals in the general population, and exercise has become one of the most effective non-drug treatments for them. Even for persons with higher levels of blood pressure, exercise has proved to be an important adjunct to drug therapy, offsetting adverse drug effects and lowering drug needs.

Diabetes

Exercise helps control diabetes, especially type 2 non–insulin-dependent diabetes mellitus (NIDDM) in obese adults. Exercise improves the action of a person's naturally produced insulin by increasing the number of insulin receptor sites (i.e., areas where insulin may be carried into cells). In managing type 1 insulin-dependent diabetes mellitus (IDDM), the type of exercise and when it is done must be balanced with food and insulin to prevent reactions caused by drops in blood sugar.

Weight Management

Exercise is extremely beneficial to weight management because it does the following: (1) helps regulate appetite, (2) increases the basal metabolic rate, and

TABLE 16-3 Target zone heart rate according to age to achieve aerobic physical effect of exercise

Age	Maximal attainable heart rate (pulse: 220 minus age)	Target zone	
		70% maximal rate	85% maximal rate
20	200	140	170
25	195	136	166
30	190	133	161
35	185	129	157
40	180	126	153
45	175	122	149
50	170	119	144
55	165	115	140
60	160	112	136
65	155	108	132
70	150	105	127
75	145	101	124

(3) reduces the genetic fat deposit set-point level (see Chapter 15). Exercise also helps reduce stress-related eating and helps "work off" the hormonal effects of adrenaline produced by stress in the body.

Bone Disease

Exercise increases calcium deposits in bone, thus increasing bone density and reducing the risk for osteoporosis.

Mental Health

Exercise stimulates the production of brain opiates, which are substances called *endorphins*. These natural substances decrease pain (this is how aspirin works, by stimulating production of endorphins) and improve the mood, including an exhilarating kind of "high."

Personal Needs

Health Status and Personal Gains

In planning a personal exercise program, it is important to check first on an individual's health status, present level of fitness, personal needs, and re-

sources required in equipment or cost. The exercise chosen should be something that is enjoyed and of some aerobic value. Also, start slowly and build gradually to avoid discouragement and injury. Moderation and regularity are the chief guides.

Aerobic Benefits

To build aerobic capacity, the level of exercise needs to raise the pulse to within 70% of an individual's maximum heart rate. You can estimate your own *cardiac rate* by subtracting your age from 220, which gives your maximum heart rate. About 70% of this figure is your *target zone rate*—the level to which you want to raise your pulse during exercise (Table 16-3). For aerobic benefits, this rate should be maintained for approximately 20 minutes about 3 times a week. Check your resting pulse before the exercise period, then again during and immediately after exercising.

Types of Physical Activity

General Exercise

It's best to have a variety of exercises in your plan. Many do not reach aerobic levels but are enjoyable

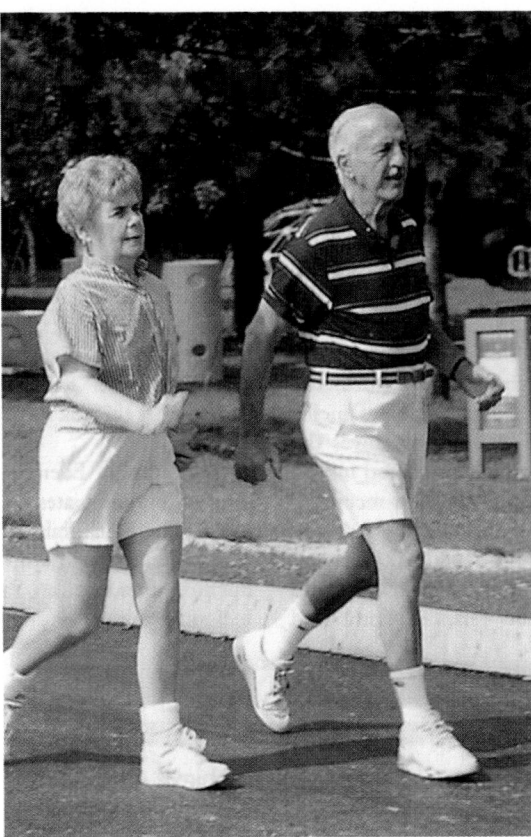

FIGURE 16-2 Aerobic walking is an enjoyable exercise that can fit into almost anyone's lifestyle. (Copyright CLG Photographics, Inc.)

and should be included. If whatever you do isn't fun, you'll soon stop, reaping no benefit.

Aerobic Exercise

Walking can be developed into an aerobic exercise. It is convenient and requires no equipment except good walking shoes. Walking is also satisfying to

TABLE 16-4 Aerobic exercises for physical fitness (maintained at aerobic level for at least 30 minutes)

Type of exercise	Aerobic forms
Ballplaying	Handball
	Raquetball
	Squash
Bicycling	Stationary
	Touring
Dancing	Aerobic routines
	Ballet
	Disco
Jumping rope	Brisk pace
Running/jogging	Brisk pace
Skating	Ice skating
	Roller skating
Skiing	Cross country
Swimming	Steady pace
Walking	Brisk pace

many people for whom other forms may not be appropriate. Start slowly and gradually increase your pace and distance. Table 16-4 provides examples of aerobic forms of exercise.

Exercise Preparation and Care

Whatever your choice of exercise, preparation and continuing care are important. Before beginning, stretch your muscles to prevent stress or injury, and take time to cool down afterward. Don't go beyond your tolerance limits; listen to your own body. When you are tired, rest. When you hurt, stop. When you want more challenge, increase your exercise level—but only then; remember, it's *your* exercise plan.

SUMMARY

Many fine muscle fibers and cells, triggered by nerve endings, work smoothly together to make all of our physical activity possible. Carbohydrate—mainly in the form of complex carbohydrate foods, or starches—is our primary fuel for energy to run this system. The constant body fuels resulting from carbohydrate metabolism are circulating blood sugar and stored glycogen in muscles and liver. Stored body fat supplies additional fuel as fatty acids. Protein, however, provides only insignificant energy for exercise. Vitamins and minerals cannot be burned for energy but are important coenzyme partners for the process of energy production.

Exercise does increase the need for kcalories and water. Cold water in small, frequent amounts is generally the best way to avoid dehydration. Electrolytes lost in sweat are replaced in the next meal. The optimal diet for athletes is 60% of the kcalories from carbohydrate (mainly complex starches), 25%

from fat, and 15% from protein. During the week before an athletic event, especially an endurance event, serious athletes may practice glycogen loading to meet the energy demands of competition. Pregame meals, however, should comprise small, mainly complex carbohydrates (starches), with little fat, protein, or fiber.

General and aerobic exercise have many benefits, which increase with practice. Excellent aerobic exercises include sustained fast walking, swimming, jogging, running, and aerobic dancing or workouts.

REVIEW QUESTIONS

1. Compare and discuss the three energy nutrients in terms of their relative roles as fuel for exercise.

2. Outline the nutrition and physical fitness principles you would discuss with a client who is an athlete. Plan a diet for this person that would meet nutrient and energy needs.

3. Why is fluid balance vital during exercise periods? How are water and electrolyte balance achieved?

4. Describe the health benefits of exercise for a person with heart disease, as well as for a person with hypertension. Also describe the benefits of exercise for an overweight person with NIDDM.

5. Describe several factors a person should consider in planning a personal exercise program. Define the term *aerobic exercise* and list its benefits.

SELF-TEST QUESTIONS

True/False

Write the correct statement for each item you answer "false."

1. Water containing electrolytes and sugar is the best way to replace these substances lost during exercise.

2. Drinking water immediately before and during an athletic event causes cramps.

3. Cold water is absorbed more quickly from the stomach.

4. Athletes need protein for extra energy.

5. Vitamins and minerals are burned for energy in workouts and training sessions.

6. Protein and fat do not contribute to glycogen stores.

7. Sweating is the main mechanism for dissipating body heat.

8. Aerobic exercise is of limited benefit in controlling heart disease and diabetes.

9. Walking can be an excellent form of aerobic exercise.

Multiple Choice

1. Which of the following general activities is most likely to provide aerobic exercise?
   a. Golf
   b. Swimming
   c. Tennis
   d. Baseball

2. To develop aerobic capacity, an exercise should:
   a. Raise the pulse to 50% of the maximum heart rate.
   b. Be maintained for alternating 10 minute periods.
   c. Be practiced consistently every day.
   d. Be practiced several times a week at an appropriate pulse rate for sustained periods of time.
3. Characteristics of a healthful exercise program should include (circle all that apply):
   a. Enjoyable activities.
   b. Moderation.
   c. Regularity.
   d. Going beyond tolerance limits.

4. Exercise is beneficial in weight management because it (circle all that apply):
   a. Helps regulate appetite.
   b. Decreases BMR.
   c. Reduces stress-related eating.
   d. Increases the set-point for fat deposit.
5. Which of these meals is the best choice for an athlete's pregame meal?
   a. Large grilled steak, fried potatoes, ice cream
   b. Fried fish, vegetable salad with cream dressing, fresh fruit
   c. Spaghetti with tomato sauce, French bread, fruit
   d. Hamburger, French fries, cola

SUGGESTIONS FOR ADDITIONAL STUDY

1. Analysis of Athletes' Diets
Interview two athletes—one male and one female—in your school or community. Ask them about food habits and attitudes, their own or ones they have observed in teammates. Ask them about the use of supplements, pregame meals, nutrition advice from coaches, and any other food- or nutrition-related practices.

Analyze your findings in terms of the total energy value of the diet (kcalories) and the relative percentages of total kcalories supplied by protein, fat, and carbohydrate. Compare the two athletes' diets and nutrition practices and beliefs. Present your findings in a class discussion. Follow-up your initial interview with any dietary counseling indicated, if appropriate.

2. Discussion Group for Athletes
Contact a school or community organization athletic director to plan an informal discussion group with team members to present nutrition information for persons involved in team sports. Discuss their questions about food and nutrition practices and beliefs. Provide a display or appropriate handouts of sound nutrition information, resources, or reference lists for sources of helpful materials.

3. Survey of Fitness Centers
Visit a variety of fitness centers in your community. Gather information and reference materials about each center's program: services offered, costs involved, staff resources, diet recommendations, or sale of any nutrition products related to their program. Compare and evaluate these programs in a follow-up class discussion.

REFERENCES

1. U.S. Department of Health and Human Services: *Healthy people 2010: Understanding and improving health*, Washington, D.C., 2000, Government Printing Office.

2. Staff: Practice points: translating research into practice: physical activity—it's not reserved for athletes, *J Am Diet Assoc* 99(2):212, 1999.

3. American Dietetic Association, Position Paper: Nutrition, aging, and continuum of care, *J Am Diet Assoc* 96(10): 1048, 1996.

4. American Dietetic Association: Position paper update for 1999, *J Am Diet Assoc* (2):234, 1999.

5. Lee I-M and others: Exercise intensity and longevity in men, the Harvard Alumni Health Study, *J Am Med Assoc* 273(15):1179, 1995.

6. Wilmore JH: Increasing physical activity: alterations in body mass and composition, *Am J Clin Nutr* 63(suppl): 456S, 1996.

7. Ryan M: Sports drinks: research asks for revelation of current recommendations, *J Am Diet Assoc* 16(1):S197, 1997.

8. Paffenbarger RS and others: Changes in physical activity and other lifeway patterns influencing longevity, *Med Sci Sports Exerc* 26(7):857, 1994.

9. Nnakwe N: Anabolic steroids and cardiovascular risk in athletes, *Nutr Today* 31(5):206, 1996.

10. Yesalis CE, Michael SB: Anabolic—androgenic steroids: current issues, *Sports Med* 19:326, 1995.

11. Franz MJ: Managing obesity in patients with comorbities, *J Am Diet Assoc* 98(suppl 2):S39-S43, 1998.

12. Rippe JM: Obesity as a chronic disease: modern medical and lifestyle management, *J Am Diet Assoc* 98(suppl 2):S9, 1998.

FURTHER READING

- Hill JO and others: Orlistat, a lipase inhibitor, for weight maintenance after conventional dieting: a 1-year study, *Am J Clin Nutr* 69(June):1108, 1999.

    Orlistat is a gastrointestinal lipase inhibitor that helps minimize regaining weight after a successful program of needed weight loss. In this study, such regain was controlled significantly with various results according to dose level.

- Schuster K: The dark side of nutrition, *Food Management* 34(June):34, 1999.

    Obsession with anything is usually unhealthy behavior, which is also true if weight control is approached unwisely, especially if used with children. This author discusses wise approaches to avoid obsession with weight control, especially with children, that can easily lead to eating disorders, inadequate nutrient intake for normal growth, and negative ideas about food. Instead, wise positive nutrition messages must promote variety, balance, moderation, enjoyment, and a wider healthy ideal weight range.

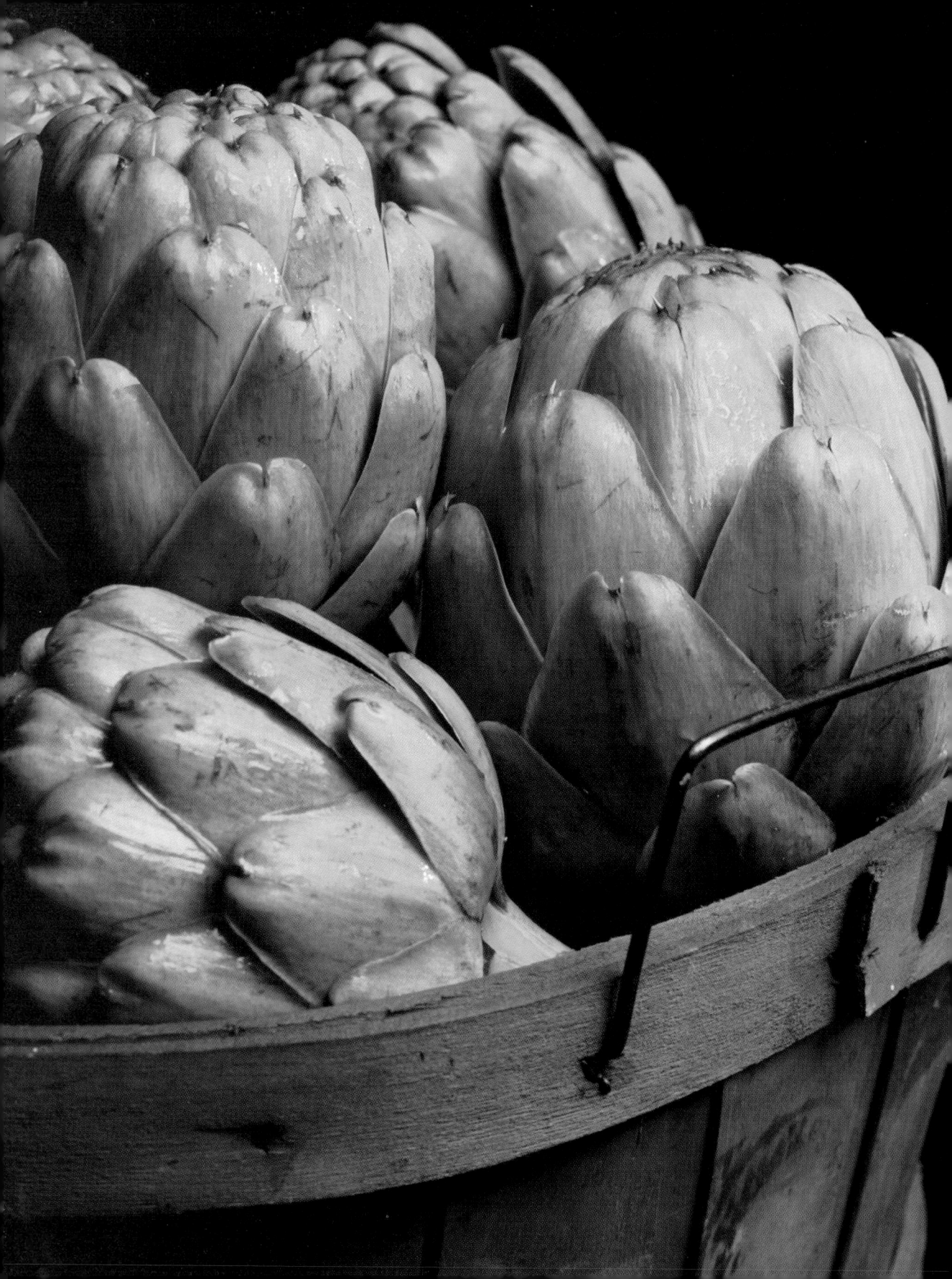

Clinical Nutrition

4

17

Nutritional Care

KEY CONCEPTS

- Valid health care is based on individual care.

- Comprehensive health care is best provided by a team of various health professionals and support staff persons.

- A personalized health care plan, based on individual needs and goals, guides actions to promote healing and health.

Persons face acute illness or chronic disease and its treatment in a variety of settings: hospital, extended-care facility, clinic, or home. Nutritional support is fundamental—and is often the primary therapy. Sensitive care is always based on an individual's needs. To meet individual nutritional needs, a broad knowledge of nutritional state, requirements, and ways of meeting the identified needs is essential. The clinical nutritionist, along with the physician, carries the major responsibility for this nutritional care. Each member of the health team helps with this person-centered care.

Here we focus on the comprehensive care of the patient's nutritional needs and explore the basic care process involved. The health care team—including the patient and family—must work together to support the healing process and promote health.

THE THERAPEUTIC PROCESS

Setting and Focus of Care

Health Care Setting

Modern hospitals are a marvel of medical technology, but these medical advances have also brought increasing confusion to many patients, whose illnesses place them in the midst of a complex system of care. Various persons come and go, and it is understandable when the course does not always run smoothly. Patients need personal advocates. Primary health care providers such as

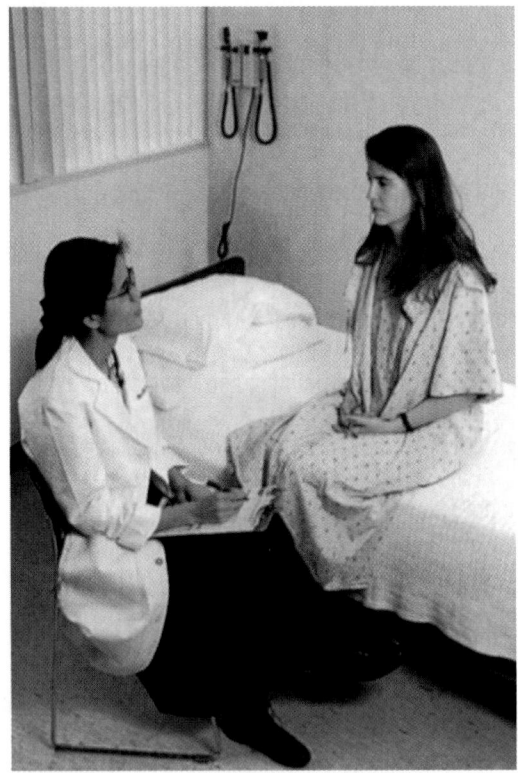

FIGURE 17-1 Interviewing patient to plan personal care. (From Seidel HM, Ball JW, Dains JE, Benedict GW: *Mosby's guide to physical examination,* ed. 3, St. Louis, 1995, Mosby. Photographer: Patrick Watson.)

the nurse and the dietitian can provide such essential support and personalized care.[1]

Health Care Team

In the area of nutritional care, the clinical nutritionist (i.e., registered dietitian [RD]) carries the major responsibility. Working closely with the physician, the nutritionist determines individual nutritional therapy needs and plan of care. Throughout this process, team support is essential. Nurses are in a unique position to provide this important nutritional support, referring patients to the clinical nutritionist (RD) when time or skills are lacking. Of all the health care team members, nurses are in the closest continuous contact with patients and their families. A real partnership with patients and their families is essential to valid care.[1,2] In developing this team relationship, all involved parties need each other's expertise and experience for a successful outcome.

Person-Centered Care

To be valid, nutritional care must be based on individual needs and must be *person-centered*. Needs must be constantly updated with the patient. Such personalized care demands a great commitment from health workers. Despite all methods, tools, and technologies described here and elsewhere, remember this basic fact: *the most healing tool you will ever use is yourself.* This is a simple yet profound truth, because it is the *human* encounter to which we bring ourselves and our skills.

Phases of the Care Process

Collecting Information

To provide person-centered care, we must collect as much information about the patient's situation as possible. We must know the nutritional status, food habits, and living situation, as well as the patient's needs, desires, and goals. The patient (Figure 17-1) and family are the primary sources of this information. Other sources include the patient's medical chart, oral or written communication with hospital staff, and related research.

Identifying Problems

A careful study of all the information you have gathered will reveal basic patient needs. Other needs will develop as the hospitalization continues. You can begin to list these needs to guide care.

Planning Care

Appropriate care is planned to meet these identified needs. This written care plan will give attention to personal needs and goals, as well as the identified requirements of medical care.

Implementing Care

Appropriate and realistic actions then carry out the personal care plan. For example, nutritional care and teaching would include an appropriate food plan with examples of food choices, food buying, or food preparation. Such activities might include family members as well.

Evaluating and Recording Results

Results must be checked to see if needs have been met so that the plan can be revised as necessary for continuing care. These actions and results must be carefully recorded in the patient's medical chart.

In the remainder of this chapter, we briefly review each of the five phases of individual health care in terms of the nutritional aspects of overall patient care. Nutritional support is an essential component of all health care.

COLLECTING AND ANALYZING NUTRITIONAL INFORMATION

Collection

Body Measures

Practice taking body measurements correctly to avoid errors. Also maintain proper equipment and careful technique. Three types of measurements are common in clinical practice, as follow:

Weight. Weigh hospital patients at consistent times (e.g., in the early morning after the bladder

is emptied and before breakfast). Weigh clinic patients without shoes in light indoor clothing or an examining gown. Ask about their usual body weight and compare it with standard weight-height tables (see Chapter 15). Ask about any recent weight loss (i.e., how much over what time period). Rapid weight loss is significant. Also ask if the cause is known, and ask about any recent weight gain, as well. Sometimes it is helpful to ask about general weight history over time (e.g., peaks and lows at what ages).

Height. Use a fixed measuring stick against the wall if possible. Otherwise, use the moveable measuring rod on the platform clinic scales. Have the person stand as straight as possible, without shoes or cap. Note the growth of children, as well as the diminishing height of older adults.

Body composition. The nutritionist usually measures various aspects of body size and composition, including the circumference of the mid-upper arm and the skinfold of the triceps, from which the circumference of the mid-upper arm muscle can be calculated. These measurements provide a good general indication of body leanness and fatness. Special calipers measure skinfold thickness (Figure 17-2).

Medical Tests

Many laboratory and radiographic tests help measure nutritional status, and reports are available in the patient's chart for study. Several of the most frequently used tests are listed here.

Plasma protein. Basic measures are hemoglobin, hematocrit, and serum albumin. Additional tests may include serum transferrin or total iron-binding capacity (TIBC) and ferritin. These tests help detect protein and iron deficiencies.

Protein metabolism. Basic 24-hour urine tests measure the products of protein metabolism (i.e., urinary creatinine and urea nitrogen). Elevated levels may indicate excess breakdown of body tissue.

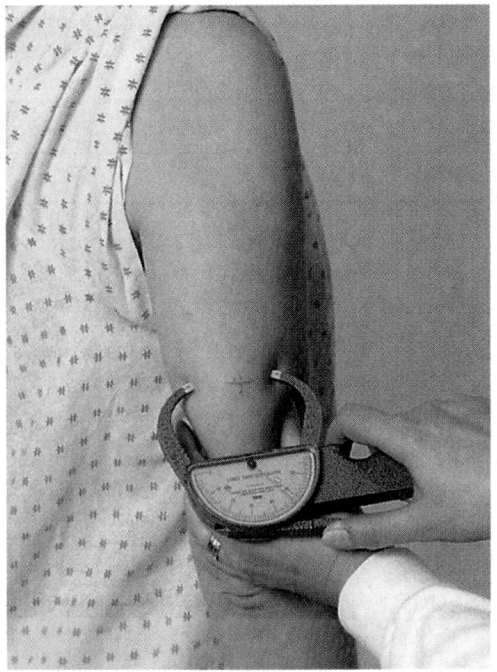

FIGURE 17-2 Assessment tools include skinfold calipers, shown above, which measure the relative amount of subcutaneous fat tissues at various body sites. (From Seidel HM, Ball JW, Dains JE, Benedict GW: *Mosby's guide to physical examination,* ed 4, St Louis, 1999, Mosby. Photographer: Patrick Watson.)

Immune system integrity. Basic tests determine the lymphocyte count, which is the ratio of these special white cells to the total white blood cell count. Skin testing may also be done to check for sensitivity to common antigens and, hence, the strength of the general immune system.

Skeletal system integrity. X-ray tests may be used, especially with older women, to determine the status of bone integrity and possible osteoporosis.

Gastrointestinal function. X-ray tests may also be used to study gastrointestinal function and prob-

lems, such as peptic ulcer disease or any malfunction along the gastrointestinal tract.

The medical tests used for nutrition assessment are generally reliable in persons of any age, but conditions in elderly patients may interfere and need to be considered in evaluating test results.[3] For example, laboratory values are affected by hydration status, presence of chronic diseases, changes in organ function, and drugs.

Observations

Careful observations of various areas of the patient's body may reveal signs of poor nutrition in comparison with signs of good nutrition. Table 17-1 lists some clinical signs of nutritional status that you should keep in mind when providing general patient care.

Diet History

General knowledge of the patient's basic eating habits helps to identify any possible nutritional deficiencies. The Clinical Applications box, "Nutrition History: Activity-Associated Food Pattern of a Typical Day"), shows an example of a general guide for a nutrition history. Sometimes a more specific food intake is obtained using a 24-hour recall; that is, going through the previous day and asking for everything consumed, food items used, and amounts and methods of preparation. A more extended 3-day food record may give further information about food habits or problems.

Analysis

Nutritional Problems

A study of all the collected nutrition information will help identify nutritional problems, which may include nutrient deficiencies (e.g., evidence of iron deficiency anemia) or underlying disease requiring a special modified diet. Signs of general malnutrition requiring rebuilding of body tissue and nutrient stores may be evidenced, and special assistance in eating and swallowing may be necessary.

TABLE 17-1 Clinical signs of nutritional status

Body area	Signs of good nutrition	Signs of poor nutrition
General apperance	Alert, responsive	Listless, apathetic, cachectic
Weight	Normal for height, age, body build	Overweight or underweight (special concern for underweight)
Posture	Erect, arms and legs straight	Sagging shoulders, sunken chest, humped back
Muscles	Well developed; firm, good tone; some fat under skin	Flaccid, poor tone; undeveloped; tender; "wasted" appearance; cannot walk properly
Nervous control	Good attention span; not irritable or restless; normal reflexes; psycho-logic stability	Inattentive, irritable, confused; burning and tingling of hands and feet (paresthesia); loss of position and vibratory sense; weakness and tenderness of muscles (may result in inability to walk); decrease or loss of ankle and knee reflexes
Gastrointestinal function	Good appetite and digestion, normal regular elimination, no palpable (per-ceptible to touch) organs or masses	Anorexia, indigestion, constipation or diarrhea, liver or spleen enlargement
Cardiovascular function	Normal heart rate and rhythm, no mur-murs, normal blood pressure for age	Rapid heart rate (greater than 100 beats/minute tachycardia), enlarged heart, abnormal rhythm, elevated blood pressure
General vitality	Endurance, energetic, sleeps well, vigorous	Easily fatigued, no energy, falls asleep easily, looks tired, apathetic
Hair	Shiny, lustrous, firm, not easily plucked, healthy scalp	Stringy, dull, brittle, dry, thin and sparse; depigmented; can be easily plucked
Skin (general)	Smooth, slightly moist, good color	Rough, dry, scaly, pale, pigmented, irritated; bruises; petechiae
Face and neck	Skin color uniform, smooth, pink, healthy appearance, not swollen	Greasy, discolored, scaly, swollen; skin dark over cheeks and under eyes; lumpiness or flakiness of skin around nose and mouth
Lips	Smooth, good color; moist; not chapped or swollen	Dry, scaly, swollen, redness and swelling (cheilosis), or angular lesions at corners of the mouth or fissures or scars (stomatitis)
Mouth, oral membranes	Reddish pink mucous membranes in oral cavity	Swollen, boggy oral mucous membranes
Gums	Good pink color, healthy, red, no swelling or bleeding	Spongy, bleed easily, marginal redness, inflamed, gums receding
Tongue	Good pink color or deep reddish in appearance, not swollen or smooth, surface papillae present, no lesion	Swelling, scarlet and raw, magenta color, beefy (glossitis), hyperemic and hypertrophic papillae, atrophic papillae
Teeth	No cavities, no pain, bright, straight, no crowding, well-shaped jaw, clean, no discoloration	Unfilled caries, absent teeth, worn surfaces, mottled (fluorosis), malpositioned

From Williams SR: Nutritional assessment and guidance in prenatal care. In Worthington-Roberts BS and Williams SR: *Nutrition in pregnancy and lactation*, ed 5, New York, 1993, McGraw-Hill.

Continued

TABLE 17-1 Clinical signs of nutritional status—cont'd

Body area	Signs of good nutrition	Signs of poor nutrition
Eyes	Bright, clear, shiny; no sores at corner of eyelids; membranes moist and healthy pink color, no prominent blood vessels or amount of tissue or sclera; no fatigue circles beneath	Eye membranes pale (pale conjunctivas), redness of membrane (conjunctival injection), dryness, signs of infection; Bitot's spots, redness and fissuring of eyelid corners (angular palpebritis), dryness of eye membrane (conjunctival xerosis), dull apearance of cornea (corneal xerosis), soft cornea (keratomalacia)
Neck (glands)	No enlargement	Thyroid enlarged
Nails	Firm, pink	Spoon-shaped (koilonychia), brittle, ridged
Legs, feet	No tenderness, weakness, or swelling, good color	Edema, tender calf, tingling weakness
Skeleton	No malformations	Bowlegs, knock-knees, check deformity at diaphragm, beaded ribs, prominent scapulas

From Williams SR: Nutritional assessment and guidance in prenatal care. In Worthington-Roberts BS and Williams SR: *Nutrition in pregnancy and lactation*, ed 5, New York, 1993, McGraw-Hill.

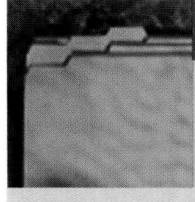

CLINICAL APPLICATIONS

Nutrition History: Activity-Associated Food Pattern of a Typical Day

Name _____ Date _____

Height _____ Weight (lb) _____ (kg) _____ Age _____

Ideal weight _____

Referral
Diagnosis
Diet order
Members of household
Occupation
Recreation, physical activity
Present food intake

	Place	Hour	Frequency, form, and amount checklist
Breakfast			Milk
			Cheese
			Meat
			Fish
			Poultry
Noon meal			Eggs
			Cream
			Butter; margarine
			Other fats
Evening meal			Vegetables, green
			Vegetables, other
			Fruits (citrus)
			Legumes
Extra meals			Potato
			Bread—kind
			Sugar
			Desserts
			Beverages
Summary			Alcohol
			Vitamins
			Candy

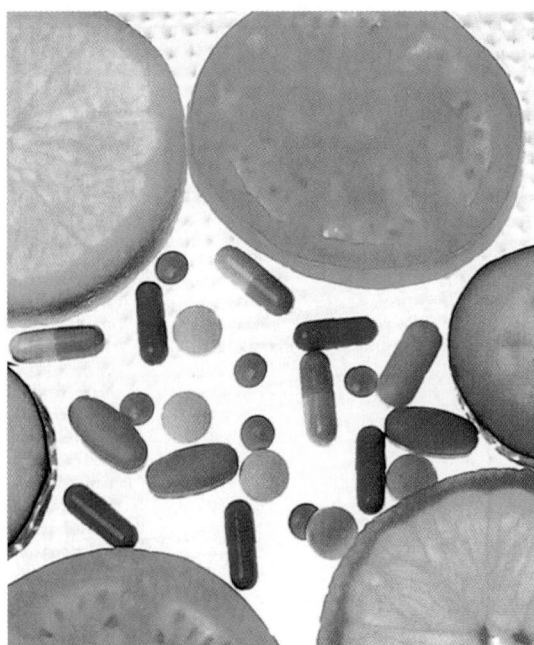

FIGURE 17-3 Many drugs, foods, and nutrients interact to cause nutritional problems. (Copyright CLG Photographics, Inc.)

Drug-Nutrient Interactions

Information about all drugs—including over-the-counter self-medications and "street drugs," as well as alcohol and prescribed drugs—is essential. Research each drug to determine any possible problems from the interaction of each with foods and nutrients (Figure17-3). Many such reactions exist and are encountered with multiple drug use, especially in elderly patients with chronic diseases.

Personal Needs and Goals

Any personal, cultural, and ethnic needs must be considered in helping a patient plan for meeting health needs. Economic needs are paramount for many persons in high-risk populations. Personal goals help establish priorities for immediate and long-term care.

PLANNING AND IMPLEMENTING NUTRITIONAL CARE
Basic Principles of Diet Therapy

Normal Nutrition Base

The primary principle of diet therapy is that it is based on a patient's normal nutritional requirements, which are important for patients to know. Any therapeutic diet is only a modification of normal nutritional needs and is only modified as an individual's specific condition requires.

Disease Modifications

Nutritional components of the normal diet may be modified in three basic ways, as follow:

1. *Nutrients*—One or more of the basic nutrients (e.g., protein, carbohydrate, fat, mineral, or vitamin) may be modified in amount or form.
2. *Energy*—The total energy value of the diet, expressed in kilocalories (kcal), may be increased or decreased.
3. *Texture*—The texture or seasoning of the diet may be modified (e.g., liquid or low-residue diets).

Personal Adaptation

Successful nutritional therapy can occur only when the diet is *personalized* (e.g., adapted to meet individual needs). This can only be done by planning *with the patient or family*. Four areas must be explored together, as follow:

1. *Personal needs*—What personal desires, concerns, goals, or life situation needs must be met?
2. *Disease*—How does the patient's disease or condition affect the body and its normal metabolic functions?
3. *Nutritional therapy*—How and why must the diet be changed to meet needs created by the patient's particular disease or condition?

4. *Food plan*—How do these necessary nutritional modifications affect daily food choices?

Routine House Diets

A schedule of routine "house" diets, based on some type of cycle menus, is usually followed in most hospitals. The basic modification is in texture, ranging from clear liquid (no milk) to full liquid (including milk) and soft food to a full regular diet. Table 17-2 summarizes details of currently liberalized routine hospital diets.

Mode of Feeding

The method of feeding used in the nutritional care plan depends on the patient's condition. The clinical nutritionist and the nurse work together to manage the diet by using oral, tube, peripheral vein, or total parenteral feeding.

Oral Feeding

As long as possible, regular oral feedings are preferred. If needed, nutrient supplements may be added.

Assisted Oral Feeding

According to the patient's condition, the nurse may need to help the patient eat. Patients usually like to help themselves as much as possible and should be encouraged to do so with whatever degree of assistance is needed. Try to learn each patient's needs and limitations so that little things (e.g., having the meat cut up or the bread buttered before bringing the tray to the bedside) can be done without making a patient feel inadequate. When complete assistance is needed, have the tray securely placed within a patient's sight. Then relax; sit down beside the bed if this is more comfortable. Make simple conversation or remain silent as a patient's condition indicates. Offer small amounts and do not rush the feeding. Give ample time for a patient to chew and swallow or rest between mouthfuls. Offer liquids between the solids, using a drinking tube if

necessary. Wipe the patient's mouth with a napkin during and after each meal. Let a patient hold the bread, if desired and able to do so. When feeding patient who is blind or has eye dressings, describe the food on the tray so that a mental image helps create a desire to eat. Sometimes it is helpful to use the face of a clock to let a patient visualize the position of certain foods on the plate (e.g., indicating that the meat is at 12 o'clock, the potatoes are at 3 o'clock, etc.). Warn the patient that the soup feels particularly hot when taken through a glass straw, and identify each food you are serving beforehand.

Assisted feeding times can provide a special opportunity for nutrition counseling and support. Important observations can be made. The nurse can closely observe the patient's physical appearance and response to the foods served and appetite and tolerance for certain foods, as well as note the meaning of food to the person. These observations can help the nurse adapt the patient's diet to meet any particular individual needs. Helping patients learn more about their diets and nutritional needs is an important part of personal care. Persons who understand the role of good food in health (i.e., that it helps them regain strength and recover from illness) are more likely to accept the diet. They also feel more encouraged to continue attention to sound eating habits after discharge from the hospital, as well as improve their eating habits in general.

Tube Feeding

When a patient cannot eat but the gastrointestinal tract can be used, an alternate form of enteral feeding by tube provides nutritional support. Various commercial formulas are available and usually preferred over locally mixed ones. A blended formula

---

enteral (Gr. *enteron,* intestine) a mode of feeding that uses the gastrointestinal tract with oral or tube feeding.

TABLE 17-2 Routine hospital diets

Food	Clear liquid	Full Liquid	Soft	Regular
Soup	Clear fat-free broth, bouillon	Same, plus strained or blended cream soups	Same, plus all cream soups	All
Cereal		Cooked refined cereal	Cooked cereal, cornflakes, rice, noodles, macaroni, spaghetti	
Bread			White bread, crackers, melba toast, zwieback	All
Protein foods		Milk, cream, milk drinks, yogurt	Same, plus eggs (not fried, mild cheese, cottage and cream cheese, fowl, fish, sweetbreads, tender beef, veal, lamb, liver, bacon, gravy	All
Vegetables			Potatoes: baked, mashed, creamed, steamed, scalloped; tender cooked whole bland vegetables; fresh lettuce, tomatoes	All
Fruit and fruit juices	Fruit juices (as tolerated), flavored fruit drinks	All	Same, plus cooked fruit: peaches, pears, applesauce, peeled apricots, white cherries; ripe peaches, pears, banana, orange and grapefruit sections without membrane	
Desserts and gelatin	Fruit-flavored gelatin, fruit ices and popsicles	Same, plus sherbet, ice cream puddings, custard, frozen yogurt	Same, plus plain sponge cakes, plain cookies, plain cake, puddings, pie made with allowed foods	All
Miscellaneous	Soft drinks (as tolerated), coffee and tea, decaffeinated coffee and tea, cereal beverages such as Postum, sugar, honey, salt, hard candy, Poly cose (Ross), residue-free supplements	Same, plus margarine, pepper, all supplements	Same, plus mild salad dressings	

may be calculated and prepared, but greater risk for contamination in preparation and storage exists.

Peripheral Vein Feeding

If a patient cannot take in food or formula through the gastrointestinal tract, intravenous (IV) feeding is required. Various solutions of dextrose, amino acids, vitamins, minerals, and lipids can be fed through peripheral veins. The nutrient and kcalorie intake is limited in this method of feeding, however, so peripheral vein feeding is only used when the nutritional need is not extensive or long-term. It is helpful for patients to understand that this is still a method of "feeding."

Total Parenteral Nutrition (TPN)

When a patient's nutritional need is great (e.g., in massive injury or debilitating disease) and assisted feeding may be required for longer time, the use of a larger central vein is needed. Total parenteral nutrition (TPN) is a special surgical procedure in which special nutrient solutions must be administered by a team of specialists (e.g., physicians, clinical dietitians, pharmacists, and nurses). Throughout this procedure the patient needs special care and support, including instruction for continued TPN use at home as needed.

EVALUATION OF NUTRITIONAL CARE

General Considerations

When the nutritional plan of care is carried out, it is evaluated in terms of the nutritional diagnosis and treatment objectives. This evaluation continues through the period of care and terminates at the point of discharge or the end of the care period. The various questions listed in the following sections are important.

Nutritional Goals

What is the effect of the diet or feeding method on the illness or the patient's situation? Is any change in the nutrients, kcalories, meal-snack pattern, or feeding method necessary?

Accuracy of Care Plan Actions

Must any of the nutritional care plan components be changed? Is it necessary to change the type of food or feeding equipment, environment for meals, counseling procedures, or types of learning activities for nutrition education?

Ability to Follow Diet

Does any hindrance or disability prevent the patient from following the treatment plan? What is the effect of the diet on the patient, family, or staff? Was all the necessary nutrition information gathered correctly? Do the patient and family understand all the self-care instructions provided? Are needed community resources available or convenient? Has any necessary food-assistance program been sufficient for the patients care?

Role of the Nurse and Clinical Dietitian

The nurse and the clinical dietitian form an important team for providing nutrition care. The clinical dietitian, who usually has an advanced degree and special clinical training, determines nutritional needs, plans and manages nutritional therapy, evaluates plan of care, and records results. Throughout this entire process, the nurse helps to develop, support, and carry out the plan of care. Successful care depends on the close teamwork of the dietitian and nurse. When necessary, the nurse may also serve as an essential coordinator, advocate, interpreter, teacher, or counselor.

---

parenteral (Gr. *para,* alongside, accessory, beyond; *enteron,* intestine) a mode of feeding that does not use the gastrointestinal tract but instead provides nutrition support by intravenous delivery of nutrient solutions.

Coordinator and Advocate

Nurses work more closely with patients than any other practitioner. They are best able to coordinate the patient's special services and treatments and can consult and refer as needed. Sometimes hospital-induced malnutrition exists because meals are often in conflict with medical procedures at mealtime or food is uneaten because of poor appetite, which are situations the nurse can help resolve.

Interpreter

The nurse can help reduce a patient's anxiety by careful, brief, easily understood explanations about various treatments and plans of care. This help includes a basic reinforcement of special diet needs, resulting food choices from menus, and illustrations of needs from foods on the tray. These activities may be difficult with uninterested or unpleasant patients, but efforts to understand such patient behaviors are important.

Teacher or Counselor

Basic health teaching and counseling are essential in nursing. Many opportunities exist during daily care for planned conversations about sound nutrition principles, which will reinforce the clinical dietitian's work with the patient. Learning about the patient's nutritional needs must begin with hospital admission or initial contact, must carry through the entire period of care, and must continue in the home environment, supported by community resources as needed.

SUMMARY

The basis for effective nutritional care begins with the patient's nutritional needs and must involve the patient and the family. Such person-centered care requires initial assessment and planning by the clinical dietitian and continuous close teamwork among all health team members providing primary care. Careful assessment of factors influencing nutritional status requires a broad foundation of pertinent information (i.e., physiologic, psychosocial, medical, and personal information). The patient's medical record is a basic means of communication among health care team members.

Nutritional therapy is based on the personal and physical needs of the patient. Successful therapy requires a close working relationship among dietetics, medical, and nursing staff in the health care facility. The nurse has a unique position to reinforce nutritional principles of the diet with the patient and family.

REVIEW QUESTIONS

1. Identify and discuss the possible effects of various psychosocial factors on the outcome of nutritional therapy.
2. List and describe commonly used measures for determining nutritional status, including the following: (1) body measures; (2) medical tests; (3) clinical observations; and (4) food habits.
3. Describe the roles of the clinical nutritionist and the nurse in nutritional care.

SELF-TEST QUESTIONS

True-False
Write the correct statement for each item you answer false.
1. Nutritional care is based on the needs of individual patients.
2. Patients' housing situations have little relation to their illnesses or continuing care.
3. History-taking is an important skill in planning nutritional care.

4. A patient's social history has little value in planning his diet.

5. Once a diet treatment plan has been established, it should be followed continuously without change.

6. Normal nutrition needs are the basis for diet therapy.

7. Patients' personal goals do not relate to their diet therapy and instruction.

8. A diet modified in energy value may be indicated for an obese patient.

9. Larger food portions stimulate ill patients with little appetite to eat.

10. The involvement of the patient's family in the diet therapy and teaching usually creates problems and is best avoided.

Multiple Choice

1. Which of the following personal details help(s) to determine a patient's nutritional needs? (Circle all that apply.)
   a. Family size
   b. Blood protein level
   c. Skinfold thickness
   d. Symptoms of illness

2. A nutrition history should include which of the following items of nutritional information? (Circle all that apply.)
   a. General food habits
   b. Food-buying practices
   c. Cooking methods
   d. Food likes and dislikes

3. Knowledge of which of the following items is necessary for carrying out valid diet therapy for a hospitalized patient? (Circle all that apply.)
   a. The specific diet and its relation to the patient's disease
   b. Foods affected by the diet modification
   c. The mode of the hospital's food service and the patient's need for any eating aids
   d. The patient's response to the diet

4. A special diet may be based on a specific nutrient modification. For example, a 30-g protein diet would include increased amounts of which of the following foods?
   a. Meat and fish
   b. Eggs and poultry
   c. Cheese and milk
   d. Fruits and vegetables

5. Which of the following actions would be helpful to a disabled patient who needs assistance in eating? (Circle all that apply.)
   a. Learning the extent of his disability and encouraging him to do as much of the feeding as he can himself
   b. Feeding the patient completely, regardless of the problem, because it saves him time and energy
   c. Hurrying the feeding to get in as much food as possible before the patient's appetite wanes
   d. Sitting comfortably by the patient's bed, offering mouthfuls of food, with ample time for chewing, swallowing, and rest as needed

SUGGESTIONS FOR ADDITIONAL STUDY

1. Group Project: The Role of the Registered Dietitian in Patient-Client Care

Form small groups of students (i.e., two or three students each) and assign visits to a number of different-sized hospitals in the community. If possible, include a large medical center, a smaller community hospital, a nursing home, and a community health center. At each of these facilities, arrange for students to interview various dietitians about their roles in patient care. Include the following types of dietitians in your interviews if possible:

- Clinic dietitian in outpatient setting
- Administrative dietitian or dietary department director
- Clinical or patient care dietitian in hospital
- Consulting dietitian to nursing homes

- Consulting dietitian in private practice
- Public health nutritionist in public health department
- Nutritionist in community health center or health agency

Include the following questions in your interviews:

- What system of food service is being used?
- What is the dietitian's role in relation to other patient care personnel such as physicians, nurses, social workers, and others?
- What types of activities does he or she conduct with patients and staff?
- What relationship does he or she have with the hospital administrator or medical chief-of-staff?

Observe the tray service in the hospital. Note the form of tray service used, the types of diets served, and the nature of the foods used in each.

2. Feeding Disabled Patients or Children

Arrange with any available health care facility in the community to assist in the feeding of a disabled patient or small child. Select a variety of community settings such as nursing homes and hospitals.

Observe the patient's reaction and attitudes toward the food. What degree of feeding assistance did the patient require? What plan of feeding assistance worked best? If a rehabilitation center is available, visit the center and observe the variety of self-feeding devices used by the patients. If visiting a pediatric ward, notice the reactions of the children to the food being served.

In a follow-up class discussion, compare the findings of various students in different settings. What recommendations can be made from these experiences?

REFERENCES

1. Belanger M-C, Dube L: The emotional experience of hospitalization: its moderators and its role in patient satisfaction with food service, *J Am Diet Assoc* 96(4):354, 1996.

2. Gallacher-Allred CR and others: Malnutrition and clinical outcome: the case for medical nutrition therapy, *J Am Diet Assoc* 96(4):361, 1996.

3. Egbert AM: The dwindles: failure to thrive in older patients, *Nutr Rev* 54(1):S25, 1996.

FURTHER READING

- American Dietetic Association, Practice Report Panel: Practice report of the American Dietetic Association: home care—an emerging practice area for dietetics, *J Am Diet Assoc* 99(11):1453, 1999.

Home care, especially for the growing numbers of older persons in our population, is increasing and the accompanying need for nutritional and nursing care reflects this pressing situation. This excellent report identifies these needs and discusses possible ways of meeting them.

- Porter C and others: Dynamics of nutrition care among nursing home residents who are eating poorly, *J Am Diet Assoc* 99(11):1444, 1999.

This article in the same journal issue provides insight into the common problem of malnutrition among nursing home residents, and the apparently haphazard ways some staff members may respond, for example: (1) using liquid supplements for vitamins but not for minerals, (2) replacing regular meals with liquid supplement drinks, or (3) resorting to unpleasant and unethical measures such as force feeding.

18

Gastrointestinal Problems

KEY CONCEPTS

- Diseases of the gastrointestinal tract and its accessory organs interrupt the body's normal cycle of digestion, absorption, and metabolism.

- Allergic conditions produce sensitivity to certain food components.

- Underlying genetic diseases cause specific metabolic defects that block the body's ability to handle specific food nutrients.

We usually take for granted our highly organized and intricate body system for handling food. When something goes wrong with the system, however, it affects our whole being.

When we consider the gastrointestinal tract and its handling of the food we eat, we are looking at much more than the physical system—we are looking at the whole person. The overall system is a sensitive mirror, both directly and indirectly, of the individual human condition.

In this chapter, we look at the sensitive system that handles our food and its nutrients to provide energy and maintain body tissues. We must base our nutritional therapy not only on the functioning of this finely integrated network but also on the person whose life it affects.

THE UPPER GASTROINTESTINAL TRACT

Problems of the Mouth

Dental Problems

Although the incidence of dental caries has declined somewhat in the past few years, tooth decay still plagues children. Some of the decline results from increased use of fluoridated public water supplies and fluoridated toothpaste, as well as better dental hygiene. The use of refined sugars (i.e., mainly as corn sweeteners in processed foods), however, continues to increase as new products are developed. In elderly persons, loss of teeth or ill-fitting dentures may cause problems with chewing and thus digestion. Sometimes a *mechanical soft diet* is helpful. In such a diet, all foods are soft-cooked and meats are ground and mixed with sauces or gravies, so that less chewing is required.

Surgical Procedures

A fractured jaw or other mouth or neck surgery poses obvious eating problems. Healing nutrients must be supplied, usually in the form of high-protein, high-caloric liquids. Table 18-1 provides an example of a simple milkshake. Other commercial formulas are also available. As healing progresses, soft foods requiring little chewing effort can be added, building to a full diet according to individual tolerance.

Oral Tissue Inflammation

The tissues of the mouth often reflect a person's general nutritional status. Malnutrition, especially severe states, causes deterioration of oral tissues, resulting in local infection or injury that brings pain and difficulty in eating. The following conditions of malnutrition in the oral cavity affect all its parts:

- **Gingivitis**—Inflammation of the gums, involving the mucous membranes and its supporting fibrosis tissue circling the base of the teeth.
- **Stomatitis**—Inflammation of the oral mucus lining the mouth.
- **Glossitis**—Inflammation of the tongue.
- **Cheilosis**—A cracking and dry scaling process at the corners of the mouth affecting the lips and corner angles, making opening the mouth to eat very difficult.

Mouth ulcers may develop from three infectious sources: (1) *Herpes simplex virus*, which causes mouth sores on the inside mucous lining of the cheeks and lips or on the lips, where they are commonly called cold sores or fever blisters; (2) *Candida albicans*, a fungus causing similar sores on the oral mucosa, which is a condition called candidiasis or thrush; or (3) *Hemolytic streptococcus*, a type of bacteria causing similar mucosal ulcers that are commonly called canker sores. These conditions are usually self-limiting and short-lived. Other causes may range from a simple toothbrush abrasion or allergies

TABLE 18-1 High-protein, high-kilocalorie formula for liquid feedings

Ingredients	Amount	Approximate food value	
Milk	1 cup	Protein	40 g
Egg substitute	Equivalent of 2 eggs	Fat	30 g
Skimmed milk powder	6 to 8 tbsp	Carbohydrates	70 g
or Casec	2 tbsp	Kilocalories	710
Sugar	2 tbsp		
Ice cream	2.5 cm (1 in) slice or 1 scoop		
Cocoa or other flavoring	2 tbsp		
Vanilla	Few drops, as desired		

to a more serious underlying illness such as cancer, which lowers the body's immune system.

In any case, eating is painful and adequate nutrition becomes a major problem. High-protein, high-caloric liquids and then soft foods (e.g., usually nonacidic or less highly spiced to avoid irritation) are generally given. Extremes of temperature are avoided if they cause pain. Colder soft or liquid foods are usually better tolerated. In severe disease, as in cancer and its treatments, using a mouthwash containing a mild topical local anesthetic before meals helps to relieve the pain of eating.

Salivary Gland Problems

Disorders of the salivary glands in the mouth also affect eating and related nutritional status. Problems may arise from infection, such as the mumps virus that attacks the parotid gland. Other problems arise from excess salivation, which occurs in numerous disorders affecting the nervous system (e.g., Parkinson's disease), from local mouth infections or injury, or from drug reactions. Conversely, lack of salivation—which causes dry mouth—may be temporary, caused by fear, infection, or drug action. Permanent dry mouth, xerostomia, is rare but sometimes occurs in middle-aged women, often associated with rheumatoid arthritis. Xerostomia may also result from radiation therapy, which causes difficulty in swallowing and speaking, taste interference, and tooth decay. More liquid food items such as beverages, soups, stews, and the use of gravies or sauces may facilitate the eating process. Extreme mouth dryness may be partially relieved by spraying an artificial saliva solution inside the mouth.

Swallowing Disorders

Swallowing is not as simple an act as it may seem. It actually involves highly integrated actions of the mouth, pharynx, and esophagus and, once started, is beyond voluntary control. Swallowing difficulty, dysphagia, is a fairly common problem with a variety of causes. It may be only temporary (e.g., a piece of food lodged in the back of the throat), for which the Heimlich manuever is appropriate first aid, or it may be associated with insufficient production of

saliva and dry mouth. Such dysfunctional swallowing often causes persons to aspirate food particles, which may or may not be evident in coughing or choking episodes. Swallowing disorders have been observed in cases of head trauma or cancer, or simply from aging.[1]

It has been estimated that dysphagia affects about 35% of nursing home residents. Subtle symptoms include an unexplained drop in food intake or repeated episodes of pneumonia, possibly related to aspiration of food particles. Watch for warning signs of dysphagia and report them immediately. These signs may include a reluctance to eat certain food consistencies or any food at all, very slow chewing or eating, fatigue from eating, frequent throat clearing, complaints of food "sticking" in the throat, holding pockets of food in the cheeks,

---

parotid glands (Gr. *para,* beyond, beside; *ous,* ear) the largest of three pairs of salivary glands situated near the ear. The parotid glands lie, one on each side, above the angle of the jaw, below and in front of the ear. They continually secrete saliva, which passes along the duct of the gland and into the mouth through an opening in the inner cheek, level with the second upper molar tooth. Normal saliva flow facilitates the chewing and swallowing of food and prevents dry mouth problems.

xerostomia (Gr. *xeros,* dry; *stoma,* mouth) dryness of the mouth from lack of normal secretions.

pharynx (Gr. *pharynx,* throat) the muscular membranous passage between the mouth and the posterior nasal passages and the larynx and esophagus.

dysphagia (Gr. *dys-,* painful; *phagein,* to eat) difficulty in swallowing.

Heimlich maneuver a first-aid maneuver to relieve a person who is choking from blockage of the breathing passageway by a swallowed foreign object or food particle. Standing behind the person, clasp the victim around the waist, placing one fist just under the sternum (breastbone) and grasping the fist with the other hand. Then make a quick, hard, thrusting movement inward and upward to dislodge the object.

painful swallowing, drooling, and/or coughing or choking during attempts to eat.[1]

The problem is usually referred to a team of specialists that includes a physician, nurse, clinical dietitian, physical therapist, and an occupational therapist, who is especially important for possessing special training in swallowing problems. Thin liquids are the most difficult food forms to swallow. Thus the diet is adapted to individual needs, in stages of adding thickened liquids and pureed foods to a regular diet.[1]

Problems of the Esophagus

Central Tube Problems

The esophagus is a long muscular tube extending from the throat to the stomach. It is bounded on both ends by circular muscles, or *sphincters*, that act as valves to control food passage. The upper sphincter muscle remains closed except during swallowing, preventing airflow into the esophagus and stomach, then opens automatically when food is swallowed and recloses immediately. Various disorders along the tube may disrupt normal swallowing, including: (1) muscle spasms or uncoordinated contractions of the tube; and (2) stricture or narrowing of the tube caused by a scar from a previous injury due to infection, ingestion of caustic chemicals, a tumor, or *esophagitis*, which is an inflammation. These problems hinder eating and require medical attention through stretching procedures or surgery to widen the tube and drug therapy to heal the inflammation. For some elderly patients who also have other morbid disease (e.g., heart problems with increased risk), gastrologists have occasionally used botulism toxin as drug therapy to reduce smooth muscle tone in the gastrointestinal tract.[2] The diet during such problems is liquid to soft in texture, depending on the extent of the closure problem.

Lower Esophageal Sphincter Problems

Defects in the operation of the lower esophageal sphincter (LES) may come from changes in the smooth muscle itself or from the nerve-muscle hormone control of *peristalsis* (see Chapter 9). Spasms occur when the LES muscles maintain an excessively high muscle tone, even while resting, thus failing to open normally when the person swallows. This condition is medically termed *achalasia*, from its unrelaxed muscle state, but is commonly called cardiospasm, from the proximity of the heart, although it does not relate to the heart at all. Symptoms include swallowing problems, frequent vomiting, a feeling of fullness in the chest, weight loss from eating difficulty, serious malnutrition, and pulmonary complications and infection caused by aspiration of food particles, especially during sleep. Surgical treatment involves dilating the LES or slitting the muscle—a *esophagomyotomy*, which improves the stricture but not the peristalsis. The postoperative course starts with oral liquids and progresses to a regular diet within a few days, depending on tolerance. Patients should avoid very hot or cold foods, citrus juices, or highly spiced foods to prevent irritation, as well as to eat frequent small meals as tolerated. Patients should eat slowly in small bites and swallows.

Gastroesophageal Reflux Disease

Ongoing LES problems lead to chronic gastroesophageal reflux disease (GERD).[3,4] This problem of the constant regurgitation of acid gastric contents into the lower part of the esophagus creates constant tissue irritation and inflammation, *esophagitis*. GERD is a serious and difficult problem that physicians graphically describe as "acid setting up shop in the esophagus." They further indicate that the problem is more widespread than the number of cases reported, because only the "tip of the iceberg" of chronic sufferers seeks medical help. The gastric acid and pepsin cause tissue erosion, resulting in the most common symptom of frequent, severe heartburn that occurs 30 to 60 minutes after eating. The pain sometimes moves into the neck or jaw or down the arms. A hiatal hernia may or may not be present. In addition, the acid reflux may be caused by pregnancy, obesity, pernicious vomiting, or nasogastric tubes. The most common complications are *stenosis*, which is a narrowing or stricture of the esophagus, and esophageal ulcer.

Treatment for GERD and its relentless esophagitis includes weight management, because obesity is often a causative factor. Other conservative measures relate to acid control (e.g., sleeping, eating, and using antacids). Patients must avoid lying down after eating and must sleep with the head of the bed elevated. Frequent use of antacids helps control the symptoms. The goals and actions of dietary care are outlined in Table 18-2.

Hiatal Hernia

The lower end of the esophagus normally enters the chest cavity through an opening in the diaphragm membrane called the *hiatus*. A hiatal hernia occurs when a portion of the upper stomach also protrudes through this opening, as shown in Figure 18-1. Hiatal hernia is not an uncommon problem, especially in obese adults, for whom weight reduction is essential. They should eat small amounts of food at a time, avoid lying down after meals, and sleep with the head of the bed elevated to prevent reflux of acidic stomach contents. Frequent use of antacids helps control the symptoms of heartburn, which is due to the acid-enzyme-food mixture tissue irritating the lower esophagus and the upper herniated area of the stomach. From 85% to 90% of persons with this esophagitis and gastritis respond to weight reduction and conservative measures. Large hiatal hernias or smaller sliding hernias may require surgical repair. Loose-fitting clothing helps to relieve discomfort.

Problems of the Stomach and Duodenum: Peptic Ulcer Disease

Incidence

Throughout the world, peptic ulcer disease affects about 10% of the population. It can occur at any age but is seen mostly in middle adulthood, between the ages of 45 and 55. Gastric and duodenal ulcers, along with the complication of perforation, occur more often in men. Other diseases and injuries such as burns may cause so-called stress ulcers.

Causes

The underlying cause of peptic ulcer disease has been identified as *Helicobacter pylori* infection.[5,6] *H. pylori* are common spiraling, rod-shaped bacteria inhabiting the gastrointestinal area around the pyloric valve. This muscular valve connects the lower part of the stomach to the head of the small

TABLE 18-2   Dietary care of gastroesophageal reflux disease (GERD)

Goal	Action
Decrease esophageal irritation	Avoid common irritants such as coffee, carbonated beverages, tomato and citrus juices, and spicy foods
	Avoid any foods such as rich desserts that may cause heartburn
Increase lower esophageal sphincter pressure	Increase protein foods
	Decrease fat to about 45 g/day or less; use nonfat milk
	Avoid strong tea, coffee, and chocolate if poorly tolerated
	Avoid peppermint and spearmint
Decrease reflux frequency and volume	Eat small, frequent meals
	Sip only a small amount of liquid with meal; drink mostly between meals
	Avoid constipation; straining increases abdominal pressure reflux
Clear food materials from the esophagus	Sit upright at the table or elevate the head of bed
	Do not recline for 2 hours or more after eating

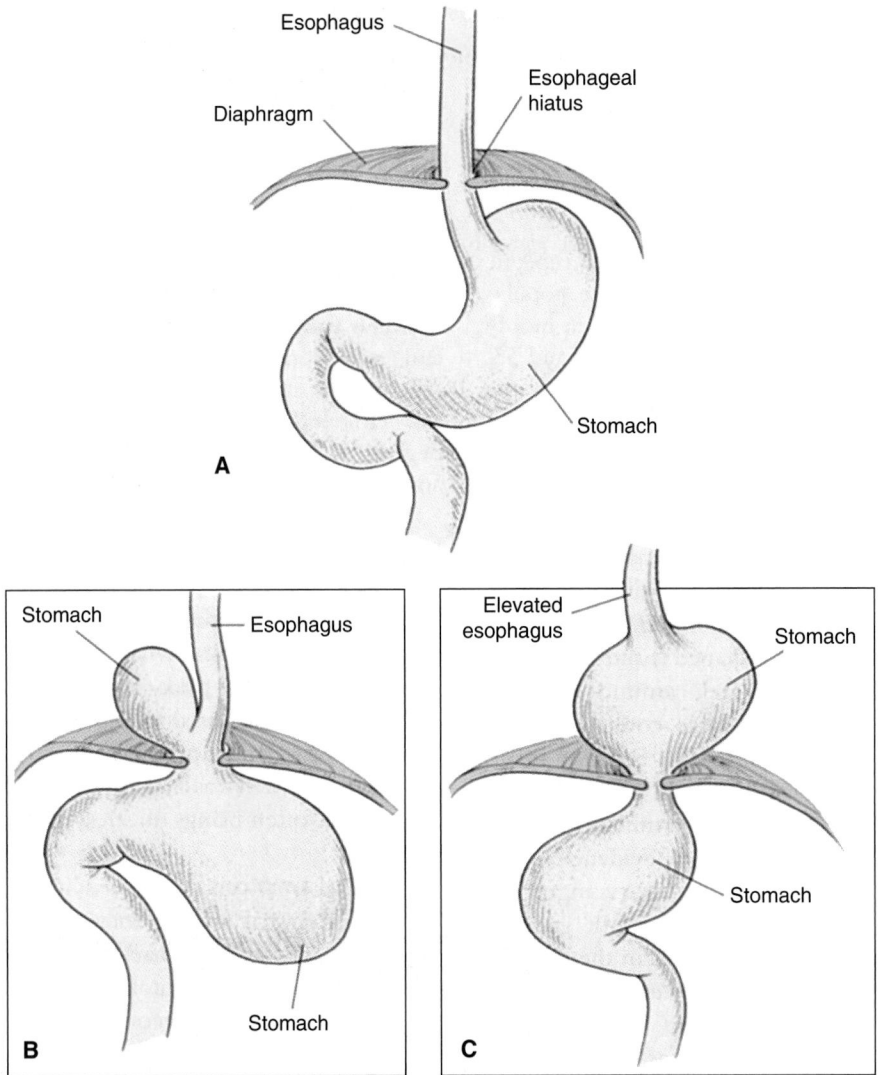

FIGURE 18-1 Hiatal hernia in comparison with normal stomach placement. **A,** Normal stomach. **B,** Paraesophageal hernia (esophagus in normal position). **C,** Esophageal hiatal hernia (elevated esophagus). (Credit: Bill Ober.)

intestine, the duodenal bulb. Infection by *H. pylori* is a major determinant of chronic active gastritis and is also a necessary ingredient, along with gastric acid and pepsin, in the ulcerative process. The third partner in the tissue damage is *nonsteroidal antiinflamatory drugs (NSAIDs)*. These widely used drugs include ibuprofen (Advil, Motrin), as well as aspirin (acethylsalicylic acid, ASA), which irritate the gastric mucosa and cause bleeding, erosion, and ulceration, especially with prolonged or excessive use. The NSAIDs, which include at least a dozen antiinflammatory drugs, are so named to distinguish

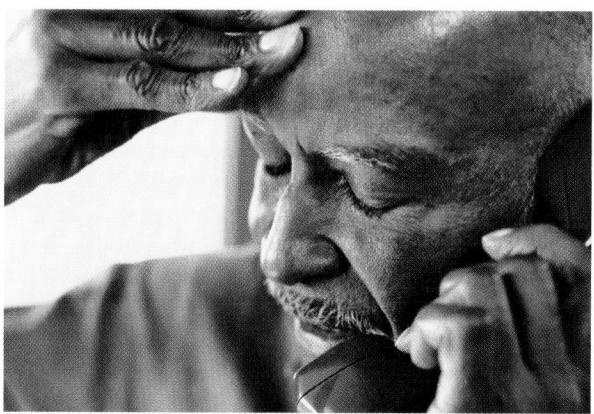

FIGURE 18-2   Stress may contribute to peptic ulcer disease in predisposed individuals. (From PhotoDisc.)

them from the steroid drugs, which are synthetic variants of the natural adrenal hormones. Some evidence also suggests a genetic factor because relatives of peptic ulcer patients have about three times as many ulcers as members of the general population. Both physical and psychologic factors, however, are clearly involved.

Physical Factors

The general term *peptic ulcer* refers to an eroded mucosal lesion in the central portion of the gastrointestinal tract. This lesion can occur in the lower esophagus, stomach, or first portion of the duodenum, the *duodenal bulb*. Most ulcers occur in the duodenal bulb, because the gastric contents emptying there are most concentrated. The lesion results from an imbalance between the following two factors: (1) the amount of gastric acid and pepsin (a powerful gastric enzyme for digestion of protein) secretions and the extent of the H. pylori infection; and (2) the degree of tissue resistance to these secretions and the infection.

Psychologic Factors

The influence of psychologic factors in the development of peptic ulcer varies. No distinct personality type is free from the disease. Stress during the young and middle adult years, however, when personal and career strivings are at a peak, may contribute to peptic ulcer development in predisposed individuals (Figure 18-2). The stress of emergency trauma and injury, as well as the long-term rehabilitation processes, often brings on stress ulcers.

Clinical Symptoms

General symptoms include increased gastric muscle tone and painful contractions when the stomach is empty. With duodenal ulcers, the amount and concentration of hydrochloric acid secretions are increased; with gastric ulcers, the secretions may be normal. Low plasma protein levels, anemia, and weight loss reveal nutritional deficiencies. Hemorrhage may be a first signal. Diagnosis is confirmed by x-ray tests and visualization by gastroscopy.

Medical Management

In treating patients with peptic ulcer disease, physicians have four basic goals, as follow: (1) to alleviate the symptoms, (2) to promote healing, (3) to prevent recurrences, and (4) to prevent complications. In addition to general traditional measures, the recently expanded knowledge base about the cause of peptic ulcer disease and the development of a number of new drugs have increased the physician's available management tools.[7]

Rest.   Adequate rest, relaxation, and sleep have long been the foundation of general care to enhance the body's natural healing process. Positive stress-coping and relaxation skills, which help patients deal with personal psychosocial stress factors, can be learned and practiced. Encouraging patients to talk about anxieties, anger, and frustrations helps them feel better. As soon as they are able, appropriate physical activity helps work out tensions. Habits that contribute to ulcer development, such as smoking and alcohol use, should be eliminated. Common drugs (e.g., aspirin) and NSAIDs (e.g., ibuprofen) should be avoided. Sometimes sedatives are prescribed to aid rest.

Drug therapy.   Advances in knowledge and therapy have currently provided physicians with four basic types of drugs for managing peptic ulcer disease.[8]

- **Blocking agents** (two types) that control acid secretion (e.g., cimetidine [Tagamet], ranitidine [Zantac]; and omeprazole [Prilosec]).
- **Mucosal protectors** that inactivate pepsin and produce a gel-like substance to cover the ulcer and protect it from acid and pepsin while it heals itself (e.g., sucralfate [Carafate]).
- **Antibiotics** that control the *H. pylori* bacterial infection (e.g., amoxicillin, tetracycline, and metronidazole).

- **Antacids** that counteract or neutralize the acid. Usually magnesium-aluminum compounds (e.g., Mylanta II or Maalox TC [therapeutic choice]) are the antacids of choice in treating peptic ulcer disease.

Maintenance drug therapy is imperative after large initial doses stabilize the growth rate of the bacteria. A continuous low dose drug therapy follows, with intermittent full-dose treatment or symptomatic self-care with the same agents used to heal the initial ulcer infection.[8] Success rates depend on the relative strengths of the risk factors that influence recurrence (Table 18-3).

Diet therapy.   Nutritional therapy for peptic ulcer has changed considerably. Its basic goal is to support healing and prevent further tissue damage.

Dietary Management

In the past, a highly restrictive, bland diet was used in the care of patients with peptic ulcer disease. A bland diet has long since proven to be ineffective and lacking in adequate nutritional support for the healing process. Such a restrictive diet is unnecessary today because newer and better drugs are available to control acid secretions and assist healing. Thus current diet therapy is based on a liberal individual approach, guided by individual responses to

TABLE 18-3   Risk factors for recurring peptic ulcer

Medical/Physical	Emotional	Behavioral
High risk		
Hypersecretion of gastric acid	Continuous, unrelieved emotional stress	Poor dietary habits
Previous recurrences of peptic ulcer with complications	Denial of emotional problems	Failure to maintain prescribed diet and drug therapy
		Cigarette smoking (10 or more per day)
Moderate risk		
Family history of peptic ulcer disease among close relatives	Emotionally stressful environment	Frequent use of aspirin and other NSAIDs
Recurring discomfort after eating	Recognition of emotional problems	Distilled alcohol consumption
		Irregular meals

any food. In this positive nutritional support for medical management, two basic goals guide food habits.

Eat a well-balanced healthy diet.   Supply a well-balanced regular healthy diet to aid tissue healing and maintenance. Nutrient-energy needs are outlined in the current RDAs and DRIs (see inside front book cover) and expressed in simple food choices in the Food Guide Pyramid (see Chapter 1). Further focus is supplied by the goals of the U.S. Dietary Guidelines (see Chapter 1).

Avoid acid stimulation.   Avoid stimulating excess gastric acid secretion, which irritates gastric mucosa. Only a few food-related habits have been shown to affect acid secretion:

- **Meal pattern**—Eat three regular meals a day without frequent snacks, especially at bedtime. Any food intake stimulates more acid output.
- **Food quantity**—Don't eat large quantities at a meal to avoid stomach distention.
- **Milk intake**—Avoid drinking milk frequently because it stimulates significant acid secretion, has only a transient buffering effect, and its animal fat content is undesirable. The milk sugar, lactose, also creates abdominal cramping, gas, and diarrhea for many persons with lactose intolerance caused by a deficiency of the enzyme lactase (see Chapter 2).
- **Seasonings**—Individual tolerance is the rule, but the following agents have caused variable results and may need to be watched: hot chili peppers, black pepper, and chili powder.
- **Dietary fiber**—There is no evidence for restricting dietary fiber. Some fibers, especially soluble forms, are beneficial.
- **Coffee**—Avoid regular and decaffeinated coffee. Coffee stimulates acid secretion and may cause indigestion. The comparative effect of regular tea and colas may be milder to some persons, but these beverages also stimulate acid secretion.

- **Citric acid juices**—These juices may cause gastric reflux and discomfort in some persons.
- **Alcohol**—Avoid alcohol in concentrated forms, such as 40% (80 proof) alcohol. Other less concentrated forms of wine, taken with food in moderation, are tolerated well by some persons. Avoid beer; it has been shown to be a potent stimulant of gastric acid. For those who find it difficult to avoid alcohol and coffee completely, a small glass of dinner wine occasionally or a small cup (*demitasse*) of coffee at the close of a meal may minimize the acid secretion.
- **Smoking**—The habit of smoking is often associated with food intake. It is best eliminated completely at any time as it hinders ulcer healing. It not only affects gastric acid secretion but also hinders the effectiveness of drug therapy.
- **Food environment**—Finally, consider the food environment. Eat slowly and savor the food in a calm environment. Respect individual responses or tolerances to specific foods. Remember that the same food may bring different responses at different times depending on stress factors.

In the long run, a wide range of foods that are attractive to the eye and taste and regular, unhurried eating habits provide the best course of action.

THE LOWER GASTROINTESTINAL TRACT
Small Intestine Diseases

Malabsorption and Diarrhea
General diarrhea usually results from basic dietary excesses. The fermentation of sugars involved or excess dietary fiber can stimulate intestinal motility. In some cases, diarrhea may result from intolerance to specific foods or nutrients, as in lactose intolerance (see Chapter 2) or acute food poisoning from a specific food-borne organism or toxin (see

Chapter 13). So-called "traveler's diarrhea," from irregular meals, unfamiliar foods, and travel tensions, is a well-known syndrome.[9] Diarrhea in infants is a more serious problem, especially if it is prolonged, that can quickly lead to dehydration and nutrient losses and is associated with infection. Intravenous fluid and electrolyte replacement may be necessary, or an oral solution of water, glucose, and electrolytes (e.g., Polycose [Ross]) may be used. As soon as it is tolerated, a regular refeeding schedule is needed to avoid malnutrition.

Malabsorption

There are multiple causes of malabsorption.[10] Some of these causes include the following:

- **Maldigestion problems**—Pancreatic disorders, biliary disease, bacterial overgrowth, ileal disease (inflammatory bowel disease)
- **Intestinal mucosal changes**—Mucosal surface alterations, intestinal surgery (e.g., as resections that shorten the bowel and absorbing surface area)
- **Genetic disease**—Cystic fibrosis with its complications of pancreatic insufficiency and lack of pancreatic enzymes
- **Intestinal enzyme deficiency**—Lactose intolerance caused by lactose deficiency (see Chapter 2)
- **Cancer and its treatment**—Absorbing surface effect of radiation and chemotherapy (see Chapter 23)
- **Metabolic defects**—Absorbing surface effects of pernicious anemia or gluten-induced mucosal disease (e.g., celiac sprue)

Four of these malabsorption conditions—celiac sprue, cystic fibrosis, inflammatory bowel disease, and short bowel syndrome—are reviewed here.

---

steatorrhea (Gr. *steatos,* fat; *rhoia,* flow) fatty diarrhea; excessive amounts of fat in the feces often caused by malabsorption diseases.

Celiac Sprue

Disease process. The childhood disorder *celiac disease* and the similar adult disease *nontropical sprue* are now known to be a single disease, so the condition is now called *celiac sprue*. In all cases, the cause is a sensitivity to the protein gluten in certain grains. The eroded mucosal surface shows villi that are malformed and deficient in number with few microvilli. This damaged mucosa effectively reduces the absorbing surface by as much as 95%. The underlying cause is as yet unknown but probably involves an enzyme deficiency and a genetic base. The major symptom of steatorrhea (e.g., about 80% of the ingested fat appears in the stools) and the progressive malnutrition are secondary effects. The primary cause is the reaction to gluten.

Nutritional management. The goal of nutritional management is to control the dietary gluten and prevent malnutrition. Wheat and rye are the main sources of gluten, but it is also present in oats and barley. Thus these grains are eliminated from the diet; corn and rice are the substitute grains used. Careful label reading is important for parents and children to learn, because many commercial products use the offending grains as thickeners or fillers. With an increasing number of processed foods and ethnic dishes now being used, it is difficult to detect all food sources of gluten, so a home test kit for gluten has been developed. A food plan generally based on the low-gluten diet given in Table 18-4 is followed.

Cystic Fibrosis

Disease process. Cystic fibrosis (CF) is the most common fatal disease in North America. It is a generalized genetic disease of childhood, occurring mainly in white populations in which 1 in 20 persons is a carrier and now 1 in 2500 newborns is affected. In past years, children with CF generally lived to about age 10, dying from complications such as damaged airways and lung infections, as well as a fibrous pancreas and lack of essential pancreatic enzymes to digest nutrients. Recent discovery of the CF gene

TABLE 18-4 Low-gluten diet for children with celiac disease

Dietary principles

- Kcalories—high, usually about 20% above normal requirement, to compensate for fecal loss
- Protein—high, usually 6 to 8 g/kg body weight
- Fat—low, but not fat-free, because of impaired absorption
- Carbohydrates—simple, easily digested sugars (fruits, vegetables) should provide about one half of the kcalories
- Feedings—small, frequent feedings during ill periods; afternoon snack for older children
- Texture—smooth, soft, avoiding irritating roughage initially, using strained foods longer than usual for age, adding whole foods as tolerated and according to age of child
- Vitamins—supplements of B vitamins, vitamins A and B in water-miscible forms, and vitamin C
- Minerals—iron supplements if anemia is present

Food groups	Foods included	Foods excluded
Milk	Milk (plain or flavored with chocolate or cocoa)	Malted milk; preparations such as Cocomalt, Hemo, Postum, Nestle's chocolate
	Buttermilk	
Meat or substitute	Lean meat, trimmed well of fat	Fat meats (sausage, pork)
	Eggs, cheese	Luncheon meats, corned beef, frankfurters, all common prepared meat products with any possible wheat filler
	Poultry, fish	
	Creamy peanut butter (if tolerated)	Duck, goose
		Smoked salmon
		Meat prepared with bread, crackers, or flour
Fruits and juices	All cooked and canned fruits and juices	Prunes, plums (unless tolerated)
	Frozen or fresh fruits as tolerated, with no skins and seeds	
Vegetables	All cooked, frozen, canned as tolerated (prepared *without* wheat, rye, oat, or barley products); raw as tolerated	Any causing individual discomfort
		All prepared with wheat, rye, oat, or barley products
Cereals	Corn or rice	Wheat, rye, oat, barley; any product containing these cereals
Breads, flours, cereal products	Breads, pancakes, or waffles made with suggested flours (cornmeal, cornstarch; rice, soybean, lima bean, potato, buckwheat)	All bread or cracker products made with gluten; wheat, rye, oat, barley, macaroni, noodles, spaghetti; any sauces, soups, or gravies prepared with gluten flour, wheat, rye, oat, or barley
Soups	Broth, bouillon (no fat or cream; no thickening with wheat, rye, oat, or barley products); soups and sauces may be thickened with cornstarch	All soups containing wheat, rye, oat, or barley products

TABLE 18-5 Levels of nutritional care for management of cystic fibrosis

Levels of care	Patient groups	Nutrition actions
Level I—Routine care	All	Diet counseling, food plans, enzyme replacement, vitamin supplements, nutrition education, exploration of problems
Level II—Anticipatory guidance	Above 90% ideal weight-height index, but at risk for energy imbalance; severe pancreatic insufficiency; frequent pulmonary infections; normal periods of rapid growth	Increased monitoring of dietary intake, complete energy-nutrient analysis, increased kcaloric density as needed; assess behavioral needs; provide counseling, nutrition education
Level III—Supportive intervention	85%-90% ideal weight-height index, decreased weight-growth velocity	Reinforce all the above actions, add energy-nutrient–dense oral supplements
Level IV—Rehabilitative care	Consistently below 85% ideal weight-height index, nutritional and growth failure	All of the above plus enteral nutrition support by nasoenteric or enterostomy tube feeding (see Chapter 22)
Level V—Resuscitative or palliative care	Below 75% ideal weight-height index, progressive nutritional failure	All of the above plus continuous enteral tube feedings or TPN (see Chapter 22)

Adapted from CFF consensus report: Ramsey B and others: Nutrition assessment and management in cystic fibrosis: a consensus report, *Am J Clin Nutr* 55:108, 1992. © Am J Clin Nutr, American Society for Clinical Nutrition.

and the underlying metabolic defect, however, has brought increased scientific knowledge, which has led to improved management of the disease and helped push the life expectancy up into the 30s or 40s.

The metabolic defect associated with CF affects the normal movement of chloride (Cl^-) and sodium (Na^+) ions in body tissue fluids (see Chapter 8). These ions become trapped in cells, causing thick mucus to form that clogs ducts and passageways. Involved organ tissues are damaged so that they no longer function normally. The classic CF symptoms include the following effects in body organ systems:

- **Thick mucus in the lungs,** which leads to damaged airways, more difficult breathing, and lung infections.
- **Pancreatic insufficiency,** which leads to lack of normal pancreatic enzymes (see Chapter 9) to digest the macronutrients and progressive loss of insulin-producing beta cells and eventual insulin-dependent diabetes mellitus (see Chapter 20).
- **Malabsorption** of undigested food nutrients, which brings about extensive malnutrition and stunted growth.

- **Liver disease** caused by clogging of bile ducts, which causes degeneration of functional liver tissue.
- **Salt (NaCl) concentration** increased in body perspiration, which brings about salt depletion.

Nutritional management. Current nutritional management of CF follows the guidelines developed by the U.S. Cystic Fibrosis Foundation. This treatment program is based on the following three factors: (1) increased knowledge of the disease process, (2) early newborn screening and diagnosis, and (3) improved pancreatic–enzyme-replacement products. These products, such as Pancrease (McNeil), contain the normal pancreatic enzymes for each energy nutrient (e.g., lipase for fat digestion, amylase for starch digestion, and the protein enzymes trypsin, chymotrypsin, and carboxypeptidase [see Chapter 9]). These enzymes are processed into very small enteric-coated beads encased in capsules that are designed not to open or dissolve until they reach the alkaline medium of the intestine. Generous doses of these special enzyme-replacement capsules, varying with a child's age (e.g., an average of about 25 to 30 capsules per

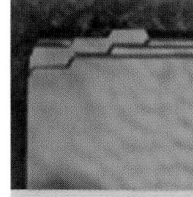

CLINICAL APPLICATIONS

Case Study: Paul's Adaptation to Cystic Fibrosis

Paul is a 12-year-old boy with cystic fibrosis. He is hospitalized with pneumonia and has difficulty breathing. Paul is a thin child with little muscle development who tires easily, although he has a large appetite. His stools are large and frequent and contain undigested food material.

Questions for Analysis

1. What is cystic fibrosis? Account for the clinical effects of the disease as evidenced by Paul's appearance and symptoms.
2. What are the basic goals of treatment in cystic fibrosis? Why is vigorous nutritional therapy

a main part of treatment? Describe the current role of enzyme-replacement therapy in this aggressive nutritional support.

3. Outline a day's food plan for Paul. Check the amount of protein and kcalories by calculating the total food values in your food plan to ensure the extra amount he needs is provided.
4. Why does Paul require therapeutic doses of multivitamins, including B complex vitamins? Why does he need to have these in water-soluble form?

---

day), are divided between the three meals and usually taken just before eating. Adequate enzyme replacement is the foundation that makes aggressive diet therapy to meet growth needs possible.

Children with CF require from 105% to 150% of the recommended nutrients for age, depending on the severity of the disease. The former low-fat diet is no longer used. Instead, a nutritionally adequate high protein, normal-to-high fat diet is recommended and provides about 20% of the kcalories as protein, 40% as carbohydrate, and 40% as fat. Routine care is based on regular nutrition assessment, diet counseling, food plans, enzyme replacement, vitamin supplements, nutrition education, and exploration of individual problems, as outlined in Table 18-5. Try applying these principles of care in the Clinical Application box, "Case Study: Paul's Adaption to Cystic Fibrosis". This specialized care is administered by the medical genetics division of community hospitals, with a team of CF specialists and their staff assistants using specific guidelines provided by the U.S. Cystic Fibrosis Foundation.

Inflammatory Bowel Disease

The term *inflammatory bowel disease* applies to both *ulcerative colitis* and *Crohn's disease*. The related condition *short-bowel syndrome* results from repeated surgical removal of parts of the small intestine as the disease progresses. All of these conditions can have severe, often devastating, nutritional results as more and more of the absorbing surface area becomes involved. Restoring positive nutrition is a basic requirement for tissue healing and health. Elemental formulas of amino acids, glucose, fat, minerals, and vitamins are more easily absorbed and support

---

elemental formula a nutrition support formula composed of simple elemental nutrient components that require no further digestive breakdown and are thus readily absorbed; formulas with the protein as free amino acids and the carbohydrate as the simple sugar glucose.

initial healing in response to antibacterial and anti-inflammatory medications. The diet is gradually advanced to restore optimal nutrient intake. The principles of continuing dietary management include the following: (1) high-protein, about 100 g/day, omitting milk at first because it causes difficulty in many patients; (2) high-energy, about 2500 to 3000 kcal; (3) increased vitamins and minerals, usually with supplements.[11,12]

The former practice of reducing fiber or residue in the diet has been questioned. The bland, low-residue diets of the past have mainly been based on tradition or anecdotal belief rather than scientific studies on humans. These diets tended to be less appetizing and nourishing than regular diets. Current study and clinical practice indicate the benefit of a regular nourishing diet, respecting individual tolerances and disease status. A close working relationship among the team of physician, clinical dietitian, and nurse is essential. The appetite is poor, but adequate nutritional intake is imperative. A range of feeding modes, including enteral and parenteral nutrition support as needed, are explored in individual cases to achieve the vigorous nutritional care required. But whatever the mode of feeding, it must always be provided with personal support, warmth, and encouragement.

Large Intestine Diseases

Diverticular Disease

Diverticulosis is an lower intestinal condition characterized by the formation of many small pouches, or pockets, along the muscular mucosal lining, usually in the colon. These little pouches are called *diverticula*. Most often they occur in older persons and develop at points of weakened muscles in the bowel wall, along the track of blood vessels entering the bowel from without. The direct cause is a progressive increase in pressure within the bowel from segmental circular muscle contractions that normally move the remaining food mass along and form the feces for elimination. When pressures become sufficiently high in one of these segments and there is insufficient fiber to maintain the necessary

bulk for preventing these high internal pressures within the colon, small diverticula develop. When these pockets become infected, a condition called *diverticulitis,* pain develops in the affected area. The commonly used collective term covering diverticulosis and diverticulitis is *diverticular disease.* As the inflammatory process grows, increased pain and tenderness are localized in the lower left side of the abdomen and are accompanied by nausea, vomiting, distention, diarrhea, intestinal spasm, and fever. Sometimes perforation occurs, and surgery is indicated. There may also often be underlying malnutrition. Aggressive nutritional therapy hastens recovery from an attack, shortens the hospital stay, and reduces costs. Current studies and clinical practice have demonstrated better management of chronic diverticular disease with an increased amount of dietary fiber rather than with the older practice of restricting fiber.[13]

Irritable Bowel Syndrome

This general stress-related disorder of the intestine occurs most frequently among women aged 45 to 64. Gastroenterologists currently estimate that 15% to 20% of the general U.S. population have problems consistent with the condition now called *irritable bowel syndrome (IBS)*. About 5% of these persons seek medical help and become patients. Although IBS is one of the most common gastrointestinal disorders, its precise nature and cause continue to puzzle practitioners. Accumulating evidence indicates, however, that IBS is a true disorder of function, with true symptoms that are neither imagined nor the result of a psychiatric disorder.[14] Medical guidelines define IBS as a functional (i.e., medical), nonorganic disorder displaying three major types of symptoms, as follow: (1) chronic and recurrent pain in any area of the abdomen; (2) small-volume bowel dysfunction, varying from constipation or diarrhea to a combination of both; and (3) excess gas formation with increased distention and bloating, accompanied by rumbling abdominal sounds, belching, and passing of gas (see Chapter 9). Patients appear tense and anxious, and stress is a major triggering factor. The transference of anxiety to body symptoms is common. A highly individual and personal approach to nutritional care is essential, based on careful nutrition assessment (see Chapter 17). Guided by this personal food and symptoms pattern, a reasonable food plan can be devised with the patient. In general, the food plan should give attention to the following basic principles:

- **Increase dietary fiber**—A regular diet with optimal energy-nutrient composition and dietary fiber food sources (e.g., whole grains, legumes, fruits, and vegetables) provides basic therapy (Table 18-6).
- **Recognize gas formers**—Some foods are recognized gas formers because of known constituents (e.g., indigestible short chains of glucose [oligsaccharides] in the case of legumes [see Chapter 2]). Others may cause gaseous discomfort on an individual basis.
- **Respect food intolerances**—Lactose intolerance, for example, in people who lack the digestive enzyme lactase is well known (see Chapter 2).
- **Reduce total fat content**—Excess fat delays gastric emptying and contributes to malabsorption problems.
- **Avoid large meals**—Large amounts of food in one meal create discomfort from gastric distention and gas. Smaller, more frequent meals usually reduce these symptoms.
- **Decrease air-swallowing habits**—These habits include eating rapidly and in large amounts, excessive fluid intake—especially of carbonated beverages, and gum-chewing.

Experienced practitioners have learned that in helping patients manage IBS, an honest and creative relationship is essential. Two such approaches include avoiding dogma and helping the patient to cope. Lifestyle and diet are highly personal and individual, and wise nutrition management involves both in realistic counseling toward a healthier life.

Constipation

This general complaint, real or imagined, is common. Americans spend a quarter of a billion dollars each year on laxatives to treat their so-called regularity problem. Intestinal elimination is highly individual, however, and a daily bowel movement is not necessary for good health. This common short-term problem usually results from various sources of nervous tension and worry, changes in routines, constant laxative use, low-fiber diets, or lack of exercise. Improved diet, exercise, and bowel habits usually remedy the situation. Any regular laxative or enema habit should be avoided. The diet should include increased fiber, naturally laxative fruits (e.g., dried prunes and figs), and adequate fluid intake, based on the assessment of current fiber and fluid intake, as well as any diuretic drug use. For example, bowel obstruction was reported in a man receiving diuretic therapy for hypertension bowel obstruction who ate excess bran cereal (e.g., a large bowl of about 20 g daily).[14] Constipation occurs at all ages but is almost epidemic among elderly persons. In all cases, a personalized approach to management is fundamental.

FOOD ALLERGIES AND INTOLERANCES

Food Allergies

The Problem of Allergy

Several conditions may cause certain food allergies or intolerances. The underlying problem is genetic or relates to the body's immune system. The word *allergy* comes from two Greek words meaning "altered

---

diverticulitis (L *divertere,* to turn aside) inflammation of pockets of tissue (diverticula) in the lining of the mucous membrane of the colon.

allergy (Gr. *allos,* other; *ergon,* work) a state of hypersensitivity to particular substances in the environment that work on the body tissues to produce problems in functions of affected tissues; the agent involved (allergen) may be a certain food eaten or a substance (e.g., pollen) inhaled.

TABLE 18-6 Dietary fiber and kilocalorie values for selected foods

Foods	Serving	Dietary fiber (g)	Kcalories
Breads and cereals			
All Bran	⅓ cup	8.5	70
Bran (100%)	½ cup	8.4	75
Bran Buds	⅓ cup	7.9	75
Corn Bran	⅔ cup	5.4	100
Bran Chex	⅔ cup	4.6	90
Cracklin' Oat Bran	⅓ cup	4.3	110
Bran Flakes	¾ cup	4.0	90
Air-popped popcorn	1 cup	2.5	25
Oatmeal	1 cup	2.2	144
Grapenuts	¼ cup	1.4	100
Whole-wheat bread	1 slice	1.4	60
Legumes, cooked			
Kidney beans	½ cup	7.3	110
Lima beans	½ cup	4.5	130
Vegetables, cooked			
Green peas	½ cup	3.6	55
Corn	½ cup	2.9	70
Parsnip	½ cup	2.7	50
Potato, with skin	1 medium	2.5	95
Brussels sprouts	½ cup	2.3	30
Carrots	½ cup	2.3	25
Broccoli	½ cup	2.2	20
Beans, green	½ cup	1.6	15
Tomato, chopped	½ cup	1.5	17
Cabbage, red & white	½ cup	1.4	15
Kale	½ cup	1.4	20
Cauliflower	½ cup	1.1	15
Lettuce (fresh)	1 cup	0.8	7
Fruits			
Apple	1 medium	3.5	80
Raisins	¼ cup	3.1	110
Prunes, dried	3	3.0	60
Strawberries	1 cup	3.0	45
Orange	1 medium	2.6	60
Banana	1 medium	2.4	105
Blueberries	½ cup	2.0	40
Dates, dried	3	1.9	70
Peach	1 medium	1.9	35
Apricot, fresh	3 medium	1.8	50
Grapefruit	½ cup	1.6	40
Apricot, dried	5 halves	1.4	40
Cherries	10	1.2	50
Pineapple	½ cup	1.1	40

Adapted from Lanza E, Butrum RR: A critical review of food fiber analysis and data, *J Am Diet Assoc* 86:732, 1986.

reactivity" and refers to the abnormal reactions of the immune system to a number of substances in our environment. A particular allergic condition results from a disorder of the immune system (i.e., immunity "gone wrong").

Common Food Allergens

Sensitivity to protein is a common basis for food allergy. The three most common food allergens are milk, egg, and wheat. Therefore the early foods of infants and children are often offenders in sensitive individuals, so substitute milk products—usually with a soy base—are used. In an allergic child's diet, solid foods are usually added slowly to the original formula, with common offenders excluded in early feedings. In some cases, a process of *food elimination* is used to identify offending foods. A core of less-often offending foods is used at first, then other single foods are gradually added to test the response. If a given food causes the allergic reaction to return, the food is then identified as an allergen and eliminated from use. The food may be tried again later to see if it still causes the same reaction, validating the initial response. If so, the food is eliminated. In the case of peanuts, however, a research team at Johns Hopkins, noting the allergic reaction encountered from the small packet of peanuts on commercial airlines, is currently developing an oral vaccine to induce tolerance in persons with peanut allergy.[15]

It is helpful to refer any person with food allergies to a clinical nutritionist (RD) to provide family support, education, and counseling. Guidance on food substitutions or special food products and modified recipes to maintain nutritional needs for growth are necessary. Children tend to become less allergic as they grow older, but family education about the label reading of all food products and cooking guides is essential from the beginning.

Genetic Disease and Food Intolerances

The Genetic Defect

Certain food intolerances stem from underlying genetic disease. In each genetic disease, the specific cell enzyme (all enzymes are proteins) controlling the cell's metabolism of a specific nutrient is missing, thus blocking the normal handling of the nutrient at that point. Three examples of genetic defects are phenylketonuria, galactosemia, and lactose intolerance.

Phenylketonuria. Phenylketonuria (PKU) results from the missing enzyme that breaks down the essential amino acid phenylalanine to tyrosine, another amino acid. If left untreated, this condition causes profound mental retardation and central nervous system damage, with irritability, hyperactivity, convulsive seizures, and bizarre behavior. Today mandatory newborn-screening programs in all areas of the United States can identify these babies, so treatment is started immediately. With treatment, these babies grow normally and have healthy lives. The treatment is a low-phenylalanine diet, using special formulas and low-protein food products. Much family counseling by the metabolic team at each care center is also needed.

Galactosemia. This genetic disease affects carbohydrate metabolism. The missing cell enzyme is one that converts galactose to glucose. Because galactose comes from the breakdown of lactose (milk sugar), all sources of lactose in an infant's diet must be eliminated. When not treated, this condition causes brain and liver damage. Newborn screening programs also identify these babies, so treatment can begin immediately to avoid such damage and enable the child to grow normally. Treatment is a galactose-free diet, with special formulas and lactose-free food guides.

Lactose intolerance. A deficiency of any one of the disaccharidases (e.g., lactase, sucrase, or maltase) in the small intestine may produce a wide range of GI problems and abdominal pain because the specific sugar involved cannot be digested. Lactose intolerance is the most common. In this condition, there is insufficient lactase to break down the milk sugar lactose, so the lactose accumulates in the intestine, causing abdominal cramping and diarrhea. Milk and all products containing lactose are carefully avoided. Milk treated with a commercial lactase product or soy milk products are substitutes.

PROBLEMS OF THE GASTROINTESTINAL ACCESSORY ORGANS

Three major accessory organs lie beside the gastrointestinal tract. These organs—the liver, gallbladder, and pancreas—produce important digestive agents that enter the intestine and aid in the handling of food substances (Figure 18-3). Diseases of these organs easily affect normal GI function and cause problems with the handling of specific types of food. The normal structure of the liver's functional units, the *lobule* and its cells, is shown in Figure 18-4.

Liver Disease

Hepatitis

Acute hepatitis is an inflammatory condition caused by viruses, alcohol, drugs, or toxins. The viral agent of the infection is transmitted by the oral-fecal route, which is common in many epidemic diseases. The carrier is usually contaminated food or water. In other cases, the virus may be transmitted by transfusions of infected blood or contaminated syringes or needles. Symptoms include anorexia and jaundice, with underlying malnu-

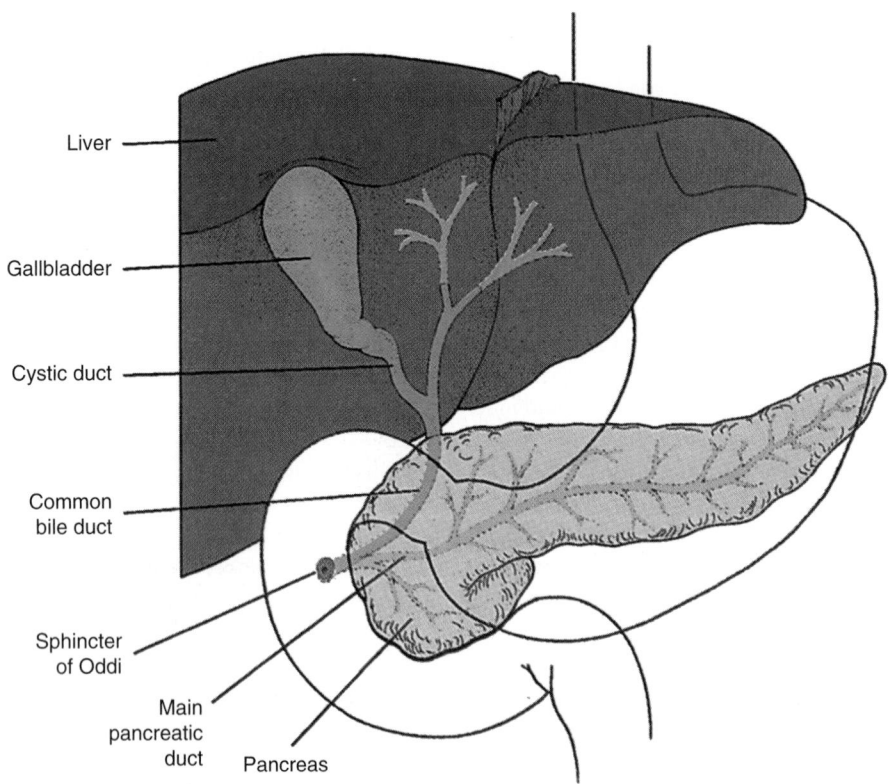

Liver

Gallbladder

Cystic duct

Common bile duct

Sphincter of Oddi

Main pancreatic duct   Pancreas

FIGURE 18-3 Biliary system organs.

trition. Treatment is based on bedrest and nutritional therapy to support healing of the involved liver tissue (Box 18-1). The following requirements govern the principles of the diet therapy and relate to the liver's function in metabolizing each nutrient:

- **High-protein**—Protein is essential for building new liver cells and tissues. It also combines with fats and removes them, preventing damage from fatty infiltration in liver tissue. The diet should supply 75 to 100 g of high quality protein daily.
- **High-carbohydrate**—Available glucose restores protective glycogen reserves in the liver. It also helps meet the energy demands of the disease process, as well as preventing the breakdown of protein for energy, thus ensuring its use for the vital tissue-building necessary for healing. The diet should supply 300 to 400 g of carbohydrate daily.

- **Moderate fat**—Some fat helps season food to encourage eating despite a poor appetite. A moderate amount of easily used fat, from milk products and vegetable oil, is beneficial. The diet should incorporate 100 to 150 g of such fat daily.
- **High-energy**—From 2500 to 3000 kcalories are needed daily to meet energy demands. This increased amount is necessary to support the healing process, to make up losses from fever and general debilitation, and to renew strength for recuperating from the disease.
- **Meals and feedings**—At first, liquid feedings (e.g., milkshakes high in protein and kcalories [see Table 18-1]) may be necessary or special formula products frequently used. As a patient's appetite and food tolerance improve, a full diet as already described is needed, observing likes and dislikes and planning ways to encourage an optimal food intake. Nutrition is the basic therapy (see the Clinical

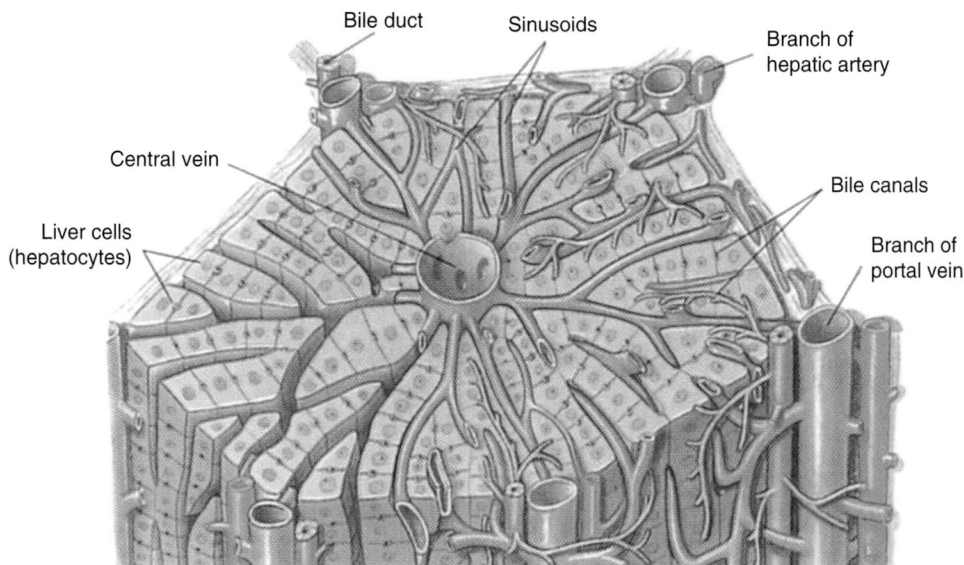

FIGURE 18-4   Liver structure showing hepatic lobule and hepatic cell. (Credit: Medical and Scientific Illustration.)

BOX 18-1 High-protein, high-carbohydrate, moderate-fat daily diet

1 L (1 qt) of milk
¼ cup egg substitute (e.g., Egg Beaters)
224 g (8 oz) lean meat, fish, poultry
4 servings vegetables:
   2 servings potato or substitute
   1 serving green leafy or yellow vegetable
   1 to 2 servings of other vegetables, including 1 raw
3 to 4 servings fruit (include juices often):
   1 to 2 citrus fruits (or other good source of ascorbic acid)
   2 servings other fruit
6 to 8 servings bread and cereal (whole grain or enriched):
   1 serving cereal
   5 to 6 slices bread, crackers
2 to 4 tbsp butter or fortified margarine
Additional jam, jelly, honey, and other carbohydrate foods as patient desires and is able to eat them
Sweetened fruit juices to increase both carbohydrate and fluid

Applications Box, "Case Study: Bill's Bout with Infectious Hepatitis").

Cirrhosis

Liver disease may advance to a chronic state of cirrhosis (Figure 18-5). The most common problem is fatty cirrhosis associated with malnutrition and alcoholism. This relentless malnutrition leads to multiple nutritional deficiencies as drinking alcohol increasingly substitutes for eating meals. Alcohol and its metabolic products can also cause direct damage to liver cells. The accompanying fatty infiltration kills liver cells, and only non-functioning fibrous scar tissue remains. Low plasma protein levels eventually fall causing *ascites*—abdominal fluid accumulation. Scar tissue impairs blood circulation, resulting in elevated venous blood pressure and esophageal *varices*. The rupture of these enlarged veins with massive hemorrhage is often the cause of death. When alcoholism is the underlying problem, treatment is difficult. Nutritional therapy focuses on as much healing support as possible.

- **Protein according to tolerance**—In the absence of impending hepatic coma, the diet should supply 80 to 100 g of protein per day to correct the severe malnutrition, heal liver tissue, and restore plasma proteins. If signs of coma begin, the protein will have to be reduced according to individual tolerance.

- **Low-sodium**—Sodium is restricted to 500 to 1000 mg per day to help reduce the fluid retention (ascites).

- **Soft texture**—If esophageal varices develop, soft foods help prevent the danger of rupture and hemorrhage.

- **Optimal general nutrition**—The remaining diet principles outlined for hepatitis are continued for cirrhosis for the same reasons. Kcalories, carbohydrates, and vitamins—especially B-complex vitamins including thiamin and folate—are important. Moderate fat is used. Alcohol is forbidden.

Hepatic Coma

One of the main functions of the liver is to remove ammonia, and hence nitrogen (see Chapter 4), from the blood by converting it to urea for

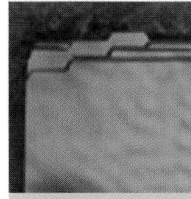

CLINICAL APPLICATIONS

Case Study: Bill's Bout with Infectious Hepatitis

Bill is a college student who spent part of his summer vacation in Mexico. Shortly after he returned home, he began to feel ill. He had little energy, no appetite, and severe headaches. Nothing he ate seemed to agree with him. He felt nauseated, began to have diarrhea, and soon developed a fever. He began to show evidence of jaundice.

Bill was hospitalized for diagnosis and treatment, and his tests indicated impaired liver function. His liver and spleen were enlarged and tender. The physician's diagnosis was infectious hepatitis. Bill's hospital diet was high in proteins, carbohydrates, and kcalories and moderately low in fats, but Bill had difficulty eating. He had no appetite, and food seemed to nauseate him even more.

Questions for Analysis

1. What are the normal functions of the liver in relation to the metabolism of carbohydrates, proteins, and fats? What other nutrient functions does the liver have?

2. What is the relationship of the normal liver functions to the effects or clinical symptoms that Bill experienced during his illness?

3. Why does vigorous nutritional therapy in liver disease (e.g., hepatitis) present a problem in planning a diet?

4. Outline a day's food plan for Bill. Calculate the amount of kcalories and protein to ensure that he is getting the necessary amount.

5. What vitamins and minerals would be significant aspects of Bill's nutritional therapy? Why?

---

urinary excretion. When cirrhosis continues and fibrous scar tissue replaces more and more normal liver tissue, the blood can no longer circulate normally through the liver. Therefore other vessels develop around this scar tissue, bypassing the liver. The blood, carrying its ammonia load, cannot get to the liver for its normal removal of the ammonia and nitrogen but instead must follow the bypass and proceed to the brain, producing ammonia intoxication and coma. The resulting *hepatic encephalopathy* brings about apathy, confusion, inappropriate behavior, and drowsiness, progressing to coma. Treatment focuses on removing the sources of excess ammonia. Because ammonia is a nitrogen compound and its main source is protein, the main dietary goal is to reduce protein intake. Table 18-7 provides a guide for reducing the diet's protein to 15 g/day, with additional increases according to individual tolerance.

Gallbladder Disease

Function

The basic function of the gallbladder is to concentrate and store bile and then release the concentrated bile into the small intestine when fat is present there. In the intestine, the bile emulsifies the fat, preparing it for initial digestion, then carries it into the cells of the intestinal wall for its continued metabolism.

Cholecystitis and Cholelithiasis

Inflammation of the gallbladder, *cholecystitis*, usually results from a low-grade chronic infection.

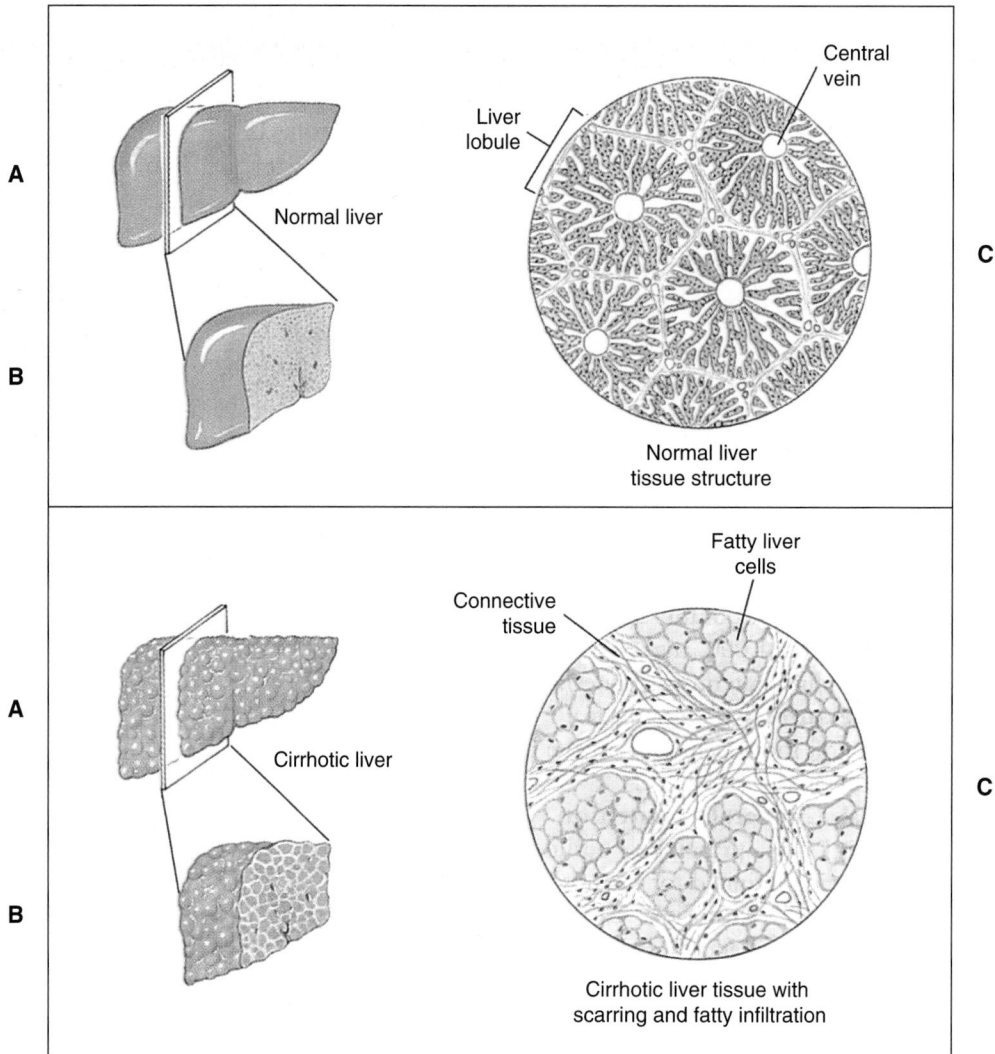

FIGURE 18-5 Comparison of normal liver and liver with cirrhotic tissue changes. **A,** Anterior view of organ. **B,** Cross-section. **C,** Tissue structure. (Credit: Medical and Scientific Illustration.)

Cholesterol in bile, which is not soluble in water, is normally kept in solution. When continued infection alters the solubility of bile ingredients, however, cholesterol separates out and forms gallstones. This condition is called *cholelithiasis*. When infection or stones or both are present, the normal con-

traction of the gallbladder, triggered by fat entering the intestine, causes pain. Thus fatty foods are usually avoided. The treatment is surgical removal of the gallbladder, a *cholecystectomy*. If a patient is obese, some weight loss before surgery may be indicated. In any case, diet therapy centers on control-

TABLE 18-7 Low-protein diets: 15 g, 30 g, 40 g, and 50 g protein

General directions
• The following diets are used when dietary protein is to be restricted.
• The patterns limit foods containing a large percentage of protein (e.g., milk, eggs, cheese, meat, fish, fowl, and legumes).
• Meat extractives, soups, broth, bouillon, gravies, and gelatin desserts should also be avoided.

Basic meal patterns (contain approximately 15 g of protein)

Breakfast	Lunch	Dinner
½ cup fruit or fruit juice	1 small potato	1 small potato
½ cup cereal	½ cup vegetable	½ cup vegetable
1 slice toast	Salad (vegetable or fruit)	Salad (vegetable or fruit)
Butter	1 slice bread	1 slice bread
Jelly	Butter	Butter
Sugar	1 serving fruit	1 serving fruit
2 tbsp cream	Sugar	Sugar
Coffee	Coffee or tea	Coffee or tea

For 30 g protein

Add: 1 cup milk
28 g (1 oz) meat, 1 egg, or equivalent

Examples of meat portions

28 g (1 oz) meat = 1 thin slice roast, 4 × 5 cm
(1½ × 2 in)
1 rounded tbsp cottage cheese
1 slice American cheese

For 40 g protein

Add: 1 cup milk
70 g (2½ oz) meat, or 1 egg and 42 g
(1½ oz) meat

70 g (2½ oz) meat = Ground beef patty
(5 from 448 g [1 lb])
1 slice roast

For 50 g protein

Add: 1 cup milk
112 g (4 oz) meat, or 2 eggs and 56 g
(2 oz) meat

112 g (4 oz) meat = 2 lamb chops
1 average steak

ling fat. Table 18-8 outlines a general low-fat diet guide, but the degree of its application depends upon individual need.

Pancreatic Disease

Pancreatitis

Acute inflammation of the pancreas, *pancreatitis*, is caused when the very enzymes the organ produces (i.e., principally trypsin [see Chapter 4]) digest the organ tissue. Obstruction of the common duct through which the inactive enzymes normally enter the intestine causes the enzymes and bile to back up into the pancreas. This mixing of digestive materials activates the powerful enzymes within the gland. In this active form, they begin to "digest" the pancreatic tissue itself, causing severe pain. Mild or moderate episodes may subside

TABLE 18-8 Low-fat and fat-free diets

Low-fat diet

General description

- This diet contains foods that are low in fat.
- Foods are prepared without the addition of fat.
- Fatty meats, gravies, oils, cream, lard, avocados, and desserts containing eggs, butter, cream, and nuts, are avoided.
- Foods should be used in the amounts specified and only as tolerated.
- The sample pattern contains approximately 85 g protein, 50 g fat, 220 g carbohydrates, and 1670 kcalories.

Foods	Allowed	Not allowed
Beverages	Skim milk, coffee, tea, carbonated beverages, fruit juices	Whole milk, cream, evaporated and condensed milk
Bread and cereals	All kinds	Rich rolls or breads, waffles, pancakes
Desserts	Gelatin, sherbet, water ices, fruit whips made without cream, angel food cake, rice and tapioca puddings made with skim milk	Pastries, pies, rich cakes, and cookies, ice cream
Fruits	All fruits, as tolerated	Avocado
Eggs	3 allowed per week, cooked any way except fried	Fried eggs
Fats	3 tsp butter or margarine daily	Salad and cooking oils, mayonnaise
Meats	Lean meat such as beef, veal, lamb, liver, lean fish and fowl, baked, broiled, or roasted without added fat	Fried meats, bacon, ham, pork, goose, duck, fatty fish, fish canned in oil, cold cuts
Cheese	Dry or fat-free cottage cheese	All other cheese
Potato or substitute	Potatoes, rice, macaroni, noodles, spaghetti, all prepared without added fat	Fried potatoes, potato chips
Soups	Bouillon or broth, without fat; soups made with skimmed milk	Cream soups
Sweets	Jam, jelly, sugar candies without nuts or chocolate	Chocolate, nuts, peanut butter
Vegetables	All kinds as tolerated	The following should be omitted if they cause distress: broccoli, cauliflower, corn, cucumber, green pepper, radishes, turnips, onions, dried peas, and beans
Miscellaneous	Salt in moderation	Pepper, spices, highly spiced food, olives, pickles, cream sauces, gravies

TABLE 18-8   Low-fat and fat-free diets—cont'd

Low-fat diet—cont'd	

Suggested menu pattern

Breakfast	Lunch and dinner
Fruit	Meat, broiled or baked
Cereal	Potato
Toast, jelly	Vegetable
1 tsp butter or margarine	Salad with fat-free dressing
Egg 3 times per week	Bread, jelly
Skim milk, 1 cup	1 tsp butter or margarine
Coffee, sugar	Fruit or dessert, as allowed
	Skim milk, 1 cup coffee, sugar

Fat-free diet	

General description

The following additional restrictions are made to the low-fat diet to make it relatively fat-free:

1. Meat, eggs, and butter or margarine are omitted.
2. A substitute for meat at the noon and evening meal is 84 g (3 oz) of fat-free cottage cheese.

completely, but the condition tends to recur. Initial care includes the following measures for acute disease involving shock: intravenous feeding, replacement of fluid and electrolytes, blood transfusion, antibiotics, pain medications, and gastric suction. As healing progresses, oral feedings are resumed. A light diet is used to reduce stimulation of pancreatic secretions. Alcohol and excess coffee should also be avoided to decrease pancreatic stimulation.

SUMMARY

Nutritional management of gastrointestinal disease is based on the degree of interference in the normal ingestion-digestion-absorption-metabolism that the disease causes. Problems in the upper GI tract relate to conditions that hinder chewing, swallowing, or transporting the food mass down the esophagus into the stomach. Esophageal problems such as muscle constriction, acid reflux causing esophagitis, or a hiatal hernia at the entry of the esophagus into the chest cavity, interfere with passage of the food into the stomach. These problems cause general acid tissue irritation and discomfort after eating. Peptic ulcer disease, a common GI problem, is an acidic erosion of the mucosal lining of the stomach or the duodenal bulb, which is where the concentrated acidic food mass enters the duodenum, the first section of the small intestine. The ulcerated tissue brings nutritional problems such as anemia and weight loss. Medical management consists of drug therapy and rest. Diet therapy is liberal and individual, with a goal of correcting malnutrition and supporting healing.

Problems of the lower GI tract include common functional disorders such as malabsorption and diarrhea, for which symptomatic and personalized treatment is indicated. Diseases such as celiac sprue, which is caused by a sensitivity to gluten in certain grains and results in malabsorption problems, and the generalized genetic disease in children, cystic fibrosis, require individualized nutritional support. The inflammatory bowel diseases Crohn's disease and ulcerative colitis involve extensive tissue damage that often requires surgical resection, as well as the resulting short bowel syndrome from the decreased absorbing surface area. Large intestine problems (e.g., diverticular disease and irritable bowel disease and constipation) involve individual anxiety and stress, as well as irregular lifestyle habits, and thus are more difficult to resolve. Nutritional therapy requires modification of the diet's protein and energy content and food texture, increased vitamins and minerals, and replacement of fluids and electrolytes. Continuous adjustment of the diet is made according to individual need.

Other food intolerances may be caused by allergies or underlying genetic disease. Specific genetic disease results from specific missing cell enzymes that control the cell metabolism of specific nutrients. The special diet in each case limits or eliminates the particular nutrient involved.

Diseases of the GI accessory organs also contribute to nutrition problems. Common liver disorders include hepatitis, which is caused by a viral infection, and cirrhosis, which is caused by progressive liver disease that damages tissue through the use of such toxins as excessive alcohol. Uncontrolled cirrhosis leads to hepatic coma and eventual liver failure and death. Nutrient and energy levels of the necessary diet therapy vary with the progression of the disease process. Gallbladder disease, infection, and stones involve some limit to fat tolerance, which is modified according to individual need. Pancreatic disease includes pancreatitis, which is a serious condition requiring immediate measures to counter the shock symptoms, followed by restorative nutritional support. Gallbladder disease requires attention to the fat content of foods. The treatment for gallstones is surgical removal of the organ, followed by moderate use of dietary fat.

REVIEW QUESTIONS

1. What general nutritional guidance would you give to a person with a hiatal hernia? What would be the basic goal of your suggestions?
2. What are the basic principles of diet planning for patients with peptic ulcer disease? How do these principles differ from the traditional therapy formerly used?
3. Describe the causes, clinical signs, and treatment of each of the following diseases: diverticular disease, celiac sprue, and inflammatory bowel disease.
4. What is the rationale for treatment in the progressive course of liver disease (i.e., hepatitis, cirrhosis, and hepatic coma)?

SELF-TEST QUESTIONS

True-False
Write the correct statement for each item you answer "false."
1. A high fiber diet is indicated for a person with dental problems.
2. Lying down after eating helps a person with hiatal hernia relieve discomfort.
3. The fundamental cause of peptic ulcer is unknown.
4. Peptic ulcer pain is reduced when the stomach is empty and can rest.
5. A low residue diet is the advocated for treatment of diverticulosis.

6. All food sources of wheat must be eliminated in the gluten-free diet for treatment of celiac disease.

7. PKU is a genetic disease requiring dietary control of the essential amino acid phenylalanine.

8. Soy products are often used for children allergic to milk.

9. The nutritional objective in cystic fibrosis is to meet growth needs and help, along with enzyme replacement therapy, compensate for nutrient losses.

Multiple Choice

1. In a gluten-free diet for celiac disease, which of the following foods is eliminated?
   a. Eggs
   b. Milk
   c. Rice
   d. Saltine crackers

2. The symptoms of anemia in malabsorption diseases are caused by poor absorption of which of the following nutrients?
   a. Vitamin K
   b. Iron and folic acid
   c. Calcium and phosphorus
   d. Fats

3. Lactose intolerance in certain population groups is caused by a genetic deficiency of which of the following enzymes?
   a. Sucrase
   b. Pepsin
   c. Lactase
   d. Maltase

4. Treatment for hepatic coma includes:
   a. Increased protein to aid healing of liver cells.
   b. Decreased protein to reduce ammonia levels in blood.
   c. Decreased kcalories to reduce the metabolic load.
   d. Increased fluid intake to stimulate output.

SUGGESTIONS FOR ADDITIONAL STUDY

Patient Nutritional Therapy Planning

Develop food plans for hospitalized patients with liver disease and gallbladder disease.

1. **Liver disease**—Write a 1-day food plan for a 45-year-old man, 183 cm (6 ft, 1 in) tall, weighing 90 kg (200 lb), with infectious hepatitis. Develop another plan for a similar patient with cirrhosis of the liver. Develop another plan for a similar patient with hepatic encephalopathy.

2. **Gallbladder disease**—Write a 1-day meal plan for a 30-year-old woman, 165 cm (5 ft, 6 in) tall, weighing 81 kg (180 lb), who has an inflamed gallbladder with stones and is awaiting a cholecystectomy.

Compare your meal plans with the plans developed by other students in the class. What principles of nutritional therapy apply in each case?

REFERENCES

1. Mann LL, Wong K: Development of an objective method for assessing viscosity of formulated foods and beverages for the dysphagic diet, *J Am Diet Assoc* 96(6):585, 1996.

2. Brzana PJ, Koch KL: Gastroesophageal reflux disease presenting with intractable nausea, *Ann Intern Med* 26(9):704, 1997.

3. Birnbaum A: Gastroesophageal reflux in children, *Food Allergy News* 8(4):1, 1999.

4. Cohen S, Parkman HP: Diseases of the esophagus. In Goldman L, Bennett JC, editors: *Cecil's Textbook of Medicine*, ed 21, vol 1, Philadelphia, 2000, W.B. Saunders.

5. Ganga-Zandzou PS and others: Natural outcome of *Helicobacter pylori* infection in asymptomatic children: a two-year follow-up study, *Pediatrics* 104(2):216, 1999.

6. Covacci A and others: *Helicobacter pylori* virulence and genetic geography, *Science* 284(5418):1328, 1999.

7. Damiamos AJ, McGarrity TJ: Treatment stratigies for Helicobacter pylori infection, *Am Fam Physician* 55(8):2765, 1997.

8. Weissman G: NSAIDS: aspirin and aspirin-like drugs. In Goldman L, Bennett JC, editors: *Cecil's Textbook of Medicine*, ed 21, vol 1, Philadelphia, 2000, W.B. Saunders.

9. Juckett G: Prevention and treatment of traveler's diarrhea, *Am Fam Physician* 60(1):119, 1999.

10. Semrad CE, Chang EB: Malabsorption syndromes. In Goldman L, Bennett JC, editors: *Cecil's Textbook of Medicine*, ed 21, vol 1, Philadelphia, 2000, W.B. Saunders.

11. Stenson WF: Chronic inflammatory bowel disease. In Goldman L, Bennett JC, editors: *Cecil's Textbook of Medicine*, ed 21, vol 1, Philadelphia, 2000, W.B. Saunders.

12. Wilcox CM: Miscellaneous inflammatory diseases of the intestine. In Goldman L, Bennett JC, editors: *Cecil's Textbook of Medicine*, ed 21, vol 1, Philadelphia, 2000, W.B. Saunders.

13. Snape WJ, Jr: Disorders of gastrointestinal motility. In Goldman L, Bennett JC, editors: *Cecil's Textbook of Medicine*, ed 21, vol 1, Philadelphia, 2000, W.B. Saunders.

14. Tally NJ: Functional gastrointestinal disorders: irritable bowel syndrome, non-ulcer dyspepsia, and non-cardiac chest pain. In Goldman L, Bennett JC, editors: *Cecil's Textbook of Medicine*, ed 21, vol 1, Philadelphia, 2000, W.B. Saunders.

15. Smith O: Fear of flying, *Science* 284(5411):61, 1999.

FURTHER READING

• Aldrich JK, Massey LK: A liberalized geriatric diet fits most dietary prescriptions for long-term-care residents, *J Am Diet Assoc* 99(4):4, 478, 1999.

This brief article describes an excellent program for care of elderly persons in a long-term care facility that focuses on quality care with an emphasis on good food that is well presented. Therapeutic diets are liberalized to encourage eating and balancing good tasting "normal food" with the necessity for diet therapy.

• Holben DH and others: Fluid intake compared with established standards and symptoms of dehydration among elderly residents of a long-term-care facility, *J Am Diet Assoc* 99(11):1447, 1999.

In this companion article, the study team of dietitians focuses on symptoms of dehydration among elderly nursing home residents, which is all too often a problem in their long-term care due to decreased thirst sensation and decreased independence.

19

Coronary Heart Disease and Hypertension

KEY CONCEPTS

- Heart disease results from several risk factors, mostly preventable ones associated with our lifestyle, that contribute to its development.

- The silent genetic risk factor without symptoms, essential hypertension, can be identified and controlled.

- Most cardiovascular risk factors are associated with nutrition and can be reduced by changing food habits and lifestyles.

Cardiovascular disease accounts for more than half of the deaths each year in the United States and is our leading health problem. This same situation exists in most other developed Western societies. Every day, thousands of people suffer heart attacks and strokes and more than a million others continue to suffer from various forms of rheumatic and congestive heart disease.

During the past 20 years, our cardiovascular death rate has declined somewhat—mostly because of improved emergency care for heart attacks, but cardiovascular disease remains our top "killer disease." Here we look at the primary underlying disease process, atherosclerosis, and the various risk factors involved and explore ways to use nutritional approaches to reduce these risk factors and help prevent disease.

CORONARY HEART DISEASE
The Basic Problem of Atherosclerosis

The Disease Process

The major cardiovascular disease and the underlying pathologic process in coronary heart disease is atherosclerosis. As much more is being learned about this disease, ongoing studies have strengthened the earlier association of key risk factors including diet to the progressive development of the atherosclerotic process.[1,2] This process is characterized by fatty fibrous plaques that begin in childhood and develop into fatty streaks, largely composed of cholesterol, on the inside lining of major blood vessels. When tissue is examined, crystals of cholesterol can be seen with the unaided eye in the softened cheesy debris of advanced disease. This fatty debris suggested its name to early investigators, from the Greek words *athera* meaning "gruel," and *sclerosis*, "hardening." This fatty fibrous process gradually thickens over time, narrowing the interior part of the blood vessel and often forming blood clots from its irritation of the vessel tissue. The thickening of the vessel or a blood clot may eventually cut off blood flow, as shown in Figure 19-1.

Cells deprived of their normal blood supply will die. The local area of dying or dead tissue is called an *infarct*. If the affected blood vessel is a major artery supplying vital blood nutrients and oxygen to the heart muscle, the *myocardium*, the result is called an acute myocardial infarction (MI) or a *heart attack*. If the affected vessel is a major artery supplying the brain, the result is called a cerebrovascular accident (CVA) or *stroke*. The major arteries and their many branches serving the heart are called *coronary* arteries because they lie across the brow of the heart muscle and resemble a crown. Thus the overall disease process is called coronary heart disease.[2,3] A common symptom of its presence is angina pectoris, or chest pain, usually radiating down the arm and sometimes brought on by excitement or effort.

Relation to Fat Metabolism

Major research studies have found elevated blood lipids to be associated with coronary heart disease and related heart attacks.[1] *Lipid* is the class name for all fats and fat-related compounds. Lipid substances involved in the disease process are described in more detail in Chapter 3. Three of these substances are emphasized in this chapter.

---

atherosclerosis (Gr. *athere,* gruel; *skleros,* hard) the underlying pathology of coronary heart disease; a common form of arteriosclerosis that is characterized by the formation, beginning in childhood in predisposed individuals, of yellow cheese-like fatty streaks containing cholesterol that develop into hardened plaques in the inner lining of major blood vessels such as the coronary arteries.

myocardial infarction (MI) (Gr. *mys,* muscle; *kardia,* heart; L. *infarcire,* to stuff in) a heart attack; caused by failure of the heart muscle to maintain normal blood circulation, due to blockage of coronary arteries with fatty cholesterol plaques that cut off delivery of oxygen to the affected part of the heart muscle.

cerebrovascular accident (CVA) (L. *cerebrum,* brain, *vas,* vessel) a stroke, caused by arteriosclerosis in a blood vessel in the brain that cuts off oxygen supply to the affected portion of brain tissue, thus paralyzing body muscle actions controlled by the affected brain area.

coronary heart disease term designating the overall medical problem resulting from the underlying disease of atherosclerosis in the coronary arteries, which serve the heart muscle tissue with blood oxygen and nutrients.

angina pectoris (L. *angina,* severe pain; *pectus,* breast) spasmodic, choking chest pain due to lack of oxygen to the heart muscle, symptom of a heart attack; may also be caused by severe effort or excitement.

lipids (Gr. *lipos,* fat) the chemical group name for fats and fat-related compounds such as cholesterol and lipoproteins.

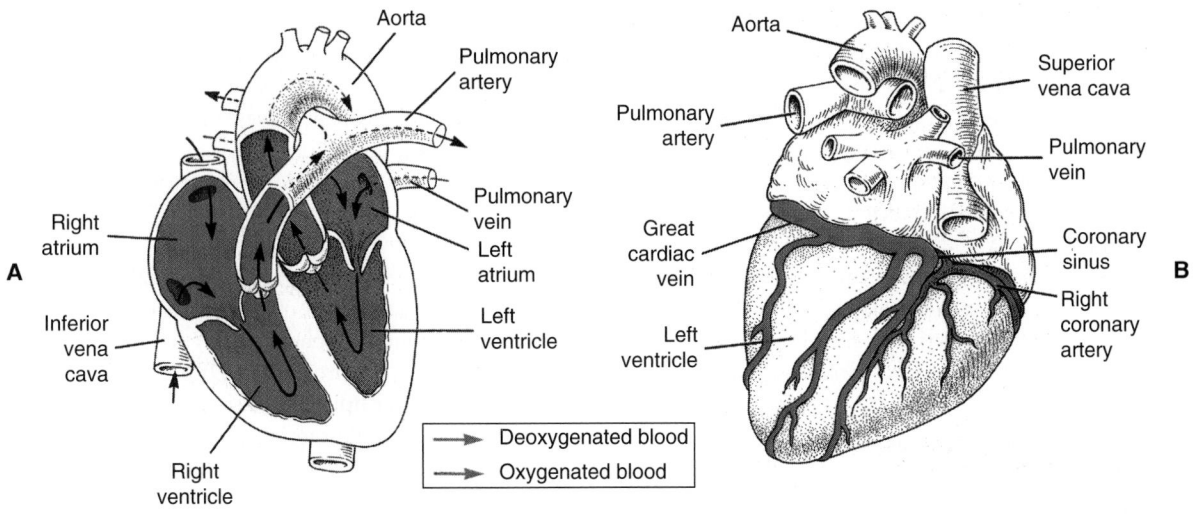

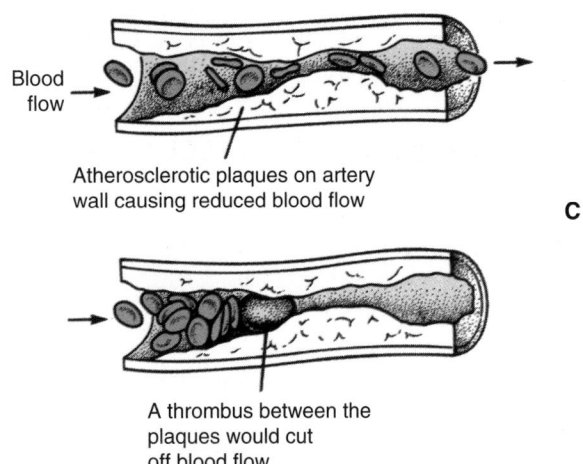

FIGURE 19-1 **A and B,** The normal human heart. **A,** Anterior view showing cardiac circulation. **B,** Posterior external view showing coronary arteries. **C,** Atherosclerotic plaque in artery.

Triglycerides. The chemical name for fat, describing its basic structure, is *triglyceride*. All simple fats, whether in our bodies or in our foods, are triglycerides. The blood test for total triglycerides measures the level circulating in our blood. Major research studies of heart disease have shown a definite association between the amount and type of dietary fat and an elevated blood lipid level. Studies of body fat distribution, especially using waist measurements in children, help to identify persons more likely to have adverse lipid levels.[1]

Cholesterol. *Cholesterol* is the fat-related compound now clearly associated with atherosclerosis and heart disease. Estimates indicate that about 60 million American adults have high blood cholesterol, many of whom have the related problems of obesity and hypertension, requiring medical advice and intervention using diet as the primary treatment.[2,3] A reduction in dietary cholesterol has been shown to lower total blood cholesterol levels and reduce the risk of heart disease in predisposed individuals. Cholesterol is produced *only* in animal tissue, thus it can *never* be found in plant foods.

Lipoproteins. Because fat is not soluble in water, it is carried in the bloodstream in small packages wrapped with protein, which are called *lipoproteins.* These compounds are produced in the intestinal wall after a meal containing fat and in the liver as part of the regular ongoing process of fat metabolism and carry fat and cholesterol to tissues for cell metabolism use and back to the liver for breakdown and excretion as needed. Lipoproteins are grouped and named according to their fat and cholesterol content (i.e., their density). Those with the highest lipid content have the lowest density. Three of these types of lipoproteins that are formed in the liver are significant in relation to heart disease risk, as follow:

- **Very low density lipoproteins (VLDL)** carry a relatively large load of fat to cells but also include about 15% cholesterol.
- **Low density lipoproteins (LDL)** carry, in addition to other lipids, at least two thirds of the total plasma cholesterol to body tissues. They are formed in the liver and in serum from catabolism of VLDL. Because LDLs constantly send cholesterol to tissues, they have been called the source of "bad cholesterol." In blood lipid tests, the total LDL is the major cholesterol of concern. A blood LDL level of up to 129 mg/dl is considered to be healthy, and the person is without risk. Borderline

---

BOX 19-1 Normal and high risk blood levels of LDL for adults

Normal—129 mg/dl or below
Borderline risk—130-159 mg/dl
High risk—160 mg/dl and above

BOX 19-2 Multiple risk factors in cardiovascular disease

Personal characteristics (no control)
Sex
Age
Family history

Learned behaviors (intervene and change)
Stress/coping
Smoking cigarettes
Sedentary life

Learned behaviors (intervene and change)—cont'd
Obesity
Food habits
    Excess fat
    Excess sugar
    Excess salt

Background conditions (screen and treat)
Hypertension
Diabetes mellitus
Hyperlipidemia (especially hypercholesterolemia)

risk occurs in the range of 130-159 mg/dl; any level above 160 mg/dl carries high risk (Box 19-1).[3]

- **High density lipoproteins (HDL)** carry less total fat and more carrier protein. They transport cholesterol from the tissues to the liver for catabolism and elimination from the body. When compared with LDL cholesterol, HDL cholesterol is often called the "good cholesterol," and higher serum levels are considered protective against cardiovascular disease. The normal HDL range is 30 to 80 mg/dl. Thus a value below 30 implies significant risk, and a value of 75 or greater contributes definite protection and decreased risk.

Risk Factors

We have learned several important facts from major studies of heart disease:

1. The underlying disease process of atherosclerosis is caused by multiple risk factors, as shown in Box 19-2. Note the personal risk factors that we cannot control but indicate need for closer attention to the remaining risks that can be controlled:
   - *Sex*—Occurs more in men than in women; after menopause women catch up with men in cholesterol level and potential heart disease risk.
   - *Age*—Occurs at an earlier age in families carrying a positive family history for heart disease; general risk increases with the aging process.
   - *Family history*—A positive family history is defined as a history of premature (before age 55 years) cardiovascular disease in a parent or grandparent or a parental high blood cholesterol above 240 mg/dl. Early screening for children and adolescents with such a high risk due to family history is important so that appropriate therapy (i.e., diet [low fat and weight control] with cholesterol-lowering drugs as needed) may be started when

the fatty streaks in coronary arteries are just beginning.[3]

2. Elevated serum cholesterol is one of the *major* risk factors for the disease process, along with hypertension, which is worsened by obesity, lack of exercise, excess food habits, stress, and smoking.

3. Dietary fat *can* affect serum cholesterol. The National Institutes of Health Consensus Group for lowering blood cholesterol has defined serum cholesterol values for persons at risk (Table 19-1) and emphasized the importance of educating the public about this preventable risk factor.

Fat-Controlled Diets

Because control of dietary fat and cholesterol has been shown to be important in reducing risks for heart disease, the dietary guidelines for healthy Americans (see Chapter 1) issued by the U.S. Departments of Agriculture and of Health and Human Services, as well as other national health agencies for heart disease, cancer, and diabetes, recommend dietary decreases in these two nutrients. The following are three primary factors in a fat-controlled diet:

1. **Reducing the total amount of fat**—No more than 30% of total energy (kcalories) intake should come from fat.

TABLE 19-1 Serum cholesterol levels identifying persons at moderate and high risk who require treatment*

Age (years)	Moderate risk	High risk
	Greater than:	Greater than:
2-19	170 mg/dl	185 mg/dl
20-29	200 mg/dl	220 mg/dl
30-39	220 mg/dl	240 mg/dl
40 and older	240 mg/dl	260 mg/dl

*Diet therapy and weight control; drug therapy only after careful maximal diet therapy.
From National Institutes of Health: *Nutr Today* 20(1):13, 1985.

TABLE 19-2 The Prudent Diet as compared with the usual American diet

	Prudent diet	Usual American diet
Total kcalories	Sufficient to maintain ideal body weight	Often excessive for need
Cholesterol	300 mg	600-800 mg
Total fats (% of kcalories)	30%-35%	40%-45%
Saturated	10% or less	15%-20%
Monounsaturated	15%	15%-20%
Polyunsaturated	10%	5%-6%
P/S ratio (polyunsaturated/saturated fat in the diet)	1-1.5/1	0.3/1
Carbohydrate (% of kcalories)	50%-55%	40%-45%
Starch (complex CHO)	30%-35%	20%-25%
Simple sugars	10%	15%-20%
Proteins (% of total kcalories)	12%-20%	12%-15%
Sodium	130 mEq (3 g)	200-250 mEq (4.5-6.0 g)

From American Heart Association Nutrition Committee: Rationale for the diet-heart statement of the American Heart Association, *Arterioscler Thromb* 4:177, 1982.

2. **Reducing the use of animal fat**—No more than approximately one third of the total fat kcalories should come from saturated animal fat, with the remainder coming from unsaturated plant fat (see Chapter 3).
3. **Reducing the intake of cholesterol**—Dietary cholesterol should be reduced to about 300 mg/day.

The Prudent Diet

This reduced amount of fat and cholesterol, together with the greater use of unsaturated plant fats than saturated animal fats, is included in the general goals of the Prudent Diet recommended by the American Heart Association and other health agencies (Table 19-2). The Step 1 and Step 2 diets provide further guidelines for lowering blood-cholesterol levels (Table 19-3). A diet mainly focused on a variety of vegetables, fruits, and grains with moderate use of polyunsaturated and monounsaturated food fats (e.g., mostly from olive oil [as used in the typical Mediterranean diet][4,5] or corn oil and other vegetable oils and products) is the basic guideline. Lesser amounts of animal foods (e.g., fish, poultry, and dairy products—particularly cheese) are used.

In general, there should be an increase in energy intake from carbohydrates—especially complex carbohydrates (e.g., starches, grains)—to about 50% to 60% of the day's total kcalories, as well as an increase in soluble fiber (see Chapter 2). When the risk factor of obesity is present, the overall excess energy value of the diet (kcalories) is also reduced accordingly, and increased exercise is encouraged (see Chapter 15). A treadmill exercise tolerance test is used to determine the exercise limit for a person with a cardiac history (Figure 19-2).

Additional Dietary Factors

Recent interest has centered on dietary fiber and *omega-3 fatty acids* as additional food factors in reducing risks involved in coronary heart disease (see Clinical Applications box, "Omega-3 Fatty Acids and Dietary Fiber in CHD Therapy"). Each of these factors may need consideration along with the primary focus on fat and cholesterol.

TABLE 19-3 Characteristics of Step 1 and Step 2 diets for lowering blood cholesterol in children and adolescents

Nutrient	Recommended intake	
	Step 1 diet	Step 2 diet
Total fat	Average of no more than 30% of total kcalories	Same
Saturated fatty acids	Less than 10% of total kcalories	Less than 7% of total kcalories
Polyunsaturated fatty acids	Up to 10% of total kcalories	Same
Monounsaturated fatty acids	Remaining total fat kcalories	Same
Cholesterol	Less than 300 mg/day	Less than 200 mg/day
Carbohydrates	About 55% of total kcalories	Same
Protein	About 15% to 20% of total kcalories	Same
Kcalories	To promote normal growth and development and to reach or maintain desirable body weight	Same

From National Cholesterol Education Program: *Report of the expert panel on blood cholesterol levels in children and adolescents,* USDHHS (PHS), National Institutes of Health, Washington, DC, 1991, US Government Printing Office.

The Problem of Acute Cardiovascular Disease

When cardiovascular disease progresses to the point of cutting off the blood supply to major coronary arteries, a critical vascular event—a heart attack or myocardial infarction (MI)—occurs (see Clinical Applications box, "Case Study: The Patient with a Myocardial Infarction (Heart Attack)"). In the initial, acute phase of the attack, additional diet modifications are required to allow for healing.

Objective: Cardiac Rest
All care, including diet, is directed toward ensuring cardiac rest so that the damaged heart may be restored to normal functioning.

Principles of Diet Therapy
The diet is modified in energy value and texture, as well as in fat and sodium.

Kcalories. A brief period of undernutrition during the first day or so after the heart attack reduces the metabolic workload on the damaged heart. The metabolic demands for digestion, absorption, and metabolism of food require a generous cardiac output volume. Thus to decrease the level of metabolic activity that the weakened heart can accommodate, small feedings are spread over the day when

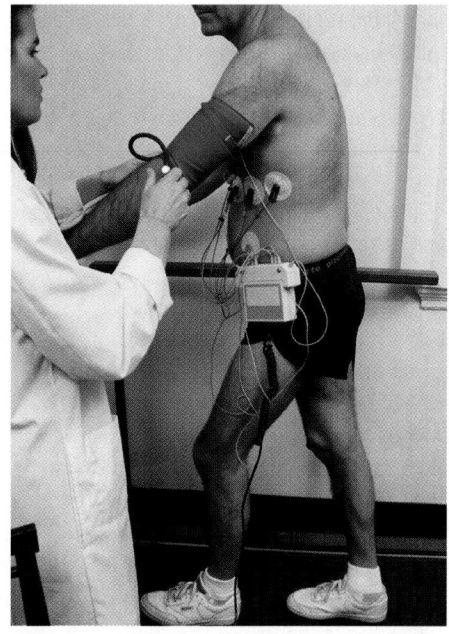

FIGURE 19-2 Patient with history of cardiac disease is evaluated for exercise tolerance with treadmill test. (Credit: PhotoDisc.)

an oral diet is started. The patient will progress to eating more as healing occurs. During the initial recovery period, the diet may be limited to about 1200 to 1500 kcalories to continue cardiac rest from metabolic workloads. Afterward, if the patient

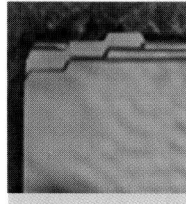

CLINICAL APPLICATIONS
Omega-3 Fatty Acids and Dietary Fiber in CHD Therapy

The primary focus of nutritional therapy for coronary heart disease (CHD) centers on controlling lipid factors, including cholesterol and saturated fats. Two additional food factors, however, play a different role and also help to protect us from CHD development.

Omega-3 fatty acids
Studies indicate that the omega-3 fatty acids *eicosapentaenoic acid (EPA)* and *docosahexaenoic acid (DHA)* may have protective functions in their capacity to hinder blood clots from forming. Scientific interest was first sparked by earlier observations among Greenland Eskimos, who eat a diet rich in fish oils but have a low incidence of heart disease. The scientists found that these fish oils contain high levels of long-chain polyunsaturated fatty acids, which they named *omega-3 fatty acids* from the nature of their chemical structure. Continuing study supports the potential nutritional and clinical importance of these fatty acids, which are found mostly in seafood and marine oils from fatty fish (e.g., cod, salmon, mackerel, and menhaden).

On the basis of current research, these omega-3 fatty acids can do the following:
- Change the pattern of plasma fatty acids to alter platelet activity and reduce the clumping of these disk-shaped blood factors to cause blood clotting, thus lowering the risk of coronary thrombosis.
- Increase antiinflammatory effects.
- Decrease synthesis of very low-density lipoproteins.

Dietary fiber
Studies indicate that water-soluble types of dietary fiber have a significant cholesterol-lowering effect. Soluble fiber includes gums, pectin, certain hemicelluloses, and storage polysaccharides. Foods rich in soluble fiber include oat bran and dried beans, with additional amounts in barley and fruits. For example, oat bran contains a primary water-soluble gum, beta-glucan, which is a lipid-lowering agent. Soluble fiber can do the following:
- Delay gastric emptying.
- Increase intestinal transit time.
- Slow glucose absorption.
- Be fermented in the colon into short-chain fatty acids that may inhibit liver cholesterol synthesis and help clear LDL-cholesterol.

Therefore it seems that factors in foods such as oats, dried beans, and fish provide valuable lipid-lowering additions to our diets.

---

is overweight, this kcalorie level may be continued to help the patient begin gradually losing excess weight.

Texture. Early feedings generally include foods that are relatively soft in texture or easily digested to avoid excess effort in eating or the discomfort of gas formation. For a time, the patient may need to be fed to reduce the physical effort of eating further and help ensure sufficient intake if appetite is poor and the patient is weak. Smaller, more frequent meals may give needed nourishment without undue strain or pressure. Depending on the patient's condition, gas-forming foods, caffeine-containing

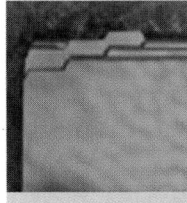

CLINICAL APPLICATIONS

Case Study: The Patient with a Myocardial Infarction (Heart Attack)

Charles Carter is a successful young businessman who works long hours and carries the major responsibility of his struggling small business. At his last physical checkup, the physician cautioned him about his pace because he was already showing some mild hypertension. His blood cholesterol was elevated, and he was overweight. In his desk job he got little exercise and found himself smoking more and eating irregularly under stress of his increasing financial pressures.

One day while commuting in the heavy freeway traffic, he felt a pain in his chest and became increasingly apprehensive. When he arrived home, the pain persisted and increased. He broke out into a cold sweat and felt nauseated. When he became more ill after trying to eat dinner, his wife called their physician and Mr. Carter was admitted to the hospital.

After emergency care and tests, the physician placed Mr. Carter in the coronary care unit at the hospital. His test results showed elevated total cholesterol, triglycerides, and lipoproteins—especially LDL, but low HDL. The electrocardiogram revealed an infarction of the posterior myocardium wall.

When Mr. Carter was first able to take oral nourishment, he had only a liquid diet. As his condition stabilized, his diet was increased to 800 kcalories (soft diet) with low cholesterol and low fat. By the end of the first week, his diet was increased again to 1200 kcalories (full diet) with low cholesterol and only 25% of the total kcalories from fat and a P/S ratio of 1/1.

Mr. Carter gradually improved over the next few weeks and was able to go home. The physician, nurse, and clinical dietitian discussed with Mr. Carter and his wife the need for care at home during a period of convalescence. They explained that he had an underlying lipid disorder and was to continue his weight loss and follow a prudent diet.

Questions for Analysis

1. Identify factors in Mr. Carter's personal and medical history that place him at high risk for coronary heart disease. Give reasons why each factor contributes to heart disease.

2. Identify as many of the laboratory tests the physician ordered as you can. Relate these tests to Mr. Carter's condition.

3. Why did Mr. Carter receive only a liquid diet at first? What is the reason for each modification in his first diet of solid food?

4. What occurs in the underlying disease process that causes a heart attack? What relation do fat and cholesterol have to this underlying process?

5. Outline a day's menu for Mr. Carter on his 1200 kcalorie Prudent Diet.

6. What needs might Mr. Carter have when he goes home? How would you help him prepare to go home? Name some community resources you might use to help him understand his illness and plan self care.

BOX 19-3 Restrictions for a mild low-sodium diet (2 to 3 g sodium/day)

Do not use

1. Salt at the table (use salt lightly in cooking)
2. Salt-preserved foods such as salted or smoked meat (bacon and bacon fat, bologna, dried or chipped beef, corned beef, frankfurters, ham, kosher meats, luncheon meats, salt pork, sausage, smoked tongue), salted or smoked fish (anchovies, caviar, salted and dried cod, herring, sardines) sauerkraut, olives

3. Highly salted foods such as crackers, pretzels, potato chips, corn chips, salted nuts, salted popcorn
4. Spices and condiments such as bouillon cubes,* catsup,* chili sauce*, celery salt, garlic salt, onion salt, monosodium glutamate, meat sauces, meat tenderizers,* pickles, prepared mustard, relishes, Worcestershire sauce, soy sauce
5. Cheese,* peanut butter*

*Dietetic low-sodium kind may be used.

beverages, hot or cold temperature extremes in foods—both solids and liquids should also generally be avoided.

Fat. The general Prudent Diet controls the amount and types of fat, as well as cholesterol (see Tables 19-2 and 19-3).

Sodium. General attention to a reduced sodium content in the foods selected is also emphasized. Usually a mild sodium restriction to about 2 to 3 g/day is sufficient (Box 19-3). This restriction can be achieved by only using salt lightly in cooking, by adding none when eating, and by avoiding salty processed foods. Appendixes D and E provide the sodium values of foods and a salt-free seasoning guide. Food labels on canned and other processed foods, as mandated by the U.S. Congress and administered by the Food and Drug Administration (FDA), provide specific information about the sodium content of such foods (see Chapter 13).

The Problem of Chronic Heart Disease

In chronic heart disease, the condition of congestive heart failure may develop over time. The pro-gressively weakened heart muscle is unable to maintain an adequate cardiac output to sustain normal blood circulation. The resulting fluid imbalances cause edema, especially pulmonary edema. This condition brings added problems in breathing and places more stress on the laboring heart.

Objective: Control of Cardiac Edema

The basic objective of diet therapy in this condition is to control the fluid imbalance that results in cardiac edema.

Principles of Diet Therapy

Because of the role of sodium in tissue fluid balance (see Chapter 8), the diet used to treat cardiac edema restricts the sodium intake. The main source of dietary sodium is common table salt, sodium chloride. The taste for salt is an acquired one. Some persons salt food heavily by habit without even tasting it first, thus habituating their taste to high salt levels. Others acquire a taste for less salt by the habit of using smaller amounts. Therefore in American diets, common daily adult intakes of sodium range widely, according to habit, from 3 to 4 g up to 10 to 12 g with heavy use. Besides the salt used in cooking or added at the table, a large amount is used in food processing. Remaining sources of sodium include that found as a naturally occurring mineral in cer-

BOX 19-4 Restrictions for a moderate low-sodium diet (1000 mg sodium/day)

Do not use

1. Salt in cooking or at the table
2. Salt-preserved foods such as salted or smoked meat (bacon and bacon fat, bologna, dried or chipped beef, corned beef, frankfurters, ham, kosher meats, luncheon meats, salt pork, sausage, smoked tongue, kidneys), salted or smoked fish (anchovies, caviar, salted and dried cod, herring, sardines, frozen fish fillets, canned salmon,* tuna*) sauerkraut, olives
3. Highly salted foods such as crackers, pretzels, potato chips, corn chips, salted nuts, salted popcorn
4. Spices and condiments such as bouillon cubes,* catsup,* chili sauce*, celery salt, garlic salt, onion salt, monosodium glutamate, meat sauces, meat tenderizers,* pickles, prepared mustard, relishes, Worcestershire sauce, soy sauce
5. Cheese,* peanut butter*
6. Buttermilk (unsalted buttermilk may be used) instead of skimmed milk
7. Canned vegetables,* canned vegetable juices*

8. Frozen peas, frozen lima beans, frozen mixed vegetables, any frozen vegetables to which salt has been added.
9. More than 1 serving of any of these vegetables in 1 day: artichokes, beet greens, beets, carrots, celery, dandelion greens, kale, mustard greens, spinach, Swiss chard, turnips (white)
10. Regular bread, rolls,* crackers*
11. Dry cereals,* except puffed rice, puffed wheat, and shredded wheat
12. Quick-cooking Cream of Wheat
13. Shellfish: clams, crab, lobster, shrimp (oysters may be used)
14. Salted butter, salted margarine, commercial French dressings,* mayonnaise,* other salad dressings*
15. Regular baking powder,* baking soda, or anything containing them; self-rising flour
16. Prepared mixes: pudding,* gelatin,* cake, biscuit
17. Commercial candies

*Dietetic low-sodium kinds may be used.

tain foods. The American Heart Association has outlined the following three main levels of sodium restriction, which can be achieved by progressively deleting the main dietary sodium sources:

1. **Mild sodium restriction (2 to 3 g)**—Salt may be used *lightly* in cooking, assuming that fresh foods are used, but *no added salt* is allowed. In addition, no salty processed foods (e.g., pickles, olives, bacon, ham, corn chips, or potato chips) are used. Box 19-3 provides a general deletion list for mild sodium restriction. Some processed foods with less salt added are beginning to appear on our food market shelves.
2. **Moderate sodium restriction (1000 mg)**— No salt is used in cooking, and no added salt

or salty foods are used. Beginning at this level, some control of foods with natural sodium is started. Vegetables higher in natural sodium are limited. Fresh foods are used, rather than those processed with salt. Salt-free baked products are generally used. Foods higher in

---

congestive heart failure chronic condition of gradually weakening heart muscle unable to pump normal blood flow through the heart-lung circulation, resulting in congestion of fluids in the lungs.

pulmonary edema (L. *pulmonis*, lung; Gr. *oidēma*, swelling) accumulation of fluid in lung tissues.

BOX 19-5 Restrictions for a strict low-sodium diet (500 mg sodium/day)

Do not use

1. Salt in cooking or at the table
2. Salt-preserved foods such as salted or smoked meat (bacon and bacon fat, bologna, dried or chipped beef, corned beef, frankfurters, ham, kosher meats, luncheon meats, salt pork, sausage, smoked tongue, kidneys), salted or smoked fish (anchovies, caviar, salted and dried cod, herring, sardines, frozen fish fillets, canned salmon,* tuna*) sauerkraut, olives
3. Highly salted foods such as crackers, pretzels, potato chips, corn chips, salted nuts, salted popcorn
4. Spices and condiments such as bouillon cubes,* catsup,* chili sauce*, celery salt, garlic salt, onion salt, monosodium glutamate, meat sauces, meat tenderizers,* pickles, prepared mustard, relishes, Worcestershire sauce, soy sauce
5. Cheese,* peanut butter*
6. Buttermilk (unsalted buttermilk may be used) instead of skimmed milk
7. More than 2 cups of skimmed milk a day, including that used on cereal
8. Any commercial foods made of milk (ice cream, ice milk, milk shakes)
9. Canned vegetables,* canned vegetable juices*
10. Frozen peas, frozen lima beans, frozen mixed vegetables, any frozen vegetables to which salt has been added.
11. The following vegetables: artichokes, beet greens, beets, carrots, celery, dandelion greens, kale, mustard greens, spinach, Swiss chard, turnips (white)
12. Regular bread,* rolls,* crackers
13. Dry cereals,* except puffed rice, puffed wheat, and shredded wheat
14. Quick-cooking Cream of Wheat
15. Shellfish: clams, crab, lobster, shrimp (oysters may be used)
16. Salted butter, salted margarine, commercial French dressings,* mayonnaise,* other salad dressings*
17. Regular baking powder,* baking soda, or anything containing them; self-rising flour
18. Prepared mixes: pudding,* gelatin,* cake, biscuit
19. Commercial candies

*Dietetic low-sodium kinds may be used.

natural sodium (e.g., meat and milk) are only used in moderate portions. Box 19-4 provides a general deletion list for moderate sodium restriction.

3. **Strict sodium restriction (500 mg)**—In addition to the mild and moderate deletions, the natural sodium food sources of meat, milk, and eggs are used in smaller portions. Milk is limited to 2 cups in any form, meat to 5 oz, and eggs to 1 oz. Higher-sodium vegetables are deleted. Box 19-5 provides a general deletion list for strict sodium restriction.

ESSENTIAL HYPERTENSION
The Problem of Hypertension

Incidence and Nature
Hypertension, or high blood pressure, is a health problem for some 60 million Americans. About 30% of American adults have high blood pressure, with the numbers increasing with age. The incidence ranges from a low of 2% for white women ages 18 to 24, to 83% for black women ages 65 to 74. When speaking of the chronic disease of elevated blood pressure, the term *hypertension* is actu-

ally more correct than *high blood pressure,* because the blood pressure may occasionally be temporarily elevated in situations such as overexertion or stress. In general, the disease hypertension means essential hypertension, and 90% of cases fall in this category. The specific cause is unknown, although injury to the inner lining of the blood vessel wall appears to be an underlying link.

Hypertension has been called the silent disease because no signs indicate its presence, but it can have serious effects if not detected, treated, and controlled. Hypertension is usually an inherited disorder; children of hypertensive parents may develop the condition at early ages, often in their adolescent years. Hypertension occurs more frequently in blacks than in whites. Obesity makes the condition worse because it forces the heart to work harder, thus maintaining higher blood pressure, to circulate blood through all the excess tissue. Smoking also increases blood pressure because the nicotine constricts the small blood vessels. Other risk factors include lack of exercise, chronic stress, certain drugs (e.g., birth control pills), and—for some sensitive persons—caffeine.

Types of Hypertensive Blood Pressure Levels

Common blood pressure measurements indicate the pressure of the blood surge in the arteries of the upper arm with each heartbeat. The power of each surge is measured in units called *millimeters of mercury (mm Hg).* Two forces are counted and represented by two numbers. The number on the top of the fraction measures the force of the blood surge when the heart contracts—the *systolic* pressure. The number on the bottom measures the pressure remaining in the arteries when the heart relaxes between beats—the *diastolic* pressure. Adult blood pressure is usually considered normal if the upper limit is recorded as 150/89 mm Hg. Current hypertension screening and treatment programs identify persons with hypertension according to degree of severity of these pressures (e.g., mild, moderate, or severe). Specific care is then outlined depending on the severity, limiting drugs as much as possible.

Mild hypertension. Diastolic pressure is 90 to 104 mm Hg. The initial focus is on approaches of diet therapy (without drugs) to reduce excess weight and restrict sodium.

Moderate hypertension. Diastolic pressure is 105 to 119 mm Hg. In addition to the diet therapy for the mild form, drugs are used according to need and usually include a diuretic agent. Continuous use of some—though not all—diuretic drugs causes loss of potassium along with the increased loss of water from the body. Because potassium is necessary for maintaining normal heart muscle action, a depletion could become dangerous. Potassium replacement is necessary. Dietary replacement by increased use of potassium-rich foods (e.g., fruits, especially bananas and orange juice, vegetables, legumes, nuts, whole grains, and meat) is an important part of therapy. Appendix D provides the sodium and potassium values of foods.

Severe hypertension. Diastolic pressure is at least 120 to 130 mm Hg. In addition to the diet for the moderate form, vigorous drug therapy is necessary. Nutritional support is important for all types of hypertension, along with other nondrug therapies of physical exercise and stress reduction.

The Principles of Nutritional Therapy

Weight Management

According to individual need, weight management requires losing excess weight and maintaining an appropriate weight for height. A sound approach to managing weight loss is given in Chapter 15, and guidance for increasing physical exercise is given in

---

essential hypertension an inherent form of high blood pressure with no specific discoverable cause, considered to be familial; also called primary hypertension.

Chapter 16. Because the overweight state has been closely associated with hypertension risk factors, a wisely planned personal program of weight reduction and physical activity is a cornerstone of therapy.

Sodium Control

In sodium-sensitive persons, additional attention is given to restricting sodium in the diet. The mild 2-g sodium level is generally sufficient (see Box 19-3). In more severe cases of hypertension, however, the moderate 1-g sodium level may be indicated (see Box 19-4).

Other Minerals

In addition to sodium control, especially for sodium-sensitive persons, other minerals have been discussed in relation to hypertension. Some evidence suggests that increased calcium intake is beneficial for some persons with hypertension. As indicated, increased potassium to replace loss with diuretic use and supply normal dietary needs is also an important part of diet therapy.

The Prudent Diet

As outlined for general coronary heart disease, the accepted diet used to control fat and cholesterol is also recommended for persons with any level of hypertension (see Tables 19-2 and 19-3). This is also a sound basic diet for general health promotion and risk reduction.

EDUCATION AND PREVENTION

Practical Food Guides

Food Planning and Purchasing

The general dietary guidelines for Americans (Chapter 1) provide a basic outline to guide food habits. The food exchange lists described in Chapter 20 and listed in Appendix F for reference give the food groups with the fat and sodium modifications discussed here. These lists also provide a guide for controlling kcalories to help plan for any needed weight management. An important part of purchasing food is reading labels carefully. The new food labels provide basic nutrition information in a boxed standard format so that it is easily recognized and clearly expressed (see Chapter 13). All processed food products that make any health claims must follow the strict guides provided by FDA. A good general guide is to use primarily fresh foods with informed selection of processed foods as necessary. Refer to Chapter 13 for background material about food supply and health.

Food Preparation

Guides for preparing primary foods while using less fat and salt are currently available because the public is more aware of these health needs. Many seasonings (e.g., herbs, spices, lemon, wine, onion, garlic, nonfat milk and yogurt, and fresh fat-free meat broth) can help train the taste for less salt and fat (see Appendix E). Less meat in leaner and smaller portions can be combined with more complex carbohydrate foods (e.g., starches such as potato, pasta, rice, bulgur, beans) to make more healthful main dishes. Whole-grain breads and cereals can provide needed fiber, and more use of fish can add healthier forms of fat in smaller quantities. A variety of vegetables may be used (e.g., in salads or steamed and lightly seasoned), and fruits add interest, taste appeal, and nourishment to meals. The American Heart Association Cookbook is an excellent guide to newer, lighter, tasteful, and healthier food preparation.

Special Needs

Individual adaptation of diet principles is important in all nutrition teaching and counseling. Special attention must be given to personal desires, ethnic diets, individual situations, and food habits as discussed in Chapter 14. Any diet must meet both personal and health needs.

Education Principles

Start Early

Prevention of hypertension and heart disease begins in childhood, especially with children in high-risk families. With close attention to normal growth needs, some preventive measures in family food habits relate to weight control and avoidance of foods high in salt and fat. For adults with heart disease and hypertension, learning should be an integral part of all therapy. When a heart attack does occur, learning should begin early in convalescence—not at hospital discharge—to give patients and their families clear and practical knowledge of positive needs.

Focus on High-Risk Groups

Education on the risks of heart disease and hypertension should be directed particularly to persons and families with these risks (see Box 19-2). For example, hypertension has been closely associated with certain high-risk groups, including blacks, persons with strong family histories, and obese individuals.

Use a Variety of Resources

As more is being learned about heart disease and hypertension, the American Heart Association and other health agencies are providing many ex- cellent resources. The American Dietetic Association provides a series of pamphlets that are helpful in client education, several of which are useful here: "Weight Expectations," "Fiber Facts," "Cholesterol Countdown," and "The Sodium Story" (P.O. Box 10960, Chicago, IL 60610). As the public and professionals have become more aware of health needs and disease prevention, an increasing number of resources and programs can also be found in most communities. These include various weight-management programs, registered dietitians in private practice or in health care centers who provide nutrition counseling, and practical food-preparation materials found in a number of recent "light cuisine" cooking classes and cookbooks. Bookstores and public libraries, as well as health education libraries in health centers and clinics, provide more materials in health promotion and self-care. For example, local health care centers teach persons with hypertension and their families how to take their own blood pressure, so they can assume more control in managing their health needs, as well as provide resources for such self-care.

SUMMARY

Coronary heart disease is the leading cause of death in the United States. Its underlying blood vessel disease is *atherosclerosis*, which involves build-up of the fatty substance containing cholesterol on the interior surfaces of blood vessels, interfering with blood flow and damaging blood vessels. If this fatty build-up becomes severe, it cuts off supplies of oxygen and nutrients to tissue cells, which in turn die. When this occurs in a major coronary artery, the result is a *myodardial infarction* or heart attack.

The risk for atherosclerosis increases with the amount and type of blood lipids (fats), or *lipoproteins*, available. Elevated *serum cholesterol* is a primary risk factor for development of atherosclerosis.

Current recommendations to help prevent coronary heart disease involve a prudent diet, weight management, and increased exercise. Such a diet limits fats to 25% to 30% of total diet kcalories, sodium intake to 2 to 3 g per day, and cholesterol intake to 300 mg/day. Dietary recommendations for acute cardiovascular disease (i.e., heart attack) include measures to ensure cardiac rest (e.g., caloric restriction, soft foods, and small meals, modified in fat, cholesterol, and sodium). Persons with chronic heart disease involving congestive heart failure benefit from a low sodium diet to control cardiac edema. Persons with hypertension can improve their condition with weight control, exercise, sodium restriction, and adequate calcium and potassium.

REVIEW QUESTIONS

1. Why are fat and cholesterol primary factors in heart disease? How are they carried in the bloodstream? Which of these "fat packages" carry so-called "good cholesterol" and which carry "bad cholesterol," the cholesterol of concern? How can we influence the relative amounts of these fat and cholesterol carriers in our blood? Describe the food changes involved.

2. Identify the risk factors for heart disease. What control do we have of these risk factors?

3. Identify four diet recommendations for a patient who has had a heart attack. Describe how each recommendation facilitates recovery.

4. Discuss the three main levels of sodium restriction, describing general food choices and preparation methods.

5. What does the term *essential hypertension* mean? Why would weight control and sodium restriction contribute to its control? What other nutrient factors may be involved in hypertension?

SELF-TEST QUESTIONS

True-False

Write the correct statement for each item you answer "false."

1. In the disease process underlying heart disease, atherosclerosis, the fatty deposits in blood vessel linings are composed mainly of cholesterol.

2. Hypertension occurs more frequently in white persons than in black persons.

3. The problem of cardiovascular disease could be solved if cholesterol could be removed entirely from the body.

4. Cholesterol is a dietary essential because humans depend entirely on food sources for their supply.

5. Lipoproteins are the major transport form of lipids in the blood.

6. The basic clinical objective in treating acute cardiovascular disease (i.e., a heart attack) is cardiac rest.

7. In chronic congestive heart disease, the heart may eventually fail because its weakened muscle must work at a faster rate to pump out the body's necessary blood supply.

8. The taste for salt is instinctive in humans to ensure a sufficient supply.

9. Sodium is an effective therapy for congestive heart failure and hypertension.

10. Essential hypertension can be cured by drugs and diet.

Multiple Choice

1. A low cholesterol diet would restrict which of the following foods? (Circle all that apply.)
   a. Fish
   b. Liver
   c. Eggs
   d. Nonfat milk

2. Helpful seasonings to use in a sodium restricted diet include which of the following? (Circle all that apply.)
   a. Lemon juice
   b. Soy sauce
   c. Herbs and spices
   d. Seasoned salt

3. Which of the following foods may be used freely on any low sodium diet?
   a. Fruits
   b. Milk
   c. Meat
   d. Spinach and carrots

SUGGESTIONS FOR ADDITIONAL STUDY

Market Survey
Visit your local market, individually or in small groups, and survey the food products in detail.

- **Fat-related foods**—Look at foods containing both saturated fats from animal sources (e.g., dairy products, meats) and unsaturated fats from plant sources (e.g., vegetable oils, dairy substitute products). Read all labels carefully and note the nutrition information given. Compare the various products in both amount and kind of fat included. Do you find the two saturated plant oils (palm and coconut oil) used in any food products? What health claims are made, and how valid do you think they are? Include food products labeled "low fat" in your survey.

- **Sodium (salt) in foods**—Make a similar survey of processed foods and their labels. Note references to salt or any other sodium compounds used. Compare any sodium-modified products you can find.
- **Sugar and fiber in foods**—Because amounts of both sugar, as a source of kcalories, and fiber, as a possible intestinal binder of cholesterol, have roles in a basic healthy diet to help reduce heart disease risks, make a survey of processed foods containing sugar and fiber. Read labels carefully and note any nutrition information given and any health claims made.

Evaluate the various products you discovered and make a summary report to present in class. Discuss your findings in comparison with those of other groups in the class.

REFERENCES

1. Freedman DS and others: Relation of circumferences and skinfold thicknesses to lipid and insulin concentrations in children and adolescents: the Bogalusa Heart Study, *Am J Clin Nutr* 69(1):108, 1999.
2. Hunink MGM and others: The recent decline in mortality from coronary heart disease, 1998-1999: the effect of secular trends in risk factors and treatment, *JAMA* 277(7): 535, 1997.
3. Anding JD and others: Blood lipids, cardiovascular fitness, obesity, and blood pressure: the presence of potential coronary heart disease risk factors in adolescents, *J Am Diet Assoc* 96(3):238, 1996.
4. Wilson CS: Mediterranean diets: once and future?, *Nutr Today* 33(6):246, 1998.
5. Roche HM and others: Effect of long-term olive oil dietary intervention on postprandial triglycerol and factor VII metabolism, *Am J Clin Nutr* 68(2):552, 1998.

FURTHER READING

- Connor WE, Connor SL: Should a low-fat, high-carbohydrate diet be recommended for everyone? The case for a low-fat, high-carbohydrate diet, *N Eng J Med* (Aug 21):562, 1997.
- Katan MB, Grundy SM, Willet WC: Should a low-fat, high-carbohydrate diet be recommended for everyone? Beyond low-fat diets, *N Engl J Med* 337(Aug 21):563, 1997.
  These well-known researchers in the field of heart disease also emphasize the role of obesity and little physical exercise as risk factors in heart disease.

- Brownson RC and others: Preventing cardiovascular disease through community-based risk reduction: the Bootheel Heart Health Project, *Am J Public Health* 86(2):206, 1996.
  This interesting heart disease reduction project in six southeastern Missouri counties—using community-based activities such as exercise groups, healthy cooking demonstrations, blood pressure and cholesterol screenings, and cardiovascular disease education—clearly shows how such a program can acheive positive results within a relatively brief period, even with modest resources.

20

Diabetes Mellitus

KEY CONCEPTS

- Diabetes mellitus is a metabolic disorder of energy balance with many causes and forms.

- A consistent sound diet is the keystone of all diabetes care and control.

- Good self-care skills practiced daily enable a person with diabetes to remain healthy and reduce risks for complications.

- A personalized care plan, balancing food intake, exercise, and insulin activity, is essential to successful diabetes management.

One in 20 Americans—nearly 11 million—have diabetes. Of these persons, about 15% are insulin-dependent and 85% are non–insulin-dependent. Diabetes complications have become our fifth-ranking cause of death from disease.

Diabetes mellitus is an ancient disease, claiming the lives of its victims at a young age. Greater knowledge of the disease and sound self-care practices have enabled many persons with diabetes to live long and fruitful lives. For the most part, with professional guidance and support, persons with diabetes can remain healthy and reduce risk of health problems by consistently practicing good self-care skills.

In this chapter, we look at diabetes to learn its nature and understand why daily self-care is essential for health.

THE NATURE OF DIABETES

History and Definition

Early History and Name

Diabetes mellitus is an ancient disease. Its symptoms were described on an Egyptian papyrus—the Ebers Papyrus, which dates to about 1500 BC. In the first century, the Greek physician Aretaeus wrote of a malady in which the body "ate its own flesh" and gave off large quantities of urine. He named it *diabetes*, from the Greek word meaning "siphon" or "to pass through." In the 17th century, the word *mellitus*, from the Latin word meaning "honey," was added because of the sweet nature of the urine. The addition of *mellitus* distinguished the disorder from another disorder, *diabetes insipidus*, in which large urine output was observed. Diabetes insipidus, however, is a much more rare and quite different disease that is caused by lack of the pituitary antidiuretic hormone (ADH). Today, the simple term *diabetes* refers to diabetes mellitus. We will follow this common usage in this chapter for simplicity.

Diabetic Dark Ages

Throughout the Middle Ages and the dawning of our scientific era, many early scientists and physicians continued to puzzle over the mystery of diabetes, but the cause remained obscure. For physicians and their patients these years could be called the "Diabetic Dark Ages." Patients had short life spans and were maintained on a variety of semistarvation and high-fat diets.

Discovery of Insulin

The first breakthrough came from a clue pointing to the pancreas's involvement in the disease process. This clue was provided by a young German medical student, Paul Langerhans (1847-1888), who found special clusters of cells scattered about the pancreas forming little "islands" of cells. Though he did not yet understand their function, Langerhans could see that these cells were different from the rest of the tissue and assumed that they must be impor-tant. When his suspicions later proved true, these little clusters of cells were named for their young discoverer—the *islands of Langerhans*. In 1922, using this important clue, two Canadian scientists, Frederick Banting and his assistant, Charles Best, together with two other research team members, physiologists J.B. Collip and J.J.R. Macleod, extracted the first insulin from animals. It proved to be a hormone that regulates the oxidation of blood sugar and helps to convert it to heat and energy. They called the new hormone *insulin*, from the Latin word *insula* meaning "island." Insulin did prove to be the effective agent for treating diabetes. The first child treated in January, 1922, Leonard Thompson, lived to adulthood but died at age 27, not from his diabetes but from coronary heart disease caused by the "diabetic diet" of the day, which was based on 70% of its total kcalories from fat! It is not surprising that his autopsy showed marked atherosclerosis.

Successful Use of Diet and Insulin

The insulin discovery team was more successful on their third try with a young girl diagnosed as having diabetes at age 11.[1] She had initially been put on a starvation diet, and her weight fell from 75 to 45 pounds (34 to 21 kg) over a 3-year period. Fortunately, however, the medical research team had learned the importance of a better regular diet for normal growth and health. Thus with good diet and the new insulin therapy, this child, Elizabeth Hughes, gained weight and vigor and lived a normal life. She married, had three children, took insulin for 58 years and died at age 73 of heart failure. No diabetes has appeared among her descendents.

Current Therapy Based on Contributory Causes

Since those early years of insulin discovery and development, continued research has increased our knowledge of diabetes and helped us develop better means of care. Diabetes is not a single disease but a syndrome of many disorders and degrees, characterized by hyperglycemia (elevated blood sugar) and, in many persons, various complications. We have also learned that diabetes has multiple causes centering around insulin activity, heredity, and excess weight, that help direct current individual therapy. Current research points to new clues, namely lack of a specific cell enzyme that creates increased insulin sensitivity and resistance to obesity.

Insulin Activity

Diabetes is an underlying metabolic disorder developing from various causes. For insulin-dependent diabetes, the underlying direct cause is an antoimmune (self-directed) attack on the insulin-producing cells of the pancreas that is genetic in origin.[2,3] All causes involve some deficiency in insulin's action in controlling the body's energy balance. It is now evident that diabetes is a condition with multiple forms, resulting from the following: (1) a lack of insulin, as in *insulin-dependent diabetes mellitus (IDDM)* or (2) insulin resistance, as in *non–insulin-dependent diabetes mellitus (NIDDM)*.

Heredity

Diabetes, especially in insulin-dependent forms, has usually been defined in terms of heredity. Now there is increasing evidence that considerable *genetic variation* exists in both major forms or classes, IDDM and NIDDM. Environmental factors, especially those contributing to obesity, play a role in bringing out the underlying genetic predisposition for diabetes.[4]

Weight

Diabetes has long been associated with weight. Early clinicians observed that diabetes in overweight persons improved with weight loss, and they described diabetes as "fat diabetes" and "thin diabetes." All of these observations preceded any knowledge about insulin or a relationship between diabetes and the pancreas. Current research has reinforced the association between overweight and NIDDM.[5]

Primary Types of Diabetes

An international work group of the National Institutes of Health has provided an improved classification for the diabetes syndrome. Two broad classes or types of primary diabetes form the basis for continued study of subtypes.

Type 1: Insulin-Dependent Diabetes Mellitus (IDDM)

In its insulin-dependent form (IDDM), which is also called type 1, diabetes develops rapidly and tends to be more severe and unstable. IDDM occurs more frequently in children, although it also occurs in young adults up to about age 40. Persons are usually underweight, and acidosis often occurs.

Type 2: Non–Insulin-Dependent Diabetes Mellitus (NIDDM)

In its non–insulin-dependent form (NIDDM), which is also called type 2, diabetes develops more slowly and is usually milder and more stable. Studies indicate that it is a genetically programmed failure of the beta cell to compensate for insulin resistance. This form of NIDDM occurs mainly in adults above age 40 but is now also being discovered in children.[4] In either case—adults or children, persons are usually overweight. As American children get heavier, the occurrence of type 2 diabetes in young people is expected to increase. Acidosis, however, appears infrequently. Most of these overweight adults and children improve with weight loss and are maintained on diet therapy alone. Sometimes an oral hypoglycemic medication is also needed for control. Currently, the 15.7 million Americans with type 2 diabetes maintain general good health with daily vigilance, strict diet and exercise, and usually oral drug control. Many persons are able to manage their diabetes with a consistent pattern of exercise balanced with diet.[6]

Secondary Forms of Diabetes

Two other secondary classes of diabetes have been recognized. One major class is *gestational diabetes*, which is induced by pregnancy. The other general class of secondary diabetes is caused by a number of conditions or agents.

Gestational Diabetes

It is not uncommon for the normal physiologic stress of pregnancy to cause *glycosuria*, or sugar in the urine. The increased metabolic work of pregnancy, with increased metabolites being produced, sometimes causes glucose to be excreted in the urine, whereas normally there is none. For this reason, prenatal clinics routinely screen pregnant women to detect any sign of diabetes. For women who do develop gestational diabetes, their blood-sugar levels are monitored carefully and they are taught to follow a tightly managed program of diet and self-testing of blood sugar levels. Monitoring tests have shown that a normal blood-sugar level can be maintained throughout the pregnancy, with very few women requiring insulin, by strict use of the following plan[7]:

- **Kcalories based on body weight**—30 kcal/kg for ideal-weight women, 24 kcal/kg for overweight women.
- **Total day's kcalories division**—40% carbohydrate, 20% protein, 40% fat.
- **Meal/snack division of total kcalories**—A 1–1–3–1–3–1/10 meal-snack pattern. This means 10% of the day's kcalories at breakfast, 10% at midmorning snack, 30% at lunch, 10% at midafternoon snack, 30% at dinner, and 10% at evening snack.
- **Blood-sugar monitoring**—Tight surveillance based on four daily self-tests of blood glucose: a fasting test each morning before eating and 1 hour after each meal, with food adjustments or insulin as needed.

Pregnant women at risk for gestational diabetes who have followed this program faithfully have produced healthy infants without the generally associated complications of macrosomia, perinatal mortality, and prematurity. These results are in sharp contrast to the generally reported rates of macrosomia in gestational diabetes (i.e., 20% to 40%). Gestational diabetes is further discussed in Chapter 10.

General Secondary Diabetes

Secondary diabetes may be caused by a number of conditions or agents affecting the pancreas. Examples include the following:

- **Pancreatic conditions or disease**—Tumor affecting the islet cells, acute viral infection by a number of agents such as the mumps virus, acute pancreatitis from biliary disease and gallstones, chronic pancreatic insufficiency such as occurs in cystic fibrosis, pancreatic surgery as may occur in cancer of the pancreas, or severe traumatic abdominal injury.
- **Alcohol**—One of the most common causes of chronic pancreatitis is alcohol abuse.
- **Drugs**—Pancreatitis may be caused by various drugs such as sulfa drugs, estrogens (including estrogen-containing contraceptive pills), thiazide diuretic drugs, tetracycline, or corticosteroids.

Symptoms of Diabetes

Initial Signs

Early signs of diabetes include three primary symptoms, as follow: (1) increased thirst—*polydipsia*, (2) increased urination—*polyuria*, and (3) increased hunger—*polyphagia*. Weight loss may occur with IDDM or obesity with NIDDM.

Laboratory Test Results

Various laboratory tests show the following results: *glycosuria* (sugar in the urine), *hyperglycemia* (elevated blood sugar), and abnormal glucose tolerance tests.

---

hyperglycemia (Gr. *hyper*, above; *glykys*, sweet) blood sugar elevated above normal limits.

macrosomia (Gr. *macro*, large; *sōma*, body) excessive fetal growth resulting in an abnormally large infant carrying high risk for perinatal mortality.

Other Possible Symptoms

Additional signs may include blurred vision, skin irritation or infection, and general weakness and loss of strength. In elderly persons with diabetes, the skin irritation may be perineal itching and the weakness may be general drowsiness.

Progressive Results

Continued symptoms may occur as the uncontrolled condition becomes more serious. These symptoms may include water and electrolyte imbalance, ketoacidosis, and coma.

THE METABOLIC PATTERN OF DIABETES

Energy Balance and Normal Blood-Sugar Controls

Energy Balance

Diabetes has been called a disease of carbohydrate metabolism, but it is a general metabolic disorder involving all three of the energy nutrients—carbohydrate, fat, and protein. Diabetes is especially related to the metabolism of the two main fuels, carbohydrate and fat, in the body's overall energy system, as described in Chapter 16. The three basic stages of normal glucose metabolism—initial interchange with glycogen and reduction to a smaller central compound (*glycolysis pathway*), joining with the other two energy nutrients fat and protein (*pyruvate link*), and final common energy production (*citrate cycle*)—are illustrated in Figure 20-1.

---

ketoacidosis **excess production of ketones; a form of metabolic acidosis as occurs in uncontrolled diabetes or starvation from burning body fat for energy fuel; a continuing, uncontrolled state can result in coma and death.**

Normal Blood-Sugar Balance

Control of blood sugar within its normal range of 70 to 120 mg/dl (3.9 to 6.6 mmol/L) is vital to life. Normal controls are "built in" to ensure that we always have sufficient circulating blood sugar, glucose, to meet our constant energy needs—even our basal metabolic energy needs during sleep—because glucose is the body's major fuel. Note the balanced sources and uses of blood glucose as shown in Figure 20-2.

Sources of blood glucose. To ensure a constant supply of the body's main fuel, the following two sources of blood glucose exist: (1) diet—the energy nutrients in our food (e.g., dietary carbohydrate, fat, and, as needed, protein); and (2) glycogen—the back-up source from constant turnover of stored glycogen in liver and muscles.

Uses of blood glucose. To prevent blood glucose from continually rising above normal range, the body "drains off" glucose as needed by using it in the following ways: (1) burning it by cell oxidation for immediate energy needs; (2) changing it to glycogen, which is briefly stored in muscles and liver, then withdrawn and changed back into glucose for short-term energy needs; and (3) changing it to fat, which is stored for longer periods as body fat.

Pancreatic Hormonal Control

The specialized cells of the islets (islands) of Langerhans in the pancreas provide three hormones that work together to regulate blood-glucose levels: (1) insulin, (2) glucagon, and (3) somatostatin. The specific arrangement of human islet cells is illustrated in Figure 20-3.

Insulin. Insulin is the major hormone controlling the level of blood glucose. It accomplishes this major function through a number of metabolic actions, as follow:

- Helping to transport circulating glucose into cells by way of specialized insulin receptors

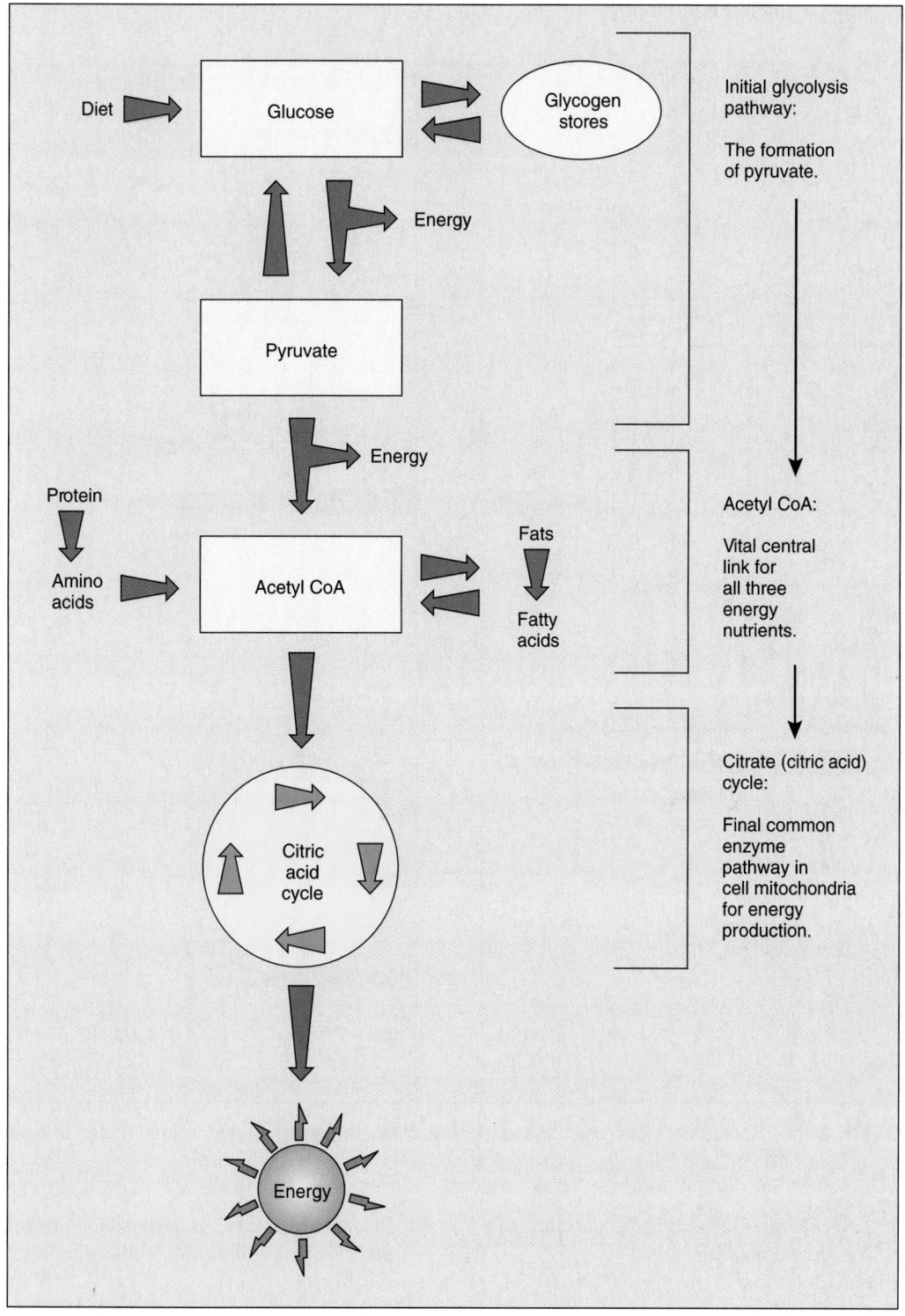

FIGURE 20-1 Basic glucose metabolism and interaction with fat and protein to yield energy.

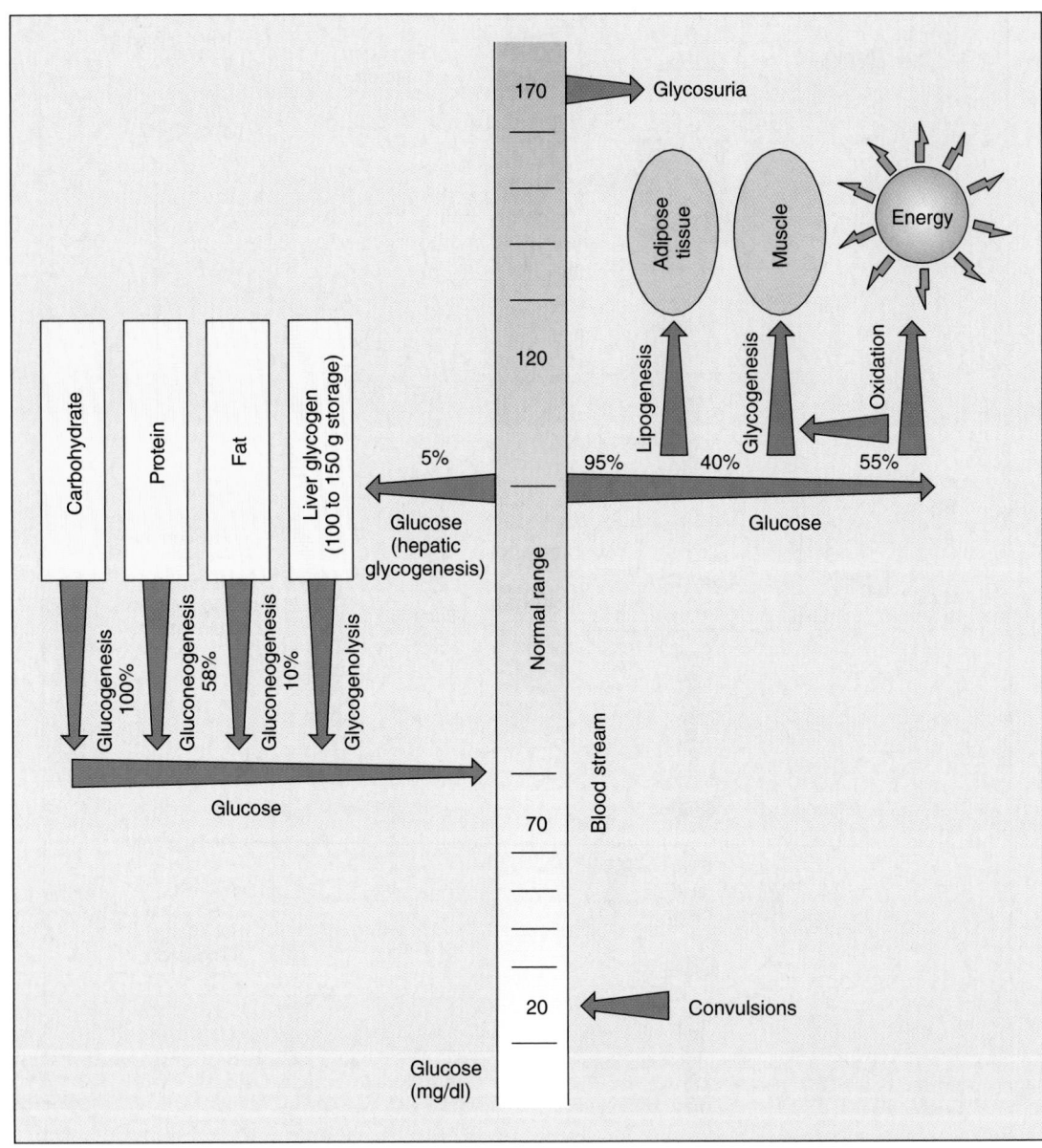

FIGURE 20-2 Sources of blood glucose (i.e., food and stored glycogen) and normal routes of control.

- Helping change glucose to glycogen and store it in liver and muscles
- Stimulating the change of glucose to fat for storage as body fat
- Inhibiting breakdown of tissue fat and protein
- Promoting uptake of amino acids by skeletal muscles, increasing tissue protein synthesis
- Influencing the burning of glucose for constant energy as needed

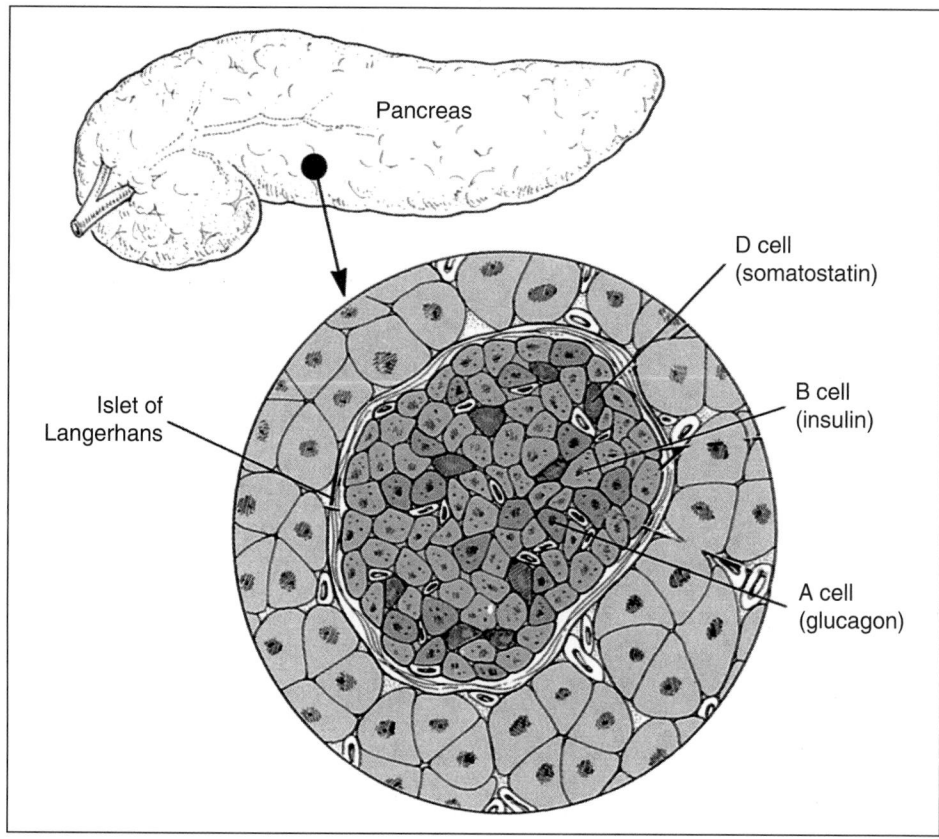

FIGURE 20-3 Islets of Langerhans, located in the pancreas.

Insulin is produced in the B cells of the islets, which fill its central zone and make up about 60% of each islet gland.

Glucagon. Glucagon is a hormone that acts in an opposite manner to insulin to balance the overall blood-glucose control. It can rapidly break down stored glycogen and, to a lesser extent, fat. This action raises blood sugar as needed to protect brain and other tissues during sleep or fasting. Glucagon is produced in the A cells of the pancreatic islets, which are arranged around the outer rim of each of these glands, making up about 30% of its total cells.

glucagon (Gr. *glykys,* sweet; *gonē,* seed) a hormone secreted by the A cells of the pancreatic islets of Langerhans in response to hyperglycemia; it has an opposite balancing effect to that of insulin, raising the blood sugar, and thus is used as a quick-acting antidote for a low blood sugar reaction of insulin. It also counteracts the overnight fast during sleep by breaking down liver glycogen to keep blood-sugar levels normal and maintain an adequate energy supply for normal nerve and brain function.

Somatostatin. Somatostatin is the pancreatic hormone that acts as a "referee" for several other hormones that affect blood-glucose levels, synthesizing their various actions. Somatostatin is produced in the D cells of the pancreatic islets, scattered among the A and B cells and making up about 10% of each islet's cells. Because it has more generalized functions in regulating circulating blood sugar, somatostatin is also produced in other parts of the body (e.g., the hypothalamus).

Abnormal Metabolism in Uncontrolled Diabetes

When normal insulin activity is lacking, such as in uncontrolled diabetes, the normal controls of blood-sugar levels do not operate. As a result, abnormal metabolic changes and imbalances occur among the three energy nutrients.

Glucose

Glucose cannot enter cells and be oxidized through its normal cell pathways to produce energy. Thus it builds up in the blood, creating hyperglycemia.

Fat

Fat tissue formation (*lipogenesis*) decreases, and fat tissue breakdown (*lipolysis*) increases. This increased fat breakdown leads to excess formation of ketones, intermediate products of fat breakdown, and their accumulation in the body, causing ketoacidosis. The appearance of one of these ketones, acetone, in the urine indicates the development of ketoacidosis.

Protein

Protein tissues are also broken down in the body's effort to secure energy sources, causing weight loss and urinary nitrogen loss.

Long-Term Complications

Poorly controlled diabetes increases risks for long-term diabetic complications. These health problems mainly relate to tissue changes affecting blood vessels in vital organs.

Retinopathy

This change in the eyes involves small hemorrhages from broken arteries in the retina, with yellow, waxy discharge or retinal detachment. This complication can eventually cause blindness. Retinopathy is not to be confused with the blurry vision that sometimes occurs as one of the first signs of diabetes. Blurry vision is caused by the increased glucose concentration in the fluids of the eye, bringing brief changes in the curved, light-refracting surface of the eye.

Nephropathy

These changes in the kidneys involve the nephrons and can lead to renal failure. This extensive intercapillary *glomerulosclerosis* (see Chapter 21) has been named the *Kimmelstiel-Wilson syndrome*, for the German-American pathologist and English physician who first described it.

Neuropathy

These changes in the nerves involve injury and disease in the peripheral nervous system—especially in the legs and feet, causing prickly sensations, increasing pain, and eventual loss of sensation due to damaged nerves. This loss of nerve reaction can lead to further tissue damage and infection from unfelt foot injuries such as bruises, burns, and deeper cellulitis.

Atherosclerosis

Coronary heart disease from underlying atherosclerosis (see Chapter 19) occurs about four times as often in persons with diabetes than in the general population. Peripheral vascular disease occurs about 40 times as often. This large risk factor accounts for the dietary recommendation to reduce dietary fats and cholesterol.

GENERAL MANAGEMENT OF DIABETES

Early Detection and Monitoring

The guiding principles for treating diabetes are early detection and prevention of complications. Community screening programs and testing of family members help to identify persons with elevated blood-sugar levels for a follow-up *glucose-tolerance test* (i.e., fasting and 2-hour tests with a measured glucose dose) and medical diagnosis of results. An additional monitoring aid is the *hemoglobin A_{1c} assay* (normal range 4% to 6%) test, which provides an effective tool for evaluating long-term management of diabetes and degree of control because the glucose attaches itself to the particular hemoglobin over the life of the red blood cell. Therefore this test reflects the level of blood glucose over the preceding 3-month period of time. Other tests such as *fructosamine* (an amino sugar formed from glucosamine) or *C-peptide* (an antibody radioimmunoassay following a special test meal to determine the type of diabetes) may sometimes be used for diagnostic purposes. But the glycosylated hemoglobin assay, Hb A_{1c}, is currently the most accurate assessment for monitoring ongoing blood-sugar control.

Basic Goals of Care

General Overall Objectives

The health care team is guided by three basic objectives in working with the person with diabetes.

Maintenance of optimal nutrition. The first objective is to sustain a high level of nutrition for general health promotion, adequate growth and development, and maintenance of an appropriate lean weight.

Avoidance of symptoms. This objective seeks to keep a person relatively free from symptoms of *hyperglycemia* and *glycosuria*, which indicate poor control.

Prevention of complications. This third objective recognizes the increased risk a person with diabetes carries for developing the significant tissue changes already described. Consistent control of blood-sugar levels helps to reduce these risks.

Special Objectives in Pregnancy

When a woman with diabetes becomes pregnant or the pregnancy induces gestational diabetes, her body metabolism changes to meet the increased physiologic needs of the pregnancy (see Chapter 10). In such a high-risk pregnancy, a team of specialists usually works closely with the mother. Careful team monitoring of the mother's diabetes management is essential to ensure her own health and healthy fetal development, as well as avoid the potential problems of fetal damage, perinatal mortality, stillbirth, prematurity, or delivery of a very large baby (*macrosomia*) who is unable to survive.

Basic Elements of Diabetes Management

Balancing three basic elements is essential in good control of diabetes.[8] First, the healthy *diet* described here forms the foundation for good management. Second, physical *exercise* provides the important balance to maintain good blood-sugar control. Third, to ensure adequate insulin activity, some persons need *drugs* (i.e., insulin injections for all children and young adults with diabetes, and oral hypoglycemic agents for older adults). In today's stressful world, however, we may well add a fourth element—*stress-coping skills*.

Importance of Good Self-Care Skills

To accomplish these objectives, a person with diabetes must learn and regularly practice good self-care. Daily self-discipline and informed self-care are necessary for sound diabetes management because all persons with diabetes must ultimately treat

---

ketones chemical name for a class of organic compounds, including three ketoacid bases that occur as intermediate products of fat metabolism, one of which is acetone.

acetone a major ketone compound that results from fat breakdown for energy in uncontrolled diabetes; persons with diabetes periodically do urinary acetone tests to monitor the status of their diabetes control.

cellulitis diffuse inflammation of soft or connective tissues (e.g., in the foot) from injury, bruises, or pressure sores that lead to infection; poor care may result in ulceration and abscess or gangrene.

themselves, with the support of a good health care team. More emphasis is now being given to comprehensive diabetes-education programs that encourage self-monitoring of blood glucose levels and more self-care responsibility.

DIET THERAPY BASED ON THE BALANCE CONCEPT

The Diabetes Control and Complications Trial

Based on the need for a more comprehensive program of care of diabetes developed on the concept of individual metabolic balance, a United States clinical research study supported by the National Institutes of Health was recently organized. This large research project, the Diabetes Control and Complications Trial (DCCT), compared the effects of intensive insulin therapy that is aimed at achieving blood glucose levels as close as possible to the normal nondiabetic range with the effects of conventional therapy on early microvascular complications of insulin dependent diabetes mellitus (IDDM)—type 1. The positive results of this important study, supported by both the American Dietetic Association and the American Diabetic Association, remain highly significant.[8] These results indicate the strength of team care, with the expanded role of the clinical dietitian, who is assisted as necessary by the diabetes team nurse (RN) and licensed vocational nurse (LVN) in individualizing the medical nutritional therapy with various diet-management tools and facilitation of insulin balance.

Application in Clinical Practice

Revised Recommendations

Based on the remarkable positive research results, the American Diabetes Association issued a revised position paper in March 1994 on nutrition recommendations and principles of care for persons with diabetes mellitus, which was immediately endorsed by the American Dietetic Association House of Delegates.[8] These guidelines outlined the goal of medical nutrition therapy: to assist patients with diabetes in making changes in nutrition and exercise habits in balance with insulin from both internal or external sources.

Core Problem

The core problem in diabetes is energy balance, the regulation of the body's primary fuel—blood glucose. Based on this concept of balance, the three main principles of nutritional therapy are as follows: (1) total energy balance, (2) nutrient balance, and (3) food-distribution balance. Personal diet is then expressed in terms of the following: (1) total kcalories required for energy; (2) ratio of these kcalories in relative amounts of the three energy nutrients carbohydrate, fat, and protein; and (3) a food distribution pattern for the day. A fundamental personal principle underlies the whole plan—*the diet for any person with diabetes is always based on the normal nutritional needs of that person for positive health.*

Total Energy Balance

Normal Growth and Weight Management

Because IDDM usually begins in childhood (average age, 11 years), the normal height-weight charts for children provide a standard for adequate growth. During adulthood, maintaining a lean weight continues to be a basic goal. Because NIDDM usually occurs in overweight adults, the major goal is weight reduction and control.

Total Kcalories

The total energy value of the diet for a person with diabetes should be sufficient kcalories to meet individual needs for normal growth and development, physical activity and exercise, and maintenance of a desirable lean weight. Exercise is always an important factor in diabetes control because it improves the body's ability to use glucose by increasing insulin-receptor sites in the tissues. Energy intake in the diet is constantly balanced with energy output in work and exercise and metabolic body work.

The RDA and DRI standards for children and adults (see inside front book cover) can serve as guides for total energy needs, with appropriate reductions in kcalories for overweight adults, as described in Chapter 15.

Nutrient Balance

The ratio of carbohydrate, fat, and protein in the diet is based on current recommendations for ideal glucose regulation and lower fat intake to reduce risks for cardiovascular complications (Table 20-1).

Carbohydrate

A more liberal use of carbohydrates, mainly in complex starch forms with fiber, is recommended. About 60% of the total kcalories of the diet should come from carbohydrates.

Complex carbohydrate. For general needs, most of the dietary carbohydrate kcalories (i.e., about 40% of the total kcalories) should come from complex forms—the starches. In most cases, these complex carbohydrates break down more slowly than simple sugars and release their available glucose over time, thus producing a smoother blood-sugar level.

Fiber. Different kinds of dietary fiber in plant foods (e.g., whole grains, vegetables, fruits) influence the rate of absorption of the carbohydrate and alter its effect on the blood-sugar level. Along with a high-carbohydrate diet, increased dietary fiber up to 40 g/day (i.e., including both soluble and insoluble forms) has been suggested by clinical researchers as an important factor in improving carbohydrate metabolism and lowering total cholesterol and LDL-cholesterol levels.

Simple carbohydrates. The remainder of the carbohydrate kcalories—about 15%—can come from simple carbohydrates (e.g., natural sugars as in fruits and milk). Sucrose-sweetened foods should be carefully controlled. These simple carbohydrates are readily absorbed and have a more immediate effect on the blood-sugar level. Honey is a form of simple sugar—mainly fructose—and is *not* a sugar substitute.

Sugar substitute sweeteners. Nutrititive and nonnutritive sweeteners may be used in the diet when used in moderation. Various sugar substitutes are available. Approved noncaloric sweeteners include products such as saccharin, aspartame,

TABLE 20-1 Distribution of major nutrients in normal and diabetic diets (as percentages of total calories)

	Starch and other polysaccharides* (%)	Sugars† and dextrins (%)	Fat (%)	Protein (%)	Alcohol (%)
Typical American diet	25-35	20-30	35-45 (⅔ saturated)	12-19	0-10
Traditional diabetic diets	25-30	10-15‡	40-45	16-21	0
Newer diabetic diets: current therapy	30-45	5-15‡	25-35 (Less than ½ saturated)	12-24	0-6

*A substantial majority of these calories are starch, but complex carbohydrates also include cellulose, hemicellulose, pentosans, and pectin.

†Monosaccharides and disaccharides—mainly sucrose, but fructose, glucose, lactose, and maltose are also included.

‡Almost exclusively natural sugars, mainly in fruit and milk (lactose).

and acesulfame-K. Aspartame is made from two amino acids, phenylalanine and aspartic acid, and is metabolized as such. Small amounts of caloric sweeteners, such as the very small amounts of sucrose, fructose, and sorbitol must be accounted for in a meal. Many persons, however, cannot tolerate sorbitol and have significant diarrhea when it is used. In summary, nutritive and nonnutritive sweeteners are safe to consume in moderation and as part of a nutritious and well-balanced diet.[9,10]

Protein

Most Americans eat much more protein than they need. Normal age requirements as outlined in the RDA standards can be a guide. For adults, 0.8 g/kg is recommended for diabetes control. In general, about 12% to 20% of the total kcalories as protein is sufficient to meet growth needs in children and maintain tissue integrity in adults. High protein intakes are generally not recommended because of their saturated fat content and unnecessary stress on the kidneys to excrete excess nitrogen.

Fat

No more than 25% to 30% of the diet's total kcalories should come from fat, with saturated fat (animal fat) composing less than 10%. Fat should always be used in moderation. Lower cholesterol intake—no more than 300 mg/day—is also recommended. Control of fat-related foods helps reduce the risk diabetes contributes to the development of atherosclerosis and coronary heart disease.

Current diet recommendations of the American Heart Association, the American Diabetes Association, and the American Dietetic Association are compared in Table 20-2.

Food Distribution Balance

As a general rule, fairly even amounts of food should be eaten at regular intervals throughout the day, adjusted to blood-glucose self-monitoring. This basic pattern helps provide a more even blood-sugar supply and prevent swings between low and high levels. Snacks between meals may be needed.

Daily Activity Schedule

Food distribution must be planned ahead, especially by persons using insulin, and adjusted according to each day's scheduled activities and blood-sugar monitoring to prevent episodes of hypoglycemia from insulin reactions. Careful distribution of food and snacks is especially important for children and adolescents with diabetes to balance with insulin during growth spurts and changing hormone patterns of puberty. Practical consideration should

TABLE 20-2 Comparison of AHA and ADA diet recommendations*

	AHA Step 1 (% total kcal)	AHA Step 2 (% total kcal)	ADA/ADA (% total kcal)
Total fat	30	30	30
Monounsaturated	10-15	10-15	12-14
Saturated	10	7	10
Polyunsaturated	Up to 10	Up to 10	6-8
Carbohydrate	50-60	50-60	55-60
Protein	15-20	15-20	0.8 g/kg
Cholesterol	300 mg/day	200 mg/day	300 mg/day

*AHA, American Heart Association; ADA, American Diabetes Association and American Dietetic Association.

be given to school and work schedules and demands, athletics, social events, and stress periods. A stressful event caused by any source—injury, anxiety, fear, pain—brings an adrenaline (epinephrine) rush, which is the common "fight or flight" effect that counteracts insulin activity and can contribute to a hypoglycemic response.

Exercise

For persons using insulin, it is especially important that any exercise period, team or individual sports, or additional physical activity is covered in the food distribution plan. This is especially important with athletes in highly competitive and physical sports such as football. Gregory and associates[11] presents the case of a college football player with diabetes and his carefully planned blood-sugar control during games. For adults with NIDDM, regular exercise is an essential part of a successful weight-management program.

Drug Therapy

The food distribution pattern will also be influenced by any form of drug therapy, type and amount and dose schedule of insulin or an oral hypoglycemic agent, that is required for control of the diabetes.[12]

Diet Management

General Planning According to Type of Diabetes

Because forms of diabetes vary widely, the nature of an individual's diabetes and its treatment largely determine the personal diet management required. Table 20-3 provides guidelines for diet strategies necessary for each of the two main types of diabetes, IDDM and NIDDM.

Individual Needs

Every person with diabetes is unique, having not only a particular form and degree of diabetes but also a different living situation, background, and food habits. All of these personal needs must be considered, as discussed in Chapters 14 and 17, if appropriate and realistic care is to be planned. The nutrition counselor, who is usually the clinical dietitian, always seeks to discover these various individual needs in a careful initial nutrition history that includes medical and psychosocial needs, as well as personal lifestyle characteristics. This information provides the basis for determining the diet prescription and calculating nutritional requirements. A personal diet plan using the balance principles described here can then be outlined.

TABLE 20-3 Dietary strategies for the two main types of diabetes mellitus

Dietary strategy	IDDM (non-obese)	NIDDM (usually obese)
Decrease energy intake (kcalories)	No	Yes
Increase frequency and number of feedings	Yes	Usually no
Have regular daily intake of kcalories of carbohydrate, protein. and fat	Very important	Not important if average caloric intake remains in low range
Plan consistent daily ratio of protein, carbohydrate and fat for each feeding	Desirable	Not necessary
Use extra or planned food to treat or prevent hypoglycemia	Very important	Not necessary
Plan regular times for meals and snacks	Very important	Not important
Use extra food for unusual exercise	Yes	Usually not necessary
During illness, use small, frequent feedings of carbohydrate to prevent starvation ketoacidosis	Important	Usually not necessary because of resistance to ketoacidosis

A major principle of diabetes management is the variety of methods and dietary guidelines that the clinical dietitian, assisted by the nutrition team, can use in planning and supporting patients with diabetes in their personal daily care of their disease. Among these various dietary guides, the familiar food exchange method—tailored by the clinical dietitian to meet individual needs—remains a commonly used approach. Materials used in the variable research methods are available from the American Dietetic Association and the American Diabetes Association.

Food Exchange System

When this method is chosen by the clinical dietitian in conference with the patient and family, it is used by both the clinical dietitian and the patient. The dietitian uses this familiar tool to calculate the patient's energy and nutrient needs, as well as to distribute foods in a balanced meal/snack plan. The food exchange system is so called because persons with diabetes use the system to select a variety of foods from the various food groups according to the personal food plan outlined by the dietitian.

In this system, commonly used foods are grouped into three basic *exchange lists* according to approximately equal food values in the portions indicated. Thus a variety of foods may be chosen from these lists to fulfill the basic food plan determined by the dietitian, while the basic diet prescription of total kcalories and balanced ratio of nutrients is maintained. The designated food values for each of the food exchange groups is shown in Table 20-4. These exchange lists are based on current principles and recommendations for wise diabetes control and health promotion. The booklet "Exchange Lists for Meal Planning" is available from both the American Diabetes Association and the American Dietetic Association. Its colorful illustrations, clear content, and style provide a helpful tool for patient and client education.[13] These exchange lists are included in Appendix F. Table 20-5 illustrates a calculated 2200 kcal diet and resulting food pattern using the exchange system. Box 20-1 gives a sample menu based on this food pattern.

Special Concerns

Special concerns come up in daily living and become an important part of ongoing diet counseling. Some suggestions for these concerns are given here.

Special diet food items. Little need exists for special "dietetic" or "diabetic" foods. Persons with diabetes should eat the regular, well-balanced diet (i.e., modified in the same areas of fat, cholesterol, sugar, fiber, and salt) that is recommended for the general population to promote health and prevent disease. This kind of a healthful diet primarily uses regular fresh foods from all the basic food groups, with limited use of processed foods (noting the grams of carbohydrate per serving on the label) and more use of nonfat seasonings. The simple principles of moderation and variety guide food choices and amounts.

Alcohol. Occasional use of alcohol in an adult diabetic diet can be planned, but caution must be the guide. Individuals with IDDM who consume alcohol must be reminded of the following: (1) to eat when they drink, because food slows alcohol absorption; and (2) to not increase insulin dose because alcohol's overall effect is lowering blood sugars. Occasional use is defined as moderate intake (i.e., less than 6% of the total kcalories on a given day) and not more than 1 or 2 equivalent portions once or twice a week. An equivalent portion is 1 oz of liquor, 4 oz of wine,

---

hypoglycemia (Gr. *hypo-,* below; *glykys,* sweet) low blood sugar; a serious condition in insulin-dependent diabetes management that requires immediate sugar intake to counteract, followed by a snack of complex carbohydrate food (e.g., bread or crackers) and a protein (e.g., lean meat, peanut butter, or cheese) to maintain the normal blood sugar

TABLE 20-4   Amount of nutrients in one serving
from each exchange list

Groups /Lists	Carbohydrate (grams)	Protein (grams)	Fat (grams)	Calories
Carbohydrate group				
Starch	15	3	0-1	80
Fruit	15	—	—	60
Milk				
Fat-free	12	8	0-3	90
Reduced-fat	12	8	5	120
Whole	12	8	8	150
Other carbohydrates	15	Varies	Varies	Varies
Vegetables	5	2	—	25
Meat and meat substitute group				
Very Lean	—	7	0-1	35
Lean	—	7	3	55
Medium-fat	—	7	5	75
High-fat	—	7	8	100
Fat group	—	—	5	45

(© 1995, American Diabetes Association and American Dietetic Association: *Exchange Lists for Meal Planning.* Used with permission.)

or 12 oz of beer. The same precautions for the use of alcohol that apply to the general public apply to people with diabetes. When a person with IDDM uses a small amount of alcohol, it should *not* be substituted for food exchanges in the diet, but only used in addition, to avoid the possibility of hypoglycemic reactions. Alcohol may be used in cooking as desired because it vaporizes in the cooking process and only contributes its flavor to the finished product.

Physical activity.   For any unusual physical activity, the person using insulin needs to make special plans ahead for snacks to cover the event. This is especially true of young persons with a sensitive brittle form of diabetes who engage in strenuous athletic competition or practice or any active individual (Table 20-6).[11] The energy demands of exercise are discussed in Chapter 16.

Hypoglycemia.   Persons with diabetes must learn how to avoid hypoglycemia, which entails drops in blood glucose levels, because it is a serious condition. The body's vital "brain food" is glucose. The brain depends on a constant supply of glucose for metabolism and proper function; a prolonged lack of glucose can lead to permanent damage.

TABLE 20-5 Calculation of diabetic diet using exchange system (2200 kcal)

Food group	Total day's exchanges	Carbohydrates: 275 g (50% kcal)	Protein: 110 g (20% kcal)	Fat: 75 g (30% kcal)	Breakfast	Lunch	Dinner	Snacks Afternoon	Snacks Bedtime
Carbohydrates									
Fruit	3	45			1	1		1	
Vegetable	4	20	8			2	2		
Other carbohydrates	1	15	Varies	Varies			1		
Milk									
Skim	2	24	16		1				1
Low-fat	—								
Whole	—								
Starch	11.5	172	34.5		3	3	3	1	1.5
Meat and meat substitutes									
Very lean	2		14	0-1				1	1
Lean	3		21	9			3		
Medium-fat	2		14	10	1	1			
High-fat	—								
Fat	11			55	3	3	3	1	1
Total g		276	107.5	75					

BOX 20-1   Sample menu prescription: 2200 kcal

275 g carbohydrate (50% kcal)
110 g protein (20% kcal)
75 g fat (30% kcal)

Breakfast

1 medium, sliced fresh peach
Shredded wheat cereal
1 poached egg on whole-grain toast
1 bran muffin
1 tsp margarine
1 cup low-fat milk
Coffee or tea

Lunch

Vegetable soup with wheat crackers
Tuna sandwich on whole-wheat bread
   Filling: Tuna (drained ½ cup)
            Mayonnaise (2 tsp)
            Chopped dill pickle
            Chopped celery
Fresh pear

Afternoon snack

10 crackers with 2 tbsp peanut butter
Orange

Dinner

Pan-broiled pork chop (trimmed well)
1 cup brown rice
½-1 cup green beans
Tossed green salad
   Italian dressing (1-2 tbsp)
½ cup applesauce
1 bran muffin

Evening snack

3 cups popped, plain popcorn
1 oz cheese
1 cup low-fat milk

Hypoglycemia can occur from too high a dose of insulin, or from hypoglycemic oral drugs that act by stimulating the islet cells in the pancreas to secrete more insulin. Hypoglycemia can also occur if a person with diabetes delays a meal or snack, does not eat enough carbohydrate, or exercises too much without sufficient food. The principle symptoms include sweating, weakness, hunger, dizziness, trembling, headache, increased heart rate, confusion, and sometimes double vision. Because behavior is often irrational and movements are uncoordinated, this state may be mistaken for drunkenness, and the person may lapse into coma.

Thus an ID bracelet or pendant is an important means of informing others of the true condition so that proper treatment—a glucose replacement in food or beverage or an injection of glucagon—can be given. Note the 15-g carbohydrate-replacement portions listed in the Bread/Cereal (Starch) and Fruit exchange groups (see Table 20-4 and Appendix F). Persons with IDDM should always carry a convenient form of sugar (e.g., sugar lumps or glucose tablets) with them to take at the first sign of a hypoglycemic attack, and then follow this sugar as soon as possible with a snack of complex carbohydrate and protein.

TABLE 20-6   Meal-planning guide for active people with IDDM

Moderate activity	Exchange needs	Sample menus
30 minutes	1 bread OR	1 bran muffin OR
	1 fruit	1 small orange
1 hour	2 bread + 1 meat OR	Tuna sandwich OR
	2 fruit + 1 milk	½ cup fruit salad + 1 cup milk
Strenuous activity	**Exchange needs**	**Sample menus**
30 minutes	2 fruit OR	1 small banana OR
	1 bread + 1 fat	½ bagel + 1 tsp cream cheese
1 hour	2 bread + 1 meat + 1 milk OR	Meat and cheese sandwich + 1 cup milk OR
	2 bread + 2 meat + 2 fruit	Hamburger + 1 cup orange juice

Illness.   When general illness occurs, food and insulin may need to be adjusted accordingly. The texture of the food can be modified to use easily digested and absorbed liquid foods (Table 20-7). This type of liquid substitution can be used for meals not eaten. In general, persons with diabetes who are ill should do the following:

- Maintain food intake every day, not skipping meals.
- Not omit insulin but follow an adjusted dosage if needed.
- Replace carbohydrate solid foods with equal liquid or soft foods.
- Monitor blood-sugar level frequently.
- Contact physician if the illness lasts more than a day or so.

Travel.   When a trip is planned, the diet counselor and the client should confer to decide on food choices depending on what will be available to the traveler. In general, preparation activities can include the following:

- Reviewing meal-planning skills, the number and type of exchanges at each meal, basic portion sizes, and tips on eating out.

- Learning about foods that will be available (e.g., ordering a diabetic diet ahead from airlines)
- Selecting appropriate snacks to carry and planning time intervals for their use.
- Planning for any time zone changes.
- Carrying some quick-acting form of carbohydrate at all times and telling companions about signs, symptoms, and treatment of hypoglycemia.
- Wearing an ID bracelet or pendant.
- Securing a physician's cover letter concerning syringes and insulin prescription.

Eating out.   In general, persons with diabetes should plan ahead so that food eaten at home before and after a meal out can be accommodated to maintain the continuing day's balance. Choosing restaurants that have the appropriate food available also makes menu selection easier.

Stress.   Any form of physiologic or psychosocial stress affects diabetes control because of the hormonal responses that are antagonistic to insulin action. Persons with diabetes, especially those using insulin, should learn useful stress-reduction exercises and activities as part of their self-care skills and practices.

TABLE 20-7 How to modify a diabetic meal plan for sick days

Usual food intake	Exchange	Carbohydrate (g)
½ chicken breast, roasted	3 meat	0
1 tsp margarine	1 fat	0
½ cup rice	1 bread	15
Tossed green salad, lemon wedge	Free food	0
¾ cup strawberries	1 fruit	10
1 cup skim milk	1 milk	12
		TOTAL 37
Sick day intake*	**Exchange**	**Carbohydrate (g)**
2 cups broth	Free food	0
1 cup gelatin	2 fruit	20
1 cup ginger ale (regular)	2 fruit	20
2 cups herbal tea	Free food	0
		TOTAL 40

*OBJECTIVE: To provide required amounts of carbohydrate for times when the person with diabetes has a poor appetite.

DIABETES EDUCATION PROGRAM

Goal: Person-Centered Self-Care

In the past few years, the traditional roles of health care professionals and their patients and clients have been changing. Patients and clients are taking a much more active and informed role in their own health care. This action is especially true in the case of persons with diabetes. By the nature of the disease process and the necessity of daily "survival" skills, persons with diabetes must practice regular, daily self-care (see Clinical Applications box, "Case Study: Richard Manages His Diabetes"). Thus any effective and successful diabetes-education program must focus on personal needs and informed self-care skills. Professional communication must reflect this personal focus and supportive concern.

Content: Tools for Self-Care

Necessary Skills

Diabetes educators and the American Diabetes Association have developed guidelines for diabetes education based on the learning needs and necessary skills and content areas required for self-care of diabetes. Persons with diabetes must have essential skills for the best possible control, as well as favorable surrounding factors related to life situations and psychosocial needs. The tools for self-care involve seven basic content areas.

Nature of diabetes. Persons should have a basic general knowledge of the nature of diabetes and how their individual form and degree of diabetes relates to this process. This means comparing the general "big picture" with their particular "personal picture." Such a comparison includes evaluating initial basic survival needs, as well as fulfillment of their own fundamental

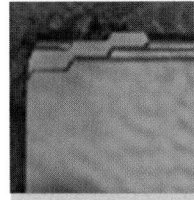

CLINICAL APPLICATIONS

Case Study: Richard Manages His Diabetes

Richard Smith, age 21, has insulin-dependent diabetes mellitus. He gives himself two injections a day, each a combination of medium-acting insulin and regular short-acting insulin. He does one injection before breakfast and one before dinner and usually tests his blood glucose level before each meal and at bedtime. Richard is a college student, who is usually active in athletics.

This is final exam week, however, and Richard's schedule is irregular. He is putting in long hours of study and is under considerable stress. On the day before a particularly difficult examination, he is reviewing his study materials at home and forgets to do his blood test or eat lunch. About midafternoon, he begins to feel faint and realizes that his blood sugar is low and an insulin reaction is imminent if he does not get a quick source of energy. He looks in the kitchen, and all he can find is orange juice, milk, butter, a loaf of bread, and a jar of peanut butter.

Questions for Analysis

1. Which of the foods should Richard eat immediately? Why?

Later, when he is feeling better, Richard makes a peanut butter and butter sandwich, pours a glass of milk, and eats his snack while he continues studying.

2. What carbohydrate food sources of energy are in his snack?

3. Are these carbohydrate sources in a form that the cells can burn for energy? What changes must Richard's body make in these sources to get them into the basic carbohydrate fuel form? What is the complex form of carbohydrate in his snack? Why is this a valuable form of carbohydrate in his diet? What is the basic form of carbohydrate fuel circulating in the blood for use by the cells?

4. What is the relationship of carbohydrate and fat in the final production of energy in the body? If Richard did not take his insulin to provide the necessary control agent for metabolizing the carbohydrate, what would happen to him as the result of improper handling of fat and accumulation of ketones?

needs—especially support for personal concerns and feelings, in dealing with their diabetes.

Nutrition. Together with their nutrition counselor (i.e., usually the clinical dietitian), persons with diabetes should develop a sound food plan based on individual nutritional needs, living and working situations, and food habits. Such planning includes understanding how the food plan relates to maintaining good diabetes control and promoting positive health.

Insulin. According to their treatment plan, persons with diabetes should understand the following about their insulin activity medications:

• *Insulin* types and duration of action (Table 20-8), as well as combinations of insulin use (see For Further Focus box, "Comparative Duration of Action of Types of Insulin"), which include learning a good insulin-injection technique (Figure 20-4), how insulin works in the body, and how its action relates to the food plan.

TABLE 20-8 Types of insulins

Insulin	Onset (hours)	Peak action (hours)	Peak duration (hours)	Species	Appearance
Rapid-acting					
Regular	½-1	2-4	5-7	Beef, pork, human	Clear
Semilente					
Intermediate-acting					
Lente	1½-4	4-12	18-24	Beef, pork, human	Cloudy
NPH					
Mixtard					
Novolin					
Long-acting					
Ultralente	2-6	10-30	36 +	Beef, pork	Cloudy
PZ1					

- *Oral hypoglycemic agents* that stimulate insulin activity, their comparative types and effects (Box 20-2), and how to regulate them.

Monitoring glucose levels. Monitoring of blood-glucose levels, as well as urinary acetone to note possible ketoacidosis, is important. This monitoring includes learning accurate self-testing procedures, as well as understanding the meaning of the results and knowing what action to take accordingly in relation to food, insulin, or exercise.

Control of emergencies. Persons should recognize the early signs of hypoglycemia and its causes and treatment. This recognition includes knowledge of hypoglycemia's relation to the interactive balances among insulin, food, and exercise as the basis of the diabetes care plan (Figure 20-5); daily diabetic care and how to prevent such episodes; the immediate emergency treatment with some form of quick-acting simple carbohydrate to counteract it; and the need to follow the emergency sugar with a snack of complex carbohydrate and protein as soon as possible to sustain a normal blood sugar.

Illness and special needs. Persons with diabetes should learn how to deal with illness and other special needs, several of which have been discussed earlier. This knowledge should include how to adjust diet and insulin, as well as planning ahead for events of daily living such as travel, eating out, exercise, or stress.

Personal ID. Persons also should learn how to obtain a personal identification bracelet or pendant by registering with Medic Alert, an international agency located in Turlock, California. Obtaining such identification should entail understanding why having it at all times is important, especially for persons using insulin.

Levels of Educational Needs

These educational needs can be organized in a diabetes-education program on the following three levels as a learning aid: (1) survival level, (2) home-management level, and (3) lifestyle level.

Resources

A number of useful resources are available from health agencies such as the American Diabetes Association and the American Heart Association,

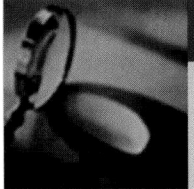

FOR FURTHER FOCUS

Comparative Duration of Action of Types of Insulin

A common method of insulin use is a mixture of short-acting and longer-acting types injected twice a day (see Table 20-8). Persons with unstable diabetes or irregular mealtimes may need to inject short-acting insulin before each meal or snack, as well as use a longer-acting type of insulin once or twice a day. Many experienced persons often self-test their blood-sugar levels with finger pricks to se- cure a blood sample and use a glucose monitor to read the result. These persons have learned to adjust their insulin dosage to their test results, food pattern, work-school-social activities, and exercise schedule. In difficult cases, a device that continu- ously delivers insulin into the bloodstream, an in- sulin pump, may be used to maintain a finer control over the body's varying insulin needs.

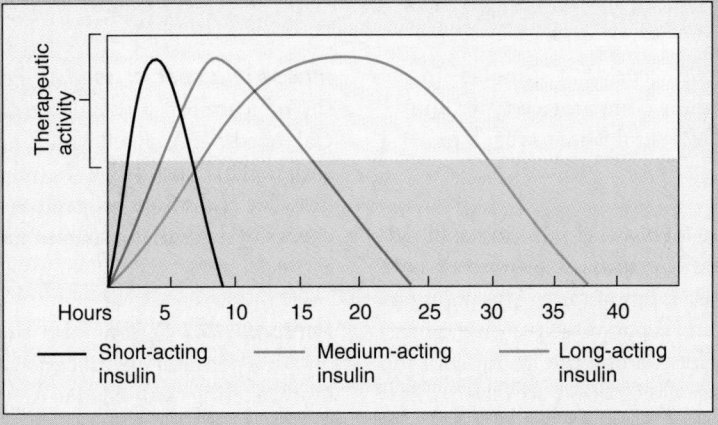

including informational materials and a useful cookbook with nutritional values of recipes. More cookbooks for consumers on the newer "light" cooking that reduces fat, sugar, and salt and suggests many alternative seasonings and methods of prep- aration are also being offered. In addition, resource persons include hospital and clinic dietitians, clini- cal nutritionists in private practice, public health nutritionists, and local chapters of the American Diabetes Association. Any resource materials used must be evaluated in terms of individual needs.

Staff Education

In the final analysis, the success of the diabetes-education program in any health care facility de- pends on the sensitivity and training of the staff conducting the program. Continuing education is essential for all professionals and their assistants. Educational games are often useful tools as part of the staff-education program, which the staff can then use in teaching their patients and clients. Many such resources can be developed.

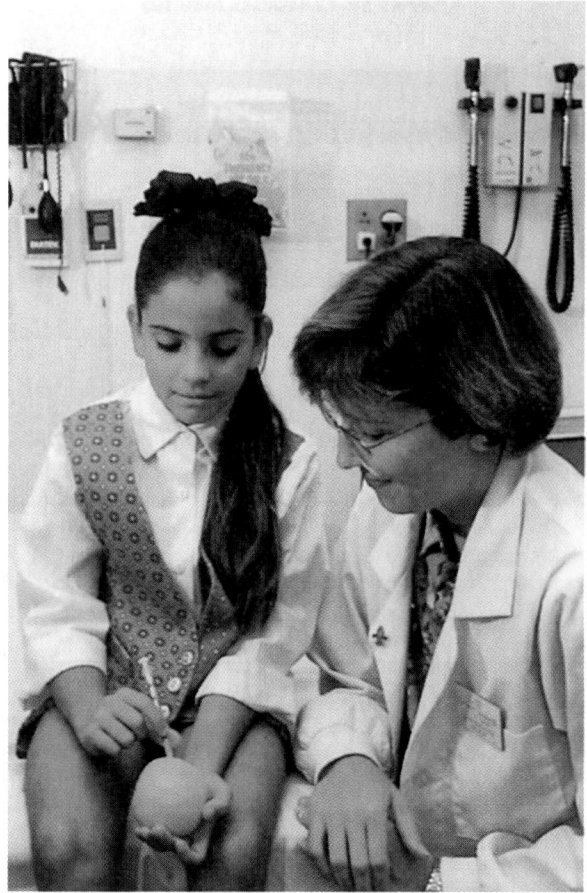

FIGURE 20-4   Young child with newly diagnosed IDDM, learning to inject her own insulin. (Copyright CLG Photographics, Inc.)

BOX 20-2   Oral hypoglycemic agents: sulfonylurea drugs

First generation

Acetohexamide (Dymelor)
Chlorpropamide (Diabinese, Glucamide)—longest acting
Tolazamide (Tolinase)
Tolbutamide (Orinase, Oramide)—shorter acting

Second generation*

Glipizide** (Glucotrol)—mild diuretic; medium-acting
Glyburide (DiaBeta, Micronase)—prolonged action

*Second generation agents are usually first line of choice because they have fewer side effects and are more effective.

**Take 30 minutes before a meal to maximize effect.

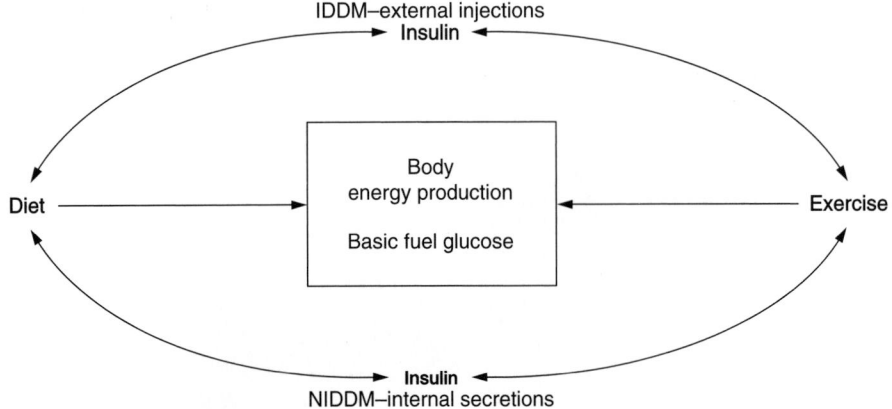

FIGURE 20-5   Basis of diabetes management: body energy balance. Interacting relations among diet (energy source), insulin (hormone controlling body use of basic fuel glucose), and exercise (physical activity using blood glucose.) *IDDM:* Insulin-dependent diabetes mellitus. *NIDDM:* Non–insulin-dependent diabetes mellitus.

SUMMARY

Diabetes mellitus is a syndrome of varying forms and degrees that have the common characteristic of hyperglycemia and other symptoms. Its underlying metabolic disorder involves all three of the energy nutrients—carbohydrate, fat, and protein—and influences energy balance. The major controlling hormone involved is insulin from the pancreas, and persons with diabetes have either a lack of insulin or a resistance to its action.

IDDM affects approximately 15% of all persons with diabetes; it occurs mostly in children and is more severe and unstable. Treatment of IDDM involves regular meals and snacks balanced with insulin and exercise. Self-monitoring of blood-glucose levels indicates that corrective actions are necessary.

NIDDM occurs mostly in adults, especially those who are overweight. Acidosis is rare. Treatment of NIDDM involves weight reduction and maintenance along with regular exercise.

For all forms of diabetes, the keystone of care is sound diet therapy. The basic food plan should be rich in complex carbohydrates and dietary fiber; low in simple sugars, fats (especially saturated fats), and cholesterol; and moderate in protein. Food should be distributed throughout the day in fairly regular amounts and at regular times and tailored to meet individual needs.

REVIEW QUESTIONS

1. Define *diabetes mellitus*. Describe the nature of the underlying metabolic disorder. What is the one common characteristic of all forms of diabetes mellitus?

2. Describe the major characteristics of the two main types of diabetes mellitus. Explain how these characteristics influence differences in nutritional therapy. List and describe medications used to control these conditions.

3. Identify and explain symptoms of uncontrolled diabetes mellitus.
4. Describe the possible long-term complications of poorly controlled diabetes mellitus.
5. In terms of the balance concept, describe the principles of a sound diet for a person with diabetes mellitus.

SELF-TEST QUESTIONS

True-False
Write the correct statement for each item you answer "false."
1. Most persons with NIDDM are underweight when the disease is discovered.
2. The two nutrients whose metabolism is most closely affected in diabetes are fat and protein.
3. Insulin is a hormone produced by the pituitary gland.
4. Insulin action is influenced by both glucagon and somatostatin.
5. Acetone in the urine of a person with diabetes usually indicates that the diabetes is in poor control.
6. Persons with diabetes are usually taught to test their own blood glucose daily and regulate their insulin, food, and exercise accordingly.
7. Coronary artery disease occurs in persons with diabetes at about four times the rate of the general population.
8. Diabetic complications occur in a relatively small number of the persons with long-term diabetes.
9. A diabetic diet is a combination of specific foods that should remain constant.
10. Persons with unstable IDDM should follow a low carbohydrate diet for better control.

Multiple Choice
1. The caloric value of the diet for a person with diabetes should be:
   a. Increased above normal requirements to meet the increased metabolic demand.
   b. Decreased below normal requirements to prevent glucose formation.
   c. Sufficient to maintain the person's appropriate lean weight.
   d. Contributed mainly by fat to spare the carbohydrate for energy needs.
2. The exchange system of diet control is based on principles of (Circle all that apply.):
   a. Equivalent food values
   b. Variety of food choices
   c. Nutritional balance
   d. Reeducation of eating habits

SUGGESTIONS FOR ADDITIONAL STUDY

1. Individual Project: Interviewing a Person with Diabetes
Have various members of the class interview persons with diabetes. Include both children and adults in the survey. Students should ask questions about the following items:

- The persons' initial symptoms
- Their feelings when they first learned they had diabetes
- Their experiences with the disease (e.g., any emergencies, complications, or hospitalizations)
- Their regular method of management at home, school, or work, as well in social situations
- The type of diet they follow

To learn more about the diet, take a diet history (see Chapter 17) if possible. Evaluate your findings in terms of total energy intake according to the person's weight and general balance of nutrients, as well as basic modifications to reduce risks for long-term complications. Have a class discussion after the interviews to compare the nature of diabetes and its management in the various persons contacted.

2. Group Project: Community Diabetes Resources
Explore any available community resources for diabetes. Investigate your local county or district chapter of the American Diabetes Association. Make an appointment with the local office direc-

tor concerning the group's activities. Collect samples of any available resource materials. If possible, visit a group meeting of the organization.

Also, interview any local clinical or community nutrition resource persons, such as your county public health nutritionist, hospital or clinic dietitian, a clinical nutrition specialist/registered dietitian in private practice. Inquire about management practices for clients with diabetes and educational materials used, as well as community resources.

REFERENCES

1. Nestle M, and others: A case of diabetes mellitus, *N Engl J Med* 81:127, October, 1982.
2. Atkinson MA, Maclaren NK: What causes diabetes?, *Sci Am* 263 (1):62, 1990.
3. Berdanier CD: Genetic errors that result in diabetes mellitus, Nutr Today 29(1):17, 1994.
4. Polonsky KS and others: Non-insulin dependent diabetes mellitus—a genetically programmed failure of the beta cell to compensate for insulin resistance, *N Engl J Med* 334(12):777, 1996.
5. Ferber D: New clues found to diabetes and obesity, *Science* 283(5407):1423, 1999.
6. Hayes C: Pattern management: a tool for improving blood glucose with exercise, *J Am Diet Assoc* 97(10 suppl 2): S167, 1997.
7. Delahanty LM: Clinical significance of medical nutrition therapy in achieving diabetes outcomes and the importance of the process, *J Am Diet Assoc* 98(1):25, 1998.
8. American Diabetes Association, American Dietetic Association: Nutrition recommendations and principles for people with diabetes mellitus, *J Am Diet Assoc* 94(5):504, 1994.
9. Drewnowski A: Intense sweeteners and control of appetite, *Nutr Res* 53(1):1, 1995.
10. Robbins DC: Acarbose: a new approach to the management of type II diabetes, *Practical Diabetol* 15:2, 1996.
11. Gregory RP and others: Nutrition management of a collegiate football player with insulin-dependent diabetes—guidelines and a case study, *J Am Diet Assoc* 94(7):775, 1994.
12. Flood TM: New oral therapy for type II diabetes, *On The Cutting Edge* 17(4):10, 1996.
13. *Exchange lists for meal-planning*, Chicago, 1995 American Dietetic Association/American Diabetes Association.

FURTHER READING

- For men only: fatherhood: will your kids get diabetes?, *The Diabetes Advisor* 1(1:Jan/Feb):21, 1999.
- Treatment topics: type 2 diabetes now threatens kids, *The Diabetes Advisor* 6(6:Nov/Dec):30, 1999.

These two regular section articles give you a taste of the helpful information in this little gem of a journal published every two months by The American Diabetes Asso-

ciation. For example, these articles indicate that type 2 diabetes, which was once considered a disease of older adults, is now becoming more common in children and teenagers. The writers indicate that the whole family will be healthier if they make eating healthful meals a family affair. Everyone benefits by being active and eating healthful meals together.

21

Renal Disease

KEY CONCEPTS

- Renal disease interferes with the normal capacity of nephrons to regulate products of body metabolism.

- Short-term renal disease requires basic nutrition support for healing rather than dietary restriction.

- The progressive degeneration of chronic renal failure requires nutrient modification according to individual disease status and dialysis treatment.

- Current therapy for renal stones depends more on the basic nutrition and health support for medical treatment than on major food and nutrient restrictions.

More than 8 million Americans suffer from some form of kidney disease, and 60,000 persons die from such diseases each year. At least another 3 million persons have related infections, many of which go undetected. These kidney problems are costly in lost work time and pay, as well as in personal quality of life. In all, they are now the fourth leading health problem in America.

In this chapter, we look at the nutritional care of persons with kidney disease, mainly the extensive problem of chronic renal failure. We see that although dialysis extends the lives of persons with this irreversible disease, it does so at tremendous personal cost—emotionally, physically, and financially. Renal disease is a serious national and personal health problem.

BASIC PHYSIOLOGY OF THE KIDNEY

Fundamental Role of the Kidneys

The kidneys perform two major functions: they make urine, through which they excrete most of the end products of body metabolism, and they control the concentrations of most of the constituents of the body fluids—especially blood. Tremendous quantities of fluid (i.e., about 180 liters) are filtered through the kidneys each day. All but 1 to 1.5 liters of this fluid is reabsorbed back into circulation to maintain necessary body fluids, particularly the circulating blood volume and all its essential components. Thus, as the blood continuously circulates through the kidneys, these marvelous twin organs repeatedly "launder" the blood to monitor and maintain its precious quantity and constituents. Indeed, the composition of the body fluids is determined not so much by what the mouth takes in as by what the kidneys keep; they are the "master chemists" of our internal environment.

Renal Nephrons

Basic Functional Unit

The basic functional unit of the kidney is the nephron. Each human kidney is made up of about 1 million nephrons, each of which can form urine by itself.[1] Many of today's advances in treating kidney disease are based on providing maximal support

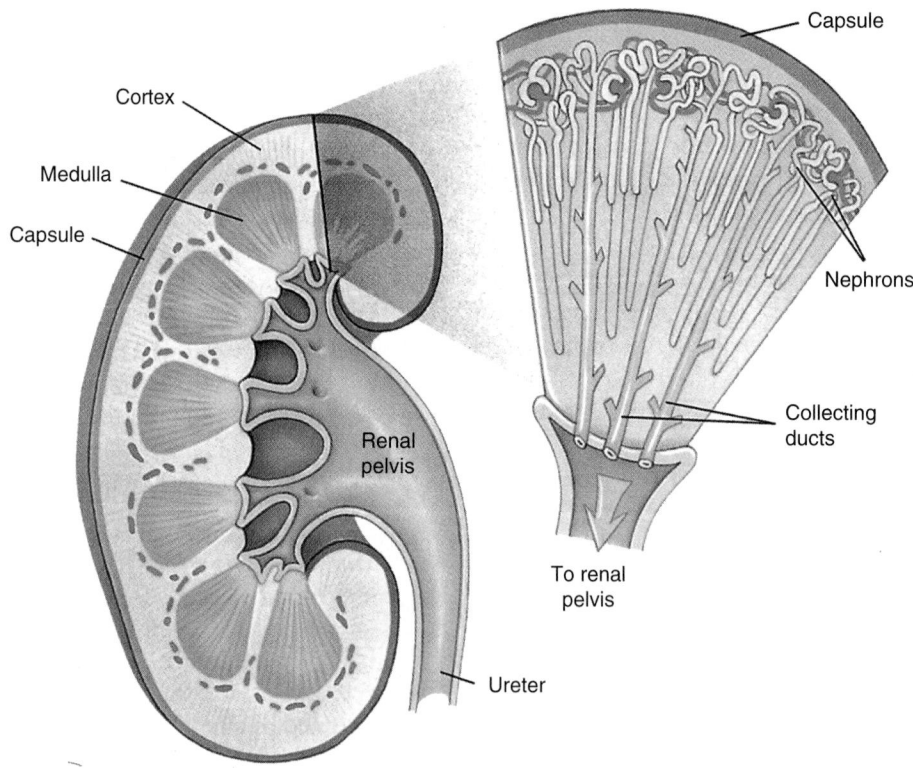

FIGURE 21-1 The nephron, the functional unit of the kidney. (Credit: Barbara Cousins; from Gottfried SS: *Human biology,* New York, 1994, McGraw-Hill.)

for the nephron's vital functions. Each minute, nephron structure is adapted in fine detail to its vital function of maintaining the balanced internal fluid environment that is necessary for life. At birth, each of us has far more nephrons than we actually need, but we begin to lose them gradually after age 30. Many researchers have related this loss to the excessive protein in a typical, Western diet, which is high in meat.

Major Nephron Functions

Each kidney contains about 1 million nephrons. While the body fluid flows through these finely built units, the following basic life-supporting tasks are performed:

1. **Filtration**—Most of the materials of the entering blood are filtered out, except for the larger components of red blood cells and proteins.
2. **Reabsorption**—As the filtrate continues through the winding tubules, substances the body needs are selectively reabsorbed and returned to the blood.
3. **Secretion**—Along the tubules, additional hydrogen ions (H+) are secreted as needed to maintain acid-base balance.
4. **Excretion**—Unneeded waste materials are excreted in the now-concentrated urine.

Special Additional Functions

In addition to major functions in regulating blood constituents and making and excreting concentrated urine, the kidneys perform the following other special functions related to maintaining body-fluid pressures, producing red blood cells, and activating vitamin D:

1. **Renin secretion**—When arteriole pressures fall, the kidneys activate and secrete *renin*, an enzyme that initiates the *renin-angiotensin-aldosterone mechanism* that operates on the kidneys' nephrons to reabsorb sodium and maintain hormonal control of body water balance (see Chapter 8).

2. **Erythropoietin secretion**—The kidneys are responsible for producing the body's major supply (i.e., 80% to 90%) of *erythropoietin*, which is a circulating hormone that is the principle factor in stimulating red blood cell production in response to decreased tissue oxygen.
3. **Vitamin D activation**—In the proximal tubules of the nephrons, the kidneys convert an intermediate inactive form of vitamin D to the final active vitamin D hormone (see Chapter 6). This action is stimulated by the parathyroid hormone.

Nephron Structures

The unique metabolic tasks that maintain body balance and life are performed by specific nephron structures. These key parts of the nephron include the glomerulus and the different tubules, as shown in Figure 21-1.

Glomerulus

At the head of each nephron, a cup-shaped membrane holds the entering blood capillary and its branching tuft of smaller vessels. This cup-shaped capsule is named Bowman's capsule, for the young English physician, Sir William Bowman, who in 1843 first clearly established the basis of plasma filtration and consequent urine secretion based on the intimate relationship of the blood-filled

---

nephron (Gr. *nephros,* kidney) microscopic anatomical and functional unit of the kidney that selectively filters and reabsorbs essential blood factors, secretes hydrogen ions as needed to maintain acid-base balance, reabsorbs water to protect body fluids, and forms and excretes a concentrated urine for elimination of wastes. There are approximately 1 million nephrons in each kidney.

glomerulus (L. *glomus,* ball, cluster) the first section of the nephron, a cluster of capillary loops cupped in the nephron head that serves as an initial filter.

glomeruli and the enveloping membrane. In this capsule, the blood is filtered across the closely held enveloping basement membrane. This cupped membrane and its tuft or cluster of branching capillaries is called the glomerulus, from the Latin word *glomus* meaning "ball." Only the larger blood proteins and cells remain behind in the circulating blood as it leaves the glomerulus.

Tubules

From the cupped head of each nephron, a small tubule carries the filtered fluid through its winding pathway and empties into the central area of the kidney. Specific materials are reabsorbed along the way in each of the four parts of these tubules.

Proximal tubule.   Most of the needed nutrients in the fluid are reabsorbed in this first part of the tubule and returned to the blood. All of the glucose and amino acids, as well as about 80% of the water and other substances, are usually reabsorbed here. Only about 20% of the filtered fluid remains to enter the next section of the tube.

Loop of Henle.   This midsection of the tubule narrows and dips down into the central part of the kidney. Here, the important exchange of sodium and water to concentrate the surrounding fluid in this central area of the kidney occurs. This concentrated fluid environment maintains the necessary *osmotic pressure* to concentrate the urine as it passes through this central area later on its way out.

Distal tubule.   This latter part of the tubule winds back up into the outer area of the kidney. Here, secretion of H+ occurs as needed to provide acid-base balance. Sodium is also reabsorbed as needed under the influence of the adrenal hormone aldosterone.

Collecting tubule.   In this final section of the tubule, a normal concentrated urine is produced by the following important water-reabsorbing actions: (1) influence of the pituitary hormone antidiuretic hormone (ADH), also called *vasopressin*; and (2) the osmotic pressure of the denser surrounding fluid in the central area of the kidney. The urine, which is now concentrated and ready for excretion, only amounts to 0.5% to 1.0% of the original fluid and materials filtered through the glomerulus at the head of the nephron.

NEPHRON DISEASE PROBLEMS

General Causes of Kidney Disease

Several disease conditions may interfere with the normal functioning of the nephrons, causing kidney disease.

Inflammatory and Degenerative Disease

The small blood vessels and membranes in the nephrons may become inflamed for a short time (e.g., in acute *glomerulonephritis*). In other cases, entire nephrons or sections of nephrons may be involved, stopping normal function and producing *nephrotic syndrome*. These nephrotic lesions may continue to affect more and more nephrons, leading to progressive *chronic renal failure*. As a result, the impaired metabolism of protein, electrolytes, and water creates nutritional disturbances.

Damage from Other Diseases

Circulatory disorders such as prolonged, poorly-controlled hypertension can cause degeneration of the small renal arteries and interfere with normal nephron function. The increased demand on other nephrons can in turn cause more hypertension and still more damage to nephrons. Uncontrolled insulin-dependent diabetes mellitus (IDDM) can also damage small renal arteries leading to *glomerulosclerosis* (i.e., loss of functioning nephrons)[2,3] and eventual chronic renal failure.[4] Kidney abnormalities present from birth may lead to poor function, infection, or obstruction.

Infection and Obstruction

Symptoms of bacterial urinary tract infection may range from occasional mild discomfort from bladder infection to more involved chronic recurrent disease and obstruction from kidney stones. Obstruction anywhere in the urinary tract blocks drainage and causes further infection and general tissue damage.

Damage from Other Agents

Various environmental agents (e.g., chemical pesticides, solvents, and similar materials) are poisons that can cause kidney damage.[5] Animal venom, certain plants, and some toxic drugs may also harm renal tissue.[6]

Genetic Defect

Congenital abnormalities of both kidneys can contribute to predisposing renal disease with extensive distortion of renal structure.

Nutritional Therapy in Renal Disease

In the treatment of renal disease, nutritional therapy in each case is based on nature of the disease process and individual responses.

Length of Disease

In short-term acute disease, medical therapy with antibiotics usually controls the disease, and nutritional therapy is largely optimal nutrition support for healing and normal growth. Long-term chronic disease involves more specific nutrient modifications.

Degree of Impaired Renal Function

In milder acute disease with few nephrons involved, less interference occurs with general renal function because the large number of back-up nephrons can meet basic needs. In progressive chronic disease, however, more and more nephrons become involved and renal failure finally results. In such cases, extensive nutritional therapy is required to help maintain renal function as long as possible.

Individual Clinical Symptoms

In continuing disease, nutrient modifications are designed to meet individual needs according to specific clinical symptoms. This personalized nutritional therapy is especially important when advanced renal disease is treated with dialysis.

In this chapter, we focus primarily on the more serious degenerative process of chronic renal failure and dialysis that requires much special nutritional therapy. Brief reviews of nutritional support for short-term conditions provide reference for general nutritional care.

Glomerulonephritis

Disease Process

This inflammatory process affects the *glomeruli*, the small blood vessels in the cupped membrane at the head of the nephron. Glomerulonephritis occurs mostly in young children and usually follows a brief course in its acute form.

Clinical Symptoms

Classic symptoms include hematuria and proteinuria, although edema and mild hypertension may

---

aldosterone a potent hormone of the outside layer of the adrenal glands that acts on the distal nephron tubule to cause reabsorption of sodium in an ion exchange with potassium. The aldosterone mechanism is essentially a sodium-conserving mechanism but also indirectly conserves water because water absorption follows the sodium resorption.

antidiuretic hormone (ADH) a hormone of the pituitary gland that acts on the distal nephron tubule to conserve water by causing its reabsorption; also called *vasopressin*.

hematuria (Gr. *haima*, blood; *ouron*, urine) the abnormal presence of blood in the urine.

proteinuria (Gr. *protos*, first, protein; *ouron*, urine) an abnormal excess of serum proteins (e.g., albumin) in the urine.

edema excess accumulation of fluids in the body tissues.

hypertension high blood pressure.

also occur. These patients usually have little appetite, which contributes to feeding problems. If the disease progresses to more renal involvement, signs of oliguria or anuria may develop.

Nutritional Therapy

General care in uncomplicated disease centers mainly on bed rest and antibiotic drug therapy. Pediatricians and clinical dietitians favor overall optimum nutrition support for growth with adequate protein. Salt is usually not restricted. In most patients with acute short-term disease—especially children with poststreptococcal disease, diet modifications are not crucial. Fluid intake is adjusted to output as a rule.

If the disease process advances, however, more specific nutritional therapy may be indicated according to individual needs, as follow:

- **Protein**—If the blood urea nitrogen (BUN) is elevated and urine output is decreased, dietary protein must be restricted. The diet is usually modified to a lowered protein intake of 0.5 g/kg ideal body weight. As long as renal function is adequate to maintain a normal BUN level, dietary protein intake may be held at 1 g/kg body weight.
- **Carbohydrate**—To provide sufficient energy in dietary kcalories, carbohydrates should be given liberally, which also helps combat catabolism of tissue protein and prevent starvation ketosis.
- **Sodium**—If low urine output indicates impaired renal function, sodium may be restricted to 500 to 1000 mg/day (see Chapter 19). As recovery occurs, the normal sodium intake of 2 to 3 g/day may be resumed.
- **Potassium**—If oliguria becomes severe, renal clearance of potassium is impaired. Thus potassium intake must be monitored carefully according to individual needs.
- **Water**—Fluid intake is restricted according to urine output. If restriction is not indicated, fluids can be consumed as desired.

Nephrotic Syndrome

Disease Process

Nephrotic syndrome, or nephrosis, results from nephron tissue damage to both the glomerulus and tubule. The primary damage is to the major filtering membrane of the glomerulus, allowing large amounts of protein to pass into the tubule. This high-protein concentration of the fluid then causes further damage to the tubule. Both filtration and reabsorption functions of the nephron are disrupted. Nephrosis may be caused by progressive glomerulonephritis, by other diseases such as diabetes or connective tissue disorders—collagen disease; or by other agents such as drugs, heavy metals, or toxic venom from stinging insects such as bees.

Clinical Symptoms

Nephrotic syndrome is characterized by a group of symptoms resulting from the nephron tissue damage and impaired function. The large protein loss leads to massive edema and ascites, as well as proteinuria. The abdomen becomes distended as the fluid accumulates. The plasma protein level is greatly reduced, especially in the albumin fraction, due to the large loss in the urine. As protein loss continues, tissue proteins are broken down and general malnutrition follows. The severe edema and ascites often mask the extent of the body-tissue wasting.

Nutritional Therapy

The former standard recommendation for patients with nephrotic syndrome was a high-protein diet, sometimes as high as 3 to 4 g/kg per day. Current evidence, however, indicates that high-protein diets may accelerate loss of renal function and moderately low-protein diets reduce albuminuria and albumin catabolism, with no change in the glomerular filtration rate (GFR). Nutritional therapy is now directed toward controlling major symptoms (i.e., edema and malnutrition), resulting from the massive protein losses. Therefore physicians and clinical dietitians are now managing these patients with diets containing less protein.

- **Protein**—Protein intake should be moderately low (i.e., 0.6 to 0.8 g/kg of body weight/day). An addition of 1 g/day of high biologic protein (see Chapter 4) is given for each gram of urinary protein lost daily. Thus individual total protein varies according to daily losses.
- **Kcalories**—Sufficient kcalories must always be provided to free protein for tissue rebuilding. High daily intakes of 50 to 60 kcal/kg may be required. Because appetite is usually poor, food must be as appetizing as possible and in a form most easily tolerated. Much kcalorie support is needed.
- **Sodium**—Dietary sodium may be moderately reduced (i.e., to approximately 1000 mg/day) if necessary to help prevent edema.
- **Other minerals and vitamins**—There is no need for potassium restriction. Iron and vitamin supplements may be helpful.

RENAL FAILURE

The two types of renal failure—acute and chronic—have a number of symptoms that reflect interference with normal nephron functions in nutrient metabolism. Both forms have similar nutritional therapy, depending on the extent of renal tissue damage.

Acute Renal Failure

Disease Process

Renal function in healthy kidneys may shut down suddenly after some metabolic insult or traumatic injury, causing a life-threatening situation. This is a medical emergency in which the clinical dietitian and the nurse play important supportive roles. There may be varying causes, as follow:

- **Severe injury,** such as extensive burns or a crushing injury involving extensive tissue damage.
- **Infectious disease,** such as peritonitis.
- **Toxic agents** in the environment, such as carbon tetrachloride or poisonous mushrooms, insect stings, or animal bites.
- **Drug reactions** in allergic or sensitive persons, such as a penicillin reaction.

Clinical Symptoms

The major sign of acute renal failure is *oliguria*, which is caused when cellular debris from the tissue damage blocks the tubules. This diminished urine output is often accompanied by proteinuria or hematuria. Water balance becomes a crucial factor. Short-term dialysis may be needed to support renal function.

Nutritional Therapy

The major challenge is the improvement of nutritional status, especially in patients with marked catabolism. Depending on a patient's condition, nutrient intake may be oral or intravenous. In the early acute phase, no protein is given and carbohydrate is

---

oliguria (Gr. *oligos,* little; *ouron,* urine) the secretion of small amounts of urine in relation to fluid intake.

anuria (Gr. *an-,* negative prefix; *ouron,* urine) an absence of urine, indicating kidney shutdown or failure.

blood urea nitrogen (BUN) a basic test of nephron function by measuring its ability to normally filter urea nitrogen, a product of protein metabolism, from the blood.

ketosis the accumulation of ketones, intermediate products of fat metabolism, in the blood.

nephrosis (Gr. *nephros,* kidney) a nephrotic syndrome caused by degenerative lesions of the renal tubules of the nephrons, especially the thin basement membrane of the glomerulus that helps support the capillary loops; marked by edema, albumuria, and decreased serum albumin.

collagen disease (Gr. *kolla,* glue; *gennan,* to produce) a disease attacking collagen tissues, the protein substance of the white fibers (collangenous fibers) of skin, tendon, bone, cartilage, and other connective tissues; any of a group of diseases that cause widespread changes in the connective tissue (e.g., rheumatoid arthritis, lupus erythematosus, scleroderma, and rheumatic fever).

ascites (Gr. *askites,* from; *askos,* bag) outflow and accumulation of serous (blood and lymph serum) fluid in the abdominal cavity; also known as abdominal or peritoneal dropsy.

increased, with additional kcalories gained from fat. Short-term dialysis for a few days during the first week may be needed, with total parenteral nutrition (TPN) used as a feeding method (see Chapter 22).[7]

Chronic Renal Failure

Disease Process

On the other hand, chronic renal failure is caused by the progressive breakdown of renal tissue, which impairs all renal functions. Few functioning nephrons remain and then gradually deteriorate. A downhill course inevitably follows. The disease process takes its toll on what researchers say is the "aging Western kidney," made vulnerable by a lifetime of large protein meals. In many Western countries, the typical adult diet averages about 3000 kcalories and over 100 g of daily protein, largely from meat.

This chronic renal insufficiency may result from a variety of diseases that involve the nephrons, as follow: (1) primary glomerular disease; (2) metabolic disease with renal involvement, such as insulin-dependent diabetes (IDDM); (3) renal vascular disease; (4) renal tubular disease; or (5) congenital abnormality of both kidneys.

Clinical Symptoms

Depending on the nature of the underlying renal disease, the chronic renal changes may involve extensive scarring of renal tissue, which distorts the kidney structure and brings vascular changes from prolonged hypertension. As the nephrons are lost one by one, the remaining ones gradually lose their ability to sustain vital body metabolic balances.

- **Water balance**—Increasingly, the kidney cannot reabsorb water and excrete a normal concentrated urine. Dehydration follows and may become critical. At other times when fluid intake exceeds output, water intoxication may occur.
- **Electrolyte balances**—Several imbalances among electrolytes result from decreasing nephron function. The failing kidney cannot appropriately respond to maintain the vital

sodium-potassium balance that guards body water (see Chapter 8). A concentration of materials (e.g., phosphate, sulfate, and organic acids) is produced by metabolism of food, which causes metabolic acidosis. The disturbed metabolism of calcium and phosphate from lack of activated vitamin D, a process that occurs in the kidneys, brings about bone pain from a disease called osteodystrophy.
- **Nitrogen retention**—Increasing loss of nephron function brings elevated amounts of nitrogenous metabolites, such as urea and creatinine.
- **Anemia**—The damaged kidney cannot accomplish its normal participation in the production of red blood cells. Therefore fewer red cells are produced, and those that are produced survive a shorter time.
- **Hypertension**—When blood flow to renal tissue is increasingly impaired, renal hypertension develops. In turn, the hypertension causes cardiovascular damage and further deterioration of the kidneys.
- **Azotemia**—The elevated BUN, serum creatinine, and serum uric acid levels are reflected in the characteristic laboratory finding of azotemia.

General Signs and Symptoms

Increasing loss of renal function causes progressive weakness, shortness of breath, general lethargy, and fatigue. Thirst, appetite loss, weight loss, diarrhea, and vomiting may occur. Increasing capillary fragility causes skin, nose, oral, and gastrointestinal bleeding. Nervous system involvement brings muscular twitching, burning sensations in the extremities, or convulsions. Irregular cyclic breathing (i.e., Cheyne-Stokes respiration) indicates acidosis, and ulceration of the mouth, a bad taste, and fetid breath also occur. Malnutrition lowers resistance to infection. Bone and joint pain continues.

Nutritional Therapy

Basic objectives. Treatment must always be individual and must be adjusted according to progres-

TABLE 21-1 Protein and nitrogen needs in chronic renal failure

Creatinine clearance (ml/min)	Nitrogen* (g/day)	Protein (g/day)
40 and above	Unrestricted	Unrestricted
10-40	9.6	60
5-20	6.4	40†
2-10	2.5-3.0 (+ 1.3-2.6)	20 (+EAA/analogues)†
8 and below	Transplantation Dialysis	
5 and below	Dialysis	

*Total protein/6.25.
†EAA, Essential amino acids/alpha-keto-, alpha-hydroxy-analogues of EAA.

sion of the illness, the type of treatment being used, and the patient's response. In general, however, basic therapy objectives in care of chronic renal failure are to do the following:

- Reduce protein breakdown.
- Avoid dehydration or excess hydration.
- Correct acidosis.
- Correct electrolyte imbalances.
- Control fluid and electrolyte losses from vomiting and diarrhea.
- Maintain optimal nutritional status.
- Maintain appetite, general morale, and sense of well-being.
- Control complications of hypertension, bone pain, and nervous system involvement.
- Retard rate of renal failure, postponing the ultimate need for dialysis.

Principles of nutritional therapy. Nutrition for chronic renal failure involves variable nutrient adjustments according to individual need.

- **Protein**—The critical problem is to provide just enough protein to maintain tissue while avoiding a damaging excess. Protein is generally limited to 0.5 to 0.6 g/kg/day, of which at least 0.35 g/kg/day is from high-biologic value protein (see Chapter 4) to ensure an adequate intake of essential amino acids. Some clinicians adjust protein according to *creatinine* clearance and indicate no need to restrict protein intake until this renal function falls below 40 ml/minute. Then dietary protein must be decreased as renal function declines (Table 21-1). A very low (e.g., 20-g) protein diet supplemented with essential amino acids is used to slow progression of renal insufficiency in advanced renal disease.
- **Amino acid supplements**—Mixtures of essential amino acids or amino acid precursors

---

osteodystrophy (Gr. *osteon,* bone; *dys,* painful, disordered, abnormal; *trephein,* to nourish) bone disease resulting from defective bone formation. The general term *dystrophy* applies to any disorder arising from faulty nutrition.

urea chief nitrogen-carrying product of dietary protein metabolism; appears in blood, lymph, and urine.

creatinine nitrogen-carrying product of tissue protein breakdown, excreted in the urine.

azotemia (Gr. *a-,* negative prefix; *zoe,* life; *azote,* nitrogen; *haima,* blood) an excess of urea and other nitrogenous substances in the blood.

provide necessary protein supplementation for low-protein diets. Commercial formulas are available for predialysis patients. Other supplements are made up of nitrogen-free "copies" of essential amino acids called *analogues*.

- **Kilocalories**—Carbohydrate and fat must supply sufficient nonprotein kcalories to spare protein for tissue protein synthesis, as well as to supply energy. Approximately 300 to 400 g of carbohydrate are needed daily. Sufficient fat (i.e., 75 to 90 g/day) is added to give a patient 2000 to 2500 total kcalories daily.
- **Water**—With predialysis patients, fluid intake should be sufficient to maintain adequate urine volume. Intake is usually balanced with output.
- **Sodium**—The need for sodium varies. If hypertension and edema are present, sodium intake must be restricted. Sodium intake usually ranges from 500 to 2000 mg/day (see Chapter 20).
- **Potassium**—The damaged kidney cannot clear potassium adequately, so the dietary intake is kept at about 1500 mg/day.
- **Phosphate and calcium**—Moderate dietary phosphorus restriction (e.g., to about 500 to 600 mg/day), along with the protein restriction, is an effective means of delaying progressive renal failure. A calcium supplement is used to correct the hypocalcemia.
- **Vitamins**—A multivitamin supplement is usually added to the diet of renal patients on protein restriction. A diet of up to 40 g of protein does not contribute the full daily need of all the vitamins (see Clinical Applications box, "Case Study: The Patient with Chronic Renal Failure").[8,9]

End-Stage Renal Disease (ESRD)

When chronic renal failure advances to an end stage, life-support decisions face the patient, family, and physician. End-stage renal disease (ESRD) occurs when the patient's glomerular filtration rate decreases to 10 ml/min.[10] This decrease is due to irreversible damage to a majority of the kidneys' nephrons. At this point, the patient has two options—chronic kidney dialysis or kidney transplant. The lives of an estimated 50,000 persons in the United States who develop kidney disease each year have been prolonged by dialysis and kidney transplants. Kidney transplantation has several advantages. Current advances in surgical techniques, immunosuppressive drugs to prevent rejection, and antibotics to control infection have helped ensure successful outcomes. In addition, the organ donor system has improved. A successful renal transplant can bring improved quality of life and is more cost-effective than dialysis.[11] Long-term effects of dialysis include bone problems, nutritional depletion, anemia, and hormonal imbalances, as well as psychologic depression and diminished quality of life from constant dependence on dialysis treatments. Dialysis, however, has become the major treatment for advanced renal disease, especially because its considerable cost—some $1.4 billion each year—is covered by Medicare. Two forms of dialysis are used: hemodialysis and ambulatory peritoneal dialysis.

Hemodialysis. Hemodialysis using an artificial kidney machine (Figure 21-2) removes toxic substances from the blood and helps restore nutrients and metabolites to normal blood levels. To prepare a patient for hemodialysis therapy, a surgical fistula is made by joining an artery and a vein on the forearm just beneath the skin. After this attachment has healed, a needle is inserted through the healed tissue and connected by tubes to the dialysis machine. A patient with chronic renal failure usually requires two to three treatments per week, each of which lasts 4 to 8 hours. During each treatment, the patient's blood makes several round trips through the dialysis solution in the machine, which removes excess waste material to maintain normal blood levels of life-sustaining substances that the patient's own kidneys can no longer accomplish. There are two compartments in the machine that are separated by a filter. One compartment contains blood from the patient that contains all the excess fluids and waste materials, and the other contains the *dialysate*, a solution that may be thought of as a

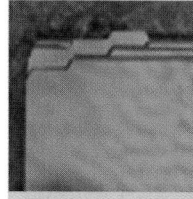

CLINICAL APPLICATIONS

Case Study: The Patient with Chronic Renal Failure

Charles Brown, age 49, is an active man working at a large company who has begun to tire more easily. He has little appetite and feels generally ill most of the time. He recently noticed some ankle swelling and some blood in his urine. At his wife's insistence, he finally decided to see his physician.

After a complete work-up, his physician's findings included the following: (1) no prior illness except a case of the flu with a throat infection during Charles' overseas service in the Army; (2) laboratory tests: albumin, red and white cells in the urine; abnormal BUN and GFR (glomerular filtration rate); (3) other symptoms: hypertension, edema, headache, occasional vision blurring, and low-grade fever. The physician discussed the findings and the serious prognosis of advanced renal disease with Charles and his wife, and together they explored the immediate medical and nutritional needs for treatment. They also discussed the ultimate need for medical management with dialysis. The physician prescribed medications to control Charles' growing symptoms and discomfort.

As time went by, Charles' symptoms increased. He lost more weight, was anemic, and experienced increased bone and joint pain. Gastrointestinal bleeding and nausea also increased, and he had occasional muscle twitching or spasms. Small mouth ulcers made eating a painful effort. Charles and his wife made visits to the clinic dietitian to learn how to manage his present predialysis diet at home.

Questions for Analysis

1. What metabolic imbalances in chronic renal failure do you think accounted for the symptoms Charles was having?
2. What are the objectives of treatment in chronic renal failure?
3. What are the basic principles of Charles' predialysis diet? Describe this type of diet. What foods would be included? Plan a 1-day menu for Charles.
4. What nutrient-related medications and supplements would Charles' physician and clinical dietitian probably use in his treatment plan? Why?

the *dialysate*, a solution that may be thought of as a "cleaning fluid." As in normal capillary filtration, the blood cells are too large to pass through the pores in the filter. The remaining smaller molecules in the blood, however, pass through the filter and are carried away by the dialysate. If the patient's blood is deficient in certain materials, these may be added to the dialysate.

The diet of a hemodialysis patient is a very im-

dialysis (Gr. *dia,* through; *lysis,* dissolution) the process of separating crystalloids (crystal-forming substances) and colloids (glue-like substances) in solution by the difference in their rates of diffusion through a semipermeable membrane; crystalloids (e.g., blood sugar and other simple metabolites) pass through readily; and colloids (e.g., plasma proteins) pass through slowly or not at all.

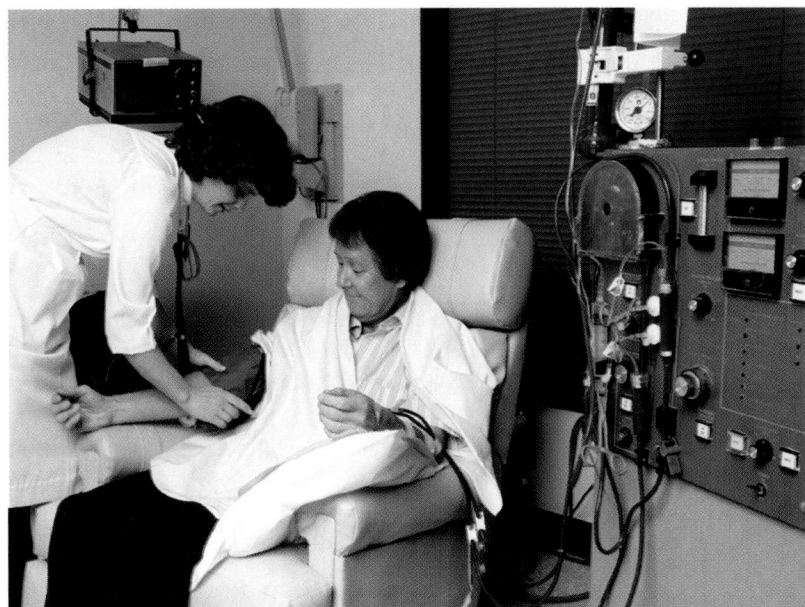

FIGURE 21-2   Patient with end-stage chronic renal disease undergoing hemodialysis treatment. (From PhotoDisc.)

Several basic objectives govern an individual's diet and are designed to do the following: (1) maintain protein and kcalorie balance, (2) prevent dehydration or fluid overload, (3) maintain normal serum potassium and sodium levels, and (4) maintain acceptable phosphate and calcium levels. Controlling infection is always an underlying goal. Nutritional therapy in most cases can be planned with more liberal nutrient allowances.

- **Protein**—For most adult dialysis patients, a standard protein allowance of 1 g/kg lean body weight is carefully calculated for each patient by the dialysis center's clinical dietitians. This amount provides for nutritional needs, maintains positive nitrogen balance, does not produce excessive nitrogenous waste, and replaces the amino acids lost during each dialysis treatment. At least 75% of this daily allowance should consist of protein foods of high biologic value, such as eggs, meat, fish,

and poultry—but little if any milk. Milk is restricted because it adds more fluid and has a high content of sodium, phosphate, and potassium.

- **Kilocalories**—A generous amount of carbohydrates with some fat will continue to supply needed kcalories for energy and protein sparing. The usual prescription is for 40 kcal per kilogram of lean body weight. Simple carbohydrate foods should supply most of the carbohydrates, and complex carbohydrates (e.g., grains and legumes) should be controlled because they contain incomplete protein and should not take up large amounts of the limited protein allowance.
- **Water balance**—Fluid is usually limited to 400 to 500 ml/day, plus an amount equal to any urine output.
- **Sodium**—To control body fluid retention and hypertension, sodium is limited to 1000 to 2000 mg/day.

- **Potassium**—To prevent potassium accumulation, which can cause cardiac problems, potassium intake is restricted to 1500 to 2000 mg/day.
- **Vitamins**—A supplement of the water-soluble vitamins (i.e., B-complex and C) is given to replace their loss during the dialysis treatment.

Ambulatory peritoneal dialysis. An alternate form of treatment some patients can use is *peritoneal dialysis*, which has the convenience of home use. In this process, the patient introduces the dialysate solution directly into the peritoneal cavity four or five times a day, where it can be exchanged for fluids that contain the metabolic waste products. Because the dialysis resulting is continuous within the body between solutions being added and drained, this process is called *continuous ambulatory peritoneal dialysis (CAPD)*. First, the patient is prepared by surgical insertion of a permanent catheter. Each treatment is then done by attaching a disposable bag containing the dialysate solution to the abdominal catheter leading into the peritoneal cavity, waiting 20 to 30 minutes for the solution exchange, and then lowering the bag to allow the force of gravity to cause the waste-containing fluid to drain into it. When the bag is empty, it can be folded around the waist or tucked into a pocket, providing the patient mobility. Intermittant use of peritoneal dialysis, self-administered at home, gives the patient more mobility and a sense of being in control. An automated device is sometimes used to provide several solution exchanges during night sleep hours and one continuous exchange during the day—a technique called *continuous cyclic peritoneal dialysis (CCPD)*. With peritoneal dialysis and good self-care, a more liberal diet may be used. The patient can do the following:

- Increase protein intake to 1.2 to 1.5 g/kg body weight.
- Limit phosphorus to 1200 mg/day by restricting phosphorus-rich foods (e.g., nuts and legumes) to 1 serving/week and dairy products—

including eggs—to a half-cup portion or one egg or its equivalent each day.
- Increase potassium by eating a wide variety of fruits and vegetables each day.
- Encourage liberal fluid intake to prevent dehydration.
- Avoid sweets and fats to control triglyceride and LDL levels.
- Maintain lean body weight by incorporating the kcalories provided by the dialysate solution into the total meal plan.

Moderate-protein oral commercial formulas are available for use by dialysis patients.

KIDNEY STONE PROBLEMS
Disease Process

The basic cause of kidney stones is unknown, but many factors relating to the nature of the urine itself or to the conditions of the urinary tract environment contribute to their formation. The four major stones formed are calcium, struvite, uric acid, and cystine stones. Figure 21-3 illustrates the formation of these various stones.

Calcium Stones

In North America, 5% to 10% of the population suffers from kidney stones, 70% to 80% of which are composed of calcium oxalate with or without phosphate.[13] Excessive urinary calcium may result from several factors, as follow: (1) excess intake from large amounts of high-calcium foods or hard water; (2) excess vitamin D, which increases calcium

---

peritoneal cavity (Gr. *per*, around; *teinein*, to stretch) a strong, smooth surface, a serous membrane lining the abdominal and pelvic walls and undersurface of the diaphragm, forming a sac enclosing the body's vital visceral organs within the *peritoneal cavity*. *Peritoneal dialysis* is a form of dialysis through the peritoneum into and out of the peritoneal cavity.

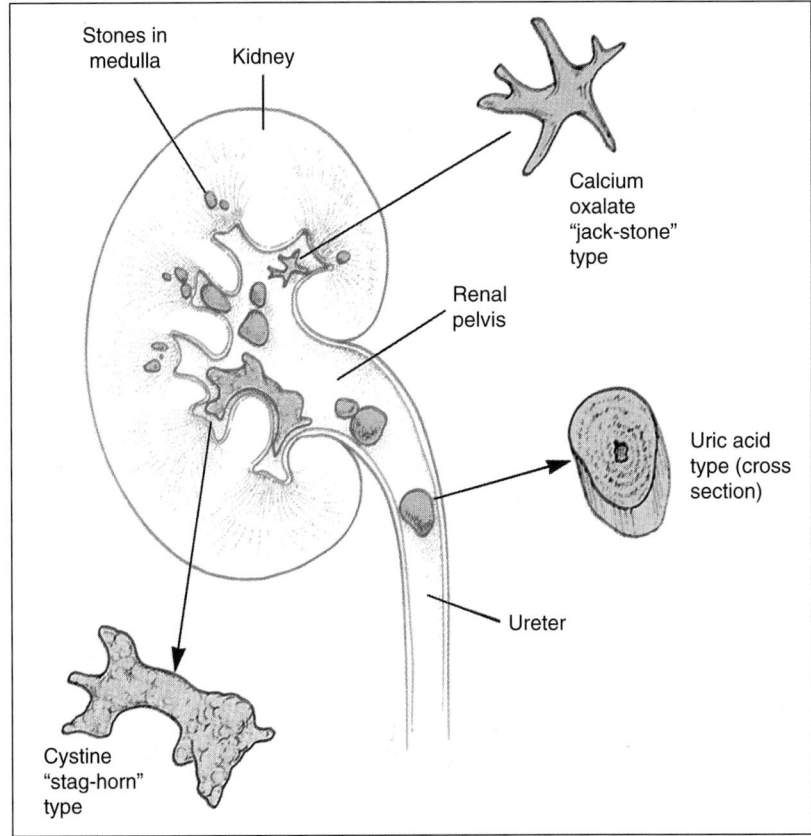

FIGURE 21-3 Renal calculi: stone in kidney, pelvis, and ureter.

absorption; (3) prolonged immobilization (e.g., in body casting or extended illness or disability), which increases calcium withdrawal from bone; or (4) hyperparathyroidism, which causes excess calcium excretion. Recent research, both salt-loading studies and reports of free-living populations, also confirms earlier observations that high intakes of salt (NaCl) result in high amounts of calcium in the urine.[14] In some persons, because of a metabolic error in handling oxalates, the oxalate forms compounds with calcium.[15,16] Oxalates only occur naturally in a few foods (Box 21-1).

Struvite Stones

Of the remaining kidney stones, struvite stones occur most frequently. These stones are composed of a single compound, magnesium ammonium phosphate ($MgNH_4PO_4$), and are often called *infection stones* because they are mainly caused by urinary tract infections—not an association with any specific nutrient. Thus no specific diet therapy is involved. Struvite stones are usually large "stag-horn" stones that are removed surgically.

Uric Acid Stones

Excess excretion of uric acid may be caused by some impairment with the metabolism of purine, from which uric acid is formed. This impairment occurs in diseases such as gout and can also occur in rapid tissue breakdown during wasting disease.

Cystine Stones

Cystine stones are the rarest kidney stones. They are caused by a genetic metabolic defect in the re-

BOX 21-1 Food sources of oxalates

Fruits
Berries, all
Currants
Concord grapes
Figs
Fruit cocktail
Plums
Rhubarb
Tangerines

Vegetables
Baked beans
Beans, green and wax
Beets
Beet greens
Celery
Chard, Swiss
Chives
Collards
Eggplant
Endive
Kale
Leeks
Mustard greens
Okra
Peppers, green

Vegetables—cont'd
Rutabagas
Spinach
Squash, summer
Sweet potatoes
Tomatoes
Tomato soup
Vegetable soup

Nuts
Almonds
Cashews
Peanuts
Peanut butter

Beverages
Chocolate
Cocoa
Draft beer
Tea

Other
Grits
Tofu, soy products
Wheat germ

nal reabsorption of the amino acid cystine. This defect results in an accumulation of cystine in the urine, a condition called *cystinuria*. Because this disorder is of genetic origin, it occurs rarely and only in children with this genetic history.

General Symptoms and Treatment

Clinical Symptoms
The main symptom of kidney stones is severe pain. Many other urinary symptoms may result from the presence of the stones. Usually, there is general weakness and sometimes fever. Laboratory examination of the urine and any passed stones help determine treatment.

Treatment
General treatment may include several considerations.

Fluid intake.   A large fluid intake is a primary therapy that helps to produce a more dilute urine and prevent accumulation of materials that form stones.

Stone composition.   In some cases, dietary control of the stone constituents may help reduce the

purines (L. *purum,* pure; Gr. *ouron,* urine) nitrogen-containing compounds that yield uric acid as a metabolic end product eliminated in the urine.

TABLE 21-2 Low-calcium diet (approximately 400 mg calcium)

Group	Foods allowed	Foods not allowed
Beverage*	Carbonated beverage, coffee, tea	Chocolate-flavored drinks, milk, milk drinks
Bread	White and light rye bread or crackers	
Cereals	Refined cereals	Oatmeal, whole-grain cereals
Desserts	Cake, cookies, gelatin desserts, pastries, pudding, sherbets, all made without chocolate, milk, or nuts; if egg yolk is used, it must be from one egg allowance	
Fat	Butter, cream (2 tbsp daily) French dressing, margarine, salad oil, shortening	Cream (except in amount allowed), mayonnaise
Fruits	Canned, cooked, or fresh fruits or juice except rhubarb	Dried fruit, rhubarb
Meat, eggs	224 g (8 oz) daily of any meat, fowl, or fish except clams, oysters, or shrimp; not more than one egg daily including those used in cooking	Clams, oysters, shrimp, cheese
Potato or substitute	Potato, hominy, macaroni, noodles, refined rice, spaghetti	Whole-grain rice
Soup	Broth, vegetable soup made from vegetables allowed	Bean or pea soup, cream or milk soup
Sweets	Honey, jam, jelly, sugar	
Vegetables	Any canned, cooked, or fresh vegetables or juice except those listed	Dried beans, broccoli, green cabbage, celery, chard, collards, endive, greens, lettuce, lentils, okra, parsley, parsnips, dried peas, rutabagas
Miscellaneous	Herbs, pickles, popcorn, relishes, salt, spices, vinegar	Chocolate, cocoa, milk gravy, nuts, olives, white sauce

*Depends on the calcium content of local water supply. In instances of high-calcium content, distilled water may be indicated.

recurrence of such stone formation, thus helping to prevent the accumulation of these metabolic substances in the urine available for stone formation.

Urinary pH. In the past, urinary pH was given much emphasis in relation to diet therapy for renal stones, but for some years now has been questioned. Research has indicated that acidification of the urine by traditional acid/alkaline ash diets may have little effect on urinary tract infections or the formation of stones in the urinary tract, because calculation methods for determining the effect of specific foods, urinary pH have not proved to be valid. It is only in general, not precise, terms that vegetables, fruits, and milk are called alkaline ash foods or that meat, cheese, eggs, and whole grains are called acid ash foods. A desired pH of the urine is better achieved by medical means than by traditional acid/alkaline ash diets.

Binding agents. Materials that bind potential stone elements in the intestine can prevent their absorption and eliminate them from the body. For example, sodium phytate is used to bind calcium, and aluminum gels are used to bind phosphate. Glycine has a similar effect on oxalates.

Nutritional Therapy

The nutritional plan of care mainly relates to the nature of the stone. The diet is designed to reduce intake of nutrients that lead to the formation of a particular type of stone.

Calcium Stones

A low-calcium diet of about 400 mg/day is usually given (Table 21-2) (i.e., about half the average adult intake of 800 mg). This lower level is mainly

BOX 21-2   Acid, alkaline, and neutral food groups

Acid ash	**Alkaline ash**	**Neutral**
Eggs	Fruits (except cranberries,	Beverages (coffee, tea)
Cheese	prunes, plums)	
Cranberries	Milk	
Prunes	Vegetables	
Plums		
Meat		
Whole grains		

achieved by removal of milk and dairy products, the main dietary sources of calcium. Other secondary calcium sources are whole grains and leafy vegetables. If a stone is calcium phosphate, additional sources of phosphorus (e.g., meats, legumes, and nuts) should be controlled. If a stone is calcium oxalate, foods high in oxalate (see Box 21-1) should be avoided.

Because calcium stones have an alkaline chemistry, an acid ash diet may also be used to create a urinary environment that is less conducive to precipitating the basic stone elements. The classification of food groups is based on the acidity (pH) of the metabolic ash produced (Box 21-2). An acid ash diet increases the amount of meat, grains, eggs, and cheese and limits the amount of vegetables, fruits, and milk. An alkaline ash diet outlines the opposite use of these foods. The use of cranberry juice has been promoted to assist in acidifying the urine, but the commercially prepared cranberry juices on the market are too dilute to be effective because they only contain about 26% cranberry juice. Therefore an enormous volume of juice is required to achieve any effectiveness as a urinary acidifying agent. Instead, to effect a sustained acidfication of urinary pH, most physicians rely on drugs.

Uric Acid Stones

About 4% of the total incidence of renal calculi are uric acid stones. Because uric acid is a metabolic product of purines, a low-purine diet is sometimes recommended. If dietary control of purines is desired, it can easily be achieved by use of a vegetar-

TABLE 21-3   Summary of dietary principles in renal stone disease

Stone chemistry	Nutrient modification	Dietary ash (urinary pH)
Calcium	Low calcium (400 mg)	Acid ash
Phosphate	Low phosphorus (1000-1200 mg)	
Oxalate	Low oxalate	
Struvite ($MgNH_4PO_4$)	Low phosphorus (1000-1200 mg) (associated with urinary infections)	Acid ash
Uric acid	Low purine	Alkaline ash
Cystine	Low methionine	Alkaline ash

ian diet that eliminates most meat—especially organ meats, concentrated meat extracts, and gravies.

Cystine Stones

Cystine is derived from the essential amino acid methionine, so a low-methionine diet is sometimes used. Because this diet is essentially a low-protein diet and the rare genetic cystinuria condition occurs mainly in children, the treatment of choice is usually a regular diet to support growth. Medical drug therapy is used to control infection or produce a more alkaline urine. General dietary principles in regard to renal stone disease are summarized in Table 21-3.

SUMMARY

The nephrons are the functional units of the kidneys. Through these unique structures, the kidney maintains life-sustaining blood levels of materials required for life and health. The nephrons accomplish their tremendous task by constantly "laundering" the blood over and over many times each day, returning necessary elements to the blood and eliminating the remainder in a concentrated urine. Various diseases that interfere with the vital function of nephrons can, if damage is extensive, cause serious renal disease.

At its end stage, chronic renal failure is treated by dialysis and kidney transplant. Dialysis patients require close monitoring for protein, water, and electrolyte balance. Renal diseases have predisposing factors (e.g., recurrent urinary tract infections may lead to renal calculi, and progressive glomerulonephritis may lead to chronic nephrotic syndrome and renal failure). The Western diet is suspect as a predisposing factor in the development of chronic renal failure. Our modern diet of excess protein may overtax human nephrons, which were not originally designed to handle a steady diet of protein-rich foods.

REVIEW QUESTIONS

1. For each of the following conditions, outline the nutritional components of therapy, explaining the effect of each on kidney function: glomerulonephritis, nephrotic syndrome, and chronic renal failure.

2. List the nutritional factors that must be monitored in persons undergoing renal dialysis.

3. Outline the medical and nutritional therapy for various types of renal stones. Why are acid/alkaline diet modifications no longer valid therapy?

SELF-TEST QUESTIONS

True-False

Write the correct statement for each item you answer "false."

1. The basic functional unit of the kidney is the nephron.
2. There are only a few nephrons in each kidney, so metabolic stress can easily cause problems.
3. The operation of the nephrons relates little to the rest of the body.
4. The glomerulus's main function is filtration.
5. The tasks of the various parts of the nephron tubules are reabsorption, secretion, and excretion.
6. Dietary modifications in acute glomerulonephritis usually involve crucial restrictions of protein and sodium.
7. The primary symptom in nephrotic syndrome is massive albuminuria.

8. The nephrotic syndrome is best treated by a moderately low protein diet.
9. The multiple symptoms of advanced chronic renal failure basically result from metabolic imbalances in the body's inability to handle protein, electrolytes, and water.
10. Prolonged immobilization (e.g., with full body casts or disability) may lead to withdrawal of bone calcium and the formation of calcium renal stones.

Multiple Choice

1. Acute glomerulonephritis is best treated by (Circle all that apply.):
   a. Reducing protein because filtration is impaired.
   b. Using a normal amount of protein for optimum tissue nutrition and growth.

c. Restricting sodium to help control edema.

d. Allowing moderate salt use in uncomplicated cases.

2. Diet therapy in nephrotic syndrome is designed to (Circle all that apply.):

a. Increase protein to replace the massive losses.

b. Decrease protein moderately to reduce albumin losses.

c. Increase kcalories to provide energy and spare protein for tissue need.

d. Restrict sodium moderately to help prevent edema.

3. The general diet needs in chronic renal failure include (Circle all that apply.):

a. Reduced protein intake.

b. Increased carbohydrate and moderate fat for needed energy.

c. Careful control of sodium and potassium according to need.

d. Increased fluids to stimulate kidney function.

SUGGESTIONS FOR ADDITIONAL STUDY

Individual or Group Project: Kidney Dialysis Center
Assign students in the class to visit a kidney dialysis center in your community. Observe the operation of the center. Interview one of the staff nurses and a clinical dietitian about the dialysis procedure and the dietary management used with the patients. If any teaching materials or diet guides are available, bring copies back to class for use in reporting your visit.

REFERENCES

1. Guyton AC, Hall JE: *Textbook of medical physiology*, ed 9, Philadelphia, 1996, W.B. Saunders.

2. Clark CM Jr, Lee DA: Prevention and treatment of the complications of diabetes mellitus, *N Engl J Med* 332(18): 1210, 1995.

3. Porte D Jr, Schwartz MW: Diabetes complications: why is glucose potentially toxic?, *Science* 272(5262):699, 1996.

4. Thadhani R and others: Acute renal failure, *N Engl J Med* 334(22):144, 1996.

5. Macias WL and others: Impact of the nutritional balance in patients with acute renal failure, *J Parenter Enter Nutr* 20(1):56, 1996.

6. Savin VJ and others: Circulation factor associated with increased glomerular permeability to albumin in recurrent focal segmented glomerulosclearosis, *N Engl J Med* 334(14):878, 1996.

7. Kopple JD: The nutrition management of the patient with acute renal failure, *J Parenter Enter Nutr* 20(1):3, 1996.

8. Forman JW and others: Nutritional intake in children with renal insufficiency: a report of Growth Failure in Children with Renal Diseases Study, *J Am Coll Nutr* 15(6):579, 1996.

9. Gillis BP and others: The MDRD Study Group: nutrition intervention program of The Modification of Diet in Renal Disease Study: a self-management approach, *J Am Diet Assoc* 95(11):1288, 1995.

10. The International Polycystic Kidney Disease Consortium: Polycystic: the complete structure of the PDK1 gene and its protein, *Cell* 81:289, 1995.

11. Fackelmann K: Megagene unmasked: huge gene leads to many tumors in the kidneys, *Sci News* 147(21):330, 1995.

12. Burtis WJ and others: Dietary hypercalciuria in patients with calcium oxalate kidney stones, *Am J Clin Nutr* 60(3):1995.

13. Massy LK, Whiting SJ: Dietary salt, urinary calcium, and kidney stone risk, *Nutr Rev* 53(5):131, 1995.

14. Dranov P: Urinary tract infection, *Am Health* 14(4):66, 1995.

15. Service RE: New vaccines may ward off urinary tract infections, *Science* 276(5312):533, 1997.

16. Langermann S and others: Prevention of mucosal *Escherichia coli* infection by FimH-adhesin-based system vaccination, *Science* 276(5312):607, 1997.

FURTHER READING

• Georgalas A and others: Nutritional strategies for the treatment of chronic renal failure in children, *Nutr Today* 28(4):24, 1993.

This article provides excellent guidelines for the nutritional care of children with chronic renal failure. The emphasis is rightly focused on the needs of the individual child. There is *no one renal diet*, but rather individual diets tailored to meet growth needs and maintain quality of life at various stages of the disease process.

• Beto JA: Which diet for which renal failure: making sense of the options, *J Am Diet Assoc* 95(8):898, 1995.

This excellent article sorts out the various types of renal diseases and their modes of treatment with a clear eye and heart for the needs of the patient. It "makes sense" of all the options.

22

Surgery and Nutritional Support

KEY CONCEPTS

- Surgical treatment requires added nutritional support for tissue healing and rapid recovery.

- The special nutritional problems of gastrointestinal surgery require diet modifications because of the surgery's effect on normal food passage.

- Diet management for surgery patients to ensure optimal nutritional support involves both oral and intravenous feeding methods.

Malnutrition continues to occur among hospitalized patients, many of whom are surgical patients. Surveys in both American and European hospitals show that almost 50% of the surgical patients have clinical signs of protein-energy malnutrition, which hinders healing. Effective nutritional support can reverse this malnutrition, greatly improve prognosis, and speed recovery. The surgical process also places physiologic and psychologic stress on patients, bringing added nutritional demands and risks for clinical problems.

In this chapter, we look at the nutritional needs of surgery patients and the enteral and parenteral feeding methods of providing nutritional support. We see that careful attention to both preoperative and postoperative nutritional support can reduce complications and provide essential resources for healing and health.

NUTRITIONAL NEEDS OF GENERAL SURGERY PATIENTS

A patient undergoing surgery faces great physiologic and psychologic stress, so nutritional demands are greatly increased during this period and deficiencies can easily develop. If these deficiencies are allowed to develop and are not met, serious malnutrition and clinical problems can occur. Therefore careful attention *must* be given to a patient's nutritional status in preparation for surgery, as well as to the individual nutritional therapy needs that follow. If these needs are met, complications are less likely to develop. Nutritional resources provide for wound healing and a more rapid recovery.

Preoperative Nutritional Care: Nutrient Reserves

When the surgery is elective (i.e., not an emergency), body nutrient stores can be built up to fortify a patient for the demands of the surgery and the period immediately following the period of limited food intake. Commercial formulas provide needed nutritional supplementation. Particular needs center on protein, energy, vitamins, and minerals.

Protein

Protein deficiencies among surgical patients are more common than one would assume. Surveys of surgical wards in large city hospitals have revealed obvious protein-energy malnutrition and multiple postsurgical complications. Every patient facing surgery needs to be fortified with adequate body protein in tissue and plasma reserves to counteract blood losses during surgery and prevent tissue breakdown in the immediate postoperative period. For example, extensive bone healing is involved in orthopedic surgery. Protein is essential for forming the sound foundation that anchors mineral matter in bone tissue and is especially important with the occurrence of bone fractures in the growing United States population of elderly persons—particularly older women.[1,2]

Energy

Sufficient kcalories must always be provided when increased protein is required for tissue building. The increased kcalories support the added energy demands and spare protein for its tissue-building work. For example, increased carbohydrate is needed to maintain optimal glycogen stores in the liver as a necessary resource for immediate energy fuel, thus directing protein to its tissue synthesis task. If a person is underweight, extra kcalories are needed to increase the weight to the ideal maintenance level before surgery. If a person is overweight and the surgery is not immediately necessary, some weight reduction may be indicated to help reduce surgical risks.

Vitamins and Minerals

When increased protein and kcalories are required for any purpose, the appropriate intake of vitamins and minerals involved in protein and energy metabolism must also be supplied. Any deficiency state (e.g., anemia) should be corrected. Water balance should be ensured because both electrolytes and fluids are necessary to prevent dehydration.

Immediate Preoperative Period

Usual preparation for surgery calls for nothing to be taken orally for at least 8 hours before the surgery. This preparation is necessary to ensure that the stomach holds no retained food at surgery. Food in the stomach may cause complications resulting from vomiting or aspiration of food particles during anesthesia or recovery from anesthesia. In addition, any food present in the stomach may interfere with the surgical procedure or increase the risk for postoperative gastric retention and expansion. Especially before gastrointestinal surgery, a nonresidue diet (see Table 22-4) may be followed for several days to clear the operative site of any food residue. Commercial nonresidue elemental formulas can provide a complete diet in liquid form. These formulas can be administered by tube or made more palatable for oral use with various flavorings.

Emergency Surgery

If the surgery is an emergency, no time is available for building up ideal nutritional reserves. Therefore it is more important for persons to maintain a good nutritional status through a healthy diet as a regular habit so that optimum nutrient reserves are available to supply needs at times of stress.

Postoperative Nutritional Care: Nutrient Needs for Healing

Nutritional support is necessary to aid recovery from surgery. In surgical disease, as well as in related surgical procedures, nutrient losses are greatly increased. At the same time, food intake is greatly diminished or even absent for a period. To supply this additional nutritional support, several nutrients require particular attention.

Protein

Optimal protein intake in the postoperative recovery period is of primary concern for all patients. Protein is needed to replace losses during surgery and supply the increased demands of the healing process. During the period immediately after surgery, the body tissues usually undergo considerable catabolism, which means that the process of tissue breakdown and loss exceeds the process of tissue buildup (see Chapter 4). A negative nitrogen balance of as much as 20 g/day may also occur during this time. This negative balance represents an actual loss of more than 0.5 kg (1 lb) of tissue protein per day. In addition to the protein losses from tissue breakdown caused by metabolic imbalances, other losses of protein from the body also occur, including plasma protein loss from hemorrhage, wound bleeding, and various body fluid losses or exudates. Increased loss of plasma protein may also occur from extensive tissue destruction, inflammation, infection, and trauma. If any degree of prior malnutrition or chronic infection existed, a patient's protein deficiency could easily become severe and cause serious complications. There are several reasons for this increased protein demand.

Building tissue. The process of wound healing requires building a great deal of new body tissue, which can only be done when enough of the essential amino acids from protein intake or body stores can be brought to the tissue by the circulating blood (see Chapter 4). The 10 essential amino acids (see Table 4-1) cannot be made by the body and must be present for tissue building. These necessary amino acids must come from diet protein or from intravenous feeding if a patient cannot eat normally for an extended period. These tissue protein deficiencies can usually be met through oral feedings, so it is important that a patient is helped to eat as soon as possible after surgery. Dietary protein intake must sometimes be increased to 100 to 150 g/day to restore lost protein and build new tissues at the wound site.

Controlling shock. A sufficient supply of plasma protein—mainly albumin—is necessary to protect the blood volume (see Chapter 8). If the plasma protein level drops, pressure to keep tissue fluid circulating between the capillaries and the cells is insufficient. If there is not enough pressure, water

---

elemental formula a nutrition support formula composed of simple elemental nutrient components that require no further digestive breakdown and are thus readily absorbed.

catabolism (Gr. *katabole,* a throwing down) the process by which body tissues are broken down, the opposite of *anabolism.* Catabolism includes all the processes in which complex substances are progressively broken down into simpler ones, usually with the release of energy. Together, anabolism and catabolism constitute metabolism, which is the coordinated operation of anabolic (building up) and catabolic (breaking down) processes into a dynamic balance of energy and substance.

exudate (L. *exsudare,* to sweat out) various materials such as cells, cellular debris, and fluids, usually resulting from inflammation, that have escaped from the blood vessels and are deposited in or on the surface tissues; protein content is high.

leaves the blood capillaries and cannot be drawn back into circulation. Shock symptoms result from a shrinking blood volume and the body's effort to restore it.

Controlling edema. When the serum protein level is low, edema develops as a result of loss of the osmotic pressure required to maintain the normal movement of fluid between the capillaries and the surrounding tissue. This condition of edema is characterized by puffiness or swelling of the tissue from the excess fluid being held there instead of being returned to circulation. Generalized edema may affect heart and lung action. Local edema at the wound site also interferes with closure of the wound and hinders the normal healing process.

Healing bone. Any bone surgery (e.g., in orthopedic problems) involves extensive bone healing. Protein, as well as mineral matter, is essential to the bone tissue for proper bone formation. Protein provides a matrix for calcium and phosphorus to be laid down to form proper bone callus and hardening. Therefore protein anchors the minerals to build strong bone tissue.

Resisting infection. Protein tissues are the major components of the body's immune system, providing its defense against infection. These defense agents include special white cells called *lymphocytes* (see Chapter 23), as well as antibodies and various other blood cells, hormones, and enzymes. Tissue strength is a major defense barrier against infection at all times.

Transporting lipids. Fat is also an important component of tissue structure, forms the center of cell walls and participating in many other necessary metabolic activities. Protein is required to carry fat in the bloodstream to all tissues (see Chapter 19) for maintaining tissue structures and activities. Protein is also necessary to carry fat to the liver for necessary work in fat metabolism. Protein in the liver combines with and removes fat, thus avoiding the danger of fatty infiltration, which would lead to liver disease.

Because protein has many important functions during recovery from surgery, protein deficiency at this time can obviously lead to many clinical problems. These problems include poor wound healing, rupture of the suture lines (dehiscence), delayed healing of fractures, depressed heart and lung action, anemia, failure of gastrointestinal stomas (see Figure 22-6) to function, reduced resistance to infection, liver damage, extensive weight loss, and increased mortality risk.

Water

Water balance after surgery is a constant concern. Sufficient fluid intake is necessary to prevent dehydration, especially in elderly persons whose thirst mechanism may be depressed and cannot be depended on to ensure adequate fluid intake. In patients who have complications or are seriously ill and have extensive drainage, as much as 7 L (almost 7.5 quarts) of fluid may be required daily. During the postoperative period, large water losses may also occur from vomiting, hemorrhage, fever, or excessive urination. The usual intravenous fluids after surgery will supply some initial needs, but oral intake should begin as soon as possible and be sufficiently maintained.

Energy

As always, when increased protein is demanded for tissue building, enough nonprotein kcalories must be supplied for energy to spare protein for its vital tissue-building function. The fuel nutrients, carbohydrate and fat, must therefore be sufficiently supplied in the total diet. Because excess fat presents general health problems, carbohydrate becomes the major source of needed fuel. The total kcalories in the postsurgery diet must be increased to 2500 to 3000 kcal/day before protein can be used entirely for tissue building and not be converted in part to fuel. In situations of acute metabolic stress (e.g., in extensive surgery or burns), kcalorie needs may increase to as much as 4000 to 5000 kcal/day. Carbohydrate not only spares protein for tissue building but also helps avoid liver damage by maintaining glycogen reserves in the liver tissue. Excessive fuel storage as body fat should be avoided, however, because fatty tissue heals poorly and is more susceptible to infection.

Vitamins

Several vitamins require particular attention in wound healing. Vitamin C is necessary for building strong tissue because it deposits a cementlike substance between the cells, thus strengthening the tissue formed. Vitamin C helps to build connective tissue, new capillary walls, and general tissue ground substance. If extensive tissue building is required, as much as 1 g vitamin C per day may be needed. As kcalories and protein are increased, the B vitamins that have important coenzyme roles in protein and energy metabolism (i.e., especially thiamin, riboflavin, and niacin) must also be increased. Other B-complex vitamins—folate, B_{12}, pyridoxine, and pantothenic acid—also play important roles in building hemoglobin and thus must be adequate to meet the demands of an increased blood supply and general metabolic stress. Vitamin K, which is essential for blood clotting, is usually present in a sufficient amount because it is synthesized by intestinal bacteria.

Minerals

Attention to any mineral deficiencies (i.e., continued adequate amounts in the diet) is essential. When tissue is broken down, as after surgery, cell potassium and phosphorus are lost. Electrolyte imbalances of sodium and chloride also result from fluid losses. Iron deficiency anemia may develop from blood loss or faulty iron absorption. Another mineral important in wound healing is zinc. An adequate amount of protein usually meets this need because most dietary zinc is found in protein foods of animal origin. Sometimes zinc supplements may be used for extensive surgery and poor zinc stores.

GENERAL DIETARY MANAGEMENT

Initial IV Fluid and Electrolytes

Most general surgical patients can and should progress to oral feedings as soon as possible to provide adequate nutrition. Remember that routine postoperative intravenous (IV) fluids are used to supply hy-

dration needs and electrolytes, not to sustain energy and nutrients. Ordinary postsurgery IVs are not designed to supply complete nutrient needs or compete with oral feedings. For example, a 5% dextrose solution (D5W) with normal saline (0.9% NaCl solution) contains only 5 g dextrose/dl (i.e., about 20 kcalories or 200 kcal/L), although the total energy need is about 10 times that amount. A rapid return to regular eating should be encouraged and maintained.

Methods of Feeding

Only two basic types of methods for dietary management are available, as follow: (1) enteral—taking in nourishment through the regular gastrointestinal route as long as it can be used, either by regular oral feedings or by tube feedings; or (2) parenteral—taking in nourishment through veins, either smaller peripheral veins or a larger central vein.

---

edema (Gr. *oidema,* swelling) an unusual accumulation of fluid in the interstitial (i.e., small structural spaces between tissue parts) tissue spaces of the body.

callus (L. *callositis,* callus, bone) unorganized meshwork of newly grown, woven bone developed on a pattern of the original clot of fibrin, formed after fracture or surgery, and normally replaced in the healing process by hard adult bone.

dehiscence (L. *dehiscere,* to gape) a splitting open; the separation of layers of a surgical wound—partial or superficial or complete—with total disruption requiring resuturing.

stoma (Gr. *stoma,* mouth, opening) the opening established in the abnormal wall, connecting with the ileum or colon, for elimination of intestinal wastes after surgical removal of diseased portions of the intestines.

enteral (Gr. *enteron,* intestine) a mode of feeding that uses the gastrointestinal tract; oral or tube feeding.

parenteral (Gr. *para-,* beyond, beside; *enteron,* intestine) a mode of feeding that does not use the gastrointestinal tract but provides nutrition by intravenous delivery of nutrient solutions.

Enteral Feedings

When the gastrointestinal tract can be used, it is the preferred route of feeding—orally by mouth if possible and if not, by tube.

Oral feeding. Most general surgical patients can and should receive oral feedings as soon as possible. Oral feedings allow more needed nutrients to be added and help to stimulate normal action of the gastrointestinal tract. Food can usually be taken orally as soon as regular bowel sounds return. When oral feedings begin, the patient usually progresses from clear to full liquids and then to a soft or regular diet. Examples of these progressive "routine house diets" used in hospitals are given in Chapter 17. Individual tolerance and needs are always the guide, but encouragement and help should be supplied in general care of postsurgery patients to enable them to eat as soon as possible. Depending on a patient's condition, a general energy-nutrient food supplement formula may be added orally, with or between meals. The energy value of foods in the regular diet may also be increased as tolerated with added sauces, seasonings, and dressings. More frequent, less bulky, concentrated small meals may be helpful, making every bite count.

Tube feeding. When regular oral feeding cannot be used, as with patients who are comatose or severely debilitated or have undergone radical neck or face surgery, nutrient formulas may be fed by tube. The most common route is the nasogastric (NG) tube, which is inserted through the nose into the stomach (Figure 22-1). Modern small-bore nasoenteric feeding tubes made of softer, more flexible polyurethane and silicone materials have replaced large-bore stiff tubing. These modern feeding tubes are more comfortable for the patient and easily carry the variety of nutrient materials now available in enteral nutrition-support formulas. With the development of improved formulas and feeding equipment, the question of using blender-mixed formulas of regular foods seldom arises now because of the following problems that they carry in relation to physical form, safety, and the digestion-absorption process:

- *Physical form*—Foods broken down and mixed in a blender yield a sticky, larger-particle mixture that does not go through the modern feeding tubes easily and thus requires the more uncomfortable large-bore tubing.
- *Safety*—Such blender-mixed formulas carry problems of bacterial growth and infection, as well as inconsistent nutrient composition because the solid components settle out.
- *Digestion and absorption*—The blended food formula requires a fully functioning digestive and absorptive system to digest the food and absorb its released nutrients. Many patients have gastrointestinal deficits that require nutrients with varying degrees of predigestion (hydrolysis) or smaller molecular structure.

In overall comparison, commercial formulas provide a sterile, homogenized solution suitable for the more comfortable, modern, small-bore feeding tubes and ensure a fixed profile of nutrients in intact or predigested form. No matter what types of feeding tube and formula are used to meet a patient's physiologic needs, however, they also contribute to psychologic stress. Much support for a patient's quality of life is an important part of patient care planning.

Alternate routes for enteral tube feeding. The nasoenteric route described is usually indicated for short-term therapy (i.e., 4 to 6 weeks) in many clinical situations. For long-term feedings, however, *enterostomies*—surgical placement of the tube at progressive points along the gastrointestinal tract—provide the preferred route.

- *Esophagostomy*—A cervical esophagostomy is often placed at the level of the cervical spine to the side of the neck after head and neck surgeries for cancer or traumatic injury. This placement removes the discomfort of the nasal route and enables the entry point to be easily concealed under clothing.

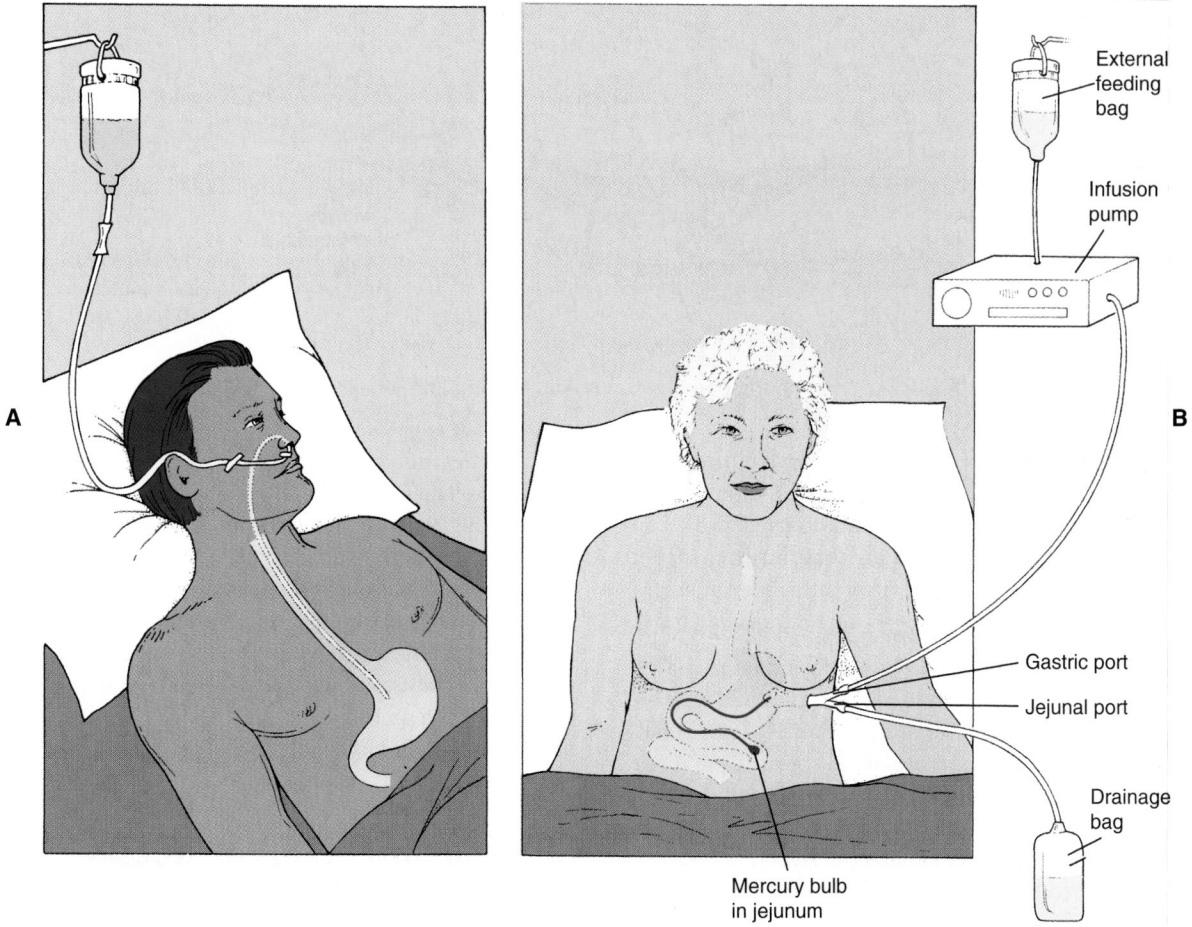

FIGURE 22-1   Types of tube feeding. **A,** Common nasogastric feeding tube. **B,** Gastrostomy-jejunal enteral feeding tube.

- *Gastrostomy*—A gastrostomy tube may be surgically placed through the abdominal wall into the stomach if a patient is not at risk for aspiration.
- *Jejunostomy*—A jejunostomy tube is surgically placed through the abdominal wall and passed through the duodenum into the jejunum, the middle section of the small intestine, if the patient is at risk for aspiration. This procedure

is indicated for patients who lack a competent gag reflex or have gastric cancer or gastric ulcerative disease.

Parenteral Feedings

Applied to nutritional therapy, *parenteral nutrition* refers to any feeding method other than the normal gastrointestinal route. In current medical and nutritional usage, *parenteral* specifically refers to the

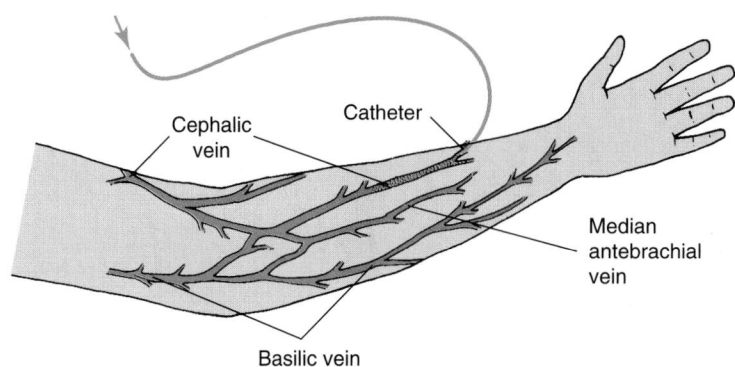

FIGURE 22-2 Peripheral parenteral nutrition feeding into small veins in the arm.

special feeding of basic predigested nutrient elements directly into the blood circulation through certain veins when the gastrointestinal tract cannot be used. Depending on the nutrition support necessary, the following two routes are available:

- *Peripheral parenteral nutrition (PPN)*—PPN is used when the energy need is no more than 2000 kcal/day and required only for a brief therapy period no longer than 10 days. Small peripheral veins, usually in the arm, are used to deliver the less concentrated solutions for brief periods (Figure 22-2).
- *Total parenteral nutrition (TPN)*—TPN is used when the energy and nutrient requirement is large and needed to supply full nutritional support for longer periods of time. A large central vein, usually the subclavian vein leading directly into the rapid flow of the superior vena cava to the heart, is used for surgical placement of the feeding catheter (Figure 22-3).

TPN is used in cases of major surgery or complications—especially those involving the gastrointestinal tract, or when the patient is unable to obtain sufficient nourishment orally. TPN provides crucial nutritional support from solutions containing large amounts of glucose, amino acids, electrolytes, minerals, and vitamins. Fat in the form of lipid emulsions is also used to supply needed kcalories and the essential fatty acid, linoleic acid. A basic TPN solution may contain 2.75% crystalline amino acids

and 25% dextrose with added electrolytes, vitamins, and trace elements (Table 22-1). The physician and clinical dietitian on the nutritional support team determine the individual formula needed based on detailed individual nutrition assessment. The pharmacist on the nutritional support team carefully mixes the solutions according to the prescription. Then the administration of the solution is an important nursing responsibility (Box 22-1). Long-term home use of TPN has been a life-saving measure for many persons but is expensive.

SPECIAL NUTRITIONAL NEEDS AFTER GASTROINTESTINAL SURGERY

Because the gastrointestinal system is uniquely designed to handle food, a surgical procedure on any part of this system requires special dietary attention or modification.

Mouth, Throat, and Neck Surgery

Surgery involving the mouth, jaw, throat, or neck requires modification in the mode of eating. A patient usually cannot chew or swallow normally, so accommodations must be made according to individual limitations.

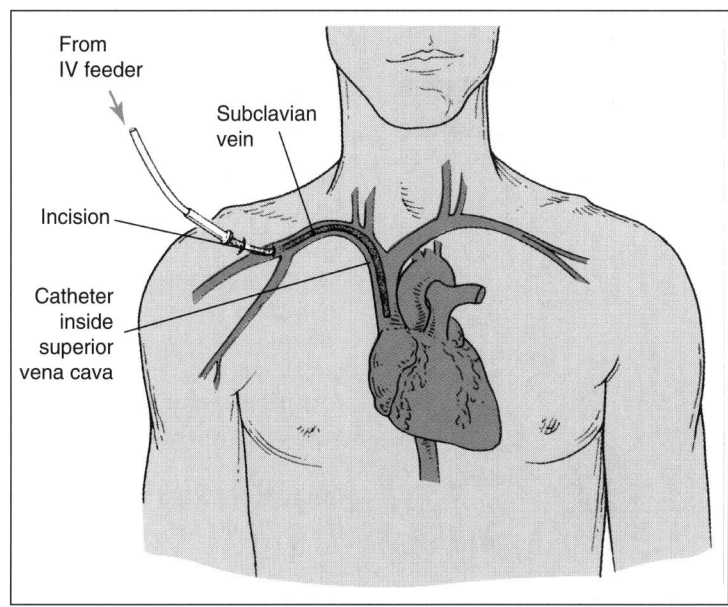

FIGURE 22-3 Catheter placement for total parenteral nutrition (TPN) made for feeding via subclavian vein to superior vena cava.

Oral Liquid Feedings

Concentrated liquid feedings should be planned to ensure adequate nutrition in a smaller amount of food. An enriched commercial formula can be used several times a day to supply needed nourishment.

Tube Feedings

In cases of radical neck or facial surgery, or when a patient is comatose or severely debilitated, tube feedings may be indicated. Current developments in small-bore feeding tubes have made tube feeding easier. For long-term need, improved equipment and standardized commercial formulas have made continued home tube feeding possible for many patients. A nasogastric tube is usually used, but if there is obstruction in the esophagus, the tube is inserted into an opening in the abdominal wall—a gastrostomy, which the surgeon makes at the time of surgery. The tube-feeding formula is generally prescribed by the physician and clinical dietitian according to the patient's nutritional need and tolerance. In any form of tube feeding, it is important to regulate the amount of formula and the rate at which it is given. Usually, 2 l is sufficient for a 24-hour period. Feedings should not exceed 240 to 360 ml (8 to 12 ounces) in each 3- to 4-hour interval. As many as 60% of ill patients receiving liquid formula diets, especially those on tube feedings, encounter diarrhea. Formulas supplemented with the soluble fiber pectin in a 1% solution (1 cc pectin/100 cc formula) have improved bowel function and reduced the incidence of diarrhea.

A wide variety of commercial formulas are available and designed to meet particular needs. These products may be made from *intact nutrients* for use with an intact system able to digest and absorb them. Others may be made from predigested *elemental nutrients*, which are readily absorbed with only minimal residue. Still others may be formulas for special problems or single-nutrient products (modules) of protein, carbohydrate, and fat mixed together as calculated by the clinical dietitian to meet a patient's specific needs. Commercial enteral formulas have the advantage of being standard in composition and immediately available for use.

TABLE 22-1 Example of basic TPN formula components

Components	Amounts
Basic solution	
Crystalline amino acids	2.75%
Dextrose	25%
Additives	
Electrolytes	
Na	50 mEq/L
Cl	50 mEq/L
K	40 mEq/L
HPO_4	25 mEq/L
Ca	5 mEq/L
Mg	8 mEq/L
Vitamins	
Multiple (MV)	1.7 ml conc./L
Vitamin C (per day)	500 mg
Trace elements solution	
(per day)	
Zn	3 mg
Cu	1.6 mg
Cr	2 μg
Se	120 μg
Mn	2 μg
I	120 μg
Fe	1.5 μg
Other additives (as needed)	
Regular insulin	0-25 U/L
Heparin	1000 U/L

These formulas are also sterile and may be stored. Some examples are given in Table 22-2.

Stomach Surgery

Nutritional Problems

Because the stomach is the first major food reservoir in the gastrointestinal tract, stomach surgery poses special problems in maintaining adequate nutrition. Some of these problems may develop immediately after the surgery, depending on the type of surgical procedure (Figure 22-4) and the individual patient's response. Other complications may occur later when the person begins to eat a regular diet.

Immediate Postoperative Period

Immediately after surgery, especially after a total gastrectomy, serious nutritional deficits may occur. If the gastric resection also involved a *vagotomy* (i.e., cutting of the vagus nerve, which supplies a major stimulus for gastric secretions), increased gastric fullness and distention may result. Lacking the normal nerve stimulus, the stomach becomes *atonic* (i.e., without normal muscle tone) and empties poorly. Food fermentation occurs, producing *flatus*, or gas, and diarrhea. Weight loss is common after extensive gastric surgery; at least half of patients fail to reach their optimal weight level.

After surgery, frequent small oral feedings are generally resumed according to a patient's tolerance. A typical pattern of simple dietary progression may

BOX 22-1 Administration of TPN formula

Careful administration of TPN formulas is essential. Specific protocols vary somewhat but usually include the following points:
- *Start slowly.* Give time to adapt to the increased glucose concentration and osmolality of the solution.
- *Schedule carefully.* During the first 24 hours, 1 to 2 L is given by continuous drip, with the slow rate usually regulated by an infusion pump.
- *Monitor closely.* Note metabolic effects of glucose (not to exceed 200 mg/dl) and electrolytes.

- *Increase volume gradually.* After first day, increase by 1 L/day to reach desired daily volume.
- *Make changes cautiously.* Watch the effect of all changes and proceed slowly.
- *Maintain a constant rate.* Keep the correct hourly infusion rate, with no "catch up" or "slow down" effort to meet original volume order.
- *Discontinue slowly.* Take patient off of TPN feeding gradually, reducing rate and daily volume about 1 L/day.

TABLE 22-2 Examples of lactose-free enteral formulas with forms macronutrient components*

Brand name	Manufacturer	Carbohydrate	Sources of:		
			Protein	Fat	
Standard complete diets: intact macronutrients					
Sustacal HC	Mead Johnson	Corn syrup, sucrose	casein	soy oil	
Isocal HCN	Mead Johnson	Corn syrup	casein	soy and MCT oils	
Magnacal	Sherwood	Maltodextrins	casein	soy oil	
Ensure	Ross	Corn syrup, sucrose	casein	corn oil	
Osmolite	Ross	Corn syrup	casein, soy protein isolate	soy, corn, MCT oils	
Travasorb	Baxter	Corn syrup, sucrose	soy protein isolate	soy oil	
Standard complete diets: hydrolyzed carbohydrate and protein					
Vital HN	Ross	Glucose oligosaccharides	small peptides	safflower oil	
Reabilan HN	O'Brien/KMI	Maltodextrin	small peptides	MCT oil, EFA	
Specialty diets: trauma					
Criticare HN	Mead Johnson	Maltodextrin	peptides	safflower oil	
Vivonex T•E•N	Norwich Eaton	Glucose oligosaccharides	crystalline amino acids	safflower oil	
Specialty diets: renal					
Amin-Aid	McGaw	Maltodextrins, sucrose	crystalline amino acids	soy oil	
Travasorb Renal	Baxter	Glucose oligosaccharides	crystalline amino acids	sunflower oil, MCT	
Specialty diets: hepatic					
Hepatic-Aid	McGaw	Maltodextrins, sucrose	crystalline amino acids	soy oil	
Travasorb Hepatic	Baxter	Glucose oligosaccharides, sucrose	crystalline amino acids	sunflower oil, MCT	
Specialty diet: pulmonary					
Pulmocare	Ross	Glucose oligosaccharides	crystalline amino acids	soy oil	
Specialty diet: protein-energy malnutrition, young children ages 1-6					
PediaSure	Ross	Corn syrup, sucrose	casein-whey	safflower-soy oils, MCT	

*All formulas are enriched with essential micronutrients—vitamins and minerals—as needed.
Abbreviations: *HC,* High calories; *HCN,* High calories and nitrogen; *MCT,* Medium chain triglycerides; *HN,* High nitrogen; *EFA,* Essential fatty acids; *T•E•N,* Total enteral nutrition.

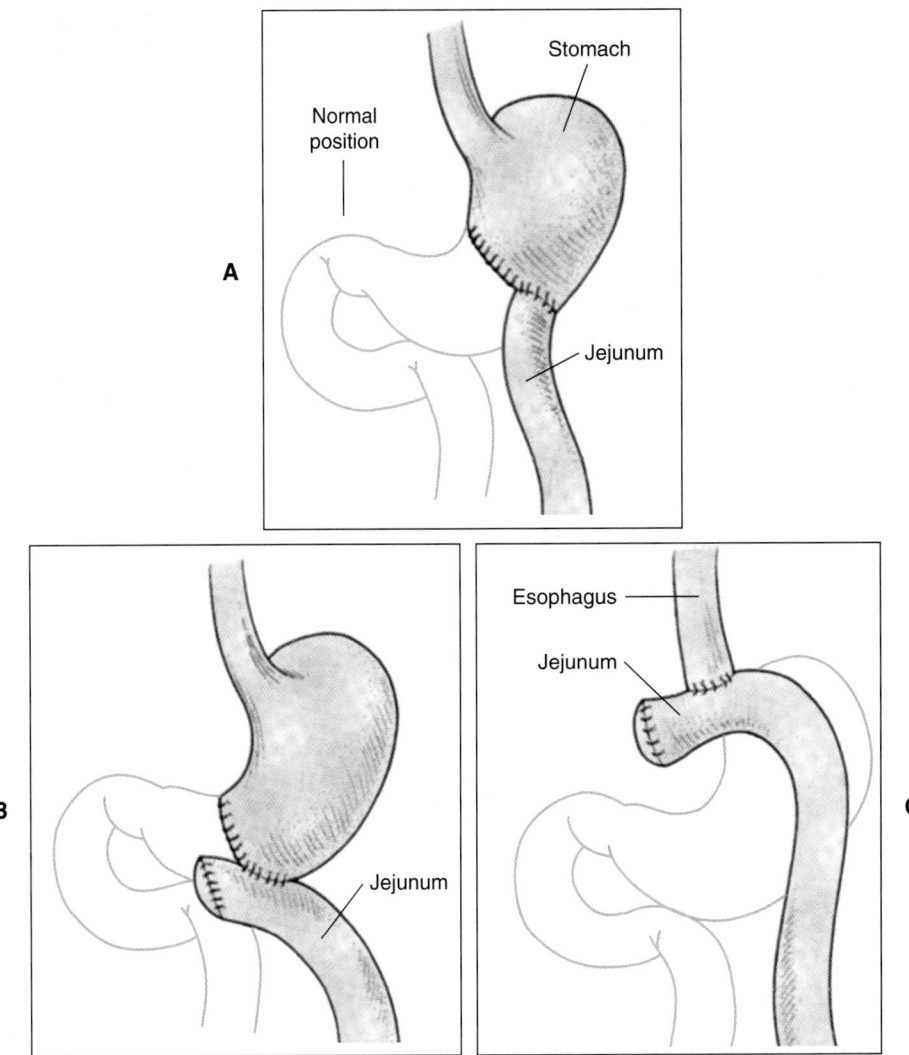

FIGURE 22-4 Gastric surgery. **A,** Partial gastrectomy, Bilroth I. **B,** Partial gastrectomy, Bilroth II. **C,** Total gastrectomy.

cover about a 2-week period. The basic principles of such general diet therapy for the immediate post-gastrectomy period involve the following: (1) size of meals—small and frequent; and (2) nature of meals—simple, easily digested, mild, low in bulk. To cover this immediate postoperative nutritional need after the gastrectomy procedure, however, surgeons leave a temporary catheter in place with a *jejunostomy* (i.e., an opening to the jejunum) through which the patient can be fed an elemental formula to ensure optimal nutritional support during this important initial period.

Later "Dumping Syndrome"

The so-called dumping syndrome is a frequently encountered complication following extensive gastric resection. After the initial recovery from surgery, when the patient begins to feel better and eats a

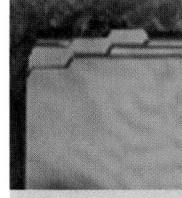

CLINICAL APPLICATIONS

Case Study: John Has a Gastrectomy

After long experience with persistent peptic ulcer disease involving more and more gastric tissue, John Riley and his physician decided that surgery was needed. John then entered the hospital for a total gastrectomy. John withstood the surgery well and received some initial nutritional support from an elemental formula fed through a tube the surgeon had placed into his jejunum. After a few days, the tube was removed and, over the next 2-week period, John was gradually able to take a soft diet in small oral feedings. He soon recovered enough to go home and gradually felt his strength returning. He was relieved to be free of his former ulcer pain and began to resume more and more of his usual activities, eating a regular diet of increasing volume and variety of foods.

As time went by, however, John began having more discomfort after meals. He felt a cramping sensation and increased heartbeat, and then a wave of weakness with sweating and dizziness. John would often become nauseated and vomit. As his anxiety increased, he began to eat less and less and his weight began to drop. He was soon in a state of general malnutrition.

John finally returned to seek medical help. The physician and clinical dietitian outlined a change in his eating habits, and a special food plan was worked out for him. Although the diet seemed strange to him, John followed it faithfully because he had felt so ill. To his surprise, he soon found that his

previous symptoms after eating had almost completely disappeared. Because he felt so much better on the new diet plan, he formed new eating habits around it. His weight gradually returned to normal, and his state of nutrition markedly improved. John found that he would always fare better if he would "nibble" on food items throughout the day rather than consume large meals as he used to do.

Questions for Analysis

1. What were John's nutritional needs immediately after surgery and over the next 2 weeks? Why was it necessary for his feedings to be resumed cautiously?
2. Why was emphasis given to postsurgical protein sources? How was this nutrient need provided?
3. Why must sufficient kcalories be consumed after surgery?
4. Why is fluid therapy paramount after surgery?
5. What minerals and vitamins need special attention after surgery? Why?
6. When John began to feel better and resumed regular eating, why did he become ill? Describe his symptoms and why they developed.
7. Outline the principles of the special diet the clinic dietitian provided to relieve John's symptoms. Plan a day's meal/snack pattern for John with basic instructions and suggestions you would discuss with him.

regular diet in greater volume and variety, discomfort may be experienced about 15 minutes after meals. A cramping, full feeling develops, the pulse becomes rapid, and a wave of weakness, cold sweating, and dizziness may follow. Persons often become

nauseated and vomit. These distressing reactions to food intake only increase anxiety. As a result, less and less food is eaten. Weight loss and general malnutrition follow (see the Clinical Applications Box, "Case Study: John Has a Gastrectomy").

This complex of symptoms constitutes a shock syndrome that results when a meal containing a large proportion of readily soluble carbohydrate rapidly enters, or "dumps" into, the small intestine. When the stomach has been removed, food passes directly from the esophagus into the small intestine (see Figure 22-4). This rapidly entering food mass is a concentrated solution in relation to the surrounding circulation of blood. Thus to achieve an osmotic balance (i.e., a state of equal concentrations of fluids within the small intestine and the surrounding blood circulation), water is drawn from the blood circulation into the intestine. This water shift rapidly shrinks the vascular fluid volume. As a result, blood pressure drops and signs of rapid heart action to rebuild the blood volume appear—rapid pulse, sweating, weakness, and tremors. In about 2 hours, a second sequence of events usually follows. The initial concentrated solution of carbohydrate has been rapidly digested and absorbed, so the blood glucose rises rapidly and stimulates an overproduction of insulin. Blood sugar eventually drops

TABLE 22-3 Diet for postoperative gastric dumping syndrome

General description

1. Five or six small meals daily
2. Relatively high-fat content to retard passage of food and help maintain weight
3. High-protein content (meat, egg, cheese) to rebuild tissue and maintain weight
4. Relatively low-carbohydrate content to prevent rapid passage of quickly used foods
5. No milk; no sugar, sweets, or desserts; no alcohol or sweet carbonated beverages
6. Liquids between meals only; avoid fluids for at least 1 hour before and after meals
7. Relatively low-roughage foods; raw foods as tolerated

Meal pattern

Breakfast	2 scrambled eggs with 1 or 2 tbsp butter or margarine
	½-1 slice bread or small serving cereal with butter or margarine
	2 crisp bacon strips
	1 serving solid fruit*
Midmorning sandwich of:	
	1 slice bread with butter or margarine
	2 oz (56 g) lean meat
Lunch	4 oz (112 g) lean meat with 1 or 2 tbsp butter or margarine
	Green or colored vegetable† with butter or margarine
	½-1 slice bread with butter or margarine
	½ banana or other solid fruit*
Midafternoon	Same snack as midmorning
Dinner	4 oz (112 g) lean meat with 1 or 2 tbsp butter or margarine
	Green or colored vegetable† with butter or margarine
	½-1 slice bread with butter or margarine (or small serving starchy vegetable substitute)
	1 serving solid fruit*
Bedtime	2 oz (56 g) meat or 2 eggs or 2 oz (56 g) cheese or cottage cheese
	1 slice bread or 5 crackers with butter or margarine

*Fruit choice: applesauce, baked apple, canned fruit (drained), banana, orange, or grapefruit sections.
†Vegetable choice: asparagus, spinach, green beans, squash, beets, carrots, green peas.

below normal levels with symptoms of mild *hypoglycemia* (low blood sugar). Dramatic relief from these distressing symptoms, as well as gradual regaining of lost weight, follows careful control of the diet (Table 22-3). Careful reintroduction of milk in small amounts may later be used to test toleration. Patients may also find that eating slowly and lying down for 15 to 30 minutes after eating helps decrease the rate of gastric emptying.

Gallbladder Surgery

For patients suffering from acute gallbladder disease, *cholecystitis*, or from gallstones, *cholelithiasis*

(Figure 22-5), the treatment is usually removal of the gallbladder, *cholecystectomy*. The modern procedure for this removal requires only minimal surgery involving small skin punctures, the common name "keyhole" or "Band-Aid" surgery, rather than the previous surgery with a long abdominal incision.[3,4] Through these small openings, the surgeon can insert needed instruments and a laparoscope fitted with a miniature camera and bright fiberoptic lighting. With only a single stitch and a small bandage closing each of the three openings, the patient can go home almost immediately and be fully recovered—and have a videotape of the whole procedure.

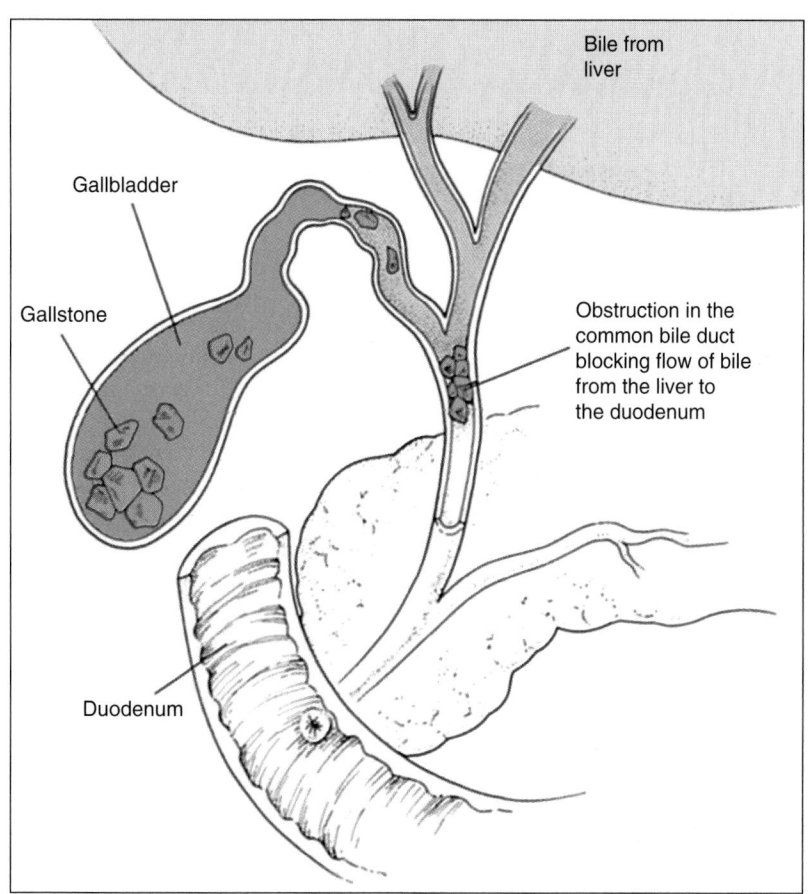

Bile from liver

Gallbladder

Gallstone

Obstruction in the common bile duct blocking flow of bile from the liver to the duodenum

Duodenum

FIGURE 22-5 Gallbladder with stone (cholelithiasis).

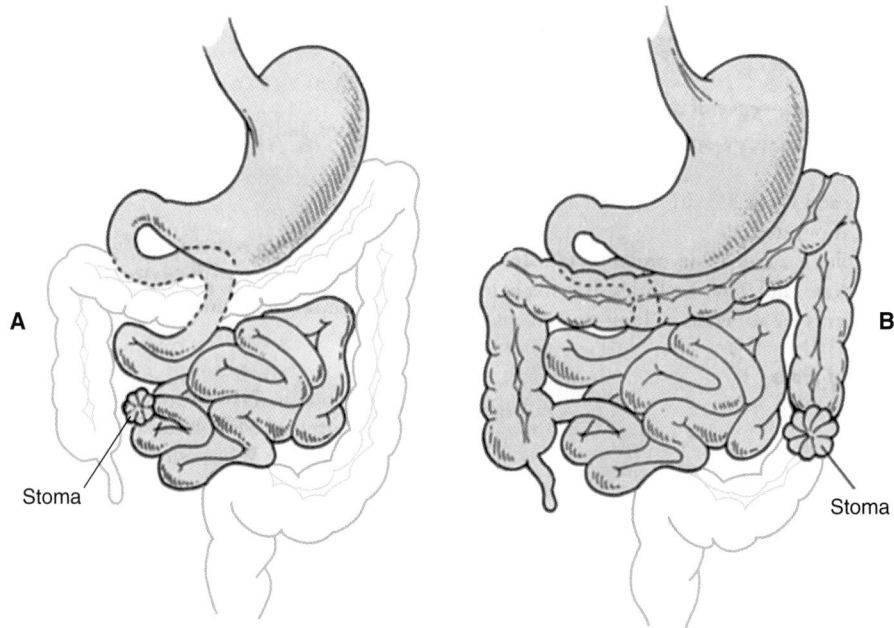

FIGURE 22-6 **A,** Ileostomy. **B,** Colostomy.

Because the function of the gallbladder is to concentrate and store bile, aiding in the digestion and absorption of fat, some moderation in dietary fat is usually indicated. After surgery, control of fat in the diet facilitates wound healing and comfort because the hormonal stimulus for bile secretion still functions in the surgical area, causing pain with intake of fatty foods. The body also needs a period of time to readjust to the more dilute supply of liver bile available to assist fat digestion and absorption. Depending on individual toleration and response, a relatively low-fat diet may be needed, such as the guide given previously for gallbladder disease (see Chapter 18).

Intestinal Surgery

In cases of intestinal disease involving tumors, lesions or obstructions, the affected intestinal area may need to be resectioned. In complicated cases involving large sections of the bowel and requiring surgical removal of most of the small intestine, nutritional support is difficult. In such cases, TPN is used to supply major support with a small allowance of oral feeding for personal food desires. After general resection for less severe cases, a diet relatively low in dietary fiber may be briefly used to allow for healing and comfort. The surgery sometimes requires making an opening in the abdominal wall to the outside from the intestine, a *stoma* (see Figure 22-6), for the elimination of fecal waste materials. If the opening is in the area of the *ileum*, the first section of the large intestine, it is called an *ileostomy*. In this area, the food mass is still fairly liquid and more problems are encountered in management. If the opening is farther along the colon in the last part of the large intestine, it is called a *colostomy*. In this area, the water is largely reabsorbed by the large intestine and the remaining feces is more formed, making management much easier. More radical surgery involving a *proctocolectomy* (i.e., removal of rectal tissue and lower colon) and construction of an *ileoanal reservoir* may be required.[5-8] For many patients, this procedure is a desirable alternative to stoma formation and care.

Coping with any ostomy is difficult at best, and patients need much support and practical help in learning about self-care. A relatively low-fiber diet may be helpful at first, but the aim is to advance as soon as possible to a regular diet. Progression to a regular diet is important both for nutritional value and emotional support. Regular food provides much psychologic help to a patient, and dietary adjustments to individual tolerances for specific foods can easily be made. Patients can revert to a low-fiber intake occasionally when diarrhea occurs.

Rectal Surgery

For a brief period after rectal surgery, or *hemorrhoidectomy*, a clear fluid or nonresidue diet (Table 22-4) may be indicated to reduce painful elimination and allow healing. In some cases, a nonresidue commercial elemental formula such as Vivonex (Sandoz) may be used to delay bowel movements until the surgical area has healed. Return to a regular diet is usually rapid.

SPECIAL NUTRITIONAL NEEDS FOR PATIENTS WITH BURNS

Nutritional Support Base

Treatment and Prognosis

Each year, more than 100,000 persons are burned severely enough to require special hospitalization and care.[7] Treatment of these extensive burns presents a tremendous nutritional challenge. In fact, nutritional care is often the determining factor in survival and healing.[7,8] The following factors influence the plan of care and its outcome:

- *Age*—Elderly persons and very young children are more vulnerable.
- *Health condition*—Any preexisting health problems or other injuries complicate care.

- *Burn severity*—The location and severity of the burns and the time elapsed before treatment are significant.

Degree and Extent of Burns

The depth of the burn affects its treatment and healing process (Figure 22-7). *First degree burns* only involve cell damage in the top layer of skin, the *epidermis*. *Second degree burns* involve cell damage in both the top and second layers of skin, the *dermis*. *Third degree burns* result in full-thickness skin loss, including the underlying fat layer. Second- and third-degree burns covering at least 15% to 20% of the total body surface—or even 10% loss in children and elderly persons—are serious and require extensive care. Burns of severe depth covering more than 50% of the body surface are often fatal. Patients with major burn injuries are usually transferred to a regional burn unit facility for specialized burn team care.

Stages of Nutritional Care

The nutritional care of adults and children with massive burns presents a great challenge and must be constantly adjusted to individual needs and responses.[7,8] At each stage, critical attention is given to amino acid needs for tissue rebuilding, fluid-electrolyte balance, and energy (kcalories) support. Three periods of care generally occur during the immediate shock, recovery, and secondary feeding periods.

Stage 1, Part 1: Immediate Shock Period

From the first hours until about the second day after a burn, massive flooding edema occurs at the burn site. Loss of protective skin leads to immediate losses of water, electrolytes (i.e., mainly sodium), and protein. As water is drawn from surrounding blood to replace the losses, general loss continues, blood volume and pressure drop, and urine output decreases. *Cell dehydration* (critical loss of cell water) follows as cell water is drawn out to balance the loss of tissue fluid. Cell potassium is also withdrawn, and circulating serum potassium levels rise.

TABLE 22-4 Nonresidue diet and postsurgical nonresidue diet

Nonresidue diet

General description

1. This diet includes only those foods free from fiber, seeds, and skins and with the minimum amount of residue.
2. Fruits and vegetables are omitted except for strained fruit juices.
3. Milk is omitted.
4. The diet is adequate in protein and calories, containing approximately 75 g protein, 100 g fat, 250 g carbohydrate, and 2260 kcalories. It is likely to be inadequate in vitamin A, calcium, and riboflavin.
5. If patients are to remain a long time on this diet, supplementary vitamins and minerals should be given.

Selection of foods

Foods	Allowed	Not allowed
Beverages	Carbonated beverages, coffee, tea	Milk, milk drinks
Bread	Crackers, melba or rusks	Whole-grain bread
Cereals	Refined as Cream of Wheat, Farina, fine cornmeal, Malt-o-Meal, pablum, rice, strained oatmeal, cornflakes, puffed rice, Rice Krispies	Whole-grain and other cereals
Cheese		None allowed
Desserts	Plain cakes and cookies, gelatin desserts, water ices, angel food cake, arrowroot cookies, tapioca puddings made with fruit juice only	Pastries, all others
Eggs	As desired, preferably hard cooked	Fried eggs
Fats	Butter or substitute, small amount cream	None
Fruits	Strained fruit juices	All others
Meat, fish, poultry	Tender beef, chicken, fish, lamb, liver, veal; crisp bacon	Fried or tough meat, pork
Potatoes or substitute	Only macaroni, noodles, spaghetti, refined rice	Potatoes, corn, hominy, unrefined rice
Soup	Bouillon and broth only	All others
Sweets	Hard candy, fondant, gumdrops, jelly, marshmallows, sugar, syrup, honey	Other candy, jam, marmalade
Vegetables	Tomato juice	All others
Miscellaneous	Salt	Pepper

Postsurgical nonresidue diet

General description

1. This diet is slightly higher in residue but has greater variety, including potatoes, white bread products, processed cheese, sauces, desserts made with milk, and cream for coffee and cereal.
2. The average daily menu will contain 85 g protein, 2300 kcalories, and is slightly higher in vitamins and minerals.

Selection of foods

To the selections listed above add

    Cheese: Processed cheese, mild cream cheeses

    Potatoes: Prepared any way, no skin

    Bread: Any kind without bran, white bread, rolls, pancakes, waffles

    Fats: 2 oz cream or half-and-half per meal, cream sauce, cream gravy

    Desserts: All desserts except those containing fruit and nuts

    Condiments: As desired.

NOTE: Fruit juice and hard candies may be taken between meals to increase caloric intake.

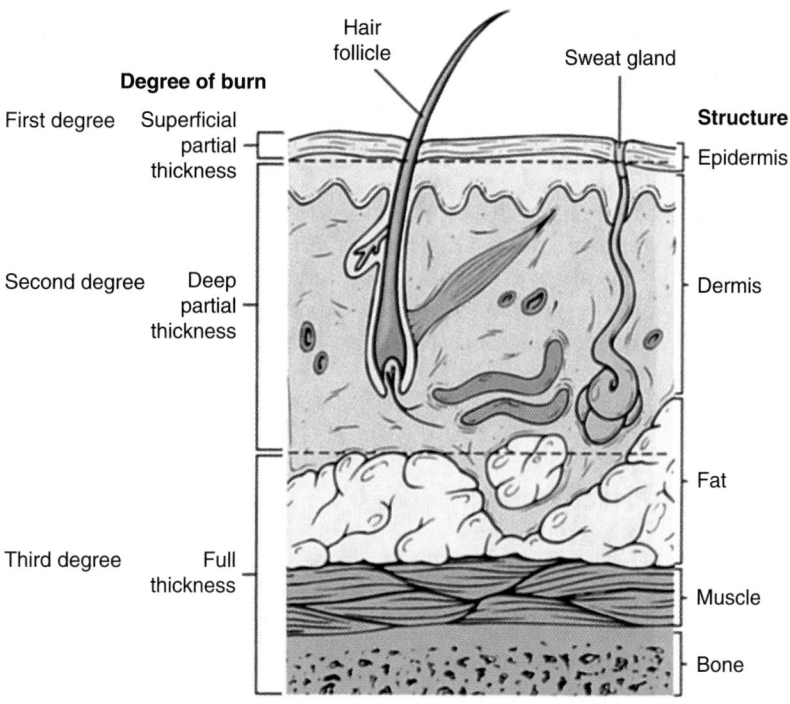

FIGURE 22-7   Depth of skin area involved in burns. (From Lewis SM, Heitkemper MM, Dirksen SR: *Medical-surgical nursing: assessment and management of clinical problems,* ed 5, St. Louis, 2000, Mosby.)

Immediate intravenous fluid therapy with a salt solution such as lactated Ringer's solution replaces water and electrolytes and helps to prevent shock. After about 12 hours when vascular permeability returns to normal and losses begin to decrease at the burn site, albumin solutions or plasma can be used to help restore blood volume. During this initial period, no attempt is made to meet protein and kcalorie requirements because of the following: (1) infusion of glucose at this time may cause *hyperglycemia* (high blood sugar), (2) amino acids would be lost at the burn site, and (3) *adynamic ileus* (i.e., obstruction of the intestines due to loss of normal bowel muscle action) develops after the injury. These factors make use of the gastrointestinal tract at this time impossible.

Stage 1, Part 2: Recovery Period
After about 48 to 72 hours, tissue fluids and electrolytes are gradually reabsorbed, balance is reestab-

lished, and the pattern of massive tissue loss is reversed. A sudden *diuresis* (i.e., increased excretion of urine) occurs, indicating successful initial therapy. Patients usually return to preinjury weight by about the end of the first week. Constant attention to fluid intake and output, with checks for any signs of dehydration or overhydration, are essential.

Stage 2, Part 1: Secondary Feeding Period
Toward the end of the first week after the burn, adequate bowel function returns and a vigorous feeding program must begin. Despite a patient's

---

lactated Ringer's solution **sterile solution of calcium chloride, potassium chloride, sodium chloride, and sodium lactate in water given to replenish fluid and electrolytes; developed by English physiologist Sidney Ringer (1835-1910)**

depression and lack of appetite, at this point life may depend on rigorous nutritional therapy. Three major reasons exist for these increased nutrient and energy demands, as follow:

1. *Tissue destruction* has brought large losses of protein and electrolytes that must be replaced.
2. *Tissue catabolism* has followed the injury with further loss of lean body mass and nitrogen.
3. *Increased metabolism* brings added nutritional needs to cover the additional energy costs of infection or fever and the increased protein metabolism of tissue replacement and skin grafting.

Stage 2, Part 2: Nutritional Therapy

Successful nutritional therapy during this critical feeding period is based on vigorous protein and energy intake.

- **High protein**—Aggressive supplementation of protein is crucial to promote early wound healing and support immune function.[7,8] Depending on the extent of the burn injury and catabolic losses, individual protein needs vary from 150 to 400 g/day. Children require 2 to 4 times the normal standards of protein for age. Most adults generally need 2 to 3 g of protein per kilogram of body weight to achieve nitrogen balance.
- **High energy**—For most adults, from 3500 to 5000 kcalories (i.e., twice the usual basal metabolic rate) are necessary to spare the protein essential for tissue rebuilding and supply the greatly increased metabolic demands for energy.[9,10] A liberal portion of the total kcalories should come from carbohydrate, with a moderate amount of fat supplying the remaining need.
- **High vitamin, high mineral**—Increased vitamin C, as much as 1 to 2 g/day, may be needed as a partner with amino acids for tissue rebuilding. Increased thiamin, riboflavin, and niacin are necessary for the increased energy and protein metabolism.

Stage 2, Part 3: Dietary Management

Either enteral or parenteral methods of feeding may be used to meet these crucial nutrient demands. With any method, a careful intake record must be maintained to measure progress toward the increased nutritional goals.

Enteral feeding. Oral feedings are desired if tolerated. Concentrated liquids are given using added protein or amino acids. Commercial formulas such as Ensure (Ross) may be used as added interval nourishment. Solid foods based on individual preferences are usually tolerated by about the second week. Some patients may require calculated tube feedings to ensure adequate intake in correct nutrient proportions. In such cases, low-bulk, defined formula solutions are given through small-bore feeding tubes. Continuous support and encouragement are always necessary, with food presented as attractively and appetizingly as possible, and well-liked items should be supplied and disliked ones avoided.

Parenteral feeding. For some patients, oral intake and tube feedings may be inadequate to meet the increased nutritional demands, or enteral feeding may be impossible because of associated injuries or complications. In such cases, parenteral feeding can provide essential nutritional support.

Stage 3: Follow-up Reconstruction

Continued nutritional support is essential to maintain tissue strength for successful skin grafting or reconstructive plastic surgery. Patients need not only the physical rebuilding of body resources any surgery requires but also much personal support to rebuild their will and spirit, because disfigurement or disability is possible. Health team members can do much to help instill courage and confidence to face the future again. Optimal physical stamina gained through persistent supportive medical, nutritional, and nursing care will help patients rebuild the personal resources needed to cope.

SUMMARY

The nutritional demands of surgery begin before a patient reaches the operating table. Before surgery, the task is to correct any existing deficiencies and build nutritional reserves to meet surgical demands. After surgery, the task is to replace losses and support recovery. The additional task of encouraging eating is often required during this period of healing.

Postsurgical feedings are given in a variety of ways. The oral route is always preferred. Inability to eat or damage to the intestinal tract, however, may require feeding through a tube or into veins. Special formulas are used for such alternate means of nourishment and are designed to meet specific individual needs. For patients undergoing surgery on the gastrointestinal tract, special diets are modified according to the surgical procedure performed. For patients with massive burns, increased nutritional support is required in successive stages in response to the burn injury and to the continuing tissue rebuilding requirements.

REVIEW QUESTIONS

1. Describe the general effect of imbalances of the following nutritional factors through the preoperative, immediate postoperative, and postoperative periods: protein, kcalories, vitamins and minerals, and fluids.
2. Describe the major surgical effects for which nutritional therapy must be planned after these procedures: mouth, throat, or neck surgery; gastric resection; cholecystectomy; and rectal surgery.
3. Write a 1-day meal plan for a person experiencing postgastrectomy "dumping syndrome." What general dietary guidelines are used?
4. How do an ileostomy and a colostomy differ? What are the dietary needs for each one?
5. Outline the nutritional care of a burn patient from treatment for immediate shock through recovery and tissue reconstruction.

SELF-TEST QUESTIONS

True-False

Write the correct statement for each item you answer "false."

1. Nothing is usually given by mouth for at least 8 hours before surgery to avoid food aspiration during anesthesia.
2. The most common nutrient deficiency related to surgery is that of protein.
3. Negative nitrogen is a rare finding after surgery.
4. Extensive drainage in complicated surgery cases increases water loss to dangerous levels if constant replacement is not provided.
5. Vitamin D is essential to wound healing because it provides a cementing substance for building strong connective tissue.
6. Regardless of the type, oral liquid feedings usually provide little nourishment.
7. Tube feedings can only be successfully prepared from complete commercial preparations.
8. A postgastrectomy patient can usually return to regular eating habits within a few days.
9. After a diseased gallbladder is surgically removed, a patient can freely tolerate any foods containing fats.
10. A careful diet record of the total food and liquid intake is important for a burned patient to ensure that increased nutrient and energy demands are met.

Multiple Choice

1. Postsurgical edema develops at the wound site as a result of:
    a. Decreased plasma protein levels.
    b. Excess water intake.
    c. Excess sodium intake.
    d. Lack of early ambulation and physical exercise.
2. In a postoperative orthopedic patient's diet, protein is essential to:
    a. Provide extra energy needed to regain strength.
    b. Provide a matrix to anchor mineral matter and form bone.
    c. Control the basal metabolic rate.
    d. Give more taste to the diet, thus increasing appetite.
3. Complete high-quality protein is essential to wound healing because it:
    a. Supplies the essential amino acids needed for tissue synthesis.
    b. Spares carbohydrate to supply the increased energy demands.
    c. Is easily digested and does not cause gastrointestinal problems.
    d. Provides the most concentrated source of kcalories.
4. A diet for postgastrectomy "dumping syndrome" should include (Circle all that apply.):
    a. Small frequent meals.
    b. No liquid with meals.
    c. No milk, sugar, sweets, or desserts.
    d. High-protein content.
5. For a burn patient, a diet high in protein and kcalories is essential to do the following for a burn patient (Circle all that apply.):
    a. Replace the extensive loss of tissue protein at the burn sites.
    b. Provide essential amino acids for extensive tissue healing.
    c. Counteract the negative nitrogen balance from loss of lean body mass.
    d. Meet added metabolic demands of infection or fever.

SUGGESTIONS FOR ADDITIONAL STUDY

Individual or Group Project: Commercial Formula Products

Take a survey to discover as many of the commercial products available for both oral and tube feeding as possible. Include both complete defined formulas such as Ensure (Ross) and elemental formulas such as Vivonex (Sandoz). To gather information, with a taste-testing session if possible, interview a clinical dietitian involved in the use of such products. Visit a pharmacy, survey the products available, and discuss each one with the pharmacist. Also survey advertisements in dietetic, nursing, and medical journals. Compare the nutritional composition, uses, and cost of the products. Prepare a report of your findings and conclusions to discuss in class.

REFERENCES

1. Zuckerman J: Hip fracture, *N Engl J Med* 334(23):1519, 1996.
2. Lipkin R: Bone fracture: treatment and risks, *Sci News* 147(12):180, 1995.
3. Frandzel S: The incredible shrinking surgery, *Am Health* 13(3):80, 1994.
4. Stix G: Boot camp for surgeons, *Sci Am* 273(3):24, 1995.
5. Tyus FJ and others: Diet tolerance and stool frequency in patients with ileoanal reservoirs, *J Am Diet Assoc* 92(7):861, 1992.
6. Alles MS and others: Bacterial fermentation of fructo-oligosaccharides and resistant starch in patients with an ileal pouch—anal anastomosis, *Am J Clin Nutr* 666 (June 1):1286, 1997.

7. Prelack K and others: Urinary urea nitrogen is imprecise as a predictor of protein balance in burned children, *J Am Diet Assoc* 97(5):489, 1997.

8. Persinger M: Burn protocol sets goals for protein balance in burned children, *J Am Diet Assoc* 97(5):495, 1997.

9. Mayes T and others: Evaluation of predicted and measured energy requirements of burned children, *J Am Diet Assoc* 96(1):24, 1996.

10. Gottschlich MM and others: Effect of lack of sleep on energy expenditure and physiologic measures in critically ill burn patients, *J Am Diet Assoc* 97(2):131, 1997.

FURTHER READING

• Mayes T and others: Evaluation of predicted and measured energy requirements of burned children, *J Am Diet Assoc* 96(1):24, 1996.

• Persinger M: Burn protocol sets goals for protein and micronutrient intake, *J Am Diet Assoc* 97(5):489, 1997.

These two articles focus on the critical postburn needs throughout the phases of healing. There is an initial need for fluid and electrolyte replacement, followed by critical energy and protein therapy with necessary vitamins and minerals, and a follow-up period of reconstructive surgery. Persistent supportive care (i.e., medical, nutritional, and nursing) is needed to help each patient rebuild the personal resources needed to cope during this difficult healing period.

23 Nutritional Support in Cancer and AIDS

KEY CONCEPTS

- Environmental agents, genetic factors, and the strength of the body's immune system relate to the development of cancer.

- The strength of the body's immune system relates to its overall nutritional status.

- Nutritional problems in the care of cancer relate to the nature of the disease process and the medical treatment methods.

- The progressive effect of the human immunodeficiency virus (HIV) through its three stages of white T-cell destruction requires strong nutrition therapy.

With the accumulating environmental problems and changing lifestyles of the past few years, cancer has become a more prevalent health problem. Because cancer is generally associated with aging, the increasing life expectancy has somewhat contributed to this increasing incidence. Although AIDS and cancer share a direct relation to the body's immune system and basic nutritional needs, their courses and fatal outcomes are unique.

In this chapter, we look at nutritional support in relation to both cancer and AIDS. We see that both conditions threaten life and have important nutritional connections in prevention and therapy.

PROCESS OF CANCER DEVELOPMENT

The Nature of Cancer

Multiple Forms

One of the problems in the study and treatment of cancer is that it is not a single problem; it has a highly varying nature and expresses itself in multiple forms. In these multiple genetic forms, cancer has become one of our major health problems—second only to heart disease—and accounts for about 20% of the total deaths in the United States each year.[1,2] The general term *cancer* is used to designate a malignant tumor or neoplasm, a term that refers to new growth. There are many forms of cancer, however, that vary worldwide and change as populations migrate to different environments. It is therefore more correct to use the plural term *cancers* in discussing this great variety of neoplasms.

Nutrition Relationships

For these reasons, no one specific treatment or special diet for cancer exists, despite various fad diets and claims. Rather, relationships of nutrition and cancer care center on two fundamental areas: (1) *prevention* in relation to the environment and the body's natural defense system, and (2) *therapy* in relation to nutritional support for medical treatment and rehabilitation.

The Normal Cell

Human life results from the process of individual cell growth and reproduction. This process goes on over and over again, almost without error, guided by a cell's *genes*. In adults, approximately 3 to 4 million cells complete the life-sustaining process of cell division every second—largely without mistake, guided by the "genetic code" contained in the specific cell nucleus material in each gene, *deoxyribonucleic acid* (DNA), which is the controlling agent. Each gene carries specific genetic information that controls the synthesis of specific proteins and transmits genetic inheritance. Thus cells only arise from cell division

of preexisting cells and carry their genetic patterns. Normal cell structures and functions operate in an orderly manner under this constant gene control, directing a cell's specific processes of protein synthesis, with regulatory genes switching on and off as needed to control normal cell activities.

The Cancer Cell

This orderly cell operation can be lost, however, with mutation or changes in the genes—especially in the regulatory genes. Cell growths may become malignant tumors when normal gene control is lost.[3,4] Thus the misguided cell and its tumor tissue represent normal cell growth that has "gone wild." Types of cancer tumors are identified by their primary site of origin and stage of growth. *Sarcomas* arise from connective tissue; *carcinomas* arise from epithelial tissue. Stages of tumor development depend on its rate of growth, degree of functional self-control, and amount of penetration or spread into surrounding tissue. Also, the incidence of cancer increases with age because a relationship exists between cancer cell development and the aging process of cells, tissues, and organ systems.

Causes of Cancer Cell Development

The underlying cause of cancer is thus the fundamental loss of cell control over normal cell reproduction. Several factors may contribute to this loss and change a normal cell into a cancer cell.

Mutations

As indicated, mutations, or changes in a cell's genes, are caused by loss of one or more of the

---

neoplasm (Gr. *neos*, new; *plasma*, formation) any new or abnormal cellular growth, specifically one that is uncontrolled and aggressive.

mutation (L. *mutare*, to change) a permanent transmissible change in a gene.

regulatory genes in the cell nucleus or damage to a specific gene that controls a specific function. Such a mutant gene may be inherited. Some cancers have strong genetic causes and tend to run in families (e.g., colon cancer).

Chemical Carcinogens

Agents that cause cancer are called *carcinogens*. Several chemical substances can interfere with the structure or function of regulatory genes. Exposure to such agents may be by individual choice (e.g., cigarette smoking)[5-8] or may result from general exposure to environmental contaminants (e.g., pesticides and industrial chemicals). The actions of such substances may result in gene mutation, damage to gene regulation, or activation of a dormant virus.

Radiation

Radiation damage to genes may come from x-rays, radioactive materials, atomic exhausts or wastes, or sunlight. Overexposure to sunlight is related to skin cancer, which is on the rise in the United States and Europe, afflicting increasingly younger persons. An estimated 750,000 Americans develop skin cancer every year from overexposure to the ultraviolet radiation of the sun. This radiation mutates the recently discovered gene called *patched (PTC)* that inhibits cell growth.[9-11] Common forms of cancer on the head and neck are usually basal cell carcinoma and are easily cured by surgical removal.

A far more lethal form of cancer, *malignant melonoma*, occurs in the skin cells that produce the pigment melanin and accounts for about 2% of all can-

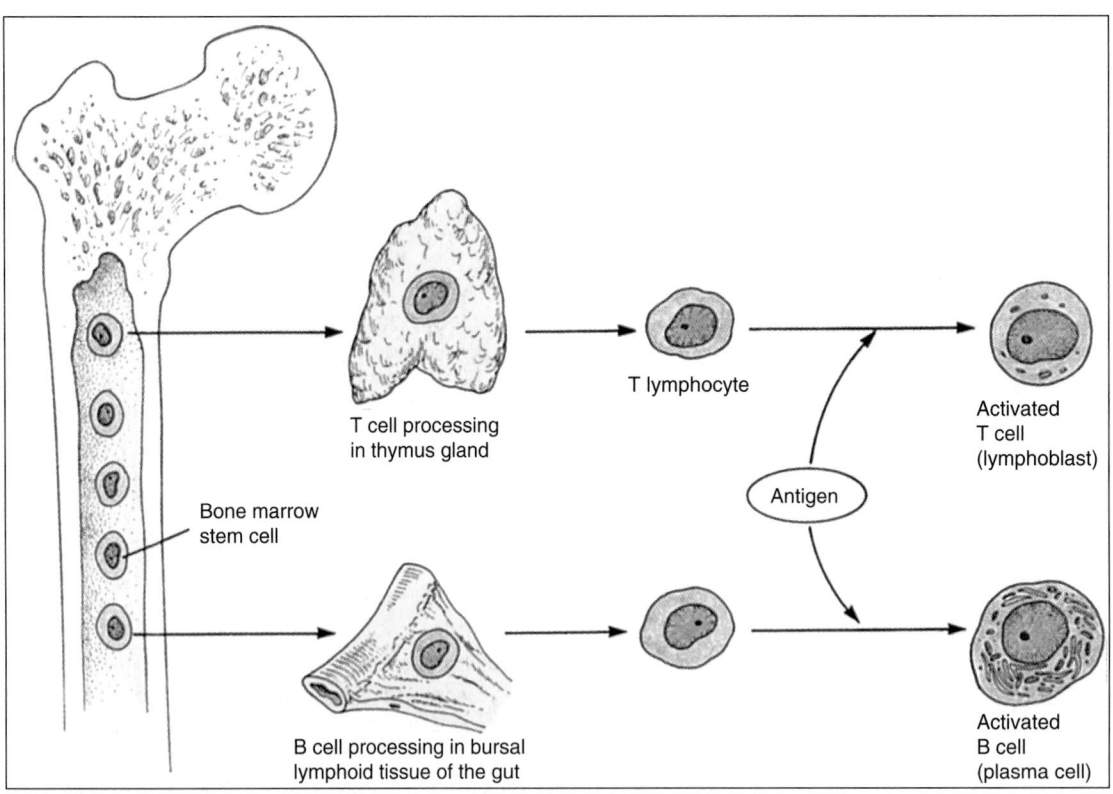

FIGURE 23-1   Development of the T and B cells, lymphocyte components of the body's immune system. (Credit [color]: Eileen Draper.)

cers. About 38,000 cases occur in the United States each year, with approximately 7000 deaths annually.[12] In the United States the incidence varies with latitude, with the greater number occurring in the southern states. The rising incidence probably results from increased exposure to sunlight during recreational, as well as general, activities.

Viruses

Oncogenic, tumor-inducing, viruses that interfere with the function of regulatory genes have been identified in animals and are the focus of much ongoing research. Although oncogenes were first found in viruses, their history indicates that they also function in normal vertebrate cells. A virus is little more than a packet of a few genes, usually fewer than five, whereas cells of complex organisms such as humans have thousands. Disease viruses act as parasites, taking over the cell machinery to reproduce themselves. Continuing study indicates that viruses must be thought of as the second most important factor for cancer development, exceeded only by tobacco use.

Epidemiologic Factors

Epidemiology is the study of disease incidence in populations. Studies of cancer distribution involve factors such as race, region, age, heredity, occupation, and diet. Racial incidence changes as population groups migrate to new environments, and then acquire the cancer characteristics of the new population. The American incidence of breast cancer, for example, has been used as a model for the diet-cancer connection in relation to obesity and the American high-fat diet.

Stress Factors

Stress is an increasing disease factor in our complex society, especially in high-risk populations that lack social and economic supports. Psychic trauma—especially the loss of central personal relationships—takes its toll. Studies of people under stress have shown measured reduction of immune response to disease, especially in the response of the "natural killer cells" of the immune system.[13] Through their influence on the integrity of the immune system, food behaviors, and nutritional status, such stressful states—enhanced at times by pain—make a person more vulnerable to other cancer-producing factors.[14]

The Body's Defense System

The human body's defense system is remarkably efficient and complex. Special cells protect us, not only against external invaders such as bacteria and viruses but also against internal "aliens" such as cancer cells.

Defensive Cells of the Immune System

Two major cell populations provide the immune system's primary "search and destroy" defense for detecting and killing alien, nonself substances that carry potential disease, including cancer cells that may arise daily in the body. These two populations of *lymphocytes*, a special type of white blood cell, develop early in life from a common stem cell in the bone marrow. The two types are called *T cells*, derived from thymus cells, and *B cells*, derived from bursal intestinal cells (Figure 23-1). A major function of T cells is to activate the *phagocytes*, special cells that destroy invaders, as well as to act as "special killer cells" that attack and kill disease-carrying antigens. A major function of B cells is to produce specialized protein known as antibodies, which also kills antigens. Specially tailored proteins called *monoclonal antibodies* have been grown in laboratory mice from specific, single-cell "clones" of original

---

antigen (antibody + Gr. *gennan,* to produce) any foreign or "nonself" substances (e.g., toxins, viruses, bacteria, and foreign proteins) that stimulate the production of antibodies specifically designed to counteract their activity.

antibody any of numerous protein molecules produced by B-cells as a primary immune defense for attaching to specific related antigens.

antibodies, giving medical researchers a tool to diagnose and treat several diseases, including cancer.

Relation of Nutrition to Immunity

Nutritional support is necessary to maintain the integrity of the human immune system. Severely malnourished persons show changes in the structure and function of their immune system. These changes are due to atrophy or losses in the basic tissues involved (i.e., liver, bowel wall, bone marrow, spleen, and lymphoid tissue). Nutrition is fundamental in maintaining normal immunity and combating sustained attacks of disease such as cancer.

The Healing Process and Nutrition

The strength of any body tissue is maintained through constant synthesis—building and rebuilding—of tissue protein. Such strong tissue is a front line of the body's defense. This process of tissue building and healing requires optimal nutritional intake. Specific nutrients—protein and key vitamins and minerals, as well as nonprotein energy sources—must be constantly supplied in the diet. Wise and early use of vigorous nutritional support for cancer patients has been shown to provide recovery of normal nutritional status, including immunocompetence, thus improving their response to therapy and prognosis.[15]

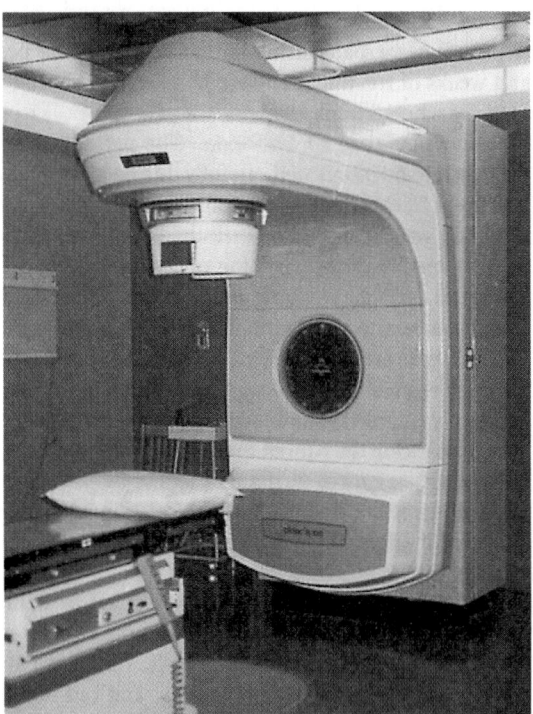

FIGURE 23-2 Radiation treatment machine. (From Lewis SM, Heitkemper MM, Dirksen SR: *Medical-surgical nursing: assessment and management of clinical problems,* ed. 5, St. Louis, 2000, Mosby.)

NUTRITIONAL SUPPORT FOR CANCER TREATMENT

Three major forms of therapy are used today as medical treatment for cancer, as follow: (1) surgery, (2) radiation, and (3) chemotherapy. Each one requires nutritional support.

Surgery

Any surgery, as discussed in Chapter 22, requires nutritional support for the healing process. This requirement is particularly true for patients with cancer because their general condition is often weakened by the disease process and its drain on the body's resources. With early diagnosis and sound nutritional support before and after surgery, many tumors can be successfully removed and recovery is often ensured. Nutritional therapy also includes any needed modifications in food texture or specific nutrients, depending on the site of the surgery or the function of the organ involved. Various methods of feeding patients after surgery are reviewed in Chapter 22.

Radiation

The site and intensity of the radiation treatment (Figure 23-2) determine the nature of the nutritional problems the patient may experience. For example, radiation to the area of the head, neck, or esophagus affects the oral mucosa and salivary secretions, thus affecting taste sensations and sensitivity to food texture and temperature, with increasing anorexia and nausea. Other means of tempting appetite through food appearance and aroma, as well as texture, must be developed. Similarly, radiation to the abdominal area affects the intestinal mucosa, causing loss of villi and absorbing surface, so malabsorption problems may follow. Ulcers or inflammation and obstruction or *fistulas* may also develop from the tissue breakdown. A fistula, from the Latin word for "pipe," is an abnormal opening or passageway within the body or to the outside. As such, it interferes with normal functioning of the involved tissue. The general malabsorption problem may be further compounded by lack of food intake resulting from loss of appetite and nausea.

Chemotherapy

Drugs have been developed to combat various cancers and are often used in combinations to achieve a desired effect in killing the cancer cells. Because these drugs are highly toxic, however, they have similar effects on normal cells and must be regulated carefully. This accounts for their side effects on rapidly growing tissues such as those of the bone marrow, gastrointestinal tract, and hair, as well as for problems in nutritional management. Other problems may relate to the use of pretreatment antidepressant drugs that have special blood pressure effects when used with certain tyramine-rich foods. These drugs are the *monoamine oxidase* (MAO) inhibitors, and their use requires a tyramine-restricted diet (Box 23-1).

- **Gastrointestinal effects**—Numerous problems may develop that interfere with food tolerance: nausea and vomiting, loss of normal taste sensations and lack of appetite, diarrhea, ulcers, malabsorption, or *stomatitis*, an inflammation of the tissues around the mouth.
- **Bone marrow effects**—Interference with the production of specific blood factors causes related problems: reduced red blood cells causing anemia, reduced white blood cells causing lowered resistance to infections, and reduced blood platelets causing bleeding.
- **Hair follicle effects**—Interference with normal hair growth results in general hair loss or baldness.

NUTRITIONAL THERAPY IN THE CANCER PATIENT
Problems Related to the Disease Process

General feeding problems pose a great challenge to the clinical dietitian planning care and the nurse providing important supportive assistance. These problems relate to the overall systemic effects of the cancer, as well as to the specific individual responses to the type of cancer involved.

General Systemic Effects

The disease process of cancer causes three basic systemic effects: (1) anorexia, or loss of appetite, (2) increased metabolism, and (3) negative nitrogen balance. These effects result in poor food intake, increased nutrient and energy needs, and more *catabolism* or breaking down of body tissues. Continuing weight loss ensues. The extent of these effects may vary widely—from a mild response to an extreme form of debilitating cachexia seen in

---

atrophy (L. *a-*, negative prefix; *trophē*, nourishment) a wasting away.

immunocompetence (L. *immunis*, free, exempt) the ability or capacity to develop an immune response (i.e., antibody production or cell-mediated immunity) following exposure to an antigen.

cachexia (Gr. *kakos*, bad; *hexis*, habit) a specific profound effect caused by malnutrition and a disturbance in glucose and fat metabolism usually seen in patients with terminal cancer or AIDS; general poor health indicated by an emaciated appearance.

BOX 23-1 Tyramine-restricted diet

General Directions

- Designed for patients on monoamine oxidase (MAO) inhibitors, drugs that have been reported to cause hypertensive crises when used with tyramine-rich foods. These include foods in which aging, protein breakdown, and putrefaction are used to increase flavor. Studies indicate that as little as 5 to 6 mg tyramine can produce a response, and 25 mg is a danger dose.
- Food sources of other pressor amines such as histamine, dihydroxyphenylalanine, and hydroxytyramine are also avoided.
- Avoid all foods listed. Limited amounts of foods with a lower tyramine amount such as yeast bread may be included in a specific diet.
- Avoid over-the-counter drugs such as decongestants, cold remedies, and antihistamines.

FOODS TO AVOID	REPRESENTATIVE TYRAMINE VALUES (μg/g OR ML)	ADDITIONAL FOODS TO AVOID
Cheeses		Other aged cheeses
N.Y. state cheddar	1416	Blue
Gruyére	516	Boursault
Stilton	466	Brick
Emmenthaler	225	Cheddars (other)
Brie	180	Gouda
Camembert	86	Mozzarella
Processed American	50	Parmesan
Wines		Provolone
Chianti	25.4	Romano
Sherry	3.6	Roquefort
Riesling	0.6	Yeast and products made with yeast
Sauterne	0.4	Homemade bread
Beer, ale—varies with brand		Yeast extracts such as soup cubes, canned meats, and marmite
Highest	4.4	Italian broad beans with pod (fava beans)
Average	2.3	Meat
Least	1.8	Aged game
		Liver
		Canned meats with yeast extracts
		Fish (salted dried)
		Herring, cod, capelin
		Pickled herring
		Other
		Cream, especially sour
		Yogurt
		Soy sauce, vanilla, chocolate
		Salad dressings

advanced disease—with individual patients. This extreme weight loss and weakness is caused by abnormalities in glucose metabolism causing a patient's body to feed off its own tissue protein.

Specific Effects Related to the Type of Cancer

In addition to the primary nutritional problems caused by the disease process itself, secondary problems in eating or use of nutrients relate to specific tumors that cause obstructions or lesions in the gastrointestinal tract or adjacent tissue. Such conditions limit food intake and digestion, as well as absorption of nutrients. Depending on the nature and location of the tumor, as well as its medical treatment, a variety of individual nutritional problems may occur and require personal attention.

Basic Objectives of Nutritional Therapy

Prevention of Catabolism

Every effort is made to meet the increased metabolic demands of the disease process, thus preventing extensive catabolic effects in tissue breakdown. It is far easier to maintain nutrition from the beginning than to rebuild the body from extensive malnutrition. The medical treatment may increase this catabolic effect.

Relief of Symptoms

The symptoms of the disease or side effects of the treatment can be devastating for a patient. Relief requires much individual and family counseling to devise ways of meeting needs and helping the patient to eat. The types of foods used, their preparation and service, or the process of feeding may have to be changed according to individual situations, responses, and needs.

Although the clinical dietitian and the physician have the primary responsibility for planning and managing the nutritional therapy program, a tremendous contribution is made by the nursing staff and other health care personnel in the day-to-day support and counsel in helping the patient to eat. It is often just this kind of constant care and support that differentiates combating the course of the disease and ensuring the comfort and well-being of the patient.

Principles of Nutritional Care

The following basic principles underlie all sound patient care, as discussed in Chapter 17: (1) identifying needs, and (2) planning care based on these needs. Only by acting upon these principles can one determine if real needs are being met. Thus nutritional assessment and care planning are primary concerns.

Nutritional Assessment

Determining and monitoring the nutritional status of each patient is the primary responsibility of the clinical dietitian, but other nursing support staff often assist in body measurements and calculations of body composition, laboratory tests and interpretation of results, physical examination and clinical observations, and complete dietary analyses. These procedures may be reviewed in Chapter 17.

Personal Care Plan

Based on the detailed information gathered about each patient, including living situation and other personal and social needs, the clinical dietitian—in consultation with the physician—develops a personal plan of nutritional therapy for each patient. This outline can then be incorporated into the nursing care plan because the nutritionist works with the nursing staff to carry it out. The day-to-day plan is constantly checked with the patient and family and changed as needed to meet the nutritional demands of the patient's condition and individual desires and tolerances.

Nutritional Needs

Although individual needs vary, guidelines for nutritional therapy must meet specific nutrient needs and goals related to the accelerated metabolism, which demands increased protein-tissue synthesis and energy production.

Energy

The hypermetabolic nature of the disease and its healing requirements place great energy demands on a cancer patient. Sufficient fuel from carbohydrate and, to a lesser extent, fat must be available to spare protein for vital tissue building. An adult patient with good nutritional status needs about 2000 kcalories, or 25 to 30 kcal/kg, for maintenance requirements. More kcalories may be needed according to the degree of individual stress or amount of weight gain needed. A malnourished patient requires 2500 to 3500 kcalories, or 35 to 40 kcal/kg, depending on the degree of malnutrition or extent of tissue injury.

Protein

Necessary tissue building for healing and to offset tissue breakdown by the disease requires essential amino acids and nitrogen. Efficient protein use depends on an optimal protein/kcalorie ratio to promote tissue building and prevent tissue catabolism. An adult patient with good nutritional status needs approximately 80 to 100 g of high-quality protein to meet maintenance requirements. A malnourished patient needs between 100 to 150 g to replenish deficits and restore positive nitrogen balance.

Vitamins and Minerals

Key vitamins and minerals control protein and energy metabolism through their coenzyme roles in specific cell enzyme pathways (see Chapters 6 and 7) and also play important roles in building and maintaining strong tissue. Therefore an optimal intake of vitamins and minerals, at least to the DRI/RDA standards but more often to higher therapeutic levels, is needed. Supplements to the dietary sources are usually indicated.

Fluid

Adequate fluid intake must be ensured for the following two reasons: (1) to replace gastrointestinal losses from fever, infection, vomiting, or diarrhea; and (2) to help the kidneys dispose of metabolic breakdown products from destroyed cancer cells and from the toxic drugs used in chemotherapy.

Some of these drugs (e.g., cyclophosphamide [Cytoxan]) require as much as 2 to 3 L of forced fluids daily to prevent hemorrhagic cystitis.

Nutritional Management

Achieving these nutritional objectives and needs in the face of frequent poor food tolerance or inability to eat presents a great challenge to the nutritional support team. The specific method of feeding depends on the patient's condition. The clinical dietitian and physician manage a particular patient's nutritional care using either enteral or parenteral modes of feeding (see Chapter 21).

Enteral: Oral Diet with Nutrient Supplementation

An oral diet with supplementation is the most desired form of feeding whenever possible. A personal food plan, based on the nutrition assessment information gathered, must be worked out with the patient and family. This food plan must include adjustments in food texture and temperature, food choices, and tolerances and should provide as much caloric and nutrient density as possible in smaller volumes of food (see Clinical Applications box, "Strategies for Improving Food Intake in Cancer or AIDS Patients"). The plan must also give special attention to eating problems with loss of appetite, mouth problems, and gastrointestinal problems.

Loss of appetite.   Anorexia is a major problem and curtails food intake when it is needed most. Anorexia often sets up a vicious cycle that can lead to the gross malnutrition of cancer cachexia if not countered by much effort. A vigorous program of eating—*not dependent on appetite for stimulus*—must be planned with the patient and family. The overall goal is to provide food with as much *nutrient density* as possible so that "every bite counts."

Mouth problems.   Various problems contributing to eating difficulties may stem from sore mouth, stomatitis, or taste changes. Decreased saliva and sore mouth often result from radiation to the head

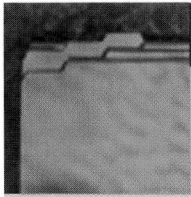

CLINICAL APPLICATIONS

Strategies for Improving Food Intake in Cancer or AIDS Patients

Suggestions for Controlling Nausea and Vomiting

- Try small, frequent meals.
- Eat more when feeling better.
- Eat drier foods with fluids in between.
- Try cold foods and saltier foods.
- Avoid fatty or overly sweet foods.
- Bypass favorite foods to prevent avoidance when feeling better.
- Do not recline right after eating.
- If vomiting, replace fluids and electrolytes with juices, broths, ginger ale, and sports drinks.
- Experiment with spices and flavoring.
- Use foods and special dishes with pleasant-smelling aromas.

Tips for Increasing Kcalories and Protein

- Fortify foods with high caloric condiments, sauces, and dressings.
- Add extra ingredients such as dry milk and cream during food preparation.

Tips for Increasing Kcalories and Protein—cont'd

- Use interval drinks of commercial food supplements.
- Use regular calorie-containing foods and beverages, not low-calorie substitutes.
- Prepare favorite foods in small quantities and freeze extra in small serving sizes for snacks.
- Eat by the clock: have a meal or snack every 1 or 2 hours.
- Eat more when appetite is good.
- Enjoy meals with pleasant surroundings, company, music.
- Keep a supply of easy-to-prepare and convenient foods on hand.
- Try mild exercise, according to physical status.
- If mouth is sore, use soft foods, avoid hot or cold temperature extremes, and check with physician or nurse for topical anesthetic mouth rinses to use before eating.

and neck area or from chemotherapy. Spraying the mouth with artificial saliva is helpful. Frequent small snacks, soft and bland and cool or cold, are often better tolerated. The treatment may often alter the tongue's taste buds, causing taste distortion, "taste blindness," and the inability to distinguish sweet, sour, salt, or bitter, bringing more food aversions. Strong food seasonings and high-protein liquid drinks may be helpful. Because the treatment may also alter salivary secretions, foods with a high liquid content should be used. Solid foods may be

swallowed more easily with the use of sauces, gravies, broth, yogurt, or salad dressings. A food processor or blender can render foods in semisolid or liquid forms for easier swallowing. Any dental problems should be corrected to help with chewing.

Gastrointestinal problems. Chemotherapy often causes nausea and vomiting, which need special individual attention (see Clinical Applications box, "Strategies for Improving Food Intake in Cancer or AIDS Patients"). Food that is hot, sweet, fatty, or spicy sometimes enhances nausea and can be avoided according to individual tolerances. Small, frequent feedings of soft to liquid cold foods, eaten slowly with rests in between, may be helpful. The physician's use of antinausea drugs such as prochlorperazine (Compazine) may help with food tolerances. Special surgical treatment involving the gastrointestinal tract requires related dietary modifications, as discussed in Chapter 22. Chemotherapy or radiation treatment can affect the mucosal cells secreting lactase and thus create lactose intolerance. In such cases, a non–milk-based nutrient supplement (e.g., Ensure [Ross], which is a soy-base product) may be used.

Pain and discomfort. Cancer patients are more able to eat if any severe pain is controlled and they are positioned as comfortably as possible. Physi-

cians previously tended to withhold pain medications for fear of addictions, but the current medical consensus is to administer as much pain control medication as needed, in close consultation with the patient and the family, and monitor responses carefully. This is especially true for children with cancer undergoing painful treatments.

Enteral: Tube Feeding

When the gastrointestinal tract can still be used but the patient is unable to eat and requires more assistance to achieve essential intake goals, tube feeding may be indicated (see Chapter 22). Many patients have negative feelings about tube feeding, however, especially about the use of a nasogastric tube. Table 23-1 lists some helpful procedures to use with such patients. On the other hand, some highly motivated patients have even learned to pass their

TABLE 23-1 Problem-solving tips for patients receiving enteral nutrition

Problem	Suggested solutions
Thirst, oral dryness	Lubricate lips
	Chew sugarless gum
	Brush teeth
	Rinse mouth frequently
	CAUTION: Use lemon drops sparingly because of cariogenic effects
Tube discomfort	Gargle with a mixture of warm water and mouthwash
	Gently blow nose
	Clean tube regularly with water or water-soluble lubricant
	If persistent, pull tube out gently, clean it, and reinsert
	Request smaller tube
Tension, fullness	Relax, breathe deeply after each feeding
Loud stomach noises	Take feedings in private
Limited mobility	Change positions in bed or chair
	Walk around the house or hospital corridor
Gustatory distress	
General dissatisfaction with feeding	Warm or chill feedings
	CAUTION: Feedings that are too cold may cause diarrhea
	Serve favorite foods that have been liquified
Persistent hunger	Chew a favorite food, then spit it out
	Chew gum
	Suck lemon drops (sparingly)
Inability to drink	Rinse mouth frequently with water and other liquids

small-caliber tubes themselves. In some instances, patients can be fed by pump-monitored slow drip during the night and be free from the tube during the day. The use of special formulas and delivery-system equipment has also made home enteral nutrition possible and practical.

Parenteral: Peripheral Vein Feeding

When the GI tract cannot be used and nutritional support is vital, intravenous feeding must be initiated. For brief periods—in cases requiring less concentrated intakes of energy and nutrients—solutions of dextrose, amino acids, vitamins, and minerals, with concurrent use of lipid emulsions, may be fed into smaller peripheral veins. Use of smaller peripheral veins carries less risk than use of a larger central vein and can supply necessary support when nutrient needs are not excessive. Peripheral vein feeding is combined with tube feeding to supply additional needs in some cases, avoiding the use of a central vein.

Parenteral: Central Vein Feeding

When nutritional needs are greater and must continue over an extended period of time, central vein feeding has often provided a life-saving alternative. This total parenteral nutrition (TPN) process requires surgical placement of the feeding catheter, along with careful assessment, monitoring, and administration. Although TPN carries risks, thus requiring skilled team management, this hyperalimentation process has provided a significant means of turning the metabolic status of cancer patients from catabolism to anabolism, often avoiding the serious development of cancer cachexia. Details of these alternate enteral and parenteral methods of feeding are discussed in Chapter 22.

CONCLUSIONS: CANCER THERAPY AND PREVENTION

Therapy

Ample evidence at this point indicates that vigorous nutritional support increases the chances for successful medical treatments in the care of cancer.

The fundamental reasons for this improved possible outcome have been briefly reviewed here. It is also evident that much effort on the part of the health care team, the patient, and the family—all working together—is absolutely necessary for vigorous nutritional support to become a reality.

Prevention

On the basis of studies concerning possible associations of nutritional factors and food forms with cancer, the National Research Council Committee on Diet, Nutrition, and Cancer has issued guidelines for the public to help persons make generally healthy food choices to reduce risks. These committee statements were intended to serve as interim guidelines until more information is available but are consistent with good nutrition and health practices and, if followed, likely to reduce the risk of cancer

Fat

Reduce fat intake from the usual American average of 40% of total kcalories to 30% to reduce the risks for breast and colon cancer associated with high-fat diets.

Fiber

Use a variety of fruits, vegetables, legumes, and whole-grain cereal products to ensure a sufficient amount and type of dietary fiber to reduce the risk for colon cancer.

Vitamins A and C

Emphasize the use of citrus fruits, carotene-rich vegetables, and fruits.

Phytochemicals

Include a wide variety of fruits and vegetables to obtain numerous compounds called phytochemicals (i.e., plant chemicals), which relate to the prevention of cancer. The American Cancer Society's dietary guidelines emphasize choosing most of our foods from plant sources, and their recent "5 a Day for Better Health" programs encourage Americans to eat five or more servings of fruits and vegetables every day.[16,17]

Processed Meats

Minimize consumption of salt-cured, pickled, or smoked foods, including smoked sausages, hot dogs, ham, and smoked fish. These smoke-cured foods have been associated with cancer in some populations.

Food Pesticides and Additives

Minimize contamination of foods by carcinogens from any source, agricultural or food industry, whether avoidable or unavoidable. Intentional food pesticides and additives, direct or indirect, should continue to be evaluated for carcinogenic activity before they are approved for use in the food supply.

Alcohol

Moderate the use of alcoholic beverages, if they are used at all.

Of these seven guidelines, the first five can be directly controlled by individual food choices. The sixth one requires action by the agricultural and food processing industries, but consumers can exercise influence through their food buying habits and support of reforms in pesticide laws. The final guideline relates to personal attitudes and habits concerning the use of alcohol; as is often the case in health habits in general, moderation is the key.

Ongoing Cancer Research

Many studies have shown that diets high in fat and low in fiber, fruits, and vegetables—major sources of vitamins A and C and phytochemicals—are associated with increased incidence and mortality from various cancers.[18] Vitamin A and its plant precursor beta-carotene have been particularly associated with protective immunity.[19] On the basis of this consistent and strong association, the U.S. National Cancer Institute has developed a current program to encourage Americans to eat five or more servings of fruits and vegetables every day,[20] which is one of the nation's health-promotion and disease-prevention objectives.[21] The "5 a Day for Better Health Program" is now underway with many associated projects through participating state public health agen-

cies and public-private partnerships with the food industry and food-service operations. The program is serving as a model for such partnerships in community nutrition.

PROCESS OF AIDS DEVELOPMENT

We will now look at acquired immunodeficiency syndrome (AIDS) and compare its relation to the body's immune system and course of development with that of cancer. Similarly, we will briefly review the process of AIDS development, its medical treatment and nutrition support, nutritional therapy, and conclusions about AIDS therapy and prevention.

It was in the late 1970s that physicians in New York City and San Francisco first puzzled over an uncommon medical problem appearing among their patients.[22] No known cause of immune suppression could be found, but persons were nonetheless suffering and dying from complications of common infections, largely pneumonia, that were ordinarily easily handled by the human immune system and the usual antibiotics or other antibacterial drugs. Its virus source and pandemic effects were soon to become alarmingly evident worldwide.

Evolution of HIV

Early Pandemic Spread

The earliest known case of AIDS was recently identified in a blood sample collected in 1959 from a Bantu man living in what is currently called the Democratic Republic of Congo, an area from which the current world epidemic is believed to have spread.[23] Early in the 1960s—first in the African country of Uganda, strange deaths began to occur from simple common infections such as pneumonia that did not respond to the usual antibiotic drugs. By the late 1970s and early 1980s, the same strange deaths were occurring in Europe and America. Similar reports of unexplained im-

BOX 23-2 Common types of microorganisms causing clinical complications in AIDS

Parasites
Pneumonia
Focal encephalitis
Malabsorption, diarrhea
Meningitis

Bacteria
Bacteremia
Diarrhea
Pneumonia
Meningitis
Tuberculosis
Encephalitis

Fungi
Fungemia
Pneumonia
Thrush, stomatitis, esophagitis
Skin lesions

Viruses
Multiple mucosal lesions, herpes simplex
Pneumonia
Non-Hodgkin's lymphomas
Multiple skin lesions, herpes zoster
Nausea, vomiting, diarrhea, fever

mune system failure increased rapidly in various parts of the world, and the pandemic spread alarmingly. These early cases were coming from quite diverse social and medical backgrounds, including heterosexual and homosexual men, intravenous drug users exchanging needles, and recipients of transfused blood and blood products (e.g., children with hemophilia and medical/surgical patients). After a feverish pace of research, the underlying infectious agent was finally discovered in May 1983. The French scientist Luc Montagnier, a leading pioneer of AIDS research, reported that he and his team at the Pasteur Institute in Paris had isolated the viral cause, now known as *human immunodeficiency virus (HIV)*.

Evolution and Spread of the Virus

Where did this new deadly virus come from and how did it gain such strength so rapidly? From studies thus far, scientists are beginning to find some answers. Apparently, HIV is not a new virus but an old one that only recently grew deadly in humans while gaining strength during the social upheavals of the 1960s and 1970s. The uprooting effect of this rapid social change, urbanization, and world travel allowed the virus to spread rapidly through world populations and reproduce aggressively in its human host.

Parasite Nature of Virus

No virus can have a life of its own. By their structure and reproductive nature, viruses are the ultimate parasites. They are mere shreds of genetic material, a small packet of genetic information encased in a protein coat. Viruses only contain a small

---

virus (L. *virus*, poison; *virion*, individual virus particle) a minute microscopic infectious organism characterized by lack of independent metabolism and the ability to reproduce with genetic continuity only within a living host. Each particle (virion) basically consists of nucleic acids (genetic material) and a protein shell that protects and contains the genetic material and any enzymes present.

pandemic (Gr. *pan*, all; *dēmos*, people) a widespread epidemic, distributed through a region, a continent, or the world.

parasite (Gr. *para*, along side; *sitos*, food, grain; *parasitos*, one who eats at another's table in ancient Greece, a term for a person who received free meals in return for amusing or flattering conversation). An organism that lives in or on an organism of another species known as the host, from whom all lifecycle nourishment is obtained.

chromosome of nucleic acids (RNA or DNA), usually with fewer than five genes. They can only live through a host, whom they invade and infect, hijacking the host's cell machinery to run off a multitude of copies of themselves. The purpose of viruses is to make as many self-copies as they can. Today's viruses are those that succeeded in this survival task over time and are, like all plants and animals, simply descendents of earlier forms. Scientists agree that HIV, which has been found to be genetically similar to viruses found in African primates (e.g., simian immunodeficiency virus [SIV]), was probably transmitted to humans in an earlier age as ancient hunters cut themselves while butchering their kills for food.[24] The rapidly increasing social-sexual changes and world travel of the past few decades have sped the transmission and rapid multiplication of HIV. The current deadly strength of HIV results from its aggressive growth within an increasing number of hosts. Today, more than 12 million people throughout the world are infected with HIV.

Stages of Disease Progression

The individual clinical course of HIV infection varies substantially, but three distinct stages mark the progression of the disease: (1) primary HIV infection and extended well period of viral incubation, (2) AIDS-related complex (ARC) of illnesses, and (3) terminal AIDS.

Stage 1: Primary HIV infection

About 2 to 4 weeks after initial exposure and infection, a mild flulike episode lasting about a week may occur. This brief mild response reflects the initial development of antibodies to the viral infection. Any subsequent HIV testing will be positive. Then for the next 8 to 10 years, the person feels perfectly well, not knowing the infection is present unless an HIV test is done. This long well period is deceptive, however, because it is actually a critical stage of viral incubation. The virus is actually "hiding away" in lymphoid tissues (e.g., lymph nodes, spleen, adenoid glands, and tonsils), where it is rapidly multiplying in its parasite lifecycle within the host, taking over more and more of its special T-helper white blood cells (CD4+) and gaining strength.[25] Researchers emphasize the crucial nature of this incubation period and the importance of earlier medical treatment intervention after an HIV-positive test to slow this viral-strengthening time while drugs and vaccines are being developed to combat its steady progression.

Stage 2: AIDS-Related Complex (ARC)

After the extended well HIV-positive stage, which may last as long as 10 years, a period of associated infectious illnesses begins. This ARC period of opportunistic illnesses is so named because by this period the HIV infection has killed enough host-protective white T-cells (i.e., T-helper lymphocytes) to severely damage the immune system and lower the body's normal disease resistance so that even the most common everyday infections have an opportunity to take root and grow. Common symptoms during this pre-AIDS period include persistent fatigue, mouth sores of thrush (i.e., oral *Candida albicans*), night sweats, diarrhea, fever over 100° F, unintentional weight loss of at least 5 kg (11 lbs), remarkable headache, new skin rash, new or unusual cough, sore throat or mouth, unusual bruises or skin discoloration, and shortness of breath.[26]

Stage 3: Final Stage of AIDS

The terminal stage of full-blown HIV infection, commonly designated as AIDS, is marked by rapidly declining T-helper lymphocyte counts from the normal healthy level of about 1000 per cubic millimeter of blood ($1000/mm^3$). Persons infected with HIV usually lose about 40 to $80/mm^3$ of T-helper lymphocytes every year.[27,28] When falling T-helper lymphocyte counts are roughly between 200 and 500 mm^3, various diseases (e.g., tuberculosis or Kaposi's sarcoma) generally occur. Kaposi's sarcoma is the most common AIDS-associated cancer, characterized by malignant, rapidly-growing tumors of the skin and the mucous linings of the gastrointestinal and respiratory tracts, where they may cause severe internal bleeding. Low-dose radiation therapy or anticancer drugs may be used to slow the spread of the tumors. At T-helper lymphocyte counts below 200/mm³, *protozoan parasites* (i.e., primitive single-cell organisms) appear and infect a number of body organs. At counts under 50/mm³, *cytomegalovirus* (CMV; a herpes virus causing lesions on mucous linings of body organs) or *lymphoma* (any cancer of the lymphoid tissue) can flourish.[29] This series of HIV effects on the body brings marked changes in body weight in both men and women, with women losing disproportionately more body fat.[30] When the AIDS virus finally kills enough white cells to overwhelm the immune system's weakened resistance to the disease complications, death follows.

NUTRITIONAL MANAGEMENT IN THE HIV/AIDS PATIENT

Support for Medical Management

Basic Current Goals

Medical management of HIV infection during all of its stages is constantly evolving. Intensive medical research for drugs and vaccines to halt this devastating virus continues. Current studies are aimed at preventing progressive immunodeficiency, stopping HIV transmission to uninfected individuals, and restoring depressed immune function to normal to prevent AIDS-associated complications. Thus, basic current medical goals are to do the following: (1) delay progression of the infection and improve the immune system, (2) prevent opportunistic illnesses, and (3) recognize the infection early and provide rapid treatment for complications, including infections and cancers.

Initial Evaluation: AIDS Team

The initial medical evaluation of a person newly diagnosed with HIV is critical in providing guidelines for ongoing comprehensive care by the AIDS team. This professional team includes medical, nutritional, nursing, and psychosocial health care specialists. Box 23-3 outlines an initial evaluation guide that emphasizes special coordinated medical care and the importance of nutritional, nursing, and psychosocial support.

Drug Therapy

The ongoing task of developing effective drugs and vaccines is difficult. One of the earliest findings

---

BOX 23-3   Initial evaluation of newly diagnosed HIV-infected patients

Routine history and physical examination include:
  History of exposure to infectious complications of AIDS
  Assessment of baseline mental status
Baseline laboratory studies
  CBC, differential, platelets
  Biochemistry screening profile
  Urinalysis
  Chest x-ray
  Tuberculin test with energy panel
  Serologic test for syphilis
  Toxoplasma serology
  T-lymphocyte subsets
  Hepatitis B serology (optional)

Nutritional assessment, counseling, support, and follow-up
Psychosocial and financial status assessment
Referral to and involvement in psychosocial support include:
  Social worker, nurse, psychologist or psychiatrist, patient support group, community support group, and agencies
Rehabilitation program for substance abusers
Planning for family members and children, including issues of testing and providing for their care.

Adapted from Gold, JWM: HIV-1 infection: diagnosis and management, *Med Clin North Am* 76(1):1, 1992.

in this drug research has been a group of compounds called *dideoxynucleosides* that inhibit the virus's necessary enzyme for copying itself, thus effectively preventing viral increase. There have been multiple toxic side effects (Box 23-4), however, some of which (e.g., nausea) may be helped by diet modifications. A second group of drugs called *protease inhibitors* have recently been added.[23,24] This class of drugs helps stop HIV by inhibiting the basic enzyme, protease, which is essential to its development.[25] The virus depends on this cell enzyme to assemble itself properly. The following drugs are currently the main protease inhibitors:

1. Saquinavir
2. Indivavir
3. Ritonavir
4. Nelfinavir
5. Nevirapine
6. Amprenavir

Vaccine Development

After disappointing research results, U.S. studies for a live AIDS vaccine have brightened. Current research for a long-awaited vaccine against HIV has been revitalized in the United States by the National Institutes of Health's (NIH) new appointment of a strong scientist to head its Vaccine Research Center in Bethesda, Maryland. An initial goal is aggressive movement toward clinical international trials.

Wasting Effects of HIV Infection on Nutritional Status

Severe Malnutrition and Weight Loss

Major weight loss is a fundamental effect of HIV infection that eventually leads to extreme cachexia similar to that seen in cancer patients. This serious, characteristic body wasting contributes to development of the full disease syndrome because malnutrition suppresses cellular immune function. The chronic, relentless body wasting of AIDS is so striking that in Africa it is called "slim disease." The attendant diseases of the wasting process play a major role in the decreased quality of life, debilitating weakness, and fatigue.

Causes of Body Wasting

The characteristic body wasting of HIV infection may be due to any of the following processes, alone or combined:

- **Inadequate food intake**—An important factor in the profound weight loss is severe *anorexia*, loss of appetite. This state is proba-

BOX 23-4 Toxic effects of AIDS drugs

AZT (azidothymidine, zidavudine)
Bone marrow suppression, decreased red and
  white blood cell counts
Anemia, muscle pain
Nausea and vomiting
Headache, malaise, fatigue, fever
Confusion, tremulousness, disordered brain function
Bluish color of fingernails and toenails

ddI (dideooxyinosine)
Painful peripheral nerves
Occasional pancreatitis

ddI (dideooxyinosine)—cont'd
Headache, insomnia, restlessness
Occasional hepatitis

ddC (dideoxycytidine)
Painful peripheral nerves
Stomatitis, fevers
Bone pain, edema

d4T (dideoxythymidine)
Painful peripheral nerves
Anemia

bly related to the patient's life-changing situation, as well as to the body's physiologic changes from the disease. Encouraging results have come with use of the drug megestrol (Megace) in treating patients with AIDS or cancer. This drug is a synthetic hormone similar to the natural hormone progesterone, which improves appetite and food intake, leading to weight gain.

- **Malabsorption of nutrients**—Diarrhea and malabsorption are common in AIDS patients. These symptoms have been related to drug-diet interactions and the progressive effects of HIV infection. The viral infection causes blunting of the intestinal villi and secretion of abnormal intestinal enzymes. In later stages of AIDS, the damaged intestinal tissues are open to opportunistic organisms, resulting in severe diarrhea and malabsorption.

- **Disordered metabolism**—In the final stage of weight loss in AIDS patients, changes in metabolism (e.g., hypermetabolism and altered energy metabolism) occur. Progressive depletion of lean body mass and increased resting energy expenditure also result.

Nutrition Assessment

A comprehensive nutrition assessment provides the baseline information necessary for starting and continuing nutritional care. The clinical dietitian on the AIDS team conducts this assessment and calculates daily kcalorie and protein needs, assessing and monitoring weight changes and evaluating laboratory tests. These tests and evaluations are especially required for certain patients on special nutrition support—enteral or parenteral. Further person-centered nutritional care required for all HIV-infected patients is evident in the ABCDs of nutrition assessment outlined in the Clinical Applications box, "The ABCDs of Nutrition Assessment of AIDS Patients." Upon first contact with a health professional, all patients should be referred to the AIDS team clinical dietitian for screening to detect the degree of any nutritional problems.

Together with the patient, the dietitian can then plan for ongoing nutritional care and support. Suggested guidelines for developing such patient-centered care plans are outlined in Table 23-2.

Nutrition Counseling, Education, and Supportive Care

Counseling Principles

An adolescent client once defined a counselor as "someone to talk to while I make up my mind," and client-centered counseling in the care of persons with HIV infection must be just that. The basic goal of nutrition counseling is to make the least amount of changes necessary in a person's lifestyle and food patterns to promote optimal nutritional status while providing maximum comfort and quality of life. In this person-centered care process, the following counseling principles are particularly important:

- *Motivation*—Changed behavior in any area requires the motivation, desire, and ability to achieve one's goals. AIDS is no exception. Until a patient perceives food patterns and behaviors as appropriate goals, it is best to wait for a better time and simply start with establishing a general supportive climate in which to continue working together. Any specific obstacle raised by the patient (e.g., time, physical limitations, money, or increased anxiety) can be met with related suggestions to think about.

- *Rationale*—Any diet or food behavior change, with possible benefits or risks, must be clearly explained to the patient. The question "Why?" is always important.

- *Provider-patient agreement*—When the patient is ready, any change must be an agreement and must fit daily routines and include any caregivers as needed. Throughout the process, the nutrition counselor should provide any necessary information and encouragement.

- *Manageable steps*—All information or actions should proceed in manageable steps, as small

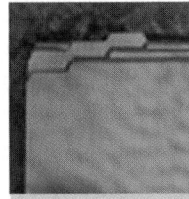

CLINICAL APPLICATIONS

The ABCDs of Nutrition Assessment of AIDS Patients

The initial nutrition-assessment visit with a patient infected with HIV is important because it sets the pattern and direction for all of the continuing nutritional care that is to follow.

This vital encounter serves both informational and relational functions. It provides the necessary baseline information for planning practical, individual nutritional support. More importantly, however, the initial visit establishes the essential provider-patient relationship, which is the very human context in which continuing nutritional care and support are provided as needed. The basic ABCDs of nutrition assessment provide a practical guide (see Chapter 17), with special EFs added for HIV-infection patients.

Anthropometry
- Age, sex, height
- Weight: current, usual, percent of usual, ideal, percent of ideal, weight loss over a defined period
- Mid-upper arm measures: circumference, triceps skinfold thickness; calculated mid-arm muscle circumference

Biochemical tests
- Serum proteins: albumin, prealbumin, transferrin
- Liver function test (evaluate liver function)
- Blood urea nitrogen, serum electrolytes (evaluate renal function)
- Urinary urea nitrogen excretion over 24 hours (nitrogen balance)

Biochemical tests—cont'd
- Creatinine height index (evaluate protein tissue breakdown)
- Complete blood count (evaluate for anemia)
- Fasting glucose (evaluate for high or low blood glucose levels)

Clinical observations
- General signs of nutritional status (see Table 17-1)
- Drug effects

Diet evaluations
- Usual intake, current intake, restrictions, modifications (use 24-hour recall and food diaries)
- Nutrition supplements, vitamin and/or mineral supplements
- Food allergies, intolerances
- Activity level (average number of kcalories expended per day)
- Support system (caregivers to help with nutritional care plan)

Environmental, behavioral, psychologic assessment
- Living situation, personal support
- Food environment, types of meals, eating assistance needed

Financial assessment
- Medical insurance
- Income, financial support through caregivers
- Ability to afford food, enteral supplements, additional vitamins and/or minerals

TABLE 23-2 Planning nutrition care for patients with AIDS

Type of problem	Possible causes	Patient care plan considerations
Food intake		
	Anorexia	Patient, caregiver roles
	Drug, food interaction	Motivation, patient decision making
	HIV, other infection	Education, counseling
	Taste alteration	Resource materials
	Food intolerances, allergies	Nutrition supplements
	Lack of access or ability to prepare food	Vitamin, mineral supplements
	Depression	Drug-food reactions
		Special enteral-parenteral nutritional support
		Monitoring, adjustments as needed
Nutrient absorption		
	HIV-related infections or cancers	Treatment of underlying disease or disorder
	Diminished gastric HCl secretion	Pancreatic enzymes supplement
	Altered mucosal absorbing surface	Drug-nutrient reactions
	Organ involvement: liver, pancreas, gallbladder, kidney	Special enteral-parenteral nutrition support, appropriate formula design
	Drug-nutrient interaction	Monitoring, adjustments as needed
Altered metabolism, excretion		
	HIV infection	Review of drug dosage, schedule
	Associated infections, diseases	Modification of diet, meal pattern
	Drug-nutrient interactions	Treatment of infection, symptoms
	Altered hormonal function	Review of diet nutrients, increase or decrease
	Organ dysfunction	Special enteral-parenteral nutrition support, appropriate formula design
		Monitoring, adjustments as needed

Adapted from Newman CF: *Practical guidelines for improving nutritional status in HIV-related disease,* University of California, David Medical School Fifth Annual Conference on Clinical Nutrition, Nutrition in the Treatment of Serious Medical Problems, Feb 28-29, 1992.

as necessary, in order of complexity and difficulty. Do simple, easy things first. Information overload can discourage anyone. In this situation, however, the stress load at any point can be intolerable for the AIDS patient. As with cancer patients at such points of stress, AIDS patients are more vulnerable to the lure of unproven therapies.

Personal Food-Management Skills

The patient's living situation and general practical skills in planning, purchasing, and preparing food must be considered. Any need for information and guidance in developing these skills or providing sources of help should be provided.

Community Programs

Information about any available community food programs (e.g., Meals-on-Wheels, for delivery of prepared meals when the patient is too ill to shop for food or prepare it) may be needed. Information about food assistance programs (e.g., Food Stamps or Food Commodities [see Chapter 13]), for which lower-income persons may qualify, may also be needed.

Psychosocial Support

In the final analysis, every aspect of care provided should be given in a form and manner that provide genuine psychosocial support. All health care providers working with HIV-infected patients must be particularly sensitive to the special psychologic and social issues that confront persons with AIDS. Major stress areas may include issues relating to autonomy and dependency, a sense of uncertainty and fear of the unknown, grief, change and loss, fear of symptoms and abandonment, and spiritual questions that arise when someone confronts a life-threatening disease. Common emotions are hostility, denial, withdrawal, depression, anxiety, guilt, and confusion. Health care providers must always be aware of how the patient and caregivers are relating to the disease, using assistance of social workers or clinical psychologists as needed. Stress-reduction groups—including exercise training—are helpful as they have proved to be in other life-threatening situations (e.g., cancer and coronary heart disease).

Most of all, however, health care workers must examine their own stresses, values, and fears about sexual orientation and behavior, intravenous drug use, and fear of AIDS transmission. Preconceived judgments are easily picked up by patients and threaten the provider-patient relationship. Before they can be effective with patients, all health care workers must first deal with their own fears and prejudices and learn to let go of judgmental behavior.

SUMMARY

The general term *cancer* is given to various abnormal, malignant tumors in different tissue sites. The cancer cell is derived from a normal cell that loses control over its growth and reproduction. Cancer cell development occurs via mutation of regulatory genes and is influenced by environmental chemical carcinogens, radiation, and special viruses. Other associated factors include diet, excessive alcohol use, and smoking, as well as physical and psychologic stress. These effects and cell development are mediated by the body's immune system, primarily through its two types of special white blood cells: T cells that can kill invading agents that cause disease, and B cells that can make specific antibodies to attack these agents.

Cancer therapy primarily consists of surgery, radiation, and chemotherapy with specific toxic drugs. Supportive nutritional care must be highly individualized according to body responses to the disease and its treatment. This care is based on nutritional assessment and provided by the following routes: oral, tube feeding, peripheral vein, and TPN through a large central vein. In any case, nutritional management must meet the physical and psychologic needs of individual patients.

Likewise, nutritional care of patients with AIDS must be built on knowledge and compassion, with a sensitivity and concern for individual patient needs. The current worldwide spread of HIV and its fatal consequences have reached epidemic proportions and are still growing. The overall disease progression follows three distinct stages: (1) HIV infection, (2) ARC with associated opportunistic illnesses, and (3) full-blown AIDS with complicating diseases leading to death.

Medical management of HIV infection, which is still without a cure or vaccine, involves supportive treatment of associated illnesses and diseases. In the terminal AIDS stage, the virus eventually gains enough strength to destroy the host's immune system (i.e., T-helper white cells), and death follows. New drugs are being used to slow the disease process, while intensive ongoing research seeks a vaccine and cure.

Nutritional management centers on providing individual nutritional support to counteract the severe body wasting and malnutrition characteris-tic of the disease. The process of nutritional care involves comprehensive nutrition assessment and evaluation of personal needs, planning care with patient and caregivers, and meeting practical food needs. Throughout the care process, nutrition coun-seling, education, and strategic services also help provide psychosocial support for each patient, ac-cording to individual needs.

REVIEW QUESTIONS

1. What is cancer? Describe several major causes of cancer cell formation. Why is cancer an in-creasing health problem?
2. In what two main ways does nutrition relate to cancer? Give examples of each.
3. Describe the major types of defense cells that are the major components of the body's im-mune system. How does nutrition relate to immunity?
4. Describe nutritional problems associated with each of the three medical treatments of cancer.
5. Outline the general procedure for nutritional management of a cancer patient.
6. List and describe the National Research Council's dietary guidelines for reducing the risk for cancer.
7. Describe the evolutionary history of HIV and its current worldwide epidemic spread. How is it transmitted, and why do you think it has spread so rapidly? Identify major population groups at risk.
8. Describe the nature of the AIDS virus and its action in the human body.
9. Describe the three stages of HIV infection from initial infection to death.
10. Outline basic parts of a comprehensive initial nutrition assessment of a patient with HIV infection, and describe the reasons for each type of information and its evaluation.
11. Describe the general process of planning nu-tritional care on the basis of the patient-assessment information and the main types of nutrition problems in patients with HIV. Devise a related plan of action for each type of problem. Give an example of how you might follow up to see what worked or did not work and make adjustments.

SELF-TEST QUESTIONS

True-False

Write the correct statement for each item you answer "false."

1. A cancer cell is unrelated to a normal cell.
2. Genes consist of cell nucleus material that controls protein synthesis and transmits hered-itary information.
3. Chemical carcinogens are substances that can cause cancer to develop.
4. The incidence of cancer is not related to age.
5. Cancer-causing mutant genes may be inher-ited, making a person more susceptible to the influence of some added environmental agent.
6. Antigens are specialized protein components of our immune systems that protect us against disease.
7. Head and neck surgery for cancer seldom re-quires diet modification in texture of foods.

8. A cancer patient treated with an MAO inhibitor for depression requires a special, low-tyramine diet.

Multiple Choice

1. Special blood cells that are major components of the immune system are:
   a. Erythrocytes.
   b. Lymphocytes.
   c. Antibodies.
   d. Platelets.

2. A serious primary problem resulting from prolonged vomiting from cancer chemotherapy relates to:
   a. Nitrogen balance.
   b. Calcium balance.
   c. Fluid and electrolyte balance.
   d. Glucose balance.

3. Side effects of cancer chemotherapy that reflect the toxic effect of the drugs on rapidly reproducing cells include:
   a. Severe headaches.
   b. Gastrointestinal symptoms.
   c. Increased urination.
   d. Decreased appetite.

4. An adequate amount of high-quality protein is essential in a cancer patient's diet to:
   a. Prevent catabolism.
   b. Meet increased energy demands.
   c. Prevent anabolism.
   d. Stimulate hypermetabolism.

5. Small amounts of which of the following types of food would most likely help treat the nausea caused by cancer chemotherapy?
   a. Hot liquids
   b. Dry, spicy foods
   c. Warm, fat-seasoned foods
   d. Soft, cold foods

SUGGESTIONS FOR ADDITIONAL STUDY

1. Individual Project: Analysis of a Cancer Patient's Diet

Interview a cancer patient being treated by chemotherapy. Collect and analyze the following data:

- Specific drugs used and the main action and side effects of each
- Symptoms experienced by the patient
- Total food intake for 1 day
- Efforts made by the patient to deal with any eating difficulties (e.g., mouth problems, GI problems, or loss of appetite)
- Any nutrient or food supplements used

Calculate the protein and kcalories in a day's food intake. Evaluate the protein/kcalorie ratio in terms of the need to prevent protein use for energy. On the basis of your findings, outline a personal food plan for the patient. Also, make a list of suggestions for helping a patient with nausea and other eating problems caused by cancer therapy. If possible, discuss the food plan with the patient.

2. Individual or Group Project: Cancer Education

Make a list of all the possible community resources for educating persons about cancer. These resources can be programs, persons, and materials designed to meet the needs of both those with cancer and the general public. The content of such resources may include any aspect of cancer, including the nature of the disease process, types and incidence of various forms of cancer, risk factors and their reduction, signs that may point to potential problems and need medical evaluation, cancer treatment and its effects, or nutrition.

Include the local chapter of the American Cancer Society as a primary resource on your list. Make an appointment to visit the office and interview a staff member about the society's work. Obtain any educational materials available. Make similar visits to community clinical facilities, hospitals, public health agencies, and private practitioners and interview any professionals (e.g., nurses, clinical nutritionists/dietitians, health educators, or physicians) involved in cancer care and education. Evaluate your findings and compare them with those of other students in a full class discussion.

REFERENCES

1. Rennie J, Rustings R: Making headway against cancer, *Sci Am* 275(3):56, 1996.
2. Cavene WK, White OL: The genetic basis of cancer, *Sci Am* 27(3):56, 1996.
3. Weinberg RA: Tumor suppressor genes, *Sci Am* 275(3):62, 1996.
4. Trichopoulos D and others: What causes cancer?, *Sci Am* 275(3):80, 1996.
5. Brennan JA and others: Association between cigarette smoking and mutation of the p53 gene in squamous-cell carcinoma of the head and neck, *N Engl J Med* 332(11): 712, 1995.
6. Kessler D and others: The Food and Drug Administration's regulation of tobacco products, *N Engl J Med* 335:988, 1998.
7. U.S. Department of Health and Human Services, Public Health Services, Centers for Disease Control, National Center for Chronic Disease Prevention and Health Promotion, Office on Smoking and Health: Projected smoking-related deaths among youth—United States, *MMWR* 45(44):971, 1996.
8. Thun MJ: Excess mortality among cigarette smokers: changes in a 20-year interval, *Am J Pub Health* 85(9):1223, 1995.
9. Pennisi E: Gene linked to commonest cancer, *Science* 272(5268):1883, 1996.
10. Johnson RL and others: Human homolog of *patched*, a candidate gene for the basal cell nervus syndrome, *Science* 272(5268):1668, 1996.
11. Travis J: Gene for the most common cancer found, *Sci News* 149(24):1996.
12. Leffel D, Brash DE: Sunlight and skin cancer, *Sci Am* 275(1):52, 1996.
13. Perera FP: Uncovering new clues to cancer risk, *Sci Am* 274(5):54, 1996.
14. Holland JC: Cancer's psychologic challenges, *Sci Am* (3):158, 1996.
15. Foley KM: Controlling the pain of cancer, *Sci Am* 275(3):164, 1996.
16. Hellman S, Vokes EE: Advancing current treatment for cancer, *Sci Am* 275(3):118, 1996.
17. Greenwald P: Chemoprevention of cancer, *Sci Am* 275(3):96, 1996.
18. Bloch AS: Nutrition and cancer: the paradox: *Diet Curr* 23(2):1996.
19. American Cancer Society: Guidelines on diet, nutrition, and health, *Nation's Health* 26(9)23, 1996.
20. Aulus J-J: Alternative cancer treatments, *Sci Am* 275(3): 162, 1996.
21. Marian M: Cancer cachexia: prevalence, mechanisms, and interventions, *Support Line* 20(April):3, 1998.
22. Piot P: AIDS: a global response (editorial), *Science* 272(5270):1855, June 28, 1996.
23. Tuofu Z and others: An African HIV-1 sequence from 1959 and implications for the origin of the epidemic, *Nature* 391(6667):594, 1998.
24. Christensen D: AIDS virus jumped from chimps, *Sci News* 155(Feb 6):84, 1999.
25. Christensen D: Why AIDS? The mystery of how HIV attacks the immune system, *Sci News* 155(13):204, 1999.
26. Kotler DP and others: Relative influences of sex, race, environment, and HIV infection on body composition in adults, *Am J Clin Nutr* 69(3): 432, 1999.
27. Ho DD: Time to hit HIV, early and hard (editorial), *N Engl J Med* 333(7):450, 1995.
28. Cohen J: Results of the new AIDS drugs brings cautious optimism, *Science* 271(5250):755, 1996.

FURTHER READING

- American Cancer Society: Guidelines on diet, nutrition, and health, *Nation's Health* 26(9): 23, 1996.
  These guidelines provide clear background for nutritional care of persons with cancer.
- Havas S and others: 5 a day for better health: a new research initiative, *J Am Diet Assoc* 94(1):32, 1994.

This article provides an interesting description and commentary of the current national project being carried out through a unique public-private partnership designed to help persons increase their intake of fruits and vegetables as encouraged in current health guidelines to decrease cancer risk.

Appendixes

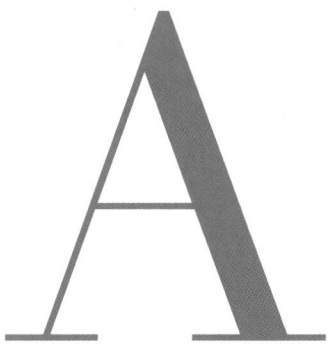

A

Food Composition Table

The following Food Composition Table was developed by Positive Input Corp. and includes all of the foods listed in *Mosby's NutriTrac Nutrition Analysis CD-ROM*, which accompanies every copy of this text. Please note, however, that you will be able to find some nutrient information in *Mosby's NutriTrac Nutrition Analysis CD-ROM* that is not listed here in the Food Composition Table.

USDA ID Code	Food Name	Weight in Grams*	Quantity of Units	Unit of Measure	Protein (gm)	Fat (gm)	Carbohydrates (gm)	Kcalories	Caffeine (gm)	Fiber (gm)	Cholesterol (mg)	Saturated Fat (gm)
3117	Babyfood, Applesauce	28.35	3	Ounce	0	0	2.92	10.49	0	0.48	0	0
3280	Babyfood, Bananas w/ Tapioca	28.35	3	Ounce	0.11	0.06	5.05	18.99	0	0.45	0	0
3681	Babyfood, Barley, Ppd w/ Whole Milk	28.35	3	Ounce	1.3	0.94	4.62	31.47	0	0	0	0
3003	Babyfood, Beef	28.35	3	Ounce	4.11	1.39	0	30.05	0	0	0	0.73
3049	Babyfood, Beef and Rice	28.35	3	Ounce	1.42	0.82	2.49	23.25	0	0	0	0
3043	Babyfood, Beef Lasagna	28.35	3	Ounce	1.19	0.6	2.84	21.83	0	0	0	0
3287	Babyfood, Beef Noodle	28.35	3	Ounce	0.71	0.54	2.1	16.16	0	0.31	0	0
3052	Babyfood, Beef Stew	28.35	3	Ounce	1.45	0.34	1.56	14.46	0	0.31	3.55	0.16
3098	Babyfood, Beets	28.35	3	Ounce	0.37	0.03	2.18	9.64	0	0.54	0	0
3100	Babyfood, Carrots	28.35	3	Ounce	0.23	0.06	2.04	9.07	0	0.48	0	0
3013	Babyfood, Chicken	28.35	3	Ounce	4.17	2.72	0	42.24	0	0	0	0.7
3069	Babyfood, Chicken Noodle	28.35	3	Ounce	0.54	0.4	2.13	14.46	0	0.31	0	0
3070	Babyfood, Chicken Soup	28.35	3	Ounce	0.45	0.48	2.04	14.18	0	0.31	0	0
3014	Babyfood, Chicken Sticks	10	3	Stick	1.46	1.44	0.14	18.8	0	0.02	0	0
3214	Babyfood, Cookies, Arrowroot	28.35	3	Ounce	2.15	4.05	20.19	125.31	0	0.06	0.3	0.94
3120	Babyfood, Corn, Creamed	28.35	3	Ounce	0.4	0.11	4.62	18.43	0	0.6	0	0
3028	Babyfood, Cottage Cheese w/ Fruit	28.35	3	Ounce	0.85	0.2	4.51	22.11	0	0	0	0
3018	Babyfood, Egg Yolks	28.35	3	Ounce	2.84	4.9	0.28	57.55	0	0	208.37	1.47
3201	Babyfood, Egg Yolks and Bacon	28.35	3	Ounce	0.71	1.42	1.76	22.4	0	0.26	0	0
3236	Babyfood, Fruit Dessert	28.35	3	Ounce	0.09	0	4.88	17.86	0	0.17	0	0
3092	Babyfood, Green Beans	28.35	3	Ounce	0.34	0.03	1.62	7.09	0	0.54	0	0
3009	Babyfood, Ham	28.35	3	Ounce	4.28	1.9	0	35.44	0	0	0	0.64
3166	Babyfood, Juice, Apple	247.791	0.75	Cup	0	0.25	28.99	116.46	0	0.25	0	0
3179	Babyfood, Juice, Mixed Fruit	247.791	0.75	Cup	0.25	0.25	28.74	116.46	0	0.25	0	0

The easiest way to look for a food is to use the "Search For" feature in *Mosby's NutriTrac Nutrition Analysis CD-ROM*. However, if you do not have access to a computer or your computer time is limited, you can easily look for a food using this Food Composition Table. The foods in the table are arranged alphabetically, within groups.

The code number before each food listing corresponds to the food data bank in *Mosby's NutriTrac*

Nutrition Analysis CD-ROM. When you input your dietary intake into the CD-ROM program, you may choose to use these code numbers. Alternatively, you may choose to enter your dietary intake into *Mosby's NutriTrac Nutrition Analysis CD-ROM* by typing a food's name or partial name and using the "Search For" option.

Column heading key: *gm* = grams; *mg* = milligrams; *mcg* = micrograms; *re* = retinol equivalent

*Please note that the "Weight in Grams" column provides the weight in grams of the serving or of one unit of measure. (For example, if a serving is 3 ounces, the "Weight in Grams" column may incidate the weight of 1 ounce.)

Monounsaturated Fat (gm)	Polyunsaturated Fat (gm)	Vitamin D (mg)	Vitamin K (mg)	Vitamin E (mg)	Vitamin A (re)	Vitamin C (mg)	Thiamin (mg)	Riboflavin (mg)	Niacin (mg)	Vitamin B6 (mg)	Folate (mg)	Vitamin B12 (mcg)	Calcium (mg)	Iron (mg)	Magnesium (mg)	Phosphorus (mg)	Potassium (mg)	Sodium (mg)	Zinc (mg)
0	0	0	0	0.17	0.28	10.72	0	0.01	0.02	0.01	0.48	0	1.42	0.06	0.85	1.7	21.83	0.57	0.01
0	0	0	0	0.17	1.13	7.29	0	0.01	0.06	0.04	1.81	0	2.27	0.09	3.4	2.55	30.62	2.55	0.02
0	0	0	0	0	0	0	0.14	0.16	1.7	0.03	2.52	0.09	65.21	3.5	8.51	42.53	54.43	13.89	0.24
0.52	0.05	0	0	0.11	8.79	0.54	0	0.05	0.93	0.03	1.62	0.42	2.27	0.47	2.55	20.41	53.87	18.71	0.57
0	0	0	0	0	22.4	1.11	0	0.02	0.38	0.04	1.7	0.14	3.12	0.2	2.27	9.92	34.02	101.21	0.26
0	0	0	0	0	44.23	0.54	0.02	0.03	0.38	0.02	1.7	0.14	5.1	0.25	3.12	11.34	34.59	128.71	0.2
0	0	0	0	0.11	24.95	0.4	0.01	0.01	0.16	0.01	1.56	0.03	2.27	0.12	1.98	8.51	13.04	4.82	0.11
0.12	0.03	0	0	0.07	65.49	0.85	0	0.02	0.37	0.02	1.7	0.14	2.55	0.2	3.12	12.47	40.26	97.81	0.25
0	0	0	0	0.15	0.85	0.68	0	0.01	0.04	0.01	8.73	0	3.97	0.09	3.97	3.97	23.53	0.03
0	0	0	0	0.15	334.81	1.56	0.01	0.01	0.14	0.02	4.9	0	6.52	0.11	3.12	5.67	57.27	13.89	0.05
1.23	0.66	0	0	0.11	15.88	0.43	0	0.05	0.97	0.05	3.15	0.11	15.59	0.28	3.12	25.52	34.59	14.46	0.29
0	0	0	0	0.07	30.33	0.34	0.01	0.01	0.15	0.01	1.5	0.04	4.82	0.11	2.55	6.8	9.92	4.82	0.08
0	0	0	0	0.07	62.65	0.28	0	0.01	0.08	0.01	1.47	0.03	10.49	0.08	1.42	6.8	18.71	4.54	0.06
0	0	0	0	0.04	95.4	0.17	0	0.02	0.2	0.01	1.11	0.04	7.3	0.16	1.4	12.1	10.6	47.9	0.1
2.55	0.24	0	0	0.13	0	1.56	0.14	0.12	1.63	0.01	2.84	0.02	9.07	0.85	6.24	32.89	44.23	104.9	0.15
0	0	0	0	0.15	2.27	0.62	0	0.01	0.14	0.01	3.6	0.01	5.1	0.08	2.27	9.36	22.96	14.74	0.07
0	0	0	0	0.17	0.57	6.75	0	0.01	0.01	0	1.45	0.02	8.79	0.04	1.13	11.06	11.91	14.46	0.05
1.96	0.64	0	0	0.22	106.6	0.4	0.02	0.08	0.01	0.05	26.11	0.44	21.55	0.78	1.98	81.36	21.83	11.06	0.54
0	0	0	0	0.08	7.94	0.26	0.01	0.02	0.08	0.01	1.16	0.03	7.94	0.13	1.42	14.18	9.92	13.61	0.08
0	0	0	0	0.07	6.8	0.85	0.01	0	0.04	0.01	0.99	0	2.55	0.06	1.42	2.27	26.93	3.69	0.01
0	0	0	0	0.15	12.19	2.38	0.01	0.03	0.09	0.01	9.27	0	18.43	0.31	6.24	36.29	0.57	0.05
0.9	0.26	0	0	0.11	2.84	0.6	0.04	0.05	0.81	0.06	0.6	0.03	1.42	0.29	3.12	25.23	59.54	18.99	0.48
0	0	0	0	1.49	4.96	143.47	0.02	0.04	0.21	0.07	0.25	0	9.91	1.41	7.43	12.39	225.49	7.43	0.07
0	0	0	0	0.5	9.91	157.59	0.06	0.03	0.3	0.11	16.6	0	19.82	0.84	12.39	12.39	250.27	9.91	0.07

USDA ID Code	Food Name	Weight in Grams*	Quantity of Units	Unit of Measure	Protein (gm)	Fat (gm)	Carbohydrates (gm)	Kcalories	Caffeine (gm)	Fiber (gm)	Cholesterol (mg)	Saturated Fat (gm)
3172	Babyfood, Juice, Orange	247.791	0.75	Cup	1.49	0.74	25.27	109.03	0	0.25	0	0
3090	Babyfood, Macaroni and Cheese	28.35	3	Ounce	0.74	0.57	2.32	17.29	0	0.09	0	0
3045	Babyfood, Macaroni and Tomato and Beef	28.35	3	Ounce	0.71	0.31	2.66	16.73	0	0.31	0	0
3021	Babyfood, Meat Sticks	10	3	Stick	1.34	1.46	0.11	18.4	0	0.02	0	0.58
3279	Babyfood, Mixed Vegetable	28.35	3	Ounce	0.28	0	2.24	9.36	0	0	0	0
3076	Babyfood, Noodles and Chicken	28.35	3	Ounce	0.48	0.62	2.58	18.14	0	0.31	0	0
3228	Babyfood, Peach Cobbler	28.35	3	Ounce	0.09	0	5.19	18.99	0	0.2	0	0
3230	Babyfood, Peach Melba	28.35	3	Ounce	0.09	0	4.65	17.01	0	0	0	0
3131	Babyfood, Peaches w/ Sugar	28.35	3	Ounce	0.14	0.06	5.36	20.13	0	0.43	0	0
3133	Babyfood, Pears	28.35	3	Ounce	0.09	0.03	3.29	12.19	0	1.02	0	0
3124	Babyfood, Peas, Buttered	28.35	3	Ounce	0.99	0.37	3.2	17.01	0	0	0	0
3135	Babyfood, Plums w/ Tapioca	28.35	3	Ounce	0.03	0	5.78	20.98	0	0.34	0	0
3694	Babyfood, Rice, Ppd w/ Whole Milk	28.35	3	Ounce	1.11	1.02	4.73	32.6	0	0	0	0
3210	Babyfood, Rice, w/ Mixed Fruit	28.35	3	Ounce	0.28	0.06	5.3	23.81	0	0.28	0	0
3050	Babyfood, Spaghetti and Tomato and Meat	28.35	3	Ounce	0.71	0.37	2.86	17.86	0	0.31	0	0
3103	Babyfood, Spinach, Creamed	28.35	3	Ounce	0.85	0.4	1.81	11.91	0	0.51	0	0
3058	Babyfood, Split Pea and Ham	28.35	3	Ounce	0.94	0.37	3.2	20.13	0	0.31	0	0
3105	Babyfood, Squash	28.35	3	Ounce	0.23	0.06	1.59	6.8	0	0.6	0	0
3109	Babyfood, Sweetpotatoes	28.35	3	Ounce	0.31	0.03	3.94	17.01	0	0.43	0	0
3216	Babyfood, Teething Biscuits	11	3	Biscuit	1.18	0.46	8.4	43.12	0	0.15	0	0
3238	Babyfood, Tropical Fruit	28.35	3	Ounce	0.06	0	4.65	17.01	0	0	0	0
3016	Babyfood, Turkey	28.35	3	Ounce	4.37	2.01	0	36.57	0	0	0	0.65
3083	Babyfood, Turkey and Rice	28.35	3	Ounce	0.51	0.4	2.04	13.89	0	0.31	0	0.12
3017	Babyfood, Turkey Sticks	10	3	Stick	1.37	1.42	0.14	18.2	0	0.05	0	0
19186	Apple Crisp	282	1	Cup	5.08	10.15	91.09	459.66	0	0	0	2.03
18001	Bagels, Blueberry	71	1	3½ In.	7.98	1.14	42.9	205.77	0	1.66	0	0.16
18005	Bagels, Cinnamon-raisin	71	1	3½ In.	6.96	1.21	39.19	194.54	0	0	0	0.19
18006	Bagels, Cinnamon-raisin, Toasted	66	1	3½ In.	7	1.19	39.14	194.04	0	0	0	0.19
18003	Bagels, Egg	71	1	3½ In.	7.53	1.49	37.63	197.38	0	0	17.04	0.3
18004	Bagels, Egg, Toasted	66	1	3½ In.	7.52	1.45	37.62	197.34	0	0	17.16	0.3
18007	Bagels, Oat Bran	71	1	3½ In.	7.6	0.85	37.84	181.05	0	0	0	0.14
18008	Bagels, Oat Bran, Toasted	66	1	3½ In.	7.59	0.86	37.82	180.84	0	0	0	0.14
18001	Bagels, Plain	71	1	3½ In.	7.46	1.14	37.91	195.25	0	1.49	0	0.16
18409	Bagels, Plain, Toasted	66	1	3½ In.	7.46	1.12	37.95	194.7	0	0	0	0.16
18009	Biscuits, Plain or Buttermilk	35	1	Each	2.17	5.78	16.98	127.4	0	0	0.35	0.87
18086	Cake, Angelfood	28.35	1	Slice	1.67	0.23	16.39	73.14	0	0.43	0	0.03
18090	Cake, Boston Cream Pie	92	1	Slice	2.21	7.82	39.47	231.84	0	1.2	34.04	2.33
18094	Cake, Carrot, w/ Cream Cheese Frosting	111	1	Slice	5.11	29.3	52.39	483.96	0	0	59.94	5.43
18096	Cake, Chocolate w/ Chocolate Frosting	64	1	Slice	2.62	10.5	34.94	234.88	0	1.79	29.44	2.97
18110	Cake, Fruitcake	43	1	Piece	1.25	3.91	26.49	139.32	0	1.51	2.15	0.48
18113	Cake, German Chocolate, w/ Frosting	111	1	Slice	3.89	20.65	55.17	404.04	0	0	53.28	5.26
18115	Cake, Gingerbread	67	1	Slice	2.68	6.83	33.97	207.03	0	2.14	23.45	1.74
18119	Cake, Pineapple Upside-down	115	1	Slice	4.03	13.92	58.08	366.85	0	0	25.3	3.35
18120	Cake, Pound	28.35	1	Slice	1.56	5.64	13.83	110	0	0	62.65	3.15
18133	Cake, Sponge	38	1	Slice	2.05	1.03	23.22	109.82	0	0	38.76	0.3
18102	Cake, White, w/ Coconut Frosting	112	1	Slice	4.93	11.54	70.78	398.72	0	0	1.12	4.36
18139	Cake, White, w/o Frosting	74	1	Slice	4	9.18	42.33	264.18	0	0	1.48	2.42
18140	Cake, Yellow, w/ Chocolate Frosting	64	1	Slice	2.43	11.14	35.46	242.56	0	1.15	35.2	3.02
18141	Cake, Yellow, w/ Vanilla Frosting	64	1	Slice	2.24	9.28	37.63	238.72	0	0	35.84	1.52
18147	Cheesecake, Commercially Prepared	85	1	Slice	4.68	19.13	21.68	272.85	0	1.79	46.75	9.79
18149	Cheesecake, Homemade	85	1	Slice	0.5	22.1	21.42	303.45	0	0	102.85	12.21
18148	Cheesecake, No-bake Type	80	1	Slice	4.4	10.16	28.4	219.2	0	1.52	33.6	5.64
18382	Cheesecake, Plain, w/ Cherry Topping	90	1	Slice	4.5	16.65	23.85	258.3	0	0	76.5	9.11
18444	Cherry Pie, Fast Food	128	1	Pie	3.84	20.61	54.53	404.48	0	0	0	3.09
18104	Coffeecake	63	1	Slice	4.28	14.68	29.42	263.34	0	2.08	20.16	3.63

Monounsaturated Fat (gm)	Polyunsaturated Fat (gm)	Vitamin D (mg)	Vitamin K (mg)	Vitamin E (mg)	Vitamin A (re)	Vitamin C (mg)	Thiamin (mg)	Riboflavin (mg)	Niacin (mg)	Vitamin B6 (mg)	Folate (mg)	Vitamin B12 (mcg)	Calcium (mg)	Iron (mg)	Magnesium (mg)	Phosphorus (mg)	Potassium (mg)	Sodium (mg)	Zinc (mg)
0	0	0	0	1.49	14.87	154.87	0.11	0.07	0.59	0.13	65.42	0	29.73	0.42	22.3	27.26	455.93	2.48	0.14
0	0	0	0	0.07	0.85	0.37	0.02	0.02	0.15	0	0.43	0.01	14.46	0.09	1.98	16.73	12.47	21.55	0.09
0	0	0	0	0.07	30.9	0.43	0.01	0.02	0.21	0.01	1.84	0.07	3.97	0.1	1.98	12.47	20.41	4.82	0.1
0.65	0.16	0	0	0.04	2.1	0.24	0.01	0.02	0.15	0.01	0.89	0.03	3.4	0.14	1.1	10.3	11.4	54.7	0.19
0	0	0	0	0	69.17	0.94	0	0.01	0.12	0.02	1.9	0	4.82	0.09	2.84	6.24	31.75	2.55	0.07
0	0	0	0	0.07	36.86	0.23	0.01	0.01	0.19	0.01	0.96	0.03	7.37	0.14	3.12	9.36	16.73	7.37	0.09
0	0	0	0	0.07	3.97	5.81	0	0	0.07	0	0.31	0	1.13	0.03	0.57	1.7	15.88	2.55	0.01
0	0	0	0	0	5.67	7.37	0	0.01	0.08	0	0.54	0	3.12	0.09	0.57	1.42	26.37	2.55	0.08
0	0	0	0	0.17	5.1	5.36	0	0.01	0.18	0.01	1.11	0	1.42	0.08	1.42	3.12	43.94	1.42	0.02
0	0	0	0	0.17	0.85	6.24	0	0.01	0.05	0	1.08	0	2.27	0.07	2.55	3.4	32.6	0.57	0.02
0	0	0	0	0	11.62	3.6	0.02	0.02	0.39	0	10.26	0	12.76	0.29	0	0	33.17	1.42	0
0	0	0	0	0.17	2.55	0.23	0	0.01	0.06	0.01	0.26	0	1.7	0.06	1.13	1.7	23.53	2.27	0.02
0	0	0	0	0	0	0	0.13	0.14	1.48	0.03	2.32	0.09	67.76	3.46	12.76	49.61	53.87	13.04	0.18
0	0	0	0	0.09	0.57	5.73	0.07	0.17	0.77	0.07	0.77	0.01	5.67	1.34	1.42	6.52	9.36	3.12	0.05
0	0	0	0	0.07	37.71	0.62	0.02	0.02	0.31	0.02	2.01	0	5.1	0.16	2.27	10.49	30.62	5.67	0.12
0	0	0	0	0.15	104.33	1.02	0.01	0.02	0.07	0.02	19.5	0.02	32.04	0.4	17.86	13.89	62.65	15.59	0.1
0	0	0	0	0.07	22.68	0.54	0.01	0.01	0.14	0.01	3.69	0	6.52	0.14	0	13.89	38.56	3.97	0.18
0	0	0	0	0.15	56.98	2.21	0	0.02	0.11	0.02	4.37	0	6.8	0.1	3.4	4.54	52.45	0.28	0.02
0	0	0	0	0.15	188.24	2.72	0.01	0.01	0.11	0.03	2.92	0	4.54	0.11	3.4	6.8	68.89	6.24	0.03
0	0	0	0	0.05	1.32	1	0.03	0.06	0.48	0.01	2.2	0.01	28.93	0.39	3.85	18.04	35.53	39.82	0.1
0	0	0	0	0	0.57	5.33	0	0.01	0.02	0.01	0.94	0	2.84	0.07	1.42	2.27	16.44	1.98	0.01
0.75	0.5	0	0	0.11	48.48	0.68	0	0.07	0.99	0.05	3.43	0.3	7.94	0.38	3.4	26.93	51.03	20.41	0.51
0.16	0.09	0	0	0.07	41.96	0.34	0	0.01	0.08	0.01	0.88	0.03	6.52	0.08	2.27	4.82	9.64	4.25	0.07
0	0	0	0	0.04	6.8	0.15	0	0.02	0.18	0.01	1.13	0.1	7.2	0.12	1.6	10.3	9.1	48.3	0.18
4.31	2.99	0	0	0	87.42	6.49	0.24	0.2	2.19	0.12	14.1	0	78.96	2.12	19.74	70.5	273.54	513.24	0.45
0.09	0.49	0	0	0	12.88	19.77	0.38	0.22	3.24	0.04	15.62	0	52.54	2.53	20.59	68.16	99.5	379.14	0.62
0.12	0.48	0	0	0	5.68	0.5	0.27	0.2	2.19	0.04	14.91	0	13.49	2.7	14.91	54.67	107.92	228.62	0.53
0.12	0.48	0	0	0	4.62	0.4	0.22	0.18	1.97	0.04	10.56	0	13.2	2.7	15.18	54.78	107.58	228.36	0.53
0.3	0.46	0	0	0	23.43	0.43	0.38	0.17	2.44	0.06	15.62	0.11	9.23	2.83	17.75	59.64	48.28	358.55	0.55
0.3	0.46	0	0	0	21.12	0.33	0.3	0.15	2.2	0.06	11.22	0.11	9.24	2.82	17.82	59.4	48.18	358.38	0.55
0.18	0.35	0	0	0	0	0.14	0.24	0.24	2.1	0.14	32.66	0	8.52	2.19	40.47	117.15	144.84	359.97	1.48
0.18	0.35	0	0	0	0	0.07	0.19	0.22	1.89	0.13	23.1	0	8.58	2.18	40.92	116.82	144.54	359.7	1.48
0.09	0.49	0	0	0	0	0	0.38	0.22	3.24	0.04	15.62	0	52.54	2.53	20.59	68.16	71.71	379.14	0.62
0.09	0.49	0	0	0	0	0	0.31	0.2	2.91	0.03	11.22	0	12.54	2.52	20.46	67.98	71.94	378.84	0.62
2.42	2.17	0	0	0	0.35	0	0.15	0.1	1.17	0.02	2.45	0.05	17.15	1.16	5.95	150.5	78.4	368.2	0.17
0.02	0.1	0	0	0	0	0	0.03	0.14	0.25	0.01	0.85	0	39.69	0.15	3.4	65.77	26.37	212.34	0.02
4.08	0.93	0	0	0	21.16	0.09	0.38	0.25	7.36	0.15	21.16	0.35	5.52	45.08	35.88	132.48	0.15		
7.24	15.1	0	0	0	426.24	1.22	0.15	0.17	1.13	0.08	13.32	0.11	27.75	1.39	19.98	78.81	124.32	273.06	0.54
5.76	1.22	0	0	0	17.92	0.06	0.02	0.09	0.37	0	5.12	0.08	27.52	1.41	21.76	78.08	128	213.76	0.44
1.79	1.39	0	0	0	8.17	0.17	0.02	0.04	0.34	0.02	1.29	0.03	14.19	0.89	6.88	22.36	65.79	116.1	0.12
8.71	5.46	0	0	0	23.31	0	0.11	0.14	1.1	0.02	4.44	0.1	53.28	1.22	18.87	173.16	150.96	368.52	0.49
3.75	0.9	0	0	0	10.72	0.07	0.13	0.12	1.05	0.03	6.7	0	46.23	2.22	10.72	112.56	161.47	306.86	0.27
5.97	3.77	0	0	0	74.75	1.38	0.18	0.18	1.37	0.04	8.05	0.09	138	1.7	14.95	94.3	128.8	366.85	0.36
1.58	0.31	0	0	0	44.23	0.03	0.04	0.06	0.37	0.01	3.12	0.05	9.92	0.39	3.12	38.84	33.74	112.83	0.13
0.36	0.17	0	0	0	17.48	0	0.09	0.1	0.73	0.02	4.94	0.09	26.6	1.03	4.18	52.06	37.62	92.72	0.19
4.14	2.42	0	0	0	12.32	0.11	0.14	0.21	1.19	0.03	5.6	0.07	100.8	1.3	13.44	78.4	110.88	318.08	0.37
3.93	2.33	0	0	0	11.84	0.15	0.14	0.18	1.13	0.02	5.18	0.06	96.2	1.12	8.88	68.82	70.3	241.98	0.24
6.19	1.34	0	0	0	17.28	0.06	0.08	0.1	0.8	0.02	5.12	0.08	23.68	1.33	19.2	103.04	113.92	215.68	0.4
3.91	3.28	0	0	0	12.16	0.13	0.06	0.04	0.32	0.02	5.76	0.13	39.68	0.68	3.84	91.52	33.92	220.16	0.16
6.58	1.17	0	0	0	136.85	0.51	0.02	0.16	0.17	0.04	12.75	0.14	43.35	0.54	9.35	79.05	76.5	175.95	0.43
6.87	1.75	0	0	0	272.85	0.34	0.03	0.18	0.34	0.04	10.2	0.21	49.3	1.06	6.8	81.6	86.7	240.55	0.47
3.12	0.52	0	0	0	79.2	0.4	0.1	0.21	0.39	0.04	14.4	0.25	137.6	0.38	15.2	187.2	168.8	304	0.37
5.21	1.38	0	0	0	216.9	0.63	0.03	0.14	0.32	0.04	9	0.15	38.7	1.11	6.3	63.9	83.7	182.7	0.36
9.53	6.92	0	0	0	21.76	1.66	0.18	0.14	1.82	0.04	3.84	0.1	28.16	1.56	12.8	55.04	83.2	478.72	0.29
8.31	1.8	0	0	0	18.27	0.19	0.13	0.14	1.06	0.02	20.16	0.07	34.02	1.2	13.86	68.04	77.49	221.13	0.51

USDA ID Code	Food Name	Weight in Grams*	Quantity of Units	Unit of Measure	Protein (gm)	Fat (gm)	Carbohydrates (gm)	Kcalories	Caffeine (gm)	Fiber (gm)	Cholesterol (mg)	Saturated Fat (gm)
18103	Coffeecake, Cheese	76	1	Slice	5.32	11.55	33.67	257.64	0	0.91	25.84	3.8
18106	Coffeecake, Fruit	50	1	Slice	2.6	5.1	25.75	155.5	0	1.25	11	1.22
18238	Cream Puffs, Shell, w/ Custard Filling	130	1	Each	8.71	20.15	29.77	335.4	0	0	174.2	4.78
18240	Croissant, Apple	57	1	Medium	4.22	4.96	21.15	144.78	0	1.43	28.5	2.53
18239	Croissant, Butter	57	1	Medium	4.67	11.97	26.11	231.42	0	1.6	42.75	6.68
18241	Croissant, Cheese	57	1	Medium	5.24	11.91	26.79	235.98	0	2.17	36.48	5.49
	Croissant, Chocolate	56	1	Medium	5.21	14.07	25.15	234.61	0	2.2	38	8.07
18245	Danish Pastry, Cheese	71	1	Each	5.68	15.55	26.41	265.54	0	0	31.95	4.94
18244	Danish Pastry, Cinnamon	65	1	Each	4.55	14.56	28.99	261.95	0	0.78	19.5	3.73
18246	Danish Pastry, Fruit,	71	1	Each	3.83	13.14	33.94	263.41	0	1.35	14.91	3.35
18433	Danish Pastry, Lemon	71	1	Each	3.83	13.14	33.94	263.41	0	0	0	3.35
18247	Danish Pastry, Nut	65	1	Each	4.62	16.38	29.71	279.5	0	1.5	29.9	3.54
18435	Danish Pastry, Raspberry	71	1	Each	3.83	13.14	33.94	263.41	0	0	0	3.35
18251	Doughnuts, Chocolate, Sugared or Glazed	42	1	Each	1.89	8.36	24.11	175.14	0	0.92	23.94	2.25
18253	Doughnuts, French Crullers, Glazed	41	1	Each	1.27	7.5	24.4	168.92	0	0	4.51	1.92
18255	Doughnuts, Glazed	60	1	Each	3.84	13.68	26.58	241.8	0	1.26	3.6	3.49
18248	Doughnuts, Plain	47	1	Each	2.35	10.76	23.36	197.87	0	0.8	17.39	1.76
18249	Doughnuts, Plain, Chocolate-coated or Frosted	43	1	Each	2.15	13.33	20.64	203.82	0	0.86	24.94	3.59
18250	Doughnuts, Plain, Sugared or Glazed	45	1	Each	2.34	10.31	22.86	191.7	0	0	14.4	2.4
18254	Doughnuts, w/ Creme Filling	85	1	Each	5.44	20.83	25.5	306.85	0	0	20.4	5.74
18256	Doughnuts, w/ Jelly Filling	85	1	Each	5.02	15.9	33.15	289	0	0	22.1	4.05
18252	Doughnuts, Whole Wheat, Sugared or Glazed	45	1	Each	2.84	8.69	19.17	162	0	0	9	1.39
18257	Eclairs, Custard-filled w/ Chocolate Glaze	62	1	Each	3.97	9.73	15	162.44	0	0	78.74	2.55
18319	Fruit Pie, Fried	128	1	Pie	3.84	20.61	54.53	404.48	0	3.33	0	3.09
18320	Lemon Meringue Pie	113	1	Slice	1.7	9.83	53.34	302.84	0	1.36	50.85	1.75
18445	Lemon Pie, Fried	128	1	Pie	3.84	20.61	54.53	404.48	0	0	0	3.09
	Muffins, Banana Nut	95	1	Each	6	12	53	340	0	2	35	0.9
18274	Muffins, Blueberry	65	1	Large	3.58	4.23	31.2	180.05	0	2.34	19.5	0.81
18279	Muffins, Corn	65	1	Large	3.84	5.46	33.09	198.25	0	0	33.15	0.98
18283	Muffins, Oat Bran	65	1	Large	4.55	4.81	31.4	175.5	0	4.88	0	0.58
18273	Muffins, Plain	65	1	Large	4.49	7.41	26.91	192.4	0	1.76	25.35	1.4
18287	Muffins, Wheat Bran	65	1	Large	4.62	7.93	27.24	183.95	0	0	21.45	1.47
18302	Pie, Apple	155	1	Slice	3.72	19.38	57.51	410.75	0	0	0	4.73
18304	Pie, Banana Cream	148	1	Slice	6.51	20.13	48.69	398.12	0	0	75.48	5.56
18305	Pie, Blueberry	125	1	Slice	2.25	12.5	43.63	290	0	0	0	2.35
18307	Pie, Butterscotch Pudding	127	1	Slice	5.97	18.16	42.29	354.33	0	0	77.47	5.09
18308	Pie, Cherry	125	1	Slice	2.5	13.75	49.75	325	0	1	0	2.5
18310	Pie, Chocolate Crème	113	1	Slice	2.94	21.92	37.97	343.52	0	2.26	5.65	5.96
18312	Pie, Chocolate Mousse	95	1	Slice	3.33	14.63	28.12	247	0	0	20.9	7.79
18313	Pie, Coconut Crème	64	1	Slice	1.34	10.62	23.81	190.72	0	0	0	4.81
18316	Pie, Coconut Custard	104	1	Slice	6.14	13.73	31.41	270.4	0	1.87	0	6
18317	Pie, Egg Custard	105	1	Slice	5.78	12.18	21.84	220.5	0	1.26	34.65	2.92
18322	Pie, Mince Meat	165	1	Slice	4.29	17.82	79.2	476.85	0	0	0	4.43
18324	Pie, Pecan	113	1	Slice	4.52	20.91	64.64	452	0	3.96	36.16	4.25
18326	Pie, Pumpkin	109	1	Slice	4.25	10.36	29.76	228.9	0	2.94	21.8	2.2
18328	Pie, Vanilla Crème	126	1	Slice	6.05	18.14	41.08	350.28	0	0	78.12	5.08
18354	Strudel, Apple	71	1	Each	2.34	7.95	29.18	194.54	0	1.56	19.88	2.08
18359	Sweet Rolls w/ Raisins and Nuts	57	1	Each	3.76	7.3	29.58	196.08	0	0	13.11	1.35
18355	Sweet Rolls, Cheese	66	1	Each	4.69	12.08	28.84	237.6	0	0	36.96	3.81
18356	Sweet Rolls, Cinnamon w/ Raisins	60	1	Each	3.72	9.84	30.54	223.2	0	0.78	39.6	2.53
14114	Beef Broth and Tomato Juice, Cnd	243.998	0.75	Cup	1.46	0.24	20.74	90.28	0	0	0	0.08
	Beer - Dark	29.5	12	Fl Oz	0.089	0	1.099	12.177	0	0.059	0	0
	Beer - Killians	29.5	12	Fl Oz	0.089	0	1.099	12.177	0	0.059	0	0
14006	Beer, Light	29.5	12	Fl Oz	0.059	0	0.383	8.26	0	0	0	0
14003	Beer, Regular	29.5	12	Fl Oz	0.089	0	1.099	12.177	0	0.059	0	0

Monounsaturated Fat (gm)	Polyunsaturated Fat (gm)	Vitamin D (mg)	Vitamin K (mg)	Vitamin E (mg)	Vitamin A (re)	Vitamin C (mg)	Thiamin (mg)	Riboflavin (mg)	Niacin (mg)	Vitamin B6 (mg)	Folate (mg)	Vitamin B12 (mcg)	Calcium (mg)	Iron (mg)	Magnesium (mg)	Phosphorus (mg)	Potassium (mg)	Sodium (mg)	Zinc (mg)
5.71	1.25	0	0	0	53.96	0.08	0.08	0.1	0.52	0.04	44.08	0.11	44.84	0.49	11.4	75.24	219.64	257.64	0.45
2.86	0.71	0	0	0	10	0.4	0.02	0.1	1.29	0.02	9.5	0.03	22.5	1.22	8.5	59	45	192.5	0.33
8.49	5.4	0	0	0	258.7	0.39	0.16	0.36	1.09	0.08	19.5	0.47	85.8	1.52	15.6	141.7	149.5	443.3	0.78
1.35	0.42	0	0	0	41.61	0.23	0.13	0.09	0.91	0.02	7.41	0.13	17.1	0.63	7.41	33.06	51.3	156.18	0.59
3.25	0.74	0	0	0	78.09	0.11	0.22	0.14	1.25	0.03	15.96	0.17	21.09	1.16	9.12	59.85	67.26	424.08	0.43
3.74	1.55	0	0	0	89.49	0.11	0.3	0.19	1.23	0.04	18.81	0.18	30.21	1.23	13.68	87re	75.24	316.35	0.54
3.31	0.89	0	0	0	76.41	0.11	0.22	0.15	1.22	0.02	16.11	0.16	23.89	1.18	10.89	63.2	69.69	376.34	0.43
7.84	1.73	0	0	0	44.02	0.07	0.13	0.18	1.42	0.04	17.75	0.17	24.85	1.14	10.65	76.68	69.58	319.5	0.56
8.1	1.86	0	0	0	7.15	0.13	0.2	0.17	1.86	0.03	21.45	0.11	46.15	1.27	12.35	69.55	81.25	241.15	0.47
7.32	1.7	0	0	0	11.36	2.77	0.19	0.16	1.41	0	11.36	0.06	32.66	1.26	10.65	63.19	58.93	251.34	0.38
7.32	1.7	0	0	0	37.63	2.77	0.05	0.07	0.55	0	11.36	0	32.66	0.53	10.65	63.19	58.93	251.34	0.38
8.19	3.74	0	0	0	9.1	1.11	0.14	0.16	1.5	0.06	17.55	0.11	61.1	1.17	20.8	71.5	61.75	235.95	0.57
7.32	1.7	0	0	0	42.6	2.77	0.05	0.07	0.55	0	11.36	0	32.66	0.53	10.65	63.19	58.93	251.34	0.38
4.61	1.03	0	0	0	10.92	0.04	0.02	0.03	0.2	0.02	7.14	0.07	89.46	0.95	14.28	68.04	49.56	142.8	0.24
4.28	0.94	0	0	0	0	0.04	0.07	0.09	0.63	0.01	3.28	0.03	10.66	0.63	4.92	50.43	31.98	141.45	0.11
7.74	1.72	0	0	0	0	0	0.22	0.13	1.71	0.03	13.2	0.05	25.8	1.22	13.2	55.8	64.8	205.2	0.46
4.53	3.83	0	0	0	7.99	0.09	0.1	0.11	0.87	0.03	3.76	0.11	20.68	0.92	9.4	126.43	59.69	256.62	0.26
7.39	1.61	0	0	0	13.33	0.04	0.05	0.05	0.56	0.02	7.31	0.16	15.05	1.06	17.2	86.86	49.02	184.47	0.26
5.38	1.17	0	0	0	1.35	0.05	0.1	0.09	0.68	0.01	5.4	0.09	27	0.48	7.65	52.65	45.9	180.9	0.2
11.46	2.53	0	0	0	6.8	0	0.29	0.13	1.91	0.02	11.9	0.08	21.25	1.56	17	64.6	68	262.65	0.68
8.98	1.99	0	0	0	6.8	1.02	0.27	0.12	1.82	0.02	14.45	0.05	21.25	1.5	17	72.25	67.15	249.05	0.64
3.6	3.11	0	0	0	8.55	0.09	0.1	0.11	0.83	0.03	6.75	0.1	22.05	0.5	9.9	46.8	66.6	159.75	0.31
4.02	2.45	0	0	0	118.42	0.19	0.07	0.16	0.5	0.04	8.68	0.21	39.06	0.73	9.3	66.34	72.54	208.94	0.38
9.53	6.92	0	0	0	3.84	1.66	0.18	0.14	1.82	0.04	3.84	0.1	28.16	1.56	12.8	55.04	83.2	478.72	0.29
4.1	3.27	0	0	0	58.76	3.62	0.07	0.24	0.73	0.03	9.04	0.17	63.28	0.69	16.95	118.65	100.57	164.98	0.55
9.53	6.92	0	0	0	3.84	0	0.18	0.14	1.82	0.04	3.84	0.1	28.16	1.56	12.8	55.04	83.2	478.72	0.29
1.5	2.4	0	0	0	21	0.033	0.18	0.12	0.035	0.01	13.2	0	44	1.01	16.1	108.2	371		0.2
1.59	1.32	0	0	0	0	0.72	0.09	0.08	0.72	0.01	10.4	0.38	37.05	1.05	10.4	128.05	79.95	290.55	0.32
2.17	1.84	0	0	0	23.4	0.07	0.18	0.21	1.32	0.05	22.1	0.12	48.1	1.83	24.05	184.6	44.85	338.65	0.47
0.92	2.96	0	0	0	0	0.33	0.17	0.06	0.27	0.1	11.7	0	40.95	2.73	102.05	244.4	329.55	255.45	1.2
1.79	3.72	0	0	0	26	0.2	0.18	0.2	1.5	0.03	8.45	0.1	130	1.55	11.05	99.45	78.65	303.55	0.36
1.91	4.09	0	0	0	162.5	5.07	0.22	0.29	2.62	0.21	33.8	0.09	121.55	2.72	50.7	185.25	206.7	382	1.79
8.36	5.17	0	0	0	18.6	2.64	0.23	0.17	1.91	0.05	6.2	0	10.85	1.74	10.85	43.4	122.45	327.05	0.29
8.46	4.87	0	0	0	103.6	2.37	0.21	0.31	1.56	0.2	16.28	0.37	111	1.54	23.68	136.16	244.2	355.2	0.71
6.69	2.43	0	0	0	42.5	3.38	0.01	0.04	0.38	0.05	5	0	10	0.38	6.25	26.25	62.5	406.25	0.2
7.64	4.35	0	0	0	106.68	0.64	0.18	0.27	1.26	0.07	13.97	0.38	128.27	1.64	21.59	134.62	220.98	335.28	0.69
7.49	2.5	0	0	0	0	0.88	0.03	0.04	0.25	0.05	10	0	15	0.6	10	36.25	101.25	307.5	0.23
12.34	2.59	0	0	0	0	0.34	0.04	0.12	0.77	0.02	7.91	0.05	40.68	1.21	23.73	76.84	143.51	153.68	0.26
4.83	0.77	0	0	0	95.95	0.48	0.05	0.14	0.57	0.03	2.85	0.2	73.15	1.03	30.4	219.45	270.75	437	0.57
4.33	0.94	0	0	0	12.8	0	0.03	0.05	0.13	0.04	3.2	0	18.56	0.51	12.8	54.4	54.4	163.2	0.41
5.79	1.24	0	0	0	28.08	0.31	0.09	0.15	0.42	0.01	4.16	0.09	84.24	0.83	18.72	126.88	182	348.4	0.71
6.05	2.02	0	0	0	52.5	0.32	0.04	0.22	0.31	0.05	21	0.45	84	0.61	11.55	117.6	111.3	252	0.55
7.68	4.69	0	0	0	3.3	9.74	0.25	0.17	1.96	0.11	8.25	0	36.3	2.46	23.1	69.3	334.95	419.1	0.36
12.14	3.35	0	0	0	53.11	1.24	0.1	0.14	0.28	0.02	6.78	0.09	39.21	1.18	20.34	87.01	83.62	479.12	0.64
5.46	1.75	0	0	0	523.2	1.64	0.06	0.17	0.2	0.06	16.35	0.43	65.4	0.86	16.35	77.39	167.86	307.38	0.49
7.61	4.33	0	0	0	107.1	0.63	0.18	0.27	1.24	0.06	13.86	0.38	113.4	1.29	16.38	131.04	158.76	327.6	0.67
4.38	1.01	0	0	0	6.39	1.21	0.03	0.02	0.23	0.03	4.26	0.11	10.65	0.3	6.39	23.43	68.87	190.99	0.13
2.66	2.85	0	0	0	60.42	0.34	0.16	0.16	1.33	0.05	17.67	0.06	36.48	1.46	15.96	62.7	123.12	185.25	0.38
6.13	1.36	0	0	0	40.92	0.13	0.1	0.09	0.55	0.04	20.46	0.11	77.88	0.5	12.54	64.68	87.12	235.62	0.42
5.46	1.27	0	0	0	38.4	1.2	0.19	0.16	1.43	0.06	14.4	0.07	43.2	0.96	10.2	45.6	66.6	229.8	0.35
0.07	0.05	0	0	0	31.72	2.2	0	0.07	0.4	0.06	10.49	0.12	26.84	1.42	7.32	31.72	234.24	319.64	0.05
0	0	0	0	0	0	0	0.002	0.008	0.135	0.015	1.782	0.006	1.485	0.009	1.782	3.564	7.425	1.485	0.006
0	0	0	0	0	0	0	0.002	0.008	0.135	0.015	1.782	0.006	1.485	0.009	1.782	3.564	7.425	1.485	0.006
0	0	0	0	0	0	0	0.003	0.009	0.116	0.015	1.209	0.003	1.475	0.012	1.475	3.54	5.31	0.885	0.009
0	0	0	0	0	0	0	0.002	0.008	0.135	0.015	1.782	0.006	1.485	0.009	1.782	3.564	7.425	1.485	0.006

USDA ID Code	Food Name	Weight in Grams*	Quantity of Units	Unit of Measure	Protein (gm)	Fat (gm)	Carbohydrates (gm)	Kcalories	Caffeine (gm)	Fiber (gm)	Cholesterol (mg)	Saturated Fat (gm)
14008	Bloody Mary	29.7	1	Fl Oz	0.15	0.03	0.98	23.17	0	0	0	0
14413	Bourbon and Soda	29	1	Fl Oz	0	0	0	26.1	0	0	0	0
14187	Clam and Tomato Juice, Cnd	241.396	0.75	Cup	1.45	0.24	26.31	111.04	0	0	0	0.02
14121	Club Soda	355.2	12	Fl Oz	0	0	0	0	0	0	0	0
14209	Coffee, Brewed	29.6	6	Fl Oz	0.03	0	0.12	0.59	17.1	0	0	0
62685	Coffee, Brewed, Decaf.	29.6	6	Fl Oz	0.03	0	0.12	0.59	0.18	0	0	0
14418	Coffee, Instant, Cappuccino Flavor	29.3	6	Fl Oz	0.06	0.32	1.64	9.38	12.16	0	0	0.28
14219	Coffee, Instant, Decaffeinated	29.858	6	Fl Oz	0.03	0	0.12	0.6	0.3	0	0	0
14420	Coffee, Instant, Mocha Flavor	29.3	6	Fl Oz	0.09	0.29	1.32	7.91	6.83	0	0	0.25
14215	Coffee, Instant, Regular	29.858	6	Fl Oz	0.03	0	0.12	0.6	9.5	0	0	0
14400	Cola	369	12	Fl Oz	0.1	0.1	38.5	151	7.6	0	0	0
62530	Cola, Diet	369	12	Fl Oz	0.2	0	0.3	2	7.6	0	0	0
14238	Cranberry-apple Juice Drink, Bottled	244.593	0.75	Cup	0.24	0	41.83	163.88	0	0.24	0	0
14240	Cranberry-apricot Juice Drink, Bottled	244.593	0.75	Cup	0.49	0	39.62	156.54	0	0.24	0	0
14241	Cranberry-grape Juice Drink, Bottled	244.593	0.75	Cup	0.49	0.24	34.24	136.97	0	0.24	0	0.08
14130	Cream Soda	371	12	Fl Oz	0	0	49.3	191	0	0	0	0
14034	Creme De Menthe, 72 Proof	33.6	1	Fl Oz	0	0.1	13.98	124.66	0	0	0	0
62635	Crystal Lite	29.575	8	Fl Oz	0	0	0	0.63	0	0	0	0
14010	Daiquiri	30.2	1	Fl Oz	0.03	0.03	2.05	56.17	0	0	0	0
14009	Daiquiri, Bottled	30.5	1	Fl Oz	0	0	4.79	38.13	0	0	0	0
14153	Dr. Pepper	360	12	Fl Oz	0	0.4	38.2	151	41	0	0	0.02
14267	Fruit Punch Drink, Cnd	247.791	0.75	Cup	0	0	29.49	116.46	0	0.25	0	0
	Gatorade Thirst Quencher	244	8	Fl Oz	0	0	14	50	0	0	0	0
	Gatorlode High Carb, Loading Recovery Drink	354	11.6	Fl Oz	0	0	71	280	0	0	0	0
	Gatorpro Sports Nutrition Sup.	336	11	Fl Oz	17	6	59	360	0	0	0	0.5
14011	Gin and Tonic	30	1	Fl Oz	0	0	2.1	22.8	0	0	0	0
14136	Ginger Ale	366	12	Fl Oz	0.1	0	31.9	124	0	0	0	0
62532	Ginger Ale, Diet	366	12	Fl Oz	0	0	0	0	0	0	0	0
14277	Grape Drink, Cnd	250.189	0.75	Cup	0	0	28.77	112.58	0	0	0	0.01
14282	Grape Juice Drink, Cnd	250.189	0.75	Cup	0.25	0	32.27	125.09	0	0.25	0	0
14142	Grape Soda	372	12	Fl Oz	0	0	41.7	161	0	0	0	0
62547	Iced Tea, Bottled, All Flavors	236.6	1	Cup	0	0	28.59	118.3	44	0	0	0
62548	Iced Tea, Bottled, All Flavors, Diet	236.6	1	Cup	0	0	0.99	0	54	0	0	0
62643	Kool-Aid	236	8	Fl Oz	0	0	25.1	98	0	0	0	0
14297	Lemonade Flavor Drink	266	1	Cup	0	0	28.73	111.72	0	0	0	0.05
14543	Lemonade, Pink	247.791	1	Cup	0.25	0	26.02	99.12	0	0	0	0.01
14290	Lemonade, Low Calorie	243.698	1	Cup	0	0	1.22	4.87	0	0	0	0
14293	Lemonade, White	247.791	1	Cup	0.25	0	26.02	99.12	0	0	0	0.01
14145	Lemon-lime Soda	355	12	Fl Oz	0	0	38.4	149	0	0	0	0
62529	Lemon-lime Soda, Diet	355	12	Fl Oz	0	0	0	0	0	0	0	0
14415	Liqueur, Coffee w/ Cream, 34 Proof	31.1	1	Fl Oz	0.87	4.88	6.5	101.7	0	0	4.67	3.01
14414	Liqueur, Coffee, 53 Proof	34.8	1	Fl Oz	0.03	0.1	16.29	116.93	0	0	0	0.04
14534	Liqueur, Coffee, 63 Proof	34.8	1	Fl Oz	0.03	0.1	11.21	107.18	0	0	0	0.04
14533	Liquor, Distilled, All 100 Proof	27.8	1	Fl Oz	0	0	0	82.01	0	0	0	0
14037	Liquor, Distilled, All 80 Proof	27.8	1	Fl Oz	0	0	0	64.22	0	0	0	0
14550	Liquor, Distilled, All 86 Proof	27.8	1	Fl Oz	0	0	0.03	69.5	0	0	0	0
14551	Liquor, Distilled, All 90 Proof	27.8	1	Fl Oz	0	0	0	73.11	0	0	0	0
14532	Liquor, Distilled, All 94 Proof	27.8	1	Fl Oz	0	0	0	76.45	0	0	0	0
14012	Manhattan	28.5	6	Fl Oz	0.03	0	0.91	63.84	0	0	0	0
62645	Margarita	29.575	6	Fl Oz	0	0	4.5	28.75	0	0	0	0
14014	Martini	28.2	6	Fl Oz	0	0	0.08	62.89	0	0	0	0
1110	Milk Shakes, Thick Chocolate	345.436	1.5	Cup	10.54	9.33	73.06	409.71	0	1.04	36.27	5.81
1111	Milk Shakes, Thick Vanilla	345.436	1.5	Cup	13.33	10.47	61.31	386.23	0	0	40.76	6.51
62659	Mountain Dew	360	12	Fl Oz	0	0	44.4	179	54	0	0	0
14327	Orange and Apricot Juice Drink, Cnd	249.389	0.75	Cup	0.75	0.25	31.67	127.19	0	0.25	0	0.02

Monounsaturated Fat (gm)	Polyunsaturated Fat (gm)	Vitamin D (mg)	Vitamin K (mg)	Vitamin E (mg)	Vitamin A (re)	Vitamin C (mg)	Thiamin (mg)	Riboflavin (mg)	Niacin (mg)	Vitamin B6 (mg)	Folate (mcg)	Vitamin B12 (mcg)	Calcium (mg)	Iron (mg)	Magnesium (mg)	Phosphorus (mg)	Potassium (mg)	Sodium (mg)	Zinc (mg)
0	0.01	0	0	0	10.1	4.1	0.01	0.01	0.13	0.02	3.95	0	2.08	0.11	2.38	4.16	43.36	66.53	0.03
0	0	0	0	0	0	0	0	0	0.01	0	0	0	0.87	0.01	0.29	0.58	0.58	4.06	0.02
0.02	0.05	0	0	0	53.11	9.9	0.1	0.07	0.46	0.2	38.38	73.87	28.97	1.45	53.11	188.29	217.26	965.58	2.61
0	0	0	0	0	0	0	0	0	0	0	0	0	1.48	0	0.3	0	0.59	6.22	0.03
0	0	0	0	0	0	0	0	0	0.07	0	0.03	0	0.59	0.01	1.48	0.3	15.98	0.59	0.01
0	0	0	0	0	0	0	0	0	0.07	0	0.03	0	0.59	0.01	1.48	0.3	15.98	0.59	0.01
0.02	0.01	0	0	0	0	0	0	0	0.05	0	0	0	1.17	0.02	1.47	4.1	18.17	15.82	0.01
0	0	0	0	0	0	0	0	0	0.08	0	0	0	0.9	0.01	1.19	0.9	10.45	0.9	0.01
0.02	0.01	0	0	0	0	0	0	0	0.04	0	0	0	1.17	0.04	1.47	4.4	18.46	5.57	0.02
0	0	0	0	0	0	0	0	0	0.08	0	0	0	0.9	0.01	1.19	0.9	10.75	0.9	0.01
0	0	0	0	0	0	0	0	0	0	0	0	0	0	0.13	3	46	4	14	0.05
0	0	0	0	0	0	0	0	0	0	0	0	0	0	0.11	4	30	0	21	0.28
0	0	0	0	0	0	78.27	0.01	0.05	0.15	0.05	0.49	0	17.12	0.15	4.89	7.34	66.04	4.89	0.1
0	0	0	0	0	112.51	0	0.01	0.02	0.29	0.05	1.47	0	22.01	0.37	7.34	12.23	149.2	4.89	0.1
0	0	0	0	0	0	78.27	0.02	0.04	0.29	0.07	1.71	0	19.57	0.02	7.34	9.78	58.7	7.34	0.1
0	0	0	0	0	0	0	0	0	0	0	0	0	19	0.19	3	0	4	43	0.24
0.01	0.06	0	0	0	0	0	0	0	0	0	0	0	0	0.02	0	0	0	1.68	0.01
0	0	0	0	0	0	0.75	0	0	0	0	0	0	0	0	0	0	0	0	0
0	0	0	0	0	0	0.48	0	0	0.01	0	0.6	0	0.91	0.05	0.6	1.81	6.34	1.51	0.02
0	0	0	0	0	0	0.4	0	0	0	0	0.24	0	0	0	0.31	0.61	3.36	12.2	0.01
0	0	0	0	0	0	0	0	0	0	0	0	0	0.92	0.01	0	3.38	0.31	3.07	0.01
0	0.01	0	0	0	2.48	73.35	0.05	0.06	0.05	0	3.22	0	19.82	0.52	4.96	2.48	61.95	54.51	0.3
0	0	0	0	0	0	0	0	0	0	0	0	0	0	0	0	0	30	110	0
0	0	2	0	3.5	160	50	1.1	0.5	6	0.64	63	0.8	280	3	70	400	1310	300	3.6
0	0	0	0	0	0	0.12	0	0	0	0	0.15	0	0.6	0.01	0.3	0.3	1.5	1.2	0.02
0	0	0	0	0	0	0	0	0	0	0	0	0	12	0.66	3	1	5	25	0.18
0	0	0	0	0	0	0	0	0	0	0	0	0	0	0	0	0	0	2.5	0
0	0.01	0	0	0	0	85.31	0.01	0.01	0.07	0.02	0.75	0	7.51	0.43	5	2.5	12.51	15.01	0.28
0	0	0	0	0	0	40.03	0.03	0.03	0.25	0.05	2	0	7.51	0.25	10.01	10.01	87.57	2.5	0.08
0	0	0	0	0	0	0	0	0	0	0	0	0	12	0.31	4	0	3	57	0.26
0	0	0	0	0	0	0	0	0	0	0	0	0	0	0	0	0	0	9.86	0
0	0	0	0	0	0	6	0	0	0	0	0	0	15	0	0	8	1	8	0
0.01	0.01	0	0	0	0	34.05	0	0	0	0	0	0	29.26	0.05	2.66	2.66	2.66	18.62	0.08
0	0.03	0	0.07	0	0	9.66	0.01	0.05	0.04	0.01	5.45	0	7.43	0.4	4.96	4.96	37.17	7.43	0.1
0	0	0	0	0	0	6.09	0	0	0	0	0.24	0	5.12	0.1	2.44	24.37	0	7.31	0.07
0	0.03	0	0	0	4.96	9.66	0.01	0.05	0.04	0.01	5.45	0	7.43	0.4	4.96	4.96	37.17	7.43	0.1
0	0	0	0	0	0	0	0	0	0.1	0	0	0	9	0.25	2	1	4	41	0.18
1.39	0.21	0	0	0	13.37	0	0	0.02	0.02	0.01	0	0.04	4.98	0.04	0.62	15.55	9.95	28.61	0.05
0.01	0.04	0	0	0	0	0	0	0	0.05	0	0	0	0.35	0.02	1.04	2.09	10.44	2.78	0.01
0.01	0.04	0	0	0	0	0	0	0	0.05	0	0	0	0.35	0.02	1.04	2.09	10.44	2.78	0.01
0	0	0	0	0	0	0	0	0	0	0	0	0	0	0.01	0	1.11	0.56	0.28	0.01
0	0	0	0	0	0	0	0	0	0	0	0	0	0	0.01	0	1.11	0.56	0.28	0.01
0	0	0	0	0	0	0	0	0	0	0	0	0	0	0.01	0	1.11	0.56	0.28	0.01
0	0	0	0	0	0	0	0	0	0	0	0	0	0	0.01	0	1.11	0.56	0.28	0.01
0	0	0	0	0	0	0	0	0	0	0	0	0	0	0.01	0	1.11	0.56	0.28	0.01
0	0	0	0	0	0	0	0	0	0.03	0	0.03	0	0.57	0.03	0.57	2	7.41	0.85	0.01
0	0	0	0	0	0	0	0	0	0	0	0	0	0	0	0	0	0	11.88	0
0	0	0	0	0	0	0	0	0	0	0	0.06	0	0.56	0.03	0.56	0.85	5.08	0.85	0.01
2.69	0.35	0	0	0.35	72.54	0	0.16	0.77	0.43	0.09	16.93	1.09	455.98	200	55.27	435.25	773.78	383.43	1.66
3.02	0.39	0	0	0.35	96.72	0	0.1	0.67	0.5	0.15	22.8	1.8	504.68	300	40.62	397.94	631.11	329.55	1.35
0.08	0.05	0	0	0	144.65	49.88	0.05	0.02	0.5	0.07	14.46	0	12.47	0.25	9.98	19.95	199.51	4.99	0.12

USDA ID Code	Food Name	Weight in Grams*	Quantity of Units	Unit of Measure	Protein (gm)	Fat (gm)	Carbohydrates (gm)	Kcalories	Caffeine (gm)	Fiber (gm)	Cholesterol (mg)	Saturated Fat (gm)
14323	Orange Drink, Cnd	247.791	0.75	Cup	0	0	31.96	126.37	0	0.25	0	0
14017	Pina Colada	31.4	6	Fl Oz	0.13	0.6	8.89	77.26	0	0	0	0.27
14334	Pineapple and Grapefruit Juice Drink, Cnd	250.189	0.75	Cup	0.5	0.25	29.02	117.59	0	0.25	0	0.02
14341	Pineapple and Orange Juice Drink, Cnd	250.189	0.75	Cup	3.25	0	29.52	125.09	0	0.25	0	0
14157	Root Beer	355	12	Fl Oz	0.1	0	39.2	152	0	0	0	0
62531	Root Beer, Diet	355	12	Fl Oz	0	0	0.355	0	0	0	0	0
14018	Screwdriver	30.4	6	Fl Oz	0.15	0	2.61	24.93	0	0	0	0
14346	Shake, Chocolate	226.4	1.5	Cup	7.7	8.38	46.41	287.53	0	0	29.43	5.24
14428	Shake, Strawberry	226.4	1.5	Cup	7.7	6.34	42.79	255.83	0	0	24.9	3.93
14347	Shake, Vanilla	226.4	1.5	Cup	7.92	6.79	40.53	251.3	0	0	24.9	4.21
14351	Strawberry Flavor Beverage	266	1	Cup	7.98	8.25	32.72	234.08	0	0	31.92	5.08
	Swiss Miss Hot Choc Mix - No Sugar	20	1	Packet	3	1.5	13	70	4	0	0	0
	Swiss Miss Hot Choc Mix - No Sugar, Fat Free	15	1	Packet	4	0	9	50	4	0	0	0
14355	Tea, Brewed	236	8	Fl Oz	0	0	0.09	0.3	48	0	0	0
14381	Tea, Herb, Brewed	236	8	Fl Oz	0	0	0.06	0.3	0	0	0	0
14371	Tea, Instant, Sweetened	236	8	Fl Oz	0.03	0	2.75	11.01	29	0	0	0
14367	Tea, Instant, Unsweetened	236	8	Fl Oz	0	0	0.06	0.3	36	0	0	0
14020	Tequila Sunrise	31.2	6	Fl Oz	0.09	0.03	2.68	34.32	0	0	0	0
14382	Thirst Quencher Drink, Bottled	236	8	Fl Oz	0	0.1	15.2	60	0	0	0	0
14023	Tom Collins	29.6	1	Fl Oz	0	0	0.38	16.28	0	0	0	0
14155	Tonic Water	29.6	12	Fl Oz	0	0	2.68	10.37	0	0	0	0
14269	Tropical Fruit Juice, Blend	246.99	0.75	Cup	0	0	28.9	113.62	0	0	0	0
	Vodka, 80 Proof	42	1.5	Fl Oz	0	0	0	97.02	0	0	0	0
	Water, Bottled, Perrier	192	6.5	Fl Oz	0	0	0	0	0	0	0	0
	Water, Municipal	240	8	Fl Oz	0	0	0	0	0	0	0	0
14032	Whiskey Sour	29.9	1	Fl Oz	0.06	0.03	1.67	40.66	0	0	0	0.01
14536	Wine, Dessert, Dry, 3.5 Oz Glass	103	1	Glass	0.206	0	12.154	157.59	0	0	0	0
14057	Wine, Dessert, Sweet, 3.5 Oz Glass	103	1	Glass	0.206	0	12.154	157.59	0	0	0	0
14084	Wine, Table, All, 3.5 Oz Glass	103	1	Glass	0.206	0	1.442	72.1	0	0	0	0
14096	Wine, Table, Red, 3.5 Oz Glass	103	1	Glass	0.206	0	1.751	74.16	0	0	0	0
14104	Wine, Table, Rose, 3.5 Oz Glass	103	1	Glass	0.206	0	1.442	73.13	0	0	0	0
14106	Wine, Table, White, 3.5 Oz Glass	103	1	Glass	0.103	0	0.824	70.04	0	0	0	0
8053	Cereals, 100% Bran	66	1	Cup	8.25	3.3	48.11	177.54	0	19.54	0	0.59
8054	Cereals, 100% Natural Cereal, Plain	104	1	Cup	12.17	22.36	65.21	488.8	0	8.84	0.66	15.05
8055	Cereals, 100% Natural Cereal, w/ apple and cinn.	104	1	Cup	10.71	19.55	69.78	477.36	0	6.86	0	15.46
	Cereals, 100% Natural Cereal, w/ oats and honey	48	0.5	Cup	5.054	7.896	32.947	213.12	0	3.6	0.48	3.466
8056	Cereals, 100% Natural Cereal, w/ raisins and dates	110	1	Cup	11.22	20.35	72.38	496.1	0	7.26	0	13.68
8028	Cereals, 40% Bran Flakes, Kellogg's	39	1	Cup	4.91	0.74	30.54	127.14	0	5.5	0	0
8029	Cereals, 40% Bran Flakes, Post	47	1	Cup	5.31	0.75	37.27	152.28	0	9.17	0	0
8153	Cereals, 40% Bran Flakes, Ralston Purina	49	1	Cup	5.64	0.69	39.1	158.76	0	6.91	0	0
8001	Cereals, All-bran	30	0.5	Cup	3.861	1.02	22.01	81.3	0	9.72	0	0.21
	Cereals, Almond Crunch	55	1	Cup	4.35	0.83	46.915	198	0	4.62	0	0.165
	Cereals, Alpha-Bits	34	1	Cup	2.584	0.782	29.444	133.28	0	1.462	0	0.128
62668	Cereals, Apple Cinnamon Cheerios	30	0.75	Cup	1.86	1.632	25.05	117.9	0	1.59	0	0.3
	Cereals, Apple Jacks	30	1	Cup	1.44	0.39	26.84	115.5	0	0.57	0	0.09
	Cereals, Apple Raisin Crisp	55	1	Cup	3.465	0.495	46.695	184.8	0	4.4	0	0.11
	Cereals, Basic 4	55	1	Cup	4.18	2.838	41.97	200.75	0	3.355	0	0.424
	Cereals, Berry Berry Kix	30	0.75	Cup	1.308	1.161	26.13	120	0	0.18	0	0.195
	Cereals, Blueberry Squares	55	0.75	Cup	4.18	0.99	43.78	181.5	0	4.84	0	0.22
8006	Cereals, Bran Chex	49	1	Cup	5.05	1.37	39.05	156.31	0	7.94	0	0.198
	Cereals, Bran Flakes, Kellogg's	29	0.75	Cup	3.016	0.638	23.159	94.83	0	4.611	0	0.116
	Cereals, Bran Flakes, Post	47	1	Cup	5.311	0.752	37.27	152.28	0	9.165	0	0.117
8008	Cereals, C.W. Post, Plain	97	1	Cup	7.95	12.804	72.653	420.98	0	7.18	0.18	1.668
8009	Cereals, C.W. Post, w/ Raisins	103	1	Cup	8.86	14.73	73.95	445.99	0	13.6	0.2	10.97
8010	Cereals, Cap'n Crunch	27	0.75	Cup	1.35	0.37	23.04	107.19	0	0.864	0	0.37

Monounsaturated Fat (gm)	Polyunsaturated Fat (gm)	Vitamin D (mg)	Vitamin K (mg)	Vitamin E (mg)	Vitamin A (re)	Vitamin C (mg)	Thiamin (mg)	Riboflavin (mg)	Niacin (mg)	Vitamin B6 (mg)	Folate (mg)	Vitamin B12 (mcg)	Calcium (mg)	Iron (mg)	Magnesium (mg)	Phosphorus (mg)	Potassium (mg)	Sodium (mg)	Zinc (mg)
0	0.01	0	0	0	4.96	84.5	0.01	0.01	0.08	0.02	5.45	0	14.87	0.69	4.96	2.48	44.6	39.65	0.22
0.05	0.11	0	0	0	0	1.48	0.01	0	0.04	0.01	3.2	0	2.51	0.07	2.51	2.2	22.29	1.88	0.04
0.03	0.07	0	0	0	10.01	115.09	0.08	0.04	0.67	0.11	26.27	0	17.51	0.78	15.01	15.01	152.61	35.03	0.15
0	0	0	0	0	132.6	56.29	0.08	0.05	0.52	0.12	27.27	0	12.51	0.68	15.01	10.01	115.09	7.51	0.15
0	0	0	0	0	0	0	0	0	0	0	0	0	19	0.18	4	2	3	49	0.26
0	0	0	0	0	0	0	0	0	0	0	0	0	0	0	0	0	0	2.5	0
0	0	0	0	0	1.82	9.48	0.02	0	0.05	0.01	10.67	0	2.13	0.02	2.43	4.26	46.51	0.3	0.01
2.43	0.32	0.91	0	0	52.07	0.91	0.13	0.55	0.36	0.11	7.92	0.77	255.83	0.7	38.49	230.93	452.8	219.61	0.93
0	0	0.45	0	0	65.66	1.81	0.1	0.44	0.4	0.1	6.79	0.7	255.83	0.25	29.43	226.4	412.05	187.91	0.82
1.95	0.25	0.45	0	0	72.45	1.81	0.1	0.41	0.42	0.12	7.47	0.82	276.21	0.2	27.17	230.93	393.94	185.65	0.82
2.36	0.3	0	0	0	74.48	2.39	0.09	0.42	0.22	0.1	12.24	0.88	292.6	0.21	31.92	228.76	369.74	127.68	0.93
0	0	0	0	0	0	0	0	0	0	0	0	0	80	0.4	0	0	0	220	0
0	0	0	0	0	0	0	0	0	0	0	0	0	80	0.2	0	0	0	180	0
0	0	0	0.01	0	0	0	0	0	0	0	1.54	0	0	0.01	0.89	0.3	10.95	0.89	0.01
0	0	0	0	0	0	0	0	0	0	0	0.18	0	0.59	0.02	0.3	0	2.66	0.3	0.01
0	0	0	0	0	0	0	0	0.01	0.01	0	1.2	0	0.65	0.01	0.65	0.32	6.15	0.97	0.01
0	0	0	0	0	0	0	0	0	0.01	0	0.09	0	0.59	0.01	0.59	0.3	5.92	0.89	0.01
0.01	0.01	0	0	0	3.12	6.02	0.01	0	0.06	0.02	3.31	0	1.87	0.09	2.18	3.12	32.45	1.25	0.02
0	0	0	0	0	0	0	0	0	0	0	0	0	0	0.12	1	22	26	96	0.05
0	0	0	0	0	0	0.5	0	0	0	0	0.21	0	1.18	0	0.3	0.3	2.37	5.03	0.02
0	0	0	0	0	0	0	0	0	0	0	0	0	0.31	0	0	0	0	1.22	0.03
0	0	0	0	0	2.47	108.43	0.02	0.03	0.05	0.01	2.22	0	9.88	0.22	4.94	2.47	32.11	9.88	0.1
0	0	0	0	0	0	0	0	0	0	0	0	0	0	0	0	2.1	0.42	0.42	0
0	0	0	0	0	0	0	0	0	0	0	0	0	26.88	0	0	0	0	1.92	0
0	0	0	0	0	0	0	0	0	0	0	0	0	0	0	0	0	0	0	0
0	0.01	0	0	0	0.3	3.77	0.06	0	0.04	0.01	1.55	0	1.79	0.02	1.2	2.09	15.85	3.29	0.01
0	0	0	0	0	0	0	0.02	0.02	0.219	0	0.412	0	8.24	0.247	9.27	9.27	94.76	9.27	0.072
0	0	0	0	0	0	0	0.02	0.02	0.219	0	0.412	0	8.24	0.247	9.27	9.27	94.76	9.27	0.072
0	0	0	0	0	0	0	0.004	0.016	0.079	0.025	1.133	0.01	8.24	0.442	10.3	14.42	91.67	8.24	0.072
0	0	0	0	0	0	0	0.005	0.029	0.083	0.035	2.06	0.01	8.24	0.443	13.39	14.42	115.36	5.15	0.093
0	0	0	0	0	0	0	0.004	0.016	0.076	0.025	1.133	0.01	8.24	0.391	10.3	15.45	101.97	5.15	0.062
0	0	0	0	0	0	0	0.004	0.005	0.069	0.014	0.206	0	9.27	0.33	10.3	14.42	82.4	5.15	0.072
0.57	1.87	0	0	1.53	0	62.7	1.58	1.78	20.92	2.11	46.86	6.27	46.2	8.12	312.18	801.24	652.08	457.38	5.74
4.27	2.01	0	0	0.73	0	0	0.31	0.56	2.37	0.19	31.2	0.13	180.96	3.07	124.8	382.72	513.76	44.72	2.35
1.83	1.33	0	0	0.73	6.24	1.04	0.33	0.57	1.87	0.11	16.64	0.3	157.04	2.89	71.76	350.48	513.76	52	2
3.475	1.042	0	0	0.548	0.48	0.144	0.168	0.077	0.85	0.086	12	0.053	46.08	1.435	50.4	148.8	210.72	12.96	1.152
3.72	1.71	0	0	0.77	6.6	0	0.31	0.65	2.09	0.17	45.1	0.15	159.5	3.12	124.3	347.6	537.9	47.3	2.11
0	0	1.37	0	0.45	516.36	0	0.51	0.58	6.86	0.7	137.67	2.07	19.11	24.76	70.98	191.88	247.65	302.64	5.15
0	0	0	0	0.54	622.28	0	0.61	0.7	8.27	0.85	165.91	2.49	20.68	7.47	101.52	296.1	250.51	430.99	2.49
0	0	0	0	0.56	648.76	25.97	0.64	0.73	8.62	0.88	172.97	2.6	22.54	7.79	117.6	272.93	286.16	456.19	2.04
0.18	0.66	2.98	0	0.55	225.3	15	0.39	0.42	5.01	0.51	105.9	1.5	105.9	4.5	128.7	294	300.3	275.4	3.75
0.22	0.44	0	0	3	47.3	0	0.523	0.594	7	0.69	99	2.101	26.4	5.99	48.95	129.8	170.5	284.35	1.43
0.26	0.291	0	0	0.02	450.16	0	0.442	0.51	5.984	0.612	120.02	1.802	9.86	3.23	20.06	61.54	65.96	215.9	1.802
0.642	0.21	0	0	0.296	225.3	15	0.375	0.426	5.001	0.501	99.9	0	35.4	4.5	20.1	65.1	60	150.3	3.75
0.12	0.18	0	0	0.049	225.3	15	0.39	0.42	5.01	0.51	105.9	0	3.3	4.5	8.7	30	31.8	134.4	3.75
0.165	0.22	0	0	0.457	233.75	0	0.385	0.44	5.17	0.495	110	1.54	14.85	1.87	9.9	85.8	85.25	373.45	1.54
0.99	1.1	0	0	0.676	375.1	14.96	0.37	0.424	4.999	0.501	99.55	0	309.65	4.499	40.15	231.55	161.7	322.85	3.751
0.462	0.06	0	0	0.171	225.3	15	0.375	0.426	5	0.501	99.9	0	22.22	4.5	5.7	37.2	23.7	184.5	3.75
0.22	0.55	0	0	0.849	0	0	0.385	0.44	5.115	0.495	110	1.54	19.25	16.5	51.15	161.7	183.15	20.35	1.54
0.254	0.671	0	0	0.56	10.78	25.97	0.64	0.26	8.62	0.88	172.97	2.6	29.4	13.99	69.09	172.97	216.09	345.45	6.48
0.116	0.406	0	0	5.365	362.79	14.993	0.377	0.435	5	0.493	102.37	1.45	13.92	8.12	60.03	149.93	175.16	226.2	3.75
0.107	0.369	0	0	0.541	622.28	0	0.611	0.705	8.272	0.846	165.91	2.491	20.68	13.442	101.52	296.1	250.51	430.99	2.491
5.995	4.656	0	0	0.679	1284.28	0	1.261	1.455	17.072	1.75	342.41	5.14	46.56	15.42	66.93	224.07	197.88	166.84	1.64
1.67	1.38	0	0	0.72	1363.72	0	1.34	1.55	18.13	1.85	363.59	5.46	50.47	16.38	74.16	231.75	260.59	160.68	1.64
0.273	0.189	0	0	0.134	3.51	0	0.375	0.424	5	0.499	100.17	0	5.4	4.504	9.45	28.62	34.56	208.44	3.753

USDA ID Code	Food Name	Weight in Grams*	Quantity of Units	Unit of Measure	Protein (gm)	Fat (gm)	Carbohydrates (gm)	Kcalories	Caffeine (gm)	Fiber (gm)	Cholesterol (mg)	Saturated Fat (gm)
8011	Cereals, Cap'n Crunch's Crunchberries	35	1	Cup	1.82	2.94	28.53	145.95	0	0.67	0.07	1.93
8012	Cereals, Cap'n Crunch's Peanut Butter	35	1	Cup	2.52	4.52	26.5	153.65	0	0.46	0	1.9
8013	Cereals, Cheerios	30	1	Cup	3.144	1.77	22.86	109.5	0	2.64	0	0.351
	Cereals, Cinnamon Life	50	1	Cup	4.355	1.735	40.4	189.5	0	2.95	0	0.325
	Cereals, Cinnamon Mini Buns	30	0.75	Cup	1.47	0.63	26.61	115.2	0	0.66	0	0.15
	Cereals, Cinnamon Oatmeal Squares	60	1	Cup	7.566	2.568	47.154	231.6	0	4.56	0	0.504
	Cereals, Cinnamon Toast Crunch	30	0.75	Cup	1.68	3.042	23.838	124.2	0	1.5	0	0.501
8014	Cereals, Cocoa Krispies	31	0.75	Cup	1.55	0.806	27.249	120.28	0	0.403	0	0.589
	Cereals, Cocoa Puffs	30	1	Cup	1.14	0.903	26.715	118.8	0	0.18	0	0.204
8017	Cereals, Cookie-crisp, Choc Chip and Van.	30	1	Cup	1.53	1.08	26.25	120	0	0.42	0	0
8018	Cereals, Corn Bran	36	1	Cup	2.45	1.26	30.35	124.56	0	6.84	0	0
8019	Cereals, Corn Chex	29	1	Cup	2059	0.116	25.433	113.68	0	0.522	0	0.016
8020	Cereals, Corn Flakes, Kellogg's	28	1	Cup	1.84	0.199	24.217	102.2	0	0.784	0	0.056
8022	Cereals, Corn Flakes, Low Sodium	25	1	Cup	1.93	0.08	22.2	99.75	0	0.28	0	0
8021	Cereals, Corn Flakes, Ralston Purina	25	1	Cup	1.95	0.1	21.65	97.5	0	0.48	0	0
	Cereals, Corn Pops	31	1	Cup	1.147	0.18	28.427	118.11	0	0.434	0	0.062
8023	Cereals, Cracklin' Oat Bran	55	0.75	Cup	4.615	6.969	40.095	224.95	0	6.545	0	2.919
8168	Cereals, Cream Of Rice, Ckd	244	1	Cup	2.2	0.24	28.06	126.88	0	0	0	0
8171	Cereals, Cream Of Wheat, Instant	241	1	Cup	4.34	0.48	31.57	154.24	0	0	0	0
8170	Cereals, Cream Of Wheat, Quick	239	1	Cup	3.59	0.48	26.77	129.06	0	0	0	0
8169	Cereals, Cream Of Wheat, Regular	251	1	Cup	3.76	0.5	27.61	133.03	0	0	0	0
8024	Cereals, Crisp Rice, Low Sodium	26	1	Cup	1.43	0.08	23.66	104.52	0	0	0	0
62634	Cereals, Crispex	29	1	Cup	2.146	0.29	24.998	108.46	0	0.638	0	0.087
8025	Cereals, Crispy Rice	28	1	Cup	1.79	0.11	24.81	110.88	0	0.34	0	0
8026	Cereals, Crispy Wheats 'n Raisins	55	1	Cup	4.466	0.759	44.33	191.4	0	3.41	0	0.154
	Cereals, Fiber One	30	0.5	Cup	2.778	0.843	24.006	61.5	0	14.25	0	0.132
8027	Cereals, Fortified Oat Flakes	48	1	Cup	8.98	0.72	34.75	177.12	0	1.44	0	0
	Cereals, Frosted Flakes	31	0.75	Cup	1.212	0.155	28.21	117.18	0	0.496	0	0.062
62637	Cereals, Frosted Mini-Wheats	55	1	Cup	5.17	0.88	45.375	186.45	0	5.885	0	0.165
8030	Cereals, Fruit Loops	30	1	Cup	1.47	0.87	26.46	117.3	0	0.57	0	0.39
	Cereals, Fruity Pebbles	32	1	Cup	1.28	1.664	27.552	129.6	0	0.416	0	1.373
8035	Cereals, Golden Grahams	30	0.75	Cup	1.596	1.08	25.689	115.5	0	0.93	0	0.177
8036	Cereals, Graham Crackos	30	1	Cup	2.25	0.18	25.92	108.3	0	1.83	0	0
8037	Cereals, Granola, Homemade	122	1	Cup	17.934	30.012	64.66	569.74	0	12.81	0	5.795
8038	Cereals, Grape-nuts	109	1	Cup	12.753	0.436	89.38	389.13	0	10.9	0	0.059
8039	Cereals, Grape-nuts Flakes	39	1	Cup	3.939	0.36	26.55	116.2	0	3.21	0	0
62639	Cereals, Great Grains	79.46	1	Cup	1.131	9	56.97	329.84	0	6	0	1.5
8040	Cereals, Heartland Natural Cereal, Plain	115	1	Cup	11.615	17.71	78.545	499.1	0	7.015	0	4.52
8041	Cereals, Heartland Natural Cereal, w/ coconut	105	1	Cup	10.92	17.12	71.3	463.05	0	7.46	0	0
8042	Cereals, Heartland Natural Cereal, w/ raisins	110	1	Cup	10.67	15.62	75.9	467.5	0	6.05	0	3.985
8043	Cereals, Honey and Nut Corn Flakes	37.867	1	Cup	2.42	2.08	31.13	150.71	0	0.45	0	0
	Cereals, Honey Graham Oh!	27	0.75	Cup	1.35	1.909	22.745	111.78	0	0.702	0	0.55
8045	Cereals, Honey Nut Cheerios	30	1	Cup	2.778	1.239	24.261	114.9	0	1.56	0	0.228
8044	Cereals, Honeybran	35	1	Cup	3.08	0.735	28.63	119.35	0	3.885	0	0.255
8046	Cereals, Honeycomb	22	1	Cup	1.28	0.4	19.6	86.02	0	0.62	0	0
62641	Cereals, Just Right	55	1	Cup	4.235	1.485	46.035	204.05	0	2.805	0	0.11
	Cereals, Just Right, Fruit & Nut	55	1	Cup	4.125	1.595	44.275	192.5	0	2.75	0	0.275
8048	Cereals, Kix	30	1.33	Cup	1.965	0.621	25.914	114.3	0	0.81	0	0.171
8049	Cereals, Life	44	1	Cup	8.1	0.84	31.5	162.36	0	2.64	0	0
	Cereals, Low Fat Granola, w/ raisins	55	0.67	Cup	4.51	2.75	43.67	201.85	0	3.3	0	0.935
	Cereals, Low Fat Granola, w/o raisins	55	0.5	Cup	4.62	3.245	44.165	213.4	0	3.245	0	0.495
62642	Cereals, Low-Fat Granola, Kellogg's	82.459	1	Cup	7.5	4.5	64.47	314.84	0	4.5	0	1.5
8050	Cereals, Lucky Charms	30	1	Cup	2.154	1.083	25.17	116.1	0	1.2	0	0.219
8178	Cereals, Malt-o-meal, Plain and Choc	240	1	Cup	3.6	0.24	25.92	122.4	0	0	0	0
8179	Cereals, Maypo, Ckd w/ water, w/ salt	240	1	Cup	5.76	2.4	31.92	170.4	0	0	0	0

Monounsaturated Fat (gm)	Polyunsaturated Fat (gm)	Vitamin D (mg)	Vitamin K (mg)	Vitamin E (mg)	Vitamin A (re)	Vitamin C (mg)	Thiamin (mg)	Riboflavin (mg)	Niacin (mg)	Vitamin B6 (mg)	Folate (mg)	Vitamin B12 (mcg)	Calcium (mg)	Iron (mg)	Magnesium (mg)	Phosphorus (mg)	Potassium (mg)	Sodium (mg)	Zinc (mg)
0.39	0.47	0	0	0.09	4.55	0	0.6	0.67	8.13	0.93	127.75	2.5	10.85	9.04	13.65	46.55	49	243.6	3.56
1.37	1.01	0	0	0.09	5.6	0	0.6	0.7	8.97	1.04	243.6	2.3	7	9.11	18.55	48.65	56.7	267.75	3.79
0.642	0.216	0.8	0	0.206	357.3	15	0.375	0.426	5	0.501	99.9	0	55.2	8.1	32.7	114	88.5	284.1	3.75
0.57	0.77	0	0	0.225	1.5	0.1	0.625	0.71	8.38	0.835	167.5	0	134.5	74.54	41.5	181	113	220	6.285
0.18	0.3	0	0	0.053	225.3	15	0.39	0.42	5.01	0.51	90	0	3.9	4.5	11.1	24	36.6	207.6	3.75
0.864	1.074	0	0	2.219	165	6.6	0.408	0.462	5.484	0.546	109.8	0	41.4	14.55	70.2	181.8	250.2	266.4	4.11
0.93	0.528	0	0	0.279	225.3	15	0.375	0.426	5.001	0.501	99.9	0	42.3	4.5	13.5	74.4	44.1	210.3	3.75
0.093	0.124	0	0	0.143	225.06	15.004	0.372	0.434	4.991	0.496	93	0	4.03	1.798	11.47	29.45	60.14	210.18	1.488
0.348	0.045	0	0	0.137	0	15	0.375	0.426	5.001	0.501	99.9	0	33	4.5	6.6	42.6	52.2	180.6	3.75
0	0	0	0	0.08	397.2	15.9	0.39	0.45	5.28	0.54	3.3	1.59	5.7	4.77	8.4	24	29.4	206.7	0.29
0	0	0	0	0.84	7.56	0	0.37	0.7	10.86	0.86	232.2	1.39	41.4	12.24	18.36	51.84	70.2	309.6	4
0.029	0.05	0	0	0.072	14.5	51.37	0.377	0.07	5.104	0.522	102.37	1.537	3.19	8.282	4.06	11.31	23.49	316.97	0.101
0.028	0.112	0.8	0	0.035	210.28	14	0.364	0.392	4.676	0.476	98.84	0	1.12	8.68	3.36	10.92	25.48	297.92	0.168
0	0	0	0	0.03	9.5	0	0	0.05	0.11	0.02	1.75	0	10.75	0.56	3.25	12.25	18.25	2.5	0.07
0	0	0	0	0.06	9.5	0	0.13	0.03	1.05	0.02	1.75	0	1.75	0.63	2.75	9.75	22	239	0.06
0.062	0.031	0	0	0.033	232.81	15.5	0.403	0.434	5.177	0.527	109.43	0	2.48	1.86	2.48	6.51	22.63	123.07	1.55
3.249	0.754	2.1	0	0.364	253	16.83	0.421	0.477	5.612	0.561	152.9	0	24.75	2.035	76.45	186.45	254.65	195.25	1.65
0	0	0	0	0	0	0			0.98	0.07	7.32	0	7.32	0.49	7.32	41.48	48.8	422.12	0.39
0	0	0	0	0	0	0	0.24	0	1.69	0.03	9.64	0	60.25	12.05	14.46	43.38	48.2	363.91	0.41
0	0	0	0	0	0	0	0.24	0	1.43	0.03	9.56	0	50.19	10.28	11.95	100.38	42.45	336.34	0.33
0	0	0	0	0	0	0	0.25	0	1.51	0.04	10.04	0	50.2	10.29	10.04	42.67	42.67	336.34	0.33
0	0	0	0	0	0	0	0	0.05	0.36	0.04	2.86	0	17.42	0.8	10.14	27.04	20.28	2.6	0.39
0.058	0.116	0.5	0	0.119	225.33	14.993	0.377	0.435	4.988	0.493	87	0	3.48	1.798	6.96	26.68	35.09	240.12	1.508
0	0	0	0	0.03	0	1.12	0.11	0.03	1.99	0.04	3.08	0.08	34.4	0.7	11.76	30.52	26.6	205.52	0.46
0.121	0.156	0	0	0.574	375.1	0	0.374	0.424	4.999	0.501	99.55	0	69.3	4.499	42.35	140.25	229.9	284.9	1.083
0.138	0.06	0	0	0.332	0	9	0.375	0.426	5.001	0.501	99.9	0	58.5	4.5	68.1	168.3	216.9	142.5	1.239
0.031	0.093	0	0	0.34	635.52	0	0.62	0.72	8.45	0.86	169.44	2.54	68.16	13.73	57.6	176.16	343.2	429.12	1.5
0.11	0.605	0	0	0.496	0	0	0.385	0.44	5.005	0.495	102.3	1.485	19.8	61.225	55.55	159.5	183.15	1.65	1.485
0.21	0.27	0.99	0	0.11	211.2	14.07	0.39	0.42	5.01	0.51	90	0	3.3	4.23	8.7	20.7	31.5	140.7	3.75
0.102	0.075	0	0	0.032	423.68	0	0.416	0.48	5.632	0.576	112.96	1.696	3.84	2.016	9.28	18.88	24.32	177.6	1.696
0.279	0.159	1.37	0	0.226	225.3	15	0.375	0.426	5.001	0.501	99.9	0	14.4	4.5	9.3	36	52.8	274.5	3.75
0	0	0	0	0.02	397.2	15.9	0.39	0.45	5.28	0.54	105.9	0	13.8	1.89	24.9	65.7	108.3	195.9	1.59
9.601	12.895	0	0	15.708	4.88	1.708	0.903	0.342	2.501	0.39	104.92	0	98.82	5.124	217.16	563.64	656.36	29.28	4.953
0.057	0.194	3.98	0	0.273	1443.16	0	1.417	1.635	19.184	1.962	384.77	5.777	10.355	31.174	73.03	273.59	364.06	757.55	2.398
0	0	0	0	0.08	429.73	0	0.42	0.49	5.71	0.58	114.57	1.72	12.98	9.28	35.7	96.72	112.95	183.06	0.65
0	0	0.75	0	0	374.81	0	0.56	0.64	7.12	0.75	74.96	0.75	35.98	2.25	52.47	179.91	179.91	224.89	1.8
4.799	7.089	0	0	0.805	6.9	1.15	0.356	0.161	1.61	0.194	64.4	0	74.75	4.336	147.2	416.3	385.25	293.25	3.036
0	0	0	0	0.74	0	1.05	0.35	0.15	1.79	0.16	56.7	0	66.15	5.39	137.55	380.1	384.3	213.15	2.74
4.228	6.241	0	0	0.77	6.6	1.1	0.319	0.143	1.54	0.198	44	0	66	4.015	140.8	376.2	414.7	205.5	2.83
0	0	0	0	0.09	501.35	20.07	0.49	0.57	6.66	0.68	133.67	0	4.54	2.39	7.57	17.42	47.71	300.66	0.14
1.064	0.276	0	0	0.109	301.32	12.042	0.375	0.472	5.017	0.499	100.44	0	12.42	4.514	12.69	41.85	45.09	177.933	13.761
0.48	0.189	1.16	0	0.312	225.3	15	0.375	0.426	5.001	0.501	99.9	0	20.4	4.5	29.4	102.9	85.2	258.9	3.75
0.08	0.262	0	0	0.812	463.4	18.55	0.455	0.525	6.16	0.63	23.45	1.855	16.1	5.565	45.85	131.95	150.5	202.3	0.903
0	0	0	0.77	0.09	291.28	0	0.29	0.33	3.87	0.4	77.66	1.17	3.74	2.09	7.48	21.78	70.4	123.86	1.17
0.275	1.045	0	0	2.238	375.65	0	0.385	0.44	5.005	0.495	102.3	1.485	14.3	16.225	34.1	106.15	121	337.7	0.88
0.77	0.55	0	0	2.997	344.3	0	0.33	0.385	4.565	0.44	110	1.375	0	14.85	33	108.9	155.65	265.65	1.045
0.147	0.036	0.66	0	0.018	375.3	15	0.375	0.426	5.001	0.501	99.9	0	43.5	8.1	9.3	42	41.1	263.1	3.75
0	0	0	0	0.31	0	0	0.95	1	11.63	0.08	36.96	0		11.62	14.08	237.6	196.68	229.24	1.45
0.66	1.155	0	0	5.533	206.25	0	0.33	0.385	4.565	0.44	110	1.375	24.2	1.925	45.65	127.05	155.65	123.75	3.465
0.66	2.09	0	0	5.533	253	0	0.44	0.495	5.61	0.55	110	1.705	22.55	2.035	46.75	134.75	137.5	134.75	4.235
0	0	0.75	0	0	224.89	0	0.56	0.64	7.12	0.75	74.96	0.75	35.98	1.5	52.47	179.91	254.87	202.4	5.62
0.393	0.15	1.12	0	0.128	225.3	15	0.375	0.426	5.001	0.501	99.9	0	32.4	4.5	19.5	75.6	54	203.1	3.75
0	0	0	0	0	0	0	0.48	0.24	5.76	0.02	4.8	0	4.8	9.6	4.8	24	31.2	324	0.17
0	0	0	0	0	703.2	28.8	0.72	0.72	9.36	0.96	9.6	2.88	124.8	8.4	50.4	247.2	211.2	259.2	1.49

USDA ID Code	Food Name	Weight in Grams*	Quantity of Units	Unit of Measure	Protein (gm)	Fat (gm)	Carbohydrates (gm)	Kcalories	Caffeine (gm)	Fiber (gm)	Cholesterol (mg)	Saturated Fat (gm)
8119	Cereals, Maypo, Ckd w/ water, w/o salt	240	1	Cup	5.76	2.4	31.92	170.4	0	5.76	0	0
	Cereals, Mueslix, Apple & Almond Crunch	55	0.75	Cup	5.39	4.95	40.865	210.65	0	4.675	0	1.045
	Cereals, Multigrain Cheerios	30	1	Cup	2.556	1.089	24.45	111.9	0	1.92	0	0.249
8052	Cereals, Nature Valley Granola	113	1	Cup	11.53	19.66	75.48	502.85	0	5.99	0	13.03
	Cereals, Nut & Honey Crunch	55	1.25	Cup	4.015	2.475	45.98	222.75	0	0.88	0	0.495
8149	Cereals, Nutri-grain, Barley	41	1	Cup	4.47	0.33	33.95	152.52	0	2.38	0	0
8150	Cereals, Nutri-grain, Corn	42	1	Cup	3.36	0.97	35.45	160.02	0	2.6	0	0
8151	Cereals, Nutri-grain, Rye	40	1	Cup	3.48	0.28	33.88	143.6	0	2.56	0	0
8152	Cereals, Nutri-grain, Wheat	30	0.75	Cup	3.03	0.99	24	100.5	0	3.78	0	0.06
	Cereals, Oat Bran Cereal	57	1.25	Cup	8.539	2.947	41.393	212.61	0	5.985	0	0.542
	Cereals, Oat Flakes	48	1	Cup	7.872	0.96	36.096	180.48	0	1.44	0	0.163
	Cereals, Oatmeal Raisin Crisp	55	1	Cup	4.351	2.447	43.703	204.05	0	3.52	0	0.385
	Cereals, Oatmeal Squares	56	1	Cup	7.274	2.587	43.316	216.16	0	4.256	0	0.476
8123	Cereals, Oats, Instant, Plain	177	1	Pkt.	4.43	1.77	18.05	104.43	0	3.01	0	0
8125	Cereals, Oats, Instant, w/ apples and cinn	149	1	Pkt.	3.87	1.64	26.37	135.59	0	0	0	0
8127	Cereals, Oats, Instant, w/ bran & rsns	195	1	Pkt.	4.88	1.95	30.42	157.95	0	0	0	0
8129	Cereals, Oats, Instant, w/ cinn and spice	161	1	Pkt.	4.83	1.93	35.1	177.1	0	2.58	0	0
8131	Cereals, Oats, Instant, w/ mapl & brn sug flav	155	1	Pkt.	4.65	1.86	31.93	162.75	0	0	0	0
8133	Cereals, Oats, Instant, w/ raisins and spice	158	1	Pkt	4.27	1.74	31.92	161.16	0	2.21	0	0
8180	Cereals, Oats, Reg and Quick and Instant	234	1	Cup	6.08	2.34	25.27	145.08	0	0	0	0.44
8058	Cereals, Product 19	30	1	Cup	2.295	0.39	25.089	109.8	0	1.23	0	0.03
	Cereals, Puffed Rice	14	1	Cup	0.98	0.126	12.288	53.62	0	0.196	0	0.045
	Cereals, Puffed Wheat	15	1.25	Cup	2.439	0.323	11.459	54.9	0	1.14	0	0.016
8059	Cereals, Quisp	30	1	Cup	1.5	2.16	24.99	124.2	0	0.54	0	1.48
8060	Cereals, Raisin Bran, Kellogg's	61	1	Cup	5.49	1.427	46.72	196.42	0	7.808	0	0.143
8061	Cereals, Raisin Bran, Post	56	1	Cup	5.208	1.064	42.336	171.92	0	7.896	0	0.176
8062	Cereals, Raisin Bran, Ralston Purina	56	1	Cup	4.368	0.28	46.48	178.08	0	7.504	0	0.046
	Cereals, Raisin Bran, Total, General Mills	55	1	Cup	3.998	1.006	42.752	178.2	0	5.005	0	0.231
	Cereals, Raisin Nut Bran	55	1	Cup	5.164	4.4	41.454	209	0	5.06	0	0.715
	Cereals, Raisin Squares	55	0.75	Cup	4.4	1.54	42.9	187	0	5.17	0	0.165
8063	Cereals, Raisins, Rice and Rye	46	1	Cup	2.62	0.14	39.28	154.56	0	2.62	0	0
	Cereals, Reese's Peanut Butter Puffs	30	0.75	Cup	2.571	3.195	22.98	129.3	0	0.39	0	0.636
8064	Cereals, Rice Chex	33	1	Cup	1.749	0.132	29.436	130.35	0	0.594	0	0.036
8065	Cereals, Rice Krispies	33	1.25	Cup	2.079	0.363	28.545	124.41	0	0.363	0	0.132
8156	Cereals, Rice, Puffed	14	1	Cup	0.88	0.07	12.57	56.28	0	0	0	0
	Cereals, Shredded Wheat, Large	23.6	1	Biscuit	2.572	0.389	19.187	84.96	0	2.313	0	0.065
	Cereals, Shredded Wheat, Small	30	1	Cup	3.3	0.495	24.12	107.1	0	2.94	0	0.083
	Cereals, S'mores Grahams	30	0.75	Cup	1.677	1.2	25.59	117	0	0.84	0	0.177
8067	Cereals, Special K	31	1	Cup	6.355	0.279	22.444	114.7	0	0.961	0	0
8068	Cereals, Sugar Corn Pops	28.4	1	Cup	1.42	0.09	25.7	108.49	0	0.23	0	0
8069	Cereals, Sugar Frosted Flakes	38	1	Cup	2.014	0.532	34.238	148.58	0	0.836	0	0.305
	Cereals, Sun Country Granola w/ almonds	57	0.5	Cup	6.709	10.271	38.304	266.19	0	2.964	0	1.265
	Cereals, Sun Country Granola, w/ raisins & dates	31	0.5	Cup	3.019	4.225	22.382	135.16	0	1.86	0	0.642
	Cereals, Super Sugar Crisp	33	1	Cup	2.145	0.297	29.766	123.42	0	0.495	0	0.052
8074	Cereals, Tasteeos	24	1	Cup	3.07	0.67	18.984	94.32	0	2.544	0	0.23
8075	Cereals, Team	42	1	Cup	2.69	0.76	36.04	164.22	0	0.55	0	0
	Cereals, Toasted Brown Sugar Squares	55	1.25	Cup	5.225	1.045	44.99	189.2	0	5.115	0	0.181
	Cereals, Toasted Oatmeal Cereal, Honey Nut	49	1	Cup	4.89	2.71	38.955	190.61	0	3.332	0.49	0.519
	Cereals, Toasted Oats Granola	55	0.75	Cup	5.803	9.691	36.234	238.05	0	3.52	0	1.271
	Cereals, Toasties	23	1	Cup	1.836	0.046	19.734	89.01	0	0.782	0	0.006
8077	Cereals, Total	30	0.75	Cup	2.988	0.696	23.88	105.3	0	2.64	0	0.18
	Cereals, Triples	30	1	Cup	2.379	1.011	24.984	116.1	0	0.84	0	0.291
8078	Cereals, Trix	30	1	Cup	0.954	1.707	26.04	122.4	0	0.72	0	0.407
	Cereals, Waffelos	30	1	Cup	1.68	1.26	25.89	121.5	0	0	0	0
8082	Cereals, Wheat Chex	46	1	Cup	4.55	1.15	37.81	168.82	0	4.09	0	0.198

Monounsaturated Fat (gm)	Polyunsaturated Fat (gm)	Vitamin D (mg)	Vitamin K (mg)	Vitamin E (mg)	Vitamin A (re)	Vitamin C (mg)	Thiamin (mg)	Riboflavin (mg)	Niacin (mg)	Vitamin B6 (mg)	Folate (mg)	Vitamin B12 (mcg)	Calcium (mg)	Iron (mg)	Magnesium (mg)	Phosphorus (mg)	Potassium (mg)	Sodium (mg)	Zinc (mg)
0	0	0	0	1.68	703.2	28.8	0.72	0.72	9.36	0.96	9.6	2.88	124.8	8.4	50.4	247.2	211.2	9.6	1.49
2.585	1.045	0	0	5.775	233.75	0	0.385	0.44	5.17	0.495	110	1.265	33.55	4.675	62.7	175.45	209	270.05	3.135
0.297	0.15	0	0	0.191	225.3	15	0.375	0.426	5	0.501	99.9	0	57	8.1	29.7	114.3	97.2	254.1	3.75
2.93	2.75	0	0	3.39	0	0	0.4	0.19	0.82	0.09	84.75	0	71.19	3.77	115.26	353.69	388.72	232.78	2.19
1.155	0.825	0	0	0.138	225.5	15.015	0.385	0.44	5.005	0.495	110	0	5.5	4.51	4.95	36.3	59.95	370.15	0.385
0	0	0	0	10.82	542.84	21.73	0.53	0.62	7.22	0.74	144.73	2.17	11.07	1.45	32.39	126.28	107.83	277.16	5.41
0	0	0	0	11.09	556.08	22.26	0.55	0.63	7.39	0.76	148.26	2.23	1.26	0.89	26.88	120.54	97.86	276.36	5.54
0	0	0	0	10.56	529.6	21.2	0.52	0.6	7.04	0.72	141.2	2.12	8.4	1.13	30.4	104	71.6	272	5.28
0.24	0.69	0	0	5.4	0	15	0.39	0.42	5.01	0.51	90	1.5	9.6	0.99	24.3	108.3	109.5	220.8	3.75
0.963	1.214	0	0	2.096	155.61	6.213	0.388	0.439	5.187	0.519	103.74	0	30.21	15.96	99.18	306.09	257.07	205.2	3.887
0.276	0.36	0	0	0.336	635.52	0	0.624	0.72	8.448	0.864	169.44	2.544	68.16	13.728	57.6	176.16	228	220.32	2.544
1.155	0.363	0	0	1.355	225.5	0	0.374	0.424	5.005	0.501	100.1	0	37.95	4.499	44.55	117.15	211.75	223.85	3.751
0.806	1.047	0	0	2.278	169.12	6.776	0.42	0.476	5.628	0.56	112.56	0	35.84	15.68	70	185.92	227.92	263.2	4.222
0	0	0	0	0.21	453.12	0	0.53	0.28	5.47	0.74	150.45	0	162.84	6.3	42.48	132.75	99.12	284.97	0.87
0	0	0	0	0	435.08	0	0.48	0.28	5.14	0.7	137.08	0	157.94	6.06	34.27	117.71	107.28	222.01	0.7
0	0	0	0	0	479.7	0	0.57	0.64	8.13	0.76	156	0	173.55	7.62	56.55	206.7	235.95	247.65	1.35
0	0	0	0	0.35	473.34	0	0.56	0.34	5.65	0.77	152.95	0	172.27	6.63	51.52	144.9	104.65	280.14	0.97
0	0	0	0	0	451.05	0	0.53	0.33	5.35	0.74	145.7	0	161.2	6.36	41.85	142.6	102.3	279	0.87
0	0	0	0	0.16	440.82	0	0.51	0.36	5.48	0.75	150.1	0	165.9	6.59	36.34	132.72	150.1	225.94	0.71
0.84	0.96	0	0	0	0	0	0.26	0.05	0.3	0.05	9.36	0	18.72	1.59	56.16	177.84	131.04	374.4	1.15
0.15	0.21	1.16	0	22.2	225.3	60	1.5	1.71	20.01	2.01	423.6	6	2.7	18	12.3	39.9	51.9	282	15
0.025	0.048	0	0	0.014	0	0	0.057	0.007	0.875	0	1.4	0	1.26	0.407	4.2	16.52	16.24	0.7	0.154
0.046	0.16	0	0	0.101	0.15	0	0.06	0.041	1.791	0.02	5.1	0.063	3.6	0.702	19.95	49.65	54.6	0.75	0.461
0.26	0.31	0	0	0.08	4.8	0	0.54	0.76	5.8	0.91	8.1	2.58	9.3	6.32	12.3	24.9	44.7	240.9	0.18
0.119	0.428	1.23	0	0.556	250.1	0	0.427	0.488	5.551	0.549	113.46	1.647	40.62	5.002	89.06	214.11	349.53	390.4	4.148
0.146	0.503	2.16	0	1.299	741.44	0	0.728	0.84	9.856	1.008	197.68	2.968	26.32	8.904	95.2	234.64	344.96	365.12	2.968
0.038	0.132	0	0	1.299	556.08	1.68	0.56	0.616	7.392	0.728	148.4	2.24	26.88	27.328	84.56	247.52	287.28	486.08	1.674
0.17	0.17	0	0	29.975	375.1	0	1.502	1.7	20.02	2.002	399.85	6.353	238.15	18.001	44.55	258.5	287.1	239.8	14.999
1.925	0.456	0	0	2.032	0	0	0.374	0.424	4.999	0.501	99.55	0	73.7	4.499	53.9	162.8	218.35	245.85	1.105
0.11	0.495	0	0	0.291	0	0	0.385	0.44	5.17	0.495	110	1.54	18.7	16.83	47.85	159.5	259.6	3.3	1.54
0	0	0	0	0.25	467.82	0.46	0.46	0.55	6.26	0.64	124.66	1.89	10.12	5.61	19.78	49.68	143.52	349.6	4.69
1.431	0.6	0	0	0.565	225.3	15	0.375	0.426	5.001	0.501	99.9	0	21	4.5	15.9	43.2	61.5	177.3	3.75
0.041	0.035	0	0	0.043	1.98	17.49	0.429	0.01	5.808	0.01	116.49	1.749	4.62	9.438	8.25	32.34	38.28	275.88	0.455
0.099	0.165	0.99	0	0.041	247.83	16.5	0.429	0.462	5.511	0.561	116.49	0	3.3	1.98	15.84	43.56	42.24	353.76	0.597
0	0	0	0	0	0	0	0.36	0.25	4.94	0.01	2.66	0	0.84	4.44	3.5	13.72	15.82	0.42	0.14
0.062	0.207	0	0	0.125	0	0	0.066	0.066	1.079	0.06	11.8	0	9.676	0.743	40.12	85.668	77.172	0.472	0.592
0.079	0.263	0	0	0.159	0	0	0.078	0.084	1.575	0.076	15	0	11.4	1.266	39.6	105.9	108.3	3	0.99
0.393	0.15	0	0	0.218	225.3	15	0.375	0.426	5.001	0.501	99.9	0	14.4	4.5	10.8	40.5	48	212.4	3.75
0	0.217	0.75	0	0.077	225.06	14.88	0.527	0.589	7.006	0.713	93	0	4.65	8.401	17.67	50.84	54.56	249.86	3.751
0	0	0.99	0	0.07	376.01	15.05	0.37	0.43	5	0.51	100.25	0	1.14	1.79	1.99	28.12	17.32	103.66	1.51
0.072	0.098	1.23	0	0.095	503.12	20.14	0.494	0.57	6.688	0.684	2.66	2.014	4.18	0.95	2.66	9.5	23.94	246.62	0.817
3.329	1.813	0	0	1.194	0	0.057	0.177	0.103	0.542	0.068	19.38	0.04	49.02	2.479	51.87	167.58	221.16	18.81	1.14
1.423	0.803	0	0	0.483	0	0.124	0.087	0.065	0.257	0.04	9.61	0.062	23.87	1.29	26.04	91.76	132.68	7.75	0.496
0.06	0.116	0	0	0.122	436.92	0	0.429	0.495	5.808	0.594	116.49	1.749	6.93	2.079	19.8	43.89	47.85	50.82	1.749
0.173	0.184	0	0	0.168	317.76	12.72	0.312	0.36	4.22	0.43	87.72	1.272	11.04	6.864	26.16	95.76	71.04	280.14	0.686
0	0	0	0	0.1	556.08	22.26	0.55	0.63	7.39	0.76	6.72	2.23	6.3	2.57	18.48	65.1	70.98	259.56	0.58
0.154	0.429	0	0	2.997	51.15	0	0.55	0.605	7.15	0.715	110	2.145	18.7	6.435	59.4	194.15	213.95	1.65	1.54
1.151	0.75	0	0	2.012	150.43	5.978	0.372	0.421	4.998	0.5	99.96	0.015	26.95	4.498	53.41	166.11	184.73	165.62	3.92
6.49	1.87	0	0	3.878	0	0	0.17	0.06	0.611	0.076	8.25	0	41.25	1.716	52.25	160.05	182.6	189.1	1.105
0.011	0.02	0	0	0.058	304.52	0	0.299	0.345	4.048	0.414	81.91	1.219	0.92	0.605	3.45	10.12	26.68	241.04	0.067
0.135	0.081	1.16	0	23.492	375.3	60	1.5	1.701	20.1	2.001	399.9	7.671	258.3	18	32.1	210.9	96.9	198.6	15
0.27	0.03	0	0	0.141	375.3	15	0.375	0.426	5.001	0.501	99.9	0	41.1	8.1	6.9	35.4	30.6	191.4	3.75
0.903	0.291	0.98	0	0.598	225.3	15	0.376	0.426	5.001	0.501	99.9	0	32.1	4.5	3.6	26.1	17.7	196.8	3.75
0	0	0	0	0	397.2	15.9	0.39	0.45	5.28	0.54	3.3	1.59	8.4	4.77	6.3	244.5	26.4	124.8	0.243
0.143	0.479	0	0	0.17	0	24.38	0.598	0.166	8.096	0.828	126.38	2.438	17.94	13.138	58.42	181.7	173.42	308.2	1.233

USDA ID Code	Food Name	Weight in Grams*	Quantity of Units	Unit of Measure	Protein (gm)	Fat (gm)	Carbohydrates (gm)	Kcalories	Caffeine (gm)	Fiber (gm)	Cholesterol (mg)	Saturated Fat (gm)
	Cereals, Wheat Germ, Toasted	28.35	1	Oz.	8.25	3.033	14.062	108.297	0	3.657	0	0.519
8080	Cereals, Wheat 'n Raisin Chex	54	1	Cup	5.08	0.43	42.98	185.22	0	3.56	0	0
8143	Cereals, Wheatena, Ckd w/ water	243	1	Cup	4.86	1.22	28.67	136.08	0	6.56	0	0
8182	Cereals, Wheatena, Ckd w/ water, w/ Salt	243	1	Cup	4.86	1.22	28.67	136.08	0	0	0	0
8089	Cereals, Wheaties	30	1	Cup	3.24	0.927	23.79	110.1	0	2.1	0	0.198
8183	Cereals, Whole Wheat Hot Natural Cereal	242	1	Cup	4.84	0.97	33.15	150.04	0	0	0	0
18268	French Toast, Frozen, Ready-to-heat	59	1	Slice	4.37	3.6	18.94	125.67	0	1.65	48.38	1.15
18269	French Toast, Made w/ Lowfat (2%) Milk	65	1	Slice	5.01	7.02	16.25	148.85	0	0	75.4	1.77
18381	French Toast, Made w/ Whole Milk	65	1	Slice	5.01	7.35	16.19	150.8	0	0	76.05	1.95
3189	Oatmeal, Dry	38.368	0.33	Cup	4.6	1.9	18.4	109	0	2.53	0	0
3689	Oatmeal, Prepared	359.999	0.75	Cup	4.5	1.8	18.9	108	0	1.6	0	0.3
18288	Pancakes Plain, Frozen	9	1	4 In.	0.47	0.3	3.92	20.61	0	0	0.81	0.07
18294	Pancakes, Blueberry	9.5	1	4 In.	0.58	0.87	2.76	21.09	0	0	5.32	0.19
18390	Pancakes, Buttermilk	9.5	1	4 In.	0.65	0.88	2.73	21.57	0	0	5.51	0.17
18298	Pancakes, Dietary	22	1	3 In.	1.12	0.18	9.28	43.78	0	0	0	0.03
18293	Pancakes, Plain	9.5	1	4 In.	0.61	0.92	2.69	21.57	0	0	5.61	0.2
18300	Pancakes, Whole-wheat	44	1	4 In.	3.74	2.86	12.94	91.52	0	0	26.84	0.77
18392	Waffles, Buttermilk	75	1	Each	6.23	10.2	24.75	216.75	0	0	50.25	1.88
18367	Waffles, Homemade, Plain	75	1	Each	5.93	10.58	24.68	218.25	0	0	51.75	2.15
18403	Waffles, Plain, Toasted	33	1	Each	2.05	2.71	13.43	87.12	0	0	7.92	0.47
62670	Cheddar Cheese, Non-Fat	28.35	1.5	Ounce	8.1		2.03	45.56	0	0	4.05	0
1150	Cheese Spread, Past. Processed, American	28.35	2	Ounce	4.65	6.02	2.47	82.35	0	0	15.65	3.78
62671	Cheese Stick, Mozzarella	28	1	Each	8	5	0	80	0	0	15	3
1147	Cheese, American, Pasteurized Processed	28.35	2	Ounce	6.28	8.86	0.45	106.44	0	0	26.76	5.58
1004	Cheese, Blue	28.35	1.5	Ounce	6.07	8.15	0.66	100.09	0	0	21.32	5.29
1005	Cheese, Brick	28.35	1.5	Ounce	6.59	8.41	0.79	105.16	0	0	26.76	5.32
1006	Cheese, Brie	28.35	1.5	Ounce	5.88	7.85	0.13	94.59	0	0	28.35	4.94
1008	Cheese, Caraway	28.35	1.5	Ounce	7.14	8.28	0.87	106.6	0	0	26.37	5.27
1009	Cheese, Cheddar	28.35	1.5	Ounce	7.06	9.4	0.36	114.13	0	0	29.74	5.98
62577	Cheese, Cheddar, Reduced Fat	28.35	1.5	Ounce	8	5	1	80	0	0	15	3
1011	Cheese, Colby	28.35	1.5	Ounce	6.74	9.1	0.73	111.6	0	0	26.9	5.73
1012	Cheese, Cottage, Creamed	28.35	1.5	Ounce	3.54	1.28	0.76	29.3	0	0	4.22	0.81
1013	Cheese, Cottage, Creamed, w/ Fruit	28.35	1.5	Ounce	2.81	0.96	3.77	35.05	0	0	3.18	0.61
62690	Cheese, Cottage, Fat Free	226	0.5	Cup	26	0	0	140	0	0	20	0
1016	Cheese, Cottage, Lowfat, 1% Fat	28.35	1.5	Ounce	3.51	0.29	0.77	20.52	0	0	1.25	0.18
1015	Cheese, Cottage, Lowfat, 2% Fat	28.35	1.5	Ounce	3.9	0.55	1.03	25.43	0	0	2.38	0.35
1014	Cheese, Cottage, Uncreamed, Dry	28.35	1.5	Ounce	4.9	0.12	0.52	23.98	0	0	1.9	0.08
1017	Cheese, Cream	28.35	1.5	Ounce	2.14	9.89	0.75	98.95	0	0	31.1	6.23
62554	Cheese, Cream, Fat Free	17.508	2	Tbsp.	2.5	0	1	17.51	0	0	2.5	0
62553	Cheese, Cream, Light	16.014	2	Tbsp.	1.5	2.5	1	35.03	0	0	7.51	1.75
	Cheese, Cream, w/Strawberry	30	1	Ounce	4		2	35	0	0	3	0
1018	Cheese, Edam	28.35	1.5	Ounce	7.08	7.88	0.41	101.1	0	0	25.29	4.98
62579	Cheese, Fat Free Slices, White	21.263	1	Slice	5	0	2	30	0	0	0	0
62578	Cheese, Fat Free Slices, Yellow	21.263	1	Slice	5	0	2	30	0	0	0	0
1019	Cheese, Feta	28.35	1.5	Ounce	4.03	6.03	1.16	74.72	0	0	25.23	4.24
1020	Cheese, Fontina	28.35	1.5	Ounce	7.26	8.83	0.44	110.29	0	0	32.89	5.44
1156	Cheese, Goat, Hard Type	28.35	1.5	Ounce	8.65	10.09	0.62	128.14	0	0	29.77	6.98
1157	Cheese, Goat, Semisoft Type	28.35	1.5	Ounce	6.12	8.46	0.72	103.19	0	0	22.4	5.85
1159	Cheese, Goat, Soft Type	28.35	1.5	Ounce	5.25	5.98	0.25	75.98	0	0	13.04	4.13
1022	Cheese, Gouda	28.35	1.5	Ounce	7.07	7.78	0.63	101.01	0	0	32.32	4.99
1023	Cheese, Gruyere	28.35	1.5	Ounce	8.45	9.17	0.1	117.07	0	0	31.19	5.36
1024	Cheese, Limburger	28.35	1.5	Ounce	5.68	7.73	0.14	92.71	0	0	25.52	4.75
1025	Cheese, Monterey	28.35	1.5	Ounce	6.94	8.58	0.19	105.84	0	0	25.23	5.41
62576	Cheese, Monterey, Reduced Fat	28.35	1.5	Ounce	8	5	1	80	0	0	15	3
1028	Cheese, Mozzarella, Part Skim Milk	28.35	1.5	Ounce	6.88	4.51	0.79	72.08	0	0	16.39	2.87

Monounsaturated Fat (gm)	Polyunsaturated Fat (gm)	Vitamin D (mg)	Vitamin K (mg)	Vitamin E (mg)	Vitamin A (re)	Vitamin C (mg)	Thiamin (mg)	Riboflavin (mg)	Niacin (mg)	Vitamin B6 (mg)	Folate (mg)	Vitamin B12 (mcg)	Calcium (mg)	Iron (mg)	Magnesium (mg)	Phosphorus (mg)	Potassium (mg)	Sodium (mg)	Zinc (mg)
0.425	1.877			5.143	0	1.701	0.473	0.232	1.585	0.277	99.792	0	12.758	2.577	90.72	324.891	268.475	1.134	4.726
0	0	0	0	0.31	0	1.62	0.54	0.59	7.13	0.7	143.1	2.16	24.3	7.72	52.92	163.08	226.8	305.64	1.19
0	0	0	0	0.9	0	0	0.02	0.05	1.34	0.05	17.01	0	9.72	1.36	48.6	145.8	187.11	4.86	1.68
0	0	0	0	0	0	0	0.02	0.05	1.34	0.05	17.01	0	9.72	1.36	48.6	145.8	187.11	578.34	1.68
0.222	0.15	1.02	0	0.369	225.3	15	0.375	0.426	5.001	0.501	99.9	0	54.6	8.1	31.8	95.4	104.1	222.3	0.708
0	0	0	0	0	0	0	0.17	0.12	2.15	0.18	26.62	0	16.94	1.5	53.24	166.98	171.82	563.86	1.16
1.23	0.7	0	0	0	31.86	0.3	0.16	0.22	1.61	0.29	14.16	0.99	63.13	1.3	10.03	82.01	79.06	292.05	0.45
2.94	1.69	0	0	0	85.8	0.2	0.13	0.21	1.06	0.05	14.95	0.2	65	1.09	11.05	76.05	87.1	311.35	0.44
3.03	1.7	0	0	0	80.6	0.2	0.13	0.21	1.06	0.05	14.95	0.2	64.35	1.09	11.05	76.05	86.45	310.7	0.44
0	0	0	0	0.15	0	1.23	0.19	0.03	0.2	0.06	29	0	14	1.08	40	128	105	1	1
0	0.7	0	0	0	0	0	0.19	0.04	0.2	0.04	7	0	15	1.19	42	133	99	1	0.86
0.11	0.09	0	0	0	2.61	0.04	0.03	0.04	0.36	0	1.26	0.01	5.58	0.31	1.26	33.48	6.57	45.81	0.06
0.22	0.4	0	0	0	4.85	0.21	0.02	0.03	0.14	0	1.14	0.02	19.57	0.16	1.52	14.35	13.11	39.14	0.05
0.22	0.43	0	0	0	2.85	0.04	0.02	0.03	0.15	0	1.24	0.02	14.92	0.16	1.43	13.21	13.78	49.59	0.06
0.03	0.08	0	0	0	2.2	0	0.04	0.02	0.37	0	1.1	0	12.76	0.39	5.94	74.8	84.92	57.64	0.15
0.24	0.42	0	0	0	5.13	0.03	0.02	0.03	0.15	0	1.14	0.02	20.81	0.17	1.52	15.11	12.54	41.71	0.05
0.77	1.06	0	0	0	28.16	0.22	0.09	0.23	1.02	0.05	9.24	0.13	110	1.37	20.24	164.12	122.76	251.68	0.46
2.52	5.09	0	0	0	26.25	0.38	0.2	0.27	1.55	0.04	11.25	0.16	136.5	1.63	13.5	123.75	128.25	450.75	0.56
2.64	5.09	0	0	0	48.75	0.3	0.2	0.26	1.55	0.04	11.25	0.19	191.25	1.73	14.25	142.5	119.25	383.25	0.51
1.06	0.92	0	0	0	120.12	0	0.13	0.16	1.46	0.3	11.55	0.83	76.56	1.48	7.26	138.6	42.24	259.71	0.19
0	0	0	0	0	60.75	0	0	0	0	0	0	0	243	0	0	0	0	283.5	0
1.76	0.18	0	0	0	53.58	0	0.01	0.12	0.04	0.03	1.98	0.11	159.3	0.09	8.09	248.06	68.58	460.69	0.73
0	0	0	0	0	40	0	0	0	0	0	0	0	240	0	0	0	0	170	0
2.54	0.28	0	0	0	82.22	0	0.01	0.1	0.02	0.02	2.21	0.2	174.49	0.11	6.31	125.87	45.93	184.28	0.85
2.21	0.23	0	0	0.18	64.64	0	0.01	0.11	0.29	0.05	10.32	0.35	149.57	0.09	6.5	109.83	72.66	395.57	0.75
2.44	0.22	0	0	0.14	85.62	0	0	0.1	0.03	0.02	5.76	0.36	190.99	0.12	6.89	127.86	38.5	158.65	0.74
2.27	0.23	0	0	0.19	51.6	0	0.02	0.15	0.11	0.07	18.43	0.47	52.16	0.14	5.67	53.3	43.09	178.43	0.67
2.35	0.24	0	0	0	81.93	0	0.01	0.13	0.05	0.02	5.16	0.08	190.88	0.18	6.27	138.92	26.37	195.62	0.83
2.66	0.27	0.09	0	0.1	85.9	0	0.01	0.11	0.02	0.02	5.16	0.23	204.49	0.19	7.88	145.18	27.9	175.91	0.88
0	0	0	0	0	60	0	0	0	0	0	0	0	240	0	0	0	23	180	0
2.63	0.27	0	0	0.1	77.96	0	0	0.11	0.03	0.02	5.16	0.23	194.08	0.22	7.32	129.42	35.86	171.29	0.87
0.36	0.04	0	0	0.03	13.61	0	0.01	0.05	0.04	0.02	3.46	0.18	17.01	0.04	1.49	37.37	23.9	114.76	0.1
0.27	0.03	0	0	0.03	10.21	0	0	0.04	0.03	0.02	2.75	0.14	13.49	0.03	1.18	29.63	18.97	114.76	0.08
0	0	0	0	0	0	0	0	0	0	0	0	0	240	0	0	0	0	840	0
0.08	0.01	0	0	0.03	3.12	0	0.01	0.05	0.04	0.02	3.52	0.18	17.27	0.04	1.51	37.93	24.24	115.1	0.11
0.16	0.02	0	0	0.02	5.67	0	0.01	0.05	0.04	0.02	3.71	0.2	19.42	0.05	1.7	42.67	27.27	115.1	0.12
0.03	0.03	0	0	0.03	2.27	0	0.01	0.04	0.04	0.02	4.2	0.23	8.99	0.07	1.12	29.48	9.19	3.63	0.13
2.79	0.36	0	0	0.27	123.89	0	0	0.06	0.03	0.01	3.74	0.12	22.65	0.34	1.83	29.6	33.85	83.77	0.15
0	0	0	0	0	50.02	0	0	0	0	0	0	0	60.03	0	0	0	0	90.04	0
0	0	0	0	0	40.02	0	0	0	0	0	0	0	24.02	0	0	0	0	75.06	0
0	0	0	0	0	10	0	0	0	0	0	0	0	24	0	0	0	0	200	0
2.3	0.19	0.26	0	0.21	71.73	0	0.01	0.11	0.02	0.02	4.59	0.44	207.24	0.12	8.44	151.84	53.21	273.58	1.06
0	0	0	0	0	40	0	0	0	0	0	0	0	120	0	0	0	18	310	0
0	0	0	0	0	40	0	0	0	0	0	0	0	120	0	0	0	18	310	0
1.31	0.17	0	0	0.01	36.29	0	0.04	0.24	0.28	0.12	9.07	0.48	139.62	0.18	5.45	95.6	17.52	316.41	0.82
2.46	0.47	0	0	0.1	82.22	0	0.01	0.06	0.04	0.02	1.7	0.48	155.93	0.07	3.97	98.18	18	226.8	0.99
2.3	0.24	0	0	0	442.26	0	0.04	0.34	0.68	0.02	1.13	0.03	253.73	0.53	15.31	206.67	13.61	98.09	0.45
1.93	0.2	0	0	0	467.78	0	0.02	0.19	0.33	0.02	0.57	0.06	84.48	0.46	8.22	106.31	44.79	146	0.19
1.36	0.14	0	0	0	385.56	0	0.02	0.11	0.12	0.07	3.4	0.05	39.69	0.54	4.54	72.58	7.37	104.33	0.26
2.2	0.19	0	0	0.1	49.33	0	0.01	0.09	0.02	0.02	5.93	0.44	198.39	0.07	8.22	154.88	34.16	232.27	1.11
2.85	0.49	0	0	0.1	85.33	0	0.02	0.08	0.03	0.02	2.95	0.45	286.62	0.05	10.18	171.6	22.96	95.26	1.11
2.44	0.14	0	0	0.18	89.59	0	0.02	0.14	0.04	0.02	16.3	0.29	140.81	0.04	5.95	111.42	36.29	226.8	0.6
2.48	0.25	0	0	0.1	71.73	0	0	0.11	0.03	0.02	5.16	0.23	211.6	0.2	7.66	125.87	22.88	152.04	0.85
0	0	0	0	0	60	0	0	0	0	0	0	0	240	0	0	0	18	180	0
1.28	0.13	0	0	0.12	50.18	0	0.01	0.09	0.03	0.02	2.49	0.23	183.06	0.06	6.58	131.26	23.73	132.11	0.78

USDA ID Code	Food Name	Weight in Grams*	Quantity of Units	Unit of Measure	Protein (gm)	Fat (gm)	Carbohydrates (gm)	Kcalories	Caffeine (gm)	Fiber (gm)	Cholesterol (mg)	Saturated Fat (gm)
1029	Cheese, Mozzarella, Part Skim Milk, Low Moisture	28.35	1.5	Ounce	7.79	4.85	0.89	79.36	0	0	15.31	3.08
1161	Cheese, Mozzarella, Substitute	28.35	1.5	Ounce	3.25	3.46	6.71	70.31	0	0	0	1.05
1026	Cheese, Mozzarella, Whole Milk	28.35	1.5	Ounce	5.51	6.12	0.63	79.77	0	0	22.23	3.73
1027	Cheese, Mozzarella, Whole Milk, Low Moisture	28.35	1.5	Ounce	6.12	6.99	0.7	90.26	0	0	25.34	4.41
1030	Cheese, Muenster	28.35	1.5	Ounce	6.64	8.52	0.32	104.43	0	0	27.1	5.42
1032	Cheese, Parmesan, Grated	5	1	Tbsp.	2.08	1.5	0.19	22.79	0	0	3.94	0.95
62608	Cheese, Parmesan, Grated, Fat Free	5.002	1	Tbsp.	0.67	0	0.67	5	0	0	1.67	0
1033	Cheese, Parmesan, Piece	28.35	1.5	Ounce	10.14	7.32	0.91	111.18	0	0	19.19	4.65
1146	Cheese, Parmesan, Shredded	28.35	1.5	Ounce	10.73	7.75	0.97	117.65	0	0	20.41	4.92
1025	Cheese, Pepper	28.35	1.5	Ounce	7.12	8.13	0.21	107.98	0	0	27.81	5.39
1035	Cheese, Provolone	28.35	1.5	Ounce	7.25	7.55	0.61	99.65	0	0	19.53	4.84
1037	Cheese, Ricotta, Part Skim Milk	28.35	1.5	Ounce	3.23	2.24	1.46	39.14	0	0	8.73	1.4
1036	Cheese, Ricotta, Whole Milk	28.35	1.5	Ounce	3.19	3.68	0.86	49.31	0	0	14.35	2.35
1038	Cheese, Romano	28.35	1.5	Ounce	9.02	7.64	1.03	109.61	0	0	29.48	4.85
1039	Cheese, Roquefort	28.35	1.5	Ounce	6.11	8.69	0.57	104.62	0	0	25.52	5.46
1040	Cheese, Swiss, Domestic	28.35	1.5	Ounce	8.06	7.78	0.96	106.53	0	0	26	5.04
1044	Cheese, Swiss, Pasteurized Processed	28.35	2	Ounce	7.01	7.09	0.6	94.56	0	0	24.04	4.55
1067	Cream Substitute, Nondairy, Liquid	15	1	Tbsp.	0.15	1.5	1.71	20.35	0	0	0	0.29
1069	Cream Substitute, Nondairy, Powdered	2	1	Tsp.	0.1	0.71	1.1	10.93	0	0	0	0.65
1049	Cream, Half and Half, Cream and Milk	15	1	Tbsp.	0.44	1.72	0.64	19.55	0	0	5.53	1.07
1053	Cream, Heavy Whipping	15	1	Tbsp.	0.31	5.55	0.42	51.72	0	0	20.56	3.45
1052	Cream, Light Whipping	15	1	Tbsp.	0.33	4.64	0.44	43.86	0	0	16.65	2.9
1050	Cream, Light, Coffee or Table	15	1	Tbsp.	0.4	2.9	0.55	29.31	0	0	9.91	1.8
1051	Cream, Medium, 25% Fat	15	1	Tbsp.	0.37	3.75	0.52	36.56	0	0	13.12	2.33
1054	Cream, Whipped, Pressurized	3	1	Tbsp.	0.1	0.67	0.37	7.72	0	0	2.28	0.41
1073	Dessert Topping, Nondairy	4	1	Tbsp.	0.05	1.01	0.92	12.73	0	0	0	0.87
1142	Egg Substitute, Frozen	240	1	Cup	27.1	26.66	7.68	383.57	0	0	4.8	4.63
1143	Egg Substitute, Liquid	251	1	Cup	30.12	8.31	1.61	210.98	0	0	2.51	1.65
1124	Egg, White Only, w/o Yolk	33.4	2	Large	3.51	0	0.34	16.7	0	0	0	0
1057	Eggnog	254	1	Cup	9.68	19	34.39	341.9	0	0	149.1	11.29
62680	Eggnog, Reduced-Fat	246	1	Cup	12	8	48	320	0	0	90	5
1128	Eggs, Chicken, Whole, Ckd, Fried	46	1	Large	6.23	6.9	0.63	91.54	0	0	211.14	1.92
1129	Eggs, Chicken, Whole, Ckd, Hard-boiled	50	1	Large	6.29	5.31	0.56	77.5	0	0	212	1.63
1130	Eggs, Chicken, Whole, Ckd, Omelet	59	1	Large	6.09	6.75	0.61	89.68	0	0	206.5	1.88
1131	Eggs, Chicken, Whole, Ckd, Poached	50	1	Large	6.22	4.99	0.61	74.5	0	0	211.5	1.54
1132	Eggs, Chicken, Whole, Ckd, Scrambled	220	0.5	Cup	24.4	26.86	4.84	365.2	0	0	774.4	8.09
1123	Eggs, Chicken, Whole, Fresh, and Frozen	50	1	Large	6.25	5.01	0.61	74.5	0	0	212.5	1.54
1075	Milk Substitutes, Fluid w/ hydr Vegetable Oils	244	1	Cup	4.27	8.32	15.03	149.95	0	0	0.49	1.87
1076	Milk Substitutes, Fluid, w/ lauric Acid Oil	244	1	Cup	4.27	8.32	15.03	149.95	0	0	0.49	7.41
1088	Milk, Buttermilk	245	1	Cup	8.11	2.16	11.74	98.99	0	0	8.57	1.34
1104	Milk, Chocolate Drink, Lowfat, 1% Fat	250	1	Cup	8.1	2.5	26.1	157.57	0	0	7.25	1.54
1103	Milk, Chocolate Drink, Lowfat, 2% Fat	250	1	Cup	8.02	5	26	178.84	0	3.75	17	3.1
1102	Milk, Chocolate Drink, Whole	250	1	Cup	7.92	8.47	25.85	208.37	0	3.75	30.5	5.26
1105	Milk, Chocolate Homemade Hot Cocoa	250	1	Cup	9.1	9.05	25.77	218.15	0	3.75	33.25	5.61
1095	Milk, Cnd, Condensed, Sweetened	305.342	0.25	Cup	24	26.4	165.6	976	0	0	26	4.2
1153	Milk, Cnd, Evaporated	251.787	0.25	Cup	17.15	19.04	25.28	338.37	0	0	74.03	11.56
1097	Milk, Cnd, Evaporated, Skim	254.984	1	Cup	19.25	0.51	28.94	198.69	0	0	9.18	0.31
1082	Milk, Light, 1% Fat	244	1	Cup	8.03	2.59	11.66	102.15	0	0	9.76	1.61
1099	Milk, Malted, Beverage	265	1	Cup	10.34	9.81	27.3	235.85	0	0	37.1	5.95
1101	Milk, Malted, Chocolate Flavor, Beverage	265	1	Cup	9.01	9.01	29.95	227.9	7.95	0	34.45	5.53
1085	Milk, Non-Fat	245	1	Cup	8.35	0.44	11.88	85.53	0	0	4.41	0.29
1079	Milk, Reduced, 2% Fat	244	1	Cup	8.13	4.68	11.71	121.2	0	0	18.3	2.92
1077	Milk, Whole, 3.3% Fat	244	1	Cup	8.03	8.15	11.37	149.92	0	0	33.18	5.07
1078	Milk, Whole, 3.7% Fat	244	1	Cup	8	8.93	11.35	156.58	0	0	34.89	5.56
1056	Sour Cream	12	1	Tbsp.	0.38	2.52	0.51	25.71	0	0	5.33	1.57

Monounsaturated Fat (gm)	Polyunsaturated Fat (gm)	Vitamin D (mg)	Vitamin K (mg)	Vitamin E (mg)	Vitamin A (re)	Vitamin C (mg)	Thiamin (mg)	Riboflavin (mg)	Niacin (mg)	Vitamin B6 (mg)	Folate (mg)	Vitamin B12 (mcg)	Calcium (mg)	Iron (mg)	Magnesium (mg)	Phosphorus (mg)	Potassium (mg)	Sodium (mg)	Zinc (mg)
1.37	0.14	0	0	0.13	54.15	0	0.01	0.1	0.03	0.02	2.81	0.26	207.32	0.07	7.45	148.58	26.89	149.6	0.89
1.77	0.49	0	0	0	123.89	0.03	0.01	0.13	0.09	0.01	3.12	0.23	172.94	0.11	11.62	165.28	128.99	194.2	0.54
1.86	0.22	0	0	0.1	68.32	0	0	0.07	0.02	0.02	1.98	0.19	146.57	0.05	5.27	105.09	19.02	105.77	0.63
1.99	0.22	0	0	0.19	77.68	0	0.08	0.03	0.02	0.02	2.21	0.21	162.98	0.06	5.86	116.89	21.15	117.65	0.7
2.47	0.19	0	0	0.13	89.59	0	0.09	0.03	0.02	0.02	3.43	0.42	203.35	0.12	7.75	132.59	38.1	177.95	0.8
0.44	0.03	0	0	0.04	8.65	0	0.02	0.02	0.02	0.01	0.4	0.07	68.79	0.05	2.54	40.36	5.36	93.08	0.16
0	0	0	0	0	0	0	0	0	0	0	0	0	16.01	0	0	0	10	15.01	0
2.13	0.16	0.2	0	0.23	42.24	0	0.01	0.09	0.08	0.03	1.96	0.34	335.52	0.23	12.39	196.86	26.14	454.03	0.78
2.48	0.19	0	0	0	49.05	0	0.01	0.1	0.08	0.03	2.27	0.4	355.23	0.25	14.4	208.37	27.5	480.82	0.9
2.46	0.24	0	0	0.1	79.89	0	0	0.12	0.03	0.02	6.13	0.22	212.76	0.2	6.23	122.77	25.76	172.77	0.81
2.1	0.22	0	0	0.1	74.84	0	0.01	0.09	0.04	0.02	2.95	0.41	214.3	0.15	7.82	140.64	39.21	248.2	0.92
0.66	0.07	0	0	0.06	32.04	0	0.01	0.05	0.02	0.01	3.71	0.08	77.11	0.12	4.19	51.77	35.44	35.35	0.38
1.03	0.11	0	0	0.1	37.99	0	0	0.06	0.03	0.01	3.46	0.1	58.68	0.11	3.2	44.82	29.65	23.84	0.33
2.22	0.17	0	0	0.21	39.97	0	0.01	0.1	0.02	0.02	1.93	0.32	301.59	0.22	11.6	215.46	24.47	340.2	0.73
2.4	0.37	0	0	0	84.77	0	0.01	0.17	0.21	0.04	13.89	0.18	187.62	0.16	8.37	111.16	25.71	512.85	0.59
2.06	0.28	0.31	0	0.14	71.73	0	0.01	0.1	0.03	0.02	1.81	0.48	272.42	0.05	10.18	171.4	31.38	73.71	1.11
2	0.18	0	0	0.19	64.92	0	0	0.08	0.01	0.01	1.67	0.35	218.83	0.17	8.26	215.89	61.09	388.48	1.02
1.13	0	0	0	0.24	1.35	0	0	0	0	0	0	0	1.4	0	0.05	9.63	28.58	11.88	0
0.02	0	0	0	0.01	0.4	0	0	0	0	0	0	0	0.45	0.02	0.08	8.44	16.24	3.62	0.01
0.5	0.06	0	0	0.02	16.05	0.13	0.01	0.02	0.01	0.01	0.37	0.05	15.73	0.01	1.53	14.28	19.44	6.1	0.08
1.6	0.21	0.19	0	0.09	63.15	0.09	0	0.02	0.01	0	0.55	0.03	9.69	0	1.05	9.36	11.31	5.64	0.03
1.36	0.13	0	0	0.09	44.25	0.09	0	0.02	0.01	0	0.55	0.03	10.41	0	1.08	9.16	14.52	5.14	0.04
0.84	0.11	0	0	0.02	27.3	0.11	0	0.02	0.01	0	0.34	0.03	14.43	0.01	1.3	11.98	18.25	5.94	0.04
1.08	0.14	0	0	0.09	34.8	0.11	0	0.02	0.01	0	0.34	0.03	13.53	0.01	1.26	10.59	17.17	5.55	0.04
0.19	0.02	0	0	0.02	6.21	0	0	0	0	0	0.08	0.01	3.03	0	0.32	2.68	4.42	3.9	0.01
0.06	0.02	0	0	0.01	3.44	0	0	0	0	0	0	0	0.25	0	0.07	0.31	0.73	1.01	0
5.84	14.98	0	0	5.07	324	1.13	0.29	0.93	0.34	0.32	39.36	0.81	174.72	4.75	35.9	172.08	511.92	478.56	2.35
2.25	4.02	0	0	1.22	542.16	0	0.28	0.75	0.28	0.01	37.4	0.75	133.03	5.27	21.89	303.71	828.3	444.27	3.26
0	0	0	0.01	0	0	0	0	0.15	0.03	0	1	1.07	2	0.01	3.67	4.34	47.76	54.78	0
5.67	0.86	0	0	0.58	203.2	3.81	0.09	0.48	0.27	0.13	2.29	1.14	330.2	0.51	46.99	277.88	419.61	138.18	1.17
0	0	0	0	0	160	2.4	0	0	0	0	0	0	480	0.4	0	0	0	280	0
2.75	1.28	0	0	1.57	114.08	0	0.03	0.24	0.04	0.07	17.48	0.42	25.3	0.72	5.06	89.24	60.72	162.38	0.55
2.04	0.71	0	0	0.98	84	0	0.03	0.26	0.03	0.06	22	0.56	25	0.6	5	86	63	62	0.53
2.69	1.26	0	0	1.54	110.33	0	0.03	0.24	0.03	0.06	17.11	0.41	24.78	0.7	5.31	87.32	59.59	159.3	0.54
1.9	0.68	0	0	0.45	95	0	0.02	0.22	0.03	0.06	17.5	0.4	24.5	0.72	5	88.5	60	140	0.55
10.49	4.73	0	0	1.85	429	0.44	0.11	0.96	0.17	0.26	66	1.69	156.2	2.64	26.4	374	303.6	616	2.2
1.9	0.68	0.65	25	1.03	95.5	0	0.03	0.25	0.04	0.07	23.5	0.5	24.5	0.72	5	89	60.5	63	0.55
4.88	1.19	0	0	2.57	0	0	0.03	0.21	0	0	0	0	79.3	250	15.57	181.05	278.89	191.05	2.88
0.43	0.02	0	0	0	0	0	0.03	0.21	0	0	0	0	79.3	250	15.57	181.05	278.89	191.05	2.88
0.62	0.08	0	0	0.15	19.6	2.4	0.08	0.38	0.14	0.08	12.25	0.54	285.18	285	26.83	218.54	370.68	257	1.03
0.75	0.09	2.5	0	0	147.5	2.32	0.09	0.41	0.32	0.1	12	0.85	286.75	285	33.32	256.5	425.5	151.75	1.03
1.47	0.18	2.5	0	0.13	142.5	2.3	0.09	0.41	0.31	0.1	12	0.85	284	285	33	254.25	422	150.5	1.03
2.47	0.31	2.5	0	0.23	72.5	2.27	0.09	0.4	0.31	0.1	11.75	0.83	280.25	280	32.57	251.25	417.25	149	1.03
2.65	0.33	0	0	0.26	85	2.4	0.1	0.43	0.36	0.11	12.25	0.87	298.25	315	55.5	270	479.75	122.75	1.23
0	0.2	0	0	0.65	62	2	0.06	0.32	0.2	0.04	8	0.34	216	108	20	194	284	98	0.98
5.88	0.62	0	0	0	135.97	4.73	0.12	0.8	0.49	0.13	19.89	0.41	656.66	0.48	60.91	509.87	763.17	266.39	1.94
0.16	0.02	5.1	0	0.01	298.33	0.06	0.11	0.79	0.44	0.14	21.93	0.61	738.18	0.74	68.85	496.96	845.27	293.23	2.29
0.75	0.1	2.44	0	0.1	143.96	2.37	0.1	0.41	0.21	0.1	12.44	0.9	300.12	0.12	33.72	234.73	380.88	123.22	0.95
2.78	0.56	0	0	0	95.4	2.92	0.2	0.59	1.31	0.19	21.73	1.03	355.1	0.27	53	302.1	530	222.6	1.14
2.57	0.38	0	0	0	79.5	2.65	0.13	0.44	0.63	0.13	16.43	0.93	304.75	0.61	47.7	265	498.2	172.25	1.09
0.12	0.02	2.45	9.8	0.1	149.45	2.4	0.09	0.34	0.22	0.1	12.74	0.93	302.33	0.1	27.83	247.2	405.72	126.17	0.98
1.35	0.17	2.44	0	0.17	139.08	2.32	0.1	0.4	0.21	0.1	12.44	0.89	296.7	0.12	33.35	232.04	376.74	121.76	0.95
2.35	0.3	2.44	9.76	0.24	75.64	2.29	0.09	0.4	0.2	0.1	12.2	0.87	291.34	0.12	32.79	227.9	369.66	119.56	0.93
2.58	0.33	0	0	0	82.96	3.59	0.09	0.39	0.2	0.1	12.2	0.87	290.36	0.12	32.7	227.16	368.44	119.07	0.93
0.73	0.09	0	0	0.07	23.4	0.1	0	0.02	0.01	0	1.3	0.04	13.97	0.01	1.35	10.19	17.28	6.4	0.03

USDA ID Code	Food Name	Weight in Grams*	Quantity of Units	Unit of Measure	Protein (gm)	Fat (gm)	Carbohydrates (gm)	Kcalories	Caffeine (gm)	Fiber (gm)	Cholesterol (mg)	Saturated Fat (gm)
62556	Sour Cream, Fat Free	16.014	1	Tbsp.	0.5	0	2.5	12.51	0	0	2.5	0
1074	Sour Cream, Imitation, Nondairy, Cultured	14.35	1	Tbsp.	0.34	2.8	0.95	29.91	0	0	0	2.55
62555	Sour Cream, Light	16.014	1	Tbsp.	0.92	1.14	0.92	16.01	0	0	4.58	0.69
62660	Sour Cream, Non-Fat	16	2	Tbsp.	0.5	0	2.5	12.5	0	0	2.5	0
	Yogurt, Dannon, 99% Fat Free	227	8	Ounce	9	3	45	240	0	0	15	1.5
	Yogurt, Dannon, Light	227	8	Ounce	9	0	45	240	0	0	15	1.5
	Yogurt, Dannon, Non Fat, No Sugar w/ Granola	227	8	Ounce	9	0	26	140	0	0	5	0
62657	Yogurt, Frozen	148	0.5	Cup	6	12	48	320	0	0	20	4
62552	Yogurt, Frozen, Fat Free	133.916	0.5	Cup	7.99	0	43.97	199.87	0	0	0	0
62658	Yogurt, Frozen, Low-Fat	148	0.5	Cup	6	6	48	280	0	0	20	4
62604	Yogurt, Fruit, Fat Free	247.957	1	Cup	10.21	0	48.13	233.37	0	0	7.29	0
62627	Yogurt, Fruit, Fat Free, Light	247.957	1	Cup	10	0	19	109.98	0	0	5	0
1121	Yogurt, Fruit, Lowfat, 10 Gm Protein Per 8 Oz	227	1	Cup	9.92	2.45	43.24	231.26	0	0	9.53	1.58
1122	Yogurt, Fruit, Lowfat, 11 Gm Protein Per 8 Oz	227	1	Cup	11.03	3.2	42.22	238.64	0	0	12.48	2.06
1120	Yogurt, Fruit, Lowfat, 9 Gm Protein Per 8 Oz	227	1	Cup	9.03	2.61	42.31	225.27	0	0	10.21	1.68
62603	Yogurt, Plain, Fat Free	247.957	1	Cup	13	0	17	119.98	0	0	5	0
1117	Yogurt, Plain, Lowfat, 12 Gm Protein Per 8 Oz	227	1	Cup	11.92	3.52	15.98	143.66	0	0	13.85	2.27
1118	Yogurt, Plain, Skim Milk, 13 Gm Protein Per 8 Oz	227	1	Cup	13.01	0.41	17.43	126.6	0	0	4.09	0.26
1116	Yogurt, Plain, Whole Milk, 8 Gm Protein Per 8 Oz	227	1	Cup	7.88	7.38	10.58	139.42	0	0	28.83	4.76
1119	Yogurt, Vanilla, Lowfat, 11 Gm Protein Per 8 Oz	227	1	Cup	11.19	2.84	31.33	193.96	0	0	11.12	1.83
4136	Butter, w/ Salt	5	1	Pat	0.05	4.06	0.01	35.85	0	0	10.95	2.53
1145	Butter, w/o Salt	5	1	Pat	0.04	4.06	0	35.84	0	0	10.95	2.52
1002	Butter, Whipped	11.011	1	Tbsp.	0.09	8.93	0.01	78.93	0	0	24.1	5.56
4002	Lard	205	0.25	Cup	0	51.2	0	460	0	0	48	20
4067	Margarine, Hard, Corn&sybn	4.7	1	Tsp.	0.04	3.78	0.04	33.78	0	0	0	0.71
4071	Margarine, Hard, Corn(hydr)	4.7	1	Tsp.	0.04	3.78	0.04	33.78	0	0	0	0.62
4128	Margarine, Imitation (appx 40% Fat)	4.805	1	Tsp.	0.02	1.86	0.02	16.59	0	0	0	0.37
4132	Margarine, Regular, w/ Salt Added	4.7	1	Tsp.	0.04	3.78	0.04	33.78	0	0	0	0.74
4131	Margarine, Regular, w/o Added Salt	4.7	1	Tsp.	0.02	3.77	0.02	33.56	0	0	0	0.71
4130	Margarine, Soft, w/ Salt Added	4.701	1	Tsp.	0.04	3.78	0.02	33.68	0	0	0	0.65
4129	Margarine, Soft, w/o Added Salt	4.701	1	Tsp.	0.04	3.78	0.04	33.68	0	0	0	0.65
4018	Mayonnaise	14.7	1	Tbsp.	0.13	4.91	3.51	57.29	0	0	3.82	0.72
62610	Mayonnaise, Fat Free	15.007	1	Tbsp.	0	0	3	10	0	0	0	0
62609	Mayonnaise, Light	15.007	1	Tbsp.	0	2	1	25.01	0	0	5	0
4053	Oil, Olive	13.511	1	Tbsp.	0	13.51	0	119.44	0	0	0	1.82
4042	Oil, Peanut	13.511	1	Tbsp.	0	13.51	0	119.44	0	0	0	2.28
4058	Oil, Sesame	13.637	1	Tbsp.	0	13.64	0	120.55	0	0	0	1.94
4044	Oil, Soybean	13.637	1	Tbsp.	0	13.64	0	120.55	0	0	0	1.96
4034	Oil, Soybean, (hydr)	13.637	1	Tbsp.	0	13.64	0	120.55	0	0	0	2.03
4543	Oil, Soybean, (hydr)&cttnsd	13.637	1	Tbsp.	0	13.64	0	120.55	0	0	0	2.45
4518	Oil, Vegetable Corn	13.637	1	Tbsp.	0	13.64	0	120.55	0	0	0	1.73
4582	Oil, Vegetable, Canola	13.637	1	Tbsp.	0	13.64	0	120.55	0	0	0	0.97
4501	Oil, Vegetable, Cocoa Butter	13.637	1	Tbsp.	0	13.64	0	120.55	0	0	0	8.14
4502	Oil, Vegetable, Cottonseed	13.637	1	Tbsp.	0	13.64	0	120.55	0	0	0	3.53
4055	Oil, Vegetable, Palm	13.637	1	Tbsp.	0	13.64	0	120.55	0	0	0	6.72
4513	Oil, Vegetable, Palm Kernel	13.637	1	Tbsp.	0	13.64	0	117.55	0	0	0	11.11
4510	Oil, Vegetable, Safflower, Linoleic	13.637	1	Tbsp.	0	13.64	0	120.55	0	0	0	1.24
4511	Oil, Vegetable, Safflower, Oleic	13.637	1	Tbsp.	0	13.64	0	120.55	0	0	0	0.83
4584	Oil, Vegetable, Sunflower	13.637	1	Tbsp.	0	13.64	0	120.55	0	0	0	1.33
62541	Salad Dressing, Blue Cheese	16.014	2	Tbsp.	0.5	3.5	2.5	45.04	0	0	5	2
62542	Salad Dressing, Blue Cheese, Fat Free	17.508	2	Tbsp.	0.25	0	6	25.01	0	0	0	0
	Salad Dressing, Ceasar	17.12	2	Tbsp.	0.17	17.12	1.31	155	0	0	1.11	3.22
	Salad Dressing, Creamy Italian	29.4	2	Tbsp.	0.03	16.12	2.33	147.43	0	0	1.22	2.43
4120	Salad Dressing, French	15.638	2	Tbsp.	0.09	6.41	2.74	67.2	0	0	9.07	1.49
62545	Salad Dressing, French, Fat Free	17.508	2	Tbsp.	0	0	6	25.01	0	0	0	0

Monounsaturated Fat (gm)	Polyunsaturated Fat (gm)	Vitamin D (mg)	Vitamin K (mg)	Vitamin E (mg)	Vitamin A (re)	Vitamin C (mg)	Thiamin (mg)	Riboflavin (mg)	Niacin (mg)	Vitamin B6 (mg)	Folate (mg)	Vitamin B12 (mcg)	Calcium (mg)	Iron (mg)	Magnesium (mg)	Phosphorus (mg)	Potassium (mg)	Sodium (mg)	Zinc (mg)
0	0	0	0	0	30.03	0	0	0	0	0	0	0	36.03	0	0	0	0	17.51	0
0.08	0.01	0	0	0.02	0	0	0	0	0	0	0	0	0.36	0.06	0.92	6.39	23.03	14.64	0.17
0	0	0	0	0	18.3	0	0	0	0	0	0	0	21.96	0	0	0	27.45	9.15	0
0	0	0	0	0	30	0	0	0	0	0	0	0	36	0	0	0	0	17.5	0
0	0	0	0	0	0	12	0	0	0	0	0	0	280	0	0	0	0	140	0
0	0	0	0	0	0	12	0	0	0	0	0	0	280	0	0	0	0	130	0
0	0	0	0	0	0	2.4	0	0	0	0	0	0	280	0.4	0	0	0	125	0
0	0	0	0	0	40	0	0	0	0	0	0	0	192	0	0	0	0	100	0
0	0	0	0	0	39.97	0	0	0	0	0	0	0	191.88	0	0	0	0	139.91	0
0	0	0	0	0	40	0	0	0	0	0	0	0	192	0	0	0	0	100	0
0	0	0	0	0	0	0	0	0	0	0	0	0	437.57	0	0	0	422.99	153.15	0
0	0	0	0	0	0	15	0	0	0	0	0	0	419.93	0.2	0	0	509.91	159.97	0
0.67	0.07	0	0	0.07	24.97	1.5	0.08	0.4	0.22	0.09	21.11	1.06	344.81	0.16	33.07	271.04	441.51	132.57	1.68
0.88	0.09	0	0	0	34.05	1.68	0.09	0.45	0.24	0.1	23.61	1.18	383.4	0.16	36.77	301.23	491	147.32	1.86
0.72	0.07	0	0	0.07	27.24	1.36	0.08	0.37	0.2	0.08	19.29	0.97	313.94	0.14	30.12	246.75	402.02	120.76	1.52
0	0	0	0	0	0	3.6	0	0.25	0	0	0	0	479.92	0	0	0.21	599.9	169.97	0
0.97	0.1	0	0	0.1	36.32	1.82	0.1	0.49	0.26	0.11	25.42	1.28	414.5	0.18	39.61	325.74	530.73	159.35	2.02
0.11	0.01	0	0	0.01	4.54	1.97	0.11	0.53	0.28	0.12	27.69	1.39	451.96	0.2	43.36	355.25	578.62	173.65	2.2
2.03	0.21	0	0	0.2	68.1	1.2	0.07	0.32	0.17	0.07	16.8	0.84	273.99	0.11	26.29	215.42	350.94	105.33	1.34
0.78	0.08	0	0	0.08	29.51	1.7	0.1	0.46	0.24	0.1	23.83	1.2	388.85	0.16	37.3	305.54	497.81	149.37	1.88
1.17	0.15	0	0	0.08	37.7	0	0	0	0	0	0.15	0.01	1.2	0.01	0.1	1.15	1.3	41.3	0
1.17	0.15	0	0	0.08	37.7	0	0	0	0	0	0.14	0.01	1.18	0.01	0.11	1.14	1.3	0.55	0
2.58	0.33	0	0	0.17	83.02	0	0	0	0	0	0.31	0.01	2.59	0.02	0.24	2.51	2.86	91.01	0.01
92.46	5.6	0	0	2.46	0	0	0	0	0	0	0	0	0.14	0	0.04	0	0.04	0.02	0.23
1.73	1.18	0	0	0.52	46.67	0.01	0	0	0	0	0.06	0	1.41	0	0.12	1.08	1.99	44.34	0
2.15	0.85	0	0	0.55	46.67	0.01	0	0	0	0	0.06	0	1.41	0	0.12	1.08	1.99	44.34	0
0.75	0.66	0	0	0.11	47.71	0	0	0	0	0	0.03	0	0.86	0	0.07	0.66	1.22	46.1	0
1.68	1.19	0	0	0.6	46.67	0.01	0	0	0	0	0.06	0	1.41	0	0.12	1.08	1.99	44.34	0
1.72	1.18	0	0	0.6	46.67	0	0	0	0	0	0.03	0	0.82	0	0.07	0.63	1.16	0.1	0
1.34	1.63	0	0	0.56	46.68	0.01	0	0	0	0	0.05	0	1.25	0	0.11	0.95	1.77	50.71	0
1.75	1.21	0	0	0.41	46.68	0.01	0	0	0	0	0.05	0	1.25	0	0.11	0.95	1.77	1.29	0
1.32	2.65	0	0	0.59	12.35	0	0	0	0	0	0.92	0.03	2.06	0.03	0.29	3.82	1.32	104.48	0.03
0	0	0	0	0	0	0	0	0	0	0	0	0	0	0	0	0	10	105.05	0
0	0	0	0	0	0	0	0	0	0	0	0	0	0	0	0	0	5	130.06	0
9.96	1.13	0	7.84	1.62	0	0	0	0	0	0	0	0	0.02	0.05	0	0.16	0	0.01	0.01
6.24	4.32	0	0.27	1.75	0	0	0	0	0	0	0	0	0.01	0	0.01	0	0	0.01	0
5.41	5.69	0	1.64	0.56	0	0	0	0	0	0	0	0	0	0	0	0	0	0	0
3.18	7.9	0	0	0.85	0	0	0	0	0	0	0	0	0.01	0	0	0.03	0	0	0
5.86	5.13	0	0	2.21	0	0	0	0	0	0	0	0	0	0	0	0	0	0	0
4.02	6.56	0	0	0.63	0	0	0	0	0	0	0	0	0	0	0	0	0	0	0
3.3	8	0	0.68	2.88	0	0	0	0	0	0	0	0	0	0	0	0	0	0	0
8.03	4.04	0	113.18	0	0	0	0	0	0	0	0	0	0	0	0	0	0	0	0
4.49	0.41	0	0	0.25	0	0	0	0	0	0	0	0	0	0	0	0	0	0	0
2.43	7.08	0	0	5.22	0	0	0	0	0	0	0	0	0	0	0	0	0	0	0
5.05	1.27	0	1.09	2.97	0	0	0	0	0	0	0	0	0	0	0	0	0.02	0	0
1.55	0.22	0	0	0.52	0	0	0	0	0	0	0	0	0	0	0	0	0	0	0
1.65	10.16	0	0.95	4.69	0	0	0	0	0	0	0	0	0	0	0	0	0	0	0
10.27	1.94	0	0	4.65	0	0	0	0	0	0	0	0	0	0	0	0	0	0	0
11.4	0.52	0	0	0	0	0	0	0	0	0	0	0	0	0	0	0	0	0	0
0	0	0	0	0	0	0	0	0	0	0	0	0	12.01	0	0	0	0	235.2	0
0	0	0	0	0.2	0	0	0	0	0	0	0	0	0	0	0	0	0	170.08	0
2.22	5.89	0	0	0.77	0.44	0	0	0	0	0	0	0	12.01	0	0	0	0	317.33	0
1.77	4.13	0	0	0.43	9.77	0	0	0	0	0	0	0	0.74	0.05	0	0	0	2.33	0
1.25	3.39	0	0	1.32	3.13	0	0	0	0	0	0.66	0.02	1.72	0.06	0	2.19	12.35	214.24	0.01
0	0	0	0	0	50.02	0	0	0	0	0	0	0	0	0	0	0	0	150.07	0

USDA ID Code	Food Name	Weight in Grams*	Quantity of Units	Unit of Measure	Protein (gm)	Fat (gm)	Carbohydrates (gm)	Kcalories	Caffeine (gm)	Fiber (gm)	Cholesterol (mg)	Saturated Fat (gm)
4020	Salad Dressing, French, Lo Fat	16.264	2	Tbsp.	0.03	0.94	3.53	21.83	0	0.05	0.98	0.13
	Salad Dressing, Honey Mustard	31.2	2	Tbsp.	0.05	6.33	14.22	102.11	0	0.23	0	1.33
4114	Salad Dressing, Italian	14.7	2	Tbsp.	0.1	7.1	1.5	68.69	0	0	0	1.03
62543	Salad Dressing, Italian, Fat Free	15.51	2	Tbsp.	0	0	1	5	0	0	0	0
4021	Salad Dressing, Italian, Lo Cal	15.013	2	Tbsp.	0.02	1.47	0.74	15.82	0	0.02	0.9	0.2
	Salad Dressing, Peppercorn	26.8	2	Tbsp.	0.02	16.22	1.1	151.22	0	0	13.11	3.11
	Salad Dressing, Poppy Seed	29.4	2	Tbsp.	0.02	12.31	6.41	130.44	0	0	0	2.33
62539	Salad Dressing, Ranch	14.519	2	Tbsp.	0	9.01	1	85.11	0	0	2.5	1.5
62540	Salad Dressing, Ranch, Fat Free	17.508	2	Tbsp.	0	0	5.5	25.01	0	0	0	0
	Salad Dressing, Raspberry Vinegrette	14.7	2	Tbsp.	0.1	7.1	1.5	68.69	0	0	0	1.03
4015	Salad Dressing, Russian	15.325	2	Tbsp.	0.25	7.79	1.59	75.71	0	0	2.76	1.12
4022	Salad Dressing, Russian, Low Cal	16.264	2	Tbsp.	0.08	0.65	4.49	23	0	0.05	0.98	0.1
4016	Salad Dressing, Sesame Seed	15.325	2	Tbsp.	0.48	6.93	1.32	67.91	0	0	0	0.95
4017	Salad Dressing, Thousand Island	15.638	2	Tbsp.	0.14	5.58	2.38	59	0	0.31	4.07	0.94
62544	Salad Dressing, Thousand Island, Fat Free	17.508	2	Tbsp.	0	0	5.5	22.51	0	0	0	0
4023	Salad Dressing, Thousand Island, Lo Cal	15.325	2	Tbsp.	0.12	1.64	2.48	24.31	0	0.18	2.3	0.25
4135	Salad Dressing, Vinegar and Oil	15.638	2	Tbsp.	0	7.83	0.39	70.18	0	0	0	1.42
11001	Alfalfa Seeds, Sprouted, Fresh	33	0.5	Cup	1.32	0.23	1.25	9.57	0	0.83	0	0.02
9007	Apples, Cnd, Sweetened	204	0.5	Cup	0.37	1	34.07	136.68	0	3.47	0	0.16
9009	Apples, Dehydrated, Sulfured	60	0.25	Cup	0.79	0.35	56.12	207.6	0	7.44	0	0.06
9003	Apples, Fresh, w/ Skin	138	1	Medium	0.26	0.5	21.05	81.42	0	3.73	0	0.08
9004	Apples, Fresh, w/o Skin	128	1	Medium	0.19	0.4	19	72.96	0	2.43	0	0.07
9028	Apricots, Cnd, Heavy Syrup Pack	258	1	Cup	1.32	0.23	55.34	214.14	0	0	0	0.02
9024	Apricots, Cnd, Juice Pack	248	1	Cup	1.56	0.1	30.6	119.04	0	3.22	0	0.01
9026	Apricots, Cnd, Light Syrup Pack	253	1	Cup	1.34	0.13	41.72	159.39	0	3.29	0	0.01
9022	Apricots, Cnd, Water Pack	243	0.5	Cup	1.73	0.39	15.53	65.61	0	3.16	0	0.03
9030	Apricots, Dehydrated, Sulfured	119	0.5	Cup	5.83	0.74	98.64	380.8	0	0	0	0.05
9032	Apricots, Dried, Sulfured	130	0.5	Cup	4.75	0.6	80.28	309.4	0	11.7	0	0.04
9021	Apricots, Fresh	35.333	3	Medium	1.5	0.4	11.8	51	0	1.4	0	0.01
9035	Apricots, Frozen, Sweetened	242	1	Cup	1.69	0.24	60.74	237.16	0	4.11	0	0.02
	Artichoke, Boiled, Hearts w/ Salt	84	0.5	Cup	2.923	0.134	9.391	42	0	4.536	0	0.031
	Artichoke, Boiled, Hearts w/o Salt	84	0.5	Cup	2.923	0.134	9.391	42	0	4.536	0	0.031
11705	Asparagus, Ckd	180	0.5	Cup	4.66	0.56	7.92	45	0	0	0	0.13
11015	Asparagus, Cnd	242	0.5	Cup	5.18	1.57	6	45.98	0	3.87	0	0.36
11011	Asparagus, Fresh	134	0.5	Cup	3.06	0.27	6.08	30.82	0	2.81	0	0.06
11019	Asparagus, Frz, Ckd	200	0.5	Cup	5.9	0.84	9.74	56	0	0	0	0.19
9037	Avocados, Fresh	201	1	Medium	3.98	30.79	14.85	323.61	0	11.86	0	4.9
11028	Bamboo Shoots, Cnd	131	0.5	Cup	2.25	0.52	4.22	24.89	0	3.93	0	0.12
11026	Bamboo Shoots, Fresh	151	0.5	Cup	3.93	0.45	7.85	40.77	0	3.32	0	0.1
	Banana, Dehydrated, Chips	100	1	Cup	3.89	1.81	88.28	346	0	7.5	0	0.698
9040	Bananas, Fresh	114	1	Medium	1.17	0.55	26.71	104.88	0	2.74	0	0.21
11924	Bean Sprouts	133.333	0.5	Cup	17.47	9.47	12.53	166.67	0	0	0	0
11056	Beans, Green, Cnd	136	0.5	Cup	1.56	0.14	6.12	27.2	0	2.58	0	0.03
11052	Beans, Green, Fresh	110	0.5	Cup	2	0.13	7.85	34.1	0	3.74	0	0.03
11061	Beans, Green, Fzn	135	0.5	Cup	1.84	0.19	8.26	35.1	0	4.46	0	0.04
11040	Beans, Lima, Fzn	180	1	Cup	11.97	0.54	35.01	189	0	0	0	0.12
11932	Beans, Yellow, Cnd	136	0.5	Cup	1.56	0.14	6.12	27.2	0	1.77	0	0.03
11722	Beans, Yellow, Fresh	110	0.5	Cup	2	0.13	7.85	34.1	0	1.98	0	0.03
11081	Beets, Ckd	170	1.5	Cup	2.86	0.31	16.93	74.8	0	2.89	0	0.05
9052	Blueberries, Cnd, Heavy Syrup	256	1	Cup	1.66	0.84	56.47	225.28	0	3.84	0	0
9050	Blueberries, Fresh	145	1	Cup	0.97	0.55	20.49	81.2	0	3.92	0	0
9055	Blueberries, Frozen, Sweetened	230	1	Cup	0.92	0.3	50.49	186.3	0	4.83	0	0
9054	Blueberries, Frozen, Unsweetened	155	1	Cup	0.65	0.99	18.86	79.05	0	4.19	0	0
11091	Broccoli, Ckd	156	0.5	Cup	4.65	0.55	7.89	43.68	0	4.52	0	0.08
11740	Broccoli, Flower Clusters, Fresh	88	1	Cup	2.62	0.31	4.61	24.64	0	0	0	0.05

Monounsaturated Fat (gm)	Polyunsaturated Fat (gm)	Vitamin D (mg)	Vitamin K (mg)	Vitamin E (mg)	Vitamin A (re)	Vitamin C (mg)	Thiamin (mg)	Riboflavin (mg)	Niacin (mg)	Vitamin B6 (mg)	Folate (mg)	Vitamin B12 (mcg)	Calcium (mg)	Iron (mg)	Magnesium (mg)	Phosphorus (mg)	Potassium (mg)	Sodium (mg)	Zinc (mg)
0.23	0.55	0	0	0.24	0	0	0	0	0	0	0	0	1.79	0.07	0	2.28	12.85	128	0.03
1.64	3.22	0	0	0.98	0	0.3	0	0	0	0	0	0	10.11	0.11	0	0	0	74.33	0
1.65	4.12	0	0	1.52	3.53	0	0	0	0	0	0.72	0.02	1.47	0.03	0.09	0.73	2.2	115.69	0.02
0	0	0	0	0	0	0	0	0	0	0	0	0	0	0	0	0	0	145.1	0
0.3	0.9	0	0	0.23	0	0	0	0	0	0	0	0	0.3	0.03	0	0.75	2.25	118.15	0.02
1.77	4.11	0	0	0	0	0.3	0	0	0	0	0	0	0.22	0.02	0	0	0	285.32	0
1.33	2.88	0	0	0	0	0.3	0	0	0	0	0	0	0.22	0.02	0	0	0	127.11	0
0	0	0	0	0	0	0	0	0	0	0	0	0	0	0	0	0	0	135.18	0
0	0	0	0	0.3	0	0	0	0	0	0	0	0	0	0	0	0	0	155.07	0
1.65	4.12	0	0	1.52	3.53	0	0	0	0	0	0.72	0.02	1.47	0.03	0.09	0.73	2.2	115.69	0.02
1.81	4.51	0	0	1.56	31.72	0.92	0.01	0.01	0.09	0	1.59	0.05	2.91	0.09	0.23	5.67	24.06	133.02	0.07
0.15	0.37	0	0	0.12	2.6	0.98	0	0	0	0	0.57	0.02	3.09	0.1	0.07	6.02	25.53	141.17	0.02
1.82	3.85	0	0	0.77	31.72	0	0	0	0	0	0	0	2.91	0	0	5.67	24.06	153.25	0.02
1.3	3.1	0	0	0.18	15.01	0	0	0	0	0	0.98	0.03	1.72	0.09	0.31	2.66	17.67	109.47	0.02
0	0	0	0	0	0	0	0	0	0	0	0	0	0	0	0	0	0	150.07	0
0.37	0.95	0	0	1.16	14.71	0	0	0	0	0	0.86	0.03	1.69	0.09	0.11	2.61	17.32	153.25	0.02
2.31	3.77	0	0	1.38	0	0	0	0	0	0	0	0	0	0	0	0	1.17	0.08	0
0.02	0.13	0	0	0.01	5.28	2.71	0.03	0.04	0.16	0.01	11.88	0	10.56	0.32	8.91	23.1	26.07	1.98	0.3
0.04	0.29	0	0	0.1	10.2	0.82	0.02	0.02	0.15	0.09	0.61	0	8.16	0.47	4.08	10.2	138.72	6.12	0.06
0.01	0.1	0	0	2.15	4.8	1.32	0.03	0.08	0.41	0.17	0.6	0	11.4	1.2	13.2	33	384	74.4	0.17
0.02	0.14	0	5.52	0.81	6.9	7.87	0.02	0.02	0.11	0.07	3.86	0	9.66	0.25	6.9	9.66	158.7	0	0.06
0.02	0.12	0	0.59	0.35	5.12	5.12	0.02	0.01	0.12	0.06	0.51	0	5.12	0.09	3.84	8.96	144.64	0	0.05
0.1	0.04	0	0	0	319.92	7.22	0.05	0.06	1.07	0.14	4.39	0	23.22	1.11	20.64	33.54	345.72	28.38	0.26
0.04	0.02	0	0	2.21	419.12	12.15	0.04	0.05	0.85	0.13	4.22	0	29.76	0.74	24.8	49.6	409.2	9.92	0.27
0.05	0.03	0	0	2.25	333.96	6.83	0.04	0.05	0.77	0.14	4.3	0	27.83	0.99	20.24	32.89	349.14	10.12	0.28
0.17	0.08	0	0	2.16	313.47	8.26	0.05	0.06	0.96	0.13	4.13	0	19.44	0.78	17.01	31.59	466.56	7.29	0.27
0.32	0.14	0	0	0	1507.73	11.31	0.05	0.18	4.26	0.62	5.24	0	72.59	7.51	74.97	186.83	2201.5	15.47	1.19
0.26	0.12	0	0	0	941.2	3.12	0.01	0.2	3.9	0.2	13.39	0	58.5	6.11	61.1	152.1	1791.4	13	0.96
0.06	0.1277	0	0	0.31	277	11	0.03	0.04	0.6	0.06	9	0	15	0.58	8	21	313	1	0.28
0.11	0.05	0	0	2.15	406.56	21.78	0.05	0.1	1.94	0.15	4.11	0	24.2	2.18	21.78	45.98	554.18	9.68	0.24
0.004	0.057	0	0	0.16	15.12	8.4	0.055	0.055	0.841	0.093	42.84	0	37.8	1.084	50.4	72.24	297.36	278.04	0.412
0.004	0.057	0	0	0.16	15.12	8.4	0.055	0.055	0.841	0.093	42.84	0	37.8	1.084	50.4	72.24	297.36	79.8	0.412
0.02	0.25	0	0	0	149.4	48.78	0.18	0.22	1.89	0.25	176.58	0	43.2	1.19	34.2	109.8	558	432	0.86
0.05	0.69	0	0	0	128.26	44.53	0.15	0.24	2.31	0.27	231.35	0	38.72	4.43	24.2	104.06	416.24	943.8	0.97
0.01	0.12	0	52.26	2.68	77.72	17.69	0.19	0.17	1.57	0.18	171.52	0	28.14	1.17	24.12	75.04	365.82	2.68	0.62
0.03	0.37	0	0	0	164	48.8	0.13	0.21	2.08	0.04	269.4	0	46	1.28	26	110	436	8	1.12
19.31	3.93	0	0	2.69	122.61	15.88	0.22	0.25	3.86	0.56	124.42	0	22.11	2.05	78.39	82.41	1203.99	20.1	0.84
0.01	0.23	0	0	0.5	1.31	1.44	0.03	0.03	0.18	0.18	4.19	0	10.48	0.42	5.24	32.75	104.8	9.17	0.85
0.01	0.2	0	0	1.51	3.02	6.04	0.23	0.11	0.91	0.36	10.72	0	19.63	0.76	4.53	89.09	804.83	6.04	1.66
0.153	0.337	0	0	0	31	7	0.18	0.24	2.8	0.44	14	0	22	1.15	108	74	1491	3	0.61
0.05	0.1	0	0.57	0.31	9.12	10.37	0.05	0.11	0.62	0.66	21.77	0	6.84	0.35	33.06	22.8	451.44	1.14	0.18
0	0	0	0	0	2.67	16	0.56	0.25	1.47	0.22	169.87	0	109.33	0.53	128	288	756	333.33	2.8
0.01	0.07	0	0	0.19	47.6	6.53	0.02	0.08	0.27	0.05	43.25	0	35.36	1.22	17.68	25.84	148.24	341.36	0.39
0.01	0.06	0	30.8	0.45	73.7	17.93	0.09	0.12	0.83	0.08	40.15	0	40.7	1.14	27.5	41.8	229.9	6.6	0.26
0.01	0.09	0	0	0.19	71.55	11.07	0.06	0.1	0.56	0.08	11.07	0	60.75	1.11	28.35	32.4	151.2	17.55	0.84
0.03	0.26	0	0	0	30.6	10.44	0.13	0.1	1.39	0.21	27.9	0	50.4	3.53	100.8	201.6	739.8	52.2	0.99
0.01	0.07	0	0	0.39	14.96	6.53	0.02	0.08	0.27	0.05	43.25	0	35.36	1.22	17.68	25.84	148.24	341.36	0.39
0.01	0.06	0	0	0.09	12.1	17.93	0.09	0.12	0.83	0.08	40.15	0	40.7	1.14	27.5	41.8	229.9	6.6	0.26
0.06	0.11	0	0	0.51	6.8	6.12	0.05	0.07	0.56	0.11	136	0	27.2	1.34	39.1	64.6	518.5	130.9	0.6
0	0	0	1.28	2.56	15.36	2.82	0.09	0.14	0.29	0.09	4.1	0	12.8	0.84	10.24	25.6	102.4	7.68	0.18
0	0	0	0	1.45	14.5	18.85	0.07	0.07	0.52	0.05	9.28	0	8.7	0.25	7.25	14.5	129.05	8.7	0.16
0	0	0	0	1.63	9.2	2.3	0.05	0.12	0.58	0.14	15.41	0	13.8	0.9	4.6	16.1	138	2.3	0.14
0	0	0	0	1.55	12.4	3.88	0.05	0.06	0.81	0.09	10.39	0	12.4	0.28	7.75	17.05	83.7	1.55	0.11
0.04	0.26	0	0	0.75	216.84	116.38	0.09	0.18	0.9	0.22	78	0	71.76	1.31	37.44	92.04	455.52	40.56	0.59
0.02	0.15	0	0	0	264	82.02	0.06	0.1	0.56	0.14	62.48	0	42.24	0.77	22	58.08	286	23.76	0.35

USDA ID Code	Food Name	Weight in Grams*	Quantity of Units	Unit of Measure	Protein (gm)	Fat (gm)	Carbohydrates (gm)	Kcalories	Caffeine (gm)	Fiber (gm)	Cholesterol (mg)	Saturated Fat (gm)
11093	Broccoli, Frz, Chopped, Ckd	184	1	Cup	5.7	0.22	9.84	51.52	0	5.52	0	0.03
11099	Brussels Sprouts, Ckd	156	1	Cup	3.98	0.8	13.53	60.84	0	6.71	0	0.16
	Cabbage, Chinese (pak-choi)	70	1	Cup	1.05	0.14	1.56	9.1	0	0.7	0	0.018
11110	Cabbage, Ckd	150	0.5	Cup	1.53	0.65	6.69	33	0	4.2	0	0.08
11749	Cabbage, Fresh	70	1	Cup	0.85	0.13	3.76	16.8	0	0	0	0.02
11960	Carrots, Baby, Fresh	10	3	Medium	0.7	0.1	7.3	31	0	1.1	0	0.1
11125	Carrots, Ckd	156	1	Cup	1.7	0.28	16.35	70.2	0	5.15	0	0.05
11128	Carrots, Cnd, Reg Pk	146	1	Cup	0.93	0.28	8.09	33.58	0	2.19	0	0.05
11124	Carrots, Fresh	60	1	Medium	0.62	0.11	6.08	25.8	0	1.8	0	0.02
11131	Carrots, Frz, Ckd	146	0.5	Cup	1.74	0.16	12.05	52.56	0	5.11	0	0.03
11136	Cauliflower, Ckd, Boiled	124	0.5	Cup	2.28	0.56	5.1	28.52	0	3.35	0	0.09
11135	Cauliflower, Fresh	100	0.5	Cup	1.98	0.21	5.2	25	0	2.5	0	0.03
11138	Cauliflower, Frz, Ckd	180	0.5	Cup	2.9	0.4	6.75	34.2	0	3.96	0	0.06
11144	Celery, Ckd	150	0.5	Cup	1.25	0.24	6.02	27	0	2.4	0	0.06
11143	Celery, Fresh	120	0.5	Cup	0.9	0.17	4.38	19.2	0	2.04	0	0.04
9066	Cherries, Sour, Red, Cnd, Heavy Syrup Pack	256	1	Cup	1.87	0.26	59.57	232.96	0	2.05	0	0.05
9065	Cherries, Sour, Red, Cnd, Light Syrup Pack	252	1	Cup	1.86	0.25	48.64	189	0	0	0	0.06
9064	Cherries, Sour, Red, Cnd, Water Pack	244	1	Cup	1.88	0.24	21.81	87.84	0	1.95	0	0.06
9067	Cherries, Sour, Red, Cnd, X-heavy Syrup Pack	261	1	Cup	1.85	0.23	76.29	297.54	0	0	0	0.05
9063	Cherries, Sour, Red, Fresh	103	0.5	Cup	1.03	0.31	12.55	51.5	0	1.24	0	0.07
9074	Cherries, Sweet, Cnd, Heavy Syrup Pack	257	1	Cup	1.54	0.39	54.66	213.31	0	1.8	0	0.09
9072	Cherries, Sweet, Cnd, Juice Pack	250	1	Cup	2.27	0.05	34.52	135	0	1.75	0	0.01
9073	Cherries, Sweet, Cnd, Light Syrup Pack	252	1	Cup	1.54	0.38	43.57	168.84	0	1.76	0	0.09
9071	Cherries, Sweet, Cnd, Water Pack	248	1	Cup	1.91	0.32	29.16	114.08	0	1.74	0	0.07
9075	Cherries, Sweet, Cnd, X-heavy Syrup Pack	261	1	Cup	1.54	0.39	68.46	266.22	0	0	0	0.09
9070	Cherries, Sweet, Fresh	145	0.5	Cup	1.74	1.39	24	104.4	0	3.34	0	0.31
9076	Cherries, Sweet, Frozen, Sweetened	259	1	Cup	2.98	0.34	57.91	230.51	0	2.59	0	0.08
	Chives, Raw	1	1	Tsp.	0.033	0.007	0.043	0.3	0	0.025	0	0.001
11159	Coleslaw	127.892	0.5	Cup	1.65	3.34	15.87	88.25	0	0	10.23	0.49
11162	Collards, Ckd	128	0.5	Cup	1.73	0.24	7.85	34.56	0	2.56	0	0
11161	Collards, Fresh	36	1	Cup	0.57	0.08	2.56	11.16	0	1.33	0	0
11164	Collards, Frz, Chopped, Ckd	170	1	Cup	5.05	0.7	12.09	61.2	0	0	0	0
20092	Corn, Ckd	140	0.5	Cup	3.68	1.02	39.07	176.4	0	6.72	0	0.14
11901	Corn, Sweet, White, Ckd	164	1	Cup	5.44	2.1	41.18	177.12	0	9.35	0	0.32
11905	Corn, Sweet, White, Cnd	164	1	Cup	4.3	1.64	30.49	132.84	0	2.3	0	0.25
11906	Corn, Sweet, White, Cnd, Cream Style	256	1	Cup	4.45	1.08	46.41	184.32	0	3.07	0	0.17
11900	Corn, Sweet, White, Fresh	154	1	Cup	4.96	1.82	29.29	132.44	0	4.93	0	0.28
11168	Corn, Sweet, Yellow, Ckd	164	1	Cup	5.44	2.1	41.18	177.12	0	4.59	0	0.32
11172	Corn, Sweet, Yellow, Cnd, Brine Pk	164	1	Cup	4.3	1.64	30.49	132.84	0	3.28	0	0.25
11174	Corn, Sweet, Yellow, Cnd, Cream Style	256	1	Cup	4.45	1.08	46.41	184.32	0	3.07	0	0.17
11167	Corn, Sweet, Yellow, Fresh	154	1	Cup	4.96	1.82	29.29	132.44	0	4.16	0	0.28
9077	Crabapples, Fresh	110	1	Cup	0.44	0.33	21.95	83.6	0	0	0	0.05
9078	Cranberries, Fresh	95	1	Cup	0.37	0.19	12.05	46.55	0	3.99	0	0
9081	Cranberry Sauce, Cnd, Sweetened	277	1	Cup	0.55	0.42	107.75	418.27	0	2.77	0	0
9082	Cranberry-orange Relish, Cnd	275	1	Cup	0.82	0.27	127.05	489.5	0	0	0	0
11205	Cucumber, Fresh	104	0.5	Cup	0.72	0.14	2.87	13.52	0	0.83	0	0.04
9087	Dates, Domestic, Natural and Dry	178	1	Cup	3.51	0.8	130.85	489.5	0	13.35	0	0
11210	Eggplant, Ckd	96	0.5	Cup	0.8	0.22	6.37	26.88	0	2.4	0	0.04
11209	Eggplant, Fresh	82	0.5	Cup	0.84	0.15	4.98	21.32	0	2.05	0	0.03
	Endive, Raw	25	0.5	Cup	0.313	0.05	0.837	4.25	0	0.775	0	0.012
9100	Fruit Hvy Syrup	255	1	Cup	0.99	0.18	48.22	186.15	0	2.81	0	0.03
9097	Fruit Juice Pack	248	1	Cup	1.14	0.02	29.41	114.08	0	2.73	0	0
9099	Fruit Lt Syrup	252	1	Cup	1.01	0.18	37.62	143.64	0	2.77	0	0.03
9105	Fruit Salad, Hvy Syrup	255	1	Cup	0.87	0.18	48.73	186.15	0	2.81	0	0.03
9103	Fruit Salad, Juice Pack	249	1	Cup	1.27	0.07	32.49	124.5	0	0	0	0.01

Monounsaturated Fat (gm)	Polyunsaturated Fat (gm)	Vitamin D (mg)	Vitamin K (mg)	Vitamin E (mg)	Vitamin A (re)	Vitamin C (mg)	Thiamin (mg)	Riboflavin (mg)	Niacin (mg)	Vitamin B6 (mg)	Folate (mg)	Vitamin B12 (mcg)	Calcium (mg)	Iron (mg)	Magnesium (mg)	Phosphorus (mg)	Potassium (mg)	Sodium (mg)	Zinc (mg)
0.01	0.1	0	0	0.88	347.76	73.78	0.1	0.15	0.84	0.24	103.78	0	93.84	1.12	36.8	101.2	331.2	44.16	0.55
0.06	0.41	0	0	1.33	112.32	96.72	0.17	0.12	0.95	0.28	93.6	0	56.16	1.87	31.2	87.36	494.52	32.76	0.51
0.011	0.067	0	0	0.084	210	31.5	0.028	0.049	0.35	0.136	45.99	0	73.5	0.56	13.3	25.9	176.4	45.5	0.133
0.05	0.29	0	0	0.16	19.5	30.15	0.09	0.08	0.42	0.17	30	0	46.5	0.26	12	22.5	145.5	12	0.14
0.01	0.06	0	0	0	9.1	35.7	0.04	0.02	0.21	0.07	39.69	0	32.9	0.39	10.5	16.1	172.2	12.6	0.13
0	0.03	0	0	0	2025	7	0.07	0.04	0.7	0.11	10	0	19	0.36	11	32	233	25	0.14
0.01	0.14	0	0	0.66	3829.8	3.59	0.05	0.09	0.79	0.38	21.68	0	48.36	0.97	20.28	46.8	354.12	102.96	0.47
0.01	0.13	0	0	0	2010.42	3.94	0.03	0.04	0.81	0.16	13.43	0	36.5	0.93	11.68	35.04	261.34	351.86	0.38
0	0.05	0	7.8	0.28	1687.8	5.58	0.06	0.04	0.56	0.09	8.4	0	16.2	0.3	9	26.4	193.8	21	0.12
0.01	0.08	0	0	0.61	2584.2	4.09	0.04	0.05	0.64	0.19	15.77	0	40.88	0.69	14.6	37.96	230.68	86.14	0.35
0.04	0.27	0	0	0.05	2.48	54.93	0.05	0.06	0.51	0.21	54.56	0	19.84	0.41	11.16	39.68	176.08	18.6	0.22
0.01	0.1	0	191	0.04	2	46.4	0.06	0.06	0.53	0.22	57	0	22	0.44	15	44	303	30	0.28
0.03	0.19	0	0	0.07	3.6	56.34	0.07	0.1	0.56	0.16	73.8	0	30.6	0.74	16.2	43.2	250.2	32.4	0.23
0.05	0.11	0	0	0.54	19.5	9.15	0.06	0.07	0.48	0.13	33	0	63	0.63	18	37.5	426	136.5	0.21
0.03	0.08	0	0	0.43	15.6	8.4	0.06	0.05	0.39	0.1	33.6	0	48	0.48	13.2	30	344.4	104.4	0.16
0.07	0.07	0	0	0.33	181.76	5.12	0.04	0.1	0.43	0.11	19.46	0	25.6	3.33	15.36	25.6	238.08	17.92	0.15
0.07	0.07	0	0	0	183.96	5.04	0.04	0.1	0.43	0.11	19.4	0	25.2	3.33	15.12	25.2	239.4	17.64	0.18
0.07	0.07	0	0	0.32	183	5.12	0.04	0.1	0.43	0.11	19.52	0	26.84	3.34	14.64	24.4	239.12	17.08	0.17
0.07	0.07	0	0	0	182.7	4.96	0.04	0.1	0.43	0.11	19.31	0	26.1	3.29	13.05	23.49	237.51	18.27	0.16
0.08	0.09	0	0	0.13	131.84	10.3	0.03	0.04	0.41	0.05	7.73	0	16.48	0.33	9.27	15.45	178.19	3.09	0.1
0.11	0.12	0	0	0.15	38.55	9.25	0.05	0.04	1.02	0.08	10.79	0	23.13	0.9	23.13	46.26	372.65	7.71	0.26
0.01	0.01	0	0	0.25	32.5	6.25	0.04	0.06	1.02	0.07	10.5	0	35	1.45	30	55	327.5	7.5	0.25
0.11	0.12	0	0	0.33	40.32	9.32	0.05	0.1	1.02	0.08	10.58	0	22.68	0.91	22.68	45.36	372.96	7.56	0.25
0.08	0.09	0	0	0.32	39.68	5.46	0.05	0.1	1.02	0.07	10.42	0	27.28	0.89	22.32	37.2	324.88	2.48	0.2
0.1	0.12	0	0	0	39.15	9.4	0.05	0.1	1.01	0.04	10.96	0	23.49	0.91	20.88	44.37	370.62	7.83	0.26
0.38	0.42	0	0	0.19	30.45	10.15	0.07	0.09	0.58	0.05	6.09	0	21.75	0.57	15.95	27.55	324.8	0	0.09
0.09	0.1	0	0	0.34	49.21	2.59	0.07	0.12	0.46	0.09	10.88	0	31.08	0.91	25.9	41.44	515.41	2.59	0.1
0.001	0.003	0	0	0.002	4.35	0.581	0.001	0.001	0.006	0.001	1.05	0	0.92	0.016	0.42	0.58	2.96	0.03	0.006
0.91	1.73	0	0	0	104.87	41.82	0.08	0.08	0.35	0.16	33.89	0	57.55	0.75	12.79	40.93	231.48	29.42	0.26
0	0	0	0	1.13	349.44	15.49	0.03	0.07	0.37	0.07	7.68	0	29.44	0.2	8.96	10.24	167.68	20.48	0.14
0	0	0	0	0.81	119.88	8.39	0.01	0.02	0.13	0.02	4.32	0	10.44	0.07	3.24	3.6	60.84	7.2	0.05
0	0	0	0	0	1016.6	44.88	0.08	0.2	1.08	0.19	129.37	0	357	1.9	51	45.9	426.7	85	0.46
0.27	0.46	0	0	0.46	8.4	0	0.07	0.03	0.78	0.08	8.4	0	1.4	0.35	50.4	106.4	43.4	0	0.88
0.61	0.99	0	0	0.15	0	10.17	0.35	0.12	2.65	0.1	76.1	0	3.28	1	52.48	168.92	408.36	27.88	0.79
0.48	0.77	0	0	0.15	0	13.94	0.05	0.13	1.96	0.08	79.7	0	8.2	1.41	32.8	106.6	319.8	529.72	0.64
0.31	0.51	0	0	0.23	0	11.78	0.06	0.14	2.46	0.16	114.69	0	7.68	0.97	43.52	130.56	343.04	729.6	1.36
0.53	0.86	0	0	0.42	0	10.47	0.31	0.09	2.62	0.08	70.53	0	3.08	0.8	56.98	137.06	415.8	23.1	0.69
0.61	0.99	0	0	0.15	36.08	10.17	0.35	0.12	2.65	0.1	76.1	0	3.28	1	52.48	168.92	408.36	27.88	0.79
0.48	0.77	0	0	0.25	26.24	13.94	0.05	0.13	1.96	0.08	79.7	0	8.2	1.41	32.8	106.6	319.8	529.72	0.64
0.31	0.51	0	0	0.23	25.6	11.78	0.06	0.14	2.46	0.16	114.69	0	7.68	0.97	43.52	130.56	343.04	729.6	1.36
0.53	0.86	0	10.78	0.14	43.12	10.47	0.31	0.09	2.62	0.08	70.53	0	3.08	0.8	56.98	137.06	415.8	23.1	0.69
0.01	0.1	0	0	0	4.4	8.8	0.03	0.02	0.11	0	0	0	19.8	0.4	7.7	16.5	213.4	1.1	0
0	0	0	0	0.1	4.75	12.83	0.03	0.02	0.1	0.06	1.62	0	6.65	0.19	4.75	8.55	67.45	0.95	0.12
0	0	0	3.88	0.28	5.54	5.54	0.04	0.06	0.28	0.04	0	0	11.08	0.61	8.31	16.62	72.02	80.33	0.14
0	0	0	0	0	19.25	49.5	0.08	0.05	0.27	0	0	0	30.25	0.55	11	22	104.5	88	0
0	0.06	0	5.2	0.08	21.84	5.51	0.02	0.02	0.23	0.04	13.52	0	14.56	0.27	11.44	20.8	149.76	2.08	0.21
0	0	0	0	0.18	8.9	0	0.16	0.18	3.92	0.34	22.43	0	56.96	2.05	62.3	71.2	1160.56	5.34	0.52
0.02	0.09	0	0	0.03	5.76	1.25	0.07	0.02	0.58	0.08	13.82	0	5.76	0.34	12.48	21.12	238.08	2.88	0.14
0.01	0.06	0	0	0.02	6.56	1.39	0.04	0.03	0.49	0.07	15.58	0	5.74	0.22	11.48	18.04	177.94	2.46	0.11
0.001	0.022	0	0	0.11	51.25	1.625	0.02	0.019	0.1	0.005	35.5	0	13	0.207	3.75	7	78.5	5.5	0.197
0.03	0.08	0	0	0.74	51	4.85	0.05	0.05	0.95	0.13	6.63	0	15.3	0.74	12.75	28.05	224.4	15.3	0.2
0.01	0.01	0	0	0.5	76.88	6.7	0.03	0.04	1	0.13	6.2	0	19.84	0.52	17.36	34.72	235.6	9.92	0.22
0.04	0.08	0	0	0.73	52.92	4.79	0.05	0.05	0.96	0.13	6.8	0	15.12	0.73	12.6	27.72	224.28	15.12	0.23
0.04	0.08	0	0	1.17	127.5	6.12	0.04	0.05	0.88	0.08	6.38	0	15.3	0.71	12.75	22.95	204	15.3	0.18
0.01	0.03	0	0	0	149.4	8.22	0.03	0.03	0.89	0.07	6.47	0	27.39	0.62	19.92	34.86	288.84	12.45	0.35

USDA ID Code	Food Name	Weight in Grams*	Quantity of Units	Unit of Measure	Protein (gm)	Fat (gm)	Carbohydrates (gm)	Kcalories	Caffeine (gm)	Fiber (gm)	Cholesterol (mg)	Saturated Fat (gm)
9104	Fruit Salad, Lt Syrup	252	1	Cup	0.86	0.18	38.15	146.16	0	0	0	0.02
9102	Fruit Salad, Water Pack	245	1	Cup	0.86	0.17	19.28	73.5	0	0	0	0.02
9096	Fruit Water Pack	245	1	Cup	1.03	0.12	20.85	78.4	0	2.69	0	0.01
9188	Fruit, Mixed, Dried	150.004	0.5	Cup	3.69	0.74	96.09	364.51	0	0	0	0.06
9189	Fruit, Mixed, Frzn, Swtnd, Thawd	250	1	Cup	3.55	0.45	60.57	245	0	4.75	0	0.06
9187	Fruit, Mixed, Hvy Syrup	255	1	Cup	0.94	0.26	47.84	183.6	0	0	0	0.04
	Garlic, Raw	3	1	Clove	0.191	0.015	0.992	4.47	0	0.063	0	0.003
9112	Grapefruit, Fresh, Pink&red	146	0.5	Medium	0.8	0.15	11.21	43.8	0	0	0	0.02
9116	Grapefruit, Fresh, White	136	0.5	Medium	0.94	0.14	11.44	44.88	0	1.5	0	0.02
9120	Grapefruit, Sections, Cnd, Juice Pack	249	1	Cup	1.74	0.22	22.93	92.13	0	1	0	0.03
9121	Grapefruit, Sections, Cnd, Light Syrup Pack	254	1	Cup	1.42	0.25	39.22	152.4	0	1.02	0	0.04
9119	Grapefruit, Sections, Cnd, Water Pack	244	1	Cup	1.42	0.24	22.33	87.84	0	0.98	0	0.03
9131	Grapes, Fresh	92	1	Cup	0.58	0.32	15.78	57.96	0	1.1	0	0.1
9400	Juice, Apple, Unsweetened	247.791	0.75	Cup	0.15	0.27	28.94	116.46	0	0	0	0.05
11655	Juice, Carrot, Cnd.	246	0.75	Cup	2.34	0.37	22.85	98.4	0	1.97	0	0.07
9080	Juice, Cranberry, Bottled	252.586	0.75	Cup	0	0.25	36.37	143.97	0	0	0	0
9135	Juice, Grape, Cnd. Or Bottle, Unsweetened	252.586	0.75	Cup	1.41	0.2	37.79	154.08	0	0.25	0	0.06
9124	Juice, Grapefruit, Cnd. Sweetened	249.389	0.75	Cup	1.45	0.22	27.76	114.72	0	0.25	0	0.03
9123	Juice, Grapefruit, Cnd. Unsweetened	246.991	0.75	Cup	1.28	0.25	22.13	93.86	0	0.25	0	0.03
9404	Juice, Grapefruit, Pink, Fresh	247	0.75	Cup	1.24	0.25	22.72	96.33	0	0	0	0.03
9128	Juice, Grapefruit, White, Fresh	247	0.75	Cup	1.24	0.25	22.72	96.33	0	0.25	0	0.03
62534	Juice, Guava	239.912	0.75	Cup	0	0	21.63	87.86	0	0	0	0
62535	Juice, Mango	239.912	0.75	Cup	0	0	21.63	87.86	0	0	0	0
9206	Juice, Orange, Fresh	248	0.75	Cup	1.74	0.5	25.79	111.6	0	0.5	0	0.06
9215	Juice, Orange, From Concentrate	248.59	0.75	Cup	1.69	0.15	26.8	111.87	0	0.5	0	0.02
62558	Juice, Orange, w/ Added Calcium	248.59	0.75	Cup	1.69	0.15	26.8	111.87	0	0.5	0	0.02
9232	Juice, Passion-fruit, Purple, Fresh	246.991	1	Cup	0.96	0.12	33.59	125.97	0	0.49	0	0
9233	Juice, Passion-fruit, Yellow, Fresh	246.991	1	Cup	1.65	0.44	35.69	148.19	0	0.49	0	0
9273	Juice, Pineapple, Cnd.	250.189	1	Cup	0.8	0.2	34.48	140.11	0	0.25	0	0.01
9294	Juice, Prune, Cnd	255.784	1	Cup	1.56	0.08	44.63	181.61	0	2.56	0	0.01
9223	Juice, Tangerine, Cnd. Sweetened	248.59	1	Cup	1.24	0.5	29.83	124.29	0	0.5	0	0.03
9221	Juice, Tangerine, Fresh	246.991	1	Cup	1.23	0.49	24.49	106.21	0	0.49	0	0.06
11886	Juice, Tomato, Cnd w/o Salt	244	1	Cup	1.85	0.15	10.32	41.48	0	1.95	0	0.02
11540	Juice, Tomato, Cnd.w/ Added Salt	244	1	Cup	1.85	0.15	10.32	41.48	0	0.98	0	0.02
62644	Juice, V-8, Low Salt	243	8	Fl Oz	1.6	0	8.2	40	0	0.25	0	0
11578	Juice, Vegetable, Cnd.	242	1	Cup	1.52	0.22	11.01	45.98	0	1.94	0	0.03
9148	Kiwifruit, Fresh	76	1	Medium	0.75	0.33	11.31	46.36	0	2.58	0	0
11247	Leeks, Ckd	104	0.5	Cup	0.84	0.21	7.92	32.24	0	0	0	0.03
11246	Leeks, Fresh	104	0.5	Cup	1.56	0.31	14.72	63.44	0	1.87	0	0.04
9150	Lemons, Fresh, w/o Peel	58	1	Medium	0.64	0.17	5.41	16.82	0	1.62	0	0.02
11250	Lettuce, Butterhead, Fresh	56	1	Cup	0.72	0.12	1.3	7.28	0	0.56	0	0.02
11252	Lettuce, Iceberg, Fresh	56	1	Cup	0.57	0.11	1.17	7.28	0	0.78	0	0.01
11253	Lettuce, Looseleaf, Fresh	56	1	Cup	0.73	0.17	1.96	10.08	0	1.06	0	0.02
11251	Lettuce, Romaine, Fresh	56	1	Cup	0.91	0.11	1.33	8.96	0	1.34	0	0.01
	Lime, Raw	67	1	Medium	0.469	0.134	7.062	20.1	0	1.876	0	0.015
9176	Mangos, Fresh	165	0.5	Cup	0.84	0.45	28.05	107.25	0	2.97	0	0.11
9185	Melon Balls, Frozen, Unthawed	173	1	Cup	1.45	0.43	13.74	57.09	0	1.21	0	0
9181	Melons, Cantaloupe, Fresh	80	1	Wedge	0.7	0.22	6.69	28	0	0.64	0	0
9183	Melons, Casaba, Fresh	164	1	Wedge	1.48	0.16	10.17	42.64	0	1.31	0	0
9184	Melons, Honeydew, Fresh	129	1	Wedge	0.59	0.13	11.84	45.15	0	0.77	0	0
11261	Mushrooms, Ckd	156	0.5	Cup	3.39	0.73	8.02	42.12	0	3.43	0	0.1
11264	Mushrooms, Cnd, Drained Solids	156	0.5	Cup	2.92	0.45	7.74	37.44	0	3.74	0	0.06
11950	Mushrooms, Enoki, Fresh	3	1	Medium	0.07	0.01	0.21	1.02	0	0	0	0
11260	Mushrooms, Fresh	70	0.5	Cup	1.46	0.29	3.26	17.5	0	0.84	0	0.04
11269	Mushrooms, Shiitake, Ckd	145	0.5	Cup	2.26	0.32	20.71	79.75	0	3.05	0	0.08

Monounsaturated Fat (gm)	Polyunsaturated Fat (gm)	Vitamin D (mg)	Vitamin K (mg)	Vitamin E (mg)	Vitamin A (re)	Vitamin C (mg)	Thiamin (mg)	Riboflavin (mg)	Niacin (mg)	Vitamin B6 (mg)	Folate (mg)	Vitamin B12 (mcg)	Calcium (mg)	Iron (mg)	Magnesium (mg)	Phosphorus (mg)	Potassium (mg)	Sodium (mg)	Zinc (mg)
0.03	0.07	0	0	0	108.36	6.3	0.04	0.05	0.92	0.08	6.55	0	17.64	0.73	12.6	22.68	206.64	15.12	0.18
0.03	0.07	0	0	0	107.8	4.65	0.04	0.05	0.92	0.08	6.37	0	17.15	0.73	12.25	22.05	191.1	7.35	0.2
0.02	0.05	0	0	0.71	61.25	5.14	0.04	0.03	0.89	0.13	6.61	0	12.25	0.61	17.15	26.95	230.3	9.8	0.22
0.35	0.17	0	0	0	366.01	5.7	0.07	0.24	2.89	0.24	5.85	0	57	4.07	58.5	115.5	1194.04	27	0.75
0.08	0.19	0	0	1.13	80	187.5	0.04	0.09	0.99	0.06	19	0	17.5	0.7	15	30	327.5	7.5	0.12
0.05	0.11	0	0	0	48.45	175.95	0.04	0.1	1.53	0.09	7.65	0	2.55	0.92	12.75	25.5	214.2	10.2	0.18
0	0.007	0	0	0	0	0.936	0.006	0.003	0.021	0.037	0.093	0	5.43	0.051	0.75	4.59	12.03	0.51	0.035
0.02	0.04	0	0	0	37.96	55.63	0.05	0.03	0.28	0.06	17.81	0	16.06	0.18	11.68	13.14	188.34	0	0.1
0.02	0.03	0	0	0.34	1.36	45.29	0.05	0.03	0.37	0.06	13.6	0	16.32	0.08	12.24	10.88	201.28	0	0.1
0.03	0.05	0	0	0.62	0	84.41	0.07	0.04	0.62	0.05	21.91	0	37.35	0.52	27.39	29.88	420.81	17.43	0.2
0.03	0.06	0	0	0.64	0	54.1	0.1	0.05	0.62	0.05	21.59	0	35.56	1.02	25.4	25.4	327.66	5.08	0.2
0.03	0.06	0	0	0.61	0	53.19	0.1	0.05	0.61	0.05	21.47	0	36.6	1	24.4	24.4	322.08	4.88	0.22
0.01	0.09	0	0	0.31	9.2	3.68	0.08	0.05	0.28	0.1	3.59	0	12.88	0.27	4.6	9.2	175.72	1.84	0.04
0.01	0.08	0	0	0.02	0	103.08	0.05	0.04	0	0.07	0.25	0	17.35	0.92	7.43	17.35	294.87	7.43	0.07
0.02	0.17	0	0	0.02	6334.5	20.91	0.23	0.14	0.95	0.53	9.35	0	59.04	1.13	34.44	103.32	718.32	71.34	0.14
0	0	0	0	0	0	89.42	0.02	0.02	0.09	0.05	0.51	0	7.58	0.38	5.05	5.05	45.47	5.05	0.18
0.01	0.06	0	0	0	2.53	0.25	0.07	0.09	0.66	0.16	6.57	0	22.73	0.61	25.26	27.78	333.41	7.58	0.13
0.03	0.05	0	0	0.12	0	67.09	0.1	0.06	0.8	0.05	25.94	0	19.95	0.9	24.94	27.43	404.01	4.99	0.15
0.03	0.06	0	0	0.12	2.47	72.12	0.1	0.05	0.57	0.05	25.69	0	17.29	0.49	24.7	27.17	377.9	2.47	0.22
0.03	0.06	0	0	0	108.68	93.86	0.1	0.05	0.49	0.11	25.19	0	22.23	0.49	29.64	37.05	400.14	2.47	0.12
0.03	0.06	0	0.05	0.12	2.47	93.86	0.1	0.05	0.49	0.11	25.19	0	22.23	0.49	29.64	37.05	400.14	2.47	0.12
0	0	0	0	0	0	40.55	0	0	0	0	0	0	0	0	0	0	0	23.65	0
0	0	0	0	0	0	40.55	0	0	0	0	0	0	0	0	0	0	0	23.65	0
0.09	0.1	0	0.1	0.22	49.6	124	0.22	0.07	0.99	0.1	75.14	0	27.28	0.5	27.28	42.16	496	2.48	0.12
0.02	0.03	0	0	0.47	19.89	96.7	0.2	0.04	0.5	0.11	108.88	0	22.37	0.25	24.86	39.77	472.32	2.49	0.12
0.02	0.03	0	0	0	19.89	96.7	0.2	0.04	0.5	0.11	108.88	0	298.31	0.25	24.86	39.77	472.32	2.49	0.12
0	0	0	0	0.12	177.83	73.6	0	0.32	3.61	0	0	0	9.88	0.59	41.99	32.11	686.64	14.82	0
0	0	0	0	0.12	595.25	44.95	0	0.25	5.53	0	0	0	9.88	0.89	41.99	61.75	686.64	14.82	0
0.02	0.07	0	0	0.05	0	26.77	0.14	0.06	0.64	0.24	57.79	0	42.53	0.65	32.52	20.02	335.25	2.5	0.28
0.05	0.02	0	0	0.03	0	10.49	0.04	0.18	2.01	0.56	1.02	0	30.69	3.02	35.81	63.95	705.96	10.23	0.54
0.04	0.06	0	0	0.22	104.41	54.69	0.15	0.05	0.25	0.08	11.44	0	44.75	0.5	19.89	34.8	442.49	2.49	0.07
0.09	0.1	0	0	0.22	103.74	76.57	0.15	0.05	0.25	0.1	11.36	0	44.46	0.49	19.76	34.58	439.64	2.47	0.07
0.02	0.06	0	0	2.22	136.64	44.65	0.11	0.08	1.64	0.27	48.56	0	21.96	1.42	26.84	46.36	536.8	24.4	0.34
0.02	0.06	0	0	2.22	136.64	44.65	0.11	0.08	1.64	0.27	48.56	0	21.96	1.42	26.84	46.36	536.8	880.84	0.34
0	0	0	0	0	62.5	39	0.04	0.05	0	0	0	0	31	1.2	0	0	439	41	0
0.03	0.09	0	0	0.77	283.14	67.03	0.1	0.07	1.76	0.34	51.06	0	26.62	1.02	26.62	41.14	467.06	883.3	0.48
0	0	0	0	0.85	13.68	74.48	0.02	0.04	0.38	0	0	0	19.76	0.31	22.8	30.4	252.32	3.8	0
0	0.12	0	0	0	5.2	4.37	0.03	0.02	0.21	0.12	25.27	0	31.2	1.14	14.56	17.68	90.48	10.4	0.06
0	0.17	0	0	0.96	10.4	12.48	0.06	0.03	0.42	0.24	66.66	0	61.36	2.18	29.12	36.4	187.2	20.8	0.12
0.01	0.05	0	0	0.14	1.74	30.74	0.02	0.01	0.06	0.05	6.15	0	15.08	0.35	4.64	9.28	80.04	1.16	0.03
0	0.07	0	0	0.25	54.32	4.48	0.03	0.03	0.17	0.03	41.05	0	17.92	0.17	7.28	12.88	143.92	2.8	0.1
0	0.06	0	63.28	0.06	18.48	2.18	0.03	0.02	0.1	0.02	31.36	0	10.64	0.28	5.04	11.2	88.48	5.04	0.12
0.01	0.09	0	0	0.25	106.4	10.08	0.03	0.04	0.22	0.03	27.89	0	38.08	0.78	6.16	14	147.84	5.04	0.16
0	0.06	0	0	0.25	145.6	13.44	0.06	0.06	0.28	0.03	75.99	0	20.16	0.62	3.36	25.2	162.4	4.48	0.14
0.013	0.037	0	0	0.161	0.67	19.49	0.02	0.013	0.134	0.029	5.49	0	22.11	0.402	4.02	12.06	68.34	1.34	0.074
0.17	0.08	0	0	1.85	641.85	45.71	0.1	0.09	0.96	0.22	0	0	16.5	0.21	14.85	18.15	257.4	3.3	0.07
0	0	0	0	0.26	306.21	10.73	0.29	0.04	1.11	0.18	44.46	0	17.3	0.5	24.22	20.76	484.4	53.63	0.29
0	0	0	0	0.12	257.6	33.76	0.03	0.02	0.46	0.09	13.6	0	8.8	0.17	8.8	13.6	247.2	7.2	0.13
0	0	0	0	0.25	4.92	26.24	0.1	0.03	0.66	0	0	0	8.2	0.66	13.12	11.48	344.4	19.68	0
0	0	0	0	0.19	5.16	31.99	0.1	0.02	0.77	0.08	0	0	7.74	0.09	9.03	12.9	349.59	12.9	0
0.01	0.29	0	0	0.19	0	6.24	0.11	0.47	6.96	0.15	28.39	0	9.36	2.71	18.72	135.72	555.36	3.12	1.36
0.01	0.18	0	0	0.19	0	0	0.13	0.03	2.49	0.1	19.19	0	17.16	1.23	23.4	102.96	201.24	663	1.12
0	0	0	0	0	0.03	0.36	0	0	0.11	0	0.9	0	0.03	0.03	0.48	3.39	11.43	0.09	0.02
0	0.12	1.33	5.6	0.08	0	2.45	0.07	0.31	2.88	0.07	14.77	0	3.5	0.87	7	72.8	259	2.8	0.51
0.1	0.04	0	0	0.17	0	0.44	0.05	0.25	2.18	0.23	30.31	0	4.35	0.64	20.3	42.05	169.65	5.8	1.93

USDA ID Code	Food Name	Weight in Grams*	Quantity of Units	Unit of Measure	Protein (gm)	Fat (gm)	Carbohydrates (gm)	Kcalories	Caffeine (gm)	Fiber (gm)	Cholesterol (mg)	Saturated Fat (gm)
11268	Mushrooms, Shiitake, Dried	3.6	1	Medium	0.34	0.04	2.71	10.66	0	0.41	0	0.01
9403	Nectar, Apricot, Cnd, w/ Added Vit C	250.988	0.75	Cup	0.93	0.23	36.12	140.55	0	0	0	0.02
9036	Nectar, Apricot, Cnd, w/o Vit C	250.988	0.75	Cup	0.93	0.23	36.12	140.55	0	1.51	0	0.02
9229	Nectar, Papaya, Cnd.	249.389	1	Cup	0.42	0.37	36.19	142.15	0	1.5	0	0.12
9251	Nectar, Peach, Cnd, wo/ Added Vit. C	248.59	1	Cup	0.67	0.05	34.6	134.24	0	1.49	0	0
	Nectarine, Raw	136	1	Medium	1.278	0.626	16.021	66.64	0	2.176	0	0.069
11279	Okra, Ckd	160	1	Cup	2.99	0.27	11.54	51.2	0	4	0	0.07
11278	Okra, Fresh	100	0.5	Cup	2	0.1	7.63	38	0	2.6	0	0.03
11281	Okra, Frz, Ckd	184	1	Cup	3.83	0.55	15.03	68.08	0	5.15	0	0.15
11280	Okra, Frz, Unprepared	142.514	0.5	Cup	2.41	0.36	9.46	42.75	0	3.14	0	0.09
62648	Olives, Green	3	5	Each	0	0.5	0	5	0	0	0	0
9194	Olives, Ripe, Canned (jumbo-super colossal)	8.3	1	Jumbo	0.08	0.57	0.47	6.72	0	0	0	0.08
9193	Olives, Ripe, Canned (small-extra large)	3.2	1	Small	0.03	0.34	0.2	3.68	0	0	0	0.05
11283	Onions, Ckd	239.797	2	Cup	3.26	0.46	24.34	105.51	0	3.36	0	0.07
11285	Onions, Cnd, Sol&liq	224	0.5	Cup	1.9	0.2	8.98	42.56	0	2.91	0	0.04
11282	Onions, Fresh	159.865	1	Cup	1.85	0.26	13.8	60.75	0	2.88	0	0.04
9200	Oranges, Fresh	131	1	Medium	1.23	0.16	15.39	61.57	0	3.14	0	0.02
9226	Papayas, Fresh	304	1	Medium	1.85	0.43	29.82	118.56	0	5.47	0	0.13
11808	Parsnips, Ckd, w/ Salt	156	0.5	Cup	2.06	0.47	30.47	126.36	0	0	0	0.08
11299	Parsnips, Ckd, w/o Salt	156	0.5	Cup	2.06	0.47	30.47	126.36	0	6.24	0	0.08
11298	Parsnips, Fresh	133	0.5	Cup	1.6	0.4	23.93	99.75	0	6.52	0	0.07
9241	Peaches, Cnd, Heavy Syrup Pack	256	1	Cup	1.15	0.26	51.05	189.44	0	2.56	0	0.03
9238	Peaches, Cnd, Juice Pack	248	1	Cup	1.56	0.07	28.69	109.12	0	2.48	0	0.01
9240	Peaches, Cnd, Light Syrup Pack	251	1	Cup	1.13	0.08	36.52	135.54	0	2.51	0	0.01
9237	Peaches, Cnd, Water Pack	244	1	Cup	1.07	0.15	14.91	58.56	0	2.44	0	0.01
9242	Peaches, Cnd, X-heavy Syrup Pack	262	1	Cup	1.23	0.08	68.28	251.52	0	0	0	0.01
9239	Peaches, Cnd, X-light Syrup	247	1	Cup	0.99	0.25	27.42	103.74	0	0	0	0.03
9244	Peaches, Dehydrated, Sulfured	116	0.25	Cup	5.67	1.19	96.49	377	0	0	0	0.13
9246	Peaches, Dried, Sulfured	160	0.25	Cup	5.78	1.22	98.13	382.4	0	13.12	0	0.13
9236	Peaches, Fresh	87	1	Medium	0.61	0.08	9.66	37.41	0	1.74	0	0.01
9250	Peaches, Frozen, Sliced, Sweetened	250	1	Cup	1.57	0.32	59.95	235	0	3.5	0	0.03
9340	Pears, Asian, Fresh	122	1	Medium	0.61	0.28	12.99	51.24	0	4.39	0	0.01
9257	Pears, Cnd, Heavy Syrup Pack	255	1	Cup	0.51	0.33	48.88	188.7	0	5.1	0	0.02
9254	Pears, Cnd, Juice Pack	248	1	Cup	0.84	0.17	32.09	124	0	4.96	0	0.01
9256	Pears, Cnd, Light Syrup Pack	251	1	Cup	0.48	0.08	38.08	143.07	0	5.02	0	0.01
9253	Pears, Cnd, Water Pack	244	1	Cup	0.46	0.07	19.06	70.76	0	4.88	0	0
9258	Pears, Cnd, X-heavy Syrup Pack	261	1	Cup	0.5	0.34	65.9	253.17	0	0	0	0.02
9255	Pears, Cnd, X-light Syrup Pack	247	1	Cup	0.74	0.25	30.13	116.09	0	0	0	0.01
9252	Pears, Fresh	166	1	Medium	0.65	0.66	25.08	97.94	0	3.98	0	0.04
11318	Peas and Carrots, Cnd	151.897	0.5	Cup	3.3	0.41	12.88	57.72	0	5.01	0	0.07
11323	Peas and Carrots, Frz, Ckd	160	0.5	Cup	4.94	0.67	16.19	76.8	0	5.76	0	0.12
11324	Peas and Onions, Cnd	120	0.5	Cup	3.94	0.46	10.28	61.2	0	0	0	0.08
11327	Peas and Onions, Frz, Ckd	180	0.5	Cup	4.57	0.36	15.53	81	0	5.4	0	0.06
11300	Peas, Edible-podded, Fresh	145	0.5	Cup	4.06	0.29	10.96	60.9	0	3.77	0	0.06
11305	Peas, Green, Ckd	160	0.5	Cup	8.58	0.35	25.02	134.4	0	8.8	0	0.06
11308	Peas, Green, Cnd	170	0.5	Cup	7.51	0.6	21.39	117.3	0	6.97	0	0.11
11310	Peas, Green, Cnd, Seasoned	170	0.5	Cup	5.25	0.46	15.73	85	0	0	0	0.08
11304	Peas, Green, Fresh	145	0.5	Cup	7.86	0.58	20.97	117.45	0	7.4	0	0.1
11313	Peas, Green, Frz, Ckd	160	0.5	Cup	8.24	0.43	22.82	124.8	0	8.8	0	0.08
11329	Peppers, Hot Chili, Green, Cnd	73	1	Each	0.66	0.07	4.45	18.25	0	1.39	0	0.01
11670	Peppers, Hot Chili, Green, Fresh	45	1	Each	0.9	0.09	4.26	18	0	0.68	0	0.01
11820	Peppers, Hot Chili, Red, Cnd	73	1	Each	0.66	0.07	4.45	18.25	0	0.95	0	0.01
11819	Peppers, Hot Chili, Red, Fresh	45	1	Each	0.9	0.09	4.26	18	0	0.68	0	0.01
11632	Peppers, Jalapeno, Cnd	136	0.25	Cup	1.09	0.82	6.66	32.64	0	0	0	0.08
11333	Peppers, Sweet, Green, Fresh	74	1	Medium	0.66	0.14	4.76	19.98	0	1.33	0	0.02

Monounsaturated Fat (gm)	Polyunsaturated Fat (gm)	Vitamin D (mg)	Vitamin K (mg)	Vitamin E (mg)	Vitamin A (re)	Vitamin C (mg)	Thiamin (mg)	Riboflavin (mg)	Niacin (mg)	Vitamin B6 (mg)	Folate (mg)	Vitamin B12 (mcg)	Calcium (mg)	Iron (mg)	Magnesium (mg)	Phosphorus (mg)	Potassium (mg)	Sodium (mg)	Zinc (mg)
0.01	0.01	1.49	0	0	0	0.13	0.01	0.05	0.51	0.03	5.88	0	0.4	0.06	4.75	10.58	55.22	0.47	0.28
0.1	0.04	0	0	0	331.3	136.54	0.02	0.04	0.65	0.06	3.26	0	17.57	0.95	12.55	22.59	286.13	7.53	0.23
0.1	0.04	0	0	0.2	331.3	1.51	0.02	0.04	0.65	0.06	3.26	0	17.57	0.95	12.55	22.59	286.13	7.53	0.23
0.1	0.09	0	0	0.05	27.43	7.48	0.01	0.01	0.37	0.02	5.24	0	24.94	0.85	7.48	0	77.31	12.47	0.37
0.02	0.03	0	0	0.02	64.63	13.18	0.01	0.03	0.72	0.02	3.48	0	12.43	0.47	9.94	14.92	99.44	17.4	0.2
0.237	0.313	0	0	1.21	100.64	7.34	0.023	0.056	1.346	0.034	5.032	0	6.8	0.099	10.88	21.76	288.32	0	0.122
0.04	0.07	0	0	1.1	92.8	26.08	0.21	0.09	1.39	0.3	73.12	0	100.8	0.72	91.2	89.6	515.2	8	0.88
0.02	0.03	0	0	0.69	66	21.1	0.2	0.06	1	0.22	87.8	0	81	0.8	57	63	303	8	0.6
0.09	0.15	0	0	1.27	93.84	22.45	0.18	0.23	1.44	0.09	267.9	0	176.64	1.23	93.84	84.64	430.56	5.52	1.14
0.06	0.09	0	0	0.98	65.56	17.67	0.13	0.15	1.01	0.06	210.35	0	115.44	0.81	61.28	59.86	300.7	4.28	0.76
0	0	0	0	0	0	0	0	0	0	0	0	0	0	0	0	0	0	13	0
0.42	0.05	0	0	0	2.91	0.12	0	0	0	0	0	0	7.8	0.28	0.33	0.25	0.75	74.53	0.02
0.25	0.03	0	0	0	1.28	0.03	0	0	0	0	0	0	2.82	0.11	0.13	0.1	0.26	27.9	0.01
0.06	0.18	0	0	0.31	0	12.47	0.1	0.06	0.4	0.31	35.97	0	52.76	0.58	26.38	83.93	398.06	7.19	0.5
0.03	0.08	0	0	0.43	0	9.63	0.07	0.01	0.14	0.31	21.73	0	100.8	0.29	13.44	62.72	248.64	831.04	0.65
0.04	0.1	0	0.83	0.21	0	10.23	0.03	0.04	0.24	0.19	30.37	0	31.97	0.35	15.99	52.76	250.99	4.8	0.3
0.03	0.03	0	1.77	0.31	27.51	69.69	0.11	0.05	0.37	0.08	39.69	0	52.4	0.13	13.1	18.34	237.11	0	0.09
0.12	0.09	0	0	3.4	85.12	187.87	0.08	0.1	1.03	0.06	115.52	0	72.96	0.3	30.4	15.2	781.28	9.12	0.21
0.17	0.07	0	0	0	0	20.28	0.13	0.08	1.13	0.15	90.79	0	57.72	0.9	45.24	107.64	572.52	383.76	0.41
0.17	0.07	0	0	1.56	0	20.28	0.13	0.08	1.13	0.15	90.79	0	57.72	0.9	45.24	107.64	572.52	15.6	0.41
0.15	0.06	0	0	1.33	0	22.61	0.12	0.07	0.93	0.12	88.84	0	47.88	0.78	38.57	94.43	498.75	13.3	0.78
0.09	0.12	0	0	2.28	84.48	7.17	0.03	0.06	1.57	0.05	8.19	0	7.68	0.69	12.8	28.16	235.52	15.36	0.23
0.03	0.04	0	7.44	3.72	94.24	8.93	0.02	0.04	1.44	0.05	8.43	0	14.88	0.67	17.36	42.16	317.44	9.92	0.27
0.03	0.04	0	0	2.23	87.85	6.02	0.02	0.06	1.49	0.05	8.28	0	7.53	0.9	12.55	27.61	243.47	12.55	0.23
0.05	0.07	0	0	2.17	129.32	7.08	0.02	0.05	1.27	0.05	8.3	0	4.88	0.78	12.2	24.4	241.56	7.32	0.22
0.03	0.04	0	0	0	34.06	3.14	0.03	0.06	1.36	0.05	8.12	0	7.86	0.76	13.1	28.82	217.46	20.96	0.24
0.09	0.12	0	0	0	66.69	7.41	0.05	0.05	1.98	0.05	8.15	0	12.35	0.74	12.35	27.17	182.78	12.35	0.22
0.44	0.58	0	0	0	164.72	12.3	0.05	0.13	5.6	0.18	7.66	0	44.08	6.39	66.12	187.92	1567.16	11.6	0.9
0.44	0.59	0	0	0	345.6	7.68	0	0.34	7	0.11	0.48	0	44.8	6.5	67.2	190.4	1593.6	11.2	0.91
0.03	0.04	0	0	0.61	46.98	5.74	0.01	0.04	0.86	0.02	2.96	0	4.35	0.1	6.09	10.44	171.39	0	0.12
0.12	0.16	0	0	2.22	70	235.5	0.03	0.09	1.63	0.04	8	0	7.5	0.92	12.5	27.5	325	15	0.12
0.06	0.07	0	0	0.61	0	4.64	0.01	0.01	0.27	0.03	9.76	0	4.88	0	9.76	13.42	147.62	0	0.02
0.07	0.08	0	0	1.28	0	2.81	0.03	0.06	0.62	0.04	3.06	0	12.75	0.56	10.2	17.85	165.75	12.75	0.2
0.03	0.04	0	1.14	1.24	2.48	3.97	0.03	0.03	0.5	0.03	2.98	0	22.32	0.72	17.36	29.76	238.08	9.92	0.22
0.02	0.02	0	0	1.26	0	1.76	0.03	0.04	0.39	0.04	3.01	0	12.55	0.7	10.04	17.57	165.66	12.55	0.2
0.01	0.02	0	0	1.22	0	2.44	0.02	0.02	0.13	0.03	2.93	0	9.76	0.51	9.76	17.08	129.32	4.88	0.22
0.07	0.08	0	0	0	0	2.87	0.03	0.06	0.62	0.04	3.13	0	13.05	0.57	10.44	18.27	167.04	13.05	0.21
0.05	0.06	0	0	0	0	4.94	0.02	0.05	0.99	0.03	2.96	0	17.29	0.49	12.35	17.29	111.15	4.94	0.17
0.14	0.16	0	0	0.83	3.32	6.64	0.03	0.07	0.17	0.03	12.12	0	18.26	0.42	9.96	18.26	207.5	0	0.2
0.03	0.2	0	0	0.64	876.45	10.03	0.11	0.08	0.88	0.13	27.8	0	34.94	1.14	21.27	69.87	151.9	394.93	0.88
0.06	0.32	0	0	0.51	1241.6	12.96	0.36	0.1	1.85	0.14	41.6	0	36.8	1.5	25.6	78.4	252.8	108.8	0.72
0.04	0.21	0	0	0	19.2	3.6	0.12	0.08	1.54	0.23	31.92	0	20.4	1.04	19.2	61.2	115.2	530.4	0.7
0.03	0.17	0	0	0.27	63	12.42	0.27	0.12	1.88	0.16	35.82	0	25.2	1.69	23.4	61.2	210.6	66.6	0.52
0.03	0.13	0	0	0.57	20.3	87	0.22	0.12	0.87	0.23	60.47	0	62.35	3.02	34.8	76.85	290	5.8	0.39
0.03	0.16	0	0	0.62	96	22.72	0.41	0.24	3.23	0.35	101.28	0	43.2	2.46	62.4	187.2	433.6	4.8	1.9
0.05	0.28	0	0	0.65	130.9	16.32	0.21	0.13	1.24	0.11	75.31	0	34	1.62	28.9	113.9	294.1	372.3	1.21
0.04	0.22	0	0	0	73.1	19.55	0.16	0.12	1.17	0.17	48.62	0	25.5	2.04	25.5	91.8	207.4	431.8	1.11
0.05	0.27	0	0	0.57	92.8	58	0.39	0.19	3.03	0.25	94.25	0	36.25	2.13	47.85	156.6	353.8	7.25	1.8
0.04	0.21	0	0	0.27	107.2	15.84	0.45	0.16	2.37	0.18	93.76	0	38.4	2.51	46.4	144	268.8	139.2	1.5
0	0.04	0	0	0.5	44.53	49.64	0.01	0.04	0.58	0.11	7.3	0	5.11	0.37	10.22	12.41	136.51	856.29	0.12
0	0.05	0	0	0.31	34.65	109.13	0.04	0.04	0.43	0.13	10.53	0	8.1	0.54	11.25	20.7	153	3.15	0.14
0	0.04	0	0	0.34	867.97	49.64	0.01	0.04	0.58	0.11	7.3	0	5.11	0.37	10.22	12.41	136.51	856.29	0.12
0	0.05	0	0	0.31	483.75	109.13	0.04	0.04	0.43	0.13	10.53	0	8.1	0.54	11.25	20.7	153	3.15	0.14
0.05	0.44	0	0	0	231.2	17.68	0.04	0.07	0.68	0.28	18.36	0	35.36	3.81	16.32	23.12	184.96	1989.68	0.26
0.01	0.08	0	0	0.51	46.62	66.08	0.05	0.02	0.38	0.18	16.28	0	6.66	0.34	7.4	14.06	130.98	1.48	0.09

USDA ID Code	Food Name	Weight in Grams*	Quantity of Units	Unit of Measure	Protein (gm)	Fat (gm)	Carbohydrates (gm)	Kcalories	Caffeine (gm)	Fiber (gm)	Cholesterol (mg)	Saturated Fat (gm)
11821	Peppers, Sweet, Red, Fresh	74	1	Medium	0.66	0.14	4.76	19.98	0	1.7	0	0.02
11951	Peppers, Sweet, Yellow, Fresh	74	1	Medium	0.74	0.16	4.68	19.98	0	0	0	0
	Persimmon, Japanese, Raw	168	1	Medium	0.974	0.319	31.23	117.6	0	6.048	0	0.034
11941	Pickle, Cucumber ,Sour	7	1	Slice	0.02	0.01	0.16	0.77	0	0.08	0	0
11937	Pickle, Cucumber, Dill	6	1	Slice	0.04	0.01	0.25	1.08	0	0.07	0	0
11947	Pickle, Cucumber, Dill, Low Sodium	6	1	Slice	0.04	0.01	0.25	1.08	0	0	0	0
11946	Pickle, Cucumber, Sour, Low Sodium	7	1	Slice	0.02	0.01	0.16	0.77	0	0.08	0	0
11940	Pickle, Cucumber, Sweet	6	1	Slice	0.02	0.02	1.91	7.02	0	0.07	0	0
11948	Pickle, Cucumber, Sweet, Low Sodium	6	1	Slice	0.02	0.02	1.91	7.02	0	0.09	0	
9270	Pineapple, Cnd, Heavy Syrup Pack	255	1	Cup	0.89	0.28	51.51	198.9	0	1.79	0	0.02
9268	Pineapple, Cnd, Juice Pack	250	1	Cup	1.05	0.2	39.25	150	0	1.75	0	0.01
9269	Pineapple, Cnd, Light Syrup Pack	252	1	Cup	0.91	0.3	33.89	131.04	0	1.76	0	0.02
9267	Pineapple, Cnd, Water Pack	246	1	Cup	1.06	0.22	20.42	78.72	0	1.72	0	0.01
9271	Pineapple, Cnd, X-heavy Syrup Pack	260	1	Cup	0.88	0.29	55.9	215.8	0	0	0	0.02
9266	Pineapple, Fresh	84	1	Slice	0.33	0.36	10.41	41.16	0	1.01	0	0.03
	Plantain, Raw	179	1	Medium	2.327	0.662	57.08	218.38	0	4.117	0	0.256
9284	Plums, Cnd, Purple, Heavy Syrup Pack	258	1	Cup	0.93	0.26	59.96	229.62	0	2.58	0	0.02
9282	Plums, Cnd, Purple, Juice Pack	252	1	Cup	1.29	0.05	38.18	146.16	0	2.52	0	0.01
9283	Plums, Cnd, Purple, Light Syrup Pack	252	1	Cup	0.93	0.25	41.03	158.76	0	2.52	0	0.02
9281	Plums, Cnd, Purple, Water Pack	249	1	Cup	0.97	0.02	27.46	102.09	0	2.49	0	0
9285	Plums, Cnd, Purple, X-heavy Syrup Pack	261	1	Cup	0.94	0.26	68.67	263.61	0	0	0	0.02
9279	Plums, Fresh	66	1	Medium	0.52	0.41	8.59	36.3	0	0.99	0	0.03
11672	Potato Pancakes, Home-prepared	28.35	1	Ounce	1.75	4.32	8.12	77.11	0	0.57	27.22	0.86
11399	Potato Puffs, Frz, Prepared	7	1	Each	0.23	0.75	2.13	15.54	0	0.22	0	0.36
11414	Potato Salad	250	0.5	Cup	6.7	20.5	27.92	357.5	0	0	170	3.57
11843	Potatoes, Au Gratin, Home-prepared	245	1	Cup	12.4	18.6	27.61	323.4	0	0	36.75	8.65
11363	Potatoes, Baked w/o Skin	202	1	Medium	3.96	0.2	43.55	187.86	0	3.03	0	0.05
11364	Potatoes, Baked, Skin only	58	1	Each	2.49	0.06	26.72	114.84	0	2.32	0	0.02
11674	Potatoes, Baked, w/ Skin	202	1	Medium	4.65	0.2	50.96	220.18	0	4.85	0	0.05
11365	Potatoes, Boiled, Ckd In Skin w/o Skin	202	1	Medium	3.78	0.2	40.66	175.74	0	3.64	0	0.05
11367	Potatoes, Boiled, Ckd w/o Skin	202	1	Medium	3.45	0.2	40.42	173.72	0	3.64	0	0.05
11366	Potatoes, Boiled, Skin only	34	1	Each	0.97	0.03	5.85	26.52	0	0	0	0.01
11376	Potatoes, Cnd, Drained Solids	180	0.5	Cup	2.54	0.38	24.5	108	0	0	0	0.1
11374	Potatoes, Cnd, Solids and Liquids	300	0.5	Cup	4.08	0.45	25.98	120	0	4.8	0	0.12
11370	Potatoes, Hashed Brown	156	0.5	Cup	3.78	21.7	11.58	238.68	0	3.12	0	8.48
11657	Potatoes, Mashed, Home-prepared	210	1	Cup	4.07	1.24	36.86	161.7	0	4.2	4.2	0.7
11930	Potatoes, Mashed, Prepared From Flakes	210	1	Cup	3.99	11.76	31.54	237.3	0	0	8.4	3.07
11368	Potatoes, Microwaved w/o Skin	156	0.5	Cup	3.28	0.16	36.32	156	0	0	0	0.04
11369	Potatoes, Microwaved, Skin only	58	1	Each	2.55	0.06	17.19	76.56	0	0	0	0.02
11675	Potatoes, Microwaved, w/ Skin	202	1	Medium	4.93	0.2	48.74	212.1	0	0	0	0.05
11671	Potatoes, O'brien, Home-prepared	194	1	Cup	4.56	2.48	30.01	157.14	0	0	7.76	1.55
11844	Potatoes, Scalloped	245	0.5	Cup	7.03	9.02	26.41	210.7	0	0	14.7	3.37
9289	Prunes, Dehydrated	132	0.5	Cup	4.88	0.96	117.57	447.48	0	0	0	0.08
9293	Prunes, Dried, Stewed, w/ Added Sugar	238	0.5	Cup	2.59	0.52	78.25	295.12	0	9.04	0	0.04
9292	Prunes, Dried, Stewed, w/o Added Sugar	212	0.5	Cup	2.48	0.49	59.53	226.84	0	13.99	0	0.04
9291	Prunes, Dried, Uncooked	161	0.5	Cup	4.2	0.84	101	384.79	0	11.43	0	0.07
11423	Pumpkin, Ckd	245	1	Cup	1.76	0.17	11.98	49	0	0	0	0.09
11424	Pumpkin, Cnd, w/o Salt	245	1	Cup	2.69	0.69	19.8	83.3	0	6.86	0	0.36
11429	Radishes, Fresh	116	0.5	Cup	0.7	0.63	4.16	19.72	0	1.86	0	0.03
11431	Radishes, Oriental, Ckd	147	0.5	Cup	0.98	0.35	5.04	24.99	0	2.35	0	0.11
11432	Radishes, Oriental, Dried	116	1	Cup	9.16	0.84	73.51	314.36	0	0	0	0.25
11430	Radishes, Oriental, Fresh	88	0.5	Cup	0.53	0.09	3.62	15.84	0	1.41	0	0.03
11637	Radishes, White Icicle, Fresh	100	0.5	Cup	1.1	0.1	2.63	14	0	0	0	0.03
9297	Raisins, Golden Seedless	145	0.66	Cup	3.4	0.5	79.5	302	0	5.8	0	0.22
9299	Raisins, Seeded	145	0.66	Cup	2.5	0.5	78.5	296	0	9.86	0	0.26

Monounsaturated Fat (gm)	Polyunsaturated Fat (gm)	Vitamin D (mg)	Vitamin K (mg)	Vitamin E (mg)	Vitamin A (re)	Vitamin C (mg)	Thiamin (mg)	Riboflavin (mg)	Niacin (mg)	Vitamin B6 (mg)	Folate (mg)	Vitamin B12 (mcg)	Calcium (mg)	Iron (mg)	Magnesium (mg)	Phosphorus (mg)	Potassium (mg)	Sodium (mg)	Zinc (mg)
0.01	0.08	0	0	0.51	421.8	140.6	0.05	0.02	0.38	0.18	16.28	0	6.66	0.34	7.4	14.06	130.98	1.48	0.09
0	0	0	0	0	17.76	135.79	0.02	0.02	0.66	0.12	19.24	0	8.14	0.34	8.88	17.76	156.88	1.48	0.13
0.062	0.072	0	0	0.991	364.56	12.6	0.05	0.034	0.168	0.168	12.6	0	13.44	0.252	15.12	28.56	270.48	1.68	0.185
0	0.01	0	0	0.01	1.05	0.07	0	0	0	0	0.05	0	0	0.03	0.28	0.98	1.61	84.56	0
0	0	0	0	0.01	1.98	0.11	0	0	0	0	0.06	0	0.54	0.03	0.66	1.26	6.96	76.92	0.01
0	0	0	0	0	1.98	0.11	0	0	0	0	0.06	0	0.54	0.03	0.66	1.26	6.96	1.08	0.01
0	0.01	0	0	0	1.05	0.07	0	0	0	0	0	0	0	0.03	0.28	0.98	1.61	1.26	0
0	0.01	0	0	0.01	0.78	0.07	0	0	0.01	0	0.06	0	0.24	0.04	0.24	0.72	1.92	56.34	0
0	0.01	0	0	0.01	0.78	0.07	0	0	0.01	0	0.06	0	0.24	0.04	0.24	0.72	1.92	1.08	0
0.03	0.1	0	0	0.26	2.55	18.87	0.23	0.06	0.73	0.19	11.73	0	35.7	0.97	40.8	17.85	265.2	2.55	0.31
0.02	0.07	0	0	0.25	10	23.75	0.24	0.05	0.71	0.18	12	0	35	0.7	35	15	305	2.5	0.25
0.03	0.1	0	0	0.25	2.52	18.9	0.23	0.06	0.74	0.19	11.84	0	35.28	0.98	40.32	17.64	264.6	2.52	0.3
0.03	0.08	0	0	0.25	4.92	18.94	0.23	0.06	0.73	0.18	11.81	0	36.9	0.98	44.28	9.84	312.42	2.46	0.3
0.03	0.1	0	0	0	2.6	18.98	0.23	0.07	0.73	0.19	11.96	0	36.4	0.99	39	18.2	265.2	2.6	0.29
0.04	0.12	0	0	0.08	1.68	12.94	0.08	0.03	0.35	0.07	8.9	0	5.88	0.31	11.76	5.88	94.92	0.84	0.07
0.057	0.124	0	0	0.483	202.27	32.936	0.093	0.097	1.228	0.535	39.38	0	5.37	1.074	66.23	60.86	893.21	7.16	0.251
0.17	0.06	0	0	1.81	67.08	1.03	0.04	0.1	0.75	0.07	6.45	0	23.22	2.17	12.9	33.54	234.78	49.02	0.18
0.04	0.01	0	0	1.76	254.52	7.06	0.06	0.15	1.19	0.07	6.55	0	25.2	0.86	20.16	37.8	388.08	2.52	0.28
0.17	0.06	0	0	1.76	65.52	1.01	0.04	0.1	0.75	0.07	6.55	0	22.68	2.17	12.6	32.76	234.36	50.4	0.2
0.01	0	0	0	1.74	226.59	6.72	0.05	0.1	0.92	0.07	6.47	0	17.43	0.4	12.45	32.37	313.74	2.49	0.2
0.17	0.05	0	0	0	65.25	1.04	0.04	0.1	0.74	0.07	6.53	0	23.49	2.14	13.05	31.32	232.29	49.59	0.18
0.27	0.09	0	0	0.4	21.12	6.27	0.03	0.06	0.33	0.05	1.45	0	2.64	0.07	4.62	6.6	113.52	0	0.07
1.32	1.85	0	0	0.04	3.97	6.24	0.04	0.05	0.61	0.11	6.8	0.05	6.8	0.44	9.36	31.47	222.83	144.02	0.24
0.3	0.06	0	0	0	0.14	0.48	0.01	0.01	0.15	0.02	1.16	0	2.1	0.11	1.33	3.36	26.6	52.22	0.02
6.2	9.34	0	0	0	82.5	25	0.19	0.15	2.22	0.35	16.75	0	47.5	1.62	37.5	130	635	1322.5	0.77
6.34	2.64	0	0	0	93.1	24.25	0.16	0.28	2.43	0.43	19.84	0	291.55	1.57	49	276.85	970.2	1060.85	1.69
0	0.09	0	0.44	0.08	0	25.86	0.21	0.04	2.82	0.61	18.38	0	10.1	0.71	50.5	101	789.82	10.1	0.59
0	0.02	0	0	0.02	0	7.83	0.07	0.06	1.78	0.36	12.53	0	19.72	4.08	24.94	58.58	332.34	12.18	0.28
0	0.09	0	1.07	0.1	0	26.06	0.22	0.07	3.32	0.7	22.22	0	20.2	2.75	54.54	115.14	844.36	16.16	0.65
0	0.09	0	0	0.1	0	26.26	0.21	0.04	2.91	0.6	20.2	0	10.1	0.63	44.44	88.88	765.58	8.08	0.61
0	0.09	0	0	0.1	0	14.95	0.2	0.04	2.65	0.54	17.98	0	16.16	0.63	40.4	80.8	662.56	10.1	0.55
0	0.01	0	0	0	0	1.77	0.01	0.01	0.42	0.08	3.3	0	15.3	2.06	10.2	18.36	138.38	4.76	0.15
0.01	0.16	0	0	0	0	9.18	0.12	0.02	1.65	0.34	11.16	0	9	2.27	25.2	50.4	412.2	468	0.5
0.01	0.19	0	0	0.12	0	37.2	0.1	0.06	2.67	0.41	13.5	0	90	2.91	42	66	729	903	1.17
9.69	2.5	0	0	0.3	0	8.89	0.12	0.03	3.12	0.43	12.01	0	12.48	1.26	31.2	65.52	500.76	37.44	0.47
0.31	0.12	0	0	0.11	39.9	14.07	0.18	0.08	2.35	0.49	17.22	0	54.6	0.57	37.8	100.8	627.9	636.3	0.61
4.84	3.26	0	0	0	44.1	20.37	0.23	0.11	1.41	0.02	15.54	0	102.9	0.46	37.8	117.6	489.3	697.2	0.38
0	0.07	0	0	0	0	23.56	0.2	0.04	2.54	0.5	19.34	0	7.8	0.64	39	170.04	641.16	10.92	0.51
0	0.02	0	0	0	0	8.87	0.04	0.04	1.29	0.29	9.63	0	26.68	3.45	21.46	47.56	377	9.28	0.3
0	0.09	0	0	0	0	30.5	0.24	0.06	3.46	0.69	24.24	0	22.22	2.5	54.54	212.1	902.94	16.16	0.73
0.67	0.11	0	0	0	110.58	32.4	0.15	0.11	1.96	0.41	16.1	0	69.84	0.91	34.92	97	516.04	420.98	0.58
3.31	1.83	0	0	0	46.55	25.97	0.17	0.23	2.58	0.44	21.31	0	139.65	1.4	46.55	154.35	926.1	820.75	0.98
0.64	0.21	0	0	0	232.32	0	0.16	0.22	3.95	0.98	2.51	0	95.04	4.65	84.48	147.84	1396.56	6.6	0.99
0.34	0.11	0	0	0	69.02	6.43	0.05	0.22	1.61	0.48	0.24	0	49.98	2.48	45.22	78.54	742.56	4.76	0.52
0.32	0.11	0	0	0	65.72	6.15	0.05	0.21	1.53	0.46	0.21	0	48.76	2.35	42.4	74.2	708.08	4.24	0.51
0.55	0.18	0	0	2.33	320.39	5.31	0.13	0.26	3.16	0.43	5.96	0	82.11	3.99	72.45	127.19	1199.45	6.44	0.85
0.02	0.01	0	0	0	264.6	11.51	0.08	0.19	1.01	0.11	20.82	0	36.75	1.4	22.05	73.5	563.5	2.45	0.56
0.09	0.04	0	36.75	2.6	5404.7	10.29	0.06	0.13	0.9	0.14	30.13	0	63.7	3.41	56.35	85.75	504.7	12.25	0.42
0.02	0.05	0	0	0	1.16	26.45	0.01	0.05	0.35	0.08	31.32	0	24.36	0.34	10.44	20.88	269.12	27.84	0.35
0.06	0.16	0	0	0	0	22.2	0	0.03	0.22	0.06	25.58	0	24.99	0.22	13.23	35.28	418.95	19.11	0.19
0.14	0.38	0	0	0	0	0	0.31	0.79	3.94	0.72	341.85	0	729.64	7.81	197.2	236.64	4053.04	322.48	2.47
0.01	0.04	0	0	0	0	19.36	0.02	0.02	0.18	0.04	24.82	0	23.76	0.35	14.08	20.24	199.76	18.48	0.13
0.02	0.05	0	0	0	0	29	0.03	0.02	0.3	0.08	14	0	27	0.8	9	28	280	16	0.13
0.03	0.2	0	0	1.02	4	3	0.1	0.19	1.1	0.32	3	0	53	1.79	35	115	746	12	0.32
0.03	0.23	0	0	1.02	0	5	0.16	0.18	1.1	0.19	3	0	28	2.59	30	79	825	28	0.18

USDA ID Code	Food Name	Weight in Grams*	Quantity of Units	Unit of Measure	Protein (gm)	Fat (gm)	Carbohydrates (gm)	Kcalories	Caffeine (gm)	Fiber (gm)	Cholesterol (mg)	Saturated Fat (gm)
9298	Raisins, Seedless	145	0.66	Cup	3.2	0.5	79.1	300	0	5.8	0	0.22
9304	Raspberries, Cnd, Red, Heavy Syrup Pack	256	1	Cup	2.12	0.31	59.8	232.96	0	8.45	0	0.01
9302	Raspberries, Fresh	123	1	Cup	1.12	0.68	14.23	60.27	0	8.36	0	0.02
9306	Raspberries, Frozen, Red, Sweetened	250	1	Cup	1.75	0.4	65.4	257.5	0	11	0	0.01
62546	Salsa	16.517	2	Tbsp.	0	0	2.5	10.01	0	0	0	0
11439	Sauerkraut, Cnd, Sol&liq	236	0.5	Cup	2.15	0.33	10.1	44.84	0	5.9	0	0.08
11640	Shallots, Freeze-dried	14.388	1	Cup	1.77	0.07	11.61	50.07	0	0	0	0.01
11677	Shallots, Fresh	159.865	1	Cup	4	0.16	26.86	115.1	0	0	0	0.03
11458	Spinach, Ckd	180	0.5	Cup	5.35	0.47	6.75	41.4	0	4.32	0	0.08
11461	Spinach, Cnd, Drained Solids	214	0.5	Cup	6.01	1.07	7.28	49.22	0	0	0	0.17
11459	Spinach, Cnd, Reg Pk, Sol&liq	234	0.5	Cup	4.94	0.87	6.83	44.46	0	5.15	0	0.14
11457	Spinach, Fresh	56	1	Cup	1.6	0.2	1.96	12.32	0	1.51	0	0.03
11464	Spinach, Frz, Ckd	190	1	Cup	5.97	0.4	10.15	53.2	0	5.7	0	0.06
11463	Spinach, Frz, Unprepared	156	0.5	Cup	4.56	0.48	6.24	37.44	0	4.68	0	0.08
11483	Squash, Acorn, Ckd. w/o Salt	205	1	Cup	2.3	0.29	29.89	114.8	0	0	0	0.06
11486	Squash, Butternut, Ckd. w/o Salt	205	1	Cup	1.85	0.18	21.5	82	0	0	0	0.04
11493	Squash, Spaghetti, Ckd. w/o Salt	155	0.5	Cup	1.02	0.4	10.01	44.95	0	2.17	0	0.1
11642	Squash, Summer, Ckd	180	0.5	Cup	1.64	0.56	7.76	36	0	2.52	0	0.12
11641	Squash, Summer, Fresh	130	0.5	Cup	1.53	0.27	5.66	26	0	2.47	0	0.06
11644	Squash, Winter, Baked	205	0.5	Cup	1.82	1.29	17.94	79.95	0	5.74	0	0.27
11643	Squash, Winter, Fresh	116	0.5	Cup	1.68	0.27	10.21	42.92	0	1.74	0	0.05
11953	Squash, Zucchini, Baby, Fresh	11	1	Medium	0.3	0.04	0.34	2.31	0	0	0	0.01
9316	Strawberries, Fresh	149	1	Cup	0.91	0.55	10.46	44.7	0	3.43	0	0.03
9320	Strawberries, Frozen, Sweetened	255	1	Cup	1.35	0.33	66.1	244.8	0	4.85	0	0.02
9318	Strawberries, Frozen, Unsweetened	149	1	Cup	0.64	0.16	13.6	52.15	0	3.13	0	0.01
11508	Sweetpotatoes, Baked In Skin	200	1	Cup	3.44	0.22	48.54	206	0	6	0	0.05
11510	Sweetpotatoes, Boiled, w/o Skin	328	1	Cup	5.41	0.98	79.64	344.4	0	8.2	0	0.21
11659	Sweetpotatoes, Candied	226.795	1	Cup	1.97	7.37	63.19	310.71	0	0	18.14	3.06
11514	Sweetpotatoes, Mashed	255	1	Cup	5.05	0.51	59.16	257.55	0	0	0	0.11
11647	Sweetpotatoes, Syrup Pack, Drained Solids	196	1	Cup	2.51	0.63	49.71	211.68	0	0	0	0.14
9219	Tangerines, Cnd, Juice Pack	249	1	Cup	1.54	0.07	23.83	92.13	0	1.74	0	0.01
9220	Tangerines, Cnd, Light Syrup Pack	252	1	Cup	1.13	0.25	40.8	153.72	0	1.76	0	0.03
9218	Tangerines, Fresh	84	1	Medium	0.53	0.16	9.4	36.96	0	1.93	0	0.02
62654	Tator Tots	2.835	10	Each	0.3	0.5	2	14	0	0.3	0	0.1
11954	Tomatillos, Fresh	34	1	Medium	0.33	0.35	1.98	10.88	0	0.65	0	0
11883	Tomatoes, Cherry	10	1	Each	0.09	0.03	0.46	2.1	0	0	0	0
11530	Tomatoes, Ckd, Boiled	240	1	Cup	2.57	0.98	13.99	64.8	0	2.4	0	0.14
11660	Tomatoes, Ckd, Stewed	101	1	Cup	1.98	2.71	13.18	79.79	0	1.72	0	0.53
11533	Tomatoes, Cnd, Stewed	255	1	Cup	2.37	0.36	16.47	66.3	0	0	0	0.05
11537	Tomatoes, Cnd, w/ Green Chilies	241	1	Cup	1.66	0.19	8.72	36.15	0	0	0	0.03
11535	Tomatoes, Cnd, Wedges In Tomato Juice	261	1	Cup	2.06	0.42	16.47	67.86	0	0	0	0.06
11531	Tomatoes, Cnd, Whole, Reg Pk	240	1	Cup	2.23	0.58	10.3	48	0	2.4	0	0.08
11529	Tomatoes, Fresh	123	1	Medium	1.05	0.41	5.71	25.83	0	1.35	0	0.06
11527	Tomatoes, Green, Fresh	123	1	Medium	1.48	0.25	6.27	29.52	0	1.85	0	0.03
11955	Tomatoes, Sun-dried	54	0.25	Cup	7.62	1.6	30.11	139.32	0	6.64	0	0.23
11956	Tomatoes, Sun-dried, Packed In Oil	110	0.25	Cup	5.57	15.49	25.66	234.3	0	0	0	2.08
11565	Turnips, Ckd	156	0.5	Cup	1.11	0.12	7.64	28.08	0	3.12	0	0.01
11564	Turnips, Fresh	130	0.5	Cup	1.17	0.13	8.1	35.1	0	2.34	0	0.01
11581	Vegetables, Mixed, Cnd	163	0.5	Cup	4.22	0.41	15.09	76.61	0	0	0	0.08
11584	Vegetables, Mixed, Frz	182	0.5	Cup	5.21	0.27	23.82	107.38	0	9.83	0	0.06
62687	Veggie Burger	90	1	Each	18	4	8	140	0	5	0	1.5
	Watercress, Raw	2.5	1	Sprig	0.058	0.003	0.032	0.275	0	0.038	0	0.001
9326	Watermelon	160	1	Cup	0.99	0.69	11.49	51.2	0	0.8	0	0
11602	Yam, Baked	136	1	Cup	2.03	0.19	37.54	157.76	0	5.3	0	0.04
20004	Barley, Cooked	193	1	Cup	3.6	0.7	44.3	157	0	31.83	0	0.1

Monounsaturated Fat (gm)	Polyunsaturated Fat (gm)	Vitamin D (mg)	Vitamin K (mg)	Vitamin E (mg)	Vitamin A (re)	Vitamin C (mg)	Thiamin (mg)	Riboflavin (mg)	Niacin (mg)	Vitamin B6 (mg)	Folate (mg)	Vitamin B12 (mcg)	Calcium (mg)	Iron (mg)	Magnesium (mg)	Phosphorus (mg)	Potassium (mg)	Sodium (mg)	Zinc (mg)
0.03	0.2	0	0	1.02	1.45	3	0.16	0.09	0.8	0.36	4.79	0	49	2.08	33	97	751	12	0.27
0.03	0.17	0	0	1.15	7.68	22.27	0.05	0.08	1.13	0.11	26.88	0	28.16	1.08	30.72	23.04	240.64	7.68	0.41
0.07	0.38	0	0	0.55	15.99	30.75	0.04	0.11	1.11	0.07	31.98	0	27.06	0.7	22.14	14.76	186.96	0	0.57
0.04	0.22	0	0	1.13	15	41.25	0.05	0.11	0.57	0.08	65	0	37.5	1.62	32.5	42.5	285	2.5	0.45
0	0	0	0	0	40.04	1.8	0	0	0	0	0	0	0	0	0	0	0	120.12	0
0.03	0.14	0	0	0.24	4.72	34.69	0.05	0.05	0.34	0.31	55.93	0	70.8	3.47	30.68	47.2	401.2	1559.96	0.45
0.01	0.03	0	0	0	807.16	5.61	0.04	0.01	0.14	0.24	16.72	0	26.33	0.86	14.96	42.59	237.4	8.49	0.28
0.02	0.06	0	0	0	1995.11	12.79	0.1	0.03	0.32	0.55	54.67	0	59.15	1.92	33.57	95.92	533.95	19.18	0.64
0.01	0.19	0	0	1.72	1474.2	17.64	0.17	0.42	0.88	0.44	262.44	0	244.8	6.43	156.6	100.8	838.8	126	1.37
0.03	0.45	0	0	0	1878.92	30.6	0.03	0.3	0.83	0.21	209.29	0	271.78	4.92	162.64	94.16	740.44	57.78	0.98
0.02	0.36	0	0	2.23	1504.62	31.59	0.04	0.25	0.63	0.19	135.72	0	194.22	3.7	131.04	74.88	538.2	746.46	0.98
0.01	0.08	0	148.96	1.06	376.32	15.74	0.04	0.11	0.41	0.11	108.86	0	55.44	1.52	44.24	27.44	312.48	44.24	0.3
0.01	0.16	0	0	1.81	1478.2	23.37	0.11	0.32	0.8	0.28	204.25	0	277.4	2.89	131.1	91.2	566.2	163.4	1.33
0.01	0.2	0	215.28	1.49	1210.56	37.91	0.13	0.24	0.68	0.22	186.58	0	173.16	3.2	90.48	63.96	503.88	115.44	0.69
0.02	0.12	0	0	0	88.15	22.14	0.34	0.03	1.81	0.4	38.34	0	90.2	1.91	88.15	92.25	895.85	8.2	0.35
0.01	0.08	0	0	0	1435	30.96	0.15	0.03	1.99	0.25	39.36	0	84.05	1.23	59.45	55.35	582.2	8.2	0.27
0.03	0.2	0	0	0.19	17.05	5.43	0.06	0.03	1.26	0.15	12.4	0	32.55	0.53	17.05	21.7	181.35	27.9	0.31
0.04	0.24	0	0	0.22	52.2	9.9	0.08	0.07	0.92	0.12	36.18	0	48.6	0.65	43.2	70.2	345.6	1.8	0.7
0.02	0.12	0	0	0.16	26	19.24	0.08	0.05	0.72	0.14	33.28	0	26	0.6	29.9	45.5	253.5	2.6	0.34
0.1	0.54	0	0	0.25	729.8	19.68	0.17	0.05	1.44	0.15	57.4	0	28.7	0.68	16.4	41	895.85	2.05	0.53
0.02	0.11	0	0	0.14	470.96	14.27	0.11	0.03	0.93	0.1	25.17	0	35.96	0.67	24.36	37.12	406	4.64	0.15
0	0.02	0	0	0	5.39	3.75	0	0	0.08	0.02	2.2	0	2.31	0.09	3.63	10.23	50.49	0.33	0.09
0.08	0.28	0	20.86	0.21	4.47	84.48	0.03	0.1	0.34	0.09	26.37	0	20.86	0.57	14.9	28.31	247.34	1.49	0.19
0.05	0.16	0	0	0.36	5.1	105.57	0.04	0.13	1.02	0.08	38	0	28.05	1.5	17.85	33.15	249.9	7.65	0.15
0.02	0.08	0	0	0.4	5.96	61.39	0.03	0.06	0.69	0.04	25.03	0	23.84	1.12	16.39	19.37	220.52	2.98	0.19
0.01	0.1	0	0	9.14	4364	49.2	0.15	0.25	1.21	0.48	45.2	0	56	0.9	40	110	696	20	0.58
0.04	0.43	0	0	14.99	5592.4	56.09	0.17	0.46	2.1	0.8	36.41	0	68.88	1.84	32.8	88.56	603.52	42.64	0.89
1.42	0.33	0	0	0	950.27	15.2	0.04	0.1	0.89	0.09	25.85	0	58.97	2.56	24.95	58.97	428.64	158.76	0.34
0.02	0.23	0	0	0	3858.15	13.26	0.07	0.23	2.44	0.6	27.29	0	76.5	3.39	61.2	132.6	535.5	191.25	0.54
0.02	0.28	0	0	0	1403.36	21.17	0.05	0.07	0.67	0.12	15.48	0	33.32	1.86	23.52	49	378.28	76.44	0.31
0.01	0.01	0	0	1.25	211.65	85.16	0.2	0.07	1.11	0.1	11.45	0	27.39	0.67	27.39	24.9	331.17	12.45	1.27
0.05	0.05	0	0	0.86	211.68	49.9	0.13	0.11	1.12	0.11	11.59	0	17.64	0.93	20.16	25.2	196.56	15.12	0.6
0.03	0.03	0	0	0.2	77.28	25.87	0.09	0.02	0.13	0.06	17.14	0	11.76	0.08	10.08	8.4	131.88	0.84	0.2
0	0	0	0	0	0	0	0	0	0	0	0	0	0	0	0	0	24	24	0
0	0	0	0	0.13	3.74	3.98	0.01	0.01	0.63	0.02	2.38	0	2.38	0.21	6.8	13.26	91.12	0.34	0.07
0.01	0.01	0	0	0.03	6.2	2.6	0.01	0	0.06	0.01	1.5	0	0.5	0.05	1.1	2.4	22.2	0.9	0.01
0.15	0.41	0	0	0.91	177.6	54.72	0.17	0.14	1.8	0.23	31.2	0	14.4	1.34	33.6	74.4	669.6	26.4	0.26
1.06	0.89	0	0	1.28	67.67	18.38	0.11	0.08	1.12	0.09	11.11	0	26.26	1.07	15.15	38.38	249.47	459.55	0.18
0.05	0.15	0	0	0	140.25	33.92	0.12	0.09	1.82	0.04	13.77	0	84.15	1.86	30.6	51	609.45	647.7	0.43
0.03	0.07	0	0	0	93.99	14.94	0.08	0.05	1.54	0.25	21.93	0	48.2	0.63	26.51	33.74	257.87	966.41	0.31
0.06	0.17	0	0	0	151.38	38.63	0.15	0.07	1.76	0.31	26.36	0	67.86	1.2	28.71	60.03	655.11	566.37	0.42
0.09	0.24	0	0	0.77	144	36.24	0.11	0.07	1.76	0.22	18.72	0	62.4	1.46	28.8	45.6	530.4	391.2	0.38
0.06	0.17	0	28.29	0.47	76.26	23.49	0.07	0.06	0.77	0.1	18.45	0	6.15	0.55	13.53	29.52	273.06	11.07	0.11
0.04	0.1	0	57.81	0.47	78.72	28.78	0.07	0.05	0.62	0.1	10.82	0	15.99	0.63	12.3	34.44	250.92	15.99	0.09
0.26	0.6	0	0	0.01	46.98	21.17	0.29	0.26	4.89	0.18	36.72	0	59.4	4.91	104.76	192.24	1850.58	1131.3	1.07
9.53	2.27	0	0	0	141.9	111.98	0.21	0.42	3.99	0.35	25.3	0	51.7	2.94	89.1	152.9	1721.5	292.6	0.86
0.01	0.07	0	0	0.05	0	18.1	0.04	0.04	0.47	0.1	14.35	0	34.32	0.34	12.48	29.64	210.6	78	0.31
0.01	0.07	0	0	0.04	0	27.3	0.05	0.04	0.52	0.12	18.85	0	39	0.39	14.3	35.1	248.3	87.1	0.35
0.03	0.19	0	0	0	1898.95	8.15	0.07	0.08	0.94	0.13	38.47	0	44.01	1.71	26.08	68.46	474.33	242.87	0.67
0.02	0.13	0	0	0.66	778.96	5.82	0.13	0.22	1.55	0.13	34.58	0	45.5	1.49	40.04	92.82	307.58	63.7	0.89
0	0.5	0	0	0	0	0	0.25	0	4	0	0	0	96	1.5	0	0	0	380	7.5
0	0.001	0	0	0.025	11.75	1.075	0.002	0.003	0.005	0.003	0.23	0	3	0.005	0.525	1.5	8.25	1.025	0.003
0	0	0	0	0.24	59.2	15.36	0.13	0.03	0.32	0.23	3.52	0	12.8	0.27	17.6	14.4	185.6	3.2	0.11
0.01	0.08	0	0	6.22	0	16.46	0.13	0.04	0.75	0.31	21.76	0	19.04	0.71	24.48	66.64	911.2	10.88	0.27
0.1	0.3	0	0	1.05	3.68	0	1.19	0.52	3.2	0.18	26	0	17	2.09	35	85	145	5	1.29

USDA ID Code	Food Name	Weight in Grams*	Quantity of Units	Unit of Measure	Protein (gm)	Fat (gm)	Carbohydrates (gm)	Kcalories	Caffeine (gm)	Fiber (gm)	Cholesterol (mg)	Saturated Fat (gm)
18080	Bread Sticks, Plain	10	1	Stick	1.2	0.95	6.84	41.2	0	0	0	0.14
18083	Bread Stuffing, Plain	232	1	Cup	8.82	16.7	51.5	389.76	0	0	0	3.39
18020	Bread, Banana	60	1	Slice	2.58	7.08	33.06	202.8	0	0	25.8	1.83
18024	Bread, Cornbread	65	1	Piece	4.36	4.62	28.28	172.9	0	0	26	1.01
18025	Bread, Cracked-wheat	25	1	Slice	2.18	0.98	12.38	65	0	1.33	0	0.23
18026	Bread, Cracked-wheat, Toasted	23	1	Slice	2.19	0.97	12.37	65.09	0	0	0	0.23
18344	Bread, Dinner Roll, Egg	35	1	Each	3.33	2.24	18.2	107.45	0	1.33	17.5	0.56
18349	Bread, Dinner Roll, French	38	1	Each	3.27	1.63	19.08	105.26	0	0	0	0.37
18345	Bread, Dinner Roll, Oat Bran	33	1	Each	3.14	1.52	13.27	77.88	0	1.35	0	0.2
18342	Bread, Dinner Roll, Plain	35	1	Each	2.94	2.56	17.64	105	0	1.05	0.35	0.61
18346	Bread, Dinner Roll, Rye	35	1	Each	3.61	1.19	18.59	100.1	0	0	0	0.21
18347	Bread, Dinner Roll, Wheat	33	1	Each	2.84	2.08	15.18	90.09	0	0	0	0.5
18348	Bread, Dinner Roll, Whole-wheat	33	1	Each	2.87	1.55	16.86	87.78	0	0	0	0.28
18027	Bread, Egg	40	1	Slice	3.8	2.4	19.12	114.8	0	0	20.4	0.59
18028	Bread, Egg, Toasted	37	1	Slice	3.89	2.44	19.46	116.55	0	0	20.72	0.6
18029	Bread, French or Vienna	25	1	Slice	2.2	0.75	12.98	68.5	0	0.7	0	0.16
18030	Bread, French or Vienna, Toasted	23	1	Slice	2.21	0.76	12.97	68.54	0	0	0	0.16
18033	Bread, Italian	30	1	Slice	2.64	1.05	15	81.3	0	0.93	0	0.26
18034	Bread, Italian, Toasted	27	1	Slice	2.62	1.05	14.85	80.46	0	0	0	0.25
18049	Bread, Lo Cal, Oat Bran	23	1	Slice	1.84	0.74	9.5	46.23	0	0	0	0.1
18050	Bread, Lo Cal, Oat Bran, Toasted	19	1	Slice	1.81	0.72	9.35	45.41	0	0	0	0.1
18051	Bread, Lo Cal, Oatmeal	23	1	Slice	1.75	0.81	9.96	48.3	0	0	0	0.14
18052	Bread, Lo Cal, Oatmeal, Toasted	19	1	Slice	1.71	0.8	9.79	47.69	0	0	0	0.14
18053	Bread, Lo Cal, Rye	23	1	Slice	2.09	0.67	9.32	46.69	0	0	0	0.08
18054	Bread, Lo Cal, Rye, Toasted	19	1	Slice	2.05	0.65	9.16	45.79	0	0	0.19	0.08
18055	Bread, Lo Cal, Wheat	23	1	Slice	2.09	0.53	10.03	45.54	0	2.6	0	0.08
18056	Bread, Lo Cal, Wheat, Toasted	19	1	Slice	2.05	0.51	9.86	44.84	0	0	0	0.08
18057	Bread, Lo Cal, White	23	1	Slice	2	0.58	10.19	47.61	0	2.14	0	0.13
18058	Bread, Lo Cal, White, Toasted	19	1	Slice	1.96	0.57	10.01	46.93	0	0	0	0.12
18035	Bread, Mixed-grain	26	1	Slice	2.6	0.99	12.06	65	0	1.85	0	0.21
18036	Bread, Mixed-grain, Toasted	24	1	Slice	2.62	0.98	12.1	65.28	0	0	0	0.21
18037	Bread, Oat Bran	30	1	Slice	3.12	1.32	11.94	70.8	0	1.35	0	0.21
18038	Bread, Oat Bran, Toasted	27	1	Slice	3.08	1.3	11.8	69.93	0	0	0	0.21
18039	Bread, Oatmeal	27	1	Slice	2.27	1.19	13.1	72.63	0	1.05	0	0.19
18040	Bread, Oatmeal, Toasted	25	1	Slice	2.3	1.2	13.18	73	0	0	0	0.19
18041	Bread, Pita, White, Enriched	60	1	Pita	5.46	0.72	33.42	165	0	0.96	0	0.1
18042	Bread, Pita, Whole-wheat	64	1	Pita	6.27	1.66	35.2	170.24	0	4.8	0	0.26
18044	Bread, Pumpernickel	32	1	Slice	2.78	0.99	15.2	80	0	1.89	0	0.14
18045	Bread, Pumpernickel, Toasted	29	1	Slice	2.76	0.99	15.14	79.75	0	0	0	0.14
18046	Bread, Pumpkin	60	1	Slice	2.4	7.68	30.72	198.6	0	0	26.4	1.23
18047	Bread, Raisin	26	1	Slice	2.05	1.14	13.6	71.24	0	1.12	0	0.28
18048	Bread, Raisin, Toasted	24	1	Slice	2.06	1.15	13.66	71.28	0	0	0	0.28
18059	Bread, Rice Bran	27	1	Slice	2.4	1.24	11.75	65.61	0	0	0	0.19
18384	Bread, Rice Bran, Toasted	25	1	Slice	2.43	1.25	11.83	66	0	0	0	0.19
18353	Bread, Rolls, Hard (includes Kaiser)	57	1	Each	5.64	2.45	30.04	167.01	0	0	0	0.35
18060	Bread, Rye	32	1	Slice	2.72	1.06	15.46	82.88	0	1.98	0	0.2
18061	Bread, Rye, Toasted	29	1	Slice	2.73	1.04	15.4	82.36	0	0	0	0.2
18064	Bread, Wheat (includes Wheat Berry)	25	1	Slice	2.28	1.03	11.8	65	0	1.08	0	0.22
18066	Bread, Wheat Bran	36	1	Slice	3.17	1.22	17.21	89.28	0	3.06	0	0.28
18067	Bread, Wheat Bran, Toasted	33	1	Slice	3.2	1.22	17.33	90.09	0	0	0	0.28
18065	Bread, Wheat, Toasted	23	1	Slice	2.28	1.01	11.8	64.86	0	0	0	0.22
18069	Bread, White	25	1	Slice	2.05	0.9	12.38	66.75	0	0.58	0.25	0.2
18070	Bread, White, Toasted	23	1	Slice	2.07	0.92	12.51	67.39	0	0	0.23	0.21
18075	Bread, Whole Wheat	25	1	Slice	2.43	1.05	11.53	61.5	0	1.73	0	0.2
18078	Bread, Whole Wheat, Toasted	25	1	Slice	2.3	1.48	14.1	76.25	0	0	0	0.22

Monounsaturated Fat (gm)	Polyunsaturated Fat (gm)	Vitamin D (mg)	Vitamin K (mg)	Vitamin E (mg)	Vitamin A (re)	Vitamin C (mg)	Thiamin (mg)	Riboflavin (mg)	Niacin (mg)	Vitamin B6 (mg)	Folate (mcg)	Vitamin B12 (mcg)	Calcium (mg)	Iron (mg)	Magnesium (mg)	Phosphorus (mg)	Potassium (mg)	Sodium (mg)	Zinc (mg)
0.37	0.36	0	0	0	0	0	0.06	0.06	0.53	0.01	3	0	2.2	0.43	3.2	12.1	12.4	65.7	0.09
7.4	4.89	0	0	0	160.08	3.94	0.39	0.33	3.69	0.12	39.44	0	148.48	3.8	34.8	113.68	303.92	1069.52	0.74
3.02	1.77	0	0	0	14.4	1.02	0.1	0.12	0.87	0.09	6.6	0.05	10.8	0.84	8.4	33.6	78.6	118.8	0.22
1.19	2.08	0	0	0	35.1	0.2	0.19	0.19	1.47	0.07	12.35	0.1	161.85	1.63	16.25	109.85	95.55	427.7	0.39
0.48	0.17	0	0	0	0	0	0.09	0.06	0.92	0.08	9.75	0.01	10.75	0.7	13	38.25	44.25	134.5	0.31
0.48	0.17	0	0	0	0	0	0.07	0.05	0.83	0.07	6.9	0.01	10.81	0.7	13.11	38.18	44.16	134.55	0.31
1.06	0.37	0	0	0	7.7	0	0.18	0.18	1.15	0.03	18.55	0.08	20.65	1.23	8.75	34.65	36.75	190.75	0.32
0.75	0.32	0	0	0	0	0	0.2	0.11	1.65	0.02	12.54	0	34.58	1.03	7.6	31.92	43.32	231.42	0.29
0.49	0.52	0	0	0	0.33	0	0.15	0.1	1.63	0.01	10.23	0	28.05	1.37	9.9	33.99	35.97	136.29	0.28
1.3	0.43	0	0	0	0	0.04	0.17	0.11	1.41	0.02	10.5	0.01	41.65	1.1	8.05	40.6	46.55	182.35	0.27
0.43	0.25	0	0	0	0	0	0.13	0.09	1.37	0.03	7.7	0	10.5	0.95	18.9	55.65	63	312.2	0.35
1.07	0.35	0	0	0	0	0	0.14	0.09	1.34	0.03	4.95	0	58.08	1.17	13.86	38.94	43.89	112.2	0.34
0.4	0.71	0	0	0	0	0	0.08	0.05	1.21	0.06	9.9	0	34.98	0.8	28.05	73.92	89.76	157.74	0.66
1.09	0.42	0	0	0	9.2	0	0.18	0.17	1.94	0.03	28	0.04	37.2	1.22	7.6	42.4	46	196.8	0.32
1.11	0.43	0	0	0	8.51	0	0.14	0.16	1.77	0.02	19.98	0.04	37.74	1.24	7.77	43.29	46.62	199.8	0.32
0.3	0.17	0	0	0	0	0	0.13	0.08	1.19	0.01	7.75	0	18.75	0.63	6.75	26.25	28.25	152.25	0.22
0.3	0.17	0	0	0	0	0	0.1	0.07	1.07	0.01	5.52	0	18.63	0.63	6.9	26.22	28.06	152.03	0.22
0.24	0.42	0	0	0	0	0	0.14	0.09	1.31	0.01	9	0	23.4	0.88	8.1	30.9	33	175.2	0.26
0.24	0.41	0	0	0	0	0	0.11	0.08	1.17	0.01	6.21	0	22.95	0.87	8.1	30.78	32.67	173.34	0.26
0.16	0.38	0	0	0	0	0	0.08	0.05	0.87	0.02	7.82	0	13.11	0.72	10.58	27.83	23.46	80.73	0.23
0.15	0.38	0	0	0	0	0	0.06	0.04	0.77	0.02	5.32	0	12.92	0.71	10.45	27.36	23.18	79.42	0.23
0.19	0.31	0	0	0	0.23	0.05	0.08	0.06	0.7	0.01	7.82	0	26.45	0.53	6.67	27.37	35.19	89.24	0.22
0.19	0.31	0	0	0	0.19	0.04	0.06	0.06	0.62	0.01	5.32	0.03	26.03	0.52	6.46	26.98	34.58	87.78	0.21
0.15	0.17	0	0	0	0	0.02	0.08	0.06	0.58	0.01	5.29	0.02	18.71	0.48	3.91	19.32	22.54	93.15	0.18
0.15	0.17	0	0	0	0	0.02	0.07	0.05	0.51	0.01	3.61	0.02	17.29	0.7	3.99	18.81	22.23	91.77	0.17
0.06	0.22	0	0	0	0	0.02	0.1	0.07	0.89	0.03	6.44	0.01	18.4	0.68	6.44	0	28.52	117.53	0.19
0.06	0.22	0	0	0	0	0.02	0.08	0.06	0.79	0.03	4.37	0.01	18.24	0.67	6.46	20.71	27.93	115.52	0.19
0.25	0.13	0	0	0	0	0.09	0.09	0.07	0.84	0.01	7.82	0.06	21.62	0.73	5.98	30.82	17.48	104.19	0.31
0.24	0.13	0	0	0	0.19	0.08	0.07	0.06	0.74	0.01	5.51	0.06	21.28	0.72	5.89	30.21	17.29	102.41	0.3
0.4	0.24	0	0	0	0	0.08	0.11	0.09	1.13	0.09	12.48	0.02	23.66	0.9	13.78	45.76	53.04	126.62	0.33
0.4	0.24	0	0	0	0	0.07	0.08	0.08	1.02	0.08	8.88	0.02	23.76	0.9	13.92	45.84	53.28	127.2	0.33
0.48	0.51	0	0	0	0	0	0.15	0.1	1.45	0.01	7.5	0	19.5	0.94	9.3	31.8	33.6	122.1	0.29
0.47	0.5	0	0	0	0	0	0.12	0.09	1.29	0.01	5.13	0	19.17	0.93	9.18	31.32	33.21	120.96	0.28
0.43	0.46	0	0	0	0.54	0.11	0.11	0.06	0.85	0.02	7.29	0	17.82	0.73	9.99	34.02	38.34	161.73	0.28
0.43	0.46	0	0	0	0.5	0.08	0.09	0.06	0.77	0.02	5.25	0.01	18	0.74	10.25	34.25	38.5	162.75	0.28
0.06	0.32	0	0	0	0	0	0.36	0.2	2.78	0.02	14.4	0	51.6	1.57	15.6	58.2	72	321.6	0.5
0.22	0.68	0	0	0	0	0	0.22	0.05	1.82	0.15	22.4	0	9.6	1.85	44.16	115.2	108.8	340.48	0.97
0.3	0.4	0	0	0	0	0	0.1	0.1	0.99	0.04	10.88	0	21.76	0.92	17.28	56.96	66.56	214.72	0.47
0.3	0.39	0	0	0	0	0	0.08	0.09	0.89	0.04	7.54	0	21.46	0.91	17.4	56.55	66.12	214.02	0.47
1.85	4.11	0	0	0	334.2	0.6	0.09	0.1	0.79	0.02	6.6	0.05	10.8	0.99	7.8	31.8	55.2	187.8	0.2
0.6	0.18	0	0	0	0	0.13	0.09	0.1	0.9	0.02	8.84	0	17.16	0.75	6.76	28.34	59.02	101.4	0.19
0.6	0.18	0	0	0	0	0.1	0.07	0.09	0.81	0.02	6.24	0	17.28	0.76	6.72	28.32	59.04	101.76	0.19
0.45	0.48	0	0	0	0	0	0.18	0.08	1.84	0.06	8.1	0	18.63	0.97	18.9	43.2	52.65	118.8	0.34
0.45	0.48	0	0	0	0	0	0.14	0.07	1.67	0.05	5.75	0	18.75	0.98	19	43.5	53	119.5	0.35
0.65	0.98	0	0	0	0	0	0.27	0.19	2.42	0.03	8.55	0	54.15	1.87	15.39	57	61.56	310.08	0.54
0.42	0.26	0	0	0	0	0	0.14	0.11	1.22	0.02	16.32	0	23.36	0.91	12.8	40	53.12	211.2	0.36
0.42	0.25	0	0	0	0	0.06	0.11	0.1	1.09	0.02	11.31	0	23.2	0.9	12.47	40.02	53.07	210.25	0.36
0.43	0.23	0	0	0	0	0	0.1	0.07	1.03	0.02	10.25	0	26.25	0.83	11.5	37.5	50.25	132.5	0.26
0.58	0.23	0	0	0	0	0	0.14	0.1	1.58	0.06	9	0	26.64	1.11	29.16	66.6	81.72	174.96	0.49
0.59	0.24	0	0	0	0	0	0.12	0.09	1.44	0.02	6.6	0	26.73	1.11	29.37	67.32	82.17	176.22	0.49
0.43	0.23	0	0	0	0	0	0.08	0.06	0.93	0.02	7.13	0	26.22	0.83	11.5	37.49	50.14	132.48	0.26
0.4	0.19	0	0	0	0	0	0.12	0.09	0.99	0.02	8.5	0	27	0.76	6	23.5	29.75	134.5	0.16
0.41	0.19	0	0	0	0	0	0.1	0.08	0.9	0.01	5.98	0	27.37	0.77	5.98	23.69	30.13	136.16	0.16
0.42	0.25	0	0	0	0	0	0.09	0.05	0.96	0.04	12.5	0	18	0.83	21.5	57.25	63	131.75	0.49
0.32	0.81	0	0	0	0	0	0.07	0.06	0.99	0.05	9	0	9	0.85	22.25	51.25	86.25	95.25	0.41

USDA ID Code	Food Name	Weight in Grams*	Quantity of Units	Unit of Measure	Protein (gm)	Fat (gm)	Carbohydrates (gm)	Kcalories	Caffeine (gm)	Fiber (gm)	Cholesterol (mg)	Saturated Fat (gm)
18351	Buns, Hamburger or Hot Dog, Mixed-grain	43	1	Each	4.13	2.58	19.18	113.09	0	1.85	0	0.61
18350	Buns, Hamburger or Hot Dog, Plain	43	1	Each	3.66	2.19	21.63	122.98	0	0	0	0.51
	Cornstarch	128	1	Cup	0.333	0.064	116.826	487.68	0	1.152	0	0.012
	Couscous, Cooked	157	1	Cup	5.95	0.251	36.455	175.84	0	2.198	0	0.046
18214	Crackers, Cheese, Regular	1	1	Each	0.1	0.25	0.58	5.03	0	0.02	0.13	0.09
18215	Crackers, Cheese, w/ Peanut Butter Filling	7	1	Each	0.88	1.62	3.99	33.74	0	0.08	0.35	0.36
62592	Crackers, Cinn. Graham Snacks, Fat Free-SnackWell	0.67	20	Each	0.04	0	0.58	2.46	0	0.02	0	0
62606	Crackers, Cracked Pepper, Fat Free-SnackWell	2.14	7	Each	0.29	0	1.85	8.56	0	0.07	0	0
18216	Crackers, Crispbread, Rye	10	1	Each	0.79	0.13	8.22	36.6	0	1.62	0	0.01
18173	Crackers, Graham, Plain or Honey	7	1	Each	0.48	0.71	5.38	29.61	0	0.19	0	0.18
18218	Crackers, Matzo, Egg	28.35	1	Each	3.49	0.6	22.28	110.85	0	0	24.95	0.16
18400	Crackers, Matzo, Egg and Onion	28.35	1	Each	2.84	1.11	21.86	110.85	0	1.42	15.03	0.27
18217	Crackers, Matzo, Plain	28.35	1	Each	2.84	0.4	23.73	111.98	0	0.85	0	0.06
18219	Crackers, Matzo, Whole-wheat	28.35	1	Each	3.71	0.43	22.37	99.51	0	3.29	0	0.07
18220	Crackers, Melba Toast, Plain	5	1	Each	0.61	0.16	3.83	19.5	0	0.33	0	0.02
18424	Crackers, Melba Toast, Plain, w/o Salt	5	1	Each	0.61	0.16	3.83	19.5	0	0	0	0.02
18221	Crackers, Melba Toast, Rye	5	1	Each	0.58	0.17	3.87	19.45	0	0.4	0	0.02
18222	Crackers, Melba Toast, Wheat	5	1	Each	0.65	0.12	3.82	18.7	0	0.37	0	0.02
18229	Crackers, Ritz	3	1	Each	0.22	0.76	1.83	15.06	0	0.06	0	0.15
18427	Crackers, Ritz, Low Sodium	3	1	Each	0.22	0.76	1.83	15.06	0	0	0	0.15
18225	Crackers, Rye, w/ Cheese Filling	7	1	Each	0.64	1.56	4.26	33.67	0	0	0.63	0.4
18226	Crackers, Rye, Wafers, Plain	25	1	Each	2.4	0.23	20.1	83.5	0	0	0	0.03
18227	Crackers, Rye, Wafers, Seasoned	22	1	Each	1.98	2.02	16.24	83.82	0	0	0	0.34
18228	Crackers, Saltines	3	1	Each	0.28	0.35	2.15	13.02	0	0.08	0	0.06
62688	Crackers, Saltines, Fat Free	3	1	Each	0.4	0	2.4	12	0	0	0	0
18425	Crackers, Saltines, Low Salt	3	1	Each	0.28	0.35	2.15	13.02	0	0	0	0.06
18230	Crackers, Snack-type, w/ Cheese Filling	7	1	Each	0.65	1.48	4.32	33.39	0	0	0.14	0.4
18231	Crackers, Snack-type, w/ Peanut Butter Filling	7	1	Each	0.78	1.67	4.11	34.16	0	0	0	0.36
62590	Crackers, Wheat, Fat Free - SnackWell	3	5	Each	0.4	0	2.4	12	0	0.2	0	0
18428	Crackers, Wheat, Low Salt	2	1	Each	0.17	0.41	1.3	9.46	0	0	0	0.07
18232	Crackers, Wheat, Regular	2	1	Each	0.17	0.41	1.3	9.46	0	0.11	0	0.07
18233	Crackers, Wheat, w/ Cheese Filling	7	1	Each	0.69	1.75	4.07	34.79	0	0	0.49	0.4
18234	Crackers, Wheat, w/ Peanut Butter Filling	7	1	Each	0.95	1.87	3.77	34.65	0	0	0	0.36
18235	Crackers, Whole-wheat	4	1	Each	0.35	0.69	2.74	17.72	0	0.42	0	0.12
18429	Crackers, Whole-wheat, Low Salt	4	1	Each	0.35	0.69	2.74	17.72	0	0	0	0.12
18260	English Muffins, Mixed-grain (includes Granola)	66	1	Each	6.01	1.19	30.56	155.1	0	0	0	0.15
18261	English Muffins, Mixed-grain, Toasted	61	1	Each	6.04	1.16	30.68	155.55	0	0	0	0.15
18258	English Muffins, Plain	57	1	Each	4.39	1.03	26.22	133.95	0	0	0	0.15
18259	English Muffins, Plain, Toasted	52	1	Each	4.37	1.04	26	132.6	0	0	0	0.15
18262	English Muffins, Raisin-cinnamon	57	1	Each	4.28	1.54	27.76	138.51	0	0	0	0.22
18263	English Muffins, Raisin-cinnamon, Toasted	52	1	Each	4.26	1.51	27.56	137.28	0	0	0	0.22
18264	English Muffins, Wheat	57	1	Each	4.96	1.14	25.54	127.11	0	0	0	0.16
18265	English Muffins, Wheat, Toasted	52	1	Each	4.89	1.09	25.32	126.36	0	0	0	0.16
18266	English Muffins, Whole-wheat	66	1	Each	5.81	1.39	26.66	133.98	0	4.16	0	0.22
18267	English Muffins, Whole-wheat, Toasted	61	1	Each	5.86	1.4	26.9	134.81	0	0	0	0.22
20081	Flour, White	125	1	Cup	12.91	1.23	95.39	455	0	4.13	0	0.19
20080	Flour, Whole Grain	120	1	Cup	16.44	2.24	87.08	406.8	0	14.64	0	0.39
20030	Grits	160	0.5	Cup	2.37	1.41	22.82	115.2	0	4	0	0.2
20330	Hominy, Cnd, Yellow	160	0.5	Cup	2.37	1.41	22.82	115.2	0	4	0	0.2
18270	Hush Puppies	22	1	Each	1.69	2.97	10.12	74.14	0	0.62	9.9	0.46
20100	Macaroni, Ckd, Enriched	140	1	Cup	6.68	0.94	39.68	197.4	0	1.82	0	0.13
20400	Macaroni, Ckd, Unenriched	140	1	Cup	6.68	0.94	39.68	197.4	0	1.82	0	0.13
20106	Macaroni, Vegetable, Ckd, Enriched	134	1	Cup	6.07	0.15	35.66	171.52	0	5.76	0	0.02
20108	Macaroni, Whole-wheat, Ckd	140	1	Cup	7.46	0.76	37.16	173.6	0	6.16	0	0.14
20113	Noodles, Chinese, Chow Mein	45	0.5	Cup	3.77	13.84	25.89	237.15	0	1.76	0	1.97

Monounsaturated Fat (gm)	Polyunsaturated Fat (gm)	Vitamin D (mg)	Vitamin K (mg)	Vitamin E (mg)	Vitamin A (re)	Vitamin C (mg)	Thiamin (mg)	Riboflavin (mg)	Niacin (mg)	Vitamin B6 (mg)	Folate (mg)	Vitamin B12 (mcg)	Calcium (mg)	Iron (mg)	Magnesium (mg)	Phosphorus (mg)	Potassium (mg)	Sodium (mg)	Zinc (mg)
1.28	0.49	0	0	0	0	0	0.2	0.13	1.92	0.04	12.04	0	40.85	1.7	20.64	52.03	64.5	196.94	0.46
1.07	0.39	0	0	0	0	0	0.21	0.13	1.69	0.02	11.61	0.01	59.77	1.36	8.6	37.84	60.63	240.8	0.27
0.02	0.032	0	0	0	0	0	0	0	0	0	0	0	2.56	0.602	3.84	16.64	3.84	11.52	0.077
0.035	0.1	0	0	0.02	0	0	0.099	0.042	1.543	0.08	23.55	0	12.56	0.597	12.56	34.54	91.06	7.85	0.408
0.09	0.05	0	0	0	0.3	0	0.01	0	0.05	0.01	0.25	0	1.51	0.05	0.36	2.18	1.45	9.95	0.01
0.85	0.31	0	0	0	0	0	0.03	0.02	0.46	0.1	1.75	0	5.53	0.2	4.06	22.68	17.15	69.44	0.08
0	0	0	0	0	0	0	0	0	0	0	0	0	0	0.01	0	0	0	2.01	0
0	0	0	0	0	0	0	0	0	0	0	0	0	3.42	0.06	0	0	0	21.4	0
0.02	0.06	0	0	0	0	0	0.02	0.01	0.1	0.02	2.2	0	3.1	0.24	7.8	26.9	31.9	26.4	0.24
0.35	0.11	0	0	0	0	0	0.02	0.02	0.29	0	1.19	0	1.68	0.26	2.1	7.28	9.45	42.35	0.06
0.17	0.13	0	0	0	3.69	0	0.18	0.18	1.44	0.02	8.22	0.14	11.34	0.77	6.52	45.08	42.53	5.95	0.21
0.28	0.28	0	0	0	5.1	0.06	0.16	0.12	1.39	0.03	2.84	0.06	10.21	1.24	8.51	25.23	23.53	80.8	0.21
0.04	0.17	0	0	0	0	0	0.11	0.08	1.1	0.03	3.97	0	3.69	0.9	7.09	25.23	31.75	0.57	0.19
0.05	0.19	0	0	0	0	0	0.1	0.08	1.53	0.05	9.92	0	6.52	1.32	37.99	86.47	89.59	0.57	0.74
0.04	0.06	0	0	0	0	0	0.02	0.01	0.21	0	1.3	0	4.65	0.19	2.95	9.8	10.1	41.45	0.1
0.04	0.06	0	0	0	0	0	0.02	0.01	0.21	0	1.3	0	4.65	0.19	2.95	9.8	10.1	0.95	0.1
0.05	0.07	0	0	0	0	0.01	0.02	0.01	0.24	0	1.1	0	3.9	0.18	1.95	9.15	9.65	44.95	0.07
0.03	0.05	0	0	0	0	0	0.02	0.01	0.25	0.01	1.2	0	2.15	0.23	2.8	8.25	7.4	41.85	0.08
0.32	0.25	0	0	0	0	0	0.01	0.01	0.12	0	0.42	0	3.6	0.11	0.81	6.84	3.99	25.41	0.02
0.32	0.25	0	0	0	0	0	0.01	0.01	0.12	0	0.42	0	3.6	0.11	0.81	6.84	10.65	11.19	0.02
0.84	0.2	0	0	0	0.14	0.01	0.04	0.03	0.25	0.01	1.12	0	15.54	0.17	2.59	23.73	23.94	73.08	0.05
0.04	0.1	0	0	0	0.5	0.03	0.11	0.07	0.4	0.07	11.25	0	10	1.49	30.25	83.5	123.75	198.5	0.7
1.05	0.37	0	0	0	0	0.02	0.07	0.05	0.54	0.04	11.44	0	9.68	0.67	23.32	67.54	99.88	195.14	0.56
0.19	0.06	0	0	0	0	0	0.02	0.01	0.16	0	0.93	0	3.57	0.16	0.81	3.15	3.84	39.06	0.02
0	0	0	0	0	0	0	0	0	0	0	0	0	0	0.12	0	0	25.6	36	0
0.19	0.06	0	0	0	0	0	0.02	0.01	0.16	0	0.93	0	3.57	0.16	0.81	3.15	21.72	19.08	0.02
0.8	0.19	0	0	0	0.49	0	0.03	0.05	0.26	0	0.98	0	17.99	0.17	2.52	28.42	30.03	98.07	0.04
0.88	0.32	0	0	0	0	0	0.03	0.02	0.41	0.01	2.38	0	6.79	0.21	3.71	16.87	15.61	65.94	0.07
0	0	0	0	0	0	0	0	0	0	0	0	0	4.8	0.08	0	0	0	34	0
0.23	0.06	0	0	0	0	0	0.01	0.01	0.1	0	0.36	0	0.98	0.09	1.24	4.4	4.06	5.66	0.03
0.23	0.06	0	0	0	0	0	0.01	0.01	0.1	0	0.36	0	0.98	0.09	1.24	4.4	3.66	15.9	0.03
0.95	0.23	0	0	0	0.63	0.11	0.03	0.03	0.22	0.02	1.33	0.01	14.28	0.18	3.78	26.74	21.42	63.91	0.06
0.98	0.36	0	0	0	0	0	0.03	0.02	0.41	0.01	2.59	0	11.9	0.19	2.66	24.29	20.79	56.49	0.06
0.38	0.11	0	0	0	0	0	0.01	0	0.18	0.01	1.12	0	2	0.12	3.96	11.8	11.88	26.36	0.09
0.38	0.11	0	0	0	0	0	0.01	0	0.18	0.01	1.12	0	2	0.12	3.96	11.8	11.88	9.88	0.09
0.55	0.37	0	0	0	0.66	0	0.28	0.21	2.36	0.06	23.1	0	129.36	1.99	29.04	98.34	102.96	274.56	0.64
0.55	0.37	0	0	0	0.61	0	0.23	0.19	2.14	0.06	16.47	0	129.93	2.01	29.28	98.82	103.09	276.33	0.64
0.17	0.51	0	0	0	0	0.06	0.25	0.16	2.21	0.02	21.09	0.02	99.18	1.43	11.97	75.81	74.67	264.48	0.4
0.17	0.5	0	0	0	0	0.05	0.2	0.14	1.98	0.02	15.08	0.02	98.28	1.41	11.44	75.4	74.36	262.08	0.4
0.29	0.78	0	0	0	0	0.17	0.22	0.17	2.03	0.04	18.24	0	83.79	1.38	8.55	43.89	118.56	254.79	0.57
0.29	0.78	0	0	0	0	0.16	0.17	0.15	1.81	0.04	13	0	82.68	1.37	8.84	43.68	117.52	252.72	0.57
0.16	0.48	0	0	0	0	0	0.25	0.17	1.91	0.05	22.23	0	101.46	1.64	22.23	65.55	106.02	217.74	0.64
0.16	0.47	0	0	0	0	0	0.2	0.15	1.71	0.05	15.6	0	100.36	1.62	21.84	64.48	105.04	215.8	0.63
0.34	0.55	0	0	0	0	0	0.2	0.09	2.25	0.11	32.34	0	174.9	1.62	46.86	186.12	138.6	420.42	1.06
0.34	0.55	0	0	0	0	0	0.16	0.08	2.03	0.1	22.57	0	175.68	1.62	46.97	187.27	139.08	422.12	1.06
0.11	0.52	0	0.63	0.46	0	0	0.98	0.62	7.38	0.06	32.5	0	18.75	5.8	27.5	135	133.75	2.5	0.88
0.28	0.93	0	1.32	1.48	0	0	0.54	0.26	7.64	0.41	52.8	0	40.8	4.66	165.6	415.2	486	6	3.52
0.37	0.64	0	0	0	0	0	0	0.01	0.05	0.01	1.6	0	16	0.99	25.6	56	14.4	336	1.68
0.37	0.64	0	0	0	17.6	0	0	0.01	0.05	0.01	1.6	0	16	0.99	25.6	56	14.4	336	1.68
0.72	1.59	0	0	0	9.46	0.04	0.08	0.07	0.61	0.02	4.4	0.04	61.16	0.67	5.28	41.58	31.68	146.96	0.15
0.11	0.38	0	0	0.04	0	0	0.29	0.14	2.34	0.05	9.8	0	9.8	1.96	25.2	75.6	43.4	1.4	0.74
0.11	0.38	0	0	0.04	0	0	0.03	0.03	0.56	0.05	9.8	0	9.8	0.7	25.2	75.6	43.4	1.4	0.74
0.02	0.06	0	0	0.05	6.7	0	0.15	0.08	1.44	0.03	8.04	0	14.74	0.66	25.46	67	41.54	8.04	0.59
0.11	0.3	0	0	0.14	0	0	0.15	0.06	0.99	0.11	7	0	21	1.48	42	124.6	61.6	4.2	1.13
3.46	7.8	0	0	0.07	4.05	0	0.26	0.19	2.68	0.05	9.9	0	9	2.13	23.4	72.45	54	197.55	0.63

USDA ID Code	Food Name	Weight in Grams*	Quantity of Units	Unit of Measure	Protein (gm)	Fat (gm)	Carbohydrates (gm)	Kcalories	Caffeine (gm)	Fiber (gm)	Cholesterol (mg)	Saturated Fat (gm)
20310	Noodles, Egg, Ckd, Enriched	160	1	Cup	7.6	2.35	39.74	212.8	0	0	52.8	0.5
20510	Noodles, Egg, Ckd, Unenriched	160	1	Cup	7.6	2.35	39.74	212.8	0	0	52.8	0.5
20112	Noodles, Egg, Spinach, Ckd, Enriched	160	1	Cup	8.06	2.51	38.8	211.2	0	3.68	52.8	0.58
20115	Noodles, Japanese, Soba, Ckd	114	0.5	Cup	5.77	0.11	24.44	112.86	0	0	0	0.02
62647	Noodles, Ramen	86	1	Each	10	16	52	380	0	2	0	8
20321	Pasta, Ckd, Enriched, w/ Added Salt	140	1	Cup	6.68	0.94	39.68	197.4	0	0	0	0.13
20121	Pasta, Ckd, Enriched, w/o Added Salt	140	1	Cup	6.68	0.94	39.68	197.4	0	2.38	0	0.13
20094	Pasta, Fresh-refrigerated, Plain, Ckd	146	1	Cup	7.52	1.53	36.4	191.26	0	0	48.18	0.22
20096	Pasta, Fresh-refrigerated, Spinach, Ckd	146	1	Cup	7.39	1.37	36.56	189.8	0	0	48.18	0.32
20097	Pasta, Homemade, Made w/ Egg, Ckd	147.2	1	Cup	7.77	2.56	34.65	191.36	0	0	60.35	0.6
20098	Pasta, Homemade, Made w/o Egg, Ckd	147.2	1	Cup	6.43	1.44	36.98	182.53	0	0	0	0.21
20127	Pasta, Spinach, Ckd	140	1	Cup	6.41	0.88	36.61	182	0	0	0	0.13
20125	Pasta, Whole-wheat, Ckd	140	1	Cup	7.46	0.76	37.16	173.6	0	6.3	0	0.14
62557	Red Beans and Rice	28.35	2	Ounce	3.98	0.5	19.89	94.5	0	3.48	0	0
20037	Rice, Brown, Long-grain, Ckd	195	1	Cup	5.03	1.76	44.77	216.45	0	3.51	0	0.35
20041	Rice, Brown, Medium-grain, Ckd	195	1	Cup	4.52	1.62	45.84	218.4	0	0	0	0.32
20045	Rice, White, Long-grain, Ckd	158	1	Cup	4.25	0.44	44.51	205.4	0	0.63	0	0.12
20049	Rice, White, Long-grain, Instant, Enriched	165	1	Cup	3.4	0.26	35.1	161.7	0	0.99	0	0.07
20051	Rice, White, Medium-grain, Ckd	186	1	Cup	4.43	0.39	53.18	241.8	0	0.56	0	0.11
20053	Rice, White, Short-grain, Ckd	186	1	Cup	4.39	0.35	53.44	241.8	0	0	0	0.09
20057	Rice, White, w/ Pasta, Ckd	202	1	Cup	5.13	5.7	43.29	246.44	0	7.88	2.02	1.09
62653	Tabouli	28.35	1	Ounce	1	2	2	30	0	1	0	0
18360	Taco Shells, Baked	13	1	Medium	0.94	2.94	8.11	60.84	0	1.05	0	0.44
18448	Taco Shells, Baked, w/o Added Salt	13	1	Medium	0.94	2.94	8.11	60.84	0	0	0	0.44
18363	Tortillas, Corn	25	1	Medium	1.43	0.63	11.65	55.5	0	1.3	0	0.08
18449	Tortillas, Corn, w/o Added Salt	25	1	Medium	1.43	0.63	11.65	55.5	0	0	0	0.08
18364	Tortillas, Flour	35	1	Medium	3.05	2.49	19.46	113.75	0	1.09	0	0.39
18450	Tortillas, Flour, w/o Added Salt	35	1	Medium	3.05	2.49	19.46	113.75	0	0	0	0.39
20089	Wild Rice, Ckd	164	1	Cup	6.54	0.56	35	165.64	0	2.95	0	0.08
62663	Wild Rice, Unkle Ben's	56	1	Cup	6	0.5	41	190	0	1	0	0
10124	Bacon	6	1	Slice	1.83	2.95	0.04	34.56	0	0	5.1	1.05
10131	Bacon, Canadian-style Bacon, Grilled	21	1	Slice	5.09	1.77	0.28	38.85	0	0	12.18	0.6
62528	Bacon, Turkey	14	1	Slice	3	2	0	25	0	0	10	0.5
7001	Barbecue Loaf, Lunch Meat	23	1	Slice	3.64	2.05	1.47	39.79	0	0	8.51	0.73
16006	Beans, Baked, Cnd, Vegetarian	254	0.5	Cup	6.1	13	54.1	382	0	13.9	13	4.9
16007	Beans, Baked, Cnd, w/ Beef	266	0.5	Cup	16.97	9.18	44.98	321.86	0	0	58.52	4.46
16008	Beans, Baked, Cnd, w/ Franks	257	0.5	Cup	17.35	16.88	39.55	364.94	0	17.73	15.42	6.04
16009	Beans, Baked, Cnd, w/ Pork	253	0.5	Cup	13.13	3.92	50.55	268.18	0	13.92	17.71	1.52
16005	Beans, Baked, Home Prepared	253	0.5	Cup	6.1	13	54.1	382	0	13.92	13	4.9
16315	Beans, Black, Ckd	256	0.5	Cup	15.2	1.2	45	214	0	0	0	0.12
16058	Beans, Garbanzo, Cnd.	240	0.5	Cup	11.9	2.7	54.3	286	0	10.6	0	0.3
16029	Beans, Kidney, Cnd	256	0.5	Cup	13.3	0.8	38.1	107	0	0	0	0.1
16073	Beans, Lima, Cnd	241	0.5	Cup	11.9	0.4	35.9	190	0	11.6	0	0.1
16039	Beans, Navy, Cnd	262	0.5	Cup	19.7	1.1	53.6	296	0	13.4	0	0.3
16044	Beans, Pinto, Cnd	240	0.5	Cup	11.7	1.9	36.6	206	0	11	0	0.4
16103	Beans, Refried, Cnd	253	0.5	Cup	13.9	3.2	39.3	238	0	13.4	0	1.2
62632	Beans, Refried,Lowfat, Cnd.	268	0.5	Cup	16	0	42	240	0	14	0	0
13347	Beef, Corned, Brisket, Ckd	28.35	3	Ounce	5.15	5.38	0.13	71.16	0	0	27.78	1.8
13353	Beef, Cured, Lunch Meat, Jellied	28.35	3	Ounce	5.39	0.94	0	31.47	0	0	9.64	0.4
13355	Beef, Cured, Pastrami	28.35	3	Ounce	4.89	8.27	0.86	98.94	0	0	26.37	2.95
13357	Beef, Cured, Sausage, Smoked	28.35	3	Ounce	4	7.63	0.69	88.45	0	0	18.99	3.24
13358	Beef, Cured, Smoked, Chopped Beef	28.35	3	Ounce	5.72	1.25	0.53	34.87	0	0	13.04	0.51
13360	Beef, Cured, Thin-sliced Beef	28.35	3	Ounce	7.97	1.09	1.62	50.18	0	0	11.62	0.47
	Beef, Filet, Tnderloin, Broiled	85	3	Ounce	23.55	9.75	0	188.7	0	0	70.55	3.681
13298	Beef, Ground, Extra Lean, Broiled	28.35	3	Ounce	7.2	4.63	0	72.58	0	0	23.81	1.82

Monounsaturated Fat (gm)	Polyunsaturated Fat (gm)	Vitamin D (mg)	Vitamin K (mg)	Vitamin E (mg)	Vitamin A (re)	Vitamin C (mg)	Thiamin (mg)	Riboflavin (mg)	Niacin (mg)	Vitamin B6 (mg)	Folate (mg)	Vitamin B12 (mcg)	Calcium (mg)	Iron (mg)	Magnesium (mg)	Phosphorus (mg)	Potassium (mg)	Sodium (mg)	Zinc (mg)
0.69	0.65	0	0	0	9.6	0	0.3	0.13	2.38	0.06	11.2	0.14	19.2	2.54	30.4	110.4	44.8	264	0.99
0.69	0.65	0	0	0	9.6	0	0.05	0.03	0.64	0.06	11.2	0.14	19.2	0.96	30.4	110.4	44.8	264	0.99
0.79	0.56	0	0	0.08	22.4	0	0.39	0.2	2.36	0.18	33.6	0.22	30.4	1.74	38.4	91.2	59.2	19.2	1.01
0.03	0.04	0	0	0	0	0	0.11	0.03	0.58	0.05	7.98	0	4.56	0.55	10.26	28.5	39.9	68.4	0.14
0	0	0	0	0	0	0	0	0	0	0	0	0	0	1.6	0	0	0	1560	0
0.11	0.38	0	0	0	0	0	0.29	0.14	2.34	0.05	9.8	0	9.8	1.96	25.2	75.6	43.4	140	0.74
0.11	0.38	0	0	0.08	0	0	0.29	0.14	2.34	0.05	9.8	0	9.8	1.96	25.2	75.6	43.4	1.4	0.74
0.18	0.63	0	0	0	8.76	0	0.31	0.22	1.45	0.05	10.22	0.2	8.76	1.66	26.28	91.98	35.04	8.76	0.82
0.43	0.31	0	0	0	20.44	0	0.26	0.2	1.48	0.16	26.28	0.2	26.28	1.62	35.04	83.22	54.02	8.76	0.92
0.75	0.77	0	0	0	25.02	0	0.25	0.26	1.85	0.05	27.97	0.15	14.72	1.71	20.61	76.54	30.91	122.18	0.65
0.28	0.75	0	0	0	0	0	0.27	0.22	1.98	0.04	25.02	0	8.83	1.66	20.61	58.88	27.97	108.93	0.54
0.1	0.36	0	0	0	21	0	0.14	0.14	2.14	0.13	16.8	0	42	1.46	86.8	151.2	81.2	19.6	1.51
0.11	0.3	0	0	0.07	0	0	0.15	0.06	0.99	0.11	7	0	21	1.48	42	124.6	61.6	4.2	1.13
0	0	0	0	0	49.74	2.98	0.11	0	1.42	0	0	0	23.87	0.75	0	0	0	392.92	0
0.64	0.63	0	0	1.4	0	0	0.19	0.05	2.98	0.28	7.8	0	19.5	0.82	83.85	161.85	83.85	9.75	1.23
0.59	0.58	0	0	0	0	0	0.2	0.02	2.59	0.29	7.8	0	19.5	1.03	85.8	150.15	154.05	1.95	1.21
0.14	0.12	0	0	0.08	0	0	0.26	0.02	2.33	0.15	4.74	0	15.8	1.9	18.96	67.94	55.3	1.58	0.77
0.08	0.07	0	0	0.08	0	0	0.12	0.08	1.45	0.02	6.6	0	13.2	1.04	8.25	23.1	6.6	4.95	0.4
0.12	0.1	0	0	0	0	0	0.31	0.03	3.41	0.09	3.72	0	5.58	2.77	24.18	68.82	53.94	0	0.78
0.11	0.09	0	0	0	0	0	0.31	0.03	2.78	0.11	3.72	0	1.86	2.72	14.88	61.38	48.36	0	0.74
2.26	1.91	0	0	0	0	0.4	0.25	0.16	3.6	0.2	14.14	0.12	16.16	1.9	24.24	74.74	84.84	1147.36	0.57
0	0	0	0	0	100	12	0	0	0	0	0	0	0	0.4	0	0	0	75	0
1.23	1.12	0	0	0	4.55	0	0.03	0.01	0.18	0.05	0.78	0	20.8	0.33	13.65	32.24	23.27	47.71	0.18
1.23	1.12	0	0	0	0	0	0.03	0.01	0.18	0	0.78	0	20.8	0.33	13.65	32.24	23.27	1.95	0.18
0.16	0.28	0	0	0	6	0	0.03	0.02	0.37	0.05	3.75	0	43.75	0.35	16.25	78.5	38.5	40.25	0.24
0.16	0.28	0	0	0	0	0	0.03	0.02	0.37	0.05	3.75	0	43.75	0.35	16.25	78.5	38.5	2.75	0.24
1.01	0.98	0	0	0	0	0	0.19	0.1	1.25	0.02	4.2	0	43.75	1.16	9.1	43.4	45.85	167.3	0.25
1.01	0.98	0	0	0	0	0	0.19	0.1	1.25	0.02	4.2	0	13.65	1.16	9.1	43.4	45.85	167.3	0.25
0.08	0.35	0	0	0	0	0	0.09	0.14	2.11	0.22	42.64	0	4.92	0.98	52.48	134.48	165.64	4.92	2.2
0	0	0	0	0	0	2.4	0	0	0	0	0	0	24	1	0	0	0	620	0
1.42	0.35	0	0	0.03	0	2.01	0.04	0.02	0.44	0.02	0.3	0.11	0.72	0.1	1.44	20.16	29.16	95.76	0.2
0.85	0.17	0	0	0.05	0	4.54	0.17	0.04	1.45	0.09	0.84	0.16	2.1	0.17	4.41	62.16	81.9	324.66	0.36
0	0	0	0	0	0	0	0	0	0	0	0	0	0	0	0	0	0	170	0
0.95	0.19	0.21	0	0	1.61	4.37	0.08	0.06	0.52	0.06	2.07	0.39	12.65	0.27	3.91	30.36	75.67	306.82	0.57
5.4	1.9	0	0	0.32	0	5.06	0.13	0.1	1.13	0.16	91.84	0	134.09	4.3	86.02	273.24	781.77	1047.42	3.69
3.68	0.55	0	0	0	55.86	4.79	0.14	0.12	2.5	0.24	115.44	0	119.7	4.26	66.5	215.46	851.2	1263.5	3.19
7.27	2.15	0	0	1.21	38.55	5.91	0.15	0.14	2.32	0.12	77.1	0	123.36	4.45	71.96	267.28	603.95	1105.1	4.81
1.7	0.5	0	0	1.37	45.54	5.06	0.13	0.1	1.13	0.16	91.84	0	134.09	4.3	86.02	273.24	781.77	1047.42	3.69
5.4	1.9	0	0	0.32	0	3	0.34	0.12	0.23	0.23	122	0	154	5.03	109	276	906	1068	1.85
0.04	0.2	0	0	0	0.86	0	0.21	0.05	0.435	0.06	128	0	46	1.8	120	240	610	408	0.97
0.6	1.2	0	0	0	5	9	0.07	0.08	0.3	1.14	160	0	77	3.24	70	216	413	718	2.54
0.1	0.4	0	0	0	0	3	0.28	0.18	1.3	0.18	126	0	69	3.15	79	134.4	658	888	1.41
0	0.2	0	0	1.74	0	0	0.13	0.08	0.6	0.22	121	0	51	4.36	94	178	530	810	1.57
0.1	0.5	0	0	1	0	2	0.37	0.14	1.3	0.27	163	0	123	4.85	123	351	755	1174	2.02
0.4	0.7	0	0	0	0	2	0.24	0.15	0.7	0.18	144	0	103	3.5	65	221	583	706	1.66
1.4	0.4	0	0	0	0	15	0.07	0.04	0.8	0.36	28	0	89	4.2	83	218	676	756	2.96
0	0	0	0	0	0	0	0	0	0	0	0	0	0	2	0	0	0	960	0
2.61	0.19	0	0	0.05	0	4.54	0.01	0.05	0.86	0.07	1.7	0.46	2.27	0.53	3.4	35.44	41.11	321.49	1.3
0.41	0.05	0	0	0	0	4.88	0.04	0.08	1.37	0.07	1.98	1.46	2.84	0.98	5.1	39.41	113.97	374.79	1.01
4.1	0.28	0	0	0.07	0	0.85	0.03	0.05	1.44	0.05	1.98	0.5	2.55	0.54	5.1	42.53	64.64	347.85	1.21
3.68	0.3	0	0	0	0	3.4	0.01	0.04	0.9	0.03	1.13	0.53	1.98	0.5	3.69	29.77	49.9	320.64	0.79
0.52	0.07	0	0	0.03	0	5.87	0.02	0.05	1.3	0.1	2.27	0.49	2.27	0.81	5.95	51.31	106.88	356.64	1.11
0.48	0.06	0	0	0.04	0	4.05	0.02	0.05	1.49	0.1	3.12	0.73	3.12	0.77	5.39	47.63	121.62	407.96	1.13
3.808	0.442	0	0	0	0	0	0.085	0.264	2.898	0.246	7.65	2.303	5.95	3.13	22.95	203.15	332.35	51.85	4.07
2.03	0.17	0	0	0.05	0	0	0.02	0.08	1.41	0.08	2.55	0.62	1.98	0.67	5.95	45.64	88.74	19.85	1.55

USDA ID Code	Food Name	Weight in Grams*	Quantity of Units	Unit of Measure	Protein (gm)	Fat (gm)	Carbohydrates (gm)	Kcalories	Caffeine (gm)	Fiber (gm)	Cholesterol (mg)	Saturated Fat (gm)
13300	Beef, Ground, Extra Lean, Pan-fried	28.35	3	Ounce	7.08	4.66	0	72.29	0	0	22.96	1.83
13305	Beef, Ground, Lean, Broiled	28.35	3	Ounce	7.01	5.23	0	77.11	0	0	24.66	2.06
13307	Beef, Ground, Lean, Pan-fried	28.35	3	Ounce	6.87	5.4	0	77.96	0	0	23.81	2.12
13312	Beef, Ground, Regular, Broiled	28.35	3	Ounce	6.82	5.87	0	81.93	0	0	25.52	2.3
13314	Beef, Ground, Regular, Pan-fried	28.35	3	Ounce	6.78	6.4	0	86.75	0	0	25.23	2.51
13326	Beef, Liver, Ckd, Braised	28.35	3	Ounce	6.91	1.39	0.97	45.64	0	0	110.28	0.54
13327	Beef, Liver, Ckd, Pan-fried	28.35	3	Ounce	7.58	2.27	2.23	61.52	0	0	136.65	0.76
7042	Beef, Loaved, Lunch Meat	28.35	1	Slice	4.08	7.43	0.82	87.32	0	0	18.14	3.17
13504	Beef, Steaks and Roasts, Ckd, 1/2 in. Fat	28.35	3	Ounce	7.07	7.62	0	98.94	0	0	25.8	3.15
13361	Beef, Steaks and Roasts, Ckd, Fat Trimmed	28.35	3	Ounce	7.75	4.92	0	77.4	0	0	24.66	1.94
13004	Beef, Steaks and Roasts, Ckd., 1/4 in. Fat	28.35	3	Ounce	7.35	6.11	0	86.47	0	0	24.95	2.42
7043	Beef, Thin Sliced	4.2	1	Slice	1.18	0.16	0.24	7.43	0	0	1.72	0.07
10126	Bologna	23	1	Slice	3.52	4.57	0.17	56.81	0	0	13.57	1.58
7007	Bologna, Beef	28.35	1	Slice	3.46	8.08	0.23	88.45	0	0	16.44	3.42
62601	Buffalo (Chicken) Wings	22.75	4	Each	4.5	3	0.5	47.5	0	0	25	0.75
5280	Chicken Roll, Light Meat	28.35	3	Ounce	5.54	2.09	0.69	45.08	0	0	14.18	0.57
5283	Chicken Salad Sandwich Spread	28.35	3	Ounce	3.3	3.83	2.1	56.7	0	0	8.51	0.98
5281	Chicken Spread, Cnd	28.35	3	Ounce	4.37	3.32	1.53	54.43	0	0	14.74	0.96
5054	Chicken, Back, Meat Only, Ckd, Fried	28.35	3	Ounce	8.5	4.34	1.61	81.65	0	0	26.37	1.17
5055	Chicken, Back, Meat Only, Ckd, Roasted	28.35	3	Ounce	7.99	3.73	0	67.76	0	0	25.52	1.02
5056	Chicken, Back, Meat Only, Ckd, Stewed	28.35	3	Ounce	7.18	3.17	0	59.25	0	0	24.1	0.86
5049	Chicken, Back, Meat&skin, Ckd, Fried, Batter	28.35	3	Ounce	6.23	6.21	2.91	93.84	0	0	24.95	1.65
5050	Chicken, Back, Meat&skin, Ckd, Fried, Flr	28.35	3	Ounce	7.88	5.88	1.84	93.84	0	0	25.23	1.59
5051	Chicken, Back, Meat&skin, Ckd, Roasted	28.35	3	Ounce	7.36	5.94	0	85.05	0	0	24.95	1.65
5052	Chicken, Back, Meat&skin, Ckd, Stewed	28.35	3	Ounce	6.29	5.14	0	73.14	0	0	22.11	1.42
5063	Chicken, Breast, Meat Only, Ckd, Fried	28.35	3	Ounce	9.48	1.34	0.14	53.01	0	0	25.8	0.37
5064	Chicken, Breast, Meat Only, Ckd, Roasted	28.35	3	Ounce	8.79	1.01	0	46.78	0	0	24.1	0.29
5065	Chicken, Breast, Meat Only, Ckd, Stewed	28.35	3	Ounce	8.22	0.86	0	42.81	0	0	21.83	0.24
5058	Chicken, Breast, Meat&skin, Ckd, Fried, Batter	28.35	3	Ounce	7.04	3.74	2.55	73.71	0	0.09	24.1	1
5059	Chicken, Breast, Meat&skin, Ckd, Fried, Flr	28.35	3	Ounce	9.03	2.51	0.46	62.94	0	0	25.23	0.69
5060	Chicken, Breast, Meat&skin, Ckd, Roasted	28.35	3	Ounce	8.45	2.21	0	55.85	0	0	23.81	0.62
5061	Chicken, Breast, Meat&skin, Ckd, Stewed	28.35	3	Ounce	7.77	2.1	0	52.16	0	0	21.26	0.59
5277	Chicken, Cnd.	28.35	3	Ounce	6.17	2.25	0	46.78	0	0	17.58	0.62
5044	Chicken, Dark Meat, Meat Only, Ckd, Fried	28.35	3	Ounce	8.22	3.29	0.73	67.76	0	0	27.22	0.88
5045	Chicken, Dark Meat, Meat Only, Ckd, Roasted	28.35	3	Ounce	7.76	2.76	0	58.12	0	0	26.37	0.75
5046	Chicken, Dark Meat, Meat Only, Ckd, Stewed	28.35	3	Ounce	7.36	2.55	0	54.43	0	0	24.95	0.69
5035	Chicken, Dark Meat, Meat&skin, Ckd, Fried, Batter	28.35	3	Ounce	6.19	5.28	2.66	84.48	0	0	25.23	1.4
5036	Chicken, Dark Meat, Meat&skin, Ckd, Fried, Flr	28.35	3	Ounce	7.72	4.79	1.16	80.8	0	0	26.08	1.3
5037	Chicken, Dark Meat, Meat&skin, Ckd, Roasted	28.35	3	Ounce	7.36	4.47	0	71.73	0	0	25.8	1.24
5038	Chicken, Dark Meat, Meat&skin, Ckd, Stewed	28.35	3	Ounce	6.66	4.16	0	66.06	0	0	23.25	1.15
5072	Chicken, Drumstick, Meat Only, Ckd, Fried	28.35	3	Ounce	8.11	2.29	0	55.28	0	0	26.65	0.6
5073	Chicken, Drumstick, Meat Only, Ckd, Roasted	28.35	3	Ounce	8.02	1.6	0	48.76	0	0	26.37	0.42
5074	Chicken, Drumstick, Meat Only, Ckd, Stewed	28.35	3	Ounce	7.8	1.62	0	47.91	0	0	24.95	0.43
5067	Chicken, Drumstick, Meat&skin, Ckd, Fried, Batter	28.35	3	Ounce	6.22	4.47	2.35	75.98	0	0	24.38	1.17
5068	Chicken, Drumstick, Meat&skin, Ckd, Fried, Flr	28.35	3	Ounce	7.64	3.89	0.46	69.46	0	0	25.52	1.04
5069	Chicken, Drumstick, Meat&skin, Ckd, Roasted	28.35	3	Ounce	7.66	3.16	0	61.24	0	0	25.8	0.86
5070	Chicken, Drumstick, Meat&skin, Ckd, Stewed	28.35	3	Ounce	7.18	3.02	0	57.83	0	0	23.53	0.82
5021	Chicken, Giblets, Ckd, Fried	28.35	3	Ounce	9.23	3.82	1.23	78.53	0	0	126.44	1.08
5022	Chicken, Giblets, Ckd, Simmered	28.35	3	Ounce	7.33	1.35	0.27	44.51	0	0	111.42	0.42
5026	Chicken, Heart, Ckd, Simmered	28.35	3	Ounce	7.49	2.25	0.03	52.45	0	0	68.61	0.64
5081	Chicken, Leg, Meat Only, Ckd, Fried	28.35	3	Ounce	8.05	2.64	0.18	58.97	0	0	28.07	0.71
5082	Chicken, Leg, Meat Only, Ckd, Roasted	28.35	3	Ounce	7.66	2.39	0	54.15	0	0	26.65	0.65
5083	Chicken, Leg, Meat Only, Ckd, Stewed	28.35	3	Ounce	7.44	2.29	0	52.45	0	0	25.23	0.62
5076	Chicken, Leg, Meat&skin, Ckd, Fried, Batter	28.35	3	Ounce	6.17	4.58	2.47	77.4	0	0	25.52	1.21
5077	Chicken, Leg, Meat&skin, Ckd, Fried, Flour	28.35	3	Ounce	7.61	4.09	0.71	72.01	0	0	26.65	1.11

Monounsaturated Fat (gm)	Polyunsaturated Fat (gm)	Vitamin D (mg)	Vitamin K (mg)	Vitamin E (mg)	Vitamin A (re)	Vitamin C (mg)	Thiamin (mg)	Riboflavin (mg)	Niacin (mg)	Vitamin B6 (mg)	Folate (mg)	Vitamin B12 (mcg)	Calcium (mg)	Iron (mg)	Magnesium (mg)	Phosphorus (mg)	Potassium (mg)	Sodium (mg)	Zinc (mg)
2.04	0.17	0	0	0.05	0	0	0.02	0.07	1.34	0.08	2.55	0.57	1.98	0.67	5.95	45.36	88.45	19.85	1.54
2.29	0.2	0	0	0.06	0	0	0.01	0.06	1.46	0.07	2.55	0.67	3.12	0.6	5.95	44.79	85.33	21.83	1.52
2.36	0.2	0	0	0.06	0	0	0.01	0.06	1.36	0.08	2.55	0.64	2.84	0.62	5.67	45.08	84.77	21.83	1.47
2.57	0.22	0	0	0.07	0	0	0.01	0.05	1.64	0.08	2.55	0.83	3.12	0.69	5.67	48.2	82.78	23.53	1.47
2.8	0.24	0	0	0.07	0	0	0.01	0.06	1.65	0.07	2.55	0.77	3.12	0.69	5.67	48.48	85.05	23.81	1.44
0.18	0.3	0	0	0	3005.67	6.52	0.06	1.16	3.04	0.26	61.52	20.13	1.98	1.92	5.67	114.53	66.62	19.85	1.72
0.46	0.48	0	0	0.18	3041.67	6.52	0.06	1.17	4.09	0.41	62.37	31.7	3.12	1.78	6.52	130.69	103.19	30.05	1.55
3.47	0.25	0	0	0.06	0	3.69	0.03	0.06	1.04	0.05	1.42	1.1	3.12	0.66	3.97	33.74	58.97	376.77	0.72
3.41	0.29	0	0	0	0	0	0.02	0.06	0.98	0.09	1.98	0.68	2.84	0.74	5.95	54.72	81.36	16.73	1.56
2.1	0.18	0	0	0.05	0	0	0.02	0.06	1.04	0.09	1.98	0.71	2.55	0.77	6.52	59.82	91.57	17.58	1.72
2.61	0.22	0	0	0.06	0	0	0.02	0.06	1.03	0.09	1.98	0.69	2.84	0.74	6.24	57.55	88.74	17.58	1.66
0.07	0.01	0	0	0.01	0	0.6	0	0.01	0.22	0.01	0.46	0.11	0.46	0.11	0.8	7.06	18.02	60.44	0.17
2.25	0.49	0	0	0.06	0	8.12	0.12	0.04	0.9	0.04	1.15	0.21	2.53	0.18	3.22	31.97	64.63	272.32	0.47
3.91	0.31	0.2	0	0.05	0	5.95	0.01	0.03	0.68	0.04	1.42	0.4	3.4	0.47	3.4	24.95	44.51	278.11	0.61
0	0	0	0	0	15	0.3	0	0	0	0	0	0	6	0.1	0	0	0	225	0
0.84	0.45	0	0	0.08	6.8	0	0.02	0.04	1.5	0.06	0.57	0.04	12.19	0.27	5.39	44.51	64.64	165.56	0.2
0.92	1.76	0	0	0	11.91	0.34	0.01	0.02	0.47	0.03	1.42	0.11	2.84	0.17	2.84	9.36	51.88	106.88	0.29
1.38	0.71	0	0	0	7.09	0	0	0.03	0.78	0.04	0.85	0.04	35.44	0.66	3.4	25.23	30.05	109.43	0.33
1.62	1.03	0	0	0	8.22	0	0.03	0.07	2.18	0.1	2.55	0.09	7.37	0.47	7.09	49.9	71.16	28.07	0.79
1.37	0.86	0	0	0.08	7.94	0	0.02	0.06	2	0.1	1.98	0.09	6.8	0.39	6.24	46.78	67.19	27.22	0.75
1.14	0.74	0	0	0.08	7.65	0	0.01	0.05	1.29	0.06	1.98	0.06	5.95	0.36	4.82	36.86	44.79	18.99	0.67
2.53	1.47	0	0	0	10.21	0	0.03	0.06	1.65	0.07	2.55	0.07	7.37	0.42	5.39	38.84	51.03	89.87	0.56
2.32	1.36	0	0	0	10.49	0	0.03	0.07	2.07	0.09	2.27	0.08	6.8	0.46	6.52	47.06	64.07	25.52	0.7
2.35	1.31	0	0	0.08	28.07	0	0.02	0.06	1.9	0.08	1.7	0.08	5.95	0.4	5.67	43.66	59.54	24.66	0.64
2.02	1.13	0	0	0.08	24.95	0	0.01	0.04	1.23	0.04	1.42	0.05	5.1	0.35	4.54	34.02	41.11	18.14	0.55
0.49	0.3	0	0	0.12	1.98	0	0.02	0.04	4.19	0.18	1.13	0.1	4.54	0.32	8.79	69.74	78.25	22.4	0.31
0.35	0.22	0	0	0.08	1.7	0	0.02	0.03	3.89	0.17	1.13	0.1	4.25	0.29	8.22	64.64	72.58	20.98	0.28
0.29	0.19	0	0	0.08	1.7	0	0.01	0.03	2.4	0.09	0.85	0.07	3.69	0.25	6.8	46.78	53.01	17.86	0.27
1.55	0.87	0	0	0.3	5.67	0	0.03	0.04	2.98	0.12	1.7	0.09	5.67	0.35	6.8	52.45	56.98	77.96	0.27
0.99	0.56	0	0	0	4.25	0	0.02	0.04	3.9	0.16	1.13	0.1	4.54	0.34	8.51	66.06	73.43	21.55	0.31
0.86	0.47	0	0	0.08	7.65	0	0.02	0.03	3.6	0.16	1.13	0.09	3.97	0.3	7.65	60.67	69.46	20.13	0.29
0.82	0.45	0	0	0.08	6.8	0	0.01	0.03	2.21	0.08	0.85	0.06	3.69	0.26	6.24	44.23	50.46	17.58	0.27
0.89	0.5	0	0	0.06	9.64	0.57	0	0.04	1.79	0.1	1.13	0.08	3.97	0.45	3.4	31.47	39.12	142.6	0.4
1.22	0.79	0	0	0	6.8	0	0.03	0.07	2	0.1	2.55	0.09	5.1	0.42	7.09	53.01	71.73	27.5	0.82
1.01	0.64	0	0	0.08	6.24	0	0.02	0.06	1.86	0.1	2.27	0.09	4.25	0.38	6.52	50.75	68.04	26.37	0.79
0.92	0.59	0	0	0.08	5.95	0	0.02	0.06	1.34	0.06	1.98	0.06	3.97	0.39	5.67	40.54	51.31	20.98	0.75
2.15	1.26	0	0	0	8.79	0	0.03	0.06	1.59	0.07	2.55	0.08	5.95	0.41	5.67	41.11	52.45	83.63	0.59
1.89	1.11	0	0	0	8.79	0	0.03	0.07	1.94	0.09	2.27	0.09	4.82	0.43	6.8	49.9	65.21	25.23	0.74
1.75	0.99	0	0	0	16.44	0	0.02	0.06	1.8	0.09	1.98	0.08	4.25	0.39	6.24	47.63	62.37	24.66	0.71
1.63	0.92	0	0	0	15.31	0	0.01	0.05	1.28	0.05	1.7	0.06	3.97	0.37	5.1	37.71	47.06	19.85	0.64
0.83	0.56	0	0	0	5.1	0	0.02	0.07	1.74	0.11	2.55	0.1	3.4	0.37	6.8	52.73	70.59	27.22	0.91
0.53	0.39	0	0	0.08	5.1	0	0.02	0.06	1.72	0.11	2.55	0.1	3.4	0.37	6.8	52.16	69.74	26.93	0.9
0.55	0.39	0	0	0.08	4.82	0	0.02	0.06	1.22	0.07	2.27	0.07	3.12	0.39	5.95	42.53	56.42	22.68	0.86
1.82	1.07	0	0	0	7.37	0	0.03	0.06	1.44	0.08	2.55	0.08	4.82	0.38	5.67	41.67	52.73	76.26	0.66
1.54	0.92	0	0	0	7.09	0	0.02	0.06	1.71	0.1	2.27	0.09	3.4	0.38	6.52	49.9	64.92	25.23	0.82
1.2	0.71	0	0	0.08	8.51	0	0.02	0.06	1.7	0.1	2.27	0.09	3.4	0.38	6.52	49.61	64.92	25.52	0.81
1.15	0.67	0	0	0.08	7.65	0	0.01	0.05	1.19	0.05	1.98	0.06	3.12	0.38	5.67	39.97	52.16	21.55	0.75
1.25	0.96	0	0	0	1014.65	2.47	0.03	0.43	3.11	0.17	107.45	3.77	5.1	2.93	7.09	81.08	93.56	32.04	1.78
0.34	0.31	0	0	0.37	631.92	2.27	0.02	0.27	1.16	0.1	106.6	2.87	3.4	1.83	5.67	64.92	44.79	16.44	1.3
0.57	0.65	0	0	0	2.55	0.51	0.02	0.21	0.79	0.09	22.68	2.07	5.39	2.56	5.67	56.42	37.42	13.61	2.07
0.97	0.63	0	0	0	5.67	0	0.02	0.07	1.9	0.11	2.55	0.1	3.69	0.4	7.09	54.72	72.01	27.22	0.84
0.86	0.56	0	0	0.08	5.39	0	0.02	0.07	1.79	0.1	2.27	0.09	3.4	0.37	6.8	51.88	68.61	25.8	0.81
0.83	0.53	0	0	0.08	5.1	0	0.02	0.06	1.36	0.06	2.27	0.07	3.12	0.4	5.95	42.24	53.87	22.11	0.79
1.87	1.09	0	0	0	7.65	0	0.03	0.06	1.54	0.08	2.55	0.08	5.1	0.4	5.67	43.09	53.58	79.1	0.62
1.61	0.94	0	0	0	7.94	0	0.02	0.07	1.86	0.1	2.27	0.09	3.69	0.41	6.8	51.6	66.06	24.95	0.76

USDA ID Code	Food Name	Weight in Grams*	Quantity of Units	Unit of Measure	Protein (gm)	Fat (gm)	Carbohydrates (gm)	Kcalories	Caffeine (gm)	Fiber (gm)	Cholesterol (mg)	Saturated Fat (gm)
5078	Chicken, Leg, Meat&skin, Ckd, Roasted	28.35	3	Ounce	7.36	3.82	0	65.77	0	0	26.08	1.05
5079	Chicken, Leg, Meat&skin, Ckd, Stewed	28.35	3	Ounce	6.85	3.66	0	62.37	0	0	23.81	1.01
5028	Chicken, Liver, Ckd, Simmered	28.35	3	Ounce	6.91	1.55	0.25	44.51	0	0	178.89	0.52
5012	Chicken, Meat Only, Ckd, Fried	28.35	3	Ounce	8.67	2.59	0.48	62.09	0	0.03	26.65	0.7
5013	Chicken, Meat Only, Roasted	28.35	3	Ounce	8.2	2.1	0	53.87	0	0	25.23	0.58
5014	Chicken, Meat Only, Stewed	28.35	3	Ounce	7.74	1.9	0	50.18	0	0	23.53	0.52
5097	Chicken, Thigh, Meat Only, Ckd, Fried	28.35	3	Ounce	7.99	2.92	0.33	61.8	0	0	28.92	0.79
5098	Chicken, Thigh, Meat Only, Ckd, Roasted	28.35	3	Ounce	7.35	3.08	0	59.25	0	0	26.93	0.86
5099	Chicken, Thigh, Meat Only, Ckd, Stewed	28.35	3	Ounce	7.09	2.78	0	55.28	0	0	25.52	0.77
5092	Chicken, Thigh, Meat&skin, Ckd, Fried, Batter	28.35	3	Ounce	6.13	4.69	2.57	78.53	0	0	26.37	1.25
5093	Chicken, Thigh, Meat&skin, Ckd, Fried, Flr	28.35	3	Ounce	7.58	4.25	0.9	74.28	0	0	27.5	1.16
5094	Chicken, Thigh, Meat&skin, Ckd, Roasted	28.35	3	Ounce	7.1	4.39	0	70.02	0	0	26.37	1.23
5095	Chicken, Thigh, Meat&skin, Ckd, Stewed	28.35	3	Ounce	6.59	4.18	0	65.77	0	0	23.81	1.17
5106	Chicken, Wing, Meat Only, Ckd, Fried	28.35	3	Ounce	8.55	2.59	0	59.82	0	0	23.81	0.71
5107	Chicken, Wing, Meat Only, Ckd, Roasted	28.35	3	Ounce	8.64	2.3	0	57.55	0	0	24.1	0.64
5108	Chicken, Wing, Meat Only, Ckd, Stewed	28.35	3	Ounce	7.71	2.04	0	51.31	0	0	20.98	0.57
5101	Chicken, Wing, Meat&skin, Ckd, Fried, Batter	28.35	3	Ounce	5.63	6.18	3.1	91.85	0	0	22.4	1.65
5102	Chicken, Wing, Meat&skin, Ckd, Fried, Flr	28.35	3	Ounce	7.4	6.28	0.68	91	0	0	22.96	1.72
5103	Chicken, Wing, Meat&skin, Ckd, Roasted	28.35	3	Ounce	7.61	5.52	0	82.22	0	0	23.81	1.55
5104	Chicken, Wing, Meat&skin, Ckd, Stewed	28.35	3	Ounce	6.46	4.77	0	70.59	0	0	19.85	1.34
16059	Chili w/ Beans, Cnd	255	0.5	Cup	14.56	14	30.37	285.6	0	11.22	43.35	6
7020	Corned Beef Loaf, Jellied	28.35	1	Slice	6.49	1.73	0	43.38	0	0	13.32	0.74
	Cornish Game Hen	110	0.5	Bird	25.63	4.257	0	147.4	0	0	116.6	1.089
5142	Duck, Domesticated, Meat Only, Roasted	28.35	3	Ounce	6.66	3.18	0	56.98	0	0	25.23	1.18
5140	Duck, Domesticated, Meat&skin, Roasted	28.35	3	Ounce	5.38	8.04	0	95.54	0	0	23.81	2.74
7021	Dutch Brand Loaf, Lunch Meat	28.35	1	Slice	3.8	5.05	1.58	68.04	0	0	13.32	1.8
7032	Ham and Cheese Loaf(or Roll), Lunch Meat	28.35	1	Slice	4.71	5.73	0.41	73.43	0	0	16.16	2.13
7033	Ham and Cheese Spread, Lunch Meat	15	1	Tbsp.	2.43	2.78	0.34	36.75	0	0	9.15	1.29
7031	Ham Salad Spread	15	1	Tbsp.	1.3	2.33	1.6	32.4	0	0	5.55	0.76
7029	Ham, Approx 11% Fat, Sliced	28.35	1	Slice	4.98	3	0.88	51.6	0	0	16.16	0.96
7027	Ham, Chopped, Not Cnd	28.35	3	Ounce	4.85	4.89	0	64.92	0	0	14.46	1.62
7026	Ham, Chopped, Spiced, Cnd	28.35	3	Ounce	4.55	5.34	0.08	67.76	0	0	13.89	1.78
7028	Ham, Extra Lean, Appx 5% Fat	28.35	1	Slice	5.49	1.41	0.27	37.14	0	0	13.32	0.46
7030	Ham, Minced	28.35	3	Ounce	4.62	5.86	0.52	74.56	0	0	19.85	2.04
62626	Hamburger Patty, Meatless	90	1	Each	18	4	8	140	0	5	0	1.5
7035	Honey Loaf, Lunch Meat	28.35	1	Slice	4.47	1.27	1.51	36.29	0	0	9.64	0.41
7022	Hot Dog, Beef	57	1	Each	6.84	16.25	1.03	179.55	0	0	34.77	6.87
7024	Hot Dog, Chicken	45	1	Each	5.82	8.77	3.06	115.65	0	0	45.45	2.49
62605	Hot Dog, Fat Free	50	1	Each	7	0	2	40	0	0	15	0
7025	Hot Dog, Turkey	45	1	Each	6.43	7.97	0.67	101.7	0	0	48.15	2.65
16137	Hummus, Fresh	246	0.5	Cup	12.1	20.8	49.6	421	0	12.5	0	3.1
17225	Lamb, Ground, Ckd, Broiled	28.35	3	Ounce	7.02	5.57	0	80.23	0	0	27.5	2.3
17016	Lamb, Leg, Shank, Meat and Fat, Ckd, Rstd	28.35	3	Ounce	7.49	3.53	0	63.79	0	0	25.52	1.44
17018	Lamb, Leg, Shank, Meat Only, Ckd, Rstd	28.35	3	Ounce	7.99	1.89	0	51.03	0	0	24.66	0.67
17020	Lamb, Leg, Sirloin, Meat and Fat, Ckd, Rstd	28.35	3	Ounce	6.98	5.86	0	82.78	0	0	27.5	2.48
17022	Lamb, Leg, Sirloin, Meat Only, Ckd, Rstd	28.35	3	Ounce	8.04	2.6	0	57.83	0	0	26.08	0.93
17012	Lamb, Leg, Whole, Meat and Fat, Ckd, Rstd	28.35	3	Ounce	7.24	4.67	0	73.14	0	0	26.37	1.95
17014	Lamb, Leg, Whole, Meat Only, Ckd, Rstd	28.35	3	Ounce	8.02	2.19	0	54.15	0	0	25.23	0.78
17024	Lamb, Loin, Meat and Fat, Ckd, Broiled	28.35	3	Ounce	7.14	6.54	0	89.59	0	0	28.35	2.79
17025	Lamb, Loin, Meat and Fat, Ckd, Roasted	28.35	3	Ounce	6.39	6.69	0	87.6	0	0	26.93	2.9
17027	Lamb, Loin, Meat Only, Ckd, Broiled	28.35	3	Ounce	8.5	2.76	0	61.24	0	0	26.93	0.99
17028	Lamb, Loin, Meat Only, Ckd, Roasted	28.35	3	Ounce	7.54	2.77	0	57.27	0	0	24.66	1.05
17002	Lamb, Meat and Fat, Ckd	28.35	3	Ounce	6.95	5.94	0	83.35	0	0	27.5	2.5
17004	Lamb, Meat Only, Ckd	28.35	3	Ounce	8	2.7	0	58.4	0	0	26.08	0.96
17030	Lamb, Rib, Meat and Fat, Ckd, Broiled	28.35	3	Ounce	6.27	8.39	0	102.34	0	0	28.07	3.6

Monounsaturated Fat (gm)	Polyunsaturated Fat (gm)	Vitamin D (mg)	Vitamin K (mg)	Vitamin E (mg)	Vitamin A (re)	Vitamin C (mg)	Thiamin (mg)	Riboflavin (mg)	Niacin (mg)	Vitamin B6 (mg)	Folate (mg)	Vitamin B12 (mcg)	Calcium (mg)	Iron (mg)	Magnesium (mg)	Phosphorus (mg)	Potassium (mg)	Sodium (mg)	Zinc (mg)
1.49	0.85	0	0	0.08	11.06	0	0.02	0.06	1.76	0.09	1.98	0.09	3.4	0.38	6.52	49.33	63.79	24.66	0.74
1.43	0.81	0	0	0.08	10.21	0	0.02	0.05	1.3	0.05	1.7	0.06	3.12	0.38	5.67	39.41	49.9	20.7	0.69
0.38	0.26	0	0	0.41	1392.84	4.48	0.04	0.5	1.26	0.16	218.3	5.5	3.97	2.4	5.95	88.45	39.69	14.46	1.23
0.95	0.61	0	0	0.13	5.1	0	0.02	0.06	2.74	0.14	1.98	0.1	4.82	0.38	7.65	58.12	72.86	25.8	0.64
0.75	0.48	0	0	0.08	4.54	0	0.02	0.05	2.6	0.13	1.7	0.09	4.25	0.34	7.09	55.28	68.89	24.38	0.6
0.68	0.44	0	0	0.08	4.25	0	0.01	0.05	1.73	0.07	1.7	0.06	3.97	0.33	5.95	42.53	51.03	19.85	0.56
1.08	0.69	0	0	0	5.95	0	0.02	0.07	2.02	0.11	2.55	0.09	3.69	0.41	7.37	56.42	73.43	26.93	0.79
1.18	0.7	0	0	0.08	5.67	0	0.02	0.07	1.85	0.1	2.27	0.09	3.4	0.37	6.8	51.88	67.47	24.95	0.73
1.05	0.64	0	0	0.08	5.39	0	0.02	0.06	1.47	0.06	1.98	0.06	3.12	0.4	5.95	42.24	51.88	21.26	0.73
1.9	1.11	0	0	0	8.22	0	0.03	0.06	1.62	0.07	2.55	0.08	5.1	0.41	5.95	43.94	54.43	81.65	0.58
1.66	0.97	0	0	0	8.22	0	0.03	0.07	1.97	0.09	2.27	0.09	3.97	0.42	7.09	53.01	67.19	24.95	0.71
1.74	0.97	0	0	0.08	13.61	0	0.02	0.06	1.8	0.09	1.98	0.08	3.4	0.38	6.24	49.33	62.94	23.81	0.67
1.66	0.92	0	0	0.08	12.47	0	0.02	0.05	1.39	0.05	1.7	0.05	3.12	0.39	5.39	39.41	48.2	20.13	0.64
0.87	0.59	0	0	0	5.1	0	0.01	0.04	2.05	0.17	1.13	0.1	4.25	0.32	5.95	46.49	58.97	25.8	0.6
0.74	0.5	0	0	0.08	5.1	0	0.01	0.04	2.07	0.17	1.13	0.1	4.54	0.33	5.95	47.06	59.54	26.08	0.61
0.65	0.45	0	0	0.08	4.54	0	0.01	0.03	1.47	0.09	0.85	0.06	3.69	0.32	5.1	37.99	43.38	20.7	0.57
2.54	1.44	0	0	0	9.64	0	0.03	0.04	1.49	0.09	1.7	0.07	5.67	0.37	4.54	34.3	39.12	90.72	0.39
2.52	1.4	0	0	0	10.77	0	0.02	0.04	1.9	0.12	0.85	0.08	4.25	0.35	5.39	42.53	50.18	21.83	0.5
2.17	1.17	0	0	0.08	13.32	0	0.01	0.04	1.88	0.12	0.85	0.08	4.25	0.36	5.39	42.81	52.16	23.25	0.52
1.87	1.01	0	0	0.08	11.34	0	0.01	0.03	1.31	0.06	0.85	0.05	3.4	0.32	4.54	34.3	39.41	18.99	0.46
5.95	0.92	0	0	1.87	86.7	4.34	0.12	0.27	0.91	0.34	57.89	0	119.85	8.75	114.75	392.7	930.75	1331.1	5.1
0.76	0.09	0	0	0.05	0	2.27	0	0.03	0.5	0.03	2.27	0.36	3.12	0.58	3.12	20.7	28.63	270.18	1.16
1.364	1.034	0	0	0.291	22	0.66	0.083	0.25	6.9	0.394	2.2	0.33	14.3	0.847	20.9	163.9	275	69.3	1.683
1.05	0.41	0	0	0.2	6.52	0	0.07	0.13	1.45	0.07	2.84	0.11	3.4	0.77	5.67	57.55	71.44	18.43	0.74
3.66	1.03	0	0	0.2	17.86	0	0.05	0.08	1.37	0.05	1.7	0.09	3.12	0.77	4.54	44.23	57.83	16.73	0.53
2.36	0.54	0.28	0	0.06	0	5.1	0.09	0.08	0.68	0.07	0.57	0.37	23.81	0.35	5.95	45.93	106.6	354.38	0.49
2.63	0.62	0.31	0	0.08	6.52	7.09	0.17	0.05	0.98	0.07	0.85	0.23	16.44	0.26	4.54	71.73	83.35	380.74	0.57
1.06	0.21	0	0	0	13.65	1.05	0.05	0.03	0.32	0.02	0.45	0.11	32.55	0.11	2.7	74.25	24.3	179.55	0.34
1.08	0.4	0	0	0.26	0	0.9	0.07	0.02	0.31	0.02	0.15	0.11	1.2	0.09	1.5	18	22.5	136.8	0.16
1.4	0.34	0	0	0.08	0	7.94	0.24	0.07	1.49	0.1	0.85	0.24	1.98	0.28	5.39	70.02	94.12	373.37	0.61
2.32	0.6	0	0	0	0	5.67	0.18	0.06	1.1	0.1	0.28	0.26	1.98	0.24	4.54	43.94	90.44	388.68	0.55
2.6	0.58	0	0	0.07	0	0.57	0.15	0.05	0.91	0.09	0.28	0.2	1.98	0.27	3.69	39.41	80.51	386.98	0.52
0.67	0.14	0	0	0.08	0	7.37	0.26	0.06	1.37	0.13	1.13	0.21	1.98	0.22	4.82	61.8	99.23	405.12	0.55
2.71	0.7	0	0	0	0	8.51	0.2	0.05	1.18	0.07	0.28	0.27	2.84	0.22	4.54	44.51	88.17	352.96	0.54
0	0.5	0	0	0	0	0	0.25	0	4	0	0	0	96	1.5	0	0	0	380	7.5
0.57	0.13	0.26	0	0.06	0	5.95	0.14	0.07	0.89	0.09	2.27	0.31	4.82	0.38	4.82	40.54	97.24	374.22	0.69
7.76	0.79	0.51	0	0.11	0	13.68	0.03	0.06	1.38	0.07	2.28	0.88	11.4	0.82	1.71	49.59	94.62	584.82	1.24
3.82	1.82	0	0	0.1	17.1	0	0.03	0.05	1.39	0.14	1.8	0.11	42.75	0.9	4.5	48.15	37.8	616.5	0.47
0	0	0	0	0	0	0	0	0	0	0	0	0	0	0.2	0	0	0	460	0
2.51	2.25	0	0	0.28	0	0	0.02	0.08	1.86	0.1	3.6	0.13	47.7	0.83	6.3	60.3	80.55	641.7	1.4
8.7	7.8	0	0	2.4	5	19	0.23	0.13	1	0.98	146	0	123	3.86	71	276	428	600	2.71
2.36	0.4	0	0	0.07	0	0	0.03	0.07	1.9	0.04	5.39	0.74	6.24	0.51	6.8	56.98	96.11	22.96	1.32
1.5	0.25	0	0	0.05	0	0	0.03	0.08	1.86	0.05	6.24	0.76	2.84	0.56	7.09	56.13	92.42	18.43	1.32
0.83	0.12	0	0	0.05	0	0	0.03	0.08	1.81	0.05	6.8	0.77	2.27	0.58	7.37	58.97	96.96	18.71	1.42
2.47	0.42	0	0	0.04	0	0	0.03	0.08	1.88	0.04	4.82	0.72	3.12	0.57	6.24	51.88	85.33	19.28	1.17
1.14	0.17	0	0	0.05	0	0	0.03	0.09	1.78	0.04	5.95	0.73	2.27	0.62	7.09	57.55	94.41	20.13	1.37
1.97	0.33	0	0	0.04	0	0	0.03	0.08	1.87	0.04	5.67	0.73	3.12	0.56	6.8	54.15	88.74	18.71	1.25
0.96	0.14	0	0	0.05	0	0	0.03	0.08	1.8	0.05	6.52	0.75	2.27	0.6	7.37	58.4	95.82	19.28	1.4
2.75	0.48	0	0	0.04	0	0	0.03	0.07	2.01	0.04	5.1	0.7	5.67	0.51	6.8	55.57	92.7	21.83	0.99
2.74	0.53	0	0	0.03	0	0	0.03	0.07	2.01	0.04	5.39	0.63	5.1	0.6	6.52	51.03	69.74	18.14	0.97
1.21	0.18	0	0	0.05	0	0	0.03	0.08	1.94	0.05	6.8	0.71	5.39	0.57	7.94	64.07	106.6	23.81	1.17
1.12	0.24	0	0	0.05	0	0	0.03	0.08	1.94	0.05	7.09	0.61	4.82	0.69	7.65	58.4	75.69	18.71	1.15
2.5	0.43	0	0	0	0	0	0.03	0.07	1.89	0.04	5.1	0.72	4.82	0.53	6.52	53.3	87.89	20.41	1.26
1.18	0.18	0	0	0.05	0	0	0.03	0.08	1.79	0.05	6.52	0.74	4.25	0.58	7.37	59.54	97.52	21.55	1.49
3.44	0.67	0	0	0.03	0	0	0.03	0.06	1.98	0.03	3.97	0.72	5.39	0.53	6.52	50.46	76.55	21.55	1.13

USDA ID Code	Food Name	Weight in Grams*	Quantity of Units	Unit of Measure	Protein (gm)	Fat (gm)	Carbohydrates (gm)	Kcalories	Caffeine (gm)	Fiber (gm)	Cholesterol (mg)	Saturated Fat (gm)
17031	Lamb, Rib, Meat and Fat, Ckd, Roasted	28.35	3	Ounce	5.99	8.45	0	101.78	0	0	27.5	3.62
17033	Lamb, Rib, Meat Only, Ckd, Broiled	28.35	3	Ounce	7.86	3.67	0	66.62	0	0	25.8	1.32
17034	Lamb, Rib, Meat Only, Ckd, Roasted	28.35	3	Ounce	7.42	3.77	0	65.77	0	0	24.95	1.35
10161	Olive Loaf, Lunch Meat	28.35	1	Slice	3.36	4.68	2.6	66.62	0	0	10.77	1.66
7051	Olive Loaf, Pork, Lunch Meat	28.35	1	Slice	3.35	4.68	2.61	66.62	0	0	10.77	1.66
10162	Pickle and Pimento Loaf, Lunch Meat	28.35	1	Slice	3.26	5.98	1.67	74.28	0	0	10.49	2.23
7058	Pickle and Pimiento Loaf, Pork, Lunch Meat	28.35	1	Slice	3.26	5.98	1.67	74.28	0	0	10.49	2.22
7062	Picnic Loaf, Lunch Meat	28.35	1	Slice	4.23	4.72	1.35	65.77	0	0	10.77	1.72
10193	Pork, Backribs	28.35	3	Ounce	6.88	8.39	0	104.9	0	0	33.45	3.12
10127	Pork, Braunschweiger	28.35	3	Ounce	3.83	9.1	0.89	101.78	0	0	44.23	3.09
7045	Pork, Cnd, Lunch Meat	21	1	Slice	2.63	6.36	0.44	70.14	0	0	13.02	2.27
10220	Pork, Ground, Ckd	28.35	3	Ounce	7.28	5.89	0	84.2	0	0	26.65	2.19
10154	Pork, Ham and Cheese Loaf or Roll	28.35	3	Ounce	4.71	5.73	0.41	73.43	0	0	16.16	2.13
10147	Pork, Ham Patties, Grilled	28.35	3	Ounce	3.77	8.75	.48	96.96	0	0	20.41	3.14
10148	Pork, Ham Salad Spread	28.35	3	Ounce	2.46	4.4	3.02	61.24	0	0	10.49	1.43
10143	Pork, Ham, Chopped, Cnd	28.35	3	Ounce	4.55	5.34	0.08	67.76	0	0	13.89	1.78
10138	Pork, Ham, Cnd, Extra Lean (appx 4% Fat), Roasted	28.35	3	Ounce	6	1.38	0.15	38.56	0	0	8.51	0.45
10185	Pork, Ham, Cnd, Extra Lean and Reg, Roasted	28.35	3	Ounce	5.94	2.39	0.14	47.34	0	0	11.62	0.8
10184	Pork, Ham, Cnd, Extra Lean and Reg, Unheated	28.35	3	Ounce	5.09	2.11	0	40.82	0	0	10.77	0.69
10140	Pork, Ham, Cnd, Regular (approx 13% Fat), Roasted	28.35	3	Ounce	5.82	4.31	0.12	64.07	0	0	17.58	1.43
10134	Pork, Ham, Extra Lean (5% Fat), Roasted	28.35	3	Ounce	5.93	1.57	0.43	41.11	0	0	15.03	0.51
10133	Pork, Ham, Extra Lean (5% Fat), Unheated	28.35	3	Ounce	5.49	1.41	0.27	37.14	0	0	13.32	0.46
10183	Pork, Ham, Extra Lean and Reg, Roasted	28.35	3	Ounce	6.23	2.17	0.14	46.78	0	0	16.16	0.74
10182	Pork, Ham, Extra Lean and Reg, Unheated	28.35	3	Ounce	5.18	2.38	0.65	45.93	0	0	15.03	0.77
10151	Pork, Ham, Meat and Fat, Roasted	28.35	3	Ounce	6.12	4.75	0	68.89	0	0	17.58	1.7
10153	Pork, Ham, Meat Only, Roasted	28.35	3	Ounce	7.1	1.56	0	44.51	0	0	15.59	0.52
10136	Pork, Ham, Regular (11% Fat), Roasted	28.35	3	Ounce	6.41	2.56	0	50.46	0	0	16.73	0.88
10135	Pork, Ham, Regular (11% Fat), Unheated	28.35	3	Ounce	4.98	3	0.88	51.6	0	0	16.16	0.96
10172	Pork, Smoked Link Sausage, Grilled	28.35	3	Ounce	6.29	9	0.6	110.28	0	0	19.28	3.21
10089	Pork, Spareribs, Meat and Fat, Ckd, Braised	28.35	3	Ounce	8.24	8.59	0	112.55	0	0	34.3	3.15
10221	Pork, Tenderloin, Meat and Fat, Ckd, Broiled	28.35	3	Ounce	8.47	2.3	0	56.98	0	0	26.65	0.83
10223	Pork, Tenderloin, Meat Only, Ckd, Broiled	28.35	3	Ounce	8.62	1.79	0	53.01	0	0	26.65	0.64
7003	Sausage, Beerwurst, Pork	23	1	Slice	3.28	4.32	0.47	54.74	0	0	13.57	1.44
7006	Sausage, Bockwurst	65	1	Link	8.66	17.92	0.31	199.55	0	0	38.35	6.58
7013	Sausage, Bratwurst	85	1	Link	11.97	21.99	1.76	255.85	0	0	51	7.92
7089	Sausage, Italian, Ckd	83	1	Link	16.62	21.33	1.25	268.09	0	0	64.74	7.53
7037	Sausage, Kielbasa, Kolbassy	85	1	Link	11.27	23.08	1.82	263.5	0	0	56.95	8.42
7038	Sausage, Knockwurst	68	1	Link	8.08	18.88	1.2	209.44	0	0	39.44	6.94
7075	Sausage, Link, Pork and Beef	68	1	Link	9.11	20.62	0.97	228.48	0	0	48.28	7.22
7057	Sausage, Pepperoni	5.5	1	Slice	1.15	2.42	0.16	27.34	0	0	4.35	0.89
7059	Sausage, Polish-style	84	1	Each	12	24.3	1.5	276	0	0	60	8.7
7064	Sausage, Pork, Links or Bulk, Ckd	13	1	Link	2.55	4.05	0.13	47.97	0	0	10.79	1.41
7072	Sausage, Salami, Beef and Pork, Dry	10	1	Slice	2.29	3.44	0.26	41.8	0	0	7.9	1.22
7068	Sausage, Salami, Beef, Ckd	23	1	Slice	3.46	4.76	0.65	60.26	0	0	14.95	2.07
7074	Sausage, Smoked Link, Pork	68	1	Link	15.1	21.56	1.43	264.52	0	0	46.24	7.7
62661	Sausage, Turkey	28.35	3	Ounce	4	2.5	1.5	45	0	0	15	1.25
5297	Turkey Bologna	21	1	Slice	2.88	3.19	0.2	41.79	0	0	20.79	1.06
7079	Turkey Breast Meat	21	1	Slice	4.73	0.33	0	23.1	0	0	8.61	0.1
5292	Turkey Burger, Breaded, Battered, Fried	28.35	3	Ounce	3.97	5.1	4.45	80.23	0	0.14	17.58	1.33
5287	Turkey Lunch Meat	28.35	1	Slice	5.37	1.44	0.1	36.29	0	0	15.88	0.48
5289	Turkey Pastrami	28.35	1	Slice	5.21	1.76	0.47	39.97	0	0	15.31	0.51
5296	Turkey Roast, Roasted	28.35	3	Ounce	6.04	1.64	0.87	43.94	0	0	15.03	0.54
5291	Turkey Roll, Light and Dark Meat	28.35	3	Ounce	5.14	1.98	0.6	42.24	0	0	15.59	0.58
5290	Turkey Roll, Light Meat	28.35	3	Ounce	5.3	2.05	0.15	41.67	0	0	12.19	0.57
5299	Turkey Salami	28.35	1	Slice	4.64	3.91	0.16	55.57	0	0	23.25	1.14

Monounsaturated Fat (gm)	Polyunsaturated Fat (gm)	Vitamin D (mg)	Vitamin K (mg)	Vitamin E (mg)	Vitamin A (re)	Vitamin C (mg)	Thiamin (mg)	Riboflavin (mg)	Niacin (mg)	Vitamin B6 (mg)	Folate (mg)	Vitamin B12 (mcg)	Calcium (mg)	Iron (mg)	Magnesium (mg)	Phosphorus (mg)	Potassium (mg)	Sodium (mg)	Zinc (mg)
3.55	0.62	0	0	0.03	0	0	0.03	0.06	1.91	0.03	4.25	0.63	6.24	0.45	5.67	47.06	76.83	20.7	0.99
1.48	0.33	0	0	0.05	0	0	0.03	0.07	1.86	0.04	5.95	0.75	4.54	0.63	8.22	60.39	88.74	24.1	1.49
1.65	0.25	0	0	0.04	0	0	0.03	0.07	1.75	0.04	6.24	0.61	5.95	0.5	6.52	55.28	89.3	22.96	1.27
2.23	0.55	0	0	0	5.67	2.49	0.08	0.07	0.52	0.07	0.57	0.36	30.9	0.15	5.39	36	84.2	420.71	0.39
2.23	0.55	0.31	0	0.07	0	2.55	0.08	0.07	0.52	0.07	0.57	0.36	30.9	0.15	5.39	36	84.2	420.71	0.39
2.72	0.73	0	0	0	1.98	3.83	0.08	0.07	0.58	0.05	1.42	0.33	26.93	0.29	5.1	39.69	96.39	393.78	0.4
2.72	0.73	0.31	0	0.07	8505	3.97	0.08	0.07	0.58	0.05	1.42	0.33	26.93	0.29	5.1	39.69	96.39	393.78	0.4
2.18	0.54	0.34	0	0	0	5.1	0.11	0.07	0.65	0.09	0.57	0.43	13.32	0.29	4.25	35.44	75.69	329.99	0.62
3.82	0.66	0	0	0	0.85	0.09	0.12	0.06	1.01	0.09	0.85	0.18	12.76	0.39	5.95	55.28	89.3	28.63	0.96
4.23	1.06	0	0	0	1196.37	2.72	0.07	0.43	2.37	0.09	12.47	5.7	2.55	2.65	3.12	47.63	56.42	324.04	0.8
3	0.75	0	0	0	0	0.21	0.08	0.04	0.66	0.04	1.26	0.19	1.26	0.15	2.1	17.22	45.15	270.69	0.31
2.62	0.53	0	0	0	0.57	0.2	0.2	0.06	1.19	0.11	1.7	0.15	6.24	0.37	6.8	64.07	102.63	20.7	0.91
2.63	0.62	0	0	0	6.52	7.12	0.17	0.07	0.98	0.07	0.85	0.23	16.44	0.26	4.54	71.73	83.35	380.74	0.57
4.16	0.94	0	0	0.07	0	0	0.1	0.05	0.92	0.05	0.85	0.2	2.55	0.46	2.84	28.63	69.17	301.36	0.54
2.04	0.77	0	0	0	0	1.7	0.12	0.03	0.59	0.04	0.28	0.22	2.27	0.17	2.84	34.02	42.53	258.55	0.31
2.6	0.58	0	0	0	0	0.51	0.15	0.05	0.91	0.09	0.28	0.2	1.98	0.27	3.69	39.41	80.51	386.98	0.52
0.71	0.12	0	0	0.07	0	7.8	0.29	0.07	1.39	0.13	1.42	0.26	1.7	0.26	5.95	59.25	98.66	321.77	0.63
1.15	0.26	0	0	0.07	0	6.49	0.27	0.07	1.43	0.11	1.42	0.24	1.98	0.3	5.67	62.65	99.51	302.78	0.66
1.01	0.22	0	0	0.07	0	7.14	0.25	0.07	1.3	0.13	1.7	0.23	1.7	0.26	4.54	58.68	94.69	361.75	0.52
2	0.5	0	0	0	0	3.97	0.23	0.07	1.5	0.09	1.42	0.3	2.27	0.39	4.82	68.89	101.21	266.77	0.71
0.74	0.15	0	0	0.07	0	5.95	0.21	0.06	1.14	0.11	0.85	0.18	2.27	0.42	3.97	55.57	81.36	341.05	0.82
0.67	0.14	0	0	0.07	0	7.46	0.26	0.06	1.37	0.13	1.13	0.21	1.98	0.22	4.82	61.8	99.23	405.12	0.55
1.06	0.3	0	0	0.07	0	6.24	0.21	0.08	1.51	0.1	0.85	0.19	2.27	0.4	5.39	70.31	102.63	392.65	0.75
1.12	0.26	0	0	0.07	0	7.71	0.25	0.07	1.44	0.11	0.85	0.23	1.98	0.26	5.1	66.91	84.2	362.31	0.58
2.23	0.51	0	0	0.07	0	0	0.17	0.06	1.26	0.11	0.85	0.18	1.98	0.25	5.39	60.67	81.08	336.51	0.66
0.72	0.18	0	0	0.07	0	0	0.19	0.07	1.42	0.13	1.13	0.2	1.98	0.27	6.24	64.35	89.59	376.2	0.73
1.26	0.4	0	0	0.07	0	6.44	0.21	0.09	1.74	0.09	0.85	0.2	2.27	0.38	6.24	79.66	115.95	425.25	0.7
1.4	0.34	0	0	0.07	0	7.85	0.24	0.07	1.49	0.1	0.85	0.24	1.98	0.28	5.39	70.02	94.12	373.37	0.61
4.15	1.07	0	0	0.09	0	0.51	0.2	0.07	1.28	0.1	1.42	0.46	8.51	0.33	5.39	45.93	95.26	425.25	0.8
3.82	0.77	0	0	0.07	0.85	0	0.12	0.11	1.55	0.1	1.13	0.31	13.32	0.52	6.8	73.99	90.72	26.37	1.3
0.95	0.21	0	0	0	0.57	0.28	0.27	0.11	1.43	0.15	1.7	0.28	1.42	0.39	9.92	82.22	125.87	18.14	0.82
0.73	0.16	0	0	0	0.57	0.28	0.28	0.11	1.46	0.15	1.7	0.28	1.42	0.41	10.21	83.63	127.86	18.43	0.84
2.07	0.54	0.21	0	0.06	0	6.67	0.13	0.04	0.75	0.08	0.69	0.2	1.84	0.17	2.99	23.69	58.19	285.2	0.4
8.45	1.94	0	0	0.09	3.9	0	0.27	0.11	2.68	0.15	3.9	0.53	10.4	0.42	11.7	94.9	175.5	718.25	1.01
10.36	2.33	0	0	0.21	0	0.85	0.43	0.16	2.72	0.18	1.7	0.81	37.4	1.1	12.75	126.65	180.2	473.45	1.96
9.92	2.73	0	0	0.21	0	1.66	0.52	0.19	3.46	0.27	4.15	1.08	19.92	1.25	14.94	141.1	252.32	765.26	1.98
11	2.62	0	0	0.19	0	17.85	0.19	0.18	2.45	0.15	4.25	1.37	37.4	1.23	13.6	125.8	230.35	914.6	1.72
8.71	1.99	0	0	0.39	0	18.36	0.23	0.1	1.86	0.12	1.36	0.8	7.48	0.62	7.48	66.64	135.32	686.8	1.13
9.65	2.22	0	0	0.15	0	12.92	0.18	0.12	2.19	0.12	1.36	1.03	6.8	0.99	8.16	72.76	128.52	642.6	1.43
1.16	0.24	0	0	0.01	0	0	0.02	0.01	0.27	0.01	0.22	0.14	0.55	0.08	0.88	6.55	19.09	112.2	0.14
11.4	2.7	0	0	0	0	0	0.42	0.12	3	0.15	3	0.84	9	1.23	12	117	201	744	1.65
1.81	0.5	0	0	0.02	0	0.26	0.1	0.03	0.59	0.04	0.26	0.22	4.16	0.16	2.21	23.92	46.93	168.22	0.33
1.71	0.32	0	0	0.03	0	2.6	0.06	0.03	0.49	0.05	0.2	0.19	0.8	0.15	1.7	14.2	37.8	186	0.32
2.17	0.24	0.28	0	0.04	0	3.98	0.02	0.04	0.74	0.04	0.46	0.7	2.07	0.5	3.22	25.99	51.52	270.48	0.5
9.96	2.56	0	0	0.17	0	1.36	0.48	0.17	3.08	0.24	3.4	1.11	20.4	0.79	12.92	110.16	228.48	1020	1.92
0	0	0	0	0	10	6	0	0	0	0	0	0	12	1.75	0	0	0	300	0
1.01	0.9	0	0	0	0	0	0.01	0.03	0.74	0.05	1.47	0.06	17.64	0.32	2.94	27.51	41.79	184.38	0.37
0.09	0.06	0	0	0	0	0	0.01	0.02	1.75	0.08	0.84	0.42	1.47	0.08	4.2	48.09	58.38	300.51	0.24
2.12	1.34	0	0	0.68	3.12	0	0.03	0.05	0.65	0.06	2.27	0.06	3.97	0.62	4.25	76.55	77.96	226.8	0.41
0.33	0.43	0	0	0.18	0	0	0.01	0.07	1	0.07	1.7	0.07	2.84	0.78	4.54	54.15	92.14	282.37	0.83
0.58	0.45	0	0	0.06	0	0	0.02	0.07	1	0.08	1.42	0.07	2.55	0.47	3.97	56.7	73.71	296.26	0.61
0.34	0.47	0	0	0.11	0	0	0.01	0.05	1.78	0.08	1.42	0.43	1.42	0.46	6.24	69.17	84.48	192.78	0.72
0.65	0.5	0	0	0.1	0	0	0.03	0.08	1.36	0.08	1.42	0.07	9.07	0.38	5.1	47.63	76.55	166.13	0.57
0.71	0.49	0	0	0	0	0	0.03	0.06	1.98	0.09	1.13	0.07	11.34	0.36	4.54	51.88	71.16	138.63	0.44
1.29	1	0	0	0	0	0	0.02	0.05	1	0.07	1.13	0.06	5.67	0.46	4.25	30.05	69.17	284.63	0.51

USDA ID Code	Food Name	Weight in Grams*	Quantity of Units	Unit of Measure	Protein (gm)	Fat (gm)	Carbohydrates (gm)	Kcalories	Caffeine (gm)	Fiber (gm)	Cholesterol (mg)	Saturated Fat (gm)
5300	Turkey Sticks, Breaded, Battered, Fried	28.35	3	Ounce	4.03	4.79	4.82	79.1	0	0	18.14	1.24
5294	Turkey Thigh, Prebasted, Meat&skin, Ckd, Roasted	28.35	3	Ounce	5.33	2.42	0	44.51	0	0	17.58	0.75
5190	Turkey, Back, Meat&skin, Ckd, Roasted	28.35	3	Ounce	7.54	4.08	0	68.89	0	0	25.8	1.19
5192	Turkey, Breast, Meat&skin, Ckd, Roasted	28.35	3	Ounce	8.14	2.1	0	53.58	0	0	20.98	0.6
5164	Turkey, Ckd, Roasted, Meat&skin&giblets&neck	28.35	3	Ounce	7.93	2.68	0.02	58.12	0	0	26.93	0.79
5188	Turkey, Dark Meat, Ckd, Roasted	28.35	3	Ounce	8.1	2.05	0	53.01	0	0	24.1	0.69
5184	Turkey, Dark Meat, Meat&skin, Ckd, Roasted	28.35	3	Ounce	7.79	3.27	0	62.65	0	0	25.23	0.99
5172	Turkey, Giblets, Ckd, Simmered, Some Giblet Fat	28.35	3	Ounce	7.53	1.44	0.59	47.34	0	0	118.5	0.44
5306	Turkey, Ground, Ckd	28.35	3	Ounce	7.76	3.73	0	66.62	0	0	28.92	0.96
5194	Turkey, Leg, Meat&skin, Ckd, Roasted	28.35	3	Ounce	7.9	2.78	0	58.97	0	0	24.1	0.87
5186	Turkey, Light Meat, Ckd, Roasted	28.35	3	Ounce	8.48	0.91	0	44.51	0	0	19.56	0.29
5182	Turkey, Light Meat, Meat&skin, Ckd, Roasted	28.35	3	Ounce	8.1	2.36	0	55.85	0	0	21.55	0.66
5168	Turkey, Meat Only, Ckd, Roasted	28.35	3	Ounce	8.31	1.41	0	48.2	0	0	21.55	0.46
5166	Turkey, Meat&skin, Ckd, Roasted	28.35	3	Ounce	7.97	2.76	0	58.97	0	0	23.25	0.81
5288	Turkey, Thin Sliced	28.35	3	Ounce	6.38	0.45	0	31.19	0	0	11.62	0.14
5196	Turkey, Wing, Meat&skin, Ckd, Roasted	28.35	3	Ounce	7.76	3.52	0	64.92	0	0	22.96	0.96
17089	Veal, Meat and Fat, Ckd	28.35	3	Ounce	8.53	3.23	0	65.49	0	0	32.32	1.21
17091	Veal, Meat Only, Ckd	28.35	3	Ounce	9.04	1.87	0	55.57	0	0	33.45	0.52
17165	Venison, Ckd, Roasted	28.35	3	Ounce	8.56	0.9	0	44.79	0	0	31.75	0.35
	Almond Butter, w/ salt	16	1	Tbsp.	2.43	9.456	3.395	101.28	0	0.592	0	0.896
	Almond Butter, w/o salt	16	1	Tbsp.	2.43	9.456	3.395	101.28	0	0.592	0	0.896
12067	Almonds, Toasted, Unblanched	141.96	0.5	Cup	28.93	72.07	32.52	836.14	0	15.9	0	6.83
12078	Brazilnuts, Dried, Unblanched	224	1	Ounce	4.1	18.8	3.6	186	0	1.5	0	4.6
12585	Cashews, Dry Roasted	112	0.5	Cup	17.2	52.4	37.2	652	0	3.6	0	10.4
12586	Cashews, Oil Roasted	112	0.5	Cup	17.2	52.4	37.2	652	0	3.6	0	10.4
12131	Macadamias, Dried	112	0.5	Cup	9.6	83.6	15.6	769	0	10.4	0	13.6
12633	Macadamias, Oil Roasted	112	0.5	Cup	9.6	83.6	15.6	769	0	10.4	0	13.6
12635	Mixed w/ Peanuts, Dry Roasted	112	0.5	Cup	20	64	24	680	0	12.33	0	8
12637	Mixed w/ Peanuts, Oil Roasted	112	0.5	Cup	19.2	64	24.4	700	0	11.2	0	10
12638	Mixed w/o Peanuts, Oil Roasted	112	0.5	Cup	19.2	64	24.4	700	0	11.2	0	10
16097	Peanut Butter, Chunk Style, w/ Salt	16.139	2	Tbsp.	3.88	8.06	3.48	95.06	0	1.07	0	1.55
16397	Peanut Butter, Chunk Style, w/o Salt	16.139	2	Tbsp.	3.88	8.06	3.48	95.06	0	1.07	0	1.55
62689	Peanut Butter, Reduced Fat	18	2	Tbsp.	4	6	7.5	95	0	1	0	1.25
16098	Peanut Butter, Smooth Style, w/ Salt	16.139	2	Tbsp.	3.97	8.07	3.34	94.9	0	0.95	0	1.55
16398	Peanut Butter, Smooth Style, w/o Salt	16.139	2	Tbsp.	3.97	8.07	3.34	94.9	0	0	0	1.55
12681	Peanut Kernels, Oil Roasted	112	0.5	Cup	37.94	70.99	27.26	836.64	0	12.67	0	9.85
16088	Peanuts, All Types, Ckd, Boiled, w/ Salt	112	0.5	Cup	6.8	7	6.8	102	0	2.8	0	1.92
16090	Peanuts, All Types, Dry-roasted, w/ Salt	112	0.5	Cup	34.57	72.5	31.4	854.1	0	11.68	0	10.06
16390	Peanuts, All Types, Dry-roasted, w/o Salt	112	0.5	Cup	34.57	72.5	31.4	854.1	0	11.68	0	10.06
16087	Peanuts, All Types, Fresh	112	0.5	Cup	37.67	71.89	23.56	827.82	0	12.41	0	9.98
16089	Peanuts, All Types, Oil-roasted, w/ Salt	112	0.5	Cup	37.94	70.99	27.26	836.64	0	13.25	0	9.85
16389	Peanuts, All Types, Oil-roasted, w/o Salt	112	0.5	Cup	37.94	70.99	27.26	836.64	0	13.25	0	9.85
16091	Peanuts, Spanish, Fresh	112	0.5	Cup	38.18	72.42	23.1	832.2	0	13.87	0	11.16
16092	Peanuts, Spanish, Oil-roasted, w/ Salt	112	0.5	Cup	41.17	72.09	25.65	851.13	0	0	0	11.11
16392	Peanuts, Spanish, Oil-roasted, w/o Salt	112	0.5	Cup	41.17	72.09	25.65	851.13	0	0	0	11.11
16093	Peanuts, Valencia, Fresh	112	0.5	Cup	36.63	69.47	30.53	832.2	0	0	0	10.7
16094	Peanuts, Valencia, Oil-roasted, w/ Salt	112	0.5	Cup	38.94	73.79	23.47	848.16	0	0	0	11.37
16394	Peanuts, Valencia, Oil-roasted, w/o Salt	112	0.5	Cup	38.94	73.79	23.47	848.16	0	0	0	11.37
16095	Peanuts, Virginia, Fresh	112	0.5	Cup	36.78	71.18	24.15	821.98	0	0	0	9.29
16096	Peanuts, Virginia, Oil-roasted, w/ Salt	112	0.5	Cup	36.99	69.53	28.4	826.54	0	0	0	9.07
16396	Peanuts, Virginia, Oil-roasted, w/o Salt	112	0.5	Cup	36.99	69.53	28.4	826.54	0	0	0	9.07
12142	Pecans, Dried	112	0.5	Cup	8.37	73.05	19.7	720.36	0	8.21	0	5.85
12147	Pine Nuts	10	1	Tbsp.	2.4	5.07	1.42	51.5	0	0.45	0	0.78
12151	Pistachios, Dried	112	0.5	Cup	26.34	61.94	31.76	738.56	0	13.82	0	7.84
12652	Pistachios, Dry Roasted	112	0.5	Cup	19.11	67.61	35.24	775.68	0	13.82	0	8.56

Monounsaturated Fat (gm)	Polyunsaturated Fat (gm)	Vitamin D (mg)	Vitamin K (mg)	Vitamin E (mg)	Vitamin A (re)	Vitamin C (mg)	Thiamin (mg)	Riboflavin (mg)	Niacin (mg)	Vitamin B6 (mg)	Folate (mg)	Vitamin B12 (mcg)	Calcium (mg)	Iron (mg)	Magnesium (mg)	Phosphorus (mg)	Potassium (mg)	Sodium (mg)	Zinc (mg)
1.96	1.24	0	0	0	3.4	0	0.03	0.05	0.6	0.06	2.55	0.07	3.97	0.62	4.25	66.34	73.71	237.57	0.41
0.72	0.67	0	0	0	0	0	0.02	0.07	0.68	0.07	1.7	0.07	2.27	0.43	4.82	48.48	68.32	123.89	1.17
1.42	1.05	0	0	0.17	0	0	0.02	0.06	0.98	0.09	2.27	0.1	9.36	0.62	6.24	53.58	73.71	20.7	1.11
0.69	0.51	0	0	0	0	0	0.02	0.04	1.8	0.14	1.7	0.1	5.95	0.4	7.65	59.54	81.65	17.86	0.58
0.86	0.69	0	0	0	19.28	0.03	0.02	0.06	1.4	0.11	5.67	0.36	7.37	0.57	6.8	56.7	77.11	18.99	0.89
0.46	0.61	0	0	0.18	0	0	0.02	0.07	1.03	0.1	2.55	0.1	9.07	0.66	6.8	57.83	82.22	22.4	1.26
1.03	0.88	0	0	0.17	0	0	0.02	0.07	1	0.09	2.55	0.1	9.36	0.64	6.52	55.57	77.68	21.55	1.18
0.33	0.33	0	0	0.41	508.88	0.48	0.01	0.26	1.28	0.09	97.81	6.81	3.69	1.9	4.82	57.83	56.7	16.73	1.04
1.39	0.92	0	0	0.1	0	0	0.02	0.05	1.37	0.11	1.98	0.09	7.09	0.55	6.8	55.57	76.55	30.33	0.81
0.81	0.77	0	0	0.18	0	0	0.02	0.07	1.01	0.09	2.55	0.1	9.07	0.65	6.52	56.42	79.38	21.83	1.21
0.16	0.24	0	0	0.03	0	0	0.02	0.04	1.94	0.15	1.7	0.1	5.39	0.38	7.94	62.09	86.47	18.14	0.58
0.81	0.57	0	0	0.04	0	0	0.02	0.04	1.78	0.13	1.7	0.1	5.95	0.4	7.37	58.97	80.8	17.86	0.58
0.29	0.41	0	0	0.09	0	0	0.02	0.05	1.54	0.13	1.98	0.1	7.09	0.5	7.37	60.39	84.48	19.85	0.88
0.9	0.7	0	0	0.1	0	0	0.02	0.05	1.44	0.12	1.98	0.1	7.37	0.51	7.09	57.55	79.38	19.28	0.84
0.13	0.08	0	0	0.03	0	0	0.01	0.03	2.36	0.1	1.13	0.57	1.98	0.11	5.67	64.92	78.81	405.69	0.32
1.32	0.83	0	0	0.05	0	0	0.01	0.04	1.63	0.12	1.7	0.1	6.8	0.41	7.09	55.85	75.41	17.29	0.6
1.25	0.23	0	0	0.11	0	0	0.02	0.09	2.26	0.09	4.25	0.45	6.24	0.33	7.37	67.76	92.14	24.66	1.35
0.67	0.17	0	0	0.12	0	0	0.02	0.1	2.39	0.09	4.54	0.47	6.8	0.33	7.94	70.88	95.82	25.23	1.45
0.25	0.18	0	0	0	0	0	0.05	0.17	1.9	0	0	0	1.98	1.27	6.8	64.07	94.97	15.31	0.78
6.14	1.984	0	0	3.242	0	0.112	0.021	0.098	0.46	0.012	10.432	0	43.2	0.592	48.48	83.68	121.28	72	0.488
6.14	1.984	0	0	3.248	0	0.112	0.021	0.098	0.46	0.012	10.432	0	43.2	0.592	48.48	83.68	121.28	1.76	0.488
46.8	15.12	0	0	22.71	0	0.99	0.19	0.85	4.02	0.11	91	0	401.75	6.98	432.98	780.78	1097.35	15.62	6.98
6.5	6.8	0	0	3.5	0	0	0.28	0.03	0.5	0.07	1	0	50	0.96	64	170	170	1	1.3
30.8	8.8	0	0	0.78	0	0	0.24	0.24	1.6	0.28	80	0	52	6.8	296	556	640	20	6.36
30.8	8.8	0	0	0.78	0	0	0.24	0.23	1.6	0.28	80	0	52	6.8	296	556	640	20	6.36
66	1.6	0	0	0.5	0	0	0.4	0.12	2.4	0.24	16	0	80	2.72	132	156	416	4	1.92
66	1.77	0	0	0.55	0	0	0.4	0.15	2.71	0.27	16	0	80	2.41	156.78	156	440.86	8	1.47
36	16	0	0	8.22	1.37	0.55	0.27	0.27	6.44	0.41	69.05	0	95.9	5.07	308.25	595.95	680	440	5.21
36	15.2	0	0	8.52	20	0	0.71	0.24	5.6	0.14	96	0	124	3.64	268	528	660	12	5.76
36	15.2	0	0	8.64	20	0	0.73	0.24	5.6	0.14	96	0	124	3.7	268	528	660	12	5.76
3.8	2.32	0	0	1.61	0	0	0.02	0.02	2.21	0.07	14.85	0	6.62	0.31	25.66	51.16	120.56	78.43	0.45
3.8	2.32	0	0	1.61	0	0	0.02	0.02	2.21	0.07	14.85	0	6.62	0.31	25.66	51.16	120.56	2.74	0.45
0	0	0	0	0	0	0	0	0	2.38	0.06	6	0	0	0.2	26.25	0	360.5	125	0.45
3.81	2.32	0	0.02	1.61	0	0	0.02	0.02	2.11	0.06	12.62	0	5.49	0.27	25.34	52.13	116.36	77.14	0.41
3.81	2.32	0	0	0	0	0	0.02	0.02	2.11	0.06	12.62	0	5.49	0.27	25.34	52.13	116.36	2.74	0.41
35.23	22.44	0	0	10.67	0	0	0.36	0.16	20.56	0.37	181.01	0	126.72	2.64	266.4	744.48	982.08	623.52	9.55
3.5	2.2	0	0	2	0	0	0.8	0.02	1.7	0.05	24	0	18	0.32	33	63	58	240	0.59
35.97	22.91	0	0	10.82	0	0	0.64	0.14	19.75	0.37	212.14	0	78.84	3.3	256.96	522.68	960.68	1186.98	4.83
35.97	22.91	0	0	11.39	0	0	0.64	0.14	19.75	0.37	212.14	0	78.84	3.3	256.96	522.68	960.68	8.76	4.83
35.67	22.72	0	0	13.33	0	0	0.93	0.2	17.62	0.51	350.11	0	134.32	6.69	245.28	548.96	1029.3	26.28	4.77
35.23	22.44	0	0	10.67	0	0	0.36	0.16	20.56	0.37	181.01	0	126.72	2.64	266.4	744.48	982.08	623.52	9.55
35.23	22.44	0	0	10.67	0	0	0.36	0.16	20.56	0.37	181.01	0	126.72	2.64	266.4	744.48	982.08	8.64	9.55
32.6	25.12	0	0	0	0	0	0.99	0.2	23.25	0.51	350.4	0	154.76	5.71	274.48	566.48	1086.24	32.12	3.1
32.45	25	0	0	0	0	0	0.47	0.12	21.95	0.38	185.07	0	147	3.35	246.96	568.89	1140.72	636.51	2.94
32.45	25	0	0	0	0	0	0.47	0.12	21.95	0.38	185.07	0	147	3.35	246.96	568.89	1140.72	8.82	2.94
31.26	24.09	0	0	0	0	0	0.93	0.44	18.8	0.5	358.43	0	90.52	3.05	268.64	490.56	484.72	1.46	4.88
33.21	25.59	0	0	0	0	0	0.13	0.22	20.65	0.35	180.72	0	77.76	2.38	230.4	459.36	881.28	1111.68	4.44
33.21	25.59	0	0	0	0	0	0.13	0.22	20.65	0.35	180.72	0	77.76	2.38	230.4	459.36	881.28	8.64	4.44
36.92	21.47	0	0	0	0	0	0.95	0.19	18.07	0.51	348.5	0	129.94	3.72	249.66	554.8	1007.4	14.6	6.47
36.07	20.98	0	0	0	0	0	0.39	0.16	21.02	0.36	179.32	0	122.98	2.39	268.84	723.58	932.36	619.19	9.47
36.07	20.98	0	0	0	0	0	0.39	0.16	21.02	0.36	179.32	0	122.98	2.39	268.84	723.58	932.36	8.58	9.47
45.53	18.09	0	0	3.35	14.04	2.16	0.92	0.14	0.96	0.2	42.34	0	38.88	2.3	138.24	314.28	423.36	1.08	5.91
1.91	2.13	0	0	0.35	0.3	0.19	0.08	0.02	0.36	0.01	5.73	0	2.6	0.92	23.3	50.8	59.9	0.4	0.43
41.82	9.36	0	0	6.67	29.44	9.22	1.05	0.22	1.38	0.32	74.24	0	172.8	8.68	202.24	643.84	1399.04	7.68	1.72
45.64	10.22	0	0	8.26	30.72	9.34	0.54	0.31	1.8	0.33	75.65	0	89.6	4.06	166.4	609.28	1241.6	998.4	1.74

USDA ID Code	Food Name	Weight in Grams*	Quantity of Units	Unit of Measure	Protein (gm)	Fat (gm)	Carbohydrates (gm)	Kcalories	Caffeine (gm)	Fiber (gm)	Cholesterol (mg)	Saturated Fat (gm)
16107	Sausage, Meatless	25	1	Link	4.63	4.54	2.46	64	0	0.7	0	0.73
	Seeds, Sesame, Toasted, w/o salt	28.35	1	Ounce	4.808	13.608	7.382	160.745	0	4.791	0	1.906
	Seeds, Sesame, Toasted, w/salt	28.35	1	Ounce	4.808	13.608	7.382	160.745	0	4.791	0	1.906
12036	Seeds, Sunflower, Dried	112	0.5	Cup	32.8	71.38	27.01	820.8	0	15.12	0	7.48
12537	Seeds, Sunflower, Dry Roasted, w/ Salt added	112	0.5	Cup	24.74	63.74	30.81	744.96	0	8.7	0	6.68
12037	Seeds, Sunflower, Dry Roasted, w/o Salt	112	0.5	Cup	24.74	63.74	30.81	744.96	0	11.52	0	6.68
12538	Seeds, Sunflower, Oil Roasted, w/ Salt added	112	0.5	Cup	28.84	77.56	19.89	830.25	0	9.18	0	8.13
12038	Seeds, Sunflower, Oil Roasted, w/o Salt	112	0.5	Cup	28.84	77.56	19.89	830.25	0	9.18	0	8.13
12539	Seeds, Sunflower, Toasted, w/ Salt added	112	0.5	Cup	23.06	76.11	27.59	829.46	0	0	0	7.98
12039	Seeds, Sunflower, Toasted, w/o Salt	112	0.5	Cup	23.06	76.11	27.59	829.46	0	0	0	7.98
	Sesame Butter, Tahini, Toasted	15	1	Tbsp.	2.55	8.064	3.179	89.25	0	1.395	0	1.129
16109	Soybeans, Boiled	172	0.5	Cup	28.62	15.43	17.06	297.56	0	10.32	0	2.23
16111	Soybeans, Dry Roasted	172	0.5	Cup	68.08	37.19	56.28	774	0	13.93	0	5.38
16126	Tofu, Fresh, Firm	28.35	1	Ounce	4.47	2.47	1.21	41.11	0	0.65	0	0.36
16127	Tofu, Fresh, Regular	28.35	1	Ounce	2.29	1.36	0.53	21.55	0	0.34	0	0.2
16129	Tofu, Fried	28.35	1	Ounce	4.87	5.72	2.98	76.83	0	1.11	0	0.83
16429	Tofu, Fried, Prepared w/ Calcium Sulfate	28.35	1	Ounce	4.87	5.72	2.98	76.83	0	0	0	0.83
16130	Tofu, Okara	28.35	1	Ounce	0.91	0.49	3.56	21.83	0	0	0	0.05
16132	Tofu, Salted and Fermented (fuyu)	28.35	1	Ounce	2.31	2.27	1.46	32.89	0	0	0	0.33
12154	Walnuts, Black, Dried	125	0.5	Cup	30.44	70.73	15.13	758.75	0	6.25	0	4.54
12155	Walnuts, English, Dried	120	0.5	Cup	17.15	74.24	22.01	770.4	0	5.76	0	6.7
	Vitamin Supplement, Centrum	1	1	Each	0	0	0	0	0	0	0	0
	Vitamin Supplement, One-A-Day	1	1	Each	0	0	0	0	0	0	0	0
	Vitamin Supplement, StressTab	1	1	Each	0	0	0	0	0	0	0	0
55188	Angel Hair Pasta, Lean Cuisine-Stouffer's	283.493	1	Each	10	5	38	240	0	0	10	1
55189	Baked Cheese Ravioli, Lean Cuisine-Stouffer's	240.969	1	Each	13	8	30	240	0	0	55	3
41297	Baked Cheese Ravioli-Healthy Choice	255.144	1	Each	14	2	44	250	0	0	20	1
55190	Baked Potato w/ Sour Cream, Lean Cuisine-Stouffer's	294.124	1	Each	9	5	38	230	0	0	15	2
41240	Banana Nut Muffin-Healthy Choice	70.873	1	Each	3	6	32	180	0	0	0	0
41276	Bean and Ham Soup-Healthy Choice	212.62	1	Each	12	4	35	220	0	0	5	1
41335	Beef and Bean Burritos (medium)-Healthy Choice	148.834	1	Each	12	7	42	270	0	0	15	3
41334	Beef and Bean Burritos (mild)-Healthy Choice	148.834	1	Each	11	5	45	250	0	0	10	1
55191	Beef and Bean Enchiladas, Lean Cuisine-Stouffer's	262.231	1	Each	15	6	32	240	0	0	45	3
41270	Beef and Potato Soup-Healthy Choice	212.62	1	Each	9	1	17	110	0	0	20	0
55192	Beef Cannelloni w/ Sauce, Lean Cuisine-Stouffer's	272.862	1	Each	14	3	28	200	0	0	25	1
62692	Beef Chow Mein	247	1	Cup	10	1.5	15	110	0	4	10	1
41249	Beef Enchilada-Healthy Choice	379.172	1	Each	15	5	66	370	0	0	30	2
55149	Beef Pie-Stouffer's	283.493	1	Each	18	27	37	460	0	0	0	0
57806	Beef Pot Pie-Swanson	198.445	1	Pie	12	19	36	370	0	0	0	0
43405	Beef Ravioli, Micro Cup-Hormel	212.62	1	Each	9	11	34	270	0	0	20	4
41251	Beef Sirloin Tips-Healthy Choice	318.93	1	Each	22	7	29	270	0	0	65	3
43413	Beef Stew, Micro Cup-Hormel	212.62	1	Each	13	15	11	230	0	0	45	5
55158	Beef Stroganoff w/ Parsley Noodles-Stouffer's	276.406	1	Each	24	20	28	390	0	0	0	0
41286	Boneless Beef Ribs w/ Barbecue Sauce-Healthy Choice	311.843	1	Each	28	6	40	330	0	0	70	2
41348	Breaded Fish-Healthy Choice	9.745	1	Stick	1	0.5	1.75	15	0	0	2.5	0
43400	Breast of Chicken w/ Spanish Rice, Top Shelf-Hormel	283.493	1	Each	27	15	38	400	0	0	75	7
41252	Breast of Turkey-Healthy Choice	297.668	1	Each	21	5	39	290	0	0	45	2
62616	Broccoli and Cheese Baked Potato-Weight Watchers	283.5	1	Each	12	7	34	230	0	6	10	2
55177	Canadian Style Bacon, French Bread Pizzas-Stouffer's	163.008	1	Each	18	15	40	370	0	0	0	0
55832	Cheddar Cheese Sauce-Stouffer's	283.92	1	Cup	26.04	60.09	22.03	731.1	0	0	130.2	0
55764	Cheddar Cheese Soup-Stouffer's	283.92	1	Cup	21.03	31.05	18.03	440.66	0	0	70.11	0
55772	Cheddar Cheese, Heat'n Serve Soup -Stouffer's	307.58	1	Cup	21.7	35.8	21.7	488.23	0	0	97.65	0
55196	Cheese Cannelloni, Lean Cuisine-Stouffer's	258.688	1	Each	23	8	27	270	0	0	25	4
55108	Cheese Enchiladas-Stouffer's	276.406	1	Each	23	29	33	490	0	0	0	0
41331	Cheese French Bread Pizza-Healthy Choice	159.465	1	Each	19	4	46	290	0	0	15	2

Monounsaturated Fat (gm)	Polyunsaturated Fat (gm)	Vitamin D (mg)	Vitamin K (mg)	Vitamin E (mg)	Vitamin A (re)	Vitamin C (mg)	Thiamin (mg)	Riboflavin (mg)	Niacin (mg)	Vitamin B6 (mg)	Folate (mg)	Vitamin B12 (mcg)	Calcium (mg)	Iron (mg)	Magnesium (mg)	Phosphorus (mg)	Potassium (mg)	Sodium (mg)	Zinc (mg)
1.12	2.32	0	0	0.53	16	0	0.59	0.1	2.8	0.21	6.5	0	15.75	0.93	9	56.25	57.75	222	0.37
5.139	5.965	0	0	0.644	1.985	0	0.342	0.132	1.542	0.041	27.159	0	37.139	2.206	98.091	219.429	115.101	11.057	2.9
5.139	5.965	0	0	0.644	1.985	0	0.342	0.132	1.542	0.041	27.159	0	37.139	2.206	98.091	219.429	115.101	166.698	2.9
13.63	47.14	0	0	72.39	7.2	2.02	3.3	0.36	6.48	1.11	327.46	0	167.04	9.75	509.76	1015.2	992.16	4.32	7.29
12.17	42.09	0	0	64.35	0	1.79	0.14	0.31	9.01	1.03	303.87	0	89.6	4.86	165.12	1478.4	1088	998.4	6.77
12.17	42.09	0	0	64.35	0	1.79	0.14	0.31	9.01	1.03	303.87	0	89.6	4.86	165.12	1478.4	1088	3.84	6.77
14.8	51.21	0	0	54	6.75	1.89	0.43	0.38	5.58	1.07	315.9	0	75.6	9.05	171.45	1537.65	652.05	814.05	7.03
14.8	51.21	0	0	67.86	6.75	1.89	0.43	0.38	5.58	1.07	315.9	0	75.6	9.05	171.45	1537.65	652.05	4.05	7.03
14.53	50.26	0	0	0	0	1.88	0.44	0.38	5.63	1.08	318.65	0	76.38	9.13	172.86	1551.72	657.94	821.42	7.1
14.53	50.26	0	0	0	0	1.88	0.44	0.38	5.63	1.08	318.65	0	76.38	9.13	172.86	1551.72	657.94	4.02	7.1
3.045	3.535	0	0	0.341	1.05	0	0.183	0.071	0.817	0.022	14.655	0	63.9	1.342	14.25	109.8	62.1	17.25	0.693
3.41	8.71	0	0	3.35	1.72	2.92	0.27	0.49	0.69	0.4	92.54	0	175.44	8.84	147.92	421.4	885.8	1.72	1.98
8.21	21	0	0	3.35	3.44	7.91	0.73	1.3	1.82	0.39	351.91	0	464.4	6.79	392.16	1116.28	2346.08	3.44	8.2
0.55	1.4	0	0	0	4.82	0.06	0.04	0.03	0.11	0.03	8.31	0	58.12	2.97	26.65	53.87	67.19	3.97	0.45
0.3	0.77	0	0	0	2.55	0.03	0.02	0.01	0.06	0.01	4.25	0	29.77	1.52	29.2	27.5	34.3	1.98	0.23
1.26	3.23	0	0	0.01	0	0	0.05	0.01	0.03	0.03	7.6	0	105.46	1.38	17.01	81.36	41.39	4.54	0.56
1.26	3.23	0	0	0	0	0	0.05	0.01	0.03	0.03	7.6	0	272.44	1.38	26.93	81.36	41.39	4.54	0.56
0.08	0.21	0	0	0	0	0	0.01	0.01	0.03	0.03	7.48	0	22.68	0.37	7.37	17.01	60.39	2.55	0.16
0.5	1.28	0	0	0	4.82	0.06	0.04	0.03	0.11	0.03	8.25	0	13.04	0.56	14.74	20.7	21.26	814.5	0.44
15.91	46.87	0	0	3.28	37.5	4	0.27	0.14	0.86	0.69	81.88	0	72.5	3.84	252.5	580	655	1.25	4.28
17.01	46.95	0	0	3.14	14.4	3.84	0.46	0.18	1.25	0.67	79.2	0	112.8	2.93	202.8	380.4	602.4	12	3.28
0	0	5	0	10	1000	60	1.5	1.7	20	2	400	6	162	18	100	109	40	0	15
0	0	5	0	10	1000	60	1.5	1.7	20	2	400	6	0	0	0	0	0	0	0
0	0	0	0	10	0	500	10	0	100	5	400	12	0	18	0	0	0	0	0
0	1	0	0	0	250	6	0.3	0.34	2.85	0	0	0	80	1.5	0	0	500	410	0
0	0	0	0	0	60	36	0.06	0.26	1.14	0	0	0	160	0.8	0	0	380	590	0
0	0	0	0	0	500	4.8	0.3	0.26	1.9	0	0	0	200	1.5	0	240	590	420	0
0	0	0	0	0	350	30	0.23	0.26	1.14	0	0	0	160	0.6	0	0	900	570	0
0	3	0	0	0	0	0	0.15	0.14	0.76	0	0	0	80	1	0	160	250	80	0
0	1	0	0	0	60	2.4	0.23	0.17	1.14	0	0	0	48	1	0	220	630	480	0
0	3	0	0	0	20	3.6	0.38	0.17	1.9	0	0	0	48	1.5	0	180	270	520	0
0	2	0	0	0	20	1.2	0.38	0.17	2.85	0	0	0	32	2	0	130	330	450	0
0	1	0	0	0	80	6	0.23	0.26	1.9	0	0	0	80	1	0	0	470	480	0
0	0	0	0	0	0	2.4	0.03	0	0.38	0	0	0	0	0.2	0	0	100	550	0
0	0	0	0	0	350	6	0.12	0.17	2.85	0	0	0	120	1.5	0	0	800	490	0
0	0	0	0	0	40	12	0	0	0	0	0	0	24	0.4	0	0	0	760	0
0	2	0	0	0	250	24	0.3	0.26	1.9	0	0	0	120	1	0	260	600	450	0
0	0	0	0	0	700	2.4	0.3	0.43	3.8	0	0	0	32	1.5	0	0	300	1130	0
0	0	0	0	0	250	0	0.23	0.17	2.85	0	0	0	16	1.5	0	0	0	730	0
5	1	0	0	0.5	100	11.4	0.15	0.27	2.47	0	0	0	48	0.9	28	0	359	920	1.05
0	2	0	0	0	700	42	0.15	0.17	2.85	0	0	0	16	1	0	190	520	360	0
4	0	0	0	0.28	320	2.4	0.05	0.1	2.28	0	0	0	16	0.9	21	0	487	1140	2.4
0	0	0	0	0	40	1.2	0.12	0.34	2.85	0	0	0	48	1.5	0	0	300	1090	0
0	2	0	0	0	60	4.8	0.23	0.26	2.85	0	0	0	48	1	0	220	670	530	0
0	0.13	0	0	0	0	0	0.01	0.02	0.1	0	0	0	0	0.1	0	0	20	31.25	0
4	3	0	0	0.07	100	3.6	0.09	0.26	7.6	0	0	0	80	0.4	35	0	584	810	1.65
0	0	0	0	0	40	48	0.45	0.26	5.7	0	0	0	32	1	0	270	540	420	0
0	0	0	0	0	200	9	0	0	0	0	0	0	300	0.8	0	0	830	550	0
0	0	0	0	0	80	6	0.6	0.43	3.8	0	0	0	160	1	0	0	300	1070	0
0	0	0	0	0	0	0	0	0.01	0	0	0	0	6.33	0.1	0	0	340.51	1392.09	0
0	0	0	0	0	0	0	0	0.01	0.19	0	0	0	4.97	0	0	0	510.77	681.02	0
0	0	0	0	0	0	0	0	0.02	0.21	0	0	0	4.95	0.11	0	0	553.33	770.32	0
0	0	0	0	0	60	21	0.12	0.26	1.52	0	0	0	240	0.4	0	0	400	590	0
0	0	0	0	0	150	6	0.09	0.34	1.52	0	0	0	480	0.8	0	0	400	550	0
0	1	0	0	0	20	0	0.45	0.26	2.85	0	0	0	240	2	0	240	310	390	0

USDA ID Code	Food Name	Weight in Grams*	Quantity of Units	Unit of Measure	Protein (gm)	Fat (gm)	Carbohydrates (gm)	Kcalories	Caffeine (gm)	Fiber (gm)	Cholesterol (mg)	Saturated Fat (gm)
41300	Cheese Manicotti-Healthy Choice	262.231	1	Each	15	3	34	220	0	0	30	2
55796	Cheese Manicotti-Stouffer's	28.35	1	Ounce	1.6	1.3	2.6	29	0	0	4	0
55822	Cheese Ravioli-Stouffer's	28.35	1	Ounce	2.8	1.9	6.4	54	0	0	14	0
55808	Cheese Stuffed Shells-Stouffer's	28.35	1	Ounce	1.5	0.9	3.4	28	0	0	3	0
55819	Cheese Tortellini w/ Egg Pasta-Stouffer's	145.29	1	Each	11.29	8.47	22.22	211.64	0	0	63.49	0
55821	Cheese Tortellini w/ Spinach Pasta-Stouffer's	28.35	1	Ounce	3	2.4	5.7	56	0	0	19	0
55109	Chicken a la King w/ Rice-Stouffer's	269.319	1	Each	18	5	38	270	0	0	0	0
43397	Chicken a la King, Top Shelf-Hormel	283.493	1	Each	18	10	49	360	0	0	37	4
57799	Chicken a la King-Swanson	250	1	Each	16.8	20.16	15.12	319.15	0	0	0	0
55197	Chicken a la Orange, Lean Cuisine-Stouffer's	226.795	1	Each	27	4	33	280	0	0	55	1
41301	Chicken a la Orange-Healthy Choice	255.144	1	Each	20	2	36	240	0	0	45	2
55792	Chicken and Dumplings-Stouffer's	220	1	Each	14.74	16.3	24.06	302.65	0	0	69.84	0
57801	Chicken and Dumplings-Swanson	200	1	Each	10.35	10.35	17.87	206.94	0	0	0	0
41253	Chicken and Pasta Divan-Healthy Choice	340.192	1	Each	25	4	41	300	0	0	50	2
55794	Chicken and Veg. Oriental-Stouffer's	220	1	Each	11.64	9.31	13.97	186.25	0	0	31.04	0
55198	Chicken and Veg. w/ Vermicelli, Lean Cuisine-Stouffer's	333.105	1	Each	18	5	30	240	0	0	30	1
41302	Chicken and Vegetables-Healthy Choice	326.017	1	Each	20	1	31	210	0	0	35	0
55199	Chicken Cacciatore, Lean Cuisine-Stouffer's	308.299	1	Each	22	7	31	280	0	0	45	2
43398	Chicken Cacciatore, Top Shelf-Hormel	283.493	1	Each	21	3	25	210	0	0	50	0
55200	Chicken Chow Mein w/ Rice, Lean Cuisine-Stouffer's	255.144	1	Each	14	5	34	240	0	0	30	1
55110	Chicken Chow Mein w/ Rice-Stouffer's	304.755	1	Each	13	5	39	250	0	0	0	0
41303	Chicken Chow Mein-Healthy Choice	240.969	1	Each	18	3	31	220	0	0	45	1
62611	Chicken Chow Mein-Weight Watchers	255.15	1	Each	12	2	34	200	0	3	25	0.5
55807	Chicken Classica -Stouffer's	28.35	1	Ounce	1.8	0.7	2.3	22	0	0	5	0
41336	Chicken Con Queso Burritos (mild)-Healthy Choice	148.834	1	Each	15	8	40	280	0	0	20	2
41254	Chicken Dijon-Healthy Choice	311.843	1	Each	21	3	40	250	0	0	40	1
55111	Chicken Divan-Stouffer's	226.795	1	Each	24	10	11	220	0	0	0	0
62618	Chicken Enchiladas Suiza-Weight Watchers	255.15	1	Each	15	8	28	250	0	4	25	3
55201	Chicken Enchiladas, Lean Cuisine-Stouffer's	279.95	1	Each	17	9	34	290	0	0	55	3
41304	Chicken Enchiladas-Healthy Choice	269.319	1	Each	14	9	44	310	0	0	35	3
55112	Chicken Enchiladas-Stouffer's	283.493	1	Each	21	31	31	490	0	0	0	0
41305	Chicken Fajitas-Healthy Choice	198.445	1	Each	17	3	25	200	0	0	35	1
55203	Chicken Fettucini, Lean Cuisine-Stouffer's	255.144	1	Each	23	6	33	280	0	0	35	3
41306	Chicken Fettucini-Healthy Choice	240.969	1	Each	19	7	39	240	0	0	45	2
62620	Chicken Fettucini-Weight Watchers	233.89	1	Each	22	9	25	280	0	2	40	3
55763	Chicken Gumbo Soup-Stouffer's	283.92	1	Cup	7.01	5.01	9.01	110.17	0	0	20.03	0
55202	Chicken in BBQ Sauce, Lean Cuisine-Stouffer's	248.057	1	Each	20	6	32	260	0	0	50	1
55204	Chicken Italiano, Lean Cuisine-Stouffer's	255.144	1	Each	22	6	33	270	0	0	40	1
55789	Chicken Italienne-Stouffer's	28.35	1	Ounce	2.2	0.9	1.2	22	0	0	7	0
55755	Chicken Noodle Soup-Stouffer's	283.92	1	Cup	7.01	7.01	10.02	130.2	0	0	20.03	0
55768	Chicken Noodle, Heat'n Serve Soup-Stouffer's	283.92	1	Cup	13.02	17.03	28.04	320.48	0	0	60.09	0
55205	Chicken Oriental, Lean Cuisine-Stouffer's	255.144	1	Each	22	7	31	280	0	0	35	2
41256	Chicken Oriental-Healthy Choice	318.93	1	Each	19	1	32	200	0	0	35	0
41257	Chicken Parmigiana-Healthy Choice	326.017	1	Each	22	4	45	280	0	0	45	2
41271	Chicken Pasta Soup-Healthy Choice	212.62	1	Each	7	2	13	100	0	0	15	0
55113	Chicken Pie-Stouffer's	283.493	1	Each	16	27	32	440	0	0	0	0
57807	Chicken Pot Pie-Swanson	198.445	1	Each	11	22	35	380	0	0	0	0
55790	Chicken Primavera-Stouffer's	28.35	1	Ounce	1.6	0.6	1.2	17	0	0	5	0
41295	Chicken Stir Fry w/ Broccoli-Healthy Choice	340.192	1	Each	21	6	35	280	0	0	55	3
55206	Chicken Tenderloins, Lean Cuisine-Stouffer's	269.319	1	Each	29	5	19	240	0	0	60	2
55820	Chicken Tortellini w/ Egg Pasta-Stouffer's	28.35	1	Ounce	3.1	1.5	6.2	51	0	0	20	0
41248	Chicken w/ Barbecue Sauce-Healthy Choice	361.454	1	Each	24	6	65	410	0	0	55	2
41277	Chicken w/ Rice Soup-Healthy Choice	212.62	1	Each	5	1	14	90	0	0	10	0
41272	Chili Beef Soup-Healthy Choice	212.62	1	Each	11	1	22	150	0	0	15	0
55114	Chili Con Carne w/ Beans-Stouffer's	248.057	1	Each	20	10	28	280	0	0	0	0

Monounsaturated Fat (gm)	Polyunsaturated Fat (gm)	Vitamin D (mg)	Vitamin K (mg)	Vitamin E (mg)	Vitamin A (re)	Vitamin C (mg)	Thiamin (mg)	Riboflavin (mg)	Niacin (mg)	Vitamin B6 (mg)	Folate (mg)	Vitamin B12 (mcg)	Calcium (mg)	Iron (mg)	Magnesium (mg)	Phosphorus (mg)	Potassium (mg)	Sodium (mg)	Zinc (mg)
0	0	0	0	0	250	6	0.3	0.26	1.9	0	0	0	120	1.5	0	210	590	310	0
0	0	0	0	0	0	2.4	0	0	0.04	0	0	0	296.01	0.02	0	0	45	108	0
0	0	0	0	0	0	0	0	0	0.02	0	0	0	336.01	0.01	0	0	16	52	0
0	0	0	0	0	0	0.6	0	0	0.06	0	0	0	248.01	0.02	0	0	53	59	0
0	0	0	0	0	0	0	0	0	0.2	0	0	0	1.52	0.07	0	0	70.55	271.61	0
0	0	0	0	0	0	0	0	0	0.06	0	0	0	0	0.02	0	0	26	79	0
0	0	0	0	0	20	1.2	0.09	0.17	2.85	0	0	0	160	0.8	0	32	260	800	0
4	2	0	0	0.17	250	1.2	0.12	0.17	8.55	0	0	0	48	0.2	28	0	476	890	1.2
0	0	0	0	0	0	0	0.05	0.23	3.19	0	0	0	53.75	0.34	0	0	0	1159.01	0
0	0	0	0	0	80	12	0.23	0.17	9.5	0	0	0	32	0.4	0	0	490	290	0
0	0	0	0	0	150	27	0.15	0.1	5.7	0	0	0	16	0.8	0	230	430	220	0
0	0	0	0	0	0	0	0	0.01	0.44	0	0	0	1.06	0.16	0	0	248.33	659.63	0
0	0	0	0	0	75.25	0	0.03	0.1	1.79	0	0	0	15.05	0.38	0	0	0	921.83	0
0	1	0	0	0	800	72	0.38	0.26	4.75	0	0	0	120	1	0	270	500	520	0
0	0	0	0	0	0	4.66	0	0	0.59	0	0	0	372.49	0.08	0	0	349.21	1078.68	0
0	1	0	0	0	150	6	0.3	0.26	5.7	0	0	0	64	1	0	0	500	500	0
0	0	0	0	0	150	9	0.3	0.17	3.8	0	0	0	32	1.5	0	190	390	490	0
0	1	0	0	0	100	9	0.23	0.17	5.7	0	0	0	32	0.8	0	0	560	570	0
0	0	0	0	0.46	100	2.4	0.15	0.26	6.65	0	0	0	80	1	0	0	0	810	0
0	1	0	0	0	60	6	0.15	0.17	4.75	0	0	0	32	0.6	0	0	350	530	0
0	0	0	0	0	80	12	0.03	0.17	1.9	0	0	0	16	0.4	0	0	340	720	0
0	1	0	0	0	80	3.6	0.15	0.14	3.8	0	0	0	16	0.8	0	290	290	440	0
0	0	0	0	0	300	36	0	0	0	0	0	0	48	0.4	0	0	360	570	0
0	0	0	0	0	0	1.2	0	0	0.1	0	0	0	112	0.01	0	0	50	83	0
0	3	0	0	0	20	6	0.45	0.34	2.85	0	0	0	80	1.5	0	170	260	500	0
0	0	0	0	0	100	9	0.23	0.14	9.5	0	0	0	16	1	0	300	350	470	0
0	0	0	0	0	60	3.6	0.45	0.17	3.8	0	0	0	200	2	0	32	490	610	0
0	0	0	0	0	40	1.2	0	0	0	0	0	0	360	0.8	0	0	470	570	0
0	2	0	0	0	250	6	0.23	0.34	2.85	0	0	0	120	1.5	0	0	450	500	0
0	1	0	0	0	80	21	0.15	0.17	4.75	0	0	0	80	0.8	0	160	380	480	0
0	0	0	0	0	60	2.4	0.09	0.34	2.85	0	0	0	240	0.6	0	0	420	860	0
0	1	0	0	0	150	9	0.23	0.17	3.8	0	0	0	64	1.5	0	210	360	310	0
0	0	0	0	0	0	0	0.3	0.43	5.7	0	0	0	120	0.8	0	0	420	500	0
0	2	0	0	0	0	0	0.23	0.17	2.85	0	0	0	64	1	0	210	190	370	0
0	0	0	0	0	40	0	0	0	0	0	0	0	240	1	0	0	730	590	0
0	0	0	0	0	0	0	0	0	0.19	0	0	0	160.24	0.1	0	0	180.27	1422.13	0
0	2	0	0	0	250	18	0.15	0.17	5.7	0	0	0	48	0.8	0	0	650	500	0
0	2	0	0	0	100	24	0.3	0.26	5.7	0	0	0	80	0.8	0	0	600	590	0
0	0	0	0	0	0	1.2	0	0	0.1	0	0	0	48	0.01	0	0	57	128	0
0	0	0	0	0	0	0	0	0	0.19	0	0	0	80.12	0.1	0	0	140.21	1281.92	0
0	0	0	0	0	0	6.01	0	0	0.57	0	0	0	240.36	0.2	0	0	310.46	1792.69	0
0	2	0	0	0	40	6	0.23	0.17	6.65	0	0	0	32	1	0	0	470	480	0
0	0	0	0	0	250	36	0.15	0.14	7.6	0	0	0	32	0.8	0	200	400	440	0
0	0	0	0	0	900	12	0.15	0.17	9.5	0	0	0	80	1	0	260	500	370	0
0	0	0	0	0	60	0	0.03	0	0.38	0	0	0	0	0	0	0	70	560	0
0	0	0	0	0	500	1.2	0.3	0.43	4.75	0	0	0	80	1	0	0	320	750	0
0	0	0	0	0	400	0	0.23	0.17	2.85	0	0	0	16	1	0	0	0	760	0
0	0	0	0	0	0	1.2	0	0	0.06	0	0	0	48	0.01	0	0	40	119	0
0	0	0	0	0	20	0	0.23	0.34	2.85	0	0	0	48	1.5	0	260	630	500	0
0	1	0	0	0	200	4.8	0.23	0.34	7.6	0	0	0	120	0.4	0	0	750	490	0
0	0	0	0	0	0	0	0	0	0.13	0	0	0	72	0.03	0	0	31	57	0
0	2	0	0	0	100	12	0.12	0.14	8.55	0	0	0	48	1.5	0	250	670	550	0
0	0	0	0	0	80	6	0.03	0.07	1.9	0	0	0	16	0.2	0	70	140	510	0
0	0	0	0	0	20	6	0.09	0.03	0.38	0	0	0	16	0.6	0	0	290	560	0
0	0	0	0	0	200	15	0.15	0.26	2.85	0	0	0	64	2	0	0	700	910	0

USDA ID Code	Food Name	Weight in Grams*	Quantity of Units	Unit of Measure	Protein (gm)	Fat (gm)	Carbohydrates (gm)	Kcalories	Caffeine (gm)	Fiber (gm)	Cholesterol (mg)	Saturated Fat (gm)
43411	Chili Mac, Micro Cup-Hormel	212.62	1	Each	10	9	18	192	0	0	22	4
43408	Chili no Beans, Micro Cup-Hormel	209.076	1	Each	18	17	15	290	0	0	60	8
55767	Chili w/ Beans Soup-Stouffer's	283.92	1	Cup	14.02	9.01	25.04	240.36	0	0	30.04	0
43409	Chili w/ Beans, Micro Cup-Hormel	209.076	1	Each	15	11	23	250	0	0	49	4
43369	Chili w/ Beans-Hormel	253.162	1	Cup	17.86	17.86	32.15	357.2	0	0	65.49	5.95
43368	Chili w/o Beans-Hormel	253.162	1	Cup	19.05	32.15	16.67	428.64	0	0	71.44	13.1
62691	Chili, Fat Free	240	0.5	Cup	14	0	30	160	0	14	0	0
43370	Chunky Chili w/ Beans-Hormel	253.162	1	Cup	17.86	16.67	29.77	345.3	0	0	59.53	0
55799	Confetti Rice-Stouffer's	28.35	1	Ounce	0.5	0.3	4.8	24	0	0	1	0
55824	Corn Pudding-Stouffer's	28.35	1	Ounce	1.2	1.7	4.5	38	0	0	15	0
55168	Corn Souffle-Stouffer's	170.096	1	Each	7	11	27	240	0	0	0	0
43366	Corned Beef Hash-Hormel	253.162	1	Cup	26.79	26.79	17.86	419.71	0	0	80.37	8.93
41278	Country Vegetable Soup-Healthy Choice	212.62	1	Each	3	1	23	120	0	0	0	0
55762	Cream of Broccoli Soup-Stouffer's	283.92	1	Cup	12.02	21.03	16.02	300.45	0	0	60.09	0
55765	Cream of Potato Soup-Stouffer's	283.92	1	Cup	11.02	13.02	34.05	300.45	0	0	30.04	0
55788	Creamed Chicken-Stouffer's	28.35	1	Ounce	2.8	3.5	1.2	48	0	0	14	0
55777	Creamed Chipped Beef-Stouffer's	28.35	1	Ounce	2.1	3.3	1.6	45	0	0	13	0
55169	Creamed Spinach-Stouffer's	127.572	1	Each	4	16	8	190	0	0	0	0
55756	Creamy Chicken Soup-Stouffer's	283.92	1	Cup	17.03	8.01	25.04	240.36	0	0	20.03	0
43375	Dinty Moore Beef Stew-Hormel	253.162	1	Cup	12.28	14.51	17.86	245.58	0	0	33.49	6.7
43376	Dinty Moore Chicken Stew-Hormel	253.162	1	Cup	13.1	21.43	17.86	309.58	0	0	95.25	4.76
43377	Dinty Moore Meatball Stew-Hormel	253.162	1	Cup	12.28	17.86	15.63	267.9	0	0	33.49	7.81
43378	Dinty Moore Vegetable Stew-Hormel	253.162	1	Cup	5.58	6.7	22.33	173.02	0	0	15.63	2.23
62636	Egg Roll	85	1	Each	7	5	21	160	0	2	10	1
41242	English Muffin Sandwich-Healthy Choice	120.484	1	Each	16	3	30	200	0	0	20	1
55170	Escalloped Apples-Stouffer's	170.096	1	Each	0	4	41	200	0	0	0	0
55117	Escalloped Chicken and Noodles-Stouffer's	283.493	1	Each	21	24	30	420	0	0	0	0
21002	Fast Food-Biscuit w/ Egg	136	1	Each	11.12	20.2	24.17	315.52	0	0	232.56	6.18
21003	Fast Food-Biscuit w/ Egg and Bacon	150	1	Each	17	31.1	28.59	457.5	0	0	352.5	9.93
21004	Fast Food-Biscuit w/ Egg and Ham	192	1	Each	20.43	27.03	30.32	441.6	0	0	299.52	8.37
21005	Fast Food-Biscuit w/ Egg and Sausage	180	1	Each	19.15	38.7	41.15	581.4	0	0	302.4	14.98
21007	Fast Food-Biscuit w/ Egg, Cheese, and Bacon	144	1	Each	16.26	31.39	33.42	476.64	0	0	260.64	11.4
21008	Fast Food-Biscuit w/ Ham	113	1	Each	13.39	18.42	43.79	386.46	0	0	24.86	11.41
21009	Fast Food-Biscuit w/ Sausage	124	1	Each	12.11	31.78	40.04	484.84	0	1.36	34.72	14.22
21010	Fast Food-Biscuit w/ Steak	141	1	Each	13.1	25.99	44.39	455.43	0	0	25.38	6.93
21001	Fast Food-Biscuit, Plain	74	1	Each	4.31	13.35	34.43	276.02	0	0	5.18	8.74
21027	Fast Food-Brownie	60	1	Each	2.74	10.1	38.97	243	0	0	9.6	3.13
21060	Fast Food-Burrito w/ Beans	108.5	1	Each	7.03	6.75	35.72	223.51	0	0	2.17	3.44
21061	Fast Food-Burrito w/ Beans and Cheese	93	1	Each	7.53	5.85	27.48	188.79	0	0	13.95	3.42
21062	Fast Food-Burrito w/ Beans and Chili Peppers	102	1	Each	8.19	7.33	29.04	206.04	0	0	16.32	3.8
21063	Fast Food-Burrito w/ Beans and Meat	115.5	1	Each	11.24	8.91	33.01	254.1	0	0	24.26	4.16
21064	Fast Food-Burrito w/ Beans, Cheese, and Beef	101.5	1	Each	7.29	6.65	19.84	165.45	0	0	61.92	3.57
21065	Fast Food-Burrito w/ Beans, Cheese, and Chili Peppers	167	1	Each	16.55	11.42	42.33	328.99	0	0	78.49	5.56
21066	Fast Food-Burrito w/ Beef	110	1	Each	13.3	10.41	29.26	261.8	0	0	31.9	5.23
21067	Fast Food-Burrito w/ Beef and Chili Peppers	100.5	1	Each	10.75	8.27	24.72	213.06	0	0	27.14	4
21068	Fast Food-Burrito w/ Beef, Cheese, and Chili Peppers	152	1	Each	20.46	12.39	31.86	316.16	0	0	85.12	5.2
21069	Fast Food-Burrito w/ Fruit (Apple or Cherry)	74	1	Each	2.5	9.52	34.98	230.88	0	0	3.7	4.57
21100	Fast Food-Cheeseburger, Large, Double Patty	258	1	Each	37.98	43.65	39.65	704.34	0	0	141.9	17.67
21098	Fast Food-Cheeseburger, Large, Single Patty	219	1	Each	28.19	32.94	38.39	562.83	0	0	87.6	15.04
21097	Fast Food-Cheeseburger, Large, Single Patty w/ Bcn&cond	195	1	Each	32	36.76	37.13	608.4	0	0	111.15	16.24
21096	Fast Food-Cheeseburger, Large, Single Patty, Plain	185	1	Each	30.14	32.99	47.42	608.65	0	0	96.2	14.84
21095	Fast Food-Cheeseburger, Regular, Double Patty	228	1	Each	29.73	35.27	53.12	649.8	0	0	93.48	12.77
21091	Fast Food-Cheeseburger, Regular, Single Patty	154	1	Each	17.83	19.79	28.14	358.82	0	0	52.36	9.19
21089	Fast Food-Cheeseburger, Regular, Single Patty, Plain	102	1	Each	14.77	15.15	31.75	319.26	0	0	49.98	6.47
21101	Fast Food-Cheeseburger, Triple Patty, Plain	304	1	Each	56.06	50.95	26.69	796.48	0	0	161.12	21.71

Monounsaturated Fat (gm)	Polyunsaturated Fat (gm)	Vitamin D (mg)	Vitamin K (mg)	Vitamin E (mg)	Vitamin A (re)	Vitamin C (mg)	Thiamin (mg)	Riboflavin (mg)	Niacin (mg)	Vitamin B6 (mg)	Folate (mg)	Vitamin B12 (mcg)	Calcium (mg)	Iron (mg)	Magnesium (mg)	Phosphorus (mg)	Potassium (mg)	Sodium (mg)	Zinc (mg)
4	0	0	0	0.17	210	0	0.08	0.17	2.09	0	0	0	0	1.5	35	0	443	977	2.1
8	1	0	0	0.01	400	0	0.08	0.24	2.47	0	0	0	48	1.6	35	0	507	830	3.9
0	0	0	0	0	0	0	0	0	0.57	0	0	0	0	0.3	0	0	711.07	991.49	0
4	0	0	0	18.9	190	0	0.14	0.15	1.71	0	0	0	48	1.9	45.5	0	677	977	2.7
7.14	1.19	0	0	0.01	250.04	0	0.11	0.2	2.04	0	0	0	57.15	1.91	58.34	0	913.25	1226.4	2.5
15.48	1.19	0	0	0.6	785.85	0	0.11	0.26	2.94	0	0	0	47.63	1.67	41.67	0	591.77	1023.98	3.21
0	0	0	0	0	2000	24	0	0	0	0	0	0	48	2	0	0	0	320	0
0	0	0	0	0	0	0	0	0	0	0	0	0	0	0	0	0	0	928.73	0
0	0	0	0	0	0	0	0	0	0.04	0	0	0	24	0	0	0	14	136	0
0	0	0	0	0	0	0.6	0	0	0.06	0	0	0	88	0.02	0	0	51	125	0
0	0	0	0	0	60	0	0.15	0.26	1.14	0	0	0	48	0.4	0	0	200	760	0
17.86	0	0	0	0.43	0	0	0	0.15	3.39	0	0	0	71.44	1.79	31.26	0	625.11	991.24	4.02
0	0	0	0	0	200	6	0.06	0.07	1.52	0	0	0	32	0.4	0	100	380	540	0
0	0	0	0	0	0	0	0	0.01	0	0	0	0	2.48	0	0	0	430.64	791.19	0
0	0	0	0	0	0	0	0	0.01	0.19	0	0	0	2.08	0.1	0	0	791.19	1422.13	0
0	0	0	0	0	0	0	0	0	0.1	0	0	0	352	0.01	0	0	37	119	0
-0	0	0	0	0	0	0	0	0	0.21	0	0	0	184	0.02	0	0	57	176	0
0	0	0	0	0	400	6	0.03	0.17	0	0	0	0	80	0.4	0	0	400	400	0
0	0	0	0	0	0	0	0.02	0.01	0.19	0	0	0	2.48	0	0	0	510.77	1281.92	0
5.58	1.12	0	0	0	814.87	2.68	0.03	0.13	2.55	0	0	0	26.79	1	23.44	0	588.27	971.15	2.85
7.14	8.33	0	0	0	476.27	2.14	0.05	0.28	3.62	0	0	0	38.1	0.71	25	0	609.63	1012.08	1.25
7.81	1.12	0	0	2.59	279.06	1.34	0.07	0.15	3.18	0	0	0	26.79	1.23	27.35	0	586.04	1093.93	2.68
1.12	2.23	0	0	0.6	714.41	2.01	0.08	0.09	1.7	0	0	0	35.72	0.67	31.26	0	509.01	948.82	0.84
0	0	0	0	0	100	1.2	0	0	0	0	0	0	24	0.2	0	0	0	350	0
0	1	0	0	0	60	3.6	0.45	0.43	2.85	0	0	0	120	2	0	220	200	510	0
0	0	0	0	0	0	30	0.03	0	0	0	0	0	0	0	0	0	90	15	0
0	0	0	0	0	20	0	0.15	0.34	3.8	0	0	0	80	0.8	0	0	300	840	0
8.19	4.22	0	0	0	178.16	0	0.34	0.34	0.71	0.08	29.92	0.75	153.68	3.13	20.4	184.96	160.48	654.16	1.1
13.28	5.7	0	0	0	52.5	2.7	0.14	0.23	2.4	0.14	30	1.04	189	3.74	24	238.5	250.5	999	1.64
11.32	5.18	0	0	0	240	0	0.67	0.6	2	0.27	32.64	1.19	220.74	4.55	30.72	316.8	318.72	1382.4	2.23
16.4	4.45	0	0	0	163.8	0	0.5	0.45	3.6	0.2	39.6	1.37	154.8	3.96	25.2	489.6	320.4	1141.2	2.16
14.23	3.49	0	0	0	165.6	1.58	0.3	0.43	2.3	0.1	37.44	1.05	164.16	2.55	20.16	459.36	230.4	1260	1.54
4.83	1.04	0	0	0	33.9	0.11	0.51	0.32	3.48	0.14	7.91	0.03	160.46	2.72	22.6	553.7	196.62	1432.84	1.65
12.82	3.03	0	0	3.08	13.64	0.12	0.4	0.29	3.27	0.11	8.68	0.51	127.72	2.58	19.84	446.4	198.4	1071.36	1.55
11.08	6.42	0	0	0	15.51	0.14	0.35	0.39	4.16	0.16	11.28	0.94	115.62	4.3	26.79	204.45	234.06	795.24	2.66
3.41	0.52	0	0	0	24.42	0	0.27	0.18	1.62	0.03	5.92	0.1	89.54	1.63	8.88	260.48	86.58	583.86	0.29
3.83	2.64	0	0	0	2.4	3.18	0.07	0.13	0.58	0.02	4.2	0.16	25.2	1.29	16.2	87.6	83.4	153	0.55
2.37	0.6	0	0	0	16.28	0.98	0.31	0.3	2.03	0.15	58.59	0.54	56.42	2.26	43.4	48.83	326.59	492.59	0.76
1.24	0.89	0	0	0	119.04	0.84	0.11	0.35	1.79	0.12	40.92	0.45	106.95	1.13	39.99	90.21	248.31	583.11	0.82
2.68	0.48	0	0	0	10.2	0.61	0.22	0.36	2.19	0.14	59.16	0.58	49.98	2.27	35.7	57.12	289.68	522.24	1.7
3.51	0.61	0	0	0	32.34	0.92	0.27	0.42	2.7	0.18	36.96	0.87	53.13	2.45	41.58	70.46	328.02	667.59	1.92
2.23	0.51	0	0	0	75.11	2.54	0.15	0.36	1.93	0.11	30.45	0.55	64.96	1.87	25.38	70.04	205.03	495.32	1.18
4.2	0.63	0	0	0	190.38	3.34	0.27	0.6	3.82	0.2	71.81	0.99	143.62	3.82	48.43	141.95	402.47	1023.71	3.02
3.7	0.43	0	0	0	14.3	0.55	0.12	0.46	3.22	0.15	19.8	0.98	41.8	3.05	40.7	86.9	369.6	745.8	2.37
3.04	0.49	0	0	0	23.12	0.8	0.2	0.4	2.54	0.15	18.09	0.64	43.22	2.22	30.15	70.35	249.24	557.78	2.16
4.97	1.11	0	0	0	56.24	1.82	0.3	0.62	4.16	0.18	28.88	1.03	110.96	3.91	34.96	158.08	332.88	1045.76	3.95
3.42	1.06	0	0	0	37	0.74	0.17	0.18	1.86	0.07	3.7	0.51	15.54	1.07	7.4	14.8	104.34	211.64	0.4
17.35	4.7	0	0	0	54.18	1.03	0.36	0.49	7.25	0.41	49.02	3.41	239.94	5.91	51.6	394.74	595.98	1148.1	6.68
12.61	2.03	0	0	1.18	129.21	7.88	0.39	0.46	7.38	0.28	28.47	2.56	205.86	4.66	43.8	310.98	444.57	1108.14	4.6
14.49	2.71	0	0	0	79.95	2.15	0.31	0.41	6.63	0.31	33.15	2.34	161.85	4.74	44.85	399.75	331.5	1043.25	6.83
12.74	2.44	0.56	0	0	148	0	0.48	0.57	11.17	0.28	38.85	2.53	90.65	5.46	38.85	421.8	643.8	1589.15	5.55
12.64	6.37	0	0	1.98	84.36	2.74	0.57	0.43	8.34	0.27	34.2	2.07	168.72	4.72	36.48	348.84	389.88	921.12	4.13
7.17	1.47	0	0	0	70.84	2.31	0.32	0.23	6.38	0.15	21.56	1.23	181.72	2.65	26.18	215.6	229.46	976.36	2.62
5.77	1.54	0.31	0	0	36.72	0	0.4	0.4	3.7	0.09	26.52	0.97	140.76	2.44	21.42	195.84	164.22	499.8	2.37
21.52	3.15	0	0	0	85.12	2.74	0.61	0.64	11.46	0.61	51.68	5.9	282.72	8.3	60.8	541.12	820.8	1212.96	10.88

USDA ID Code	Food Name	Weight in Grams*	Quantity of Units	Unit of Measure	Protein (gm)	Fat (gm)	Carbohydrates (gm)	Kcalories	Caffeine (gm)	Fiber (gm)	Cholesterol (mg)	Saturated Fat (gm)
21103	Fast Food-Chicken Fillet Sandwich w/ Cheese	228	1	Each	29.41	38.76	41.59	631.56	0	0	77.52	12.45
21102	Fast Food-Chicken Fillet Sandwich, Plain	182	1	Each	24.12	29.45	38.69	515.06	0	0	60.06	8.53
21037	Fast Food-Chicken Nuggets, Plain	17	1	Each	2.82	2.95	2.58	48.28	0	0.07	10.2	0.92
21038	Fast Food-Chicken Nuggets, w/ Barb. Sauce	17	1	Each	2.24	2.35	3.27	43.18	0	0	7.99	0.73
21039	Fast Food-Chicken Nuggets, w/ Honey	17	1	Each	2.48	2.59	3.97	48.62	0	0	9.01	0.81
21040	Fast Food-Chicken Nuggets, w/ Must. Sauce	17	1	Each	2.28	2.48	2.73	42.16	0	0	7.99	0.75
21041	Fast Food-Chicken Nuggets, w/ Sweet and Sour	17	1	Each	2.22	2.35	3.79	45.22	0	0	7.99	0.72
21042	Fast Food-Chili Con Carne	252.999	1	Cup	24.62	8.27	21.93	255.53	0	0	134.09	3.43
21070	Fast Food-Chimichanga, w/ Beef	174	1	Each	19.61	19.68	42.8	424.56	0	0	8.7	8.51
21071	Fast Food-Chimichanga, w/ Beef and Cheese	183	1	Each	20.06	23.44	39.33	442.86	0	0	51.24	11.18
21030	Fast Food-Chocolate Chip Cookies	55	1	Box	2.89	12.14	36.22	232.65	0	0	11.55	5.34
21043	Fast Food-Clams, Breaded and Fried	28.35	3	Ounce	3.16	6.51	9.57	111.13	0	0	21.55	1.63
21128	Fast Food-Corn On The Cob w/ Butter	146	1	Each	4.47	3.43	31.94	154.76	0	0	5.84	1.64
21045	Fast Food-Crab, Soft-shell, Fried	125	1	Each	10.99	17.86	31.2	333.75	0	0	45	4.4
21011	Fast Food-Croissant w/ Egg and Cheese	127	1	Each	12.79	24.7	24.31	368.3	0	0	215.9	14.07
21012	Fast Food-Croissant w/ Egg, Cheese, and Bacon	129	1	Each	16.23	28.35	23.65	412.8	0	0	215.43	15.43
21013	Fast Food-Croissant w/ Egg, Cheese, and Ham	152	1	Each	18.92	33.58	24.2	474.24	0	0	212.8	17.48
21014	Fast Food-Croissant w/ Egg, Cheese, and Sausage	160	1	Each	20.3	38.16	24.72	523.2	0	0	216	18.23
21015	Fast Food-Danish Pastry, Cheese	91	1	Each	5.83	24.62	28.69	353.08	0	0	20.02	5.12
21016	Fast Food-Danish Pastry, Cinnamon	88	1	Each	4.8	16.72	46.85	349.36	0	0	27.28	3.48
21017	Fast Food-Danish Pastry, Fruit	94	1	Each	4.76	15.93	45.06	334.64	0	0	18.8	3.32
21104	Fast Food-Egg and Cheese Sandwich	146	1	Each	15.61	19.42	25.93	340.18	0	0	290.54	6.63
21018	Fast Food-Egg, Scrambled	47	2	Eggs	13.2	14.7	2.5	175	0	0	346	2.89
21074	Fast Food-Enchilada w/ Cheese	163	1	Each	9.63	18.84	28.54	319.48	0	0	44.01	10.59
21075	Fast Food-Enchilada w/ Cheese and Beef	192	1	Each	11.92	17.64	30.47	322.56	0	0	40.32	9.05
21076	Fast Food-Enchirito w/ Cheese, Beef, and Beans	193	1	Each	17.89	16.08	33.79	343.54	0	0	50.18	7.95
21019	Fast Food-Eng. Muffin w/ Butter	63	1	Each	4.87	5.76	30.36	189	0	0	12.6	2.43
21020	Fast Food-Eng. Muffin w/ Cheese and Sausage	115	1	Each	15.34	24.27	29.16	393.3	0	0	58.65	9.85
21021	Fast Food-Eng. Muffin w/ Egg, Cheese, and Can. Bacon	146	1	Each	19.81	19.75	31.45	382.52	0	0	233.6	9.05
21022	Fast Food-Eng. Muffin w/ Egg, Cheese, and Sausage	165	1	Each	21.66	30.86	30.97	486.75	0	0	273.9	12.42
21047	Fast Food-Fish Fillet, Battered and Fried	91	1	Each	13.34	11.18	15.44	211.12	0	0	30.94	2.57
21105	Fast Food-Fish Sandwich w/ Tartar Sauce	158	1	Each	16.94	22.77	41.02	431.34	0	0	55.3	5.23
21106	Fast Food-Fish Sandwich w/ Tartar Sauce and Cheese	183	1	Each	20.61	28.6	47.63	523.38	0	0	67.71	8.14
21023	Fast Food-French Toast w/ Butter	67.5	1	Slice	5.17	9.38	18.02	178.2	0	0	58.05	0
21031	Fast Food-Fried Pie, Fruit (Apple, Cherry, or Lemon)	85	1	Each	2.41	14.37	33.05	266.05	0	0	12.75	6.51
21077	Fast Food-Frijoles w/ Cheese	28.35	3	Ounce	1.93	1.32	4.87	38.27	0	0	6.24	0.69
21116	Fast Food-Ham and Cheese Sandwich	146	1	Each	20.69	15.48	33.35	351.86	0	0	58.4	6.44
21117	Fast Food-Ham, Egg, and Cheese Sandwich	143	1	Each	19.25	16.3	30.95	347.49	0	0	245.96	7.4
21114	Fast Food-Hamburger, Double Patty w/ Cond and Veg	226	1	Each	34.28	26.56	40.27	540.14	0	0	122.04	10.52
21111	Fast Food-Hamburger, Double Patty w/ Condiments	215	1	Each	31.82	32.47	38.74	576.2	0	0	103.2	12
21110	Fast Food-Hamburger, Double Patty, Plain	176	1	Each	29.92	27.9	42.93	543.84	0	0	98.56	10.38
21113	Fast Food-Hamburger, Large, Single Patty w/ Cond&veg	218	1	Each	25.83	27.36	40	512.3	0	0	87.2	10.42
21112	Fast Food-Hamburger, Large, Single Patty, Plain	137	1	Each	22.62	22.92	31.73	426.07	0	0	71.24	8.38
21108	Fast Food-Hamburger, Single Patty w/ Condiments	107	1	Each	13.6	10.23	32.68	274.99	0	0	42.8	3.51
21107	Fast Food-Hamburger, Single Patty, Plain	90	1	Each	12.32	11.82	30.51	274.5	0	0	35.1	4.14
21115	Fast Food-Hamburger, Triple Patty w/ Condiments	259	1	Each	49.99	41.47	28.59	691.53	0	0	142.45	15.92
21119	Fast Food-Hot Dog w/ Chili	114	1	Each	13.51	13.44	31.29	296.4	0	0	51.3	4.85
21120	Fast Food-Hot Dog w/ Corn Flour Coating (corndog)	175	1	Each	16.8	18.9	55.79	460.25	0	0	78.75	5.16
21118	Fast Food-Hot Dog, Plain	98	1	Each	10.39	14.54	18.03	242.06	0	0	44.1	5.11
21028	Fast Food-Ice Milk, Vanilla, Soft-serve w/ Cone	103	1	Each	3.89	6.12	24.11	163.77	0	0	27.81	3.53
21078	Fast Food-Nachos w/ Cheese	28.35	3	Ounce	2.28	4.75	9.11	86.75	0	0	4.54	1.95
21079	Fast Food-Nachos w/ Cheese and Jalapeno Peppers	28.35	3	Ounce	2.34	4.75	8.35	84.48	0	0	11.62	1.95
21080	Fast Food-Nachos w/ Cheese, Beans, Ground Beef	28.35	3	Ounce	2.2	3.41	6.21	63.22	0	0	2.27	1.39
21081	Fast Food-Nachos w/ Cinnamon and Sugar	28.35	3	Ounce	1.87	9.36	16.49	153.94	0	0	10.21	4.74
21130	Fast Food-Onion Rings, Breaded and Fried	10	1	Each	0.45	1.87	3.77	33.2	0	0	1.7	0.84

Monounsaturated Fat (gm)	Polyunsaturated Fat (gm)	Vitamin D (mg)	Vitamin K (mg)	Vitamin E (mg)	Vitamin A (re)	Vitamin C (mg)	Thiamin (mg)	Riboflavin (mg)	Niacin (mg)	Vitamin B6 (mg)	Folate (mg)	Vitamin B12 (mcg)	Calcium (mg)	Iron (mg)	Magnesium (mg)	Phosphorus (mg)	Potassium (mg)	Sodium (mg)	Zinc (mg)
13.65	9.95	0	0	0	127.68	2.96	0.41	0.46	9.07	0.41	45.6	0.46	257.64	3.63	43.32	405.84	332.88	1238.04	2.9
10.41	8.38	0	0	0	30.94	8.92	0.33	0.24	6.81	0.2	29.12	0.38	60.06	4.68	34.58	232.96	353.08	957.32	1.87
1.45	0.37	0	0	0.33	5.1	0.07	0.02	0.02	1.14	0.05	1.87	0.05	2.72	0.21	3.4	34	41.82	90.44	0.18
1.15	0.31	0	0	0	6.12	0.1	0.01	0.02	0.92	0.04	3.57	0.04	2.72	0.19	3.23	28.05	41.65	108.46	0.15
1.27	0.33	0	0	0	4.42	0.07	0.01	0.02	1.01	0.05	1.7	0.04	2.55	0.2	2.89	29.92	37.74	79.39	0.16
1.18	0.38	0	0	0	4.25	0.05	0.02	0.02	0.91	0.04	1.53	0.04	3.23	0.19	3.4	28.56	36.55	103.36	0.15
1.13	0.29	0	0	0	9.52	0.1	0.01	0.03	0.9	0.04	1.53	0.05	2.72	0.19	3.06	27.54	36.21	88.57	0.14
3.41	0.53	0	0	0	166.98	1.52	0.13	1.14	2.48	0.33	30.36	1.14	68.31	5.19	45.54	197.34	690.69	1006.94	3.57
8.06	1.14	0	0	0	15.66	4.7	0.49	0.64	5.78	0.28	31.32	1.51	62.64	4.54	62.64	123.54	586.38	910.02	4.96
9.43	0.73	0	0	0	126.27	2.75	0.38	0.86	4.67	0.22	32.94	1.3	237.9	3.84	60.39	186.66	203.13	957.09	3.37
5.05	1.03	0	0	0.37	14.85	0.55	0.09	0.19	1.39	0.03	15.95	0.1	19.8	1.47	16.5	52.25	81.95	188.1	0.34
2.82	1.67	0	0	0	9.07	0	0.05	0.07	0.71	0.01	2.27	0.27	5.1	0.75	7.65	58.68	65.49	205.54	0.4
1	0.61	0	0	0	96.36	6.86	0.25	0.1	2.18	0.32	43.8	0	4.38	0.88	40.88	108.04	359.16	29.2	0.91
7.69	4.88	0	0	0	3.75	0.75	0.1	0.08	1.75	0.15	20	4.48	55	1.81	25	131.25	162.5	1117.5	1.06
7.54	1.37	0	0	0	255.27	0.13	0.19	0.38	1.51	0.1	36.83	0.77	243.84	2.2	21.59	347.98	173.99	551.18	1.75
9.18	1.76	0	0	0	119.97	2.19	0.35	0.34	2.19	0.12	34.83	0.86	150.93	2.19	23.22	276.06	201.24	888.81	1.9
11.39	2.36	0	0	0	117.04	11.4	0.52	0.3	3.19	0.23	36.48	1	144.4	2.13	25.84	335.92	272.08	1080.72	2.17
14.25	3.01	0	0	0	108.8	0.16	0.99	0.32	4	0.11	38.4	0.9	144	3.04	24	289.6	283.2	1115.2	2.14
15.6	2.42	0	0	0	42.77	2.64	0.26	0.21	2.55	0.05	14.56	0.23	70.07	1.85	15.47	80.08	116.48	319.41	0.63
10.59	1.65	0	0	0	5.28	2.55	0.26	0.19	2.2	0.05	14.08	0.22	36.96	1.8	14.08	73.92	95.92	326.48	0.48
10.1	1.57	0	0	0	24.44	1.6	0.29	0.21	1.8	0.06	15.04	0.24	21.62	1.4	14.1	68.62	109.98	332.76	0.48
8.27	2.58	0	0	0	181.04	1.46	0.26	0.57	2.07	0.13	36.5	1.14	224.84	2.98	21.9	302.22	188.34	804.46	1.65
2.77	0.93	0.8	0	0.45	125.96	1	0.08	0.6	0.3	0.19	63	0.95	60	2.59	13	230	154	226	1.64
6.31	0.82	0	0	0	185.82	0.98	0.08	0.42	1.91	0.39	34.23	0.75	324.37	1.32	50.53	133.66	239.61	784.03	2.51
6.15	1.39	0	0	0	142.08	1.34	0.1	0.4	2.52	0.27	192	1.02	228.48	3.07	82.56	167.04	574.08	1319.04	2.69
6.52	0.33	0	0	0	133.17	4.63	0.17	0.69	2.99	0.21	252.83	1.62	218.09	2.39	71.41	223.88	559.7	1250.64	2.76
1.53	1.35	0	0	0.13	33.39	0.76	0.25	0.32	2.61	0.04	17.01	0.02	102.69	1.59	13.23	85.05	69.3	386.19	0.42
10.08	2.69	0	0	0	86.25	1.27	0.7	0.25	4.14	0.15	18.4	0.68	167.9	2.25	24.15	186.3	215.05	1036.15	1.68
6.76	2.06	1.17	0	0.6	157.68	1.31	0.48	0.53	3.93	0.16	43.8	0.8	207.32	3.29	33.58	319.74	213.16	784.02	1.81
12.75	3.32	0	0	0	171.6	1.49	0.84	0.5	4.46	0.2	54.45	1.37	196.35	3.47	29.7	287.1	293.7	1135.2	2.36
2.35	5.71	0	0	0	10.92	0	0.1	0.1	1.91	0.09	50.96	1.01	16.38	1.92	21.84	155.61	291.2	484.12	0.4
7.69	8.25	0	0	0.87	30.02	2.84	0.33	0.22	3.4	0.11	44.24	1.07	83.74	2.61	33.18	211.72	339.7	614.62	1
8.92	9.43	0.92	0	1.83	96.99	2.75	0.46	0.42	4.23	0.11	31.11	1.08	184.84	3.5	36.6	311.1	353.19	938.79	1.17
0	0	0	0	0	72.9	0.07	0.29	0.25	1.96	0.03	14.85	0.18	36.45	0.95	8.1	72.9	88.43	256.5	0.3
5.83	1.16	0	0	0.37	33.15	1.11	0.1	0.08	0.98	0.03	4.25	0.08	12.75	0.88	7.65	37.4	51	324.7	0.17
0.44	0.12	0	0	0	11.91	0.26	0.02	0.06	0.25	0.03	18.99	0.12	32.04	0.38	14.46	29.77	102.63	149.69	0.29
6.74	1.38	0	0	0.29	75.92	2.77	0.31	0.48	2.69	0.2	71.54	0.54	129.94	3.24	16.06	151.84	290.54	770.88	1.37
5.74	1.69	0	0	0	148.72	2.72	0.43	0.56	4.2	0.16	42.9	1.23	211.64	3.1	25.74	346.06	210.21	1005.29	1.99
10.33	2.8	0	0	0	11.3	1.13	0.36	0.38	7.57	0.54	27.12	4.07	101.7	5.85	49.72	314.14	569.52	791	5.67
14.13	2.76	0	0	0	4.3	1.08	0.34	0.41	6.73	0.37	45.15	3.33	92.45	5.55	45.15	283.8	526.75	741.75	5.81
12.11	2.34	0.7	0	1.32	0	0	0.33	0.37	8.25	0.32	36.96	2.92	86.24	4.56	36.96	234.08	362.56	554.4	5.72
11.42	2.2	0	0	0	32.7	2.62	0.41	0.37	7.28	0.33	37.06	2.38	95.92	4.93	43.6	233.26	479.6	824.04	5.72
9.88	2.14	0.55	0	0	0	0	0.29	0.29	6.25	0.23	31.51	2.06	73.98	3.58	27.4	175.36	267.15	474.02	4.11
3.72	1.77	0	0	0.43	12.84	2.57	0.26	0.32	4.7	0.13	17.12	0.83	51.36	2.46	22.47	110.21	215.07	563.89	2.05
5.46	0.92	0.27	0	0.5	0	0	0.33	0.27	3.72	0.06	25.2	0.89	63	2.4	18.9	102.6	144.9	387	2
18.23	2.74	0	0	0	15.54	1.3	0.31	0.54	10.96	0.62	31.08	4.92	64.75	8.31	54.39	393.68	784.77	712.25	10.75
6.59	1.19	0	0	0	5.7	2.74	0.22	0.4	3.74	0.1	50.16	0.3	19.38	3.28	10.26	191.52	166.44	479.94	0.78
9.11	3.5	0	0	0	36.75	0	0.28	0.7	4.17	0.09	59.5	0.44	101.5	6.18	17.5	166.25	262.5	973	1.31
6.85	1.71	0	0	0	0	0.1	0.24	0.27	3.65	0.05	29.4	0.51	23.52	2.31	12.74	97.02	143.08	670.32	1.98
1.82	0.36	0.21	0	0.38	51.5	1.13	0.05	0.26	0.31	0.06	5.15	0.21	153.47	0.15	15.45	139.05	168.92	91.67	0.57
2.01	0.56	0	0	0	22.96	0.31	0.05	0.09	0.39	0.05	2.55	0.21	68.32	0.32	13.89	69.17	43.09	204.69	0.45
2	0.56	0	0	0	65.49	0.14	0.02	0.07	0.39	0.05	2.55	0.14	86.18	0.34	15.03	54.72	40.82	241.26	0.4
1.22	0.63	0	0	0	52.16	0.54	0.03	0.08	0.37	0.05	4.25	0.11	42.81	0.31	10.77	43.09	50.18	200.15	0.41
3.08	1.07	0	0	0	2.84	2.07	0.05	0.12	1.02	0.05	1.98	0.45	22.11	0.75	5.1	8.51	20.41	114.25	0.15
0.8	0.08	0	0	0.04	0.1	0.07	0.01	0.01	0.11	0.01	1.4	0.02	8.8	0.1	1.9	10.4	15.6	51.8	0.04

USDA ID Code	Food Name	Weight in Grams*	Quantity of Units	Unit of Measure	Protein (gm)	Fat (gm)	Carbohydrates (gm)	Kcalories	Caffeine (gm)	Fiber (gm)	Cholesterol (mg)	Saturated Fat (gm)
21048	Fast Food-Oysters, Battered or Breaded, and Fried	28.35	3	Ounce	2.56	3.66	8.13	75.13	0	0	22.11	0.93
21025	Fast Food-Pancakes w/ Butter and Syrup	74	1	Each	2.63	4.46	28.99	165.76	0	0	18.5	1.87
21049	Fast Food-Pizza w/ Cheese	63	1	Slice	7.68	3.21	20.5	140.49	0	0	9.45	1.54
21050	Fast Food-Pizza w/ Cheese, Sausage, and Vegetables	79	1	Slice	13.01	5.36	21.29	184.07	0	0	20.54	1.53
21051	Fast Food-Pizza w/ Pepperoni	71	1	Slice	10.12	6.96	19.87	181.05	0	0	14.2	2.24
21131	Fast Food-Potato, Baked w/ Cheese Sauce	296	1	Each	14.62	28.74	46.5	473.6	0	0	17.76	10.56
21132	Fast Food-Potato, Baked w/ Cheese Sauce and Bacon	299	1	Each	18.42	25.89	44.43	451.49	0	0	29.9	10.13
21133	Fast Food-Potato, Baked w/ Cheese Sauce and Broccoli	339	1	Each	13.66	21.42	46.58	403.41	0	0	20.34	8.51
21134	Fast Food-Potato, Baked w/ Cheese Sauce and Chili	395	1	Each	23.23	21.84	55.85	481.9	0	0	31.6	13.04
21135	Fast Food-Potato, Baked w/ Sour Cream and Chives	302	1	Each	6.67	22.32	50.01	392.6	0	0	24.16	10.01
21136	Fast Food-Potato, French Fried In Beef Tallow	115	1	Large	4.59	18.5	44.36	358.8	0	0	20.7	8.52
21137	Fast Food-Potato, French Fried In Beef Tallow and Veg Oil	115	1	Large	4.59	18.5	44.36	357.65	0	0	16.1	7.63
21138	Fast Food-Potato, French Fried In Vegetable Oil	115	1	Large	4.59	18.5	44.36	355.35	0	0	0	5.74
21139	Fast Food-Potato, Mashed	240.024	0.5	Cup	5.54	2.9	38.69	199.22	0	0	4.8	1.15
21026	Fast Food-Potatoes, Hashed Brown	144	0.5	Cup	3.89	18.43	32.3	302.4	0	0	18.72	8.65
21122	Fast Food-Roast Beef Sandwich w/ Cheese	176	1	Each	32.23	18	45.37	473.44	0	0	77.44	9.03
21121	Fast Food-Roast Beef Sandwich, Plain	139	1	Each	21.5	13.76	33.44	346.11	0	0	51.43	3.61
21052	Fast Food-Salad, w/o Dressing	138.667	0.5	Cup	1.73	0.1	4.47	22.19	0	0	0	0.01
21053	Fast Food-Salad, w/o Dressing, w/ Cheese and Egg	144.666	0.5	Cup	5.84	3.86	3.17	67.99	0	0	65.1	1.98
21054	Fast Food-Salad, w/o Dressing, w/ Chicken	145.333	0.5	Cup	11.63	1.45	2.49	69.76	0	0	47.96	0.39
21055	Fast Food-Salad, w/o Dressing, w/ Pasta and Seafood	277.998	0.5	Cup	10.95	13.9	21.32	252.98	0	0	33.36	1.71
21056	Fast Food-Salad, w/o Dressing, w/ Shrimp	157.333	0.5	Cup	9.68	1.65	4.41	70.8	0	0	119.57	0.43
21058	Fast Food-Scallops, Breaded and Fried	24	1	Each	2.63	3.23	6.42	64.32	0	0	18	0.81
21059	Fast Food-Shrimp, Breaded and Fried	28.35	1	Ounce	3.26	4.3	6.91	78.53	0	0	34.59	0.93
21123	Fast Food-Steak Sandwich	140	1	Each	20.82	9.66	35.66	315	0	0	50.4	2.62
21124	Fast Food-Submarine Sandwich w/ Coldcuts	228	1	Each	21.84	18.63	51.05	456	0	0	36.48	6.81
21125	Fast Food-Submarine Sandwich w/ Roast Beef	216	1	Each	28.64	12.96	44.3	410.4	0	0	73.44	7.09
21126	Fast Food-Submarine Sandwich w/ Tuna Salad	256	1	Each	29.7	27.98	55.37	583.68	0	0	48.64	5.33
21032	Fast Food-Sundae, Caramel	155	1	Each	7.3	9.27	49.31	303.8	0	0	24.8	4.51
21033	Fast Food-Sundae, Hot Fudge	158	1	Each	5.64	8.63	47.67	284.4	0	0	20.54	5.02
21034	Fast Food-Sundae, Strawberry	153	1	Each	6.26	7.85	44.65	267.75	0	0	21.42	3.74
21082	Fast Food-Taco	263	1	Large	31.77	31.61	41.11	568.08	0	0	86.79	17.48
21083	Fast Food-Taco Salad	132	0.5	Cup	8.82	9.85	15.72	186.12	0	0	29.04	4.55
21084	Fast Food-Taco Salad w/ Chili Con Carne	174	0.5	Cup	11.61	8.75	17.71	193.14	0	0	3.48	4
21088	Fast Food-Tostada w/ Guacamole	28.35	1	Ounce	1.36	2.53	3.48	39.12	0	0	4.25	1.07
21085	Fast Food-Tostada, w/ Beans and Cheese	144	1	Each	9.6	9.86	26.52	223.2	0	0	30.24	5.37
21086	Fast Food-Tostada, w/ Beans, Beef, and Cheese	225	1	Each	16.09	16.94	29.66	333	0	0	74.25	11.48
21087	Fast Food-Tostada, w/ Beef and Cheese	163	1	Each	18.99	16.35	22.77	314.59	0	0	40.75	10.39
62621	Fettucini Alfredo with Broccoli-Weight Watchers	240.975	1	Each	15	6	24	220	0	6	15	2.5
55208	Fettucini Alfredo, Lean Cuisine-Stouffer's	255.144	1	Each	14	7	41	280	0	0	15	3
55171	Fettucini Alfredo-Stouffer's	141.746	1	Each	8	14	22	245	0	0	0	0
55209	Fettucini Primavera, Lean Cuisine-Stouffer's	283.493	1	Each	14	8	32	260	0	0	45	3
55831	Fettucini Sauce (Alfredo Style)-Stouffer's	283.92	1	Cup	14.02	67.1	11.02	701.05	0	0	180.27	0
41288	Fettucini w/ Turkey and Vegetables-Healthy Choice	354.367	1	Each	29	6	45	350	0	0	60	3
62612	Fiesta Chicken-Weight Watchers	240.975	1	Each	12	2	38	220	0	5	25	0.5
55773	Fiesta Mexicali Heat'n Serve Soup -Stouffer's	283.92	1	Cup	3	3	18.03	110.17	0	0	10.02	0
55210	Filet of Fish Divan, Lean Cuisine-Stouffer's	294.124	1	Each	27	5	13	210	0	0	65	2
55211	Filet of Fish Florentine, Lean Cuisine-Stouffer's	272.862	1	Each	26	7	13	220	0	0	65	3
55178	French Bread Pizza, Cheese-Stouffer's	145.29	1	Each	16	14	40	350	0	0	0	0
41332	French Bread Pizza, Deluxe-Healthy Choice	180.727	1	Each	23	7	41	330	0	0	35	3
55181	French Bread Pizza, Deluxe-Stouffer's	173.639	1	Each	21	19	40	420	0	0	0	0
55180	French Bread Pizza, Double Cheese-Stouffer's	166.552	1	Each	22	18	43	420	0	0	0	0
55182	French Bread Pizza, Hamburger-Stouffer's	173.639	1	Each	23	18	39	410	0	0	0	0
55183	French Bread Pizza, Pepperoni-Stouffer's	159.465	1	Each	19	19	39	400	0	0	0	0
55185	French Bread Pizza, Sausage-Stouffer's	170.096	1	Each	20	21	40	430	0	0	0	0

Monounsaturated Fat (gm)	Polyunsaturated Fat (gm)	Vitamin D (mg)	Vitamin K (mg)	Vitamin E (mg)	Vitamin A (re)	Vitamin C (mg)	Thiamin (mg)	Riboflavin (mg)	Niacin (mg)	Vitamin B6 (mg)	Folate (mg)	Vitamin B12 (mcg)	Calcium (mg)	Iron (mg)	Magnesium (mg)	Phosphorus (mg)	Potassium (mg)	Sodium (mg)	Zinc (mg)
1.41	0.95	0	0	0	22.11	0.85	0.06	0.07	0.9	0.01	2.55	0.21	5.67	0.91	4.82	39.97	37.14	138.06	3.19
1.68	0.62	0	0	0.44	22.2	1.11	0.13	0.18	1.08	0.04	11.1	0.07	40.7	0.84	15.54	151.7	79.92	352.24	0.33
0.99	0.49	0	0	0	73.71	1.26	0.18	0.16	2.48	0.04	58.59	0.33	116.55	0.58	15.75	112.77	109.62	335.79	0.81
2.54	0.91	0	0	0	101.12	1.58	0.21	0.17	1.96	0.09	26.86	0.36	101.12	1.53	18.17	131.14	178.54	382.36	1.11
3.14	1.17	0	0	0	54.67	1.63	0.13	0.23	3.05	0.06	52.54	0.18	64.61	0.94	8.52	75.26	152.65	266.96	0.52
10.7	6.04	0	0	0	227.92	26.05	0.24	0.21	3.34	0.71	26.64	0.18	310.8	3.02	65.12	319.68	1166.24	381.84	1.89
9.71	4.75	0	0	0	173.42	28.7	0.27	0.24	3.98	0.75	29.9	0.33	307.97	3.14	68.77	346.84	1178.06	971.75	2.15
7.68	4.18	0	0	0	277.98	48.48	0.27	0.27	3.59	0.34	61.02	0.34	335.61	3.32	77.97	345.78	1440.75	484.77	2.03
6.84	0.9	0	0	0	173.8	31.6	0.28	0.36	4.19	0.95	51.35	0.24	410.8	6.12	110.6	497.7	1572.1	699.15	3.79
7.87	3.32	0	0	0	277.84	33.82	0.27	0.18	3.71	0.79	33.22	0.21	105.7	3.11	69.46	184.22	1383.16	181.2	0.91
8.03	0.93	0	0	0.02	3.45	6.1	0.16	0.05	2.6	0.3	37.95	0.14	18.4	1.55	37.95	152.95	818.8	187.45	0.6
8.23	1.99	0	0	0	3.45	6.1	0.16	0.05	2.6	0.3	37.95	0.14	18.4	1.55	37.95	152.95	818.8	187.45	0.6
9.11	2.84	0	0	0.22	3.45	6.1	0.16	0.05	2.6	0.3	37.95	0.14	18.4	1.55	37.95	152.95	818.8	187.45	0.6
0.84	0.7	0	0	0	24	0.96	0.22	0.12	2.88	0.55	19.2	0.12	50.4	1.13	43.2	132.01	705.67	544.85	0.77
7.72	0.94	0	0	0.24	5.76	10.94	0.16	0.03	2.15	0.33	15.84	0.03	14.4	0.96	31.68	138.24	534.24	580.32	0.43
3.66	3.5	0	0	0	45.76	0	0.39	0.46	5.9	0.33	40.48	2.06	183.04	5.05	40.48	401.28	344.96	1633.28	5.37
6.8	1.71	0	0	0	20.85	2.09	0.38	0.31	5.87	0.26	40.31	1.22	54.21	4.23	30.58	239.08	315.53	792.3	3.39
0.01	0.05	0	0	0	158.08	32.17	0.04	0.07	0.76	0.11	51.31	0	18.03	0.87	15.25	54.08	238.51	36.05	0.29
1.17	0.32	0	0	0	76.67	6.51	0.06	0.12	0.65	0.07	56.42	0.2	66.55	0.45	15.91	88.25	247.38	79.57	0.67
0.45	0.37	0	0	0	63.95	11.63	0.07	0.09	3.92	0.29	45.05	0.13	24.71	0.73	21.8	113.36	297.93	139.52	0.6
3.21	6.05	0	0	0	425.34	25.58	0.19	0.14	2.36	0.22	66.72	1.14	47.26	2.11	33.36	136.22	400.32	1048.05	1.11
0.55	0.32	0	0	0	51.92	6.14	0.08	0.11	0.77	0.09	58.21	2.52	39.33	0.6	25.17	106.99	269.04	325.68	0.85
2.09	0.1	0	0	0	6.96	0	0.03	0.14	0	0.01	6.72	0.07	3.12	0.34	5.28	48.72	48.96	153.12	0.18
3	0.11	0	0	0	6.24	0	0.04	0.16	0	0.01	8.22	0.03	14.46	0.51	6.8	59.54	31.75	250.05	0.21
3.67	2.3	0	0	0	30.8	3.78	0.28	0.25	5.01	0.25	61.6	1.08	63	3.54	33.6	204.4	359.8	547.4	3.11
8.23	2.28	0	0	0	79.8	12.31	1	0.8	5.49	0.14	54.72	1.09	189.24	2.51	68.4	287.28	394.44	1650.72	2.58
1.84	2.61	0	0	0	49.68	5.62	0.41	0.41	5.96	0.32	45.36	1.81	41.04	2.81	66.96	192.24	330.48	844.56	4.38
13.4	7.3	0	0	0	40.96	3.58	0.46	0.33	11.34	0.23	56.32	1.61	74.24	2.64	79.36	220.16	335.36	1292.8	1.87
3.03	1.01	0.31	0	0.9	68.2	3.41	0.06	0.29	0.95	0.05	12.4	0.6	189.1	0.22	27.9	217	317.75	195.3	0.82
2.33	0.81	0.47	0	0.66	56.88	2.37	0.06	0.3	1.07	0.13	9.48	0.65	206.98	0.58	33.18	227.52	395	181.7	0.95
2.66	1.02	0.46	0	0.78	58.14	1.99	0.06	0.28	0.9	0.08	18.36	0.64	160.65	0.32	24.48	154.53	270.81	91.8	0.66
10.11	1.48	0	0	0	226.18	3.42	0.24	0.68	4.94	0.37	36.82	1.6	339.27	3.71	107.83	312.97	728.51	1233.47	6.05
3.44	1.17	0	0	0	51.48	2.38	0.07	0.24	1.64	0.15	26.4	0.42	128.04	1.52	34.32	95.04	277.2	508.2	1.8
3.03	1.02	0	0	0	142.68	2.26	0.1	0.33	1.69	0.35	41.76	0.49	163.56	1.77	34.8	102.66	261	589.86	2.19
0.92	0.33	0	0	0	23.53	0.4	0.01	0.06	0.22	0.03	11.91	0.11	45.93	0.18	7.94	25.23	70.59	86.75	0.44
3.05	0.75	0	0	0	84.96	1.3	0.1	0.33	1.32	0.16	74.88	0.69	210.24	1.89	59.04	116.64	403.2	542.88	1.9
3.51	0.6	0	0	0	173.25	4.05	0.09	0.5	2.86	0.25	96.75	1.13	189	2.45	67.5	173.25	490.5	870.75	3.17
3.34	0.97	0	0	0	96.17	2.61	0.1	0.55	3.15	0.23	14.67	1.17	216.79	2.87	63.57	179.3	572.13	896.5	3.68
0	0	0	0	0	60	1.2	0	0	0	0	0	0	300	1.5	0	0	510	540	0
0	0	0	0	0	0	0	0.3	0.43	1.52	0	0	0	200	0.8	0	0	270	570	0
0	0	0	0	0	0	0	0.15	0.26	0.95	0	0	0	120	0.4	0	0	100	400	0
0	0	0	0	0	400	18	0.3	0.43	1.52	0	0	0	240	0.8	0	0	400	510	0
0	0	0	0	0	0	0	0	0.01	0	0	0	0	2.72	0	0	0	340.51	1812.72	0
0	2	0	0	0	150	0	0.45	0.51	3.8	0	0	0	120	1.5	0	310	450	480	0
0	0	0	0	0	450	42	0	0	0	0	0	0	72	1.5	0	0	490	480	0
0	0	0	0	0	0	6.01	0	0	0.19	0	0	0	2.4	1	0	0	430.64	711.07	0
0	1	0	0	0	20	27	0.15	0.34	1.9	0	0	0	120	0.4	0	0	800	490	0
0	2	0	0	0	500	1.2	0.15	0.34	1.9	0	0	0	120	0.4	0	0	780	590	0
0	0	0	0	0	60	3.6	0.45	0.34	2.85	0	0	0	200	1.5	0	0	300	630	0
0	1	0	0	0	80	6	0.45	0.34	3.8	0	0	0	200	2.5	0	280	350	500	0
0	0	0	0	0	100	6	0.45	0.43	3.8	0	0	0	160	1.5	0	0	350	950	0
0	0	0	0	0	40	6	0.45	0.51	3.8	0	0	0	360	1.5	0	0	320	850	0
0	0	0	0	0	60	6	0.38	0.34	3.8	0	0	0	160	1.5	0	0	340	650	0
0	0	0	0	0	100	6	0.53	0.43	3.8	0	0	0	160	1.5	0	0	300	880	0
0	0	0	0	0	80	6	0.6	0.43	3.8	0	0	0	160	1.5	0	0	340	840	0

USDA ID Code	Food Name	Weight in Grams*	Quantity of Units	Unit of Measure	Protein (gm)	Fat (gm)	Carbohydrates (gm)	Kcalories	Caffeine (gm)	Fiber (gm)	Cholesterol (mg)	Saturated Fat (gm)
55187	French Bread Pizza, Vegetable Deluxe-Stouffer's	180.727	1	Each	18	20	41	420	0	0	0	0
55761	French Onion Soup-Stouffer's	283.92	1	Cup	4.01	4.01	10.02	100.15	0	0	0	0
41337	Garden Potato Casserole-Healthy Choice	262.231	1	Each	12	4	23	180	0	0	20	2
55774	Garden Tomato Heat'n Serve Soup-Stouffer's	283.92	1	Cup	4.01	3	16.02	110.17	0	0	10.02	0
41273	Garden Vegetable Soup-Healthy Choice	212.62	1	Each	3	1	18	100	0	0	0	0
43399	Glazed Breast of Chicken, Top Shelf-Hormel	283.493	1	Each	19	2	19	170	0	0	35	1
55212	Glazed Chicken w/ Veg. Lean Cuisine-Stouffer's	240.969	1	Each	21	7	24	250	0	0	50	2
41307	Glazed Chicken-Healthy Choice	240.969	1	Each	21	3	27	220	0	0	45	1
55784	Glazed Chicken-Stouffer's	28.35	1	Ounce	2.9	1.1	1	26	0	0	9	0
55172	Green Bean Mushroom Casserole-Stouffer's	134.659	1	Each	5	10	13	160	0	0	0	0
55118	Green Pepper Steak w/ Rice-Stouffer's	297.668	1	Each	20	10	35	310	0	0	0	0
55780	Green Pepper Steak-Stouffer's	28.35	1	Ounce	2.6	1.4	1.3	28	0	0	7	0
62617	Grilled Salisbury Steak-Weight Watchers	240.975	1	Each	19	9	24	250	0	4	30	3
55159	Ham and Asparagus Bake-Stouffer's	269.319	1	Each	18	35	32	520	0	0	0	0
62683	Hamburger Helper, Beef Noodle	220	1	Cup	4	10.5	23	260	0	1	5	4
62682	Hamburger Helper, Cheesy Italian	220	1	Cup	5	21	30	330	0	1	5	2
62681	Hamburger Helper, Chili Mac	220	1	Cup	3	16	30	290	0	1	4	4
55809	Heartland Medley-Stouffer's	28.35	1	Ounce	1.4	0.4	1.8	17	0	0	3	0
41279	Hearty Beef Soup-Healthy Choice	212.62	1	Each	9	1	17	120	0	0	20	0
41280	Hearty Chicken Soup-Healthy Choice	212.62	1	Each	7	2	17	110	0	0	25	0
41258	Herb Roasted Chicken-Healthy Choice	347.279	1	Each	22	5	50	300	0	0	40	2
41311	Homestyle Turkey w/ Vegetables-Healthy Choice	269.319	1	Each	26	2	34	260	0	0	30	0
55214	Honey Mustard Chicken, Lean Cuisine-Stouffer's	212.62	1	Each	18	4	30	230	0	0	40	1
41312	Honey Mustard Chicken-Healthy Choice	269.319	1	Each	26	4	41	310	0	0	45	1
43371	Hot Chili no Beans-Hormel	212.62	1	Each	16	27	14	360	0	0	60	11
43410	Hot Chili w/ Beans, Micro Cup-Hormel	209.076	1	Each	15	11	24	250	0	0	49	4
43372	Hot Chili w/ Beans-Hormel	212.62	1	Each	15	15	27	300	0	0	55	5
62622	Italian Cheese Lasagna-Weight Watchers	311.85	1	Each	29	8	28	300	0	7	25	3
43395	Italian Lasagna, Top Shelf-Hormel	283.493	1	Each	23	16	30	350	0	0	60	8
55798	Italian Style Vegetables-Stouffer's	28.35	1	Ounce	0.3	0.3	1.6	10	0	0	0	0
62613	Lasagna Florentine-Weight Watchers	283.5	1	Each	13	2	37	210	0	5	10	0.5
55215	Lasagna w/ Meat Sauce, Lean Cuisine-Stouffer's	290.581	1	Each	20	6	36	280	0	0	25	3
41308	Lasagna w/ Meat Sauce-Healthy Choice	283.493	1	Each	18	5	37	260	0	0	20	2
62623	Lasagna with Meat Sauce-Weight Watchers	290.59	1	Each	24	7	34	290	0	7	15	2.5
43403	Lasagna, Micro Cup-Hormel	212.62	1	Each	8	13	25	250	0	0	23	6
55134	Lasagna-Stouffer's	283.493	1	Each	18	12	40	340	0	0	0	0
41259	Lemon Pepper Fish-Healthy Choice	304.755	1	Each	13	5	52	300	0	0	40	1
41274	Lentil Soup-Healthy Choice	212.62	1	Each	8	1	23	140	0	0	0	0
55216	Linguini w/ Clam Sauce, Lean Cuisine-Stouffer's	272.862	1	Each	17	8	36	280	0	0	30	2
	Macaroni & Cheese, Deluxe Light, Kraft	90	1	Serving	14	4.5	48	290	0	0	15	2.5
	Macaroni & Cheese, Kraft	70	1	Serving	12	18.5	50	420	0	0	15	5
55217	Macaroni and Beef in Sauce, Lean Cuisine-Stouffer's	283.493	1	Each	14	6	35	250	0	0	25	1
55137	Macaroni and Beef w/ Tomatoes-Stouffer's	326.017	1	Each	21	12	38	340	0	0	0	0
41338	Macaroni and Beef-Healthy Choice	240.969	1	Each	12	3	32	200	0	0	15	1
62533	Macaroni and Cheese	111.912	1	Cup	1	12.99	43.97	359.72	0	15.99	39.97	7.99
57808	Macaroni and Cheese Pot Pie-Swanson	198.445	1	Each	7	8	24	200	0	0	0	0
55218	Macaroni and Cheese, Lean Cuisine-Stouffer's	255.144	1	Each	15	9	37	290	0	0	30	4
43406	Macaroni and Cheese, Micro Cup-Hormel	212.62	1	Each	12	11	28	260	0	0	45	6
41339	Macaroni and Cheese-Healthy Choice	255.144	1	Each	12	6	45	280	0	0	20	3
55155	Macaroni and Cheese-Stouffer's	170.096	1	Each	11	13	23	250	0	0	0	0
62624	Macaroni and Cheese-Weight Watchers	255.15	1	Each	11	7	49	300	0	7	20	2
41309	Mandarin Chicken-Healthy Choice	311.843	1	Each	23	2	39	260	0	0	50	0
55830	Marinara Sauce-Stouffer's	283.92	1	Cup	3	11.02	18.03	180.27	0	0	0	0
55219	Meatloaf w/ Mac. and Cheese, Lean Cuisine-Stouffer's	265.775	1	Each	26	8	26	280	0	0	55	3
41260	Meatloaf-Healthy Choice	340.192	1	Each	17	8	48	340	0	0	40	3

Monounsaturated Fat (gm)	Polyunsaturated Fat (gm)	Vitamin D (mg)	Vitamin K (mg)	Vitamin E (mg)	Vitamin A (re)	Vitamin C (mg)	Thiamin (mg)	Riboflavin (mg)	Niacin (mg)	Vitamin B6 (mg)	Folate (mcg)	Vitamin B12 (mcg)	Calcium (mg)	Iron (mg)	Magnesium (mg)	Phosphorus (mg)	Potassium (mg)	Sodium (mg)	Zinc (mg)
0	0	0	0	0	250	3.6	0.45	0.43	3.8	0	0	0	280	1.5	0	0	230	830	0
0	0	0	0	0	0	0	0.02	0.02	0	0	0	0	240.36	0	0	0	170.26	2073.11	0
0	0	0	0	0	0	0	0	0	0	0	0	0	0	0	0	0	600	360	0
0	0	0	0	0	0	0	0	0	0.19	0	0	0	240.36	0.3	0	0	430.64	1051.58	0
0	0	0	0	0	350	9	0.09	0.07	0.76	0	0	0	16	0.4	0	0	230	560	0
1	1	0	0	0.76	400	3.6	0.06	0.17	7.6	0	0	0	32	0.4	35	0	804	780	1.05
0	4	0	0	0	20	3.6	0.15	0.17	7.6	0	0	0	16	0.2	0	0	580	590	0
0	1	0	0	0	0	1.2	0.15	0.14	6.65	0	0	0	0	0.6	0	240	370	510	0
0	0	0	0	0	0	0	0	0	0.23	0	0	0	24	0.01	0	0	45	105	0
0	0	0	0	0	40	2.4	0.06	0.17	0.38	0	0	0	64	0.2	0	0	200	550	0
0	0	0	0	0	40	6	0.15	0.17	3.8	0	0	0	16	1	0	0	410	700	0
0	0	0	0	0	0	3.6	0	0	0.1	0	0	0	48	0.02	0	0	51	164	0
0	0	0	0	0	60	0	0	0	0	0	0	0	120	1.5	0	0	450	590	0
0	0	0	0	0	60	36	0.53	0.51	2.85	0	0	0	160	0.8	0	0	360	1100	0
0	0	0	0	0	60	0	0.23	0.17	3.8	0	0	0	24	1	0	0	240	900	0
0	0	0	0	0	60	0	0.3	0.34	3.8	0	0	0	120	1.5	0	0	400	900	0
0	0	0	0	0	200	0	0.3	0.26	4.75	0	0	0	24	1.5	0	0	0	900	0
0	0	0	0	0	0	0.6	0	0	0.06	0	0	0	40	0.02	0	0	60	85	0
0	0	0	0	0	150	9	0.06	0.1	1.9	0	0	0	32	0.4	0	90	280	540	0
0	0	0	0	0	200	2.4	0.09	0.17	1.9	0	0	0	32	0.4	0	90	190	520	0
0	1	0	0	0	250	24	0.15	0.14	7.6	0	0	0	32	0.8	0	280	370	560	0
0	0	0	0	0	100	4.8	0.03	0.07	0	0	0	0	32	0	0	0	100	550	0
0	1	0	0	0	200	2.4	0.15	0.17	3.8	0	0	0	16	0.4	0	0	340	540	0
0	0	0	0	0	100	3.6	0.15	0.03	1.52	0	0	0	16	0.8	0	0	110	520	0
13	1	0	0	10.56	330	0	0.05	0.22	2.47	0	0	0	40	1.4	35	0	497	860	2.7
4	0	0	0	1.95	190	0	0.14	0.15	1.71	0	0	0	48	1.9	45.5	0	677	977	2.7
6	1	0	0	0	210	0	0.09	0.17	1.71	0	0	0	48	1.8	49	0	777	1030	2.25
0	0	0	0	0	350	15	0	0	0	0	0	0	780	1.5	0	0	720	560	0
5	1	0	0	0.7	100	2.4	0.3	0.51	3.8	0	0	0	240	1.5	49	0	728	840	3.15
0	0	0	0	0	0	1.8	0	0	0.02	0	0	0	72	0.01	0	0	62	147	0
0	0	0	0	0	300	15	0	0	0	0	0	0	300	1.5	0	0	440	420	0
0	0	0	0	0	100	6	0.15	0.26	2.85	0	0	0	120	1	0	0	700	560	0
0	1	0	0	0	150	2.4	0.3	0.26	1.9	0	0	0	80	1.5	0	210	500	420	0
0	0	0	0	0	250	12	0	0	0	0	0	0	480	1.5	0	0	720	580	0
4	2	0	0	0	100	1.8	0.12	0.2	1.9	0	0	0	40	0.8	24.5	0	331	949	1.05
0	0	0	0	0	150	6	0.15	0.34	6.65	0	0	0	200	1	0	0	570	840	0
0	2	0	0	0	80	48	0.23	0.14	1.14	0	0	0	32	0.6	0	180	410	370	0
0	0	0	0	0	60	2.4	0.06	0.03	0.38	0	0	0	0	0.6	0	0	160	480	0
0	2	0	0	0	0	0	0.3	0.17	1.9	0	0	0	32	1.5	0	0	90	560	0
0	0	0	0	0	0	0	0	0	0	0	0	0	160	1.5	0	0	0	810	0
0	0	0	0	0	0	0	0	0	0	0	0	0	120	1.5	0	0	0	760	0
0	1	0	0	0	100	3.6	0.15	0.17	2.85	0	0	0	48	1.5	0	0	450	540	0
0	0	0	0	0	60	6	0.06	0.1	1.9	0	0	0	32	0.8	0	0	300	1440	0
0	0	0	0	0	200	15	0.3	0.26	0	0	0	0	32	1	0	0	530	420	0
0	0	0	0	0	99.92	0	0	0	0	0	0	0	239.81	1.5	0	0	0	1029.19	0
0	0	0	0	0	80	0	0.09	0.17	0.76	0	0	0	120	0.6	0	0	0	740	0
0	0	0	0	0	0	0	0.3	0.43	1.52	0	0	0	200	0.8	0	0	160	550	0
3	1	0	0	0	80	6	0.09	0.26	1.14	0	0	0	80	0.6	24.5	0	209	650	1.05
0	1	0	0	0	0	0	0.3	0.26	1.14	0	0	0	120	1	0	230	220	520	0
0	0	0	0	0	20	0	0.15	0.26	0.38	0	0	0	160	0.4	0	0	140	640	0
0	0	0	0	0	100	0	0	0	0	0	0	0	300	1	0	0	410	570	0
0	0	0	0	0	250	9	0.15	0.17	4.75	0	0	0	16	1	0	200	400	400	0
0	0	0	0	0	0	66.1	0	0	0.38	0	0	0	0	0.2	0	0	681.02	1221.83	0
0	1	0	0	0	60	9	0.23	0.43	3.8	0	0	0	120	2	0	0	550	540	0
0	1	0	0	0	0	0	0	0	0	0	0	0	0	0	0	240	690	560	0

USDA ID Code	Food Name	Weight in Grams*	Quantity of Units	Unit of Measure	Protein (gm)	Fat (gm)	Carbohydrates (gm)	Kcalories	Caffeine (gm)	Fiber (gm)	Cholesterol (mg)	Saturated Fat (gm)
55779	Meatloaf-Stouffer's	28.35	1	Ounce	4.4	3.4	2.1	57	0	0	15	0
55812	Mexicali Chicken-Stouffer's	28.35	1	Ounce	1.4	0.8	1.8	20	0	0	5	0
55770	Minestrone Heat'n Serve Soup-Stouffer's	283.92	1	Cup	5.01	4.01	18.03	130.2	0	0	0	0
41281	Minestrone Soup-Healthy Choice	212.62	1	Each	6	1	30	160	0	0	0	0
55760	Minestrone Soup-Stouffer's	283.92	1	Cup	6.01	3	20.03	140.21	0	0	10.02	0
41313	Mushroom Gravy over Beef Sirloin Tips-Healthy Choice	269.319	1	Each	22	5	43	310	0	0	35	2
62619	Nacho Grande Chicken Enchiladas-Weight Watchers	255.15	1	Each	15	8	42	290	0	4	20	2.5
41340	Nacho Macaroni and Cheese-Healthy Choice	255.144	1	Each	13	5	44	280	0	0	20	3
55754	Navy Bean w/ Ham Soup-Stouffer's	283.92	1	Cup	11.02	8.01	31.05	240.36	0	0	20.03	0
55757	New England Clam Chowder Soup-Stouffer's	283.92	1	Cup	14.02	23.03	21.03	340.51	0	0	40.06	0
55829	Newburg Sauce Supreme-Stouffer's	283.92	1	Cup	7.01	41.06	20.03	480.72	0	0	120.18	0
43407	Noodles and Chicken, Micro Cup-Hormel	212.62	1	Each	7	7	19	174	0	0	29	2
55804	Noodles Romanoff-Stouffer's	283.92	1	Cup	17.03	25.04	36.05	440.66	0	0	40.06	0
41282	Old Fashioned Chicken Noodle Soup-Healthy Choice	212.62	1	Each	5	2	11	90	0	0	20	0
55806	Old-Fashion Stuff'n-Stouffer's	283.92	0.5	Cup	11.02	37.06	61.09	620.93	0	0	10.02	0
55220	Oriental Beef w/ Veg., Lean Cuisine-Stouffer's	244.513	1	Each	20	9	31	290	0	0	40	2
41314	Oriental Chicken w/ Spicy Peanut Sauce-Healthy Choice	269.319	1	Each	33	5	40	340	0	0	45	1
55221	Oven Baked Chicken, Lean Cuisine-Stouffer's	226.795	1	Each	17	5	21	200	0	0	35	2
	Pasta Accents - Primavera	175	1	Serving	9	10	27	230	0	0	0	0
55800	Pasta Florentine-Stouffer's	283.92	0.5	Cup	16.02	21.03	32.05	380.57	0	0	50.07	0
41294	Pasta Italiano-Healthy Choice	340.192	1	Each	16	5	59	350	0	0	30	2
55810	Pasta Roma-Stouffer's	283.92	0.5	Cup	16.02	7.01	31.05	260.39	0	0	30.04	0
41292	Pasta Shells w/ Tomato Sauce-Healthy Choice	340.192	1	Each	24	3	53	330	0	0	35	2
55142	Pasta Shells, Cheese w/ Sauce-Stouffer's	262.231	1	Each	17	13	28	300	0	0	0	0
41287	Pasta w/ Cacciatore Chicken-Healthy Choice	354.367	1	Each	26	3	47	310	0	0	35	0
41293	Pasta w/ Teriyaki Chicken-Healthy Choice	357.91	1	Each	24	3	58	350	0	0	45	1
41333	Pepperoni French Bread Pizza-Healthy Choice	170.096	1	Each	20	7	38	310	0	0	30	3
62625	Pepperoni Pizza-Weight Watchers	157.626	1	Each	23	12	46	390	0	4	45	4
55827	Pesto Sauce-Stouffer's	283.92	0.25	Cup	35.05	61.09	21.03	771.16	0	0	70.11	0
	Pizza, DiGiorno, 3 Meat	154	1	Slice	19	16	40	380	0	3.11	40	8
	Pizza, DiGiorno, 4 Cheese	139	1	Slice	16	11	39	320	0	3.11	25.1	6.1
	Pizza, Red Baron, Pepperoni	154	1	Slice	19	24	40	450	0	2	35	9
	Pizza, Red Baron, Special Deluxe	129	1	Slice	13	18	32	340	0	2	25	7
	Pizza, Tombstone, Sausage & Pepperoni	132	1	Slice	19	19	25	340	0	2	45	9
	Pizza, Tony's, Supreme, Sausage & Pepperoni	122	1	Slice	13	20	28	340	0	2	25	7
	Pizza, Totino's, Microwave for One Cheese	104	1	Each	10	11	25	240	0	1	15	3.5
	Pizza, Totino's, Microwave for One Pepperoni	104	1	Each	10	16	25	280	0	1	15	3.5
	Pizza, Totino's, Party Cheese	277	1	Slice	15	5	33	320	0	2	20	5
	Pizza, Totino's, Party Pepperoni	289	1	Slice	14	21	33	380	0	2	20	5
	Pizza, Totino's, Party Supreme	309	1	Slice	15	20	34	380	0	2	20	4.5
55174	Potatoes Au Gratin-Stouffer's	163.008	1	Each	5	9	17	170	0	0	0	0
62536	Ravioli, Beef	243.935	1	Cup	9	5	35.99	229.94	0	4	19.99	2.5
62537	Ravioli, Cheese	243.935	1	Cup	9	3	37.99	219.94	0	4	15	1.5
62662	Rice-a-Roni Wild Rice	56	1	Cup	5	1	43	240	0	1	0	0
55222	Rigatoni Bake, Lean Cuisine-Stouffer's	276.406	1	Each	18	8	27	250	0	0	25	3
41341	Rigatoni in Meat Sauce-Healthy Choice	269.319	1	Each	16	6	34	260	0	0	30	2
55782	Rigatoni w/ Meat Sauce-Stouffer's	283.92	0.5	Cup	16.02	11.02	31.05	290.44	0	0	30.04	0
62614	Roast Turkey Medallions-Weight Watchers	240.975	1	Each	10	2	34	190	0	4	20	0.5
41310	Roasted Turkey and Mushrooms in Gravy-Healthy Choice	240.969	1	Each	18	3	26	200	0	0	40	1
41290	Salisbury Steak w/ Mushroom Gravy-Healthy Choice	311.843	1	Each	21	6	35	280	0	0	55	3
43402	Salisbury Steak, Top Shelf-Hormel	283.493	1	Each	25	15	22	320	0	0	70	7
41262	Salsa Chicken-Healthy Choice	318.93	1	Each	20	2	36	240	0	0	50	1
43412	Scalloped Potatoes and Ham, Micro Cup-Hormel	212.62	1	Each	8	16	21	260	0	0	33	6
55175	Scalloped Potatoes-Stouffer's	163.008	1	Each	4	6	16	130	0	0	0	0
41263	Shrimp Marinara-Healthy Choice	297.668	1	Each	10	1	51	260	0	0	60	0

Monounsaturated Fat (gm)	Polyunsaturated Fat (gm)	Vitamin D (mg)	Vitamin K (mg)	Vitamin E (mg)	Vitamin A (re)	Vitamin C (mg)	Thiamin (mg)	Riboflavin (mg)	Niacin (mg)	Vitamin B6 (mg)	Folate (mg)	Vitamin B12 (mcg)	Calcium (mg)	Iron (mg)	Magnesium (mg)	Phosphorus (mg)	Potassium (mg)	Sodium (mg)	Zinc (mg)
0	0	0	0	0	0	0	0	0	0.13	0	0	0	48	0.06	0	0	4.4	193	0
0	0	0	0	0	0	4.2	0	0	0.11	0	0	0	88	0.02	0	0	68	48	0
0	0	0	0	0	0	0	0	0	0	0	0	0	0	0.2	0	0	310.46	1191.79	0
0	0	0	0	0	60	15	0.12	0.14	1.52	0	0	0	32	0.6	0	130	440	520	0
0	0	0	0	0	0	0	0	0	0.19	0	0	0	0	0.2	0	0	370.56	1281.92	0
0	0	0	0	0	60	2.4	0	0.03	0.38	0	0	0	0	0.2	0	0	80	500	0
0	0	0	0	0	300	12	0	0	0	0	0	0	360	0.6	0	0	600	560	0
0	0	0	0	0	0	0	0.6	0.51	0	0	0	0	160	0.8	0	0	420	560	0
0	0	0	0	0	0	0	0	0	0.19	0	0	0	70.11	3	0	0	570.86	1251.88	0
0	0	0	0	0	0	0	0	0.01	0.19	0	0	0	2.48	0.1	0	0	570.86	961.44	0
0	0	0	0	0	0	0	0	0.01	0	0	0	0	1.84	0	0	0	370.56	1051.58	0
3	2	0	0	0	270	8.4	0.08	0.12	1.71	0	0	0	32	0.7	21	0	254	1009	0.75
0	0	0	0	0	0	0	0	0.01	0.19	0	0	0	1.6	0.2	0	0	260.39	1992.99	0
0	0	0	0	0	80	12	0.03	0.1	1.9	0	0	0	16	0.2	0	60	130	540	0
0	0	0	0	0	0	0.84	0.01	0.01	0.74	0	0	0	0	0.33	0	0	200.3	1121.68	0
0	0	0	0	0	150	1.2	0.09	0.17	2.85	0	0	0	16	1	0	0	400	590	0
0	1	0	0	0	0	2.4	0	0	0.38	0	0	0	0	0.2	0	0	50	470	0
0	0	0	0	0	350	6	0.15	0.17	7.6	0	0	0	16	0.8	0	0	550	480	0
0	0	0	0	0	0	20	0	0	0	0	0	0	160	1.2	0	0	0	450	0
0	0	0	0	0	0	0.54	0	0.01	0.19	0	0	0	3.45	0.1	0	0	400.6	891.34	0
0	3	0	0	0	60	0	0.53	0.51	2.85	0	0	0	48	2	0	180	540	530	0
0	0	0	0	0	0	6.01	0.11	0.01	0.95	0	0	0	1.04	0.3	0	0	600.9	781.17	0
0	0	0	0	0	100	21	0.53	0.43	2.85	0	0	0	320	1.5	0	240	640	470	0
0	0	0	0	0	150	9	0.12	0.26	1.9	0	0	0	280	1	0	0	480	820	0
0	1	0	0	0	100	6	0.45	0.43	6.65	0	0	0	32	1.5	0	250	660	430	0
0	2	0	0	0	100	6	0.3	0.34	3.8	0	0	0	48	1.5	0	200	390	370	0
0	1	0	0	0	150	0	0.53	0.34	3.8	0	0	0	160	2.5	0	240	350	470	0
0	0	0	0	0	80	4.8	0	0	0	0	0	0	540	1	0	0	320	650	0
0	0	0	0	0	0	12.02	0	0.02	0.38	0	0	0	5.69	0.3	0	0	620.93	1362.04	0
0	1	0	0	0	138.3	0	0.5	0.3	3	0	0	0	330	1	0	200	330	1100	0
0	1	0	0	0	138.3	0	0.5	0.3	3	0	0	0	350	0.9	0	200	330	870	0
0	1	0	0	0	90	0	0	0	0	0	0	0	330	1.9	0	200	330	920	0
0	1	0	0	0	78	0	0	0	0	0	0	0	220	2.7	0	200	330	690	0
0	1	0	0	0	150	1.2	0	0	0	0	0	0	350	0.9	0	200	330	820	0
0	1	0	0	0	40	2.4	0	0	0	0	0	0	200	1.5	0	200	330	610	0
0	1	0	0	0	0	0	0	0	0	0	0	0	220	1.5	0	180	290	530	0
0	1	0	0	0	0	0	0	0	0	0	0	0	200	1.5	0	180	290	710	0
0	1	0	0	0	0	0	0	0	0	0	0	0	300	1.5	0	200	330	630	0
0	1	0	0	0	0	0	0	0	0	0	0	0	280	1.5	0	200	330	920	0
0	1	0	0	0	0	0	0	0	0	0	0	0	280	1.5	0	200	330	890	0
0	0	0	0	0	20	3.6	0	0.1	0.76	0	0	0	48	0.8	0	0	260	670	0
0	0	0	0	0	149.96	2.4	0	0	0	0	0	0	0	1.5	0	0	0	1149.69	0
0	0	0	0	0	59.98	1.2	0	0	0	0	0	0	23.99	1.5	0	0	0	1279.66	0
0	0	0	0	0	80	6	0.15	0.1	1.52	0	0	0	48	0.8	0	0	0	1110	0
0	1	0	0	0	200	6	0.23	0.34	3.8	0	0	0	160	1.5	0	0	620	430	0
0	0	0	0	0	200	2.4	0.3	0.26	2.85	0	0	0	120	1.5	0	200	700	540	0
0	0	0	0	0	0	48.07	0	0.01	0.76	0	0	0	2.08	0.3	0	0	620.93	851.28	0
0	0	0	0	0	100	4.8	0	0	0	0	0	0	24	1	0	0	220	530	0
0	1	0	0	0	200	0	0.12	0.14	2.85	0	0	0	16	0.8	0	150	260	380	0
0	0	0	0	0	0	0	0	0	0	0	0	0	0	0	0	260	630	500	0
8	1	0	0	0.03	0	3.6	0.03	0.26	4.75	0	0	0	16	1.5	35	0	801	910	5.7
0	0	0	0	0	200	66	0.23	0.17	3.8	0	0	0	64	0.6	0	200	540	450	0
8	2	0	0	0.39	0	11.4	0.09	0.1	2.09	0	0	0	32	0.4	21	0	425	768	0.9
0	0	0	0	0	0	2.4	0.03	0.14	0.76	0	0	0	80	0.2	0	0	375	610	0
0	0	0	0	0	100	114	0.23	0.14	1.14	0	0	0	48	1.5	0	130	390	320	0

USDA ID Code	Food Name	Weight in Grams*	Quantity of Units	Unit of Measure	Protein (gm)	Fat (gm)	Carbohydrates (gm)	Kcalories	Caffeine (gm)	Fiber (gm)	Cholesterol (mg)	Saturated Fat (gm)
62615	Shrimp Marinara-Weight Watchers	255.15	1	Each	9	2	35	190	0	4	40	0.5
55143	Single Serving Stuffed Pepper-Stouffer's	283.493	1	Each	10	8	28	220	0	0	0	0
41264	Sirloin Beef w/ Barbecue Sauce-Healthy Choice	311.843	1	Each	17	4	44	280	0	0	25	2
41291	Sliced Turkey Breast w/ Gravy and Dressing-Healthy Choice	283.493	1	Each	27	4	30	270	0	0	50	2
41296	Sliced Turkey Breast w/ Gravy-Healthy Choice	340.192	1	Each	19	3	46	290	0	0	20	1
55225	Sliced Turkey w/ Dressing, Lean Cuisine-Stouffer's	223.251	1	Each	16	5	23	200	0	0	25	1
41265	Southwestern Style Chicken-Healthy Choice	354.367	1	Each	25	5	51	340	0	0	60	2
43404	Spaghetti and Meatballs, Micro Cup-Hormel	212.62	1	Each	10	7	27	210	0	0	20	3
55226	Spaghetti w/ Meat Sauce, Lean Cuisine-Stouffer's	326.017	1	Each	15	6	45	290	0	0	20	2
43396	Spaghetti w/ Meat Sauce, Top Shelf-Hormel	283.493	1	Each	14	6	37	260	0	0	20	2
41342	Spaghetti w/ Meat Sauce-Healthy Choice	283.493	1	Each	14	6	42	280	0	0	20	2
55247	Spaghetti w/ Meat Sauce-Stouffer's	364.998	1	Each	16	12	38	320	0	0	0	0
55150	Spaghetti w/ Meatballs, -Stouffer's	276.406	1	Each	14	9	37	290	0	0	0	0
55176	Spinach Souffle-Stouffer's	170.096	1	Each	9	15	11	220	0	0	0	0
41283	Split Pea and Ham Soup-Healthy Choice	212.62	1	Each	10	3	25	170	0	0	10	1
55766	Split Pea Soup w/ Ham-Stouffer's	283.92	1	Cup	15.02	3	35.05	220.33	0	0	10.02	0
55781	Stuffed Cabbage no Sauce-Stouffer's	28.35	1	Ounce	2	2.1	3.1	39	0	0	5	0
55228	Stuffed Cabbage w/ Meat, Lean Cuisine-Stouffer's	269.319	1	Each	13	6	26	210	0	0	30	2
55778	Stuffed Cabbage-Stouffer's	28.35	1	Ounce	1.4	1.4	2.7	29	0	0	4	0
55157	Stuffed Green Peppers-Stouffer's	219.707	1	Each	9	8	22	200	0	0	0	0
55229	Swedish Meatballs w/ Pasta, Lean Cuisine-Stouffer's	258.688	1	Each	23	8	31	290	0	0	55	3
55148	Swedish Meatballs w/ Pasta-Stouffer's	262.231	1	Each	24	21	32	420	0	0	0	0
41266	Sweet and Sour Chicken-Healthy Choice	326.017	1	Each	20	2	52	280	0	0	35	0
43438	Taco Shells, Chi-Chi's-Hormel	20	1	Each	1.41	4.94	11.99	98.77	0	0	0	0
43401	Tender Beef Roast, Top Shelf-Hormel	283.493	1	Each	28	6	19	240	0	0	60	2
41267	Teriyaki Chicken-Healthy Choice	347.279	1	Each	24	4	39	290	0	0	55	1
55811	Three Bean Chili-Stouffer's	283.92	1	Cup	10.02	5.01	32.05	210.32	0	0	20.03	0
41284	Tomato Garden Soup-Healthy Choice	212.62	1	Each	4	3	22	130	0	0	5	1
62538	Tortellini, Beef	257.894	1	Cup	5	1	45.98	229.91	0	9	14.99	0
55160	Tortellini-Cheese in Alfredo Sauce-Stouffer's	251.6	1	Each	26	37	35	580	0	0	0	0
55161	Tortellini-Cheese w/ Tomato Sauce-Stouffer's	262.231	1	Each	18	15	39	360	0	0	0	0
55162	Tuna Noodle Casserole-Stouffer's	283.493	1	Each	17	15	33	280	0	0	0	0
55814	Turkey and Gravy-Stouffer's	255	1	Each	11.99	2.47	2.12	77.6	0	0	23.28	0
55232	Turkey Dijon, Lean Cuisine-Stouffer's	269.319	1	Each	20	6	20	210	0	0	45	2
55791	Turkey Dijonnaise-Stouffer's	260	1	Each	8.47	5.29	7.05	112.88	0	0	28.22	0
55163	Turkey Pie-Stouffer's	283.493	1	Each	16	24	33	410	0	0	0	0
57809	Turkey Pot Pie-Swanson	198	1	Each	5.54	10.58	18.14	191.49	0	0	0	0
41243	Turkey Sausage Omelet on English Muffin-Healthy Choice	134.659	1	Each	16	4	30	210	0	0	20	2
41268	Turkey Tetrazzini-Healthy Choice	357.91	1	Each	23	6	49	340	0	0	40	3
55164	Turkey Tetrazzini-Stouffer's	283.493	1	Each	22	23	26	400	0	0	0	0
41275	Turkey Vegetable Soup-Healthy Choice	212.62	1	Each	4	3	17	110	0	0	15	1
41285	Vegetable Beef Soup-Healthy Choice	212.62	1	Each	8	1	21	130	0	0	15	0
55759	Vegetable Beef w/ Barley Soup-Stouffer's	283.92	1	Cup	4.01	13.02	15.02	190.29	0	0	10.02	0
55797	Vegetable Chow Mein-Stouffer's	28.35	1	Ounce	0.3	0.7	1.6	14	0	0	0	0
55166	Vegetable Lasagna-Stouffer's	274.042	1	Each	23	20	33	400	0	0	0	0
41343	Vegetable Pasta Italiano-Healthy Choice	283.493	1	Each	7	1	46	220	0	0	0	0
55758	Vegetarian Vegetable Soup-Stouffer's	283.92	1	Cup	6.01	2	20.03	120.18	0	0	0	0
55828	Veloute Sauce Supreme-Stouffer's	307.58	1	Cup	8.68	49.91	20.61	564.18	0	0	97.65	0
55167	Welsh Rarebit-Stouffer's	141.746	1	Each	13	20	9	270	0	0	0	0
41244	Western Style Omelet on English Muffin-Healthy Choice	134.659	1	Each	16	3	29	200	0	0	15	2
55826	Whipped Sweet Potatoes-Stouffer's	283.92	0.5	Cup	3	18.03	60.09	410.61	0	0	60.09	0
41269	Yankee Pot Roast-Healthy Choice	311.843	1	Each	19	4	36	260	0	0	55	2
55233	Zucchini Lasagna, Lean Cuisine-Stouffer's	311.843	1	Each	17	6	34	260	0	0	20	2
41344	Zucchini Lasagna-Healthy Choice	326.017	1	Each	14	3	41	250	0	0	15	2
32391	Arby's-Beef'N Cheddar Sandwich	194	1	Each	35.27	19.84	29.76	443.11	0	1.21	84.88	9.92

Monounsaturated Fat (gm)	Polyunsaturated Fat (gm)	Vitamin D (mg)	Vitamin K (mg)	Vitamin E (mg)	Vitamin A (re)	Vitamin C (mg)	Thiamin (mg)	Riboflavin (mg)	Niacin (mg)	Vitamin B6 (mg)	Folate (mg)	Vitamin B12 (mcg)	Calcium (mg)	Iron (mg)	Magnesium (mg)	Phosphorus (mg)	Potassium (mg)	Sodium (mg)	Zinc (mg)
0	0	0	0	0	150	6	0	0	0	0	0	0	120	1	0	0	440	400	0
0	0	0	0	0	20	6	0.23	0.17	2.85	0	0	0	32	1	0	0	400	1010	0
0	1	0	0	0	0	0	0	0	0	0	0	0	0	0	0	190	630	240	0
0	1	0	0	0	150	0	0.3	0.34	7.6	0	0	0	48	1	0	310	590	530	0
0	1	0	0	0	150	27	0.15	0.1	1.52	0	0	0	16	0.6	0	0	360	520	0
0	2	0	0	0	500	6	0.23	0.26	4.75	0	0	0	32	0.8	0	0	400	590	0
0	2	0	0	0	0	0	0	0	0	0	0	0	0	0	0	260	560	550	0
3	1	0	0	0	140	3.6	0.12	0.26	2.28	0	0	0	32	1.1	24.5	0	341	930	1.05
0	2	0	0	0	100	6	0.3	0.34	3.8	0	0	0	48	2	0	0	500	500	0
2	1	0	0	0.11	100	2.4	0.23	0.26	3.8	0	0	0	48	1.5	45.5	0	879	980	2.4
0	2	0	0	0	250	4.8	0.38	0.26	1.9	0	0	0	48	2	0	160	540	480	0
0	12	0	0	0	150	6	0.15	0.17	3.8	0	0	0	80	1.5	0	0	800	560	0
0	0	0	0	0	100	6	0.3	0.26	3.8	0	0	0	64	1.5	0	0	550	790	0
0	0	0	0	0	200	6	0.12	0.34	0.38	0	0	0	120	0.4	0	0	345	820	0
0	0	0	0	0	100	6	0.15	0.14	1.9	0	0	0	16	0.6	0	190	450	460	0
0	0	0	0	0	0	0	0.01	0	0.38	0	0	0	240.36	0.2	0	0	570.86	1191.79	0
0	0	0	0	0	0	0.6	0	0	0.08	0	0	0	72	0.04	0	0	48	150	0
0	1	0	0	0	80	6	0.12	0.17	3.8	0	0	0	64	1.5	0	0	600	560	0
0	0	0	0	0	0	3	0	0	0.06	0	0	0	48	0.02	0	0	51	145	0
0	0	0	0	0	60	6	0.12	0.14	2.85	0	0	0	32	0.8	0	0	380	650	0
0	1	0	0	0	20	0	0.23	0.34	3.8	0	0	0	48	1.5	0	0	450	550	0
0	0	0	0	0	20	1.2	0.15	0.26	2.85	0	0	0	48	1.5	0	0	350	740	0
0	0	0	0	0	250	30	0.15	0.17	8.55	0	0	0	32	1	0	220	480	320	0
0	0	0	0	0.09	0	0	0.06	0.07	0.54	0	0	0	0	0.14	0	0	0	3.53	0
2	1	0	0	0	400	2.4	0.75	0.43	5.7	0	0	0	16	1.5	42	0	933	880	4.5
0	2	0	0	0	20	6	0.09	0.1	7.6	0	0	0	32	0.8	0	250	520	560	0
0	0	0	0	0	0	6.01	0	0.01	0.57	0	0	0	1.2	0.4	0	0	891.34	861.29	0
0	0	0	0	0	100	6	0.06	0.1	1.14	0	0	0	32	0.4	0	70	440	510	0
0	0	0	0	0	149.94	3.6	0	0	0	0	0	0	95.96	1.5	0	0	0	769.68	0
0	0	0	0	0	40	3.6	0.3	0.51	1.9	0	0	0	320	0.8	0	0	270	830	0
0	0	0	0	0	150	6	0.23	0.34	1.9	0	0	0	240	1	0	0	420	720	0
0	0	0	0	0	20	0	0.15	0.34	3.8	0	0	0	120	0.6	0	0	380	1090	0
0	0	0	0	0	0	0.42	0	0	0.87	0	0	0	84.66	0.03	0	0	405.65	296.3	0
0	0	0	0	0	400	2.4	0.23	0.34	4.75	0	0	0	120	0.4	0	0	640	590	0
0	0	0	0	0	0	0.63	0	0	0.27	0	0	0	0	0.07	0	0	176.37	356.27	0
0	0	0	0	0	250	0	0.3	0.43	3.8	0	0	0	80	1	0	0	290	750	0
0	0	0	0	0	176.37	0	0.11	0.09	1.44	0	0	0	8.06	0.5	0	0	0	362.82	0
0	1	0	0	0	60	0	0.38	0.51	2.85	0	0	0	160	2	0	250	590	470	0
0	2	0	0	0	0	72	0.23	0.34	3.8	0	0	0	80	1	0	250	510	490	0
0	0	0	0	0	20	0	0.15	0.43	2.85	0	0	0	80	0.8	0	0	300	960	0
0	1	0	0	0	150	4.8	0.03	0.03	0.38	0	0	0	16	0.2	0	0	140	540	0
0	0	0	0	0	150	15	0.09	0.1	1.9	0	0	0	32	0.4	0	120	360	530	0
0	0	0	0	0	0	0	0	0	0.19	0	0	0	240.36	0.1	0	0	340.51	1251.88	0
0	0	0	0	0	0	0.6	0	0	0.02	0	0	0	24	0.01	0	0	26	156	0
0	0	0	0	0	250	0	0.12	0.43	0.76	0	0	0	160	0.6	0	0	350	760	0
0	0	0	0	0	250	0	0.45	0.26	1.52	0	0	0	32	2.5	0	0	380	330	0
0	0	0	0	0	0	0	0	0	0.19	0	0	0	0	0.1	0	0	400.6	911.37	0
0	0	0	0	0	0	0	0	0.01	0	0	0	0	2.26	0	0	0	368.89	1410.45	0
0	0	0	0	0	40	0	0.03	0.34	0	0	0	0	280	0.2	0	0	140	460	0
0	0	0	0	0	100	3.6	0.45	0.51	1.9	0	0	0	160	2	0	240	220	480	0
0	0	0	0	0	0	0	0	0	0.19	0	0	0	0	0.1	0	0	400.6	1111.67	0
0	0	0	0	0	100	9	0.15	0.17	1.52	0	0	0	32	1	0	150	350	400	0
0	0	0	0	0	150	6	0.15	0.26	1.9	0	0	0	200	0.8	0	0	650	520	0
0	0	0	0	0	350	6	0.38	0.26	1.9	0	0	0	200	1.5	0	250	830	400	0
4.08	3.86	0	0	0.44	63.93	1.32	0.42	0.51	6.5	0.37	45.19	2.26	201.72	5.62	44.09	442.01	380.28	1801.11	5.95

USDA ID Code	Food Name	Weight in Grams*	Quantity of Units	Unit of Measure	Protein (gm)	Fat (gm)	Carbohydrates (gm)	Kcalories	Caffeine (gm)	Fiber (gm)	Cholesterol (mg)	Saturated Fat (gm)
32433	Arby's-Boston Clam Chowder	226.795	1	Each	10	11	18	207	0	1.4	28	4
32400	Arby's-Chicken Breast Fillet Sandwich	204	1	Each	25.5	27.72	53.22	546.59	0	1.77	100.89	5.65
	Arby's-Chicken Cordon Bleu	240	1	Each	38	33	46	623	0	5	77	5.65
	Arby's-Chicken Fingers	102	1	Each	16	16	20	290	0	0.5	32	2
32434	Arby's-Cream of Broccoli Soup	226.795	1	Each	9	8	19	180	0	1.8	3	5
32413	Arby's-Curly Fries	99.223	1	Each	4.2	17.7	43.2	337	0	0	0	7.4
32405	Arby's-Fish Fillet Sandwich	221	1	Each	23	27	50	526	0	0	43.8	7
32411	Arby's-French Fries	70.873	1	Each	2.1	13.2	29.8	246	0	0	0	3
	Arby's-Grilled Chicken BBQ	201	1	Each	23	13	47	388	0	2	43	3
	Arby's-Grilled Chicken Delux	230	1	Each	23	20	47	430	0	3	61	4
32406	Arby's-Ham'N Cheese Sandwich	170.096	1	Each	24.47	18.64	38.45	411.26	0	1.17	67.57	7.46
32390	Arby's-Regular Roast Beef	155.921	1	Each	24.68	15.7	38.14	388.12	0	1.12	58.33	4.04
	Arby's-Roast Chicken Delux	195	1	Each	20	6	33	276	0	4	33	2
32393	Arby's-Super Roast Beef	240.969	1	Each	25.74	22.66	51.49	515.92	0	1.65	41.19	8.75
32410	Arby's-Turkey Sub	277	1	Each	32.86	28.17	53.99	598.6	0	0	82.16	6.22
32438	Arby's-Wisconsin Cheese Soup	226.795	1	Each	9	19	19	287	0	1.8	31	8
34858	Burger King Bacon Double Cheeseburger	218	1	Each	44	39	28	640	0	1	145	18
	Burger King Barbecue Dipping Sauce	28	1	Each	0	0	9	35	0	0	0	0
	Burger King Biscuit With Bacon, Egg and Cheese	171	1	Each	19	31	39	280	0	1	225	10
	Burger King Biscuit with Sausage	151	1	Each	16	40	41	360	0	1	45	13
	Burger King BK Big Fish sandwich	255	1	Each	26	41	56	700	0	3	90	6
	Burger King BK Broiler- chicken sandwich	248	1	Each	30	29	41	550	0	2	80	6
	Burger King Broiled Chicken Salad	302	1	Each	21	10	7	90	0	3	60	4
34856	Burger King Cheeseburger	138	1	Each	23	16	28	380	0	1	65	9
	Burger King Chicken Sandwich	229	1	Each	26	43	54	710	0	2	60	9
	Burger King Chicken Tenders - 8 piece	117	1	Each	21	17	19	310	0	3	50	4
	Burger King Chocolate Shake - Medium	397	1	Each	12	10	75	440	0	4	30	6
	Burger King Coated French Fries, medium, salted	102	1	Each	3	17	43	340	0	3	0	5
	Burger King Coca Cola Classic - medium	360	1	Each	0	0	70	280	3.08	0	0	0
	Burger King Croissan'Wich, w/ sausage, egg and cheese	176	1	Each	22	46	25	600	0	1	260	16
	Burger King Diet Coke - medium	360	1	Each	0	0	0	1	3.08	0	0	0
34857	Burger King Double Cheeseburger	210	1	Each	41	36	28	600	0	1	135	17
	Burger King Double Whopper	351	1	Each	33	46	46	730	0	3	115	16
	Burger King Double Whopper w/ cheese	375	1	Each	52	63	46	960	0	3	195	24
	Burger King Dutch Apple Pie	113	1	Each	3	15	39	300	0	2	0	3
	Burger King French Dressing	30	1	Each	0	10	11	140	0	0	0	2
	Burger King French Fries, medium, salted	116	1	Each	5	20	43	180	0	3	0	5
	Burger King French Toast Sticks	141	1	Each	4	27	60	500	0	1	0	27
	Burger King Garden Salad	255	1	Each	6	5	8	100	0	4	15	3
	Burger King Grape Jam	12	1	Each	0	0	8	30	0	0	0	0
34855	Burger King Hamburger	126	1	Each	20	15	28	330	0	1	55	6
	Burger King Hash Browns	71	1	Each	2	12	25	110	0	2	0	3
	Burger King Honey Dipping Sauce	28	1	Each	0	0	21	80	0	0	0	0
	Burger King Ketchup	14	1	Each	0	0	4	15	0	0	0	0
	Burger King Onion Rings	124	1	Each	4	14	41	310	0	6	0	2
	Burger King Ranch Dressing	30	1	Each	0	19	2	180	0	0	10	4
	Burger King Reduced Calorie light Italian Dressing	30	1	Each	0	0.5	3	15	0	0	0	0
34843	Burger King Salad w/ 1000 Island	176	1	Each	2	12	9	145	0	0	17	0
34842	Burger King Salad w/ Bleu Cheese	176	1	Each	3	16	7	184	0	0	22	0
34844	Burger King Salad w/ French	176	1	Each	2	11	13	152	0	0	0	0
34845	Burger King Salad w/ Golden Italian	176	1	Each	2	14	7	162	0	0	0	0
34841	Burger King Salad w/ House Dressing	176	1	Each	3	13	8	159	0	0	11	0
34846	Burger King Salad w/ Reduced-Calorie Italian	176	1	Each	2	1	7	42	0	0	0	0
	Burger King Side Salad	133	1	Each	3	3	4	60	0	2	5	2
	Burger King Strawberry Jam	12	1	Each	0	0	8	30	0	0	0	0

Monounsaturated Fat (gm)	Polyunsaturated Fat (gm)	Vitamin D (mg)	Vitamin K (mg)	Vitamin E (mg)	Vitamin A (re)	Vitamin C (mg)	Thiamin (mg)	Riboflavin (mg)	Niacin (mg)	Vitamin B6 (mg)	Folate (mg)	Vitamin B12 (mcg)	Calcium (mg)	Iron (mg)	Magnesium (mg)	Phosphorus (mg)	Potassium (mg)	Sodium (mg)	Zinc (mg)
5	2	0	0	0.1	100	4	0.06	0.22	0.9	0.12	9	9.38	170	1.4	20	143	319	1157	0.7
10.64	11.42	0	0	2.88	16.63	0	0.5	0.43	16.41	0.72	35.48	0.38	123.07	3.88	51	321.52	365.87	1129.76	1.88
10.64	11.42	0	0	2.88	16.63	0	0.5	0.43	16.41	0.72	35.48	0.38	123.07	3.88	51	321.52	365.87	1594	1.88
4	4.1	0	0	1.4	2.6	0	0	0	0	0.09	17	0.19	92	1.9	22	140	190	677	0.3
2	1	0	0	1.4	50	9	0.11	0.42	0.8	0.18	46	0.59	237	0.8	55	193	455	1113	0.7
7.6	1.5	0	0	0	0	0	0.06	0.07	1.9	0	0	0	16	0.8	0	0	724	167	0
9.2	10.6	0	0	0	0	1.2	0.35	0.31	5.32	0	0	0	72	2.1	0	0	450	872	0
5.5	4.7	0	0	0	0	3.6	0.06	0	1.9	0	0	0	0	0.6	0	0	240	114	0
2	1	0	0	0	16.63	0	0.5	0.43	16.41	0.72	35.48	0.38	123.07	3.88	51	321.52	365.87	1002	1.88
2	1	0	0	0	16.63	0	0.5	0.43	16.41	0.72	35.48	0.38	123.07	3.88	51	321.52	365.87	848	1.88
7.81	1.63	0	0	1.28	111.84	3.5	0.36	0.57	3.15	0.23	82.72	0.63	151.46	3.84	18.64	177.09	337.86	899.41	1.63
7.63	1.91	0	0	0.22	70.67	2.24	0.43	0.35	6.62	0.3	44.87	1.37	60.57	4.71	34.77	268.09	354.47	888.41	3.81
2	1	0	0	0	16.63	0	0.5	0.43	16.41	0.72	35.48	0.38	123.07	3.88	51	321.52	365.87	777	1.88
8.44	5.56	0	0	0.41	0	0	0.65	0.62	9.68	0.49	42.22	4.42	118.42	6.59	59.73	413.97	517.98	821.77	11.02
7.04	8.22	0	0	0	0	0	0.53	0.4	9.39	0	0	0	93.9	3.17	0	0	0	1431.95	0
8	3	0	0	0.4	90	2	0.03	0.24	0.7	0.05	7	0	252	1.3	7	241	441	1129	1.1
14.5	6.22	0	0	1.55	73.54	8.29	0.31	0.4	8.39	0.38	32.11	3.36	161.59	4.14	39.36	386.37	479.59	1240	6.63
0	0	0	0	0	0	0	0	0	0	0	0	0	0	0	0	0	0	400	0
0	0	0	0	0	0	0	0	0	0	0	0	0	0	0	0	0	0	1530	0
0	0	0	0	0	0	0	0	0	0	0	0	0	0	0	0	0	0	1390	0
0	0	0	0	0	0	0	0	0	0	0	0	0	0	0	0	0	0	980	0
0	0	0	0	0	0	0	0	0	0	0	0	0	0	0	0	0	0	4803	0
0	0	0	0	0	0	0	0	0	0	0	0	0	0	0	0	0	0	110	0
0	0	0	0	0	0	0	0	0	0	0	0	0	0	0	0	0	0	770	0
0	0	0	0	0	0	0	0	0	0	0	0	0	0	0	0	0	0	1400	0
0	0	0	0	0	0	0	0	0	0	0	0	0	0	0	0	0	0	710	0
0	0	0	0	0	0	0	0	0	0	0	0	0	0	0	0	0	0	330	0
0	0	0	0	0	0	0	0	0	0	0	0	0	0	0	0	0	0	680	0
0	0	0	0	0	0	0	0	0	0	0	0	0	0	0	0	0	0	0	0
0	0	0	0	0	0	0	0	0	0	0	0	0	0	0	0	0	0	1140	0
12.24	2.23	0	0	2	111.25	6.68	0.24	0.34	5.45	0.27	34.49	2.01	210.27	3.34	34.49	339.33	382.72	1060	4.45
0	0	0	0	0	0	0	0	0	0	0	0	0	0	0	0	0	0	1350	0
0	0	0	0	0	0	0	0	0	0	0	0	0	0	0	0	0	0	1420	0
0	0	0	0	0	0	0	0	0	0	0	0	0	0	0	0	0	0	230	0
0	0	0	0	0	0	0	0	0	0	0	0	0	0	0	0	0	0	190	0
0	0	0	0	0	0	0	0	0	0	0	0	0	0	0	0	0	0	240	0
0	0	0	0	0	0	0	0	0	0	0	0	0	0	0	0	0	0	490	0
0	0	0	0	0	0	0	0	0	0	0	0	0	0	0	0	0	0	115	0
0	0	0	0	0	0	0	0	0	0	0	0	0	0	0	0	0	0	0	0
0	0	0	0	0	0	0	0	0	0	0	0	0	0	0	0	0	0	530	0
0	0	0	0	0	0	0	0	0	0	0	0	0	0	0	0	0	0	320	0
0	0	0	0	0	0	0	0	0	0	0	0	0	0	0	0	0	0	20	0
0	0	0	0	0	0	0	0	0	0	0	0	0	0	0	0	0	0	180	0
0	0	0	0	0	0	0	0	0	0	0	0	0	0	0	0	0	0	810	0
0	0	0	0	0	0	0	0	0	0	0	0	0	0	0	0	0	0	170	0
0	0	0	0	0	0	0	0	0	0	0	0	0	0	0	0	0	0	50	0
0	0	0	0	0	0	25.8	0	0	0.19	0	0	0	336	0.14	98	528	405	251	0.08
0	0	0	0	0	0	25.2	0	0	0.19	0	0	0	528	0.13	101.5	664	382	333	0.09
0	0	0	0	0	0	25.8	0	0	0.19	0	0	0	320	0.14	98	480	410	330	0.07
0	0	0	0	0	0	25.2	0	0	0.19	0	0	0	320	0.13	98	480	389	292	0.06
0	0	0	0	0	0	25.2	0	0	0.19	0	0	0	352	0.13	94.5	592	402	293	0.08
0	0	0	0	0	0	25.2	0	0	0.19	0	0	0	320	0.14	105	472	390	430	0.06
0	0	0	0	0	0	0	0	0	0	0	0	0	0	0	0	0	0	55	0
0	0	0	0	0	0	0	0	0	0	0	0	0	0	0	0	0	0	5	0

USDA ID Code	Food Name	Weight in Grams*	Quantity of Units	Unit of Measure	Protein (gm)	Fat (gm)	Carbohydrates (gm)	Kcalories	Caffeine (gm)	Fiber (gm)	Cholesterol (mg)	Saturated Fat (gm)
	Burger King Sweet & Sour Dipping Sauce	28	1	Each	0	0	11	45	0	0	0	0
	Burger King Thousand Island Dressing	30	1	Each	0	12	7	140	0	0	15	3
	Burger King Vanilla Shake - medium	397	1	Each	13	9	73	430	0	2	30	5
34859	Burger King Whopper	270	1	Each	27	39	45	640	0	3	90	11
	Burger King Whopper Jr.	164	1	Each	21	24	29	420	0	2	60	8
	Burger King Whopper Jr. with cheese	177	1	Each	23	28	29	460	0	2	75	10
37167	Dunkin' Donuts-Almond Croissant	105	1	Each	8	27	38	420	0	3	0	0
37146	Dunkin' Donuts-Apple Filled w/ Cinnamon Sugar	79	1	Each	5	11	33	250	0	1	0	0
37160	Dunkin' Donuts-Apple 'n Spice Muffin	100	1	Each	6	8	52	300	0	2	25	0
37159	Dunkin' Donuts-Banana Nut Muffin	103	1	Each	7	10	49	310	0	3	30	0
37147	Dunkin' Donuts-Bavarian Filled /w Chocolate	79	1	Each	5	11	32	240	0	2	0	0
37149	Dunkin' Donuts-Blueberry Filled	67	1	Each	4	8	29	210	0	2	0	0
37156	Dunkin' Donuts-Blueberry Muffin	101	1	Each	6	8	46	280	0	2	30	0
37157	Dunkin' Donuts-Bran Muffin w/ Raisins	104	1	Each	6	9	51	310	0	4	15	0
37151	Dunkin' Donuts-Cake Ring, Plain	62	1	Each	4	17	25	270	0	1	0	0
37163	Dunkin' Donuts-Chocolate Chunk Cookie	43	1	Each	3	10	25	200	0	1	30	0
37164	Dunkin' Donuts-Chocolate Chunk Cookie w/ Nuts	43	1	Each	3	11	23	210	0	2	30	0
37168	Dunkin' Donuts-Chocolate Croissant	94	1	Each	7	29	38	440	0	3	0	0
37145	Dunkin' Donuts-Chocolate Frosted Yeast Ring	55	1	Each	4	10	25	200	0	1	0	0
37158	Dunkin' Donuts-Corn Muffin	96	1	Each	7	12	51	340	0	1	40	0
37161	Dunkin' Donuts-Cranberry Nut Muffin	98	1	Each	6	9	44	290	0	2	25	0
37166	Dunkin' Donuts-Croissant, Plain	72	1	Each	7	19	27	310	0	2	0	0
37153	Dunkin' Donuts-Glazed Buttermilk Ring	74	1	Each	4	14	37	290	0	1	10	0
37152	Dunkin' Donuts-Glazed Chocolate Rings	71	1	Each	3.5	21	34	324	0	1.9	0	0
37144	Dunkin' Donuts-Glazed Coffee Roll	81	1	Each	5	12	37	280	0	2	0	0
37155	Dunkin' Donuts-Glazed French Cruller	38	1	Each	2	8	16	140	0	0	30	0
37143	Dunkin' Donuts-Glazed Yeast Ring	55	1	Each	4	9	26	200	0	1	0	0
37150	Dunkin' Donuts-Jelly Filled	67	1	Each	4	9	31	220	0	1	0	0
37148	Dunkin' Donuts-Lemon Filled	79	1	Each	4	12	33	260	0	1	0	0
37162	Dunkin' Donuts-Oat Bran Muffin	100	1	Each	7	11	50	330	0	3	0	0
37165	Dunkin' Donuts-Oatmeal Pecan Raisin Cookie	46	1	Each	3	9	28	200	0	1	25	0
40349	Hardee's-Big Cheese	141.75	1	Each	30	30	28	495	0	0	0	0
40350	Hardee's-Big Deluxe	248.1	1	Each	31	41	46	675	0	0	0	0
40356	Hardee's-Big Fish Sandwich	191.358	1	Each	20	26	49	514	0	0	0	0
40353	Hardee's-Big Roast Beef	163.008	1	Each	21.9	13.38	38.93	364.94	0	1.09	54.74	6.08
40351	Hardee's-Big Twin	141.746	1	Each	18.84	20.48	27.86	368.7	0	1.39	45.06	9.01
40358	Hardee's-Biscuit	77.961	1	Each	5	13	35	275	0	0	0	0
40348	Hardee's-Cheeseburger	100.631	1	Each	17	17	29	335	0	0	0	0
40357	Hardee's-Chicken Fillet	191.358	1	Each	27	26	42	510	0	0	0	0
40347	Hardee's-Hamburger	100.063	1	Each	17	13	29	305	0	0	0	0
40354	Hardee's-Hot Dog	50	1	Each	11	22	26	346	0	0	0	0
40355	Hardee's-Hot Ham & Cheese	141.746	1	Each	23	15	37	376	0	0	0	0
40352	Hardee's-Roast Beef Sandwich	141.746	1	Each	18.65	11.19	38.54	323.28	0	0.99	43.52	4.97
44118	Jack In The Box-Bacon Cheeseburger	242	1	Each	35	45	41	705	0	0	113	14.9
44101	Jack In The Box-Breakfast Jack	126	1	Each	18.74	13.54	29.16	313.44	0	0	189.52	5.31
44141	Jack In The Box-Cheesecake	99	1	Each	8	18	29	309	0	0	63	9.4
44115	Jack In The Box-Jumbo Jack	222	1	Each	25.27	26.17	40.61	497.24	0	0	72.2	10.29
44116	Jack In The Box-Jumbo Jack w/ Cheese	242	1	Each	28.47	31.14	40.04	558.74	0	0	97.87	13.35
44136	Jack In The Box-Regular French Fries	109	1	Each	4	17	45	351	0	0	0	4
44135	Jack In The Box-Small French Fries	68	1	Each	3	11	28	219	0	0	0	2.5
47265	K.F.C.-Colonel's Chicken Sandwich	166	1	Each	20.8	27	39	482	0	1.4	47	6
47261	K.F.C.-French Fries	77	1	Each	3.2	12	31	244	0	0	2	3
47260	K.F.C.-Mashed Potatoes and Gravy	98	1	Each	2.4	2	12	71	0	0	0	1
47239	K.F.C.-Original Recipe Center Breast	103	1	Each	25.18	15.26	9.16	260.93	0	0.08	86.98	3.81
47240	K.F.C.-Original Recipe Drumstick	57	1	Each	11.57	11.57	4.96	168.52	0	0	58.65	2.48

Monounsaturated Fat (gm)	Polyunsaturated Fat (gm)	Vitamin D (mg)	Vitamin K (mg)	Vitamin E (mg)	Vitamin A (re)	Vitamin C (mg)	Thiamin (mg)	Riboflavin (mg)	Niacin (mg)	Vitamin B6 (mg)	Folate (mg)	Vitamin B12 (mcg)	Calcium (mg)	Iron (mg)	Magnesium (mg)	Phosphorus (mg)	Potassium (mg)	Sodium (mg)	Zinc (mg)
0	0	0	0	0	0	0	0	0	0	0	0	0	0	0	0	0	0	50	0
0	0	0	0	0	0	0	0	0	0	0	0	0	0	0	0	0	0	190	0
0	0	0	0	0	0	0	0	0	0	0	0	0	0	0	0	0	0	330	0
14.99	2.39	0	0	4.24	208.55	14.12	0.02	0.03	5.65	0.34	33.67	3.05	112.96	6.52	54.31	338.89	564.81	870	5.76
0	0	0	0	0	0	0	0	0	0	0	0	0	0	0	0	0	0	530	0
0	0	0	0	0	0	0	0	0	0	0	0	0	0	0	0	0	0	770	0
0	0	0	0	0	0	0	0	0	0	0	0	0	0	0	0	0	0	280	0
0	0	0	0	0	0	0	0	0	0	0	0	0	0	0	0	0	0	280	0
0	0	0	0	0	0	0	0	0	0	0	0	0	0	0	0	0	0	360	0
0	0	0	0	0	0	0	0	0	0	0	0	0	0	0	0	0	0	410	0
0	0	0	0	0	0	0	0	0	0	0	0	0	0	0	0	0	0	260	0
0	0	0	0	0	0	0	0	0	0	0	0	0	0	0	0	0	0	240	0
0	0	0	0	0	0	0	0	0	0	0	0	0	0	0	0	0	0	340	0
0	0	0	0	0	0	0	0	0	0	0	0	0	0	0	0	0	0	560	0
0	0	0	0	0	0	0	0	0	0	0	0	0	0	0	0	0	0	330	0
0	0	0	0	0	0	0	0	0	0	0	0	0	0	0	0	0	0	110	0
0	0	0	0	0	0	0	0	0	0	0	0	0	0	0	0	0	0	100	0
0	0	0	0	0	0	0	0	0	0	0	0	0	0	0	0	0	0	220	0
0	0	0	0	0	0	0	0	0	0	0	0	0	0	0	0	0	0	190	0
0	0	0	0	0	0	0	0	0	0	0	0	0	0	0	0	0	0	560	0
0	0	0	0	0	0	0	0	0	0	0	0	0	0	0	0	0	0	360	0
0	0	0	0	0	0	0	0	0	0	0	0	0	0	0	0	0	0	240	0
0	0	0	0	0	0	0	0	0	0	0	0	0	0	0	0	0	0	370	0
0	0	0	0	0	0	0	0	0	0	0	0	0	0	0	0	0	0	383	0
0	0	0	0	0	0	0	0	0	0	0	0	0	0	0	0	0	0	310	0
0	0	0	0	0	0	0	0	0	0	0	0	0	0	0	0	0	0	130	0
0	0	0	0	0	0	0	0	0	0	0	0	0	0	0	0	0	0	230	0
0	0	0	0	0	0	0	0	0	0	0	0	0	0	0	0	0	0	230	0
0	0	0	0	0	0	0	0	0	0	0	0	0	0	0	0	0	0	280	0
0	0	0	0	0	0	0	0	0	0	0	0	0	0	0	0	0	0	450	0
0	0	0	0	0	0	0	0	0	0	0	0	0	0	0	0	0	0	100	0
0	0	0	0	0	0	0	0	0	0	0	0	0	0	0	0	0	0	1251	0
0	0	0	0	0	0	0	0	0	0	0	0	0	0	0	0	0	0	1063	0
0	0	0	0	0	0	0	0	0	0	0	0	0	0	0	0	0	0	314	0
6.08	2.43	0	0	0.24	0	0	0.36	0.41	6.57	0.34	29.2	2.98	80.29	4.5	40.14	279.79	389.27	1070.5	7.42
7.37	4.1	0	0	0.74	13.93	2.46	0.23	0.25	5.49	0.22	27.86	1.86	65.55	3.28	28.68	161.41	229.42	475.22	3.77
0	0	0	0	0	0	0	0	0	0	0	0	0	0	0	0	0	0	650	0
0	0	0	0	0	0	2	0.51	0.32	5.5	0	0	0	0	0	0	0	0	789	0
0	0	0	0	0	0	0	0	0	0	0	0	0	0	0	0	0	0	360	0
0	0	0	0	0	0	2	0.55	0.58	6.4	0	0	0	0	0	0	0	0	682	0
0	0	0	0	0	0	0	0	0	0	0	0	0	0	0	0	0	0	744	0
0	0	0	0	0	0	0	0	0	0	0	0	0	0	0	0	0	0	1067	0
4.97	2.49	0	0	0.25	0	0	0.32	0.36	5.72	0.3	24.87	2.6	69.63	3.85	34.81	243.7	323.28	907.67	6.47
15.7	8.7	0	0	0.6	70	7.8	0.24	0.48	8.36	0	0	0	200	2.8	0	0	0	1240	0
5.21	2.6	0	0	0.14	138.5	3.12	0.43	0.49	5.31	0.15	0	1.15	184.31	2.6	24.99	322.81	197.85	1079.85	1.87
7.4	1.6	0	0	0.32	0	0	0.05	0.24	1.9	0	0	0	88	0.3	0	0	0	208	0
11.37	2.17	0	0	0.18	66.78	3.61	0.42	0.31	10.47	0.27	0	2.42	120.93	4.06	39.71	235.54	444	1023.37	3.79
11.21	1.78	0	0	0.21	195.74	4.45	0.46	0.34	10.05	0.28	0	2.71	242.89	4.09	43.6	365.67	443.96	1482.25	4.27
7	0	0	0	5.31	0	25.8	0.18	0.03	3.61	0	0	0	0	0.7	0	0	0	194	0
7	0	0	0	10.36	0	16.2	0.11	0	2.28	0	0	0	0	0.4	0	0	0	121	0
3.9	9	0	0	2.3	14	0	0.39	0.27	10.64	0.59	29	0.31	100	3.1	41	261	297	1060	1.5
7	1	0	0	0	0	15.6	0.15	0.05	1.9	0	0	0	0	0.3	0	0	0	139	0
0	0	0	0	0	0	0	0	0.03	1.14	0	0	0	16	0.2	0	0	0	339	0
3.59	1.53	0	0	0.46	15.26	0	0.08	0.13	14.04	0.59	3.81	0.35	16.02	1.22	30.52	238.04	264.75	602.74	1.14
3.06	1.65	0	0	0.41	14.04	0	0.05	0.13	3.39	0.2	4.96	0.18	6.61	0.74	13.22	99.13	129.7	267.65	1.65

USDA ID Code	Food Name	Weight in Grams*	Quantity of Units	Unit of Measure	Protein (gm)	Fat (gm)	Carbohydrates (gm)	Kcalories	Caffeine (gm)	Fiber (gm)	Cholesterol (mg)	Saturated Fat (gm)
47241	K.F.C.-Original Recipe Thigh	95	1	Each	15.97	23.95	11.18	324.12	0	0.08	102.98	6.39
47237	K.F.C.-Original Recipe Wing	53	1	Each	11.8	11	5	172	0	0	59	3
48215	McDonald's-Apple Danish	105	1	Each	5	16	51	360	0	1.6	25	4
	McDonald's-Arch Deluxe	239	1	Each	28	31	39	550	0	4	90	11
	McDonald's-Arch Deluxe w/Bacon	247	1	Each	32	34	39	590	0	4	100	12
48204	McDonald's-Bacon, Egg and Cheese Biscuit	153	1	Each	18	28	36	470	0	1	235	8.04
48174	McDonald's-Big Mac	215	1	Each	25	32	43	560	0	0	103	10.1
48205	McDonald's-Biscuit w/ Spread	75	1	Each	5	13	32	260	0	1	1	3
	McDonald's-Breakfast Burrito	117	1	Each	13	19	23	320	0	1	195	7
48170	McDonald's-Cheeseburger	116	1	Each	15	13	35	320	0	0	50	5
48181	McDonald's-Chicken McNuggets	18.5	1	Each	3.33	2.5	2.83	45	0	0	9.17	0.58
48226	McDonald's-Chocolate Lowfat Milk Shake	294.124	1	Each	11.04	1.71	66.25	321.23	0	0	10.04	0.7
	McDonald's-Cinnamon Roll	95	1	Each	7	20	47	400	0	2	75	5
	McDonald's-Crispy Chicken Deluxe	223	1	Each	26	25	43	0	0	3	55	4
48198	McDonald's-Egg McMuffin	135	1	Each	17.61	10.76	27.39	283.7	0	1.37	221.09	3.72
48201	McDonald's-English Muffin w/ Spread	58	1	Each	5	4	26	170	0	1.6	9	2.4
48175	McDonald's-Fish Filet Deluxe	141	1	Each	27	28	54	560	0	1.09	49.65	5.16
48188	McDonald's-Garden Salad	189	1	Each	4	2	6	50	0	0	65	0.6
	McDonald's-Grilled Chicken Deluxe	223	1	Each	27	20	38	300	0	3	50	1
	McDonald's-Grilled Chicken Sld Deluxe	257	1	Each	21	1.5	7	120	0	0	45	0
48169	McDonald's-Hamburger	102	1	Each	13	9	34	260	0	0	30	3.5
48209	McDonald's-Hash Brown Potatoes	53	1	Each	1	7	15	130	0	0	0	1
48210	McDonald's-Hotcakes w/ Margarine and Syrup	174	1	Each	13	19	100	570	0	0	15	3
48216	McDonald's-Iced Cheese Danish	110	1	Each	7	22	47	410	0	0	47	6
48180	McDonald's-Large French Fries	122	1	Each	6	22	57	450	0	0	0	5
	McDonald's-Lowfat Apple Bran Muffin	114	1	Each	6	3	61	300	0	3	0	0.5
48223	McDonald's-McDonaldland Cookies	56.699	1	Each	3	5	32	180	0	0	0	1
48171	McDonald's-Quarter Pounder	166	1	Each	23	21	37	420	0	0	85	8
	McDonald's-Quarter Pounderw/Chse	200	1	Each	28	30	38	530	0	2	95	13
48207	McDonald's-Sausage Biscuit	118	1	Each	11	31	35	470	0	0	44	8
48203	McDonald's-Sausage Biscuit w/ Egg	175	1	Each	19	28	27	440	0	0	260	10
48199	McDonald's-Sausage McMuffin	135	1	Each	15	20	27	345	0	0	57	7
48200	McDonald's-Sausage McMuffin w/ Egg	159	1	Each	21	25	27	430	0	0	270	8
48208	McDonald's-Scrambled Eggs	100	1	Each	12	10	1	140	0	0	425	3
48178	McDonald's-Small French Fries	68	1	Each	3	12	26	220	0	0	0	2.5
48227	McDonald's-Strawberry Lowfat Milk Shake	294.124	1	Each	11	9	60	360	0	0	10	0.6
	McDonald's-Super Size Fries	176	1	Each	8	26	68	540	0	6	0	4.5
48225	McDonald's-Vanilla Lowfat Milk Shake	294.124	1	Each	11	9	60	360	0	0	10	0.6
	McDonald's-Vanilla RF Ice Crm Cone	90	1	Each	4	4.5	23	150	0	0	20	3
52366	Pizza Hut-Cheese Pizza, Hand Tossed	70	1	Slice	17	10	27.5	259	0	0	27.5	6.8
52359	Pizza Hut-Cheese Pizza, Pan	70	1	Slice	15	9	28.5	246	0	0	17	4.5
53322	Pizza Hut-Cheese Pizza, Thin'n Crispy	70	1	Slice	14	8.5	18.5	199	0	0	16.5	5.2
52370	Pizza Hut-Pepperoni Personal Pan Pizza	250	1	Each	37	29	76	675	0	0	53	12.5
52367	Pizza Hut-Pepperoni Pizza, Hand Tossed	70	1	Slice	14	11.5	25	250	0	0	25	6.45
52360	Pizza Hut-Pepperoni Pizza, Pan	70	1	Slice	14.5	11	31	270	0	0	21	4.5
52363	Pizza Hut-Pepperoni Pizza, Thin'n Crispy	70	1	Slice	13	10	18	206.5	0	0	23	5.3
52365	Pizza Hut-Super Sprm Pizza, Thin'n Crispy	70	1	Slice	14.5	10.5	22	231.5	0	0	28	5.15
52362	Pizza Hut-Super Supreme Pizza, Pan	70	1	Slice	16.5	13	26.5	281.5	0	0	27.5	6
52369	Pizza Hut-Super Supreme, Hand Tossed	70	1	Slice	16.5	12.5	27	278	0	0	27	6.5
52371	Pizza Hut-Supreme Personal Pan Pizza	250	1	Each	33	28	76	647	0	0	49	11.2
52368	Pizza Hut-Supreme Pizza, Hand Tossed	70	1	Slice	16	13	25	270	0	0	27.5	6.1
52361	Pizza Hut-Supreme Pizza, Pan	70	1	Slice	16	15	26.5	294.5	0	0	24	7
52364	Pizza Hut-Supreme Pizza, Thin'n Crispy	70	1	Slice	14	11	20.5	229.5	0	0	21	5.5
54494	Red Lobster-Atlantic Ocean Perch, Lunch	141.746	1	Each	24	4	1	130	0	0	75	1.1
54506	Red Lobster-Calamari, Brded and Fried, Lunch	141.746	1	Each	13	21	30	360	0	0	140	5.6

Monounsaturated Fat (gm)	Polyunsaturated Fat (gm)	Vitamin D (mg)	Vitamin K (mg)	Vitamin E (mg)	Vitamin A (re)	Vitamin C (mg)	Thiamin (mg)	Riboflavin (mg)	Niacin (mg)	Vitamin B6 (mg)	Folate (mcg)	Vitamin B12 (mcg)	Calcium (mg)	Iron (mg)	Magnesium (mg)	Phosphorus (mg)	Potassium (mg)	Sodium (mg)	Zinc (mg)
5.59	3.19	0	0	0.48	27.94	0	0.09	0.23	6.55	0.32	7.98	0.29	12.77	1.44	23.15	176.43	223.53	549.24	2.39
6	2	0	0	0	0	0	0.03	0.07	2.85	0	0	0	24	0.3	0	0	0	383	0
11	2	0	0	3.8	35	15	0.3	0.17	2.2	0.03	3	0	14	1.4	8	31	69	290	0.2
0	0	0	0	0	10	0	0	0	0	0	0	0	6	25	0	0	0	1010	0
0	0	0	0	0	10	0	0	0	0	0	0	0	6	6	0	0	0	1150	0
15.79	1.96	0	0	1.47	156.92	0	0.35	0.32	2.45	0.17	17.65	0.58	181.44	2.55	30.4	442.33	232.44	1250	1.67
20.1	1.5	0	0	0	106	2	0.48	0.41	6.8	0.27	21	1.8	256	4	38	314	237	950	4.7
9	1	0	0	1.8	0	0	0.23	0.1	1.52	0.03	6	0.1	75	1.3	14	168	100	730	0.7
0	0	0	0	0	10	15	0	0	0	0	0	0	8	10	0	0	0	600	0
7.7	1	0	0	0.5	118	2	0.29	0.21	3.9	0.12	18	0.94	199	2.3	21	177	223	750	2.1
1.67	0.25	0	0	0	0	0	0.02	0.02	1.27	0	0	0	0	0.1	0	0	0	96.67	0
0.9	0.1	0	0	0	92.35	0	0.13	0.5	0.4	0	0	0	333.27	0.8	0	0	0	240.92	0
0	0	0	0	0	10	0	0	0	0	0	0	0	8	8	0	0	0	340	0
0	0	0	0	0	6	8	0	0	0	0	0	0	6	15	0	0	0	1060	0
5.97	1.27	0	0	1.76	146.74	0.98	0.46	0.32	3.62	0.16	43.04	0.78	250.43	2.74	32.28	312.07	208.37	723.91	1.76
2	1	0	0	0.1	37	0	0.33	0.14	2.5	0.1	51	1.6	151	1.6	12	60	74	285	0.4
10.13	10.72	0	0	0	43.69	0	0.3	0.14	2.68	0.1	19.86	0.81	163.84	1.79	26.81	227.39	148.94	1060	0.89
1	0.4	0	0	0	900	21	0.09	0.1	0.38	0	0	0	32	0.8	0	0	0	70	0
0	0	0	0	0	6	8	0	0	0	0	0	0	6	15	0	0	0	930	0
0	0	0	0	0	120	40	0	0	0	0	0	0	4	8	0	0	0	240	0
5	1	0	0	0	40	4	0.3	0.17	3.8	0	0	0	15	1.5	0	0	0	580	0
4	2	0	0	0	0	1.2	0.06	0	0.76	0	0	0	0	0	0	0	0	330	0
5	5	0	0	0	40	0	0.3	0.34	2.85	0	0	0	80	1	0	0	0	750	0
13	2	0	0	0	40	0	0.3	0.26	1.9	0	0	0	32	0.8	0	0	0	420	0
15	2	0	0	0	0	15	0.23	0	2.85	0	0	0	0	0.6	0	0	0	290	0
0	0	0	0	0	0	0	0	0	0	0	0	0	10	8	0	0	0	380	0
7	1	0	0	0	0	0	0.23	0.17	1.9	0	0	0	0	1	0	0	0	190	0
11	1	0	0	0	40	3.6	0.38	0.26	6.65	0	0	0	120	2	0	0	0	645	0
0	0	0	0	0	10	4	0	0	0	0	0	0	15	25	0	0	0	1290	0
17	3	0	0	0	0	0	0.45	0.17	3.8	0	0	0	64	1	0	0	0	1080	0
20	3	0	0	0	60	0	0.45	0.34	3.8	0	0	0	80	2	0	0	0	1210	0
11	2	0	0	0	40	0	0.53	0.26	4.75	0	0	0	160	1.5	0	0	0	770	0
14	3	0	0	0	100	0	0.53	0.43	4.75	0	0	0	200	2	0	0	0	920	0
5	2	0	0	0	100	0	0.06	0.26	0	0	0	0	48	1	0	0	0	290	0
8	1	0	0	0	0	9	0.15	0	1.9	0	0	0	0	0.2	0	0	0	110	0
0.6	0.1	0	0	0	60	0	0.12	0.51	0.38	0	0	0	280	0	0	0	0	170	0
0	0	0	0	0	0	0	0	0	0	0	0	0	35	8	0	0	0	350	0
0.6	0.1	0	0	0	60	0	0.12	0.51	0	0	0	0	280	0	0	0	0	170	0
0	0	0	0	0	6	2	0	0	0	0	0	0	10	2	0	0	0	75	0
3.2	0	0	0	0	50	4.8	0.24	0.25	2.57	0	0	0.3	300	1.5	31.5	220	198	638	2.33
4.5	0	0	0	0	45	3.6	0.28	0.3	2.47	0	0	0.3	252	1.5	26.25	188	160	470	2.03
3.3	0	0	0	0	35	2.4	0.2	0.2	2.28	0	0	0.25	264	0.9	21	188	130.5	433.5	1.8
16.5	0	0	0	0	120	10.2	0.56	0.66	7.79	0	0	0.44	584	3.2	52.5	360	408	1335	3.75
5.05	0	0	0	0	50	3.6	0.27	0.26	2.66	0	0	0.33	176	1.4	26.25	156	207.5	633.5	1.88
6.5	0	0	0	0	50	4.2	0.32	0.25	2.57	0	0	0.3	208	1.75	24.5	176	202.5	563.5	2.1
4.7	0	0	0	0	35	3	0.21	0.21	2.47	0	0	0.25	180	0.9	19.25	148	143.5	493	1.73
5.35	0	0	0	0	50	4.2	0.29	0.22	2.57	0	0	0.35	184	1.35	26.25	168	231.5	668	2.25
7	0	0	0	0	60	5.4	0.38	0.33	3.04	0	0	0.4	216	1.85	31.5	188	266	723.5	2.7
6	0	0	0	0	55	6	0.35	0.29	3.52	0	0	0.41	176	1.9	33.25	168	258	824	2.4
16.8	0	0	0	0	120	10.8	0.59	0.66	7.6	0	0	0.46	416	3.7	52.5	320	487	1313	3.75
6.9	0	0	0	0	55	6	0.35	0.26	3.42	0	0	0.4	192	2.25	35	184	289	735	2.85
8	0	0	0	0	60	4.8	0.41	0.4	2.85	0	0	0.38	200	1.4	33.25	184	290	831.5	2.78
5.5	0	0	0	0	50	4.8	0.3	0.25	2.57	0	0	0.3	172	1.65	29.75	160	272	664	2.33
0	1.2	0	0	0	0	0	0.06	0.1	1.52	0	0	0.3	0	0	21	160	0	190	0.3
0	1.5	0	0	0	0	0	0.23	0.14	1.52	0	0	2	0	0.6	21	360	0	1150	0.9

USDA ID Code	Food Name	Weight in Grams*	Quantity of Units	Unit of Measure	Protein (gm)	Fat (gm)	Carbohydrates (gm)	Kcalories	Caffeine (gm)	Fiber (gm)	Cholesterol (mg)	Saturated Fat (gm)
54486	Red Lobster-Catfish, Lunch Portion	141.746	1	Each	20	10	0	170	0	0	85	2.5
54514	Red Lobster-Chicken Breast, Skinless, Lunch	113.397	1	Each	26	3	0	140	0	0	70	1
54487	Red Lobster-Cod, Atlantic, Lunch Portion	141.746	1	Each	23	1	0	100	0	0	70	0.3
54510	Red Lobster-Deep Sea Scallops, Lnch Portion	141.746	1	Each	26	2	2	130	0	0	50	0.4
54488	Red Lobster-Flounder, Lunch Portion	141.746	1	Each	21	1	1	100	0	0	70	0.3
54489	Red Lobster-Grouper, Lunch Portion	141.746	1	Each	26	1	0	110	0	0	65	0.3
54490	Red Lobster-Haddock, Lunch Portion	141.746	1	Each	24	1	2	110	0	0	85	0.3
54491	Red Lobster-Halibut, Lunch Portion	141.746	1	Each	25	1	1	110	0	0	60	0.3
54513	Red Lobster-Hamburger, Lunch Portion	151.181	1	Each	37	28	0	410	0	0	130	11
54504	Red Lobster-King Crab Legs, Lunch Portion	453.59	1	Each	32	2	6	170	0	0	100	0.5
54507	Red Lobster-Langostino, Lunch Portion	141.746	1	Each	26	1	2	120	0	0	210	0.2
54500	Red Lobster-Lemon Sole, Lunch Portion	141.746	1	Each	27	1	1	120	0	0	65	0.3
54524	Red Lobster-Live Maine Lobster	510.288	1	Each	36	8	5	240	0	0	310	1.9
54492	Red Lobster-Mackerel, Lunch Portion	141.746	1	Each	20	12	1	190	0	0	100	3.6
54493	Red Lobster-Monkfish, Lunch Portion	141.746	1	Each	24	1	0	110	0	0	80	0.2
54498	Red Lobster-Norwegian Salmon, Lunch	141.746	1	Each	27	12	3	230	0	0	80	2.7
54495	Red Lobster-Pollock, Lunch Portion	141.746	1	Each	28	1	1	120	0	0	90	0.3
54502	Red Lobster-Rainbow Trout, Lunch Portion	141.746	1	Each	23	9	0	170	0	0	90	2.5
54496	Red Lobster-Red Rockfish, Lunch Portion	141.746	1	Each	21	1	0	90	0	0	85	0.3
54497	Red Lobster-Red Snapper, Lunch Portion	141.746	1	Each	25	1	0	110	0	0	70	0.4
54509	Red Lobster-Rock Lobster, Lunch Portion	368.541	1	Each	49	3	2	230	0	0	200	0.7
54511	Red Lobster-Shrimp, Lunch Portion	198.445	1	Each	25	2	0	120	0	0	230	0.5
54505	Red Lobster-Snow Crab Legs, Lunch Portion	453.59	1	Each	33	2	1	150	0	0	130	0.6
54499	Red Lobster-Sockeye Salmon, Lunch Portion	141.746	1	Each	28	4	3	160	0	0	50	1.1
54512	Red Lobster-Strip Steak, Lunch Portion	255.144	1	Each	47	40	0	560	0	0	150	17
54501	Red Lobster-Swordfish, Lunch Portion	141.746	1	Each	17	4	0	100	0	0	100	1.2
54503	Red Lobster-Yellow Fin Tuna, Lunch Portion	141.746	1	Each	32	2	6	180	0	0	70	0.5
	Subway B.L.T. - 6" white	191	1	Each	14	10	38	311	0	3	16	3
	Subway BMT - 6" Italian	213	1	Each	44	55	83	982	0	5	133	20
	Subway BMT - 6" Wheat	253	1	Each	21	22	45	460	0	3	56	7
	Subway Bologna - Deli Sandwich	171	1	Each	10	12	38	292	0	2	20	4
	Subway Chicken Taco Sub - 6" white	286	1	Each	24	16	43	421	0	3	52	5
	Subway Classic Italian B.M.T. - 6" white	246	1	Each	21	21	39	445	0	3	56	8
	Subway Club - 6" white	246	1	Each	21	5	40	297	0	3	26	1
	Subway Club Salad	331	1	Each	14	3	12	126	0	1	26	1
	Subway Club Sandwich - 12" Italian	213	1	Each	46	22	83	693	0	5	84	7
	Subway Club Sandwich - 12" Wheat	220	1	Each	47	23	89	722	0	6	84	7
	Subway Cold Cut Combo - 12" Italian	184	1	Each	46	40	83	853	0	5	166	12
	Subway Cold Cut Combo - 12" Wheat	184	1	Each	48	41	88	853	0	6	166	12
	Subway Cold Cut Trio - 6" white	246	1	Each	19	13	39	362	0	3	64	4
	Subway Cold Cut Trio Salad	330	1	Each	13	11	11	191	0	1	64	3
	Subway Ham - 6" white	232	1	Each	18	5	39	287	0	3	28	1
	Subway Ham - Deli Sandwich	171	1	Each	11	4	37	234	0	2	14	1
	Subway Ham and Cheese - 12" Italian	184	1	Each	38	18	81	643	0	5	73	7
	Subway Ham and Cheese - 12" Italian	239	1	Each	19	5	45	302	0	3	28	1
	Subway Meat Ball Sandwich - 12" Italian	215	1	Each	42	44	96	918	0	3	88	17
	Subway Meat Ball Sandwich - 12" Wheat	224	1	Each	44	45	101	947	0	0	88	17
	Subway Meatballs - 6" white	260	1	Each	18	16	44	404	0	3	33	6
	Subway Melt - 6" white	251	1	Each	22	12	40	366	0	3	42	5
	Subway Pizza Sub - 6" white	250	1	Each	19	22	41	448	0	3	50	9
	Subway Roast Beef - 12" Italian	184	1	Each	42	23	84	689	0	5	83	8
	Subway Roast Beef - 12" Wheat	189	1	Each	41	24	89	717	0	6	75	8
	Subway Roast Beef - 6" white	232	1	Each	19	5	39	288	0	3	20	1
	Subway Roast Beef - Deli Sandwich	180	1	Each	13	4	38	245	0	2	13	1
	Subway Roast Beef Salad	316	1	Each	12	3	11	117	0	1	20	1

Monounsaturated Fat (gm)	Polyunsaturated Fat (gm)	Vitamin D (mg)	Vitamin K (mg)	Vitamin E (mg)	Vitamin A (re)	Vitamin C (mg)	Thiamin (mg)	Riboflavin (mg)	Niacin (mg)	Vitamin B6 (mg)	Folate (mg)	Vitamin B12 (mcg)	Calcium (mg)	Iron (mg)	Magnesium (mg)	Phosphorus (mg)	Potassium (mg)	Sodium (mg)	Zinc (mg)
0	1.9	0	0	0	0	0	0.3	0.14	1.9	0	0	0.04	0	0	21	160	0	50	0.3
0	1	0	0	0	0	0	0.06	0.1	11.4	0	0	0.08	0	0.4	21	160	0	60	0.9
0	0.6	0	0	0	0	0	0.03	0.07	0.76	0	0	0.6	0	0	28	200	0	200	0.3
0	1.5	0	0	0	0	0	0	0.1	1.9	0	0	0.4	0	0	52.5	240	0	260	1.5
0	0.7	0	0	0	0	0	0.03	0	1.52	0	0	0.3	16	0	21	48	0	95	0.3
0	0.5	0	0	0	0	0	0.06	0.03	1.52	0	0	0.08	32	0	28	200	0	70	0.3
0	1.1	0	0	0	0	0	0.03	0.07	2.85	0	0	0.2	0	0	21	160	0	180	0.3
0	0.7	0	0	0	0	0	0.15	0	2.85	0	0	0.3	0	0	28	240	0	105	0
0	1	0	0	0	0	0	0.06	0.34	7.6	0	0	1.2	0	1.5	28	200	0	115	7.5
0	1.6	0	0	0	0	0	0.09	0.17	1.9	0	0	1.6	48	0	70	320	0	900	6
0	0.6	0	0	0	0	0	0.12	0	1.14	0	0	2	16	0.8	35	160	0	410	1.5
0	0.4	0	0	0	0	0	0.06	0.1	0.38	0	0	0.4	0	0	21	64	0	90	0.3
0	4.1	0	0	0	0	0	0.15	0.17	2.85	0	0	2	320	0.8	52.5	320	0	550	6.75
0	5.4	0	0	0	0	0	0.15	0.43	5.7	0	0	0.8	16	0.8	21	200	0	250	1.2
0	0.7	0	0	0	40	0	0.06	0.14	0.76	0	0	0.2	0	1	14	64	0	95	0.3
0	4.6	0	0	0	0	0	0.23	0.07	6.65	0	0	0.2	16	0	35	240	0	60	0.3
0	1	0	0	0	0	0	0.06	0.17	0.38	0	0	1	0	0	28	160	0	90	0.3
0	4	0	0	0	0	0	0.12	0.17	2.85	0	0	1	80	0	21	200	0	90	0.9
0	0.5	0	0	0	0	0	0.09	0.1	0.76	0	0	0.6	0	0	21	120	0	95	0.3
0	0.6	0	0	0	0	0	0.06	0.03	4.75	0	0	0.3	0	0	21	120	0	140	0.3
0	1.4	0	0	0	0	0	0	0.07	3.8	0	0	0.5	48	0	87.5	400	0	1090	6
0	1.1	0	0	0	0	0	0	0.03	1.9	0	0	0.5	32	0	35	120	0	110	1.5
0	1.8	0	0	0	0	0	0.03	0.1	1.9	0	0	1.6	80	0.2	70	200	0	1630	6
0	1.8	0	0	0	0	0	0.38	0.14	7.6	0	0	2	0	0	35	280	0	60	0.3
0	2	0	0	0	0	0	0.15	0.34	7.6	0	0	1.2	0	2	35	280	0	115	9
0	1	0	0	0	20	0	0.06	0.07	3.8	0	0	0.3	0	0	28	80	0	140	0.6
0	1.6	0	0	0	0	0	0.06	0.03	13.3	0	0	1.6	0	0.6	35	240	0	70	0.3
0	0	0	0	0	601	15	0	0	0	0	0	0	27	3	0	0	0	945	0
24	7	0	0	5.1	67	5	0.27	0.34	5.1	0.48	63	2.33	64	4.3	66	308	917	3139	6.1
25	7	0	0	0	753	15	0	0	0	0	0	0	44	4	0	0	1002	3199	0
0	0	0	0	0	565	14	0	0	0	0	0	0	39	3	0	0	0	744	0
0	0	0	0	0	1044	18	0	0	0	0	0	0	118	4	0	0	0	1264	0
0	0	0	0	0	753	15	0	0	0	0	0	0	44	4	0	0	0	1652	0
0	0	0	0	0	601	15	0	0	0	0	0	0	29	4	0	0	0	1341	0
0	0	0	0	0	1363	32	0	0	0	0	0	0	26	2	0	0	0	1067	0
8	4	0	0	1.3	74	20	0.48	0.33	12.5	0.58	47	0.95	58	3.1	66	384	971	2717	2.5
9	4	0	0	4.2	83	15	0.49	0.35	9.3	0.46	43	0.44	96	3.2	40	247	1055	2777	1.4
15	10	0	0	0.9	87	17	0.36	0.33	3.8	0.2	39	1.23	227	2.9	28	315	876	2218	2.7
15	10	0	0	0.9	90	18	0.37	0.35	3.9	0.21	41	1.28	235	3	29	327	1010	2278	2.8
0	0	0	0	0	649	16	0	0	0	0	0	0	49	4	0	0	0	1401	0
0	0	0	0	0	1412	33	0	0	0	0	0	0	46	2	0	0	0	1127	0
0	0	0	0	0	601	15	0	0	0	0	0	0	28	3	0	0	0	1308	0
0	0	0	0	0	565	14	0	0	0	0	0	0	24	3	0	0	0	773	0
8	4	0	0	3.8	174	17	0.53	0.39	3.6	0.34	45	0.76	304	2.2	50	527	834	1710	2.8
8	4	0	0	0	0	0	0	0	0	0	0	0	35	3	0	0	918	1319	0
17	4	0	0	1	72	19	0.33	0.39	9.4	0.4	35	3.21	78	5	47	263	1210	2022	6.2
18	4	0	0	0	0	0	0	0	0	0	0	0	0	0	0	0	1498	2082	0
0	0	0	0	0	712	16	0	0	0	0	0	0	32	4	0	0	0	1035	0
0	0	0	0	0	777	15	0	0	0	0	0	0	93	4	0	0	0	1735	0
0	0	0	0	0	1190	16	0	0	0	0	0	0	103	4	0	0	0	1609	0
9	4	0	0	4.4	58	5	0.23	0.29	4.4	0.42	54	2.01	55	3.7	57	266	910	2288	5.3
9	4	0	0	4.5	59	5	0.24	0.3	4.5	0.43	56	2.07	56	3.8	59	273	994	2348	5.4
0	0	0	0	0	601	15	0	0	0	0	0	0	25	4	0	0	0	928	0
0	0	0	0	0	565	14	0	0	0	0	0	0	23	3	0	0	0	638	0
0	0	0	0	0	1363	32	0	0	0	0	0	0	23	2	0	0	0	654	0

USDA ID Code	Food Name	Weight in Grams*	Quantity of Units	Unit of Measure	Protein (gm)	Fat (gm)	Carbohydrates (gm)	Kcalories	Caffeine (gm)	Fiber (gm)	Cholesterol (mg)	Saturated Fat (gm)
	Subway Roasted Chicken Breast - 6" hot	246	1	Each	26	6	41	332	0	3	48	1
	Subway Seafood - 12" Italian	210	1	Each	29	57	94	986	0	0	56	11
	Subway Seafood - 12" Wheat	219	1	Each	31	58	100	1015	0	2.5	56	11
	Subway Seafood & Crab - 6" white	246	1	Each	19	19	38	415	0	3	34	3
	Subway Seafood & Crab Salad	331	1	Each	13	17	10	244	0	2	34	3
	Subway Spicy Italian - 12" Italian	213	1	Each	42	63	83	1043	0	5	137	23
	Subway Spicy Italian - 6" white	232	1	Each	20	24	38	467	0	3	57	9
	Subway Steak & Cheese - 6" white	257	1	Each	29	10	41	383	0	3	70	6
	Subway Steak and Cheese - 12" Italian	213	1	Each	43	32	83	765	0	6	82	12
	Subway Tuna - 6" white	246	1	Each	18	32	38	527	0	3	36	5
	Subway Tuna - Deli Sandwich, lite mayo	178	1	Each	11	9	38	279	0	2	16	2
	Subway Turkey Breast - 12" Italian	192	1	Each	42	20	88	674	0	7	67	6
	Subway Turkey Breast - 6" white	232	1	Each	17	4	40	273	0	3	19	1
	Subway Turkey Breast - Deli sandwich	180	1	Each	12	4	38	235	0	2	12	1
	Subway Turkey Breast & Ham - 6" white	232	1	Each	18	5	39	280	0	3	24	1
	Subway Turkey Breast Salad	316	1	Each	11	2	12	316	0	1	19	1
	Subway Veggie Delight - 6" white	175	1	Each	9	3	38	222	0	3	0	0
	Subway Veggie Delite - 6" wheat	182	1	Each	9	3	44	237	0	3	0	0
	Subway Veggie Delite Salad	260	1	Each	2	1	10	51	0	1	0	0
58318	Taco Bell-Bean Burrito	206	1	Each	15	14	63	387	0	3	9	4
58319	Taco Bell-Beef Burrito	206	1	Each	25	21	48	431	0	2	57	8
58321	Taco Bell-Burrito Supreme	198	1	Each	20	22	55	440	0	3	33	8
62585	Taco Bell-Light 7-Layer Burrito	276	1	Each	19	9	67	440	0	0	5	0
62583	Taco Bell-Light Bean Burrito	198	1	Each	14	6	55	330	0	0	5	0
62586	Taco Bell-Light Burrito Supreme	248	1	Each	20	8	50	350	0	0	25	0
62584	Taco Bell-Light Chicken Burrito	170	1	Each	12	6	45	290	0	0	30	0
62587	Taco Bell-Light Chicken Burrito Supreme	248	1	Each	18	10	62	410	0	0	65	0
62582	Taco Bell-Light Chicken Soft Taco	120	1	Each	9	5	26	180	0	0	30	0
62575	Taco Bell-Light Soft Taco	99	1	Each	13	5	19	180	0	2	25	4
62581	Taco Bell-Light Soft Taco Supreme	128	1	Each	14	5	23	200	0	0	25	0
62574	Taco Bell-Light Taco	78	1	Each	11	5	11	140	0	1	20	4
62588	Taco Bell-Light Taco Salad	464	1	Each	30	9	35	330	0	0	50	0
62580	Taco Bell-Light Taco Supreme	106	1	Each	14	5	23	160	0	0	20	0
58328	Taco Bell-Mexican Pizza	223	1	Each	21	37	40	575	0	3	52	11
58325	Taco Bell-Nachos	106	1	Each	7	18	37	346	0	1	9	6
58323	Taco Bell-Nachos Bell Grande	287	1	Each	22	35	61	649	0	4	36	12
58329	Taco Bell-Pintos 'N Cheese	128	1	Each	9	9	19	190	0	2	16	4
58337	Taco Bell-Salsa	10	1	Each	1	0	4	18	0	0.4	0	0
58314	Taco Bell-Soft Taco	92	1	Each	12	12	18	225	0	2	32	5
58313	Taco Bell-Taco	78	1	Each	10	11	11	183	0	1	32	5
58332	Taco Bell-Taco Salad	575	1	Each	34	61	55	905	0	4	80	19
58333	Taco Bell-Taco Salad w/o Shell	520	1	Each	28	31	22	484	0	3	80	14
58316	Taco Bell-Tostada	156	1	Each	9	11	27	243	0	2	16	4
	Wendy's Big Bacon Classic	285	1	Each	34	30	46	580	0	3	100	12
61273	Wendy's Big Classic	251	1	Each	27	23	44	480	0	0	75	7
62322	Wendy's Bkd Potato w/ Bacon and Cheese	380	1	Each	17	17	75	510	0	0	15	4
61287	Wendy's Bkd Potato w/ Broccoli and Cheese	411	1	Each	9	14	77	450	0	0	0	2
62524	Wendy's Bkd Potato w/ Cheese	383	1	Each	14	24	74	550	0	0	30	8
	Wendy's Breaded Chicken Sandwich	208	1	Each	28	18	44	440	0	2	60	3.5
	Wendy's Cheeseburger, Kids' Meal	123	1	Each	17	13	33	320	0	2	45	6
61281	Wendy's Chicken Club Sandwich	216	1	Each	31	20	44	470	0	2	70	4
61292	Wendy's Chili, Large	340	1	Each	28	9	31	290	0	0	60	4
61291	Wendy's Chili, Small	227	1	Each	19	6	21	190	0	0	40	2
61285	Wendy's French Fries, Biggie	170	1	Each	7	23	61	450	0	0	0	5
61284	Wendy's French Fries, Medium	136	1	Each	5	17	50	360	0	0	0	4

Monounsaturated Fat (gm)	Polyunsaturated Fat (gm)	Vitamin D (mg)	Vitamin K (mg)	Vitamin E (mg)	Vitamin A (re)	Vitamin C (mg)	Thiamin (mg)	Riboflavin (mg)	Niacin (mg)	Vitamin B6 (mg)	Folate (mg)	Vitamin B12 (mcg)	Calcium (mg)	Iron (mg)	Magnesium (mg)	Phosphorus (mg)	Potassium (mg)	Sodium (mg)	Zinc (mg)
0	0	0	0	0	617	15	0	0	0	0	0	0	35	3	0	0	0	967	0
15	28	0	0	2.5	107	5	0.51	0.38	7	0.26	91	6.54	230	4.4	32	336	641	2027	5.3
16	28	0	0	0	0	0	0	0	0	0	0	0	0	0	0	0	557	1967	0
0	0	0	0	0	604	15	0	0	0	0	0	0	28	3	0	0	0	849	0
0	0	0	0	0	1366	32	0	0	0	0	0	0	25	2	0	0	0	575	0
28	7	0	0	0	0	0	0	0	0	0	0	0	0	0	0	0	880	2282	0
0	0	0	0	0	845	15	0	0	0	0	0	0	40	4	0	0	0	1592	0
0	0	0	0	0	877	18	0	0	0	0	0	0	88	5	0	0	0	1106	0
12	4	0	0	0.8	119	6	0.33	0.46	5.1	0.38	36	2.54	231	4.2	43	456	909	1556	6.8
0	0	0	0	0	627	15	0	0	0	0	0	0	32	3	0	0	0	875	0
0	0	0	0	0	628	14	0	0	0	0	0	0	26	3	0	0	0	583	0
7	7	0	0	0	0	0	0	0	0	0	0	0	0	0	0	0	605	2520	0
0	0	0	0	0	601	15	0	0	0	0	0	0	30	4	0	0	0	1391	0
0	0	0	0	0	565	14	0	0	0	0	0	0	26	3	0	0	0	944	0
0	0	0	0	0	601	15	0	0	0	0	0	0	29	3	0	0	0	1350	0
0	0	0	0	0	1363	32	0	0	0	0	0	0	28	2	0	0	0	1117	0
0	0	0	0	0	601	15	0	0	0	0	0	0	25	0	0	0	0	3	0
0	0	0	0	0	601	15	0	0	0	0	0	0	32	3	0	0	0	593	0
0	0	0	0	0	1363	32	0	0	0	0	0	0	23	1	0	0	0	308	0
0	2	0	0	0	0	53	0.4	2	2.8	0	0	0	190	4	0	0	495	1148	0
0	2	0	0	0	0	2	0.4	0.3	3.2	0	0	0	150	3	0	0	380	1311	0
0	2	0	0	0	0	26	0.4	2.1	3.6	0	0	0	190	4	0	0	501	1181	0
0	0	0	0	0	350	4.8	0	0	0	0	0	0	300	2.5	0	0	0	1130	0
0	0	0	0	0	300	2.4	0	0	0	0	0	0	120	2	0	0	0	1340	0
0	0	0	0	0	600	9	0	0	0	0	0	0	96	1.5	0	0	0	1160	0
0	0	0	0	0	200	3.6	0	0	0	0	0	0	72	1.5	0	0	0	900	0
0	0	0	0	0	250	4.8	0	0	0	0	0	0	72	1.5	0	0	0	1190	0
0	0	0	0	0	150	4.8	0	0	0	0	0	0	48	0.8	0	0	0	570	0
0	1	0	0	0	40	0	0.4	0.2	2.8	0	0	0	48	0.6	0	0	196	554	0
0	0	0	0	0	100	2.4	0	0	0	0	0	0	48	0.6	0	0	0	610	0
0	1	0	0	0	40	0	0.1	0.1	1.2	0	0	0	0	0	0	0	159	276	0
0	0	0	0	0	1200	27	0	0	0	0	0	0	120	1.5	0	0	0	1610	0
0	0	0	0	0	100	2.4	0	0	0	0	0	0	0	0	0	0	0	340	0
0	10	0	0	0	0	31	0.3	0.3	3	0	0	0	257	4	0	0	408	1031	0
0	2	0	0	0	0	2	0	0.2	0.6	0	0	0	191	1	0	0	159	399	0
0	3	0	0	0	0	58	0.1	0.3	2.2	0	0	0	297	3	0	0	674	997	0
0	1	0	0	0	0	52	0.1	0.2	0.4	0	0	0	156	1	0	0	384	642	0
0	0	0	0	0	0	0	0	0.1	0	0	0	0	36	1	0	0	376	376	0
0	1	0	0	0	0	1	0.4	0.2	2.8	0	0	0	116	2	0	0	196	554	0
0	1	0	0	0	0	1	0.1	0.1	1.2	0	0	0	84	1	0	0	159	276	0
0	12	0	0	0	0	75	0.5	0.6	4.8	0	0	0	320	6	0	0	673	910	0
0	2	0	0	0	0	74	0.2	0.4	3.2	0	0	0	290	4	0	0	612	680	0
0	1	0	0	0	0	45	0.1	0.2	0.6	0	0	0	180	2	0	0	401	596	0
0	0	0	0	0	15	25	0	0	0	0	0	0	25	30	0	0	0	1460	0
8	7	0	0	0	60	12	0.45	0.26	6.65	0	0	0	120	3.5	0	0	500	850	0
3	8	0	0	0	100	36	0.45	0.17	6.65	0	0	0	80	2.5	0	0	1370	1170	0
3	7	0	0	0	200	60	0.3	0.14	4.75	0	0	0	80	2.5	0	0	1310	450	0
6	7	0	0	0	150	36	0.3	0.17	3.8	0	0	0	240	2	0	0	1210	640	0
0	0	0	0	0	4	10	0	0	0	0	0	0	10	16	0	0	0	840	0
0	0	0	0	0	6	0	0	0	0	0	0	0	17	18	0	0	0	830	0
7	9	0	0	0	20	9	0.6	0.43	15.2	0	0	0	80	8	0	0	470	970	0
2	1	0	0	0	150	12	0.15	0.17	2.85	0	0	0	80	4.5	0	0	660	1000	0
1	1	0	0	0	100	6	0.09	0.14	1.9	0	0	0	64	3	0	0	440	670	0
15	1	0	0	0	0	12	0.3	0.07	3.8	0	0	0	16	0.8	0	0	950	280	0
12	1	0	0	0	0	9	0.23	0.03	2.85	0	0	0	16	0.6	0	0	760	220	0

USDA ID Code	Food Name	Weight in Grams*	Quantity of Units	Unit of Measure	Protein (gm)	Fat (gm)	Carbohydrates (gm)	Kcalories	Caffeine (gm)	Fiber (gm)	Cholesterol (mg)	Saturated Fat (gm)
61283	Wendy's French Fries, Small	91	1	Each	3	12	33	240	0	0	0	2
61302	Wendy's Frosty Dairy Dessert, Large	402.22	1	Each	15	17	91	570	0	0	70	9
61301	Wendy's Frosty Dairy Dessert, Medium	321.776	1	Each	12	13	76	460	0	0	55	7
61300	Wendy's Frosty Dairy Dessert, Small	241.332	1	Each	9	10	57	340	0	0	40	5
	Wendy's Grilled Chicken Sandwich	189	1	Each	27	8	35	310	0	2	65	1.5
	Wendy's Hamburger, Kids' Meal	111	1	Each	15	10	33	270	0	2	30	3.5
	Wendy's Jr. Bacon Cheeseburger	166	1	Each	20	19	34	380	0	2	60	7
	Wendy's Jr. Cheesburger	130	1	Each	17	13	34	320	0	2	45	6
	Wendy's Jr. Cheesburger Deluxe	180	1	Each	18	17	36	360	0	3	50	6
	Wendy's Jr. Hamburger	118	1	Each	15	10	34	270	0	2	30	3.5
61271	Wendy's Plain Single	133	1	Each	24	16	31	360	0	2	65	6
61272	Wendy's Single w/ everything	219	1	Each	25	20	37	420	0	3	70	6
	Wendy's Spicy Chicken Sandwich	213	1	Each	28	15	43	410	0	2	65	2.5
62477	White Castle-Cheeseburger Sandwich	64.8	1	Each	7.8	11.2	15.53	199.58	0	2.7	0	0
62481	White Castle-Chicken Sandwich	63.786	1	Each	7.99	7.45	20.49	185.75	0	1.73	0	0
62478	White Castle-Fish Sandwich, w/o Tartar	59.333	1	Each	5.78	4.98	20.87	155.44	0	1.41	0	0
62483	White Castle-French Fries	96.83	1	Each	2.49	14.7	37.73	301.14	0	4.64	0	0
62476	White Castle-Hamburger Sandwich	58.5	1	Each	5.88	7.94	15.38	161.27	0	2.13	0	0
62485	White Castle-Onion Chips	92.135	1	Each	3.72	16.55	38.83	328.66	0	3.52	0	0
62484	White Castle-Onion Rings	60.17	1	Each	2.91	13.38	26.62	245.49	0	2.61	0	0
62479	White Castle-Sausage and Egg Sandwich	96.25	1	Each	12.55	22.02	16.05	322.37	0	3.03	0	0
62480	White Castle-Sausage Sandwich	48.667	1	Each	6.67	12.29	13.3	196.1	0	1.95	0	0
15002	Anchovy, European, Cnd In Oil	28.35	3	Ounce	8.19	2.75	0	59.54	0	0	24.1	0.62
15187	Bass, Freshwater, Ckd, Dry Heat	28.35	3	Ounce	6.86	1.34	0	41.39	0	0	24.66	0.28
15188	Bass, Striped, Ckd, Dry Heat	28.35	3	Ounce	6.44	0.85	0	35.15	0	0	29.2	0.18
15189	Bluefish, Ckd, Dry Heat	28.35	3	Ounce	7.28	1.54	0	45.08	0	0	21.55	0.33
15235	Catfish, Channel, Farmed, Ckd, Dry Heat	28.35	3	Ounce	5.31	2.27	0	43.09	0	0	18.14	0.51
15233	Catfish, Channel, Wild, Ckd, Dry Heat	28.35	3	Ounce	5.24	0.81	0	29.77	0	0	20.41	0.21
15011	Catfish, Fried	28.35	3	Ounce	5.13	3.78	2.28	64.92	0	0	22.96	0.93
15012	Caviar, Black and Red, Granular	16	1	Tbsp.	3.94	2.86	0.64	40.32	0	0	94.08	0.65
15158	Clam, Ckd, Breaded and Fried	28.35	3	Ounce	4.04	3.16	2.93	57.27	0	0	17.29	0.76
15159	Clam, Ckd, Moist Heat	28.35	3	Ounce	7.24	0.55	1.45	41.96	0	0	18.99	0.05
15160	Clam, Cnd, Drained Solids	28.35	3	Ounce	7.24	0.55	1.45	41.96	0	0	18.99	0.05
15016	Cod, Atlantic, Ckd, Dry Heat	28.35	3	Ounce	6.47	0.24	0	29.77	0	0	15.59	0.05
15017	Cod, Atlantic, Cnd	28.35	3	Ounce	6.45	0.24	0	29.77	0	0	15.59	0.05
15137	Crab, Alaska King, Ckd, Moist Heat	28.35	3	Ounce	5.49	0.44	0	27.5	0	0	15.03	0.04
15138	Crab, Alaska King, Imitation	28.35	3	Ounce	3.41	0.37	2.9	28.92	0	0	5.67	0.07
15140	Crab, Blue, Ckd, Moist Heat	28.35	3	Ounce	5.73	0.5	0	28.92	0	0	28.35	0.06
15141	Crab, Blue, Cnd	28.35	3	Ounce	5.82	0.35	0	28.07	0	0	25.23	0.07
15142	Crab, Blue, Crab Cakes	28.35	3	Ounce	5.73	2.13	0.14	43.94	0	0	42.53	0.42
15226	Crab, Dungeness, Ckd, Moist Heat	28.35	3	Ounce	6.33	0.35	0.27	31.19	0	0	21.55	0.05
15227	Crab, Queen, Ckd, Moist Heat	28.35	3	Ounce	6.72	0.43	0	32.6	0	0	20.13	0.05
15243	Crayfish, Farmed, Ckd, Moist Heat	28.35	3	Ounce	4.97	0.37	0	24.66	0	0	38.84	0.06
15146	Crayfish, Wild, Ckd, Moist Heat	28.35	3	Ounce	4.75	0.34	0	24.95	0	0	37.71	0.05
15027	Fish Fillets and Sticks, Fried	28.35	3	Ounce	4.44	3.47	6.73	77.11	0	0	31.75	0.89
15029	Flounder, Ckd, Dry Heat	28.35	3	Ounce	6.85	0.43	0	33.17	0	0	19.28	0.1
15032	Grouper, Ckd, Dry Heat	28.35	3	Ounce	7.04	0.37	0	33.45	0	0	13.32	0.08
15034	Haddock, Ckd, Dry Heat	28.35	3	Ounce	6.87	0.26	0	31.75	0	0	20.98	0.05
15035	Haddock, Smoked	28.35	3	Ounce	7.15	0.27	0	32.89	0	0	21.83	0.05
15037	Halibut, Ckd, Dry Heat	28.35	3	Ounce	7.57	0.83	0	39.69	0	0	11.62	0.12
15196	Halibut, Greenland, Ckd, Dry Heat	28.35	3	Ounce	5.22	5.03	0	67.76	0	0	16.73	0.88
15040	Herring, Ckd, Dry Heat	28.35	3	Ounce	6.53	3.29	0	57.55	0	0	21.83	0.74
15042	Herring, Kippered	28.35	3	Ounce	6.97	3.51	0	61.52	0	0	23.25	0.79
15197	Herring, Pacific, Ckd, Dry Heat	28.35	3	Ounce	5.96	5.04	0	70.88	0	0	28.07	1.18
15041	Herring, Pickled	28.35	3	Ounce	4.02	5.1	2.73	74.28	0	0	3.69	0.68

Monounsaturated Fat (gm)	Polyunsaturated Fat (gm)	Vitamin D (mg)	Vitamin K (mg)	Vitamin E (mg)	Vitamin A (re)	Vitamin C (mg)	Thiamin (mg)	Riboflavin (mg)	Niacin (mg)	Vitamin B6 (mg)	Folate (mg)	Vitamin B12 (mcg)	Calcium (mg)	Iron (mg)	Magnesium (mg)	Phosphorus (mg)	Potassium (mg)	Sodium (mg)	Zinc (mg)
8	1	0	0	0	0	6	0.15	0.03	1.9	0	0	0	0	0.4	0	0	510	150	0
4	1	0	0	0	100	0	0.23	1.36	0.76	0	0	0	400	1	0	0	1040	330	0
3	1	0	0	0	100	0	0.15	1.02	0.76	0	0	0	320	0.8	0	0	830	260	0
3	0	0	0	0	80	0	0.12	0.77	0.38	0	0	0	240	0.6	0	0	630	200	0
0	0	0	0	0	4	10	0	0	0	0	0	0	10	15	0	0	0	790	0
0	0	0	0	0	2	0	0	0	0	0	0	0	11	17	0	0	0	610	0
0	0	0	0	0	8	10	0	0	0	0	0	0	17	19	0	0	0	850	0
0	0	0	0	0	6	2	0	0	0	0	0	0	17	18	0	0	0	830	0
0	0	0	0	0	10	10	0	0	0	0	0	0	18	19	0	0	0	890	0
0	0	0	0	0	2	2	0	0	0	0	0	0	11	17	0	0	0	610	0
7	2	0	0	0	0	0	0.38	0.17	5.7	0	0	0	80	3	0	0	280	580	0
7	7	0	0	0	60	9	0.38	0.17	6.65	0	0	0	80	3	0	0	430	920	0
0	0	0	0	0	4	10	0	0	0	0	0	0	11	15	0	0	0	1280	0
0	0	0	0	0	0	0	0	0	0	0	0	0	0	0	0	0	0	361	0
0	0	0	0	0	0	0	0	0	0	0	0	0	0	0	0	0	0	497	0
0	0	0	0	0	0	0	0	0	0	0	0	0	0	0	0	0	0	201	0
0	0	0	0	0	0	0	0	0	0	0	0	0	0	0	0	0	0	193	0
0	0	0	0	0	0	0	0	0	0	0	0	0	0	0	0	0	0	266	0
0	0	0	0	0	0	0	0	0	0	0	0	0	0	0	0	0	0	823	0
0	0	0	0	0	0	0	0	0	0	0	0	0	0	0	0	0	0	566	0
0	0	0	0	0	0	0	0	0	0	0	0	0	0	0	0	0	0	698	0
0	0	0	0	0	0	0	0	0	0	0	0	0	0	0	0	0	0	488	0
1.07	0.73	0	0	1.42	5.95	0	0.02	0.1	5.64	0.06	3.54	0.25	65.77	1.31	19.56	71.44	154.22	1039.88	0.69
0.52	0.39	0	0	0	9.92	0.6	0.02	0.03	0.43	0.04	4.82	0.65	29.2	0.54	10.77	72.58	129.28	25.52	0.24
0.24	0.28	0	0	0	8.79	0	0.03	0.01	0.73	0.1	2.84	1.25	5.39	0.31	14.46	72.01	92.99	24.95	0.14
0.65	0.38	0	0	0	39.12	0	0.02	0.03	2.05	0.13	0.57	1.76	2.55	0.18	11.91	82.5	135.23	21.83	0.29
1.18	0.39	0	0	0	4.25	0.23	0.12	0.02	0.71	0.05	1.98	0.79	2.55	0.23	7.37	69.46	91	22.68	0.3
0.31	0.18	0	0	0	4.25	0.23	0.06	0.02	0.68	0.03	2.84	0.82	3.12	0.1	7.94	86.18	118.79	14.18	0.17
1.59	0.94	0	0	0	2.27	0	0.02	0.04	0.65	0.05	4.68	0.54	12.47	0.41	7.65	61.24	96.39	79.38	0.24
0.74	1.19	0.93	0	1.12	89.6	0	0.03	0.1	0.02	0.05	8	3.2	44	1.9	48	56.96	28.96	240	0.15
1.29	0.81	0	0	0	25.52	2.84	0.03	0.07	0.59	0.02	5.16	11.42	17.86	3.94	3.97	53.3	92.42	103.19	0.41
0.05	0.16	0	0	0	48.48	6.27	0.04	0.12	0.95	0.03	8.16	28.03	26.08	7.93	5.1	95.82	178.04	31.75	0.77
0.05	0.16	0	0	0.28	48.48	6.27	0.04	0.12	0.95	0.03	8.16	28.03	26.08	7.93	5.1	95.82	178.04	31.75	0.77
0.04	0.08	0	0	0.09	3.97	0.28	0.02	0.02	0.71	0.08	2.3	0.3	3.97	0.14	11.91	39.12	69.17	22.11	0.16
0.04	0.08	0.6	0	0.06	3.97	0.28	0.02	0.02	0.71	0.08	2.3	0.3	5.95	0.14	11.62	73.71	149.69	61.8	0.16
0.05	0.15	0	0	0	2.55	2.15	0.02	0.02	0.38	0.05	14.46	3.26	16.73	0.22	17.86	79.38	74.28	303.91	2.16
0.06	0.19	0	0	0	5.67	0	0.01	0.01	0.05	0.01	0.45	0.45	3.69	0.11	12.19	79.95	25.52	238.42	0.09
0.08	0.19	0	0	0.28	0.57	0.94	0.03	0.01	0.94	0.05	14.4	2.07	29.48	0.26	9.36	58.4	91.85	79.1	1.2
0.06	0.12	0	0	0.28	0.57	0.77	0.02	0.02	0.39	0.04	12.05	0.13	28.63	0.24	11.06	73.71	106.03	94.41	1.14
0.8	0.64	0	0	0	22.96	0.79	0.03	0.02	0.82	0.05	11.77	1.68	29.77	0.31	9.36	60.39	91.85	93.56	1.16
0.06	0.12	0	0	0	8.79	1.02	0.02	0.06	1.03	0.05	11.91	2.94	16.73	0.12	16.44	49.61	115.67	107.16	1.55
0.09	0.15	0	0	0	14.74	2.04	0.03	0.07	0.82	0.05	11.91	2.94	9.36	0.82	17.86	36.29	56.7	195.9	1.02
0.07	0.12	0	0	0	4.25	0.14	0.01	0.02	0.47	0.04	3.12	0.88	14.46	0.31	9.36	68.32	67.47	27.5	0.42
0.07	0.1	0	0	0.43	4.25	0.26	0.01	0.02	0.65	0.02	12.47	0.61	17.01	0.24	9.36	76.55	83.92	26.65	0.5
1.44	0.9	0	0	0	8.79	0	0.04	0.05	0.6	0.02	5.16	0.51	5.67	0.21	7.09	51.31	73.99	165	0.19
0.09	0.12	0	0	0	3.12	0	0.02	0.03	0.62	0.07	2.61	0.71	5.1	0.1	16.44	81.93	97.52	29.77	0.18
0.08	0.11	0	0	0	14.18	0	0.02	0	0.11	0.1	2.89	0.2	5.95	0.32	10.49	40.54	134.66	15.03	0.14
0.04	0.09	0	0	0	5.39	0	0.01	0.01	1.31	0.1	3.77	0.39	11.91	0.38	14.18	68.32	113.12	24.66	0.14
0.04	0.09	0	0	0.11	6.24	0	0.01	0.01	1.44	0.11	4.34	0.45	13.89	0.4	15.31	71.16	117.65	216.31	0.14
0.27	0.27	0	0	0	15.31	0	0.02	0.03	2.02	0.11	3.91	0.39	17.01	0.3	30.33	80.8	163.3	19.56	0.15
3.05	0.5	0	0	0	5.1	0	0.02	0.03	0.55	0.14	0.28	0.27	1.13	0.24	9.36	59.54	97.52	29.2	0.14
1.36	0.78	0	0	0.38	8.79	0.2	0.03	0.08	1.17	0.1	3.26	3.73	20.98	0.4	11.62	85.9	118.79	32.6	0.36
1.45	0.83	0.85	0	0.28	11.06	0.28	0.04	0.09	1.25	0.12	3.88	5.3	23.81	0.43	13.04	92.14	126.72	260.25	0.39
2.5	0.88	0	0	0	9.92	0	0.02	0.07	0.8	0.15	1.7	2.73	30.05	0.41	11.62	82.78	153.66	26.93	0.19
3.39	0.48	4.82	0	0.28	73.14	0	0.01	0.04	0.94	0.05	0.68	1.21	21.83	0.35	2.27	25.23	19.56	246.65	0.15

USDA ID Code	Food Name	Weight in Grams*	Quantity of Units	Unit of Measure	Protein (gm)	Fat (gm)	Carbohydrates (gm)	Kcalories	Caffeine (gm)	Fiber (gm)	Cholesterol (mg)	Saturated Fat (gm)
15148	Lobster, Northern, Ckd, Moist Heat	28.35	3	Ounce	5.81	0.17	0.36	27.78	0	0	20.41	0.03
15228	Lobster, Spiny, Ckd, Moist Heat	28.35	3	Ounce	7.49	0.55	0.88	40.54	0	0	25.52	0.09
15056	Mullet, Striped, Ckd, Dry Heat	28.35	3	Ounce	7.03	1.38	0	42.53	0	0	17.86	0.41
15165	Mussel, Blue, Ckd, Moist Heat	28.35	3	Ounce	6.75	1.27	2.1	48.76	0	0	15.88	0.24
15168	Oyster, Eastern, Breaded and Fried	28.35	3	Ounce	2.49	3.57	3.29	55.85	0	0	22.96	0.91
15170	Oyster, Eastern, Cnd	28.35	3	Ounce	2	0.7	1.11	19.56	0	0	15.59	0.18
15245	Oysters, Raw	28.35	3	Ounce	1.48	0.44	1.57	16.73	0	0	7.09	0.13
15058	Perch, Atlantic, Ckd, Dry Heat	28.35	3	Ounce	6.77	0.59	0	34.3	0	0	15.31	0.09
15061	Perch, Ckd, Dry Heat	28.35	3	Ounce	7.05	0.33	0	33.17	0	0	32.6	0.07
15063	Pike, Northern, Ckd, Dry Heat	28.35	3	Ounce	7	0.25	0	32.04	0	0	14.18	0.04
15204	Pike, Walleye, Ckd, Dry Heat	28.35	3	Ounce	6.96	0.44	0	33.74	0	0	31.19	0.09
15205	Pollock, Atlantic, Ckd, Dry Heat	28.35	3	Ounce	7.06	0.36	0	33.45	0	0	25.8	0.05
15069	Pompano, Florida, Ckd, Dry Heat	28.35	3	Ounce	6.72	3.44	0	59.82	0	0	18.14	1.28
15071	Rockfish, Pacific, Ckd, Dry Heat	28.35	3	Ounce	6.82	0.57	0	34.3	0	0	12.47	0.13
15232	Roughy, Orange, Ckd, Dry Heat	28.35	3	Ounce	5.34	0.26	0	25.23	0	0	7.37	0.01
15209	Salmon, Atlantic, Wild, Ckd, Dry Heat	28.35	3	Ounce	7.21	2.3	0	51.6	0	0	20.13	0.36
15210	Salmon, Chinook, Ckd, Dry Heat	28.35	3	Ounce	7.29	3.79	0	65.49	0	0	24.1	0.91
15211	Salmon, Chum, Ckd, Dry Heat	28.35	3	Ounce	7.32	1.37	0	43.66	0	0	26.93	0.31
15087	Salmon, Cnd.	28.35	3	Ounce	5.8	2.07	0	43.38	0	0	12.47	0.47
15239	Salmon, Coho, Farmed, Ckd, Dry Heat	28.35	3	Ounce	6.89	2.33	0	50.46	0	0	17.86	0.55
15247	Salmon, Coho, Wild, Ckd, Dry Heat	28.35	3	Ounce	6.65	1.22	0	39.41	0	0	15.59	0.3
15082	Salmon, Coho, Wild, Ckd, Moist Heat	28.35	3	Ounce	7.76	2.13	0	52.16	0	0	16.16	0.45
15212	Salmon, Pink, Ckd, Dry Heat	28.35	3	Ounce	7.25	1.25	0	42.24	0	0	18.99	0.2
15088	Sardine, Atlantic, Cnd In Oil	28.35	3	Ounce	6.98	3.25	0	58.97	0	0	40.26	0.43
15173	Scallop, Breaded and Fried	28.35	3	Ounce	5.12	3.1	2.87	60.95	0	0	17.29	0.76
15174	Scallop, Imitation	28.35	3	Ounce	3.62	0.12	3.01	28.07	0	0	6.24	0.02
62652	Scallops, Sauteed	28.35	3	Ounce	9.67	0.33	0.67	50	0	0	20	0
15092	Sea Bass, Ckd, Dry Heat	28.35	3	Ounce	6.7	0.73	0	35.15	0	0	15.03	0.19
15096	Shark, Ckd, Batter-dipped and Fried	28.35	3	Ounce	5.28	3.92	1.81	64.64	0	0	16.73	0.91
15150	Shrimp, Ckd, Breaded and Fried	28.35	3	Ounce	6.06	3.48	3.25	68.61	0	0	50.18	0.59
15151	Shrimp, Ckd, Moist Heat	28.35	3	Ounce	5.93	0.31	0	28.07	0	0	55.28	0.08
15152	Shrimp, Cnd	28.35	3	Ounce	6.54	0.56	0.29	34.02	0	0	49.05	0.11
15149	Shrimp, Fresh	28.35	3	Ounce	5.76	0.49	0.26	30.05	0	0	43.09	0.09
15153	Shrimp, Imitation	28.35	3	Ounce	3.51	0.42	2.59	28.63	0	0	10.21	0.08
15100	Smelt, Rainbow, Ckd, Dry Heat	28.35	3	Ounce	6.41	0.88	0	35.15	0	0	25.52	0.16
15102	Snapper, Ckd, Dry Heat	28.35	3	Ounce	7.46	0.49	0	36.29	0	0	13.32	0.1
15176	Squid, Fried	28.35	3	Ounce	5.09	2.12	2.21	49.61	0	0	73.71	0.53
15218	Sunfish, Ckd, Dry Heat	28.35	3	Ounce	7.05	0.26	0	32.32	0	0	24.38	0.05
15111	Swordfish, Ckd, Dry Heat	28.35	3	Ounce	7.2	1.46	0	43.94	0	0	14.18	0.4
15219	Trout, Ckd, Dry Heat	28.35	3	Ounce	7.55	2.4	0	53.87	0	0	20.98	0.42
15241	Trout, Rainbow, Farmed, Ckd, Dry Heat	28.35	3	Ounce	6.88	2.04	0	47.91	0	0	19.28	0.6
15116	Trout, Rainbow, Wild, Ckd, Dry Heat	28.35	3	Ounce	6.5	1.65	0	42.53	0	0	19.56	0.46
15128	Tuna Salad	28.35	3	Ounce	4.55	2.63	2.67	53.01	0	0	3.69	0.44
15183	Tuna, Light Meat, Cnd In Oil	28.35	3	Ounce	8.26	2.33	0	56.13	0	0	5.1	0.43
15184	Tuna, Light Meat, Cnd In Water	28.35	3	Ounce	8.39	0.14	0	37.14	0	0	5.1	0.05
15121	Tuna, Light, Cnd In Water	28.35	3	Ounce	7.23	0.23	0	32.89	0	0	8.51	0.07
15220	Tuna, Skipjack, Ckd, Dry Heat	28.35	3	Ounce	8	0.37	0	37.42	0	0	17.01	0.12
15185	Tuna, White Meat, Cnd In Oil	28.35	3	Ounce	7.52	2.29	0	52.73	0	0	8.79	0.47
15186	Tuna, White Meat, Cnd In Water	28.35	3	Ounce	7.56	0.7	0	38.56	0	0	11.91	0.19
15221	Tuna, Yellowfin, Ckd, Dry Heat	28.35	3	Ounce	8.5	0.35	0	39.41	0	0	16.44	0.09
15223	Whitefish, Ckd, Dry Heat	28.35	3	Ounce	6.94	2.13	0	48.76	0	0	21.83	0.33
15131	Whitefish, Smoked	28.35	3	Ounce	6.63	0.26	0	30.62	0	0	9.36	0.06
15225	Yellowtail, Ckd, Dry Heat	28.35	3	Ounce	8.41	1.91	0	53.01	0	0	20.13	0
15135	Yellowtail, Fresh	28.35	3	Ounce	6.56	1.49	0	41.39	0	0	15.59	0.36
19065	Almond Joy Candy Bar	50	1	Bar	2.35	13.85	29.2	232	0	0	1	8.31

Monounsaturated Fat (gm)	Polyunsaturated Fat (gm)	Vitamin D (mg)	Vitamin K (mg)	Vitamin E (mg)	Vitamin A (re)	Vitamin C (mg)	Thiamin (mg)	Riboflavin (mg)	Niacin (mg)	Vitamin B6 (mg)	Folate (mg)	Vitamin B12 (mcg)	Calcium (mg)	Iron (mg)	Magnesium (mg)	Phosphorus (mg)	Potassium (mg)	Sodium (mg)	Zinc (mg)
0.05	0.03	0	0	0.28	7.37	0	0	0.02	0.3	0.02	3.15	0.88	17.29	0.11	9.92	52.45	99.79	107.73	0.83
0.1	0.21	0	0	0	1.7	0.6	0	0.02	1.39	0.05	0.28	1.15	17.86	0.4	14.46	64.92	58.97	64.35	2.06
0.39	0.26	0	0	0	11.91	0.34	0.03	0.03	1.79	0.14	2.78	0.07	8.79	0.4	9.36	69.17	129.84	20.13	0.25
0.29	0.34	0	0	0.24	25.8	3.86	0.09	0.12	0.85	0.03	21.43	6.8	9.36	1.91	10.49	80.8	75.98	104.61	0.76
1.33	0.94	0	0	0	25.52	1.08	0.04	0.06	0.47	0.02	3.86	4.43	17.58	1.97	16.44	45.08	69.17	118.22	24.7
0.07	0.21	0	0	0.24	25.52	1.42	0.04	0.05	0.35	0.03	2.52	5.42	12.76	1.9	15.31	39.41	64.92	31.75	25.78
0.04	0.17	0	0	0	2.27	1.33	0.03	0.02	0.36	0.02	5.1	4.59	0	1.64	9.36	26.37	35.15	50.46	10.75
0.23	0.16	0	0	0	3.97	0.23	0.04	0.04	0.69	0.08	2.95	0.33	38.84	0.33	11.06	78.53	99.23	27.22	0.17
0.06	0.13	0	0	0	2.84	0.48	0.02	0.03	0.54	0.04	1.64	0.62	28.92	0.33	10.77	72.86	97.52	22.4	0.41
0.06	0.07	0	0	0	6.8	1.08	0.02	0.02	0.79	0.04	4.9	0.65	20.7	0.2	11.34	79.95	93.84	13.89	0.24
0.11	0.16	0	0	0	6.8	0	0.09	0.06	0.79	0.04	4.82	0.65	39.97	0.47	10.77	76.26	141.47	18.43	0.22
0.04	0.18	0	0	0	3.4	0	0.02	0.06	1.13	0.09	0.85	1.04	21.83	0.17	24.38	80.23	129.28	31.19	0.17
0.94	0.41	0	0	0	10.21	0	0.19	0.04	1.08	0.07	4.9	0.34	12.19	0.19	8.79	96.67	180.31	21.55	0.2
0.13	0.17	0	0	0	18.71	0	0.01	0.02	1.11	0.08	2.95	0.34	3.4	0.15	9.64	64.64	147.42	21.83	0.15
0.17	0	0	0	0	6.8	0	0.03	0.05	1.04	0.1	2.27	0.65	10.77	0.07	10.77	72.58	109.15	22.96	0.27
0.76	0.92	0	0	0	3.69	0	0.08	0.14	2.86	0.27	8.22	0.86	4.25	0.29	10.49	72.58	178.04	15.88	0.23
1.63	0.75	0	0	0	42.24	1.16	0.01	0.04	2.85	0.13	9.92	0.81	7.94	0.26	34.59	105.18	143.17	17.01	0.16
0.56	0.33	0	0	0	9.64	0	0.03	0.06	2.42	0.13	1.42	0.98	3.97	0.2	7.94	102.91	155.93	18.14	0.17
0.79	0.65	0	0	0.45	15.03	0	0	0.05	1.55	0.09	2.78	0.09	67.76	0.3	8.22	92.42	106.88	152.52	0.29
1.03	0.56	0	0	0	16.73	0.43	0.03	0.03	2.1	0.16	3.97	0.9	3.4	0.11	9.64	94.12	130.41	14.74	0.13
0.45	0.36	0	0	0	11.06	0.4	0.02	0.04	2.25	0.16	3.69	1.42	0	0.17	9.36	91.29	123.04	16.44	0.16
0.77	0.71	0	0	0	9.07	0.28	0.03	0.05	2.21	0.16	2.55	1.27	13.04	0.2	9.92	84.48	128.99	15.03	0.15
0.34	0.49	0	0	0	11.62	0	0.06	0.02	2.42	0.07	1.42	0.98	4.82	0.28	9.36	83.63	117.37	24.38	0.2
1.1	1.46	1.93	0	0.09	18.99	0	0.02	0.06	1.49	0.05	3.35	2.53	108.3	0.83	11.06	138.92	112.55	143.17	0.37
1.28	0.81	0	0	0	6.24	0.65	0.01	0.03	0.43	0.04	5.16	0.37	11.91	0.23	16.73	66.91	94.41	131.54	0.3
0.02	0.06	0	0	0	5.67	0	0	0	0.09	0.01	0.45	0.45	2.27	0.09	12.19	79.95	29.2	225.38	0.09
0	0	0	0	0	0	0.6	0	0	0	0	0	0	8	0	0	0	0	91.67	0
0.15	0.27	0	0	0	18.14	0	0.04	0.04	0.54	0.13	1.64	0.09	70.31	0.1	15.03	70.31	92.99	24.66	0.15
1.68	1.05	0	0	0	15.31	0	0.02	0.03	0.79	0.09	1.47	0.34	14.18	0.31	12.19	55	43.94	34.59	0.14
1.08	1.44	0	0	0	15.88	0.43	0.04	0.04	0.87	0.03	2.3	0.53	18.99	0.36	11.34	61.8	63.79	97.52	0.39
0.06	0.12	0	0	1.03	18.71	0.62	0.01	0.01	0.73	0.04	0.99	0.42	11.06	0.88	9.64	38.84	51.6	63.5	0.44
0.08	0.21	0	0	0.71	5.1	0.65	0.01	0.01	0.78	0.03	0.51	0.32	16.73	0.78	11.62	66.06	59.54	47.91	0.36
0.07	0.19	1.08	0	0.81	15.31	0.57	0.01	0.01	0.72	0.03	0.85	0.33	14.74	0.68	10.49	58.12	52.45	41.96	0.31
0.06	0.21	0	0	0	5.67	0	0.01	0.01	0.05	0.01	0.45	0.45	5.39	0.17	12.19	79.95	25.23	199.87	0.09
0.23	0.32	0	0	0	4.82	0	0	0.04	0.5	0.05	1.3	1.13	21.83	0.33	10.77	83.63	105.46	21.83	0.6
0.09	0.17	0	0	0	9.92	0.45	0.02	0	0.1	0.13	1.64	0.99	11.34	0.07	10.49	56.98	147.99	16.16	0.12
0.78	0.61	0	0	0	3.12	1.19	0.02	0.13	0.74	0.02	1.5	0.35	11.06	0.29	10.77	71.16	79.1	86.75	0.49
0.04	0.09	0	0	0	4.82	0.28	0.03	0.02	0.41	0.04	4.82	0.65	29.2	0.44	10.77	65.49	127.29	29.2	0.56
0.56	0.34	0	0	0	11.62	0.31	0.01	0.03	3.34	0.11	0.65	0.57	1.7	0.29	9.64	95.54	104.61	32.6	0.42
1.18	0.54	0	0	0	5.39	0.14	0.12	0.12	1.64	0.07	4.25	2.12	15.59	0.54	7.94	89.02	131.26	18.99	0.24
0.59	0.66	0	0	0	24.38	0.94	0.07	0.02	2.49	0.11	6.8	1.41	0	0.09	9.07	75.41	125.02	11.91	0.14
0.49	0.52	0	0	0	4.25	0.57	0.04	0.03	1.64	0.1	5.39	1.79	0	0.11	8.79	76.26	127.01	15.88	0.14
0.82	1.17	0	0	0	7.65	0.62	0.01	0.02	1.9	0.02	2.07	0.34	4.82	0.28	5.39	50.46	50.46	113.97	0.16
0.84	0.82	0	0	0.34	6.52	0	0.01	0.03	3.52	0.03	1.5	0.62	3.69	0.39	8.79	88.17	58.68	14.18	0.26
0.04	0.04	0	0	0.15	6.52	0	0.01	0.03	3.52	0.11	1.33	0.62	3.4	0.91	8.22	52.73	89.02	14.18	0.12
0.05	0.1	0	0	0.15	4.82	0	0.01	0.02	3.76	0.1	1.13	0.85	3.12	0.43	7.65	46.21	67.19	95.82	0.22
0.07	0.11	0	0	0	5.1	0.28	0.01	0.03	5.32	0.28	2.84	0.62	10.49	0.45	12.47	80.8	147.99	13.32	0.3
0.7	0.96	0	0	0	6.8	0	0	0.02	3.32	0.12	1.3	0.62	1.13	0.18	9.64	75.69	94.41	14.18	0.13
0.18	0.26	0	0	0	6.8	0	0	0.01	1.64	0.12	1.16	0.62	1.13	0.17	9.64	75.69	80.23	14.18	0.13
0.06	0.1	0	0	0	5.67	0.28	0.14	0.02	3.38	0.29	0.57	0.17	5.95	0.27	18.14	69.46	161.31	13.32	0.19
0.73	0.78	0	0	0	11.06	0	0.05	0.04	1.09	0.1	4.82	0.27	9.36	0.13	11.91	98.09	115.1	18.43	0.36
0.08	0.08	0	0	0.06	16.16	0	0.01	0.03	0.68	0.11	2.07	0.92	5.1	0.14	6.52	37.42	119.92	288.89	0.14
0	0	0	0	0	8.79	0.82	0.05	0.01	2.47	0.05	1.13	0.35	8.22	0.18	10.77	56.98	152.52	14.19	0.14
0.56	0.4	0	0	0	8.22	0.79	0.04	0.01	1.93	0.05	1.05	0.37	6.52	0.14	8.51	44.51	119.07	11.06	0.15
2.63	1.19	0	0	0	2	0.1	0.02	0.08	0.24	0.03	4	0.06	39.5	0.6	33	70	185.5	67	0.4

USDA ID Code	Food Name	Weight in Grams*	Quantity of Units	Unit of Measure	Protein (gm)	Fat (gm)	Carbohydrates (gm)	Kcalories	Caffeine (gm)	Fiber (gm)	Cholesterol (mg)	Saturated Fat (gm)
19066	Alpine White Bar w/ Almonds	35	1	Bar	3.5	12.92	17.64	197.4	0	1.89	4.2	6.67
62631	Bagel Chips	28.35	1	Ounce	4	6	20	150	0	1	0	1
19400	Banana Chips	28.35	1	Ounce	0.65	9.53	16.56	147.14	0	2.18	0	8.21
19002	Beef Jerky, Chopped and Formed	28.35	3	Ounce	11.25	3.69	4.11	95.82	0	0.03	32.04	1.66
18151	Brownies	56	1	Each	2.69	9.13	35.78	226.8	0	1.34	9.52	2.42
18155	Butter Cookies	5	1	Each	0.31	0.94	3.45	23.35	0	0.12	4.35	0.54
19069	Butterfinger Bar	61	1	Bar	4.7	11.29	40.5	266.57	2.44	1.65	0.61	5.17
19070	Butterscotch Candy	6	1	Piece	0.01	0.21	5.72	23.7	0	0	0.54	0.07
19074	Caramels	8	1	Piece	0.37	0.65	6.16	30.56	0	0.1	0.56	0.53
	Carefree Bubble Gum	3	1	Each	0	0	2	10	0	0	0	0
	Carefree Gum	3	1	Each	0	0	2	8	0	0	0	0
19163	Chewing Gum	3	1	Stick	0	0.01	2.9	10.23	0	0	0	0
	Chewing Gum - Cinnamon	3	1	Each	0	0	2	10	0	0	0	0
	Chewing Gum - Mint Flavors	3	1	Each	0	0	2	10	0	0	0	0
62672	Chewing Gum, Sugar-Free	1.7	1	Stick	0	0	1	5	0	0	0	0
19033	Chex Mix	42.525	1	Cup	4.68	7.36	27.68	180.73	0	0	0	0
18198	Chocolate Chip Cookies, Dietary	7	1	Each	0.27	1.18	5.14	31.5	0	0	0	0.57
18159	Chocolate Chip Cookies, Higher Fat, Enr	10	1	Each	0.54	2.26	6.68	48.1	0	0.25	0	0.78
18158	Chocolate Chip Cookies, Lower Fat	10	1	Each	0.58	1.54	7.33	45.3	0	0	0	0.45
18160	Chocolate Chip Cookies, Soft-type	15	1	Each	0.53	3.65	8.87	68.7	0	0.48	0	1.12
18157	Chocolate Wafers	6	1	Each	0.4	0.85	4.34	25.98	0	0	0.12	0.22
19119	Chunky Bar	35	1	Bar	3.15	10.22	19.99	173.25	10.15	1.68	3.85	8.13
19219	Coconut Cream Pudding	280	1	Cup	8.68	7	49.84	291.2	0	0	19.6	5.04
19049	Combos Snacks Cheddar Pretzel	28.35	1	Ounce	2.78	5.53	18.43	135.51	0	0	2.55	0
62589	Cookie Cakes, Devils Food, Fat Free-SnackWell	16	1	Each	1	0	13	50	0	0.5	0	0
62591	Cookie Cakes, Double Fudge, Fat Free-SnackWell	16	1	Each	1	0	12	50	0	0.5	0	0
62656	Corn Chips	2.231	13	Chips	0.15	0.85	1.15	12.31	0	0.08	0	0.12
19401	Cornnuts, Barbecue-flavor	28.35	1	Ounce	2.55	4.05	20.33	123.61	0	2.38	0	0.73
19402	Cornnuts, Nacho-flavor	28.35	1	Ounce	2.66	4.03	20.3	124.17	0	2.27	0.57	0.73
19009	Cornnuts, Plain	28.35	1	Ounce	2.41	4	20.78	124.46	0	1.96	0	0.72
18150	Crackers, Animal	2.5	1	Each	0.17	0.35	1.85	11.15	0	0	0	0.09
19032	Doo Dads Snack Mix, Original Flavor	56.7	1	Cup	5.84	10.49	36.46	258.55	0	3.86	0.57	0
	Doritos - Cool Ranch	28	1	Ounce	2	7	18	140	0	0	0	1
	Doritos - Nacho Cheese	28	1	Ounce	2	7	17	140	0	0	0	1
62686	Doughnut Holes	15	1	Each	0.78	3.44	7.62	63.9	0	0	4.8	0.8
19168	Egg Custards	282	1	Cup	14.38	13.25	30.17	296.1	0	0	245.34	6.63
19098	Fifth Avenue Bar	60	1	Bar	4.74	12.72	40.8	279.6	0	0	2.4	0
18170	Fig Bars	16	1	Each	0.59	1.17	11.34	55.68	0	0.74	0	0.21
	Fig Newton - Fat Free	29	2	Each	1	0	22	100	0	0	0	0
	Fritos	28	1	Ounce	2	10	15	160	0	0	0	1.5
	Fritos-Barbecue	28	1	Ounce	2	9	16	160	0	0	0	1.5
62638	Frosted Pop Tart, Fruit	52	1	Each	2	5	38	200	0	1	0	1.5
19226	Frostings, Chocolate, Creamy	28.35	1	Ounce	0.31	4.99	17.92	112.55	0	0	0	1.57
19713	Frostings, Cream Cheese-flavor	28.35	1	Ounce	0.03	4.9	18.91	117.09	0	0	0	1.43
19229	Frostings, Sour Cream-flavor	28.35	1	Ounce	0.03	4.88	19.16	116.8	0	0	0	1.42
19230	Frostings, Vanilla, Creamy	28.35	1	Ounce	0.03	4.76	19.67	118.79	0	0	0	1.39
41319	Frozen Dessert, Bordeaux Cherry-Healthy Choice	132.969	1	Cup	6	4	46	240	0	0	10	0
41320	Frozen Dessert, Butter Pecan Crunch-Healthy Choice	132.969	1	Cup	6	4	52	280	0	0	10	0
41321	Frozen Dessert, Chocolate Chip-Healthy Choice	132.969	1	Cup	6	4	48	260	0	0	10	0
41322	Frozen Dessert, Coffee Toffee-Healthy Choice	132.969	1	Cup	6	4	50	260	0	0	10	0
41323	Frozen Dessert, Cookies 'n Cream-Healthy Choice	132.969	1	Cup	8	4	48	260	0	0	10	0
41324	Frozen Dessert, Double Fudge Swirl-Healthy Choice	132.969	1	Cup	6	4	48	260	0	0	10	0
41325	Frozen Dessert, Fudge Brownie-Healthy Choice	132.969	1	Cup	6	4	54	280	0	0	10	0
41326	Frozen Dessert, Mint Chocolate Chip-Healthy Choice	132.969	1	Cup	6	4	50	280	0	0	10	0
41327	Frozen Dessert, Neapolitan-Healthy Choice	132.969	1	Cup	6	4	44	240	0	0	10	0

Monounsaturated Fat (gm)	Polyunsaturated Fat (gm)	Vitamin D (mg)	Vitamin K (mg)	Vitamin E (mg)	Vitamin A (re)	Vitamin C (mg)	Thiamin (mg)	Riboflavin (mg)	Niacin (mg)	Vitamin B6 (mg)	Folate (mg)	Vitamin B12 (mcg)	Calcium (mg)	Iron (mg)	Magnesium (mg)	Phosphorus (mg)	Potassium (mg)	Sodium (mg)	Zinc (mg)
4.81	0.88	0	0	0	8.75	0.14	0.03	0.15	0.03	0.03	4.55	0.3	80.85	0.2	13.3	81.55	146.3	25.55	0.4
3	2	0	0	0	0	0	0	0	0	0	0	0	0	0.4	0	0	0	190	0
0.55	0.18	0	0	1.53	2.27	1.79	0.02	0	0.2	0.07	3.97	0	5.1	0.35	21.55	15.88	151.96	1.7	0.21
1.51	0.16	0	0	0.04	0	0	0.03	0.26	2.61	0.13	4.82	1.13	3.12	1.56	14.46	107.73	169.25	815.06	2.3
4.73	1.44	0	0	0	11.2	0.06	0.14	0.12	0.96	0.02	6.72	0.08	16.24	1.26	17.36	56.56	83.44	174.72	0.4
0.26	0.05	0	0	0	7.55	0	0.02	0.02	0.16	0	0.3	0.01	1.45	0.11	0.6	5.1	5.55	17.55	0.02
3.82	1.81	0	0	0.81	11.59	1.71	0.09	0.03	2.01	0.04	18.91	0.09	14.64	0.64	27.45	57.95	129.32	82.96	0.45
0.03	0	0	0	0	2.04	0	0	0	0	0	0	0	0.18	0	0.06	0.18	0.24	2.58	0
0.07	0.01	0	0	0.04	0.64	0.04	0	0.01	0.02	0	0.4	0	11.04	0.01	1.36	9.12	17.12	19.6	0.04
0	0	0	0	0	0	0	0	0	0	0	0	0	0	0	0	0	0	0	0
0	0	0	0	0	0	0	0	0	0	0	0	0	0	0	0	0	0	0	0
0	0	0	0	0	0	0	0	0	0	0	0	0	0	0	0	0	0.12	0.18	0
0	0	0	0	0	0	0	0	0	0	0	0	0	0	0	0	0	0	0	0
0	0	0	0	0	0	0	0	0	0	0	0	0	0	0	0	0	0	0	0
0	0	0	0	0	0	0	0	0	0	0	0	0	0	0	0	0	0	0	0
0	0	0	0	0	5.95	20.2	0.66	0.21	7.16	0.66	0	5.27	14.88	10.5	26.79	79.52	114.39	432.48	0.89
0.47	0.07	0	0	0	0	0	0.02	0.01	0.18	0	0.42	0	2.31	0.24	1.75	6.23	13.93	0.77	0.04
1.15	0.22	0	0	0	0	0	0.02	0.03	0.27	0.01	0.9	0	2.5	0.28	3.1	10.8	13.5	31.5	0.06
0.79	0.17	0	0	0	0	0.03	0.03	0.03	0.28	0.03	0.6	0	1.9	0.31	2.8	8.4	12.3	37.7	0.07
1.95	0.4	0	0	0	0.15	0	0.02	0.03	0.24	0.02	0.75	0	2.25	0.36	5.25	7.5	13.95	48.9	0.07
0.45	0.1	0	0	0	0.12	0	0.01	0.02	0.17	0	0.66	0	1.86	0.24	3.18	7.92	12.6	34.8	0.07
0.11	1.54	0	0	0	3.85	0.11	0.03	0.14	0.67	0.04	7.7	0.13	50.05	0.44	25.55	72.8	186.9	18.55	0.64
1.46	0.2	0	0	0	140	1.96	0.09	0.41	0.25	0.41	11.2	0.73	316.4	0.56	44.8	249.2	445.2	456.4	1.04
0	0	0	0	0	1.98	0	0.03	0.16	0.9	0.01	2.27	0.03	54.15	0.86	6.24	40.54	36.86	316.67	0.21
0	0	0	0	0	0	0	0	0	0	0	0	0	0	0	0	0	0	25	0
0	0	0	0	0	0	0	0	0	0	0	0	0	0	0.2	0	0	0	70	0
0	0	0	0	0	0	0	0	0	0	0	0	0	5.54	0.02	0	0	0	15.38	0
2.09	0.91	0	0	0	9.64	0.11	0.1	0.04	0.43	0.05	0	0	4.82	0.48	30.9	80.23	81.08	276.7	0.53
2.07	0.91	0	0	0	1.13	4.39	0.1	0.02	0.34	0.06	4.25	0	9.92	0.48	30.9	87.6	88.17	179.74	0.51
2.06	0.9	0	0	0.29	0	0	0.01	0.04	0.48	0.06	0	0	2.55	0.47	32.04	77.96	78.81	155.64	0.5
0.19	0.05	0	0	0	0	0	0.01	0.01	0.09	0	0.35	0	1.08	0.07	0.45	2.85	2.5	9.83	0.02
0	0	0	0	0	24.38	0.06	0.2	0.15	3.04	0.12	22.68	0.01	41.96	1.42	34.02	167.83	157.06	720.66	1.28
0	0	0	0	0	0	0	0	0	0	0	0	0	32	0.2	0	0	0	170	0
0	0	0	0	0	0	0	0	0	0	0	0	0	32	0.2	0	0	0	200	0
1.79	0.39	0	0	0	0.45	0.02	0.03	0.03	0.23	0	1.8	0.03	9	0.16	2.55	17.55	15.3	60.3	0.07
4.26	0.99	0	0	0	169.2	1.41	0.09	0.64	0.24	0.14	28.2	0.87	315.84	0.85	39.48	318.66	431.46	217.14	1.49
0	0	0	0	0	4.8	0	0.01	0.13	1.96	0.06	33	0.11	42	0.6	37.8	90	196.8	111.6	0.65
0.64	0.2	0	0	0	0.64	0.03	0.03	0.03	0.3	0.01	1.6	0	10.24	0.46	4.32	9.92	33.12	56	0.06
0	0	0	0	0	0	0	0	0	0	0	0	0	0	0	0	0	0	115	0
0	0	0	0	0	0	0	0	0	0	0	0	0	0	0	0	0	0	160	0
0	0	0	0	0	0	0	0	0	0	0	0	0	0	0	0	0	0	310	0
0	0	0	0	0	100	0	0.15	0.17	1.9	0.2	20	0	0	1	0	16	0	170	0
2.56	0.6	0	0	0	56.13	0	0	0	0.03	0	0	0	2.27	0.4	5.95	22.4	55.57	51.88	0.08
2.56	0.67	0	0	0	0	0	0	0	0	0	0	0	0.85	0.05	0.57	0.85	9.92	11.06	0
2.55	0.66	0	0	0	34.59	0	0	0.01	0.19	0	0.28	0	0.57	0.02	0.57	1.13	55	57.83	0
2.49	0.65	0	0	0	64.07	0	0	0	0	0	0	0	0.85	0.03	0.28	11.06	10.49	25.52	0
0	2	0	0	0	0	0	0.06	0.34	0	0	0	0	160	0	0	200	300	100	0
0	2	0	0	0	0	2.4	0.12	0.34	0	0	0	0	160	0	0	160	300	160	0
0	2	0	0	0	0	2.4	0.12	0.27	0	0	0	0	160	0.4	0	160	320	140	0
0	2	0	0	0	0	2.4	0.12	0.34	0	0	0	0	160	0	0	160	320	160	0
0	2	0	0	0	0	0	0.06	0.34	0	0	0	0	240	0	0	200	360	160	0
0	2	0	0	0	0	0	0.12	0.27	0	0	0	0	160	0.8	0	200	420	140	0
0	2	0	0	0	0	0	0.06	0.27	0	0	0	0	160	0.4	0	160	380	140	0
0	4	0	0	0	0	0	0.12	0.27	0	0	0	0	160	0.4	0	0	340	160	0
0	2	0	0	0	0	0	0.06	0.34	0	0	0	0	160	0	0	200	320	120	0

USDA ID Code	Food Name	Weight in Grams*	Quantity of Units	Unit of Measure	Protein (gm)	Fat (gm)	Carbohydrates (gm)	Kcalories	Caffeine (gm)	Fiber (gm)	Cholesterol (mg)	Saturated Fat (gm)
41328	Frozen Dessert, Praline and Caramel-Healthy Choice	132.969	1	Cup	6	4	52	260	0	0	10	0
41329	Frozen Dessert, Rocky Road-Healthy Choice	132.969	1	Cup	6	4	64	320	0	0	10	0
41330	Frozen Dessert, Vanilla-Healthy Choice	132.969	1	Cup	8	4	42	240	0	0	10	0
	Frozen Yogurt - low fat	72	0-Jan	Cup	3	3	22	120	0	0	10	2
19263	Fruit and Juice Bars	77	1	Bar	0.92	0.08	15.55	63.14	0	0	0	0
19381	Fudge, Brown Sugar w/ Nuts	14	1	Piece	0.41	1.41	10.86	55.44	0	0	0.84	0.25
19100	Fudge, Chocolate	17	1	Piece	0.29	1.45	13.52	64.77	0	0.14	2.38	0.88
19101	Fudge, Chocolate w/ Nuts	19	1	Piece	0.65	3.06	13.83	80.94	0	0.25	2.66	1.07
19102	Fudge, Peanut Butter	16	1	Piece	0.59	1.04	12.53	59.36	0	0	0.64	0.24
19103	Fudge, Vanilla	16	1	Piece	0.18	0.86	13.17	59.04	0	0	2.56	0.54
19104	Fudge, Vanilla w/ Nuts	15	1	Piece	0.44	2	11.28	62.25	0	0.09	2.1	0.56
19215	Gelatin Pops	44	1	Each	0.53	0.04	7.35	30.8	0	0	0	0
18172	Gingersnaps	7	1	Each	0.39	0.69	5.38	29.12	0	0.15	0	0.12
19105	Goobers	1	1	Piece	0.14	0.34	0.49	5.13	0.22	0	0.09	0.12
62684	Granola Bar, Low-Fat	28	1	Each	2	2	21	110	0	1	0	0
19016	Granola Bars, Hard, Almond	28.35	1	Each	2.18	7.23	17.58	140.33	0	0	0	3.55
19017	Granola Bars, Hard, Chocolate Chip	28.35	1	Each	2.07	4.62	20.44	124.17	0	1.25	0	3.23
19019	Granola Bars, Hard, Peanut	28.35	1	Each	3.12	6.07	18.06	135.8	0	0	0	0.71
19420	Granola Bars, Hard, Peanut Butter	28.35	1	Each	2.78	6.75	17.66	136.93	0	0	0	0.91
19015	Granola Bars, Hard, Plain	28.35	1	Each	2.86	5.61	18.26	133.53	0	1.5	0	0.67
19404	Granola Bars, Soft, Chocolate Chip	28.35	1	Each	2.07	4.71	19.59	119.07	0	1.36	0.28	2.89
19406	Granola Bars, Soft, Nut and Raisin	28.35	1	Each	2.27	5.78	18.03	128.71	0	1.59	0.28	2.7
19021	Granola Bars, Soft, Peanut Butter	28.35	1	Each	2.98	4.48	18.26	120.77	0	1.22	0.28	1.03
19027	Granola Bars, Soft, Peanut Butter and Choc Chip	28.35	1	Each	2.78	5.67	17.63	122.47	0	1.19	0.28	1.58
19020	Granola Bars, Soft, Plain	28.35	1	Each	2.1	4.88	19.08	125.59	0	1.3	0.28	2.05
19022	Granola Bars, Soft, Raisin	28.35	1	Each	2.15	5.05	18.82	127.01	0	1.19	0.28	2.71
19106	Gumdrops	3.5	1	Each	0	0	3.46	13.51	0	0	0	0
	Ice Cream - fat free	72	0.5	Cup	4	0	23	100	0	0	0	0
	Ice Cream - Haagen Dazs - Low Fat	92	0.5	Cup	7	2.5	29	170	0	0	0	0
	Ice Cream - light	67	0.5	Cup	3	4.5	18	130	0	0	35	2.5
	Ice Cream - Starbucks	99	0.5	Cup	4	13	30	250	0	0	60	8
	Ice Cream - Starbucks - Low Fat	99	0.5	Cup	5	3	31	170	0	0	10	1.5
18271	Ice Cream Cones, Cake or Wafer-type	4	1.5	Each	0.32	0.28	3.16	16.68	0	0.16	0	0.04
18272	Ice Cream Cones, Sugar, Rolled-type	10	1.5	Each	0.79	0.38	8.41	40.2	0	0.46	0	0.06
62640	Ice Cream Sandwich	63	1	Each	3	6	27	170	0	1	10	3
19270	Ice Cream, Chocolate	91	0.5	Cup	4.2	14.9	20.2	232	1.5	0	0	0
19090	Ice Cream, French Vanilla, Soft-serve	88	0.5	Cup	4.3	11.2	19.2	185	0	0	78	6.4
19271	Ice Cream, Strawberry	90	0.5	Cup	4.22	11.09	36.43	253.44	0	0	38.28	0
19095	Ice Cream, Vanilla	90	0.5	Cup	4.62	14.52	31.15	265.32	0	0	58.08	8.96
19089	Ice Cream, Vanilla, Rich	90	0.5	Cup	4.65	21.54	29.79	320.46	0	0	81.11	13.26
19088	Ice Milk, Vanilla	66	0.5	Cup	2.5	2.8	15	92	0	0	9	1.7
19096	Ice Milk, Vanilla, Soft Serve	88	0.5	Cup	4.3	2.3	19.2	111	0	0	11	1.4
19283	Ice Pops	52	1	Bar	0	0	9.83	37.44	0	0	0	0
19717	Ice Pops, w/ Added Ascorbic Acid	52	1	Bar	0	0	9.83	37.44	0	0	0	0
19173	Jello	140	0.5	Cup	1.7	0	19.6	83	0	0	0	0
19108	Jellybeans	1.1	1	Each	0	0.01	1.02	4.04	0	0	0	0
19109	Kit Kat Wafer Bar	46	1	Bar	3.08	13.11	28.47	234.6	5.06	0.41	11.5	7.67
19110	Krackel Chocolate Bar	47	1	Bar	2.91	13.07	29.09	235.94	8.46	0	8.93	5.55
19107	Lollipop	6	1	Each	0	0	5.89	22.38	0	0	0	0
19140	M&M's Peanut	49	1	Pkg	5.24	13.18	28.91	242.55	0	1.57	6.37	0
19141	M&M's Plain	48	1	Pkg	3.02	10.66	32.74	228.48	0	1.49	7.2	0
62667	M&M's, Almond	42	1	Pkg	4	13	25	230	0	2	5	4
19116	Marshmallows	46	1	Cup	0.83	0.09	37.4	146.28	0	0.05	0	0
19120	Milk Chocolate	44	1	Bar	3.04	13.46	26.09	225.72	11	1.54	9.68	8.09
19126	Milk Chocolate Coated Peanuts	28.35	1	Ounce	3.71	9.5	14	147.14	6.24	1.19	2.55	4.14

Monounsaturated Fat (gm)	Polyunsaturated Fat (gm)	Vitamin D (mg)	Vitamin K (mg)	Vitamin E (mg)	Vitamin A (re)	Vitamin C (mg)	Thiamin (mg)	Riboflavin (mg)	Niacin (mg)	Vitamin B6 (mg)	Folate (mg)	Vitamin B12 (mcg)	Calcium (mg)	Iron (mg)	Magnesium (mg)	Phosphorus (mg)	Potassium (mg)	Sodium (mg)	Zinc (mg)
0	2	0	0	0	0	0	0.06	0.34	0	0	0	0	160	0	0	200	320	140	0
0	2	0	0	0	0	0	0.06	0.34	0	0	0	0	160	0	0	200	380	140	0
0	2	0	0	0	0	0	0.12	0.51	0	0	0	0	240	0	0	200	360	120	0
0	0	0	0	0	0	0	0	0	0	0	0	0	64	0	0	0	0	55	0
0	0	0	0	0	2.31	7.32	0.01	0.01	0.12	0.02	4.62	0	3.85	0.15	3.08	4.62	40.81	3.08	0.04
0.34	0.76	0	0	0	2.38	0.08	0.01	0.01	0.03	0.01	1.54	0	15.54	0.25	6.86	12.04	52.36	13.72	0.09
0.44	0.05	0	0	0.02	7.82	0.03	0	0.01	0.02	0	0.34	0.01	7.14	0.08	4.25	9.86	17.51	10.54	0.07
0.82	1.03	0	0	0.08	8.93	0.11	0.01	0.02	0.04	0.02	1.9	0.01	9.5	0.14	8.55	17.67	30.02	11.4	0.14
0.48	0.27	0	0	0	1.6	0.03	0	0.01	0.24	0.01	1.76	0.01	6.72	0.04	3.52	10.4	20.96	11.68	0.07
0.25	0.03	0	0	0.03	8	0.03	0	0.01	0	0	0.16	0.01	6.24	0.01	0.8	5.12	8	10.72	0.02
0.5	0.83	0	0	0.07	6.9	0.09	0.01	0.01	0.03	0.01	1.5	0.01	7.05	0.06	4.05	10.65	16.95	9.15	0.08
0	0	0	0	0	0	0	0	0	0	0	0	0	0.88	0.01	0.44	0	0.88	20.24	0.01
0.39	0.1	0	0	0	0	0	0.01	0.02	0.23	0.01	0.42	0	5.39	0.45	3.43	5.81	24.22	45.78	0.04
0.15	0.05	0	0	0	0	0	0	0	0.05	0	0.08	0	1.27	0.01	1.19	2.96	5.02	0.41	0.02
0	0	0	0	0	0	0	0	0	0	0	0	0	0	0.2	0	0	0	70	0
2.19	1.07	0	0	0	1.13	0	0.08	0.02	0.17	0.01	3.4	0	9.07	0.71	22.96	64.64	77.4	72.58	0.45
0.75	0.36	0	0	0	1.13	0.03	0.05	0.03	0.16	0.02	3.69	0	21.83	0.86	20.41	57.83	71.16	97.52	0.55
1.63	3.37	0	0	0	0.85	0	0.05	0.02	0.41	0.02	6.52	0	11.06	0.71	31.19	85.05	86.47	78.81	0.59
1.98	3.42	0	0	0	0.57	0.06	0.06	0.03	0.56	0.03	5.1	0	11.62	0.68	15.59	39.41	82.5	80.23	0.35
1.24	3.42	0	0	0	4.25	0.26	0.07	0.03	0.45	0.02	6.52	0	17.29	0.84	27.5	78.53	95.26	83.35	0.43
1	0.56	0	0	0	1.42	0	0.06	0.04	0.27	0.03	6.24	0.05	26.37	0.72	22.11	65.21	96.39	77.11	0.43
1.2	1.56	0	0	0	1.13	0	0.05	0.05	0.74	0.03	8.51	0.07	23.81	0.62	25.8	68.32	111.13	72.01	0.45
1.87	1.21	0	0	0	0.57	0	0.06	0.04	0.89	0.03	9.07	0.06	25.8	0.6	24.38	70.88	82.5	115.95	0.53
2.37	1.31	0	0	0	0.57	0	0.03	0.03	0.89	0.03	9.36	0.13	22.68	0.55	24.95	74.28	106.88	92.99	0.48
1.08	1.51	0	0	0	0	0	0.08	0.05	0.15	0.03	6.8	0.11	29.77	0.73	20.98	65.21	92.14	78.81	0.43
0.81	0.91	0	0	0	0	0	0.07	0.05	0.31	0.03	5.95	0.05	28.63	0.69	20.41	62.37	102.63	79.95	0.37
0	0	0	0	0	0	0	0	0	0	0	0	0	0.11	0.01	0.04	0.04	0.18	1.54	0
0	0	0	0	0	0	0	0	0	0	0	0	0	120	0	0	0	0	65	0
0	0	0	0	0	0	0	0	0	0	0	0	0	160	0	0	0	0	50	0
0	0	0	0	0	0	0	0	0	0	0	0	0	80	0	0	0	0	50	0
0	0	0	0	0	0	0	0	0	0	0	0	0	120	0	0	0	0	15	0
0	0	0	0	0	0	0	0	0	0	0	0	0	80	0	0	0	0	65	0
0.11	0.1	0	0	0	0	0	0.01	0.01	0.18	0	0.2	0	1	0.14	1.04	3.88	4.48	5.72	0.03
0.15	0.15	0	0	0	0	0	0.05	0.04	0.51	0.01	0.5	0	4.4	0.44	3.1	10.3	14.5	32	0.08
0	0	0	0	0	20	0	0	0	0	0	0	0	48	0.4	0	0	0	140	0
0	0	0	0	0	0	0	0.01	0.19	0	0.6	0	0	84	0.46	0	96	200	45	0
3	0.4	0	0	0	132	1	0.04	0.16	0.1	0.06	8	0.43	113	0.19	10	100	152	52	0.45
0	0	0	0	0	102.96	10.16	0.06	0.34	0.22	0.07	15.84	0.4	158.4	0.28	18.48	132	248.16	79.2	0.45
4.18	0.54	0	0	0	154.44	0.79	0.05	0.32	0.15	0.06	6.6	0.51	168.96	0.12	18.48	138.6	262.68	105.6	0.91
6.2	0.8	0	0	0	244.66	0.93	0.05	0.22	0.11	0.05	6.65	0.48	155.57	0.07	14.63	126.32	211.42	74.46	0.53
0.8	0.1	0	0	0	31	1	0.04	0.17	0.1	0.04	4	0.44	92	0.07	10	72	139	56	0.29
0.7	0.1	0	0	0	26	1	0.07	0.17	0.1	0.04	5	0.44	138	0.05	12	106	194	62	0.47
0	0	0	0	0	0	0	0	0	0	0	0	0	0	0	0.52	0	2.08	6.24	0.01
0	0	0	0	0	0	5.56	0	0	0	0	0	0	0	0	0.52	0	2.08	6.24	0.01
0	0	0	0	0	0	0	0	0	0	0	0	0	3	0.04	1	31	1	59	0.04
0	0	0	0	0	0	0	0	0	0	0	0	0	0.03	0.01	0.02	0.04	0.41	0.28	0
3.58	0.22	0	0	0.36	13.8	0.83	0.03	0.12	0.19	0.02	0	0.32	82.8	0.39	20.24	80.04	141.68	46.46	0.46
3.3	2.6	0	0	0	5.64	0.19	0.02	0.14	0.21	0.02	3.76	0.27	84.13	0.38	25.85	103.87	160.74	63.92	0.57
0	0	0	0	0	0	0	0	0	0	0	0	0	0.18	0.02	0.18	0.18	0.3	2.28	0
0	0	0	0	2.72	4.41	0	0.03	0.1	1.56	0.09	27.44	0.17	65.17	0.73	40.18	134.26	191.1	45.57	0.74
0	0	0	0	0.6	12.48	0	0.03	0.12	0.26	0.03	3.84	0.2	81.12	0.73	32.16	93.6	187.68	48.96	0.61
0	0	0	0	0	0	0	0	0	0	0	0	0	72	0.4	0	0	0	20	0
0	0	0	0	0	0	0	0	0	0.04	0	0.46	0	1.38	0.11	0.92	3.68	2.3	21.62	0.02
4.39	0.4	0	0	0.55	21.12	0.18	0.03	0.13	0.14	0.02	3.08	0.17	84.04	0.61	26.4	95.04	169.4	36.08	0.61
3.66	1.23	0	0	0.72	0	0	0.03	0.05	1.2	0.06	2.27	0.13	29.48	0.37	25.52	60.1	142.32	11.62	0.53

USDA ID Code	Food Name	Weight in Grams*	Quantity of Units	Unit of Measure	Protein (gm)	Fat (gm)	Carbohydrates (gm)	Kcalories	Caffeine (gm)	Fiber (gm)	Cholesterol (mg)	Saturated Fat (gm)
19127	Milk Chocolate Coated Raisins	28.35	1	Ounce	1.16	4.2	19.36	110.57	7.09	1.19	0.85	2.49
19132	Milk Chocolate w/ Almonds	41	1	Bar	3.69	14.1	21.81	215.66	9.02	2.54	7.79	6.96
19135	Milky Way Bar	60	1	Bar	2.7	9.12	43.5	251.4	0	0.96	12	4.73
18177	Molasses Cookies	15	1	Each	0.84	1.92	11.07	64.5	0	0	0	0.35
19142	Mounds Candy Bar	20	1	Bar	0.72	4.32	11.58	72.2	0	0.64	0	2.3
19143	Mr. Goodbar Chocolate Bar	50	1	Bar	6.3	16.15	25.65	257	5	2.15	10	9.03
19145	Nestle Crunch	40	1	Bar	2.48	10.4	25.68	197.6	9.6	1.04	7.6	5.74
18200	Oatmeal Cookies, Dietary	7	1	Each	0.34	1.26	4.89	31.43	0	0	0	0.56
18178	Oatmeal Cookies, Regular	18	1	Each	1.12	3.26	12.37	81	0	0.56	0	0.6
18179	Oatmeal Cookies, Soft-type	15	1	Each	0.92	2.21	9.86	61.35	0	0.41	1.35	0.43
18199	Oreos, Dietary	10	1	Each	0.45	2.21	6.77	46.1	0	0	0	1.04
18166	Oreos, Regular	10	1	Each	0.47	2.06	7.03	47.2	0	0.3	0	0.41
18168	Oreos, w/ Extra Creme Filling	13	1	Each	0.47	3.28	8.85	65	0	0	0	0.63
19031	Oriental Mix, Rice-based	28.35	1	Ounce	5.67	11.54	9.38	154.51	0	3.74	0	5.04
19147	Peanut Bar	40	1	Bar	6.2	13.48	18.96	208.8	0	1.32	2.8	1.72
19148	Peanut Brittle	28.35	1	Ounce	2.13	5.41	19.65	128.43	0	0.57	3.69	1.42
18185	Peanut Butter Cookies, Regular	15	1	Each	1.44	3.54	8.84	71.55	0	0	0.15	0.8
18186	Peanut Butter Cookies, Soft-type	15	1	Each	0.8	3.66	8.66	68.55	0	0.26	0	0.81
18201	Peanut Butter Sandwich Cookies, Dietary	10	1	Each	1	3.4	5.08	53.5	0	0	0	1.18
18190	Peanut Butter Sandwich Cookies, Regular	14	1	Each	1.23	2.95	9.18	66.92	0	0	0	0.63
19034	Popcorn, Air-popped	8	1	Cup	0.96	0.34	6.23	30.56	0	1.21	0	0.05
19806	Popcorn, Air-popped, White Popcorn	8	1	Cup	0.96	0.34	6.23	30.56	0	0	0	0.05
19036	Popcorn, Cakes	10	1	Cake	0.97	0.31	8.01	38.4	0	0.29	0	0.05
19038	Popcorn, Caramel-coated, w/ Peanuts	35.182	1	Cup	2.25	2.74	28.39	140.73	0	1.34	0	0.37
19039	Popcorn, Caramel-coated, w/o Peanuts	35.2	1	Cup	1.34	4.51	27.84	151.71	0	1.83	1.76	1.27
19040	Popcorn, Cheese-flavor	6	1	Cup	1.02	3.65	5.68	57.86	0	1.09	1.21	0.71
62649	Popcorn, Microwave	14	4	Cup	0.75	3	4.25	42.5	0	0.75	0	0.75
62650	Popcorn, Microwave, Low-Fat	14	4	Cup	0.67	1	3.67	23.33	0	0.5	0	0.17
	Popcorn, Microwave-Pop Secret-94% Fat Free	5	1	Serving	1	0	4	20	0	0	0	0
19035	Popcorn, Oil-popped	11	1	Cup	0.99	3.09	6.29	55	0	1.1	0	0.54
19807	Popcorn, Oil-popped, White Popcorn	11	1	Cup	0.99	3.09	6.29	55	0	0	0	0.54
62602	Popsicles	56	1	Each	0	0	11	40	0	0	0	0
19408	Pork Skins, Barbecue-flavor	28.35	1	Ounce	16.41	9.02	0.45	152.52	0	0	32.6	3.28
19041	Pork Skins, Plain	28.35	1	Ounce	17.38	8.87	0	154.51	0	0	26.93	3.22
	Potato Chips - Baked Lays	28	1	Ounce	2	1.5	23	110	0	0	0	0
	Potato Chips - Barbeque	28	1	Ounce	2	10	15	160	0	0	0	1.5
19042	Potato Chips, Barbecue-flavor	28.35	1	Ounce	2.18	9.19	14.97	139.2	0	1.25	0	2.28
19421	Potato Chips, Cheese-flavor	28.35	1	Ounce	2.41	7.71	16.36	140.62	0	0	1.13	2.44
19422	Potato Chips, Light	28.35	1	Ounce	2.01	5.9	18.97	133.53	0	0	0	1.18
19411	Potato Chips, Plain, Salted	28.35	1	Ounce	1.98	9.81	15	151.96	0	1.28	0	3.11
19811	Potato Chips, Plain, Unsalted	28.35	1	Ounce	1.98	9.81	15	151.96	0	0	0	3.11
19412	Potato Chips, Pringles, Cheese-flavor	28.35	1	Ounce	1.98	10.49	14.35	156.21	0	0	1.13	2.71
19045	Potato Chips, Pringles, Light	28.35	1	Ounce	1.59	7.29	18.4	142.03	0	1.02	0	1.45
19410	Potato Chips, Pringles, Plain	28.35	1	Ounce	1.67	10.89	14.46	158.19	0	1.02	0	2.68
19046	Potato Chips, Pringles, Sour-cream&onion-flavor	28.35	1	Ounce	1.87	10.49	14.54	155.07	0	0	0.85	2.68
19043	Potato Chips, Sour-cream-and-onion-flavor	28.35	1	Ounce	2.3	9.61	14.6	150.54	0	1.47	1.98	2.52
11920	Potato Chips, w/o Salt Added	28.35	1	Ounce	1.82	10.03	14.7	148.27	0	1.36	0	2.57
19415	Potato Sticks	28.35	1	Ounce	1.9	9.75	15.11	147.99	0	0.96	0	2.52
62693	Power Bar	65	1	Each	10	2.5	45	230	0	3	0	0.5
19216	Praline	39	1	Piece	1.09	9.48	24.18	177.06	0	0	0	0.73
19047	Pretzels, Hard, Plain, Salted	28.35	1	Ounce	2.58	0.99	22.45	108.01	0	0.91	0	0.21
19814	Pretzels, Hard, Plain, Unsalted	28.35	1	Ounce	2.58	0.99	22.45	108.01	0	0.79	0	0.21
19050	Pretzels, Hard, Whole-wheat	28.35	1	Ounce	3.15	0.74	23.02	102.63	0	0	0	0.16
19072	Pudding Pops, Chocolate	47	1	Each	1.88	2.21	11.94	71.91	0	0.19	0.94	0
19073	Pudding Pops, Vanilla	47	1	Each	1.88	2.07	12.6	74.73	0	0	0.94	0

Monounsaturated Fat (gm)	Polyunsaturated Fat (gm)	Vitamin D (mg)	Vitamin K (mg)	Vitamin E (mg)	Vitamin A (re)	Vitamin C (mg)	Thiamin (mg)	Riboflavin (mg)	Niacin (mg)	Vitamin B6 (mg)	Folate (mcg)	Vitamin B12 (mcg)	Calcium (mg)	Iron (mg)	Magnesium (mg)	Phosphorus (mg)	Potassium (mg)	Sodium (mg)	Zinc (mg)
1.34	0.14	0	0	0.27	1.98	0.06	0.02	0.05	0.11	0.03	1.42	0.06	24.38	0.48	12.76	40.54	145.72	10.21	0.22
5.53	0.93	0	0	5.18	5.74	0.08	0.02	0.18	0.3	0.02	4.51	0.22	91.84	0.67	36.9	108.24	182.04	30.34	0.55
3.28	0.32	0	0	0.39	28.2	0.54	0.02	0.13	0.21	0.03	5.4	0.31	78	0.46	20.4	98.4	144.6	144	0.43
1.11	0.27	0	0	0	0	0	0.05	0.04	0.45	0.04	1.05	0	11.1	0.96	7.8	14.25	51.9	68.85	0.07
1.33	0.15	0	0	0.38	0.2	0.02	0	0.01	0.01	0.01	0.6	0	4.6	0.75	13.6	24	42	25	0.21
5.65	0.76	0	0	0.62	5	0	0.03	0.14	2.36	0.06	36	0.23	55.5	0.6	47.5	140	225	17	0.9
3.81	0.4	0	0	0	6	0.12	0.02	0.11	0.2	0.03	3.6	0.15	67.6	0.26	18.4	71.2	137.6	59.2	0.44
0.53	0.11	0	0	0	0.14	0.04	0.02	0.01	0.14	0	0.56	0	3.22	0.23	2.24	10.08	12.25	0.63	0.05
1.87	0.49	0	0	0	0.36	0.07	0.05	0.04	0.4	0.01	1.26	0	6.66	0.46	5.94	24.84	25.56	68.94	0.14
1.22	0.35	0	0	0	0.6	0.05	0.03	0.03	0.27	0.01	1.2	0	13.5	0.42	4.5	31.35	20.25	52.35	0.07
0.91	0.15	0	0	0	0.1	0	0.04	0.03	0.31	0	1	0.01	5.8	0.52	6.6	17.7	29.5	24.3	0.11
1.18	0.27	0	0	0	0	0	0.01	0.02	0.21	0	0.5	0	2.6	0.39	4.5	9.8	17.5	60.4	0.08
1.91	0.43	0	0	0	0	0	0.01	0.02	0.2	0	0.52	0	3.12	0.37	4.42	11.83	15.86	64.09	0.08
2.96	2.66	0	0	0	1.42	0.23	0.08	0.04	2.98	0.05	24.66	0	21.83	0.78	39.69	111.98	146.57	235.02	1.3
6.71	4.27	0	0	0.39	20.4	0	0.04	0.06	3.17	0.04	24	0.01	31.2	0.39	29.6	61.2	162.8	96.4	0.55
2.4	1.33	0	0	0.46	13.32	0	0.05	0.01	0.99	0.03	19.85	0	8.51	0.39	14.18	31.47	58.97	128.14	0.27
1.32	1.22	0	0	0	1.35	0	0.03	0.03	0.64	0.01	4.8	0.01	5.25	0.38	6.75	12.9	25.05	62.25	0.08
1.99	0.66	0	0	0	0	0	0.04	0.02	0.32	0.01	0.75	0	1.8	0.13	4.8	13.05	16.05	50.4	0.08
1.53	0.51	0	0	0	0	0	0.02	0.01	0.5	0.01	3.3	0	5.4	0.23	5	18.8	9.4	41.2	0.18
1.54	0.58	0	0	0	0.14	0.01	0.05	0.04	0.52	0.01	2.1	0.01	7.42	0.36	6.86	26.32	26.88	51.52	0.15
0.09	0.15	0	0	0.01	1.6	0	0.02	0.02	0.16	0.02	1.84	0	0.8	0.21	10.48	24	24.08	0.32	0.28
0.09	0.15	0	0	0	0.24	0	0.02	0.02	0.16	0.02	1.84	0	0.8	0.21	10.48	24	24.08	0.32	0.28
0.09	0.14	0	0	0.07	0.7	0	0.01	0.02	0.6	0.02	1.8	0	0.9	0.19	15.9	27.7	32.7	28.8	0.4
0.96	1.15	0	0	0.53	2.11	0	0.02	0.04	0.7	0.07	5.63	0	23.22	1.38	28.15	44.68	124.9	103.79	0.44
1.01	1.58	0	0	0.42	3.52	0	0.02	0.02	0.77	0.01	0.7	0	15.14	0.61	12.32	29.22	38.37	72.51	0.2
1.07	1.69	0	0	0.01	4.84	0.06	0.01	0.03	0.16	0.03	1.21	0.06	12.43	0.25	10.01	39.71	28.71	97.79	0.22
0	0	0	0	0	0	0	0	0	0	0	0	0	0	0.05	0	0	0	72.5	0
0	0	0	0	0	0	0	0	0	0	0	0	0	0	0.07	0	0	0	55	0
0	0	0	0	0	0	0	0	0	0	0	0	0	0	0	0	0	0	40	0
0.9	1.48	0	0	0.01	1.65	0.03	0.01	0.01	0.17	0.02	1.87	0	1.1	0.31	11.88	27.5	24.75	97.24	0.29
0.9	1.48	0	0	0	0.22	0.03	0.01	0.01	0.17	0.02	1.87	0	1.1	0.31	11.88	27.5	24.75	97.24	0.29
0	0	0	0	0	0	1.2	0	0	0	0	0	0	0	0	0	0	0	10	0
4.26	0.98	0	0	0	51.6	0.43	0.02	0.12	0.95	0.04	8.79	0.04	12.19	0.29	0	62.37	51.03	756.09	0.2
4.19	1.03	0	0	0	11.06	0.14	0.03	0.08	0.44	0.01	0	0.18	8.51	0.25	3.12	24.1	36	521.07	0.16
0	0	0	0	0	0	0	0	0	0	0	0	0	48	0.4	0	0	0	150	0
0	0	0	0	0	0	6.4	0	0	0	0	0	0	0	0.2	0	0	0	300	0
1.85	4.64	0	0	1.42	6.24	9.61	0.06	0.06	1.33	0.18	23.53	0	14.18	0.55	21.26	52.73	357.49	212.63	0.27
2.19	2.71	0	0	0	2.27	15.34	0.04	0.04	1.42	0.1	0	0	20.41	0.52	21.26	84.77	433.19	224.82	0.26
1.36	3.1	0	0	0	0	7.29	0.06	0.08	1.98	0.19	7.65	0	5.95	0.38	25.23	54.72	494.42	139.48	0.02
2.79	3.45	0	0	1.38	0	8.82	0.05	0.06	1.08	0.19	12.76	0	6.8	0.46	18.99	46.78	361.46	168.4	0.31
2.79	3.45	0	0	0	0	8.82	0.05	0.06	1.08	0.19	12.76	0	6.8	0.46	18.99	46.78	361.46	2.27	0.31
2.02	5.29	0	0	0	0	2.41	0.05	0.03	0.74	0.15	5.1	0	31.19	0.45	15.03	46.21	108.01	214.04	0.18
1.68	3.82	0	0	1.42	0	3.4	0.05	0.02	1.19	0.22	6.52	0	9.64	0.43	17.86	43.66	284.92	121.34	0.17
2.06	5.66	0	0	1.38	0	2.32	0.06	0.03	0.89	0.04	1.98	0	6.8	0.43	16.44	44.51	285.77	185.98	0.17
2.02	5.32	0	0	0	27.78	2.69	0.05	0.03	0.71	0.13	6.52	0	18.14	0.4	15.59	47.91	140.62	204.12	0.2
1.74	4.94	0	0	0	5.95	10.57	0.05	0.06	1.14	0.19	17.58	0.28	20.41	0.45	20.98	49.9	377.34	177.19	0.28
1.77	5.15	0	0	2.23	0	11.79	0.04	0.01	1.19	0.14	12.81	0	6.8	0.34	16.73	43.38	367.98	2.27	0.3
1.75	5.07	0	0	1.38	0	13.41	0.03	0.03	1.36	0.09	11.34	0	5.1	0.64	18.14	48.76	350.69	70.88	0.28
1.5	0.5	0	0	0	0	0	1.5	1.7	19	2	200	2	360	3.5	122.5	280	0	90	5.25
5.92	2.35	0	0	0	1.95	0.27	0.12	0.02	0.13	0.03	5.46	0	12.09	0.46	20.28	42.51	82.29	24.18	0.79
0.39	0.35	0	0	0.06	0	0	0.13	0.18	1.49	0.03	23.53	0	10.21	1.22	9.92	32.04	41.39	486.2	0.24
0.39	0.35	0	0	0.06	0	0	0.13	0.18	1.49	0.03	23.53	0	10.21	1.22	9.92	32.04	41.39	81.93	0.24
0.29	0.24	0	0	0	0	0.28	0.12	0.08	1.85	0.08	15.31	0	7.94	0.76	8.51	35.44	121.91	57.55	0.18
0	0	0	0	0.01	15.51	0.19	0.02	0.08	0.06	0.01	1.41	0.25	66.27	0.22	9.87	52.64	105.28	77.55	0.17
0	0	0	0	0.01	24.44	0.14	0.02	0.09	0.02	0.02	2.35	0.17	60.63	0.03	5.17	47.47	64.86	49.82	0.16

USDA ID Code	Food Name	Weight in Grams*	Quantity of Units	Unit of Measure	Protein (gm)	Fat (gm)	Carbohydrates (gm)	Kcalories	Caffeine (gm)	Fiber (gm)	Cholesterol (mg)	Saturated Fat (gm)
19311	Pudding, Banana	298.116	1	Cup	7.15	10.73	63.2	378.61	0	0	0	1.67
19167	Pudding, Bread	252	1	Cup	13.1	14.87	61.99	423.36	0	0	166.32	5.77
19183	Pudding, Chocolate	298.116	1	Cup	8.05	11.92	67.97	396.49	14.91	2.98	8.94	2.12
19380	Pudding, Lemon	298.116	1	Cup	0.3	8.94	74.53	372.65	0	0	0	1.34
19193	Pudding, Rice	298.116	1	Cup	5.96	22.36	65.59	485.93	0	0	2.98	3.49
19218	Pudding, Tapioca	298.116	1	Cup	5.96	11.03	57.83	354.76	0	0.3	2.98	1.79
19201	Pudding, Vanilla	298.116	1	Cup	6.86	10.73	65.29	387.55	0	0.3	20.87	1.7
18191	Raisin Cookies, Soft-type	15	1	Each	0.62	2.04	10.2	60.15	0	0	0.3	0.53
19149	Raisinets	1	10	Piece	0.05	0.16	0.71	4.12	0.25	0	0.04	0.07
62607	Reduced Fat Chocolate Chip Cookies	0.448	2	Each	1	1.25	10.5	50	0	0.02	0	0.02
62595	Reduced Fat Chocolate Sandwich Cookies-SnackWell	12.5	2	Each	0.5	1.25	10.5	50	0	0.5	0	0.25
62593	Reduced Fat Classic Golden Crackers-SnackWell	2.33	6	Each	0.17	0.17	1.83	9.99	0	0	0	0
62594	Reduced Fat Creme Sandwich Cookies-SnackWell	13	2	Each	0.5	1.25	10.5	55	0	0.5	0	0.25
62597	Reduced Fat French Onion Snack Crackers-SnackWell	0.938	32	Each	0.06	0.06	0.72	3.75	0	0.03	0.72	0
62598	Reduced Fat Oatmeal Raisin Cookies-SnackWell	13.5	2	Each	1	1.25	10	55	0	0.5	0	0.25
62525	Reduced Fat Zesty Cheese Snack Crackers-SnackWell	0.938	32	Each	0.09	0.06	0.72	3.75	0	0.03	0.16	0.02
19150	Reese's Peanut Butter Cups	7	1	Each	0.77	2.18	3.35	33.95	0.77	0.29	1.05	1.61
19151	Reese's Pieces Candy	55	1	Pkg	7.21	11.39	34.16	257.95	0	2.26	2.2	0
19052	Rice Cakes, Brown Rice, Buckwheat	9	1	Cake	0.81	0.32	7.21	34.2	0	0.34	0	0.06
19817	Rice Cakes, Brown Rice, Buckwheat, Unsalted	9	1	Cake	0.81	0.32	7.21	34.2	0	0	0	0.06
19413	Rice Cakes, Brown Rice, Corn	9	1	Cake	0.76	0.29	7.31	34.65	0	0.26	0	0.06
19414	Rice Cakes, Brown Rice, Multigrain	9	1	Cake	0.77	0.32	7.21	34.83	0	0.27	0	0.05
19818	Rice Cakes, Brown Rice, Multigrain, Unsalted	9	1	Cake	0.77	0.32	7.21	34.83	0	0	0	0.05
19051	Rice Cakes, Brown Rice, Plain	9	1	Cake	0.74	0.25	7.34	34.83	0	0.38	0	0.05
19816	Rice Cakes, Brown Rice, Plain, Unsalted	9	1	Cake	0.74	0.25	7.34	34.83	0	0.38	0	0.05
19416	Rice Cakes, Brown Rice, Rye	9	1	Cake	0.73	0.34	7.19	34.74	0	0.36	0	0.05
62669	Rice Krispie Treats	40	1	Cup	1.33	2	33.33	160	0	0	0	0
	Ruffles - Reduced Fat	28	1	Ounce	2	6.7	18	140	0	0	0	1
19418	Sesame Sticks, Wheat-based, Salted	28.35	1	Ounce	3.09	10.4	13.18	153.37	0	0.79	0	1.84
19820	Sesame Sticks, Wheat-based, Unsalted	28.35	1	Ounce	3.09	10.4	13.18	153.37	0	0	0	1.84
19097	Sherbet, All Flavors	192	1	Cup	2.11	3.84	58.37	264.96	0	0	9.6	2.23
18193	Shortbread Cookies, Pecan	14	1	Each	0.69	4.55	8.16	75.88	0	0.25	4.62	0.99
18192	Shortbread Cookies, Plain	8	1	Each	0.49	1.93	5.16	40.16	0	0	1.6	0.49
19370	Skittles Bite Size Candies	65	1	Pkg	0.2	1.95	62.4	254.8	0	0	0	0
19407	Slim Jims, Smoked	28.35	1	Ounce	6.1	14.06	1.53	155.93	0	0	37.71	5.9
19155	Snickers Bar	61	1	Bar	5.86	13.6	36.78	277.55	0	1.83	7.32	7.29
	Sorbet - Ben & Jerry's	110	0.5	Cup	0	0	32	130	0	0	0	0
62599	Sorbet, All Flavors	180.053	0.5	Cup	0	0	50.01	200.06	0	2	0	0
19164	Special Dark Sweet Chocolate Bar	79	1	Bar	3.71	23.86	48.66	376.04	60.04	4.35	0	0
18203	Sugar Cookies, Dietary	7	1	Each	0.81	0.91	4.85	30.17	0	0	0	0.16
18204	Sugar Cookies, Regular (includes Vanilla)	15	1	Each	0.77	3.17	10.19	71.7	0	0	7.65	0.81
	Sun Chips - original	28	1	Ounce	1	6	20	140	0	0	0	1
19093	Symphony Milk Chocolate Bar	68	1	Bar	5.3	22.03	38.62	354.96	0	0	19.04	0
19113	Syrup, Pancake, w/ Butter	20	1	Tbsp.	0	0.32	14.82	59.2	0	0	0.8	0.2
19382	Taffy	15	1	Piece	0.02	0.5	13.71	56.4	0	0	1.35	0.31
19524	Taro Chips	28.35	1	Ounce	0.65	7.06	19.31	141.18	0	2.04	0	1.82
19159	Three Musketeers Bar	60	1	Bar	1.92	7.74	46.08	249.6	0	0.96	6.6	3.9
18361	Toaster Pastries, Brown-sugar-cinn.	52	1	Each	2.65	7.38	35.41	214.24	0	0	0	1.87
18362	Toaster Pastries, Fruit	52	1	Each	2.44	5.3	36.97	204.36	0	0	0	0.8
19383	Toffee	12	1	Piece	0.13	3.94	7.72	65.04	0	0	12.6	2.45
62655	Tortilla Chips, Low-Fat, Baked	2.181	13	Chips	0.23	0.08	1.85	8.46	0	0.15	0	0
19057	Tortilla Chips, Nacho-flavor	28.35	1	Ounce	2.21	7.26	17.69	141.18	0	1.5	0.85	1.39
19424	Tortilla Chips, Nacho-flavor, Light	28.35	1	Ounce	2.47	4.31	20.3	126.16	0	0	0.85	0.82
19056	Tortilla Chips, Plain	28.35	1	Ounce	1.98	7.43	17.83	142.03	0	1.87	0	1.42
19058	Tortilla Chips, Ranch-flavor	28.35	1	Ounce	2.15	6.75	18.31	138.92	0	0	0.28	1.29

Monounsaturated Fat (gm)	Polyunsaturated Fat (gm)	Vitamin D (mg)	Vitamin K (mg)	Vitamin E (mg)	Vitamin A (re)	Vitamin C (mg)	Thiamin (mg)	Riboflavin (mg)	Niacin (mg)	Vitamin B6 (mg)	Folate (mg)	Vitamin B12 (mcg)	Calcium (mg)	Iron (mg)	Magnesium (mg)	Phosphorus (mg)	Potassium (mg)	Sodium (mg)	Zinc (mg)
4.56	3.96	0	0	0	89.43	1.49	0.06	0.44	0.49	0.06	5.96	0.54	253.4	0.39	23.85	205.7	327.93	584.31	0.83
5.42	2.39	0	0	0	163.8	2.02	0.23	0.56	1.58	0.19	32.76	0	287.28	2.77	47.88	274.68	564.48	582.12	1.31
5.07	4.26	0	0	0.37	32.79	5.37	0.08	0.46	1.03	0.08	8.94	0	268.3	1.52	62.6	238.49	536.61	384.57	1.25
3.88	3.4	0	0	0	0	0.3	0	0.01	0.01	0	0	0	5.96	0.21	2.98	14.91	2.98	417.36	0.09
9.57	8.32	0	0	0	104.34	1.49	0.05	0.21	0.48	0.09	8.94	0.63	155.02	0.89	23.85	202.72	178.87	253.4	1.46
4.71	4.05	0	0	0.27	0	2.09	0.07	0.29	0.93	0.29	11.92	0.33	250.42	0.69	23.85	235.51	310.04	351.78	0.8
4.59	3.99	0	0	0.37	17.89	0	0.07	0.41	0.75	0.03	0	0.3	262.34	0.39	23.85	202.72	336.87	402.46	0.75
1.12	0.27	0	0	0	1.8	0.05	0.03	0.03	0.3	0.01	1.35	0.02	6.9	0.34	3.15	12.45	21	50.7	0.05
0.06	0.02	0	0	0	0.09	0	0	0	0	0	0.05	0	1.08	0.01	0.45	1.44	5.14	0.36	0.01
0.02	0	0	0	0	0	0	0	0	0	0	0	0	0	0.01	0	0	0	2.63	0
0.25	0	0	0	0	0	0	0	0	0	0	0	0	0	0.2	0	0	0	95	0
0	0	0	0	0	0	0	0	0	0	0	0	0	3.99	0.07	0	0	0	23.3	0
0.5	0	0	0	0	0	0	0	0	0	0	0	0	12	0.1	0	0	0	47.5	0
0.02	0	0	0	0	0	0	0	0	0	0	0	0	1.5	0.02	0	0	0	9.06	0
0.25	0.25	0	0	0	0	0	0	0	0	0	0	0	12	0.2	0	0	0	67.5	0
0.02	0	0	0	0	0	0	0	0	0	0	0	0	1.5	0.02	0	0	0	10.94	0
0.15	0.15	0	0	0.09	1.33	0	0	0.01	0.28	0.01	1.96	0.03	5.46	0.08	5.95	16.8	28	20.3	0.1
0	0	0	0	0.73	2.2	0.28	0.03	0.13	3.14	0.07	30.8	0.18	73.15	0.83	44.55	126.5	242	82.5	0.61
0.1	0.1	0	0	0	0	0	0.01	0.01	0.73	0.01	1.89	0	0.99	0.1	13.59	34.2	26.91	10.44	0.23
0.1	0.1	0	0	0	0	0	0.01	0.01	0.73	0.01	1.89	0	0.99	0.1	13.59	34.2	26.91	0.36	0.23
0.1	0.1	0	0	0	0	0	0.01	0.01	0.58	0.01	1.71	0	0.81	0.11	10.26	28.8	24.75	26.19	0.2
0.1	0.13	0	0	0	0	0	0.01	0.02	0.59	0.01	1.8	0	1.89	0.18	12.33	33.3	26.46	22.68	0.23
0.1	0.13	0	0	0	0	0	0.01	0.02	0.59	0.01	1.8	0	1.89	0.18	12.33	33.3	26.46	0.36	0.23
0.09	0.09	0	0	0.06	0.45	0	0.01	0.01	0.7	0.01	1.89	0	0.99	0.13	11.79	32.4	26.1	29.34	0.27
0.09	0.09	0	0	0.01	0.45	0	0.01	0.01	0.7	0.01	1.89	0	0.99	0.13	11.79	32.4	26.1	2.34	0.27
0.12	0.14	0	0	0	0	0	0.01	0.01	0.63	0.01	0.45	0	1.89	0.16	12.96	34.2	27.99	9.9	0.27
1.33	0	0.67	0	0	200	20	0.5	0.57	6.33	0.67	0	0.67	0	1.33	0	21.33	26.67	226.67	0
0	0	0	0	0	0	0	0	0	0	0	0	0	0	0.2	0	0	0	130	0
3.09	4.94	0	0	1.11	2.55	0	0.03	0.02	0.44	0.02	6.24	0	48.2	0.21	12.76	39.12	50.18	421.85	0.33
3.09	4.94	0	0	0	2.55	0	0.03	0.02	0.44	0.02	6.24	0	48.2	0.21	12.76	39.12	50.18	8.22	0.33
1.02	0.15	0	0	0	26.88	8.26	0.05	0.13	0.18	0.07	7.68	0.25	103.68	0.27	15.36	76.8	184.32	88.32	0.92
2.65	0.68	0	0	0	0.28	0.03	0.04	0.03	0.35	0	1.12	0	4.2	0.34	2.52	11.9	10.22	39.34	0.08
1.08	0.25	0	0	0	0.96	0	0.03	0.03	0.27	0	0.72	0.01	2.8	0.22	1.36	8.64	8	36.4	0.04
0	0	0	0	0	0	0	0	0	0	0	0	0	1.95	0.07	0.65	1.95	14.95	29.9	0.01
5.8	1.25	0	0	0	47.91	1.93	0.04	0.12	1.29	0.06	0	0.28	19.28	0.96	5.95	51.03	72.86	419.58	0.69
4.11	0.52	0	0	3.39	18.91	0.18	0.03	0.11	1.82	0.11	24.4	0.25	70.15	0.48	36.6	128.71	198.86	163.48	0.7
0	0	0	0	0	0	0	0	0	0	0	0	0	80	0	0	0	0	10	0
0	0	0	0	0	0	24.01	0	0	0	0	0	0	0	0	0	0	0	20.01	0
0	0	0	0	0.8	1.58	0	0.02	0.19	0.53	0.04	3.16	0	15.01	1.66	90.85	126.4	268.6	7.9	1.19
0.53	0.13	0	0	0	0	0	0.03	0.01	0.22	0	0.49	0	2.1	0.27	0.63	5.67	7.28	0.21	0.02
1.76	0.4	0	0	0	4.05	0.02	0.03	0.03	0.4	0.01	1.65	0.02	3.15	0.32	1.8	12	9.45	53.55	0.06
0	0	0	0	0	0	1.2	0	0	0	0	0	0	0	0	0	0	0	115	0
0	0	0	0	0	8.84	0.27	0.06	0.26	0.22	0.03	4.76	0.27	159.8	0.68	37.4	170	261.8	58.48	0.77
0.09	0.01	0	0	0	3	0	0	0	0	0	0	0	0.4	0.02	0.4	2	0.6	19.6	0.01
0.14	0.02	0	0	0	4.95	0	0	0	0	0	0	0	0.45	0.01	0.15	0.45	0.6	13.35	0
1.26	3.65	0	0	1.39	0	1.42	0.05	0.01	0.15	0.12	5.67	0	17.01	0.34	23.81	37.14	214.04	96.96	0.11
2.57	0.27	0	0	0.28	15.6	0.24	0.02	0.08	0.14	0.01	0	0.13	50.4	0.44	17.4	54.6	79.8	116.4	0.33
4.15	0.96	0	0	0	116.48	0.1	0.19	0.3	2.38	0.22	41.6	0.06	17.68	2.1	12.48	69.16	59.28	220.48	0.33
2.14	2.01	0	0	0	55.12	0.16	0.15	0.19	2.05	0.2	41.6	0.03	13.52	1.81	9.36	57.72	58.24	217.88	0.34
1.14	0.15	0	0	0	38.16	0.02	0	0	0.24	0.01	0	0	4.08	0.01	0.48	3.96	6	22.44	0.02
0	0	0	0	0	0	0	0	0	0	0	0	0	3.69	0	0	0	0	10.77	0
4.28	1	0	0	0	11.62	0.51	0.04	0.05	0.41	0.08	3.97	0.01	41.67	0.41	23.25	69.17	61.24	200.72	0.34
2.54	0.6	0	0	0	11.91	0.06	0.06	0.08	0.12	0.07	7.37	0	45.08	0.46	27.5	90.15	77.11	284.35	0
4.38	1.03	0	0	0.39	5.67	0	0.02	0.05	0.36	0.08	3.12	0	43.66	0.43	24.95	58.12	55.85	149.69	0.43
3.98	0.94	0	0	0	7.65	0.26	0.03	0.07	0.41	0.06	4.82	0	39.97	0.41	25.23	67.76	69.17	173.5	0.35

USDA ID Code	Food Name	Weight in Grams*	Quantity of Units	Unit of Measure	Protein (gm)	Fat (gm)	Carbohydrates (gm)	Kcalories	Caffeine (gm)	Fiber (gm)	Cholesterol (mg)	Saturated Fat (gm)
19063	Tortilla Chips, Taco-flavor	28.35	1	Ounce	2.24	6.86	17.89	136.08	0	0	1.42	1.32
	Tostitos - Baked	28	1	Ounce	2	1	24	110	0	0	0	0
	Tostitos - Baked, salsa & sour cream	28	1	Ounce	2	3	21	120	0	0	0	0.5
19059	Trail Mix, Regular	150	1	Cup	20.7	44.1	67.35	693	0	0	0	8.33
19821	Trail Mix, Regular, Unsalted	150	1	Cup	20.7	44.1	67.35	693	0	0	0	8.33
19062	Trail Mix, Regular, w/ Chocolate Chips	146	1	Cup	20.73	46.57	65.55	706.64	0	0	5.84	8.91
19061	Trail Mix, Tropical	140	1	Cup	8.82	23.94	91.84	569.8	0	0	0	11.87
62673	Triscuits	4.429	7	Each	0.43	0.71	3	20	0	0.57	0	0.14
62674	Triscuits, Low-Fat	4	8	Each	0.38	0.38	3	16.25	0	0.5	0	0.06
19138	Truffles	12	1	Piece	0.68	4.12	5.4	58.56	0	0	6.24	2.58
19160	Twix	57	1	Each	3.08	13.4	37.45	272.46	1.71	0.97	5.13	0
19112	Twizzlers Strawberry Candy	71	1	Pkg	2.34	1.14	65.82	262.7	0	0	0	0
18210	Vanilla Sandwich Cookies w/ Creme Filling	10	1	Each	0.45	2	7.21	48.3	0	0.15	0	0.36
18213	Vanilla Wafers, Higher Fat	6	1	Each	0.26	1.16	4.27	28.38	0	0	0	0.3
18212	Vanilla Wafers, Lower Fat	4	1	Each	0.2	0.61	2.94	17.64	0	0	2.32	0.14
62675	Wheat Thins	1.813	16	Each	0.13	0.38	1.19	8.75	0	0.13	0	0.06
62676	Wheat Thins, Low-Fat	1.611	18	Each	0.11	0.22	1.17	6.67	0	0.11	0	0.03
19393	Yogurt, Soft-serve, Chocolate	144.089	1	Cup	5.76	8.65	35.88	230.54	0	0	7.2	5.23
19293	Yogurt, Soft-serve, Vanilla	144.089	1	Cup	5.76	8.07	34.87	229.1	0	0	2.88	4.93
	York Peppermint Pattie (large)	42	1	Lg Patty	0.92	2.98	33.64	165.06	0	0.84	0.42	1.81
19091	York Peppermint Pattie (small)	17	1	Sm Patty	0.37	1.2	13.61	66.81	0	0.34	0.17	0.73
6474	Soup, Bean w/ Bacon	253	1	Cup	7.9	5.9	22.8	172	0	8.6	3	1.5
6007	Soup, Bean w/ Ham	256	1	Cup	12.61	8.51	27.12	230.85	0	11.18	21.87	3.33
6406	Soup, Bean w/ Hot Dogs	-256	1	Cup	9.97	6.97	22	187.5	0	0	12.5	2.12
6404	Soup, Bean w/ Pork	253	1	Cup	7.89	5.95	22.8	172.04	0	8.6	2.53	1.52
6008	Soup, Beef Broth or Bouillon	240	1	Cup	3	0.53	1	30	0	0	0	0.5
6547	Soup, Beef Mushroom	244	1	Cup	5.8	3	6.3	73	0	0	7	1.5
6409	Soup, Beef Noodle	244	1	Cup	4.83	3.07	8.98	82.96	0	0.73	4.88	1.15
6070	Soup, Beef, Chunky	230	1	Cup	11.74	5.14	19.56	170.4	0	1.44	14.4	2.54
6402	Soup, Black Bean	247	1	Cup	5.63	1.51	19.81	116.09	0	4.45	0	0.4
6478	Soup, Cauliflower	253	1	Cup	2.89	1.72	10.73	69.15	0	0	0	0.26
6411	Soup, Cheese	247	1	Cup	5.41	10.47	10.52	155.61	0	0	29.64	6.67
6480	Soup, Chicken Broth or Bouillon	244	1	Cup	1.34	1.1	1.44	21.96	0	0	0	0.27
6417	Soup, Chicken Gumbo	244	1	Cup	2.64	1.44	8.37	56.12	0	1.95	4.88	0.32
6549	Soup, Chicken Mushroom	244	1	Cup	4.39	9.15	9.27	131.76	0	0	9.76	2.39
6419	Soup, Chicken Noodle	241	1	Cup	4.05	2.46	9.35	74.71	0	0.72	7.23	0.65
6018	Soup, Chicken Noodle, Chunky	240	1	Cup	12.72	6	17.04	175.2	0	3.84	19.2	1.39
6485	Soup, Chicken Rice	241	1	Cup	2.45	1.44	9.25	60.67	0	0.76	2.53	0.33
6022	Soup, Chicken Rice, Chunky	243	1	Cup	12.26	3.19	12.98	127.2	0	0.96	12	0.96
6425	Soup, Chicken Vegetable	241	1	Cup	3.62	2.84	8.58	74.71	0	0.96	9.64	0.84
6024	Soup, Chicken Vegetable, Chunky	240	1	Cup	12.31	4.82	18.89	165.6	0	0	16.8	1.44
6412	Soup, Chicken w/ Dumplings	241	1	Cup	5.62	5.52	6.05	96.4	0	0.72	33.74	1.3
6423	Soup, Chicken w/ Rice	241	1	Cup	3.54	1.9	7.16	60.25	0	0.72	7.23	0.46
6015	Soup, Chicken, Chunky	251	1	Cup	12.7	6.63	17.27	178.21	0	1.51	30.12	1.98
6426	Soup, Chili Beef	250	1	Cup	6.7	6.6	21.45	170	0	9.5	12.5	3.35
6027	Soup, Clam Chowder, Manhattan Style	244	1	Cup	2.2	2.2	12.2	78	0	1.5	2	0.4
6230	Soup, Clam Chowder, New England	248	1	Cup	4.8	2.9	12.4	95	0	1.5	5	0.4
6034	Soup, Crab	240	1	Cup	5.49	1.51	10.3	75.64	0	0.73	9.76	0.39
6201	Soup, Cream Of Asparagus	248	1	Cup	6.32	8.18	16.39	161.2	0	0.74	22.32	3.32
6210	Soup, Cream Of Celery	248	1	Cup	5.68	9.7	14.53	163.68	0	0.74	32.24	3.94
6216	Soup, Cream Of Chicken	248	1	Cup	7.46	11.46	14.98	190.96	0	0.25	27.28	4.64
6243	Soup, Cream Of Mushroom	248	1	Cup	6.05	13.59	15	203.36	0	0.5	19.84	5.13
6246	Soup, Cream Of Onion	248	1	Cup	6.8	9.37	18.35	186	0	0.74	32.24	4.04
6253	Soup, Cream Of Potato	248	1	Cup	5.78	6.45	17.16	148.8	0	0.5	22.32	3.77
6256	Soup, Cream Of Shrimp	248	1	Cup	6.82	9.3	13.91	163.68	0	0.25	34.72	5.78

Monounsaturated Fat (gm)	Polyunsaturated Fat (gm)	Vitamin D (mg)	Vitamin K (mg)	Vitamin E (mg)	Vitamin A (re)	Vitamin C (mg)	Thiamin (mg)	Riboflavin (mg)	Niacin (mg)	Vitamin B6 (mg)	Folate (mg)	Vitamin B12 (mcg)	Calcium (mg)	Iron (mg)	Magnesium (mg)	Phosphorus (mg)	Potassium (mg)	Sodium (mg)	Zinc (mg)
4.05	0.95	0	0	0	25.8	0.26	0.07	0.06	0.57	0.08	5.95	0	43.94	0.57	24.95	67.76	61.52	223.11	0.36
0	0	0	0	0	0	0	0	0	0	0	0	0	32	0.2	0	0	0	200	0
0	0	0	0	0	0	0	0	0	0	0	0	0	32	0.2	0	0	0	190	0
18.8	14.48	0	0	0	3	2.1	0.69	0.3	7.07	0.45	106.5	0	117	4.58	237	517.5	1027.5	343.5	4.83
18.8	14.48	0	0	0	3	2.1	0.69	0.3	7.07	0.45	106.5	0	117	4.58	237	517.5	1027.5	15	4.83
19.77	16.48	0	0	0	7.3	1.9	0.6	0.33	6.43	0.38	94.9	0	159.14	4.95	235.06	565.02	946.08	176.66	4.58
3.49	7.22	0	0	0	7	10.64	0.63	0.16	2.07	0.46	58.8	0	79.8	3.7	134.4	260.4	992.6	14	1.64
0.07	0.21	0	0	0	0	0	0	0	0	0	0	0	0	0.11	0	11.43	0	24.29	0
0	0.13	0	0	0	0	0	0	0	0	0	0	0	0	0.13	0	15	0	22.5	0
1.22	0.13	0	0	0	17.16	0.05	0.01	0.03	0.03	0	0.12	0.04	18.6	0.12	5.64	21.24	36.6	8.52	0.13
0	0	0	0	0.4	18.24	0.11	0.03	0.11	0.21	0.02	3.99	0.22	67.26	0.38	16.53	76.38	117.42	114.57	0.39
0	0	0	0	0	0	0	0.01	0.03	0.07	0.01	0	0	24.85	0.36	4.26	220.1	45.44	196.67	0.11
1.18	0.28	0	0	0	0	0	0.03	0.02	0.27	0	0.4	0	2.7	0.22	1.4	7.5	9.1	34.9	0.04
0.66	0.15	0	0	0	0	0	0.02	0.01	0.18	0	0.48	0	1.5	0.13	0.72	3.84	6.42	18.36	0.02
0.24	0.15	0	0	0	0.72	0	0.01	0.01	0.12	0	0.36	0	1.92	0.1	0.56	4.16	3.88	12.48	0.01
0.03	0.16	0	0	0	0	0	0	0	0	0	0	0	1.5	0.03	0	0	0	10.63	0
0	0.08	0	0	0	0	0	0	0	0	0	0	0	1.33	0.02	0	4.44	0	12.22	0
2.52	0.32	0	0	0	61.96	0.43	0.05	0.3	0.44	0.11	15.85	0.42	211.81	1.8	38.9	200.28	376.07	141.21	0.71
2.29	0.3	0	0	0.07	82.13	1.15	0.05	0.32	0.41	0.12	8.65	0.42	206.05	0.43	20.17	185.88	304.03	125.36	0.61
1.05	0.084	0	0	0	0	0	0	0	0	0	0	0	6.3	0.42	0	0	54.18	10.08	0
0.43	0.034	0	0	0	0.11	0	0	0.01	0.09	0	0.44	0	2.55	0.17	0	0	21.93	4.08	0
2.2	1.8	0	0	0.26	89	2	0.09	0.03	0.6	0.04	32	0.05	81	2.05	46	132	402	951	1.03
3.84	0.95	0	0	0.07	396.09	4.37	0.15	0.15	1.7	0.12	29.16	0.07	77.76	3.23	46.17	143.37	425.25	972	1.07
2.72	1.65	0	0	0	87.5	1	0.11	0.06	1.03	0.13	30	0.07	87.5	2.35	47.5	165	477.5	1092.5	1.18
2.18	1.82	0	0	0.08	88.55	1.52	0.09	0.03	0.57	0.04	31.88	0.05	80.96	2.05	45.54	131.56	402.27	951.28	1.03
0.44	0.04	0	0	0	0	0	0	0.1	3.74	0.04	9.6	0.34	40	0.8	9.6	62	260	1800	0
1.2	0.1	0	0	0	0	5	0.04	0.06	1	0.05	10	0.2	5	0.88	10	34	154	942	1.46
1.24	0.49	0	0	0	63.44	0.24	0.07	0.06	1.07	0.04	4.39	0.2	14.64	1.1	4.88	46.36	100.04	915.6	1.54
2.14	0.22	0	0	0.17	261.6	6.96	0.06	0.15	2.7	0.13	13.44	0.62	31.2	2.33	4.8	120	336	866.4	2.64
0.54	0.47	0	0	0.07	49.4	0.74	0.08	0.05	0.53	0.09	24.7	0.02	44.46	2.15	41.99	106.21	274.17	1197.95	1.41
0.74	0.64	0	0	0	0	2.56	0.08	0.08	0.51	0.03	2.56	0.18	10.24	0.51	2.56	51.22	105	842.57	0.26
2.96	0.3	0	0	0	108.68	0	0.02	0.14	0.4	0.02	4.94	0	140.79	0.74	4.94	135.85	153.14	958.36	0.64
0.41	0.37	0	0	0.02	12.2	0	0.01	0.03	0.2	0	2.44	0.02	14.64	0.07	4.88	12.2	24.4	1483.52	0.01
0.66	0.34	0	0	0.04	14.64	4.88	0.02	0.05	0.66	0.06	4.88	0.02	24.4	0.9	4.88	24.4	75.64	954.04	0.38
4.03	2.32	0	0	0	112.24	0	0.02	0.11	1.63	0.05	0.24	0.05	29.28	0.88	9.76	26.84	153.72	941.84	0.98
1.11	0.55	0	0	0.07	72.3	0.24	0.05	0.06	1.39	0.03	2.17	0.14	16.87	0.77	4.82	36.15	55.43	1106.19	0.4
2.66	1.51	0	0	0.79	122.4	0	0.07	0.17	4.32	0.05	4.8	0.31	24	1.44	9.6	72	108	849.6	0.96
0.63	0.43	0	0	0.04	0	0	0	0	0.36	0.03	0.51	0.08	7.58	0	0	10.11	10.11	980.86	0.13
1.44	0.67	0	0	0.09	585.6	3.84	0.02	0.1	4.1	0.05	3.84	0.31	33.6	1.87	9.6	72	108	888	0.96
1.28	0.6	0	0	0.08	265.1	0.96	0.04	0.06	1.23	0.05	4.82	0.12	16.87	0.87	7.23	40.97	154.24	944.72	0.37
2.16	1.01	0	0	0	600	5.52	0.04	0.17	3.29	0.1	12	0.24	26.4	1.46	9.6	105.6	367.2	1068	2.16
2.53	1.3	0	0	0.14	53.02	0	0.02	0.07	1.75	0.04	2.41	0.17	14.46	0.63	4.82	60.25	115.68	860.37	0.37
0.92	0.41	0	0	0.05	65.07	0.24	0.02	0.02	1.13	0.02	0.96	0.14	16.87	0.75	0	21.69	101.22	814.58	0.26
2.96	1.38	0	0	0.18	130.52	1.26	0.09	0.17	4.42	0.05	4.52	0.25	25.1	1.73	7.53	112.95	175.7	888.54	1
2.8	0.27	0	0	0.17	150	4	0.06	0.07	1.07	0.16	17.5	0.32	42.5	2.12	30	147.5	525	1035	1.4
0.4	1.3	0	0	0.1	98	4	0.03	0.04	0.8	0.1	10	4.05	27	1.63	12	41	188	578	0.98
1.2	1.1	0	0	0.15	0	2	0.02	0.04	1	0.08	4	8	44	1.49	7	54	146	915	0.75
0.68	0.39	0	0	0.1	51.24	0	0.2	0.07	1.34	0.12	14.64	0.2	65.88	1.22	14.64	87.84	326.96	1234.64	1.46
2.08	2.23	0	0	0.84	84.32	3.97	0.1	0.28	0.88	0.06	29.76	0.5	173.6	0.87	19.84	153.76	359.6	1041.6	0.93
2.46	2.65	0	0	0.97	66.96	1.49	0.07	0.25	0.44	0.06	8.43	0.5	186	0.69	22.32	151.28	310	1009.36	0.2
4.46	1.64	0	0	0.24	94.24	1.24	0.07	0.26	0.92	0.07	7.69	0.55	181.04	0.67	17.36	151.28	272.8	1046.56	0.67
2.98	4.61	0	0	1.34	37.2	2.23	0.08	0.28	0.91	0.06	9.92	0.5	178.56	0.6	19.84	156.24	270.32	1076.32	0.64
3.27	1.59	0	0	0.07	66.96	2.48	0.1	0.27	0.61	0.07	12.4	0.5	178.56	0.69	22.32	153.76	310	1004.4	0.62
1.74	0.57	0	0	0.1	66.96	1.24	0.08	0.24	0.64	0.09	9.18	0.5	166.16	0.55	17.36	161.2	322.4	1061.44	0.67
2.68	0.35	0	0	0.87	54.56	1.24	0.06	0.23	0.53	0.45	9.92	1.04	163.68	0.6	22.32	146.32	248	1036.64	0.8

USDA ID Code	Food Name	Weight in Grams*	Quantity of Units	Unit of Measure	Protein (gm)	Fat (gm)	Carbohydrates (gm)	Kcalories	Caffeine (gm)	Fiber (gm)	Cholesterol (mg)	Saturated Fat (gm)
6501	Soup, Cream Of Vegetable	260.1	1	Cup	1.9	5.7	12.3	106.64	0	0.52	0	1.43
6036	Soup, Gazpacho	244	1	Cup	8.69	2.24	0.78	56.12	0	3.66	0	0.29
	Soup, Hot and Sour	244	1	Cup	15	8	5	162	0	0.5	34	3
	Soup, Instant	240	1	Cup	3	1	7	50	0	0.7	2	0.001
6037	Soup, Lentil w/ ham	248	1	Cup	9.28	2.78	20.24	138.88	0	0	7.44	1.12
6440	Soup, Minestrone	241	1	Cup	4.27	2.51	11.23	81.94	0	0.96	2.41	0.55
6039	Soup, Minestrone, Chunky	240	1	Cup	5.11	2.81	20.74	127.2	0	1.92	4.8	1.49
6493	Soup, Mushroom	253	1	Cup	2.23	4.86	11.13	96.14	0	0.76	0	0.81
6445	Soup, Onion	241	1	Cup	3.76	1.74	8.17	57.84	0	0.96	0	0.27
6249	Soup, Pea, Green	254	1	Cup	12.62	7.04	32.23	238.76	0	2.79	17.78	4.01
6451	Soup, Pea, Split w/ Ham	253	1	Cup	10.32	4.4	27.96	189.75	0	0	7.59	1.77
6050	Soup, Pea, Split w/ Ham, Chunky	240	1	Cup	11.09	3.98	26.81	184.8	0	4.08	7.2	1.58
	Soup, Sweet & Sour	244	1	Cup	3	1	14	72	0	1.6	5	0.001
6359	Soup, Tomato	248	1	Cup	6.1	6	22.3	161.2	0	0.5	17.36	2.9
6461	Soup, Tomato Beef w/ noodle	244	1	Cup	4.47	4.29	21.15	139.08	0	1.46	4.88	1.59
6463	Soup, Tomato Rice	247	1	Cup	2.1	2.72	21.93	118.56	0	1.48	2.47	0.52
6499	Soup, Tomato Vegetable	253	1	Cup	2	0.86	10.22	55.66	0	0.51	0	0.38
6465	Soup, Turkey Noodle	244	1	Cup	3.9	2	8.64	68.32	0	0.73	4.88	0.56
6466	Soup, Turkey Vegetable	241	1	Cup	3.08	3.04	8.63	72.3	0	0.48	2.41	0.89
6064	Soup, Turkey, Chunky	236	1	Cup	10.22	4.41	14.07	134.52	0	0	9.44	1.23
6500	Soup, Vegetable Beef	253.1	1	Cup	2.94	1.11	8.02	53.15	0	0.51	0	0.56
6067	Soup, Vegetable, Chunky	240	1	Cup	3.5	3.7	19.01	122.4	0	1.2	0	0.55
6468	Soup, Vegetarian Vegetable	241	1	Cup	2.1	1.93	11.98	72.3	0	0.48	0	0.29
	Soup, Won-Ton	241	1	Cup	14	7	14	182	0	0.9	53	2
19294	Apple Butter	18	1	Tbsp.	0.02	0.05	8.59	33.12	0	0.23	0	0
9020	Applesauce, Sweetened	255	1	Cup	0.46	0.46	50.77	193.8	0	3.06	0	0.08
9019	Applesauce, Unsweetened	244	1	Cup	0.41	0.12	27.55	104.92	0	2.93	0	0.02
62678	Bean Dip	15	2	Tbsp.	0.5	0	2	10	0	0.5	0	0
11935	Catsup	15	1	Tbsp.	0.23	0.05	4.09	15.6	0	0.19	0	0.01
11949	Catsup, Low Sodium	15	1	Tbsp.	0.23	0.05	4.09	15.6	0	0.24	0	0.01
18242	Croutons, Plain	30	0.5	Cup	3.57	1.98	22.05	122.1	0	1.53	0	0.47
18243	Croutons, Seasoned	40	0.5	Cup	4.32	7.32	25.4	186	0	2	1.2	2.01
62677	French Onion Dip	15	2	Tbsp.	0.5	2.5	1	30	0	0	7.5	1.5
6114	Gravy, Au Jus, Cnd	149	0.25	Cup	2.86	0.48	5.96	38.14	0	0	0	0.24
6116	Gravy, Beef, Cnd	234	0.25	Cup	8.8	5.6	11.2	124	0	1	8	2.6
6119	Gravy, Chicken, Cnd	238	0.25	Cup	4.6	13.61	12.92	188.34	0	0.95	4.77	3.36
6121	Gravy, Mushroom, Cnd	298	0.25	Cup	3	6.46	13.04	119.2	0	0.95	0	0.95
6125	Gravy, Turkey, Cnd	298	0.25	Cup	6.2	5.01	12.16	121.58	0	0.95	4.77	1.48
6527	Gravy, Unspecified Type	298	0.25	Cup	3.22	1.99	14.38	86.26	0	0	0	0.71
19296	Honey	21	1	Tbsp.	0.06	0	17.3	63.84	0	0.04	0	0
19297	Jams and Preserves	20	1	Tbsp.	0.14	0.04	12.88	48.4	0	0.22	0	0
19300	Jellies	19	1	Tbsp.	0.08	0.02	13.45	51.49	0	0.19	0	0
19303	Marmalade, Orange	20	1	Tbsp.	0.06	0	13.26	49.2	0	0.04	0	0
62646	Mustard	5	1	Tbsp.	0	0	0	0	0	0	0	0
62679	Nacho Cheese Dip	16.5	2	Tbsp.	0	1.25	2	20	0	0	0	0.25
11958	Pickle Relish, Hamburger	15	1	Tbsp.	0.09	0.08	5.17	19.35	0	0.48	0	0.01
11944	Pickle Relish, Hot Dog	15	1	Tbsp.	0.22	0.07	3.5	13.65	0	0	0	0.01
11945	Pickle Relish, Sweet	15	1	Tbsp.	0.06	0.07	5.26	19.5	0	0	0	0.01
62651	Salt Substitute	4.8	0.25	Tsp.	0	0	0	0	0	0	0	0
2047	Salt, Table	6	1	Tsp.	0	0	0	0	0	0	0	0
	Sauce, A-1 Steak	31.3	2	Tbsp.	0.003	0.005	5	19	0	0.5	0	0.002
6150	Sauce, Barbecue	250	0.5	Cup	4.5	4.5	32	187.5	0	3	0	0.67
	Sauce, Chinese Mustard	15	1	Tbsp.	1	1	1	11	0	0.4	0	0.002
11256	Sauce, Marinara	250	0.5	Cup	4	8.37	25.45	170	0	0	0	1.2
6134	Sauce, Soy (Tamari)	18	1	Tbsp.	0.93	0.01	1.53	9.54	0	0	0	0

Monounsaturated Fat (gm)	Polyunsaturated Fat (gm)	Vitamin D (mg)	Vitamin K (mg)	Vitamin E (mg)	Vitamin A (re)	Vitamin C (mg)	Thiamin (mg)	Riboflavin (mg)	Niacin (mg)	Vitamin B6 (mg)	Folate (mcg)	Vitamin B12 (mcg)	Calcium (mg)	Iron (mg)	Magnesium (mg)	Phosphorus (mg)	Potassium (mg)	Sodium (mg)	Zinc (mg)
2.55	1.48	0	0	1.24	2.6	3.9	1.22	0.11	0.52	0.03	7.8	0.13	31.21	0.52	10.4	54.62	96.24	1170.45	0.26
0.54	1.32	0	0	0.46	19.52	3.17	0.05	0.02	0.93	0.15	9.76	0	24.4	0.98	7.32	36.6	224.48	1183.4	0.24
0.3	0.68	0	0	0.3	0.03	0.6	0	0	0	0	0	0	32	1.65	0	0	0	1011	0
0	0	0	0	0	0.03	0.03	0	0	0	0	0	0	27	0.45	0	0	0	1222	0
1.29	0.32	0	0	0	34.72	4.22	0.17	0.11	1.35	0.22	49.6	0.3	42.16	2.65	22.32	183.52	357.12	1319.36	0.74
0.7	1.11	0	0	0.07	233.77	1.21	0.05	0.04	0.94	0.1	16.15	0	33.74	0.92	7.23	55.43	313.3	910.98	0.74
0.91	0.26	0	0	0.72	434.4	4.8	0.06	0.12	1.18	0.24	31.2	0	60	1.78	14.4	110.4	612	864	1.44
2.25	1.54	0	0	0.63	0	1.01	0.28	0.11	0.5	0.03	5.06	0.25	65.78	0.51	5.06	75.9	199.87	1019.59	0.09
0.75	0.65	0	0	0.29	0	1.21	0.03	0.02	0.6	0.05	15.18	0	26.51	0.67	2.41	12.05	67.48	1053.17	0.61
2.18	0.53	0	0	0.18	58.42	2.79	0.15	0.27	1.34	0.1	7.87	0.43	172.72	2.01	55.88	238.76	375.92	1046.48	1.76
1.8	0.63	0	0	0	45.54	1.52	0.15	0.08	1.47	0.07	2.53	0.25	22.77	2.28	48.07	212.52	399.74	1006.94	1.32
1.63	0.58	0	0	0.14	487.2	6.96	0.12	0.09	2.52	0.22	4.56	0.24	33.6	2.14	38.4	177.6	304.8	964.8	3.12
0	0	0	0	0	30	16.8	0	0	0	0	0	0	27	0.45	0	0	0	1292	0
1.61	1.12	0	0	2.6	109.12	67.7	0.13	0.25	1.52	0.16	20.83	0.45	158.72	1.81	22.32	148.8	448.88	932.48	0.29
1.73	0.68	0	0	0.78	53.68	0	0.08	0.09	1.87	0.09	7.32	0.2	17.08	1.12	7.32	56.12	219.6	917.44	0.75
0.59	1.36	0	0	0.79	76.57	14.82	0.06	0.05	1.05	0.08	13.58	0	22.23	0.79	4.94	34.58	330.98	815.1	0.51
0.3	0.08	0	0	0.81	20.24	6.07	0.06	0.05	0.79	0.05	10.12	0	7.59	0.63	20.24	30.36	103.73	1146.09	0.17
0.81	0.49	0	0	0.06	29.28	0.24	0.07	0.06	1.4	0.04	2.2	0.15	12.2	0.95	4.88	48.8	75.64	814.96	0.58
1.33	0.67	0	0	0.14	243.41	0	0.03	0.04	1	0.05	4.82	0.17	16.87	0.77	4.82	40.97	175.93	906.16	0.61
1.77	1.09	0	0	0	715.08	6.37	0.04	0.11	3.59	0.31	11.09	2.12	49.56	1.91	23.6	103.84	361.08	922.76	2.12
0.46	0.05	0	0	0.03	22.78	1.27	0.03	0.04	0.46	0.05	7.59	0.25	12.65	0.86	22.78	35.43	75.93	1002.28	0.27
1.58	1.39	0	0	0.6	588	6	0.07	0.06	1.2	0.19	16.56	0	55.2	1.63	7.2	72	396	1010.4	3.12
0.82	0.72	0	0	0.8	301.25	1.45	0.05	0.05	0.92	0.06	10.6	0	21.69	1.08	7.23	33.74	209.67	821.81	0.46
0.001	0.003	0	0	0	100	3.6	0	0	0	0	0	0	29	1.5	0	0	0	543	0
0	0	0	0	0	0	0.32	0	0	0.01	0.01	0	0	0.9	0.02	0.54	1.08	16.38	0	0.01
0.02	0.14	0	0	0.13	2.55	4.34	0.03	0.07	0.48	0.07	1.53	0	10.2	0.89	7.65	17.85	155.55	7.65	0.1
0	0.03	0	0	0.12	7.32	2.93	0.03	0.06	0.46	0.06	1.46	0	7.32	0.29	7.32	17.08	183	4.88	0.07
0	0	0	0	0	0	0	0	0	0	0	0	0	0	0.1	0	0	0	75	0
0.01	0.02	0	0	0.22	15.3	2.26	0.01	0.01	0.21	0.03	2.25	0	2.85	0.1	3.3	5.85	72.15	177.9	0.03
0.01	0.02	0	0	0.22	15.3	2.26	0.01	0.01	0.21	0.03	2.25	0	2.85	0.1	3.3	5.85	72.15	3	0.03
1.01	0.32	0	0	0	0	0	0.19	0.08	1.63	0.01	6.6	0	22.8	1.22	9.3	34.5	37.2	209.4	0.27
3.82	1	0	0	0	2	0	0.2	0.17	1.86	0.03	16	0.03	38.4	1.13	16.8	56	72.4	495.2	0.38
0	0	0	0	0	20	0.6	0	0	0	0	0	0	12	0	0	0	0	52.5	0
0.19	0.02	0	0	0	0	2.38	0.05	0.14	2.15	0.02	4.77	0.24	9.54	1.43	4.77	71.52	193.1	119.2	2.38
2.2	0.2	0	0	0.3	0	0	0.08	0.08	1.6	0.02	4	0.24	14	1.64	4	70	190	1330	2.34
6.08	3.58	0	0	0.37	264.62	0	0.04	0.1	1.06	0.02	4.77	0.24	47.68	1.12	4.77	69.14	259.86	1375.57	1.91
2.79	2.43	0	0	0.15	0	0	0.08	0.15	1.6	0.05	28.61	0	16.69	1.57	4.77	35.76	252.7	1358.88	1.67
2.15	1.17	0	0	0.14	0	0	0.05	0.19	3.1	0.05	4.77	0.24	9.54	1.67	4.77	69.14	259.86	1375.57	1.91
0.78	0.39	0	0	0	0	1.83	0.05	0.11	0.78	0.03	3.4	0.18	36.6	0.26	10.46	49.67	65.35	1422.02	0.26
0	0	0	0	0	0	0.11	0	0.01	0.03	0.01	0.42	0	1.26	0.09	0.42	0.84	10.92	0.84	0.05
0.02	0	0	0	0	0.2	1.76	0	0	0.01	0	6.6	0	4	0.1	0.8	2.2	15.4	8	0.01
0	0	0	0	0	0.38	0.17	0	0	0.01	0	0.19	0	1.52	0.04	1.14	0.95	12.16	6.84	0.01
0	0	0	0	0	1	0.96	0	0	0.01	0	7.2	0	7.6	0.03	0.4	1.2	7.4	11.2	0.01
0	0	0	0	0	0	0	0	0	0	0	0	0	0	0	0	0	0	75	0
0	0	0	0	0	0	0	0	0	0	0	0	0	12	0	0	0	0	100	0
0.04	0.02	0	0	0	4.05	0.34	0	0.01	0.09	0	0.15	0	0.6	0.17	1.05	2.55	11.4	164.4	0.02
0.03	0.02	0	0	0	2.55	0.15	0.01	0.01	0.07	0	0.15	0	0.75	0.19	2.85	6	11.7	163.65	0.03
0.03	0.02	0	0	0	2.4	0.15	0	0	0.03	0	0.15	0	0.45	0.13	0.75	2.1	3.75	121.65	0.02
0	0	0	0	0	0	0	0	0	0	0	0	0	0	0	0	0	0	2440	0
0	0	0	0	0	0	0	0	0	0	0	0	0	2.7	0.01	0.12	0	0.48	2325.48	0
0	0	0	0	0	32	4.8	0	0	0	0	0	0	12	0.3	0	0	0	454	0
1.92	1.7	0	0	2.77	217.5	17.5	0.07	0.05	2.25	0.19	10	0	47.5	2.25	45	50	435	2037.5	0.5
0	0	0	0	0	0	0	0	0	0	0	0	0	12	0.3	0	0	0	188	0
4.28	2.29	0	0	0	240	32	0.11	0.15	3.97	0.62	33.75	0	45	2	60	87.5	1060	1572.5	0.67
0	0.01	0	0	0	0	0	0.01	0.02	0.6	0.03	2.79	0	3.06	0.36	6.12	19.8	32.4	1028.7	0.07

USDA ID Code	Food Name	Weight in Grams*	Quantity of Units	Unit of Measure	Protein (gm)	Fat (gm)	Carbohydrates (gm)	Kcalories	Caffeine (gm)	Fiber (gm)	Cholesterol (mg)	Saturated Fat (gm)
11455	Sauce, Spaghetti	249	0.5	Cup	4.53	11.88	39.67	271.41	0	8.47	0	1.7
6112	Sauce, Teriyaki	18	1	Tbsp.	1.07	0	2.87	15.12	0	0.02	0	0
6313	Sauce, White	263.8	0.5	Cup	10.21	13.45	21.39	240.06	0	0	34.29	6.41
	Sauce, Worcestershire	34	2	Tbsp.	0	0	6	23	0	0	0	0
62666	Spaghetti Sauce w/garlic and herbs, Healthy Choice	113	1	Cup	2	0.59	9	40		0		
62665	Spaghetti Sauce, Prego	146	1	Cup	3.56	4.15	26.11	154.31	0	3.56	0	1.19
62664	Spaghetti Sauce, Ragu	146	1	Cup	3.56	4.75	20.18	130.57	0	3.56	0	1.78
19334	Sugar, Brown	5	1	Tsp.	0	0	4.87	18.8	0	0	0	0
19335	Sugar, Granulated	4	1	Tsp.	0	0	4	15.48	0	0	0	0
19336	Sugar, Powdered	8	1	Tbsp.	0	0.01	7.96	31.12	0	0	0	0
19349	Syrup, Corn, Dark	20	1	Tbsp.	0	0	15.32	56.4	0	0	0	0
19351	Syrup, Corn, High-fructose	19	1	Tbsp.	0	0	14.44	53.39	0	0	0	0
19350	Syrup, Corn, Light	20	1	Tbsp.	0	0	15.32	56.4	0	0	0	0
19352	Syrup, Malt	24	1	Tbsp.	1.49	0	17.11	76.32	0	0	0	0
19353	Syrup, Maple	20	1	Tbsp.	0	0.04	13.44	52.4	0	0	0	0
19128	Syrup, Pancake, Lo Cal	19.98	1	Tbsp.	0	0	8.85	32.77	0	0	0	0
19360	Syrup, Pancake, w/ 2% Maple	20	1	Tbsp.	0	0.02	13.92	53	0	0	0	0
19364	Toppings, Butterscotch or Caramel	20.513	1	Tbsp.	0.31	0.02	13.52	51.69	0	0	0.21	0.02
62550	Toppings, Caramel	16.68	1	Tbsp.	0.27	0	13.01	51.71	0	0	0	0
19348	Toppings, Chocolate	21	1	Tbsp.	0.92	2.81	12.37	72.66	1.89	0.25	2.52	1.18
62549	Toppings, Hot Fudge	19.018	1	Tbsp.	1	2	11.01	70.07	0	0	0	0.5
19365	Toppings, Marshmallow Cream	20.513	1	Tbsp.	0.35	0.04	16.31	63.59	0	0	0	0
19367	Toppings, Nuts in Syrup	20.513	1	Tbsp.	0.92	4.51	10.95	83.69	0	0.33	0	0.4
19366	Toppings, Pineapple	21.268	1	Tbsp.	0.02	0.02	14.12	53.81	0	0.21	0	0
19137	Toppings, Strawberry	21.268	1	Tbsp.	0.04	0.02	14.1	54.02	0	0.21	0	0

Monounsaturated Fat (gm)	Polyunsaturated Fat (gm)	Vitamin D (mg)	Vitamin K (mg)	Vitamin E (mg)	Vitamin A (re)	Vitamin C (mg)	Thiamin (mg)	Riboflavin (mg)	Niacin (mg)	Vitamin B6 (mg)	Folate (mg)	Vitamin B12 (mcg)	Calcium (mg)	Iron (mg)	Magnesium (mg)	Phosphorus (mg)	Potassium (mg)	Sodium (mg)	Zinc (mg)
6.07	3.25	0	0	6.22	306.27	27.89	0.14	0.15	3.75	0.88	53.78	0	69.72	1.62	59.76	89.64	956.16	1235.04	0.52
0	0	0	0	0	0	0	0.01	0.01	0.23	0.02	3.6	0	4.5	0.31	10.98	27.72	40.5	689.94	0.02
4.7	1.69	0	0	0	92.33	2.64	0.08	0.45	0.53	0.07	15.83	1.06	424.72	0.26	263.8	255.89	443.18	796.68	0.55
0	0	0	0	0	0.003	4.2	0	0	0	0	0	0	43	1.5	0	0	0	333	0
0	0	0	0	0	56	18	0	0	0	0	0	0	24	0.8	0	0	0	390	0
0	0	0	0	0	356.1	21.37	0	0	0	0	0	0	85.46	0.71	0	0	0	724.07	0
0	0	0	0	0	178.05	1.42	0	0	0	0	0	0	56.98	0.71	0	0	0	652.85	0
0	0	0	0	0	0	0	0	0	0	0	0.05	0	4.25	0.1	1.45	1.1	17.3	1.95	0.01
0	0	0	0	0	0	0	0	0	0	0	0	0	0.04	0	0	0.08	0.08	0.04	0
0	0	0	0	0	0	0	0	0	0	0	0	0	0.08	0	0	0.16	0.16	0.08	0
0	0	0	0	0	0	0	0	0	0	0	0	0	3.6	0.07	1.6	2.2	8.8	31	0.01
0	0	0	0	0	0	0	0	0	0	0	0	0	0	0.01	0	0	0	0.38	0
0	0	0	0	0	0	0	0	0	0	0	0	0	0.6	0.01	0.4	0.4	0.8	24.2	0
0	0	0	0	0	0	0	0	0.09	1.95	0.12	2.88	0	14.64	0.23	17.28	56.64	76.8	8.4	0.03
0	0	0	0	0	0	0	0	0	0.01	0	0	0	13.4	0.24	2.8	0.4	40.8	1.8	0.83
0	0	0	0	0	0	0	0	0	0	0	0	0	0.2	0	0	8.59	0.6	39.96	0
0	0	0	0	0	0	0	0	0	0	0	0	0	1	0.01	0.4	2	1.2	12.2	0.05
0	0	0	0	0	5.54	0.06	0	0.02	0.01	0	0.41	0.02	10.87	0.04	1.44	9.64	17.23	71.59	0.04
0	0	0	0	0	0	0	0	0	0	0	0	0	2.34	0	0	4.67	5.67	11.01	0.03
0.77	0.68	0	0	0	4.62	0.11	0.01	0.05	0.04	0.01	0.84	0.06	21	0.25	10.08	35.7	45.15	27.3	0.17
0	0	0	0	0	0	0	0	0	0	0	0	0	36.03	0.2	0	0	0	35.03	0
0	0	0	0	0	0	0	0	0	0.02	0	0.21	0	0.62	0.05	0.41	1.64	1.03	9.44	0.01
1.02	2.82	0	0	0.18	0.82	0.23	0.04	0.02	0.08	0.04	4.31	0	8.21	0.22	12.92	22.77	42.87	8.62	0.21
0	0	0	0	0	0.43	12.46	0.01	0	0.02	0	0.64	0	4.68	0.1	0.43	1.7	67.42	13.4	0.1
0	0	0	0	0.03	0.43	5.3	0	0	0.05	0	0.43	0	5.1	0.21	0.85	2.76	15.53	4.47	0.1

B Cholesterol Content of Foods

Item	Amount of cholesterol		
	100 g edible portion* (mg)	Edible portion of 450 g (1 lb) as purchased (mg)	Refuse from item as purchased (%)
Beef, raw			
With bone†	70	270	15
Without bone†	70	320	0
Brains, raw	>2000	>9000	0
Butter	250	1135	0
Caviar or fish roe	>300	>1300	0
Cheese			
Cheddar	100	455	0
Cottage, creamed	15	70	0
Cream	120	545	0
Other (25%-30% fat)	85	385	0
Cheese spread	65	295	0
Chicken, flesh only, raw	60	—	0
Crab			
In shell†	125	270	52
Meat only†	125	565	0
Egg, whole	550	2200	12
Egg white	0	0	0
Egg yolk			
Fresh	1500	6800	0
Frozen	1280	5800	0
Dried	2950	13,380	0
Fish			
Steak†	70	265	16
Fillet†	70	320	0

	Amount of cholesterol		
Item	100 g edible portion* (mg)	Edible portion of 450 g (1 lb) as purchased (mg)	Refuse from item as purchased (%)
Heart, raw	150	680	0
Ice cream	45	205	0
Kidney, raw	375	1700	0
Lamb, raw			
With bone†	70	265	16
Without bone†	70	320	0
Lard and other animal fat	95	430	0
Liver, raw	300	1360	0
Lobster			
Whole†	200	235	74
Meat only†	200	900	0
Margarine			
All vegetable fat	0	0	0
Two-thirds animal fat, one-third vegetable fat	65	295	0
Milk			
Fluid, whole	11	50	0
Dried, whole	85	385	0
Fluid, skim	3	15	0
Mutton			
With bone†	65	250	16
Without bone†	65	295	0
Oysters			
In shell†	>200	>90	90
Meat only†	>200	>900	0
Pork			
With bone†	70	260	18
Without bone†	70	320	0
Shrimp			
In shell†	125	390	31
Flesh only†	125	565	0
Sweetbreads (thymus)	250	1135	0
Veal			
With bone†	90	320	21
Without bone†	90	410	0

From Watt, BK, Merrill, AL: *Composition of foods—raw, processed, prepared,* U.S. Department of Agriculture, Agriculture Handbook No 8, Dec 1963.

*Data apply to 100 g of edible portion of the item, although it may be purchased with the refuse indicated and described or implied in the first column.

†Items that have the same chemical composition for the edible portion but differ in the amount of refuse.

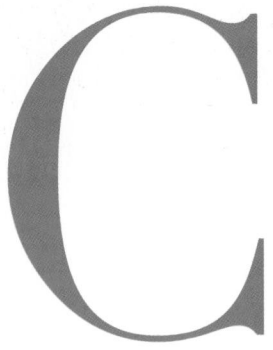

Dietary Fiber in Selected Plant Foods

Food	Amount	Weight (g)	Total dietary fiber (g)	Noncellulose polysaccharides (g)	Cellulose (g)	Lignin
Apple	1 med					
Flesh		138	1.96	1.29	0.66	0.01
Skin		100	3.71	2.21	1.01	0.49
Banana	1 small	119	2.08	1.33	0.44	0.31
Beans						
Baked	1 cup	255	18.53	14.45	3.59	0.48
Green, cooked	1 cup	125	4.19	2.31	1.61	0.26
Bread						
White	1 slice	25	0.68	0.50	0.18	Trace
Whole meal	1 slice	25	2.13	1.49	0.33	0.31
Broccoli, cooked	1 cup	155	6.36	4.53	1.78	0.05
Brussels sprouts, cooked	1 cup	155	4.43	3.08	1.24	0.11
Cabbage, cooked	1 cup	145	4.10	2.55	1.00	0.55
Carrots, cooked	1 cup	155	5.74	3.44	2.29	Trace
Cauliflower, cooked	1 cup	125	2.25	0.84	1.41	Trace
Cereals						
All-Bran	1 oz	30	8.01	5.35	1.80	0.86
Corn Flakes	1 cup	25	2.75	1.82	0.61	0.33
Grapenuts	¼ cup	30	2.10	1.54	0.38	0.17
Puffed Wheat	1 cup	15	2.31	1.55	0.39	0.37
Rice Krispies	1 cup	30	1.34	1.04	0.23	0.07
Shredded Wheat	1 biscuit	25	3.07	2.20	0.66	0.21
Special K	1 cup	30	1.64	1.10	0.22	0.32
Cherries	10 cherries	68	0.84	0.63	0.17	0.05
Cookies						
Ginger	4 snaps	28	0.56	0.41	0.08	0.07

Food	Amount	Weight (g)	Total dietary fiber (g)	Noncellulose polysaccharides (g)	Cellulose (g)	Lignin
Oatmeal	4 cookies	52	2.08	1.64	0.21	0.22
Plain	4 cookies	48	0.80	0.68	0.05	0.06
Corn	1 cup	165	7.82	7.11	0.51	0.20
Canned	1 cup	165	9.39	8.20	1.06	0.13
Flour						
Bran	1 cup	100	44.00	32.70	8.05	3.23
White	1 cup	115	3.62	2.90	0.69	0.03
Whole meal	1 cup	120	11.41	7.50	2.95	0.96
Grapefruit	½ cup	100	0.44	0.34	0.04	0.06
Jam, strawberry	1 tbsp	20	0.22	0.17	0.02	0.03
Lettuce	⅛ head	100	1.53	0.47	1.06	Trace
Marmalade, orange	1 tbsp	20	0.14	0.13	0.01	Trace
Onions, raw, sliced	1 cup	100	2.10	1.55	0.55	Trace
Orange	1 cup	200	0.58	0.44	0.08	0.06
Parsnips, raw, diced	1 cup	100	4.90	3.77	1.13	Trace
Peach, flesh and skin	1 med	100	2.28	1.46	0.20	0.62
Peanuts	1 oz	30	2.79	1.92	0.51	0.36
Peanut butter	1 tbsp	16	1.21	0.90	0.31	Trace
Pear	1 med					
Flesh		164	4.00	2.16	1.10	0.74
Skin		100	8.59	3.72	2.18	2.67
Peas, canned	1 cup	170	13.35	8.85	3.91	0.60
Peas, raw or frozen	1 cup	100	7.75	5.48	2.09	0.18
Plums	1 plum	66	1.00	0.65	0.15	0.20
Potato, raw	1 med	135	4.73	3.36	1.38	Trace
Raisins	1 oz	30	1.32	0.72	0.25	0.35
Strawberries	1 cup	149	2.65	1.39	1.04	0.22
Tomato						
Raw	1 med	135	1.89	0.88	0.61	0.41
Canned, drained	1 cup	240	2.04	1.08	0.89	0.07
Turnips, raw	1 med	100	2.20	1.50	0.70	Trace

Adapted from Southgate, DAT, et al: A guide to calculating intakes of dietary fiber, *J Hum Nutr* 30:303, 1976.

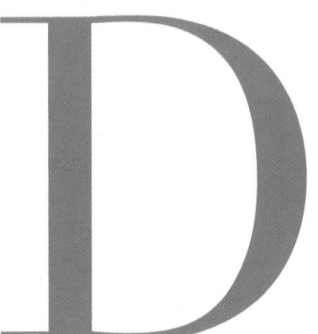

Sodium and Potassium Content of Foods, 100 g, Edible Portion

Food and description	Sodium (mg)	Potassium (mg)
Almonds		
Dried	4	773
Roasted and salted	198	773
Apple brown betty	153	100
Apple butter	2	252
Apple juice, canned or bottled	1	101
Apples		
Raw, pared	1	110
Frozen, sliced, sweetened	14	68
Applesauce, canned, sweetened	2	65
Apricot nectar, canned (approx. 40% fruit)	Trace	151
Apricots		
Raw	1	281
Canned, syrup pack, light	1	239
Dried, sulfured, cooked, fruit, and liquid	8	318

Numbers in parentheses denote values inputed, usually from another form of the food or from a similar food. Dashes denote lack of reliable data for a constituent believed to be present in measurable amount. Values are selected from Watt, BK, Merril, AL: *Composition of foods—raw, processed, prepared,* U.S. Department of Agriculture, Agriculture Handbook No 8, Dec 1963.

For notes see end of table.

Food and description	Sodium (mg)	Potassium (mg)
Asparagus		
Cooked spears, boiled, drained	1	183
Canned spears, green		
Regular pack, solids and liquid	236[1]	166
Special dietary pack (low sodium), solids and liquid	3	166
Frozen		
Cuts and tips, cooked, boiled, drained	1	220
Spears, cooked, boiled, drained	1	238
Avocados, raw, all commercial varieties	4	604
Bacon, cured, cooked, broiled or fried, drained	1021	236
Bacon, Canadian, cooked, broiled or fried, drained	2555	432
Baking powders		
Home use		
Straight phosphate	8220	170
Special low-sodium preparations	6	10,948
Bananas, raw, common	1	370
Barbecue sauce	815	174
Bass, black sea, raw	68	256
Beans, common, mature seeds, dry		
White		
Cooked	7	416
Canned, solids and liquid, with pork and tomato sauce	463	210
Red, cooked	3	340
Beans, lima		
Immature seeds		
Cooked, boiled, drained	1	422
Canned		
Regular pack, solids and liquid	236[1]	222
Special dietary pack (low sodium), solids and liquid	4	222
Frozen, thin-seeded types, commonly called baby limas cooked, boiled, drained	129	394
Mature seeds, dry, cooked	2	612
Beans, mung, sprouted seeds, cooked, boiled, drained	4	156
Beans, snap		
Green		
Cooked, boiled, drained	4	151
Canned		
Regular pack, solids and liquid	236[1]	95
Special dietary pack (low sodium), solids and liquid	2	95
Frozen, cut, cooked, boiled, drained	1	152
Yellow or wax		
Cooked, boiled, drained	3	151
Canned		

Food and description	Sodium (mg)	Potassium (mg)
Regular pack, solids and liquid	236[1]	95
Special dietary pack (low sodium), solids and liquid	2	95
Frozen, cut, cooked, boiled, drained	1	164
Beans and frankfurters, canned	539	262
Beef		
Retail cuts, trimmed to retail level		
Round	60	370
Rump	60	370
Hamburger, regular ground, cooked	47	450
Beef and vegetable stew, canned	411	174
Beef, corned, boneless		
Cooked, medium fat	1740	150
Canned corned-beef hash (with potato)	540	200
Beef, dried, cooked, creamed	716	153
Beef potpie, commercial, frozen, unheated	366	93
Beet greens, common, cooked, boiled, drained	76	332
Canned		
Regular pack, solids and liquid	236[1]	167
Special dietary pack (low sodium), solids and liquid	46	167
Beverages, alcoholic		
Beer, alcohol 4.5% by volume (3.6% by weight)	7	25
Gin, rum, vodka, whisky		
80 proof (33.4% alcohol by weight)	1	2
86 proof (36.0% alcohol by weight)	1	2
90 proof (37.9% alcohol by weight)	1	2
94 proof (39.7% alcohol by weight)	1	2
100 proof (42.5% alcohol by weight)	1	2
Wines		
Dessert, alcohol 18.8% by volume (15.3% by weight)	4	75
Table, alcohol 12.2% by volume (9.9% by weight)	5	92
Biscuit dough, commercial, frozen	910	86
Biscuit mix, with enriched flour, and biscuits baked from mix		
Dry form	1300	80
Made with milk	973	116
Biscuits, baking powder, made with enriched flour	626	117
Blackberries, including dewberries, boysenberries, and youngberries, raw	1	170
Blackberries, canned, solids and liquid		
Water pack, with or without artificial sweetener	1	115
Syrup pack, heavy	1	109
Blueberries		
Raw	1	81
Frozen, not thawed, sweetened	1	66

Food and description	Sodium (mg)	Potassium (mg)
Bluefish, cooked		
Baked or broiled	104	—
Fried	146	—
Boston brown bread	251	292
Bouillon cubes or powder	24,000	100
Boysenberries, frozen, not thawed, sweetened	1	105
Bran, added sugar and malt extract	1060	1070
Bran flakes (40% bran), added thiamine	925	—
Bran flakes with raisins, added thiamine	800	—
Brazil nuts	1	715
Bread crumbs, dry, grated	736	152
Bread stuffing mix and stuffings prepared from mix, dry form	1331	172
Breads		
Cracked wheat	529	134
French or Vienna, enriched	580	90
Italian, enriched	585	74
Raisin	365	233
Rye, American ($\frac{1}{3}$ rye, $\frac{2}{3}$ clear flour)	557	145
White enriched, made with 3%-4% nonfat dry milk	507	105
Whole wheat, made with 2% nonfat dry milk	527	273
Broccoli		
Cooked spears, boiled, drained	10	267
Frozen, spears, cooked, boiled, drained	12	220
Brussels sprouts, frozen, cooked, boiled, drained	14	295
Buffalo fish, raw	52	293
Bulgur (parboiled wheat), canned, made from hard red winter wheat		
Unseasoned[2]	599	87
Seasoned[3]	460	112
Butter[4]	987	23
Buttermilk, fluid, cultured (made from skim milk)	130	140
Cabbage		
Common varieties (Danish, domestic, and pointed types)		
Raw	20	233
Cooked, boiled until tender, drained, shredded, cooked in small amount of water	14	163
Red, raw	26	268
Cabbage, Chinese (also called celery cabbage or petsai)	23	253
Cakes		
Baked from home recipes		
Angel food	283	88
Fruit cake, made with enriched flour, dark	158	496
Gingerbread, made with enriched flour	237	454
Plain cake or cupcake, without icing	300	79

Food and description	Sodium (mg)	Potassium (mg)
Pound, modified	178	78
Frozen, commercial, devil's food, with chocolate icing	420	119
Candy		
Caramels, plain or chocolate	226	192
Chocolate, sweet	33	269
Chocolate coated, chocolate fudge	228	193
Gum drops, starch jelly pieces	35	5
Hard	32	4
Marshmallows	39	6
Peanut bars	10	448
Carp, raw	50	286
Carrots		
Raw	47	341
Canned		
Regular pack, solids and liquid	236[1]	120
Special dietary pack (low sodium), solids and liquid	39	120
Cashew nuts	15[5]	464
Catfish, freshwater, raw	60	330
Cauliflower		
Cooked, boiled, drained	9	206
Frozen, cooked, boiled, drained	10	207
Caviar, sturgeon, granular	2200	180
Celery, all, including green and yellow varieties		
Raw	126	341
Cooked, boiled, drained	88	239
Chard, Swiss, cooked, boiled, drained	86	321
Cheese straws	721	63
Cheeses		
Natural cheeses		
Cheddar (domestic type, commonly called American)	700	82
Cottage (large or small curd)		
Creamed	229	85
Uncreamed	290	72
Cream	250	74
Parmesan	734	149
Swiss (domestic)	710	104
Pasteurized process cheese, American	1136[6]	80
Pasteurized process cheese spread, American	1625[6]	240
Cherries		
Raw, sweet	2	191
Canned		
Sour, red, solids and liquid, water pack	2	130

Food and description	Sodium (mg)	Potassium (mg)
Sweet, solids and liquid, syrup pack, light	1	128
Frozen, not thawed, sweetened	2	130
Chicken, all classes		
Light meat without skin, cooked, roasted	64	411
Dark meat without skin, cooked, roasted	86	321
Chicken potpie, commercial, frozen, unheated	411	153
Chicory, Witloof (also called French or Belgian endive), bleached head (forced), raw	7	182
Chili con carne, canned, with beans	531	233
Chocolate, bitter or baking	4	830
Chocolate syrup, fudge type	89	284
Chop suey, with meat, canned	551	138
Chow mein, chicken (without noodles), canned	290	167
Citron, candied	290	120
Clams, raw		
Soft, meat only	36	235
Hard or round, meat only	205	311
Clams, canned, including hard, soft, razor, and unspecified solids and liquid	—	140
Cocoa and chocolate-flavored beverage powders		
Cocoa powder with nonfat dry milk	525	800
Mix for hot chocolate	382	605
Cocoa, dry powder, high-fat or breakfast		
Plain	6	1522
Processed with alkali	717	651
Coconut cream (liquid expressed from grated coconut meat)	4	324
Coconut meat, fresh	23	256
Cod		
Cooked, broiled	110	407
Dehydrated, lightly salted	8100	160
Coffee, instant, water-soluble solids		
Dry powder	72	3256
Beverage	1	36
Coleslaw, made with French dressing (commercial)	268	205
Collards, cooked, boiled, drained, leaves, including stems, cooked in small amount of water	25	234
Cookie dough, plain, chilled in roll, baked	548	48
Cookies		
Assorted, packaged, commercial	365	67
Butter, thin, rich	418	60
Gingersnaps	571	462
Molasses	386	138
Oatmeal with raisins	162	370
Sandwich type	483	38

Food and description	Sodium (mg)	Potassium (mg)
Vanilla wafer	252	72
Corn, sweet		
Cooked, boiled, drained, white and yellow, kernels, cut off cob before cooking	Trace	165
Canned		
Regular pack, cream style, white and yellow, solids and liquid	236[1]	(97)
Special dietary pack (low sodium), cream style, white and yellow, solids and liquid	2	(97)
Frozen, kernels cut off cob, cooked, boiled, drained	1	184
Corn fritters	477	133
Corn grits, degermed, enriched, dry form	1	80
Corn products used mainly as ready-to-eat breakfast cereals		
Corn flakes, added nutrients	1005	120
Corn, puffed, added nutrients	1060	—
Corn, rice, and wheat flakes, mixed, added nutrients	950	—
Cornbread, baked from home recipes, southern style, made with degermed cornmeal, enriched		
Cornbread mix and cornbread baked from mix, cornbread, made with egg, milk	744	127
Cornmeal, white or yellow, degermed, enriched, dry form	1	120
Cornstarch	Trace	Trace
Cowpeas, including blackeye peas		
Immature seeds, canned, solids and liquid	236[1]	352
Young pods, with seeds, cooked, boiled, drained	3	196
Crab, canned	1000	110
Crackers		
Butter	1092	113
Graham, plain	670	384
Saltines	(1100)	(120)
Sandwich type, peanut-cheese	992	226
Soda	1100	120
Cranberries, raw	2	82
Cranberry juice cocktail, bottled (approx. 33% cranberry juice)	1	10
Cranberry sauce, sweetened, canned, strained	1	30
Cream, fluid, light, coffee, or table, 20% fat	43	122
Cream substitutes, dried, containing cream, skim milk (calcium reduced), and lactose	575	—
Cream puffs with custard filling	83	121
Cress, garden, raw	14	606
Croaker, Atlantic, cooked, baked	120	323
Cucumbers, raw, pared	6	160
Custard, baked	79	146
Dates, domestic, natural and dry	1	648
Doughnuts, cake type	501	90
Duck, domesticated, raw, flesh only	74	285

Food and description	Sodium (mg)	Potassium (mg)
Eggplant, cooked, boiled, drained	1	150
Eggs, chicken		
Raw		
Whole, fresh and frozen	122	129
Whites, fresh and frozen	146	139
Yolks, fresh	52	98
Endive (curly endive and escarole), raw	14	294
Farina		
Enriched		
Regular		
Dry form	2	83
Cooked	144	9
Quick-cooking, cooked	165	10
Instant-cooking, cooked	188	13
Nonenriched, regular, dry form	2	83
Figs, canned, solids and liquid, syrup pack, light	2	152
Flatfishes (flounders, soles, sand dabs), raw	78	342
Fruit cocktail, canned, solids and liquid, water pack, with or without artificial sweetener	5	168
Garlic, cloves, raw	19	529
Ginger root, fresh	6	264
Gizzard, chicken, all classes, cooked, simmered	57	211
Goose, domesticated, flesh only, cooked, roasted	124	605
Gooseberries, canned, solids and liquid, syrup pack, heavy	1	98
Grapefruit		
Raw, pulp, pink, red, white, all varieties	1	135
Canned, juice, sweetened	1	162
Grapefruit juice and orange juice blended, canned, sweetened	1	184
Grapes, raw, American type (slip skin), such as Concord, Delaware, Niagara,		
Catawba, and Scuppernong	3	158
Grapejuice, canned or bottled	2	116
Guavas, whole, raw, common	4	289
Haddock, cooked, fried	177	348
Hake, including Pacific hake, squirrel hake, and silver hake or whiting; raw	74	363
Halibut, Atlantic and Pacific, cooked, broiled	134	525
Ham croquette	342	83
Heart, beef, lean, cooked, braised	104	232
Herring		
Raw, Pacific	74	420
Smoked, hard	6231	157
Honey, strained or extracted	5	51
Horseradish, prepared	96	290
Ice cream and frozen custard, regular, approximately 17% fat	63[7]	181

Food and description	Sodium (mg)	Potassium (mg)
Ice cream cones	232	244
Ice milk	68[7]	195
Jams and preserves	12	88
Kale, cooked, boiled, drained, leaves including stems	43	221
Kingfish; southern, gulf, and northern (whiting); raw	83	250
Lake herring (cisco), raw	47	319
Lamb, retail cuts	70	290
Lemon juice, canned or bottled, unsweetened	1	141
Lettuce, raw crisphead varieties such as Iceberg, New York, and Great Lakes strains	9	175
Lime juice, canned or bottled, unsweetened	1	104
Liver, beef, cooked, fried	184	380
Lobster, northern, canned or cooked	210	180
Loganberries, canned, solids and liquid, syrup pack, light	1	111
Macadamia nuts	—	164
Macaroni, unenriched, dry form	2	197
Macaroni and cheese, canned	304	58
Margarine[8]	987	23
Marmalade, citrus	14	33
Milk, cow		
Fluid (pasteurized and raw)		
Whole, 3.7% fat	50	144
Skim	52	145
Canned, evaporated (unsweetened)	118	303
Dry, skim (nonfat solids), regular	532	1745
Malted		
Dry powder	440	720
Beverage	91	200
Chocolate drink, fluid, commercial		
Made with skim milk	46	142
Made with whole (3.5% fat) milk	47	146
Molasses, cane		
First extraction or light	15	917
Third extraction or blackstrap	96	2927
Muffin mixes, corn, and muffins baked from mixes		
Made with egg, milk	479	110
Made with egg, water	346	104
Mushrooms		
Raw	15	414
Canned, solids and liquid	400	197
Muskmelons, raw, cantaloupes, other netted varieties	12	251
Mussels, Atlantic and Pacific, raw, meat only	289	315
Mustard greens, cooked, boiled, drained	18	220

Food and description	Sodium (mg)	Potassium (mg)
Mustard, prepared		
Brown	1307	130
Yellow	1252	130
Nectarines, raw	6	294
New Zealand spinach, cooked, boiled, drained	92	463
Noodles, egg noodles, enriched, cooked	2	44
Oat products used mainly as hot breakfast cereals, oatmeal or rolled oats		
Dry form	2	352
Cooked	218	61
Oat products used mainly as ready-to-eat breakfast cereals, with or without corn, puffed, added nutrients	1267	—
Ocean perch, Atlantic (redfish)		
Raw	79	269
Cooked, fried	153	284
Ocean perch, Pacific, raw	63	390
Oils, salad or cooking	0	0
Okra		
Raw	3	249
Cooked, boiled, drained	2	174
Olives, pickled; canned or bottled		
Green	2400	55
Ripe, Ascolano (extra large, mammoth, giant jumbo)	813	34
Ripe, salt-cured, oil-coated, Greek style	3288	—
Onions, mature (dry), raw	10	157
Onions, young green (bunching varieties), raw, bulb and entire top	5	231
Oranges, raw, peeled fruit, all commercial varieties	1	200
Orange juice		
Raw, all commercial varieties	1	200
Canned, unsweetened	1	199
Frozen concentrate, unsweetened, diluted with 3 parts water, by volume	1	186
Oysters		
Raw, meat only, Eastern	73	121
Cooked, fried	206	203
Frozen, solids and liquid	380	210
Oyster stew, commercial frozen, prepared with equal volume of milk	366	176
Pancake and waffle mixes and pancakes baked from mixes, plain and buttermilk, made with egg, milk	564	154
Parsnips, cooked, boiled, drained	8	379
Peaches		
Raw	1	202
Canned, solids and liquid, water pack, with or without artificial sweetener	2	137
Frozen, sliced, sweetened, not thawed	2	124

Food and description	Sodium (mg)	Potassium (mg)
Peanut butters made with small amounts of added fat, salt	607	670
Peanuts		
Roasted with skins	5	701
Roasted and salted	418	674
Pears		
Raw, including skin	2	130
Canned, solids and liquid, syrup pack, light	1	85
Peas, green, immature		
Cooked, boiled, drained	1	196
Canned, Alaska (early or June peas)		
Regular pack, solids and liquid	236[1]	96
Special dietary pack (low sodium), solids and liquid	3	96
Frozen, cooked, boiled, drained	115	135
Peas, mature seeds, dry, whole, raw	35	1005
Peas and carrots, frozen, cooked, boiled, drained	84	157
Pecans	Trace	603
Peppers, hot, chili, mature, red, raw, pods excluding seeds	25	564
Peppers, sweet, garden varieties, immature, green, raw	13	213
Perch, yellow, raw	68	230
Pickles, cucumber, dill	1428	200
Piecrust or plain pastry, made with enriched flour, baked	611	50
Pies, baked, piecrust made with unenriched flour		
Apple	301	80
Cherry	304	105
Mincemeat	448	178
Pumpkin	214	160
Pike, walleye, raw	51	319
Pineapple		
Raw	1	146
Frozen chunks, sweetened, not thawed	2	100
Pizza, with cheese, from home recipe, baked		
With cheese topping	702	130
With sausage topping	729	168
Plate dinners, frozen, commercial, unheated		
Beef pot roast, whole oven-browned potatoes, peas, corn	259	244
Chicken, fried; mashed potatoes; mixed vegetables (carrots, peas, corn, beans)	344	112
Meat loaf with tomato sauce, mashed potatoes, peas	393	115
Turkey, sliced; mashed potatoes, peas	400	176
Plums		
Raw, Damson	2	299
Canned, solids and liquid, purple (Italian prunes), syrup pack, light	1	145
Popcorn, popped		

Food and description	Sodium (mg)	Potassium (mg)
Plain	(3)	—
Oil and salt added	1940	—
Pork, fresh, retail cuts, trimmed to retail level, loin	65	390
Pork, lightly cured, commercial, ham, medium-fat class, separable, lean, cooked, roasted	930	326
Pork, cured, canned ham, contents of can	(1100)	(340)
Potatoes		
Cooked, boiled in skin	3[9]	407
Dehydrated mashed, flakes without milk		
Dry form	89	1600
Prepared, water, milk, table fat added	231	286
Pretzels	1680[10]	130
Prunes, dried, "softenized," cooked (fruit and liquid), with added sugar	3	262
Pudding mixes and puddings made from mixes, with starch base		
With milk, cooked	129	136
With milk, without cooking	124	129
Pumpkin, canned	2	240
Radishes, raw, common	18	322
Raisins, natural (unbleached), cooked, fruit and liquid, added sugar	13	355
Raspberries		
Canned, solids and liquid, water pack, with or without artificial sweetener, red	1	114
Frozen, red, sweetened, not thawed	1	100
Rennin products		
Tablet (salts, starch, rennin enzyme)	22,300	—
Dessert mixes and desserts prepared from mixes		
Chocolate, dessert made with milk	52	125
Other flavors (vanilla, caramel, fruit flavorings)		
Mix, dry form	6	—
Dessert, made with milk	46	128
Rhubarb, cooked, added sugar	2	203
Rice		
Brown		
Raw	9	214
Cooked	282	70
White (fully milled or polished), enriched, common commercial varieties, all types		
Raw	5	92
Cooked	374	28
Rice products used mainly as ready-to-eat breakfast cereals		
Rice flakes, added nutrients	987	180
Rice, puffed; added nutrients, without salt	2	100
Rice, puffed or open-popped, presweetened, honey and added nutrients	706	—
Rockfish, including black, canary, yellowtail, rasphead, and bocaccio, cooked,	68	446

Food and description	Sodium (mg)	Potassium (mg)
oven-steamed		
Roe, cooked, baked or broiled, cod and shad[11]	73	132
Rolls and buns, commercial, ready-to-serve		
Danish pastry	366	112
Hard rolls, enriched	625	97
Plain (pan rolls), enriched	506	95
Sweet rolls	389	124
Rusk	246	161
Rutabagas, cooked, boiled, drained	4	167
Rye, flour, medium	(1)	203
Rye wafers, whole grain	882	600
Salad dressings, commercial[12]		
Blue and Roquefort cheese		
Regular	1094	37
Special dietary (low calorie), low fat (approx. 5 kcal/tsp)	1108	34
French		
Regular	1370	79
Special dietary (low calorie), low fat (approx. 5 kcal/tsp)	787	79
Mayonnaise	597	34
Thousand Island		
Regular	700	113
Special dietary (low calorie, approx. 10 kcal/tsp)	700	113
Salmon, coho (silver)		
Raw	48[13]	421
Canned, solids and liquid	351[14]	339
Salt pork, raw	1212	42
Salt sticks, regular type	1674	92
Sandwich spread (with chopped pickle)		
Regular	626	92
Special dietary (low calorie, approx. 5 kcal/tsp)	626	92
Sardines, Atlantic, canned in oil, drained solids	823	590
Sardines, Pacific, in tomato sauce, solids and liquid	400	320
Sauerkraut, canned, solids and liquid	747[15]	140
Sausage, cold cuts, and luncheon meats		
Bologna, all samples	1300	230
Frankfurters, raw, all samples	1100	220
Luncheon meat, pork, cured ham or shoulder, chopped, spiced or unspiced, canned	1234	222
Pork sausage, links or bulk, cooked	958	269
Scallops, bay and sea, cooked, steamed	265	476
Soups, commercial, canned		
Beef broth, bouillon, and consomme, prepared with equal volume of water	326	54

Food and description	Sodium (mg)	Potassium (mg)
Chicken noodle, prepared with equal volume of water	408	23
Tomato		
Prepared with equal volume of water	396	94
Prepared with equal volume of milk	422	167
Vegetable beef, prepared with equal volume of water	427	66
Soy sauce	7325	366
Spaghetti, enriched, cooked, tender stage	1	61
Spaghetti, in tomato sauce with cheese, canned	382	121
Spinach		
Cooked, boiled, drained	50	324
Canned		
Regular pack, drained solids	236[1]	250
Special dietary pack (low sodium), solids and liquid	34	250
Frozen, chopped, cooked, boiled, drained	52	333
Squash, summer, all varieties, cooked, boiled, drained	1	141
Squash, frozen		
Summer, yellow crookneck, cooked, boiled, drained	3	167
Winter, heated	1	207
Strawberries		
Raw	1	164
Frozen, sweetened, not thawed, sliced	1	112
Sturgeon, cooked, steamed	108	235
Succotash (corn and lima beans), frozen, cooked, boiled, drained	38	246
Sugars, beet or cane, brown	30	344
Sweet potatoes		
Cooked, all, baked in skin	12	300
Canned, liquid pack, solids and liquid, regular pack in syrup	48	(120)
Dehydrated flakes, prepared with water	45	140
Tangerines, raw (Dancy variety)	2	126
Tapioca, dry	3	18
Tapioca desserts, tapioca cream pudding	156	135
Tartar sauce, regular	707	78
Tea, instant (water-soluble solids), carbohydrate added		
Dry powder	—	4530
Beverage	—	25
Tomato catsup, bottled	1042[16]	363
Tomato juice, canned or bottled		
Regular pack	200	227
Special dietary pack (low sodium)	3	227
Tomato juice cocktail, canned or bottled	200	221
Tomato puree, canned		
Regular pack	399	426

Food and description	Sodium (mg)	Potassium (mg)
Special dietary pack (low sodium)	6	426
Tomatoes, ripe		
Raw	3	244
Canned, solids and liquid, regular pack	130	217
Tongue, beef, medium fat, cooked, braised	61	164
Tuna, canned		
In oil, solids and liquid	800	301
In water, solids and liquid	41[17]	279[17]
Turkey, all classes		
Light meat, cooked, roasted	82	411
Dark meat, cooked, roasted	99	398
Turkey potpie, commercial, frozen, unheated	369	114
Turnips, cooked, boiled, drained	34	188
Turnip greens, leaves, including stems		
Canned, solids and liquid	236[1]	243
Frozen, cooked, boiled, drained	17	149
Veal, retail cuts, untrimmed	80	500
Vinegar, cider	1	100
Waffles, frozen, made with enriched flour	644	158
Walnuts		
Black	3	460
Persian or English	2	450
Watercress leaves including stems, raw	52	282
Watermelon, raw	1	100
Wheat flours		
Whole (from hard wheats)	3	370
Patent		
All-purpose or family flour, enriched	2	95
Self-rising flour, enriched (anhydrous monocalcium phosphate used as a baking acid)[18]	1079	—[19]
Wild rice, raw	7	220
Yeast		
Baker's, compressed	16	610
Brewer's, debittered	121	1894
Yogurt, made from whole milk	47	132
Zweiback	250	150

FOOTNOTES

[1]Estimated average based on addition of salt in the amount of 0.6% of the finished product.

[2]Processed, partially debranned, whole-kernel wheat with salt added.

[3]Processed, partially debranned, whole-kernel wheat with chicken fat, chicken stock base, dehydrated onion flakes, salt, monosodium glutamate, and herbs.

[4]Values apply to salted butter. Unsalted butter contains less than 10 mg of either sodium or potassium per 100 g. Value for vitamin A is the year-round average.

[5]Applies to unsalted nuts. For salted nuts, value is approximately 200 mg per 100 g.

[6]Values for phosphorus and sodium are based on use of 1.5% anhydrous disodium phosphate as the emulsifying agent. If emulsifying agent does not contain either phosphorus (P) or sod (Na), the content of these two nutrients in milligrams per 100 g is as follows:

	Na	P
American process cheese	650	444
Swiss process cheese	681	540
American cheese food	—	427
American cheese spread	1139	548

[7]Value for product without added salt.

[8]Values apply to salted margarine. Unsalted margarine contains less than 10 mg/100 g of either sodium or potassium. Vitamin A value based on the minimum required to meet federal specifications for margarine with vitamin A added, 15,000 IUA/lb.

[9]Applies to product without added salt. If salt is added, an estimated average value for sodium is 236 mg/100 g.

[10]Sodium content is variable. For example, very think pretzel sticks contain about twice the average amount listed.

[11]Prepared with butter or margarine, lemon juice or vinegar.

[12]Values apply to products containing salt. For those without salt, sodium content is low, ranging from less than 10 to50 mg/100 g; the amount usually is indicated on the label.

[13]Sample dipped in brine contained 215 mg sodium/100 g.

[14]For product canned without added salt, value is approximately the same as for raw salmon.

[15]Values for sauerkraut and sauerkraut juice are based on salt content of 1.9% and 2.0%, respectively, in the finished products. The amounts in some samples may vary significantly from the estimate.

[16]Applies to regular pack. For special dietary pack (low sodium), values range from 5-35 mg/100 g.

[17]One sample with salt added contained 875 mg of sodium/100 g and 275 mg of potassium.

[18]The acid ingredient most commonly used in self-rising flour. When sodium acid pyrophosphate in combination with either anhydrous monocalcium phosphate or calcium carbonate is used, the value for calcium is approximately 120 mg/100 g; for phosphorus, 540 mg; for sodium, 1360 mg.

[19]90 mg of potassium/100 g contributed by flour. Small quantities of additional potassium may be provided by other ingredients.

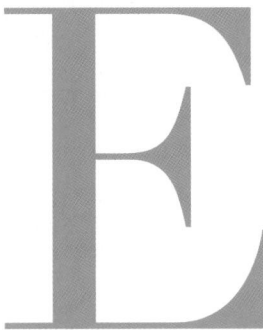 **Salt-Free Seasoning Guide**

Fish	Beef	Poultry and veal	Gravies and sauces
Breaded, battered fillets	Swiss steak	Fried chicken	Barbecue
Dry mustard, onion; oregano, basil, garlic; thyme	Rosemary, black pepper; bay leaf, thyme; clove	Basil, oregano, garlic; onion, dill; sesame seed, nutmeg	Bay leaf, thyme, red pepper; cinnamon, ginger, allspice, dry mustard, red pepper; chili powder
Broiled steaks or fillets	Roast beef	Roast chicken or turkey	Brown
Chili or curry powder; tarragon	Basil, oregano; bay leaf; nutmeg; tarragon, marjoram	Ginger, garlic; onion, thyme, tarragon	Chervil, onion; onion, bay leaf, thyme; onion, nutmeg; tarragon
Fillets in butter sauce	Beef stew	Chicken croquettes	Chicken
Thyme, chervil; dill; fennel	Chili powder; bay leaf, tarragon; caraway; marjoram	Dill; curry; chili, cumin; tarragon, oregano	Dry mustard; ginger, garlic; marjoram, thyme, bay leaf
Fish soup	Meatballs	Veal patties	Cream
Italian seasoning; bay leaf, thyme, tarragon	Garlic, thyme; basil, oregano, onion; thyme, garlic; black pepper, dry mustard	Italian seasoning; tarragon; dill, onion, sesame seed	White pepper, dry mustard; curry powder; dill, onion, paprika; tarragon, thyme
Fish cakes	Beef stroganoff	Barbecue chicken	
Tarragon, savory; dry mustard, white pepper; red pepper, oregano	Red pepper, onion, garlic; nutmeg, onion; curry powder	Garlic, dry mustard; clove, allspice, dry mustard; basil, garlic, and oregano	

Soups	Salads	Pasta, beans, and rice	Vegetables
Chicken	Chicken	Baked beans	Asparagus
Thyme, savory; ginger; clove, white pepper, allspice	Curry or chili powder; Italian seasoning; thyme, tarragon	Dry mustard; chili powder; clove, onion; ginger, dry mustard	Ginger; sesame seed; basil, onion
Clam chowder	Coleslaw	Rice and vegetables	Broccoli
Basil, oregano; nutmeg, white pepper; thyme, garlic powder	Dill; caraway; poppy; dry mustard, ginger	Curry; thyme, onion, paprika; rosemary, garlic; ginger, onion, garlic	Italian seasoning; marjoram, basil; nutmeg, onion; sesame seed
Mushroom	Fish or seafood	Spanish rice	Cabbage
Ginger; oregano; thyme, tarragon; bay leaf, black pepper; chili powder	Dill; tarragon, ginger, dry mustard, red pepper; ginger, onion, garlic	Cumin, oregano, basil; Italian seasoning	Caraway; onion, nutmeg; allspice, clove
Onion	Macaroni	Spaghetti	Carrots
Curry, carraway; marjoram, garlic; cloves	Dill; basil, thyme, oregano; dry mustard, garlic	Italian seasoning, nutmeg; oregano, basil, nutmeg; red pepper, tarragon	Ginger; nutmeg; onion, dill
Tomato	Potato	Rice pilaf	Cauliflower
Bay leaf, thyme; Italian seasoning; oregano, onion; nutmeg	Chili powder; curry; dry mustard, onion	Dill; thyme, savory, black pepper	Dry mustard; basil; paprika, onion
Vegetable			Tomatoes
Italian seasoning; paprika, caraway; rosemary, thyme; fennel, thyme			Oregano; chili powder; dill, onion
			Spinach
			Savory, thyme; nutmeg; garlic, onion

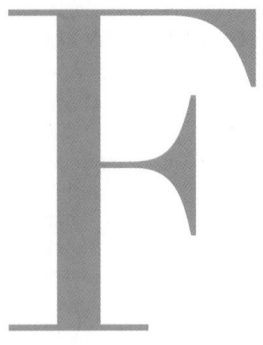

Exchange Lists

Groups/Lists	Carbohydrate (grams)	Protein (grams)	Fat (grams)	kCalories
Carbohydrate Group				
Starch	15	3	1 or less	80
Fruit	15	—	—	60
Milk				
Skim	12	8	0-3	90
Low-fat	12	8	5	120
Whole	12	8	8	150
Other carbohydrates	15	varies	varies	varies
Vegetables	5	2	—	25
Meat and Meat Substitute Group				
Very lean	—	7	0-1	35
Lean	—	7	3	55
Medium-fat	—	7	5	75
High-fat	—	7	8	100
Fat Group	—	—	5	45

From American Diabetes Association, American Dietetic Association: *Exchange lists for meal planning,* rev, Chicago, 1995, ADA/ADA.

Common Measurements

3 tsp = 1 Tbsp

4 Tbsp = ¼ cup

5⅓ Tbsp = ⅓ cup

4 oz = ½ cup

8 oz = 1 cup

1 cup = ½ pint

The Exchange Lists are the basis of a meal planning system designed by a committee of the American Diabetes Association and The American Dietetic Association. While designed primarily for people with diabetes and others who must follow special diets, the Exchange Lists are based on principles of good nutrition that apply to everyone. 1995 American Diabetes Association, Inc., The American Dietetic Association.

Starch

One starch exchange equals 15 g carbohydrate, 3 g protein, 0-1 g fat, and 80 kcalories.

Bread

Bagel	½ (1 oz)
Bread, reduced-calorie	2 slices (1½ oz)
Bread, white, whole-wheat, pumpernickel, rye	1 slice (1 oz)
Bread sticks, crisp, 4 in long × ½ in	2 (⅔ oz)
English muffin	½
Hot dog or hamburger bun	½ (1 oz)
Pita, 6 in across	½
Roll, plain, small	1 (1 oz)
Raisin bread, unfrosted	1 slice (1 oz)
Tortilla, corn, 6 in across	1
Tortilla, flour, 7 to 8 in across	1
Waffle, 4½ in square, reduced-fat	1

Cereals and Grains

Bran cereals	½ cup
Bulgur	½ cup
Cereals	½ cup
Cereals, unsweetened, ready-to-eat	¾ cup
Cornmeal (dry)	3 Tbsp
Couscous	⅓ cup
Flour (dry)	3 Tbsp
Granola, low-fat	¼ cup
Grape-Nuts	¼ cup
Grits	½ cup
Kasha	½ cup
Millet	¼ cup
Muesli	¼ cup
Oats	½ cup
Pasta	½ cup
Puffed cereal	1½ cups
Rice milk	½ cup
Rice, white or brown	⅓ cup
Shredded wheat	½ cup
Sugar-frosted cereal	½ cup
Wheat germ	3 Tbsp

Starchy Vegetables

Baked beans	⅓ cup
Corn	½ cup
Corn on cob, medium	1 (5 oz)
Mixed vegetables with corn, peas, or pasta	1 cup
Peas, green	½ cup
Plantain	½ cup
Potato, backed or boiled	1 small (3 oz)
Potato, mashed	½ cup
Squash, winter (acorn, butternut)	1 cup
Yam, sweet potato, plain	½ cup

Crackers and Snacks

Animal crackers	8
Graham crackers, 2½ in square	3
Matzoh	¾ oz
Melba toast	4 slices
Oyster crackers	24
Popcorn (popped, no fat added or low-fat microwave)	3 cups
Pretzels	¾ oz
Rice cakes, 4 in across	2
Saltine-type crackers	6
Snack chips, fat-free (tortilla, potato)	15-20 (¾ oz)
Whole-wheat crackers, no fat added	2-5 (¾ oz)

Dried Beans, Peas, and Lentils

Count as 1 starch exchange, plus 1 very lean meat exchange.

Beans and peas (garbanzo, pinto, kidney, white, split, black-eyed)	½ cup
Lima beans	⅔ cup
Lentils	½ cup
Miso*	3 Tbsp

Starchy Foods Prepared with Fat

Count as 1 starch exchange, plus 1 fat exchange.

Biscuit, 2½ in across	1
Chow mein noodles	½ cup
Corn bread, 2 in-cube	1 (2 oz)
Crackers, round butter type	6
Croutons	1 cup
French-fried potatoes	16-25 (3 oz)
Granola	¼ cup
Muffin, small	1 (1½ oz)
Pancake, 4 in across	2
Popcorn, microwave	3 cups
Sandwich crackers, cheese or peanut butter filling	3
Stuffing, bread (prepared)	⅓ cup
Taco shell, 6 in across	2

*400 mg or more of sodium per serving.

| Waffle, 4½ in square | | 1 |
| Whole-wheat crackers, fat added | | 4-6 (1 oz) |

Food (Starch Group)	Uncooked	Cooked
Oatmeal	3 Tbsp	½ cup
Cream of Wheat	2 Tbsp	½ cup
Grits	3 Tbsp	½ cup
Rice	2 Tbsp	⅓ cup
Spaghetti	¼ cup	½ cup
Noodles	⅓ cup	½ cup
Macaroni	¼ cup	½ cup
Dried beans	¼ cup	½ cup
Dried peas	¼ cup	½ cup
Lentils	3 Tbsp	½ cup

Fruits

One fruit exchange equals 15 g carbohydrate and 60 kcalories. The weight includes skin, core, seeds, and rind.

Fruit

Apple, unpeeled, small	1 (4 oz)
Applesauce, unsweetened	½ cup
Apples, dried	4 rings
Apricots, fresh	4 whole (5½ oz)
Apricots, dried	8 halves
Apricots, canned	½ cup
Banana, small	1 (4 oz)
Blackberries	¾ cup
Blueberries	¾ cup
Cantaloupe, small	⅓ melon (11 oz) or 1 cup cubes
Cherries, sweet, fresh	12 (3 oz)
Cherries, sweet, canned	½ cup
Dates	3
Figs, fresh	1½ large or 2 medium (3½ oz)
Figs, dried	1½
Fruit cocktail	½ cup
Grapefruit, large	½ (11 oz)
Grapefruit sections, canned	¾ cup
Grapes, small	17 (3 oz)
Honeydew melon	1 slice (10 oz) or 1 cup cubes
Kiwi	1 (3½ oz)
Mandarin oranges, canned	¾ cup
Mango, small	½ fruit (5½ oz) or ½ cup
Nectarine, small	1 (5 oz)
Orange, small	1 (6½ oz)
Papaya	½ fruit (8 oz) or 1 cup cubes
Peach, medium, fresh	1 (6 oz)
Peaches, canned	½ cup
Pear, large, fresh	½ (4 oz)
Pears, canned	½ cup
Pineapple, fresh	¾ cup
Pineapple, canned	½ cup
Plums, small	2 (5 oz)
Plums, canned	½ cup
Prunes, dried	3
Raisins	2 Tbsp
Raspberries	1 cup
Strawberries	1¼ cup whole berries
Tangerines, small	2 (8 oz)
Watermelon	1 slice (13½ oz) or 1¼ cup cubes

Fruit Juice

Apple juice/cider	½ cup
Cranberry juice cocktail	⅓ cup
Cranberry juice cocktail, reduced-calorie	1 cup
Fruit juice blends, 100% juice	⅓ cup
Grape juice	⅓ cup
Grapefruit juice	½ cup
Orange juice	½ cup
Pineapple juice	½ cup
Prune juice	⅓ cup

Milk

One milk exchange equals 12 g carbohydrate and 8 g protein.

	Carbohydrate (grams)	Protein (grams)	Fat (grams)	Calories
Skim/very low-fat	12	8	0-3	90
Low-fat	12	8	5	120
Whole	12	8	8	150

Skim and Very Low-Fat Milk

0–3 g fat per serving

Skim milk	1 cup
½% milk	1 cup
1% milk	1 cup
Nonfat or low-fat buttermilk	1 cup
Evaporated skim milk	½ cup
Nonfat dry milk	⅓ cup dry
Plain nonfat yogurt	¾ cup
Nonfat or low-fat fruit-flavored yogurt sweetened with aspartame or with a nonnutritive sweetener	1 cup

Low Fat

5 g fat per serving

2% milk	1 cup
Plain low-fat yogurt	¾ cup
Sweet acidophilus milk	1 cup

Whole Milk

8 g fat per serving

Whole milk	1 cup
Evaporated whole milk	½ cup
Goat's milk	1 cup
Kefir	1 cup

Other Carbohydrates

Substitutes for a starch, fruit, or milk exchange. One exchange equals 15 g carbohydrate, or 1 starch, or 1 fruit, or 1 milk.

Food	*Serving Size*	*Exchanges Per Serving*
Angel food cake, unfrosted	1/12th cake	2 carbohydrates
Brownie, small, unfrosted	2 in square	1 carbohydrate, 1 fat
Cake, unfrosted	2 in square	1 carbohydrate, 1 fat
Cake, frosted	2 in square	2 carbohydrates, 1 fat
Cookie, fat-free	2 small	1 carbohydrate
Cookie or sandwich cookie with cream filling	2 small	1 carbohydrate, 1 fat
Cupcake, frosted	1 small	2 carbohydrates, 1 fat
Cranberry sauce, jellied	1/4 cup	2 carbohydrates
Doughnut, plain cake	1 medium (1½ oz)	1½ carbohydrates, 2 fats
Doughnut, glazed	3¾ in across (2 oz)	2 carbohydrates, 2 fats
Fruit juice bars, frozen, 100% juice	1 bar (3 oz)	1 carbohydrate
Fruit snacks, chewy (pureed fruit concentrate)	1 roll (¾ oz)	1 carbohydrate
Fruit spread, 100% fruit	1 Tbsp	1 carbohydrate
Gelatin, regular	½ cup	1 carbohydrate
Gingersnaps	3	1 carbohydrate
Granola bar	1 bar	1 carbohydrate, 1 fat
Granola bar, fat-free	1 bar	2 carbohydrates
Hummus	⅓ cup	1 carbohydrate, 1 fat
Ice cream	½ cup	1 carbohydrate, 2 fats
Ice cream, light	½ cup	1 carbohydrate, 1 fat
Ice cream, fat-free, no sugar added	½ cup	1 carbohydrate
Jam or jelly, regular	1 Tbsp	1 carbohydrate
Milk, chocolate, whole	1 cup	2 carbohydrates, 1 fat
Pie, fruit, 2 crusts	⅙ pie	3 carbohydrates, 2 fats
Pie, pumpkin or custard	⅛ pie	1 carbohydrate, 2 fats
Potato chips	12-18 (1 oz)	1 carbohydrate, 2 fats
Pudding, regular (made with low-fat milk)	½ cup	2 carbohydrates
Pudding, sugar-free (made with low-fat milk)	½ cup	1 carbohydrate

Salad dressing, fat-free*	¼ cup	1 carbohydrate
Sherbet, sorbet	½ cup	2 carbohydrates
Spaghetti or pasta sauce, canned*	½ cup	1 carbohydrate, 1 fat
Sweet roll or Danish	1 (2½ oz)	2½ carbohydrates, 2 fats
Syrup, light	2 Tbsp	1 carbohydrate
Syrup, regular	1 Tbsp	1 carbohydrate
Syrup, regular	¼ cup	4 carbohydrates
Tortilla chips	6-12 (1 oz)	1 carbohydrate, 2 fats
Yogurt, frozen, low-fat, fat-free	⅓ cup	1 carbohydrate, 0-1 fat
Yogurt, frozen, fat-free, no sugar added	½ cup	1 carbohydrate
Yogurt, low-fat with fruit	1 cup	3 carbohydrates, 0-1 fat
Vanilla wafers	5	1 carbohydrate, 1 fat

Vegetables

One vegetable exchange equals 5 g carbohydrate, 2 g protein, 0 g fat, and 25 kcalories.

Artichoke
Artichoke hearts
Asparagus
Beans (green, wax, Italian)
Bean sprouts
Beets
Broccoli
Brussels sprouts
Cabbage
Carrots
Cauliflower
Celery
Cucumber
Eggplant

Green onions or scallions
Greens (collard, kale, mustard, turnip)
Kohlrabi
Leeks
Mixed vegetables (without corn, peas, or pasta)
Mushrooms
Okra
Onions
Pea pods
Peppers (all varieties)
Radishes

Salad greens (endive, escarole, lettuce, romaine, spinach)
Sauerkraut*
Spinach
Summer squash
Tomato
Tomatoes, canned
Tomato sauce*
Tomato/vegetable juice*
Turnips
Water chestnuts
Watercress
Zucchini

Meat and Meat Substitutes

	Carbohydrate (grams)	Protein (grams)	Fat (grams)	Calories
Very lean	0	7	0-1	35
Lean	0	7	3	55
Medium-fat	0	7	5	75
High-fat	0	7	8	100

Very Lean Meat and Meat Substitutes List

One exchange equals 0 g carbohydrate, 7 g protein, 0-1 g fat, and 35 kcalories.

Poultry: Chicken or turkey (white meat, no skin), Cornish hen (no skin)   1 oz

Fish: Fresh or frozen cod, flounder, haddock, halibut, trout, tuna, fresh or canned in water   1 oz

Shellfish: Clams, crab, lobster, scallops, shrimp, imitation shellfish   1 oz

Game: Duck or pheasant (no skin), venison, buffalo, ostrich 1 oz
Cheese with 1 g or less fat per ounce:
  Nonfat or low-fat cottage cheese ¼ cup
  Fat-free cheese 1 oz
Other: Processed sandwich meats with 1 g or less fat per ounce, such as deli thin,
  shaved meats, chipped beef,* turkey ham 1 oz
  Egg whites 2
  Egg substitutes, plain ¼ cup
  Hot dogs with 1 g or less fat per ounce* 1 oz
  Kidney (high in cholesterol) 1 oz
Sausage with 1 g or less fat per ounce 1 oz
Count as one very lean meat and one starch exchange.
Dried beans, peas, lentils (cooked) ½ cup

Lean Meat and Meat Substitutes List
One exchange equals 0 g carbohydrate, 7 g protein, 3 g fat, and 55 kcalories.
Beef: USDA Select or Choice grades of lean beef trimmed of fat, such as round, sirloin,
  and flank steak; tenderloin; roast (rib, chuck, rump); steak (T-bone, porterhouse, cubed),
  ground round 1 oz
Pork: Lean pork, such as fresh ham; canned, cured, or boiled ham; Canadian bacon;*
  tenderloin, center loin chop 1 oz
Lamb: Roast, chop, leg 1 oz
Veal: Lean chop, roast 1 oz
Poultry: Chicken, turkey (dark meat, no skin), chicken white meat (with skin), domestic
  duck or goose (well-drained of fat, no skin) 1 oz
Fish:
  Herring (uncreamed or smoked) 1 oz
  Oysters 6 medium
  Salmon (fresh or canned), catfish 1 oz
  Sardines (canned) 2 medium
  Tuna (canned in oil, drained) 1 oz
Game: Goose (no skin), rabbit 1 oz
Cheese:
  4.5%-fat cottage cheese ¼ cup
  Grated Parmesan 2 Tbsp
  Cheeses with 3 g or less fat per ounce 1 oz
Other:
  Hot dogs with 3 g or less fat per ounce* 1½ oz
  Processed sandwich meat with 3 g or less fat per ounce, such as turkey pastrami or kielbasa 1 oz
  Liver, heart (high in cholesterol) 1 oz

Medium-Fat Meat and Meat Substitutes List
One exchange equals 0 g carbohydrate, 7 g protein, 5 g fat, and 75 kcalories.
Beef: Most beef products fall into this category (ground beef, meatloaf, corned beef,
  short ribs, prime grades of meat trimmed of fat, such as prime rib) 1 oz
Pork: Top loin, Boston butt, cutlet 1 oz
Lamb: Rib roast, ground 1 oz

Veal: Cutlet (ground or cubed, unbreaded)   1 oz
Poultry: Chicken dark meat (with skin), ground turkey or ground chicken, fried chicken
  (with skin)   1 oz
Fish: Any fried fish product   1 oz
Cheese: With 5 g or less fat per ounce
  Feta   1 oz
  Mozzarella   1 oz
  Ricotta   ¼ cup (2 oz)
Other:
  Egg (high in cholesterol, limit to 3 per week)   1
  Sausage with 5 g or less fat per ounce   1 oz
  Soy milk   1 cup
  Tempeh   ¼ cup
Tofu   4 oz or ½ cup

High-Fat Meat and Meat Substitutes List

One exchange equals 0 g carbohydrate, 7 g protein, 8 g fat, and 100 kcalories.
Pork: Spareribs, ground pork, pork sausage   1 oz
Cheese: All regular cheeses, such as American,* cheddar, Monterey Jack, Swiss   1 oz
Other: Processed sandwich meats with 8 g or less fat per ounce, such as bologna,
  pimento loaf, salami   1 oz
  Sausage, such as bratwurst, Italian, knockwurst, Polish, smoked   1 oz
  Hot dog (turkey or chicken)*   1 (10/lb)
  Bacon   3 slices (20 slices/lb)
Count as one high-fat meat plus one fat exchange.
Hot dog (beef, pork, or combination)*   1 (10/lb)
Peanut butter (contains unsaturated fat)   2 Tbsp

Fats

Monounsaturated Fats List

One fat exchange equals 5 g fat and 45 kcalories.
Avocado, medium   ⅛ (1 oz)
Oil (canola, olive, peanut)   1 tsp
Olives: ripe (black)   8 large
  green, stuffed*   10 large
Nuts
  almonds, cashews   6 nuts
  mixed (50% peanuts)   6 nuts
  peanuts   10 nuts
  pecans   4 halves
Peanut butter, smooth or crunchy   2 tsp
Sesame seeds   1 Tbsp
Tahini paste   2 tsp

Polyunsaturated Fats List

One fat exchange equals 5 g fat and 45 kcalories.
Margarine: stick, tub, or squeeze   1 tsp

lower-fat (30% to 50% vegetable oil)	1 Tbsp
Mayonnaise: regular	1 tsp
reduced-fat	1 Tbsp
Nuts, walnuts, English	4 halves
Oil (corn, safflower, soybean)	1 tsp
Salad dressing: regular*	1 Tbsp
reduced-fat	2 Tbsp
Miracle Whip Salad Dressing: regular	2 tsp
reduced-fat	1 Tbsp
Seeds: pumpkin, sunflower	1 Tbsp

Saturated Fats List

One fat exchange equals 5 g of fat and 45 kcalories.

Bacon, cooked	1 slice (20 slices/lb)
Bacon, grease	1 tsp
Butter: stick	1 tsp
whipped	2 tsp
reduced-fat	1 Tbsp
Chitterlings, boiled	2 Tbsp ($\frac{1}{2}$ oz)
Coconut, sweetened, shredded	2 Tbsp
Cream, half and half	2 Tbsp
Cream cheese: regular	1 Tbsp ($\frac{1}{2}$ oz)
reduced-fat	2 Tbsp (1 oz)
Fatback or salt pork, see below†	
Shortening or lard	1 tsp
Sour cream: regular	2 Tbsp
reduced-fat	3 Tbsp

Free Foods

> 20 kcalories or >5 g carbohydrates per serving

Fat-Free or Reduced-Fat Foods

Limit to 3 servings/day

Cream cheese, fat-free	1 Tbsp
Creamers, nondairy, liquid	1 Tbsp
Creamers, nondairy, powdered	2 tsp
Mayonnaise, fat-free	1 Tbsp
Mayonnaise, reduced-fat	1 tsp
Margarine, fat-free	4 Tbsp
Margarine, reduced-fat	1 tsp
Miracle Whip, nonfat	1 Tbsp
Miracle Whip, reduced-fat	1 tsp
Nonstick cooking spray	
Salad dressing, fat-free	1 Tbsp
Salad dressing, fat-free, Italian	2 Tbsp

†Use a piece 1 inch × 1 inch × 1/4 inch if you plan to eat the fatback cooked with vegetables. Use a piece 2 inches × 1 inch × 1/2 inch when eating only the vegetables with the fatback removed.

Salsa	¼ cup
Sour cream, fat-free, reduced-fat	1 Tbsp
Whipped topping, regular or light	2 Tbsp
Sugar-Free or Low-Sugar Foods	
Candy, hard, sugar-free	1 candy
Gelatin dessert, sugar-free	
Gelatin, unflavored	
Gum, sugar-free	
Jam or jelly, low-sugar or light	2 tsp
Sugar substitutes‡	
Syrup, sugar-free	2 Tbsp
Drinks	
Bouillon, broth, consomme*	
Bouillon or broth, low-sodium	
Carbonated or mineral water	
Cocoa powder, unsweetened	1 Tbsp
Coffee	
Club soda	
Diet soft drinks, sugar-free	
Drink mixes, sugar-free	
Tea	
Tonic water, sugar-free	
Condiments	
Ketchup	1 Tbsp
Horseradish	
Lemon juice	
Lime juice	
Mustard	
Pickles, dill*	1½ large
Soy sauce, regular or light*	
Taco sauce	1 Tbsp
Vinegar	

Seasonings

Be careful with seasonings that contain sodium or are salts, such as garlic or celery salt, and lemon pepper.

Flavoring extracts
Garlic
Herbs, fresh or dried
Pimento
Spices
Tobasco or hot pepper sauce
Wine, used in cooking
Worcestershire sauce

‡Sugar substitutes, alternatives, or replacements that are approved by the Food and Drug Administration (FDA) are safe to use. Common brand names include: Equal (aspartame), Sprinkle Sweet (saccharin), Sweet One (acesulfame K), Sweet-10 (saccharin), Sugar Twin (saccharin), and Sweet 'n Low (saccharin).

Combination Foods

Food	Serving Size	Exchanges Per Serving
Entrees		
Tuna noodle casserole, lasagna, spaghetti with meatballs, chili with beans, macaroni and cheese*	1 cup (8 oz)	2 carbohydrates, 2 medium-fat meats
Chow mein (without noodles or rice)	2 cups (16 oz)	1 carbohydrate, 2 lean meats
Pizza, cheese, thin crust*	¼ of 10 in (5 oz)	2 carbohydrates, 2 medium-fat meats, 1 fat
Pizza, meat topping, thin crust*	¼ of 10 in (5 oz)	2 carbohydrates, 2 medium-fat meats, 2 fats
Pot pie*	1 (7 oz)	2 carbohydrates, 1 medium-fat meat, 4 fats
Frozen entrees		
Salisbury steak with gravy, mashed potato*	1 (11 oz)	2 carbohydrates, 3 medium-fat meats, 3-4 fats
Turkey with gravy, mashed potato, dressing*	1 (11 oz)	2 carbohydrates, 2 medium-fat meats, 2 fats
Entree with less than 300 calories*	1 (8 oz)	2 carbohydrates, 3 lean meats
Soups		
Bean*	1 cup	1 carbohydrate, 1 very lean meat
Cream (made with water)*	1 cup (8 oz)	1 carbohydrate, 1 fat
Split pea (made with water)*	½ cup (4 oz)	1 carbohydrate
Tomato (made with water)*	1 cup (8 oz)	1 carbohydrate
Vegetable beef, chicken noodle, or other broth type	1 cup (8 oz)	1 carbohydrate

Fast Foods

Food	Serving Size	Exchanges Per Serving
Burritos with beef*	2	4 carbohydrates, 2 medium-fat meats, 2 fats
Chicken nuggets*	6	1 carbohydrate, 2 medium-fat meats, 1 fat
Chicken breast and wing, breaded and fried*	1 each	1 carbohydrate, 4 medium-fat meats, 2 fats
Fish sandwich/tartar sauce*	1	3 carbohydrates, 1 medium-fat meat, 3 fats
French fries, thin	20-25	2 carbohydrates, 2 fats
Hamburger, regular	1	2 carbohydrates, 2 medium-fat meats
Hamburger, large*	1	2 carbohydrates, 3 medium-fat meats, 1 fat
Hot dug with bun*	1	1 carbohydrate, 1 high-fat meat, 1 fat
Individual pan pizza*	1	5 carbohydrates, 3 medium-fat meats, 3 fats
Soft-serve cone	1 medium	2 carbohydrates, 1 fat
Submarine sandwich*	1 sub (6 in.)	3 carbohydrates, 1 vegetable, 2 medium-fat meats, 1 fat
Taco, hard shell*	1 (6 oz)	2 carbohydrates, 2 medium-fat meats, 2 fats
Taco, soft shell*	1 (3 oz)	1 carbohydrate, 1 medium-fat meat, 1 fat

Meal Plan

Meal Plan for: _____

Dietitian: _____

Date: _____

Phone: _____

Carbohydrate _____ Grams _____ Percent _____

Protein _____ _____ _____

Fat _____ _____ _____

Calories _____ _____ _____

Time	Number of Exchanges/Choices	Menu Ideas	Menu Ideas
	Carbohydrate group ____ ____ Starch ____ Fruit ____ Milk ____ Meat group ____ Fat group ____ ____ ____		
	Carbohydrate group ____ ____ Starch ____ Fruit ____ Milk ✓ Vegetables ____ Meat group ____ Fat group ____ ____ ____		
	Carbohydrate group ____ ____ Starch ____ Fruit ____ Milk ✓ Vegetables ____ Meat group ____ Fat group ____ ____ ____		

PLANNING INDIVIDUALIZED DIETS USING EXCHANGE LISTS

Step 1: Conduct Nutrition History

A 4-hour or 3-day recall (see Chapter 14) can be used to determine usual food intake. Categorize intake into exchanges (or servings) from each list at each meal and snack. Translate into kcalories and grams of carbohydrate, protein, and fat from exchanges. Round off kcalorie level to the nearest 50 or 100 kcalories. Calculations of food intake are not precise enough to allow more accuracy, and patients may consume an extra 50 to 60 kcalories/day from free foods (see Exchange Lists). When in doubt, round up instead of down. Determine percentages of carbohydrate, protein, and fat in current intake.

To determine total kcalories, add up the number of exchanges actually consumed from each Exchange Group. Multiply the number of exchanges by the number of kcalories in each Exchange Group.

Number of exchanges from starch list	= ____	×	80 kcal	= ____
Number of exchanges from fruit list	= ____	×	60 kcal	= ____
Number of exchanges from milk list	= ____	×	80 kcal (skim)	= ____
	= ____	×	120 kcal (low-fat)	= ____
	= ____	×	150 kcal (whole)	= ____
Number of exchanges from vegetable list	= ____	×	25 kcal	= ____
Number of exchanges from meat groups	= ____	×	35 kcal (very lean)	= ____
	= ____	×	55 kcal (lean)	= ____
	= ____	×	75 kcal (medium-fat)	= ____
	= ____	×	100 kcal (high-fat)	= ____
Number of exchanges from fat list	= ____	×	45 kcal	= ____
			Total kcal	____

Using the total number of each Exchange Group, calculate the grams of carbohydrate (CHO), protein (PRO) and fat (FAT).

	Number of Exchanges CHO			Number of Exchanges PRO			Number of Exchange FAT		
Bread list	____ × 15g	= ____ g		____ × 2g	= ____ g		____ × 0-3g	= ____ g
Fruit list	____ × 15g	= ____ g		____ × 0g	= ____ g		____ × 0g	= ____ g
Milk list								
Skim	____ × 12g	= ____ g		____ × 8g	= ____ g		____ × 0g	= ____ g
Low-fat	____ × 12g	= ____ g		____ × 8g	= ____ g		____ × 5g	= ____ g
Whole	____ × 12g	= ____ g		____ × 8g	= ____ g		____ × 8g	= ____ g
Vegetable list	____ × 5g	= ____ g		____ × 2g	= ____ g		____ × 0g	= ____ g
Meat list								
Very lean	____ × 0g	= ____ g		____ × 7g	= ____ g		____ × 0-1g	= ____ g
Lean	____ × 0g	= ____ g		____ × 7g	= ____ g		____ × 3g	= ____ g
Medium-fat	____ × 0g	= ____ g		____ × 7g	= ____ g		____ × 5g	= ____ g
High-fat	____ × 0g	= ____ g		____ × 7g	= ____ g		____ × 8g	= ____ g
Fat group	____ × 0g	= ____ g		____ × 0g	= ____ g		____ × 5g	= ____ g
	Total ____			Total ____			Total ____	

Take total kcalories from above and determine the percentage of the diet that is carbohydrate, protein, and fat:

A.

Multiply total grams CHO $\times$ 4 kcal = _____ kcal
Multiply total grams PRO $\times$ 4 kcal = _____ kcal
Multiply total grams FAT $\times$ 9 kcal = _____ kcal
                                                          Total   _____ kcal

B. Divide each nutrient's total kcalories by the total kcalories for the day, and multiply by 100 to get the percentage of kcalories.

Kcal from CHO $\times$ 100 = % kcal from CHO   _____ $\times$ 100 = _____ Total kcal
Kcal from PRO $\times$ 100 = % kcal from PRO   _____ $\times$ 100 = _____ Total kcal
Kcal from FAT $\times$ 100 = % kcal from FAT   _____ $\times$ 100 = _____ Total kcal

Step 2: Calculate Daily Kilocalorie Requirements

Kcalorie needs are based on age, weight, and activity level. Use the Harris-Benedict equation to calculate energy needs. Round figure to nearest 100 kcalories. Subtract kcalories if weight loss is desired. Reducing kcaloric intake by 500 kcal/day will theoretically produce a 1 lb weight loss per week. Never reduce kcaloric level to below that required for basal energy needs.

Example: CG is a 62-year-old female with NIDDM. She is 5'5" tall (medium frame), and weighs 140 lb. CG walks 10 to 12 miles per week at the mall.

$$655.1 + [9.6 \times \text{wt (kg)}] + [1.8 \times \text{ht (cm)}] - [4.7 \times \text{age (yrs)}]$$
$$655.1 + [9.6 \times 63.6 \text{ kg}] + [1.8 \times 165.1 \text{ cm}] - [4.7 \times 62]$$
$$655.1 + 610.6 + 297.2 - 291.4 = 1271.5 \text{ kcalories}$$
$$1271.5 \text{ kcalories} \times 1.3 \text{ (activity factor)} = 1652.95 \text{ kcalories}$$
$$\text{Round off to 1700 kcalories}$$

If weight loss is desired, subtract 500 kcalories: 1700 − 500 = 1200 kcalories, which is below her basal energy needs of 1271.5 kcalories. Adjust to 1300 kcalories if weight loss is determined to be a treatment goal.

Step 3: Determine Distribution of Carbohydrate, Protein, and Fat Kcalories

This should be based on the patient's usual intake, blood glucose levels, blood lipid levels, and treatment goals.

Example: CG's 24-hr recall indicates an intake of approximately 1500 kcalories distributed into 17% protein, 30% fat, and 53% carbohydrate. Her pertinent lab values: glycosylated hemoglobin is 6%, cholesterol 210 mg/dl, LDL-cholesterol 179 mg/dl, HDL-cholesterol 55 mg/dl. Although her lipid levels are at the high end of normal or just slightly above normal, her exercise and eating habits appear to be sufficient to control her blood glucose levels. In this case, you would distribute her kcalories in the same pattern as found in her diet recall:

$$\text{Carbohydrate: } 1500 \text{ kcal} \times .53 = 795 \text{ kcal} \div 4\text{kcal/gm} = 199 \text{ gm}$$
$$\text{Protein: } 1500 \text{ kcal} \times .17 = 255 \text{ kcal} \div 4 \text{ kcal/gm} = 64 \text{ gm}$$
$$\text{Fat: } 1500 \text{ kcal} \times .30 = 450 \text{ kcal} \div 9 \text{ kcal/gm} = 50 \text{ gm}$$

Step 4: Determine Servings from Each Exchange List

These calculations are based on the amount of carbohydrate, protein, and fat in each exchange list and the patient's preferences for foods within each list or group. The type of milk the patient uses should be calculated into the meal plan. Skim milk and low-fat milks are recommended, but whole milk can be used if the patient will not drink the others. Although lean meats should be encouraged, when calculating fat grams per meat serving, use the fat value that best represents actual intake. People do not need to add or subtract fat exchanges when using different meat categories.

Example: CG's usual eating pattern indicates she uses the following amounts from the milk, vegetable, and fruit exchange groups:

	Servings	Carbohydrate (gm)	Protein (gm)	Fat (gm)	Kcal
Milk, skim	1	12	8	1	90
Vegetables	4	20	8	0	100
Fruits	4	60	0	0	240
Carbohydrate Subtotal		92	16	1	430

The starch exchange list is the only group remaining that provides carbohydrates. To determine the number of servings to be used from this group, subtract the total grams of carbohydrate (92 gm) from the milk, vegetable, and fruit lists from the total grams of carbohydrate (199 gm) in the meal plan. This amount is divided by 15 gm carbohydrate/serving in the starch list.

	Servings	Carbohydrate (gm)	Protein (gm)	Fat (gm)	Kcal
Carbohydrate Subtotal		92	24	1	460
Starches	7	105	21	7	560
Protein Subtotal		197	45	8	1020

The meat exchange list is the only group remaining that provides protein. To determine the number of servings to be used from this group, subtract the total grams of protein (48 gm) from the milk, vegetable, and starch lists from the total grams of protein (56 gm) in the meal plan. This amount is divided by 7 gm protein/serving in the meat list.

	Servings	Carbohydrate (gm)	Protein (gm)	Fat (gm)	Kcal
Protein Subtotal		197	45	8	1020
Meat/lean	4	0	28	12	220
Fat Subtotal		197	73	20	1240

The fat exchange list is the only group remaining that provides fat. To determine the number of servings to be used from this group, subtract the total grams of fat (20 gm) from the milk, starch, and meat lists from the total grams of fat (50 gm) in the meal plan. This amount is divided by 5 gm fat/serving in the fat list.

	Servings	Carbohydrate (gm)	Protein (gm)	Fat (gm)	Kcal
Fat Subtotal		197	73	20	1240
Fats	6	0	0	30	270
TOTAL		197	73	50	1510

Note: When calculating the number of servings from each exchange list, round to the nearest whole number. It is usually impractical to calculate and plan half servings from the lists.

The daily distribution of servings from the exchange list is as follows. These servings can now be divided into the appropriate number of meals and snacks per day.

Exchange List Group	Servings	Carbohydrate (gm)	Protein (gm)	Fat (gm)	Kcalories
Carbohydrates	12				
Starches	7	105	21	7	560
Fruit	4	60	0	0	240
Milk (skim)	1	0	0	30	270
Vegetables	4	20	8	1	90
Meats/lean	4	0	28	12	220
Fats	6	0	0	30	270

Modified from American Dietetic Association: *Exchange lists for meal planning,* Alexandria Va, 1995, American Diabetes Association; American Dietetic Association, *Handbook of clinical dietetics,* ed 2, New Haven, 1992, Yale University Press; Davis JR, Sherer K: *Applied nutrition and diet therapy for nurses,* ed 2, Philadelphia, 1994, WB Saunders; American Dietetic Association: Nutrition recommendations and principles for people with diabetes mellitus, *J Am Diet Assoc* 94:504, 1994; and Tinker LF, Heins JM, Holler HJ: Commentary and translation: 1994 nutrition recommendations for diabetes, *J Am Diet Assoc* 94:507, 1994.

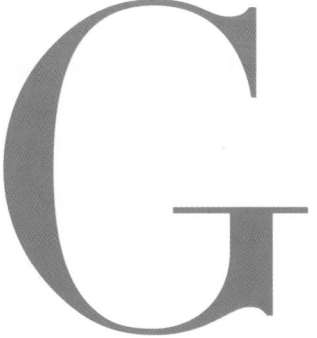

G Recommended Nutrient Intakes for Canadians

Summary examples of recommended nutrient intake based on age and body weight expressed as daily rates

Age	Sex	Energy (kcal)	Thiamin (mg)	Riboflavin (mg)	Niacin NE	n-3 PUFA (g)	n-6 PUFA (g)	Weight (kg)	Protein (g)	Vitamin A RE
0-4 months	Both	600	0.3	0.3	4	0.5	3	6.0	12*	400
5-12 months	Both	900	0.4	0.5	7	0.5	3	9.0	12	400
1 year	Both	1100	0.5	0.6	8	0.6	4	11	13	400
2-3 years	Both	1300	0.6	0.7	9	0.7	4	14	16	400
4-6 years	Both	1800	0.7	0.9	13	1.0	6	18	19	500
7-9 years	M	2200	0.9	1.1	16	1.2	7	25	26	700
	F	1900	0.8	1.0	14	1.0	6	25	26	700
10-12 years	M	2500	1.0	1.3	18	1.4	8	34	34	800
	F	2200	0.9	1.1	16	1.2	7	36	36	800
13-15 years	M	2800	1.1	1.4	20	1.5	9	50	49	900
	F	2200	0.9	1.1	16	1.2	7	48	46	800
16-18 years	M	3200	1.3	1.6	23	1.8	11	62	58	1000
	F	2100	0.8	1.1	15	1.2	7	53	47	800
19-24 years	M	3000	1.2	1.5	22	1.6	10	71	61	1000
	F	2100	0.8	1.1	15	1.2	7	58	50	800
25-49 years	M	2700	1.1	1.4	19	1.5	9	74	64	1000
	F	1900	0.8	1.0	14	1.1	7	59	51	800
50-74 years	M	2300	0.9	1.2	16	1.3	8	73	63	1000
	F	1800	0.8§	1.0§	14§	1.1§	7§	63	54	800
75+ years	M	2000	0.8	1.0	14	1.1	7	69	59	1000
	F**	1700	0.8§	1.0§	14§	1.1§	7§	64	55	800
Pregnancy (additional)										
1st Trimester		100	0.1	0.1	0.11	0.05	0.3		5	0
2nd Trimester		300	0.1	0.3	0.22	0.16	0.9		20	0
3rd Trimester		300	0.1	0.3	0.22	0.16	0.9		24	0
Lactation (additional)		450	0.2	0.4	0.33	0.25	1.5	20	400	

Vitamin D (µg)	Vitamin E (mg)	Vitamin C (mg)	Folate (µg)	Vitamin B₁₂ (µg)	Calcium (mg)	Phosphorus (mg)	Magnesium (mg)	Iron (mg)	Iodine (µg)	Zinc (mg)
10	3	20	25	0.3	250†	150	20	0.3‡	30	2‡
10	3	20	40	0.4	400	200	32	7	40	3
10	3	20	40	0.5	500	300	40	6	55	4
5	4	20	50	0.6	550	350	50	6	65	4
5	5	25	70	0.8	600	400	65	8	85	5
2.5	7	25	90	1.0	700	500	100	8	110	7
2.5	6	25	90	1.0	700	500	100	8	95	7
2.5	8	25	120	1.0	900	700	130	8	125	9
2.5	7	25	130	1.0	1100	800	135	8	110	9
2.5	9	30	175	1.0	1100	900	185	10	160	12
2.5	7	30	170	1.0	1000	850	180	13	160	9
2.5	10	40¶	220	1.0	900	1000	230	10	160	12
2.5	7	30¶	190	1.0	700	850	200	12	160	9
2.5	10	40¶	220	1.0	800	1000	240	9	160	12
2.5	7	30¶	180	1.0	700	850	200	13	160	9
2.5	9	40¶	230	1.0	800	1000	250	9	160	12
2.5	6	30¶	185	1.0	700	850	200	13	160	9
5	7	40¶	230	1.0	800	1000	250	9	160	12
5	6	30¶	195	1.0	800	850	210	8	160	9
5	6	40¶	215	1.0	800	1000	230	9	160	12
5	5	30¶	200	1.0	800	850	210	8	160	9
2.5	2	0	200	1.2	500	200	15	0	25	6
2.5	2	10	200	1.2	500	200	45	5	25	6
2.5	2	10	200	1.2	500	200	45	10	25	6
2.5	3	25	100	0.2	500	200	65	0	50	6

From Scientific Review Committee: Nutrition recommendations, *Health and Welfare,* Ottawa, 1990.

NE, Niacin equivalents; *PUFA,* polyunsaturated fatty acids; *RE,* retinol equivalents.

*Protein is assumed to be from breast milk and must be adjusted for infant formula.

†Infant formula with high phosphorus should contain 375 mg of calcium.

‡Breast milk is assumed to be the source of the mineral.

¶Smokers should increase vitamin C by 50%.

§Level below which intake should not fall.

**Assumes moderate physical activity.

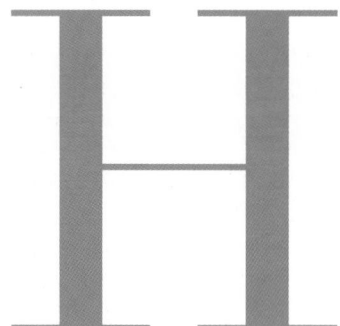# Calculation Aids and Conversion Tables

More than 185 years ago a group of French scientists set up the metric system of weights and measures. Today, with refinements over years of use, it is called the "Système International" (SI). Here are a few conversion factors to help you make transitions in your necessary calculations.

Metric System of Measurement

Like our money system, this is a simple decimal system based on units of 10. It is uniform and used internationally.

Weight units:

1 kilogram (kg) = 1000 grams (gm or g)
1 g = 1000 milligrams (mg)
1 mg = 1000 micrograms (mcg or μg)

Length units:

1 meter (m) = 100 centimeters (cm)
1000 meters = 1 kilometer (km)

Volume units:

1 liter (l) = 1000 milliliters (ml)
1 milliliter = 1 cubic centimeter (cc)

Temperature units: Celcius (C) scale, based on 100 equal units between 0° C (freezing point of water) and 100° C (boiling point of water); this scale is used entirely in all scientific work.

Energy units:

Kilocalorie (kcal) = Amount of energy required to raise 1 kg water 1° C
Kilojoule (kJ) = Amount of energy required to move 1 kg mass 1 m by a force of 1 newton
1 kcal = 4.184 kJ

British/American System of Measurement

Our customary system is a confusion of units with no uniform relationships. It is not a decimal system, but rather a jumbled collection of different units collected in usage and language over time. It is used mainly in America.

Weight units: 1 pound (lb) = 16 ounces (oz)

Length units: 1 foot (ft) = 12 inches (in)
1 yard (yd) = 3 feet (ft)

Volume units:

3 teaspoons (tsp) = 1 tablespoon (tbsp)
16 tbsp = 1 cup
1 cup = 8 fluid ounces (fl oz)
4 cups = 1 quart (qt)
5 cups = 1 imperial quart (qt), Canada

Temperature units: Fahrenheit (F) scale, based on 180 equals units between 32° F (freezing point of water) and 212° F (boiling point of water) at standard atmospheric pressure

Conversions Between Measurement Systems

Weight: 1 oz = 28.35 g (usually used as 28 or 30 g)
            2.2 lb = 1 kg
Length: 1 in = 2.54 cm
            1 ft = 30.48 cm
            39.37 in = 1 m
Volume: 1.06 qt = 1 L
            0.85 imperial qt = 1 L (Canada)
Temperature: Boiling point of   100° C   212° F
            water
            Body temperature   37° C   98.6° F
            Freezing point of water   0° C   32° F
    Interconversion formulas:
Fahrenheit temperature (°F) = $\frac{9}{5}$ (°C) + 32
    Celsius temperature (°C) = $\frac{5}{9}$ (°F − 32)

Retinol Equivalents

The following definitions and equivalences that are internationally agreed on provide a basis for calculating retinol equivalent conversions.

   Definitions: International units (IU) and retinol equivalents (RE) are defined as follows:
      1 IU = 0.3 μg retinol (0.0003 mg)
      1 IU = 0.6 μg beta-carotene (0.0006 mg)
      1 RE = 6 μg retinol
      1 RE = 6 μg beta-carotene
      1 RE = 12 μg other provitamin A carotenoids
      1 RE = 3.33 IU retinol
      1 RE = 10 IU beta-carotene
   Conversion formulas: On the basis of weight, beta-carotene is one-half as active as retinol; on the basis of structure, the other provitamin carotenoids are one-fourth as active as retinol. In addition, retinol is more completely absorbed in the intestine, whereas the provitamin carotenoids are much less well utilized, with an average absorption of about one-third. Therefore in overall activity beta-carotene is one-sixth as active as retinol, and the other carotenoids are one-twelfth as active. These differences in utilization provide the basis for the 1:6:12 relationship shown in the equivalences given and in the following formulas for calculating retinol equivalents from values of vitamin A, beta-carotene, and other active carotenoids, expressed either as international units or micrograms:
If retinol and beta-carotene are given in micrograms:
      Micrograms of retinol + (Micrograms of beta-carotene ÷ 6) = RE
      If both are given as IU:
   International units of retinol ÷ 3.33) +
(International units of beta-carotene ÷ 10) =RE
If beta-carotene and other carotenoids are given in micrograms:
      (Micrograms of beta-carotene ÷ 6) +
(Micrograms of other carotenoids ÷ 12) =RE

Approximate metric conversions

When you know	Multiply by	to find
Weight		
Ounces	28	Grams
Pounds	0.45	Kilograms
Length		
Inches	2.5	Centimeters
Feet	30	Centimeters
Yards	0.9	Meters
Miles	1.6	Kilometers
Volume		
Teaspoons	5	Millimeters
Tablespoons	15	Millimeters
Fluid ounces	30	Millimeters
Cups	0.24	Liters
Pints	0.47	Liters
Quarts	0.95	Liters
Temperature		
Fahrenheit temperature	$\frac{5}{9}$ (after subtracting 32)	Celsius temperature

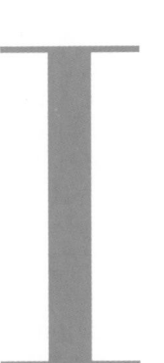

Recommended Dietary Allowances (RDAs) and Dietary Reference Intakes (DRIs)

Food and Nutrition Board, National Academy of Sciences—National Research Council Recommended Dietary Allowances, Revised 1989

Designed for the maintenance of good nutrition of practically all healthy people in the United States

Category	Age (years) or condition	Weight† (kg)	Weight† (lb)	Height† (cm)	Height† (in)	Protein (g)	Vitamin A (µg RE)‡	Vitamin D (µg)¶	Vitamin E (mg α-TE)§	Vitamin K (µg)	Vitamin C (mg)	Thiamin (mg)	Riboflavin (mg)	Niacin (mg NE)**	Vitamin B6 (mg)	Folate (µg)	Vitamin B12 (µg)	Calcium (mg)	Phosphorus (mg)	Magnesium (mg)	Iron (mg)	Zinc (mg)	Iodine (µg)	Selenium (µg)
Infants	0.0-0.5	6	13	60	24	13	375	7.5	3	5	30	0.3	0.4	5	0.3	25	0.3	400	300	40	6	5	40	10
	0.5-1.0	9	20	71	28	14	375	10	4	10	35	0.4	0.5	6	0.6	35	0.5	600	500	60	10	5	50	15
Children	1-3	13	29	90	35	16	400	10	6	15	40	0.7	0.8	9	1.0	50	0.7	800	800	80	10	10	70	20
	4-6	20	44	112	44	24	500	10	7	20	45	0.9	1.1	12	1.1	75	1.0	800	800	120	10	10	90	20
	7-10	28	62	132	52	28	700	10	7	30	45	1.0	1.2	13	1.4	100	1.4	800	800	170	10	10	120	30
Males	11-14	45	99	157	62	45	1000	10	10	45	50	1.3	1.5	17	1.7	150	2.0	1200	1200	270	12	15	150	40
	15-18	66	145	176	69	59	1000	10	10	65	60	1.5	1.8	20	2.0	200	2.0	1200	1200	400	12	15	150	50
	19-24	72	160	177	70	58	1000	10	10	70	60	1.5	1.7	19	2.0	200	2.0	1200	1200	350	10	15	150	70
	25-50	79	174	176	70	63	1000	5	10	80	60	1.5	1.7	19	2.0	200	2.0	800	800	350	10	15	150	70
	51+	77	170	173	68	63	1000	5	10	80	60	1.2	1.4	15	2.0	200	2.0	800	800	350	10	15	150	70
Females	11-14	46	101	157	62	46	800	10	8	45	50	1.1	1.3	15	1.4	150	2.0	1200	1200	280	15	12	150	45
	15-18	55	120	163	64	44	800	10	8	55	60	1.1	1.3	15	1.5	180	2.0	1200	1200	300	15	12	150	50
	19-24	58	128	164	65	46	800	10	8	60	60	1.1	1.3	15	1.6	180	2.0	1200	1200	280	15	12	150	55
	25-50	63	138	163	64	50	800	5	8	65	60	1.1	1.3	15	1.6	180	2.0	800	800	280	15	12	150	55
	51+	65	143	160	63	50	800	5	8	65	60	1.0	1.2	13	1.6	180	2.0	800	800	280	10	12	150	55
Pregnant						60	800	10	10	65	70	1.5	1.6	17	2.2	400	2.2	1200	1200	300	30	15	175	65
Lactating	1st 6 months					65	1300	10	12	65	95	1.6	1.8	20	2.1	280	2.6	1200	1200	355	15	19	200	75
	2nd 6 months					62	1200	10	11	65	90	1.6	1.7	20	2.1	260	2.6	1200	1200	340	15	16	200	75

*The allowances, expressed as average daily intakes over time, are intended to provide for individual variations among most normal persons as they live in the United States under usual environmental stresses. Diets should be based on a variety of common foods in order to provide other nutrients for which human requirements have been less well defined. See text for detailed discussion of allowances and of nutrients not tabulated.

†Weights and heights of reference adults are actual medians for the U.S. population of the designated age, as reported by NHANES II. The median weights and heights of those under 19 years of age were taken from Hamill et al. (1979). The use of these figures does not imply that the height-to-weight ratios are ideal.

‡Retinol equivalents. 1 retinol equivalent = 1 µg retinol or 6 µg β-carotene. See text for calculation of vitamin A activity of diets as retinol equivalents.

¶As cholecalciferol. 10 µg cholecalciferol = 400 IU of vitamin D.

§α-Tocopherol equivalents. 1 mg d-α tocopherol = 1 α-TE. See text for variation in allowances and calculation of vitamin E activity of the diet as α-tocopherol equivalents.

**1 NE (niacin equivalent) is equal to mg of niacin or 60 mg of dietary tryptophan.

From Food and Nutrition Board, National Academy of Sciences, National Research Council: *Recommended dietary allowances*, ed 10, Washington, D.C. 1989, National Academy Press.

Food and Nutrition Board, Institute of Medicine–National Academy of Sciences Dietary Reference Intakes: Recommended Intakes for Individuals

Life-Stage Group	Calcium (mg/d)	Phosphorus (mg/d)	Magnesium (mg/d)	Vitamin D (μg/d)a-b	Fluoride (mg/d)	Thiamin (mg/d)	Riboflavin (mg/d)	Niacin (mg/d)c	Vitamin B6 (mg/d)	Folate (μg/d)d	Vitamin B12 (μg/d)	Pantothenic Acid (mg/d)	Biotin (μg)	Choline e (mg/d)	Vitamin C† (mg/d)	Vitamin E† (as alpha-Tocopherol) (mg/d)	Selenium† (μg/d)
Infants																	
0-6 mo	210*	100*	30*	5*	0.01*	0.2*	0.3*	2*	0.1*	65*	0.4*	1.7*	5*	125*	40*	4*	15*
7-12 mo	270*	275*	75*	5*	0.5*	0.3*	0.4*	4*	0.3*	80*	0.5*	1.8*	6*	150*	50*	6*	20*
Children																	
1-3 yr	500*	**460**	**80**	5*	0.7*	**0.5**	**0.5**	**6**	**0.5**	**150**	**0.9**	2*	8*	200*	**15**	**6**	**20**
4-8 yr	800*	**500**	**130**	5*	1*	**0.6**	**0.6**	**8**	**0.6**	**200**	**1.2**	3*	12*	250*	**25**	**8**	**30**
Males																	
9-13 yr	1300*	**1250**	**240**	5*	2*	**0.9**	**0.9**	**12**	**1.0**	**300**	**1.8**	4*	20*	375*	**45**	**11**	**40**
14-18 yr	1300*	**1250**	**410**	5*	3*	**1.2**	**1.3**	**16**	**1.3**	**400**	**2.4**	5*	25*	550*	**75**	**15**	**55**
19-30 yr	1000*	**700**	**400**	5*	4*	**1.2**	**1.3**	**16**	**1.3**	**400**	**2.4**	5*	30*	550*	**90**	**15**	**55**
31-50 yr	1000*	**700**	**420**	5*	4*	**1.2**	**1.3**	**16**	**1.3**	**400**	**2.4**	5*	30*	550*	**90**	**15**	**55**
51-70 yr	1200*	**700**	**420**	10*	4*	**1.2**	**1.3**	**16**	**1.7**	**400**	**2.4f**	5*	30*	550*	**90**	**15**	**55**
>70 yr	1200*	**700**	**420**	15*	4*	**1.2**	**1.3**	**16**	**1.7**	**400**	**2.4f**	5*	30*	550*	**90**	**15**	**55**
Females																	
9-13 yr	1300*	**1250**	**240**	5*	2*	**0.9**	**0.9**	**12**	**1.0**	**300**	**1.8**	4*	20*	375*	**45**	**11**	**40**
14-18 yr	1300*	**1250**	**360**	5*	3*	**1.0**	**1.0**	**14**	**1.2**	**400g**	**2.4**	5*	25*	400*	**65**	**15**	**55**
19-30 yr	1000*	**700**	**310**	5*	3*	**1.1**	**1.1**	**14**	**1.3**	**400g**	**2.4**	5*	30*	425*	**75**	**15**	**55**
31-50 yr	1000*	**700**	**320**	5*	3*	**1.1**	**1.1**	**14**	**1.3**	**400g**	**2.4**	5*	30*	425*	**75**	**15**	**55**
51-70 yr	1200*	**700**	**320**	10*	3*	**1.1**	**1.1**	**14**	**1.5**	**400**	**2.4f**	5*	30*	425*	**75**	**15**	**55**
>70 yr	1200*	**700**	**320**	15*	3*	**1.1**	**1.1**	**14**	**1.5**	**400**	**2.4f**	5*	30*	425*	**75**	**15**	**55**
Pregnancy																	
≤18 yr	1300*	**1250**	**400**	5*	3*	**1.4**	**1.4**	**18**	**1.9**	**600h**	**2.6**	6*	30*	450*	**80**	**15**	**60**
19-30 yr	1000*	**700**	**350**	5*	3*	**1.4**	**1.4**	**18**	**1.9**	**600h**	**2.6**	6*	30*	450*	**85**	**15**	**60**
31-50 yr	1000*	**700**	**360**	5*	3*	**1.4**	**1.4**	**18**	**1.9**	**600h**	**2.6**	6*	30*	450*	**85**	**15**	**60**
Lactation																	
≤18 yr	1300*	**1250**	**360**	5*	3*	**1.5**	**1.6**	**17**	**2.0**	**500**	**2.8**	7*	35*	550*	**115**	**19**	**70**
19-30 yr	1000*	**700**	**310**	5*	3*	**1.5**	**1.6**	**17**	**2.0**	**500**	**2.8**	7*	35*	550*	**120**	**19**	**70**
31-50 yr	1000*	**700**	**320**	5*	3*	**1.5**	**1.6**	**17**	**2.0**	**500**	**2.8**	7*	35*	550*	**120**	**19**	**70**

NOTE: This table presents Recommended Dietary Allowances (RDAs) in **bold type** and Adequate Intakes (AIs) in ordinary type followed by an asterisk (*). RDAs and AIs may both be used as goals for individual intake. RDAs are set to meet the needs of almost all (97% to 98%) individuals in a group. For healthy breastfed infants, the AI is the mean intake. The AI for other life-stage and gender groups is thought to cover needs of all individuals in the group, but lack of data or uncertainty in the data prevent being able to specify with confidence the percentage of individuals covered by this intake.

a As cholecalciferol. 1 μg cholecalciferol = 40 IU vitamin D.

b In the absence of adequate exposure to sunlight.

c As niacin equivalents (NE). 1 mg of niacin = 60 mg tryptophan; 0-6 months = preformed niacin (not NE).

d As dietary folate equivalents (DFE). 1 DFE = 1 μg food folate = 0.6 μg of folic acid (from fortified food or supplement) consumed with food = 0.5 μg of synthetic (supplemental) folic acid taken on an empty stomach.

e Although AIs have been set for choline, there are few data to assess whether a dietary supply of choline is needed at all stages of the life cycle, and it may be that the choline requirement can be met by endogenous synthesis at some of these stages.

f Because 10 to 30 percent of older people may malabsorb food bound B12, it is advisable for those older than 50 years to meet their RDA mainly by consuming foods fortified with B12 or a supplement containing B12.

g In view of evidence linking folate intake with neural tube defects in the fetus, it is recommended that all women capable of becoming pregnant consume 400 μg of synthetic folic acid from fortified foods and/or supplements in addition to intake of food folate from a varied diet.

h It is assumed that women will continue consuming 400 μg of folic acid until their pregnancy is confirmed and they enter prenatal care, which ordinarily occurs after the end of the periconceptional period—the critical time for formation of the neural tube.

†From Food and Nutrition Board, Institute of Medicine: *Dietary reference intakes for vitamin C, vitamin E, selenium, and carotenoids,* Washington, DC, 2000, National Academy Press.

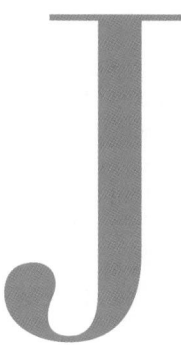

Cultural Dietary Patterns

Only foods that are specifically associated with these cultural groups are noted. Individuals may also consume typical American foods as well; assumptions of dietary patterns cannot be made, but knowledge of these unique foods provides a common understanding of the range of possible food choices.

Native American

Each tribe may have specific foods; commonly consumed foods are listed here.

1. Bread, Cereal, Rice, and Pasta Group
Blue corn flour (ground dried blue corn kernels) used to make cornbread, mush dumplings; fruit dumplings (walakshi); fry bread (biscuit dough deep fried); ground sweet acorn; tortillas; wheat or rye used to make cornmeal and flours.

2. Vegetable Group
Cabbage, carrots, cassava, dandelion greens, eggplant, milkweed, onions, pumpkin, squash (all varieties), sweet and white potatoes, turnips, wild tullies (a tuber), yellow corn.

3. Fruit Group
Dried wild cherries and grapes; wild banana, berries, and yucca.

4. Milk, Yogurt, and Cheese Group
None.

5. Meat, Poultry, Fish, Dry Beans, Eggs, and Nuts Groups
Duck, eggs, fish eggs (roe), geese, groundhog, kidney beans, lentils, peanuts, pinenuts, pinto beans, all nuts, venison, wild rabbit.

6. Fats, Oils, and Sweets
None.

African–American

1. Bread, Cereal, Rice, and Pasta Group
Biscuits, cornbread as spoon bread, cornpone or hush puppies, grits.

2. Vegetable Group
Leafy greens including dandelion greens, kale, mustard greens, collard greens, turnips.

3. Fruit Group
None.

4. Milk, Yogurt, and Cheese Group
Buttermilk.

5. Meat, Poultry, Fish, Dry Beans, Eggs, and Nuts Group

Pork and pork products, scrapple (cornmeal and pork), chitterlings (pork intestines), bacon, pig's feet, pig ears, souse, pork neck bones, fried meats and poultry, organ meats (kidney, liver, tongue, tripe), venison, rabbit, catfish, buffalo fish, mackerel, legumes (black-eyed peas, kidney, navy, chickpeas).

6. Fats, Oils, and Sweets

Lard.

Japanese

1. Bread, Cereal, Rice, and Pasta Group

Rice and rice products, rice flour (mochiko), noodles (comen/soba), seaweed around rice with or without fish (sushi).

2. Vegetable Group

Bamboo shoots (takenoko), burdock (gobo), cabbage (nappa), dried mushrooms (shiitake), eggplant, horseradish (wasabi), Japanese parsley (seri), lotus root (renkon), mustard greens, pickled cabbage (kimchee), pickled vegetables, seaweed (laver, nori, wakame, kombu), vegetable soup (mizutaki), white radish (daikon).

3. Fruit Group

Pear-like apple (nasi), persimmons.

4. Milk, Yogurt, and Cheese Group

None.

5. Meat, Poultry, Fish, Dry Beans, Eggs, and Nuts Group

Fish and shellfish including dried fish with bones, raw fish (sashimi), and fish cake (kamaboko); soybeans as soybean curd (tofu), fermented soy bean paste (miso), and sprouts; red beans (azuki).

6. Fats, Oils, and Sweets

Soy and rice oil.

Chinese

1. Bread, Cereal, Rice, and Pasta Group

Rice and related products (flour, cakes, and noodles); noodles made from barley, corn, and millet; wheat and related products (breads, noodles, spaghetti, stuffed noodles [won ton] and filled buns [bow]).

2. Vegetable Group

Bamboo shoots; cabbage (napa); Chinese celery; Chinese parsley (coriander); Chinese turnips (lo bok); dried day lillies; dry fungus (Black Juda's ear); leafy green vegetables including kale, Chinese cress, Chinese mustard greens (gai choy), Chinese chard (bok choy), amaranth greens (yin choy), wolfberry leaves (gou gay), and Chinese broccoli (gai lan); lotus tubers; okra; snow peas; stir-fried vegetables (chow yuk); taro roots, white radish (daikon).

3. Fruit Group

Kumquat.

4. Milk, Yogurt, and Cheese Group

None.

5. Meat, Poultry, Fish, Dry Beans, Eggs, and Nuts Group

Fish and seafood (all kinds, dried and fresh), hen, legumes, nuts, organ meats, pigeon eggs, pork and pork products, soybean curd (tofu), steamed stuffed dumplings (dim sum).

6. Fats, Oils, and Sweets

Peanut, soy, sesame and rice oil; lard.

Filipino

1. Bread, Cereal, Rice, and Pasta Group

Noodles, rice, rice flour (mochiko), stuffed noodles (won ton), white bread (pan de sal).

2. Vegetable Group

Bamboo shoots, dark green leafy vegetables (malunggay and salvyot), eggplant, sweet potatoes (camotes), okra, palm, peppers, turnips, root crop (gabi).

3. Fruit Group

Avocado, bitter melon (ampalaya), guavas, jackfruit, limes, mangoes, papaya, pod fruit (tamarind), pomelos, tangelo (naranghita).

4. Milk, Yogurt, and Cheese Group

Custards.

5. Meat, Poultry, Fish, Dry Beans, Eggs, and Nuts Group

Fish in all forms; dried fish (dilis); egg roll (lumpia); fish sauce (alamang and bagoong); legumes such as mung beans, bean sprouts, chickpeas, organ meats (liver, heart, intestines); pork with chicken in soy sauce (adobo); pork sausage; soybean curd (tofu).

6. Fats, Oils, and Sweets

None.

Southeastern Asians: (Laos, Cambodia, Thailand, Vietnam, the Hmong and the Mien)

1. Bread, Cereal, Rice, and Pasta Group

Rice (long and short grain) and related products such as noodles; Hmong cornbread or cake.

2. Vegetable Group

Bamboo shoots, broccoli, Chinese parsley (coriander), mustard greens, pickled vegetables, water chestnuts, Thai chili peppers.

3. Fruit Group

Apple pear (Asian pear), bitter melon, coconut cream and milk, guava, jackfruit, mango.

4. Milk, Yogurt, and Cheese Group

Sweetened condensed milk.

5. Meat, Poultry, Fish, Dry Beans, Eggs, and Nuts Group

Beef; chicken; deer; eggs; fish and shellfish (all kinds of freshwater and saltwater); legumes including black-eyed peas, peanuts, kidney beans, and soybeans, organ meats (liver, stomach); pork; rabbit; soybean curd (tofu).

6. Fats, Oils, and Sweets

Lard, peanut oil.

Mexican

1. Bread, Cereal, Rice and Pasta Group

Corn and related products; taco shells (fried corn tortillas); tortillas (corn and flour); white bread.

2. Vegetable Group

Cactus (nopoles), chili peppers, salsa, tomatoes, yambean root (jicama), yucca root (cassava or manioc).

3. Fruit Group

Avocado, guacamole (mashed avocado, onion, cilantro [coriander], and chilis), papaya.

4. Milk, Yogurt, and Cheese Group

Cheese, flan, sour cream.

5. Meat, Poultry, Fish, Dry Beans, Eggs, and Nuts Group

Black or pinto beans (reijoles); refried beans (frijoles refritos); flour tortilla stuffed with beef, chicken, eggs, or beans (burrito); corn tortilla stuffed with chicken, cheese, or beef topped with chili sauce (enchilada); Mexican sausage (chorizo).

6. Fats, Oils, and Sweets

Bacon fat, lard (manteca), salt port.

Puerto Rican and Cuban

1. Bread, Cereal, Rice, and Pasta Group

Rice; starchy green bananas, usually fried (plantain).

2. Vegetable Group

Beets; eggplant; tubers (yucca); white yams (boniato).

3. Fruit Group

Coconuts, guava, mango, oranges (sweet and sour), prune and mango paste.

4. Milk, Yogurt, and Cheese Group

Flan, hard cheese (queso de mano).

5. Meat, Poultry, Fish, Dry Beans, Eggs, and Nuts Group

Chicken, fish, (all kinds and preparations including smoked, salted, canned, and fresh), legumes (all kinds especially black beans), pork (fried), sausage (chorizo).

6. Fats, Oils, and Sweets

Olive and peanut oil, lard.

Jewish

The foods below reflect both religious and cultural customs of Jewish people. Adherence to religious dietary patterns by followers of the different forms of Judaism (Orthodox, Conservative, Reform, and Reconstructionist) vary. Generally, Orthodox Jews and many Conservative Jews follow kosher dietary rules both at home and when out. Others may only observe when in their own homes. These rules of "keeping kosher" are reviewed in the next section on religious dietary patterns.

1. Bread, Cereal, Rice, and Pasta Group

Bagel, buckwheat groats (kasha), dumplings made with matzoh meal (matzoh balls or knaidelach), egg bread (challah), noodle or potato pudding (kugel), crepe filled with farmer cheese and/or fruit (blintz), unleavened bread or large cracker made with wheat flour and water (matzoh).

2. Vegetable Group

Potato pancakes (latkes); a vegetable stew made with sweet potatoes, carrots, prunes, and sometimes brisket (tzimmes); beet soup (borscht).

3. Fruit Group

None.

4. Milk, Yogurt, and Cheese Group

None.

5. Meat, Poultry, Fish, Dry Beans, Eggs, and Nuts Group

A mixture of fish formed into balls and poached (gefilte fish); smoked salmon (lox).

6. Fats, Oils, and Sweets

Chicken fat.

Religious Dietary Patterns

Beliefs of several major religions include practices that affect or prescribe specific dietary patterns or prohibit consumption of certain types of foods. Individuals practicing these religions may or may not adhere to all of the prescribed customs. Following is a brief review of some of these practices.

Moslem

Pork and pork-related products are not eaten. Meats that are consumed must be slaughtered by prescribed rituals; these procedures are similar to the Judaic kosher slaughtering of animals, so Moslems may eat kosher meats. Coffee, tea, and alcohol are not consumed. During the month of Ramadan, Muslims fast during the day from dawn to sunset.

Christianity

Some sects may not eat meat on holy days; others prohibit alcohol consumption.

Hinduism

Animal foods of beef, pork, lamb, and poultry are not eaten. Followers are lactovegetarians or vegans.

Judaism

Food consumption is guided by religious doctrines; no pork or pork-related products nor seafood or fish without scales and fins are eaten. Dairy foods are not consumed with meat or animal-related foods (excludes fish). If meat or dairy is eaten, 6 hours must pass for the other to be acceptable for consumption. Animals are slaughtered according to a ritual in which blood is drained and the carcass is salted and rinsed; meat prepared in this manner is "kosher." The preparation of all processed foods must also adhere to these guidelines. Because meat and dairy must not mix, two sets of dishes and utensils are used at home and in kosher restaurants. Foods that are neither meat nor dairy are called parve and are often so labeled by food manufacturers. Additional customs affect food consumption on Saturday, the Sabbath, during which no cooking occurs. Special foods are associated with each religious holiday. Fasting (no water or food) for 24 hours occurs during Yom Kippur (Day of Atonement). During Passover, an 8-day holiday, no leavened bread is consumed, only matzoh (made from flour and water) and products made from matzoh flour; other symbolic food restrictions are also observed.

Seventh Day Adventist

General restrictions of pork and pork-related products, shellfish, alcohol, coffee, and tea are followed. Some followers are ovo-lacto-vegetarians, whereas others are vegans.

From Grodner M, Long Anderson S, DeYoung S: *Foundations and clinical applications of nutrition: a nursing approach,* ed 2, St. Louis, 2000, Mosby.

Answers to Self-Test Questions

Chapter 1
True-False
1. T
2. F
3. F
Multiple Choice
1. a
2. d
3. a

Chapter 2
True-False
1. F
2. T
3. F
4. T
5. F
6. T
Multiple Choice
1. d
2. b

Chapter 3
True-False
1. F
2. T
3. F
4. F
5. T
Multiple Choice
1. a
2. a, d
3. b

Chapter 4
True-False
1. F
2. T
3. F
4. F
5. F
6. F
7. T
8. T
9. T

10. F
11. T
Multiple Choice
1. a
2. d
3. c

Chapter 5
True-False
1. F
2. F
3. T
4. F
5. F
6. F
Multiple Choice
1. b
2. c
3. c
4. c
5. d
6. c

Chapter 6
True-False
1. F
2. F
3. T
4. F
5. T
6. T
Multiple Choice
1. b, c, e
2. c
3. d

Chapter 7
True-False
1. F
2. T
3. F
4. T
5. F
6. F
7. F

8. T
Multiple Choice
1. c
2. a
3. b

Chapter 8
Matching
1. k
2. g
3. n
4. a
5. l
6. b
7. f
8. h
9. i
10. p
11. d
12. o
13. j
14. c
15. e
16. m

Chapter 9
True-False
1. F
2. T
3. F
4. T
5. F
6. F
7. T
Multiple Choice
1. d
2. a, c, d
3. c
4. b
5. d
6. a

Chapter 10
True-False
1. T

2. F
3. F
4. T
5. F
6. F
7. T
8. T
9. T
10. T
Multiple Choice
1. a
2. b
3. b
4. d

Chapter 11
True-False
1. F
2. F
3. F
4. F
5. F
Multiple Choice
1. a, b, e
2. c
3. b

Chapter 12
True-False
1. F
2. F
3. F
4. F
5. T
6. F
7. F
Multiple Choice
1. d
2. a, b, c
3. b, d
4. a, b, c, d

Chapter 13
True-False
1. F

2. F
3. F
4. T
5. F
6. T
7. F
8. T
Multiple Choice
1. a, b, c, d, e
2. c

Chapter 14
True-False
1. F
2. T
3. T
4. T
5. F
6. F
Multiple Choice
1. d
2. a, c, d
3. a, b
4. b
5. c

Chapter 15
True-False
1. F
2. F
3. F
4. T
5. F
Multiple Choice
1. c, e
2. b
3. b, c

Chapter 16
True-False
1. F
2. F
3. T
4. F
5. F
6. T
7. T
8. F
9. T

Multiple Choice
1. b
2. d
3. a, b, c
4. a, c
5. c

Chapter 17
True-False
1. T
2. F
3. T
4. F
5. F
6. T
7. F
8. T
9. F
10. F
Multiple Choice
1. a, b, c, d
2. a, b, c, d
3. a, b, c, d
4. d
5. a, d

Chapter 18
True-False
1. F
2. F
3. T
4. F
5. F
6. T
7. T
8. T
9. T
Multiple Choice
1. d
2. b
3. c
4. b

Chapter 19
True-False
1. T
2. F
3. F
4. F

5. T
6. T
7. T
8. F
9. F
10. F
Multiple Choice
1. b
2. a
3. a

Chapter 20
True-False
1. F
2. F
3. F
4. T
5. T
6. T
7. T
8. F
9. F
10. F
Multiple Choice
1. c
2. a, b, c, d

Chapter 21
True-False
1. T
2. F
3. F
4. T
5. T
6. F
7. T
8. F
9. T
10. T
Multiple Choice
1. b, d
2. b, c, e
3. a, b, c

Chapter 22
True-False
1. T
2. T
3. F

4. T
5. F
6. F
7. F
8. F
9. F
10. T
Multiple Choice
1. a
2. b
3. a
4. a, b, c, d, e
5. a, b, c, d

Chapter 23
True-False
1. F
2. T
3. T
4. F
5. T
6. F
7. F
8. T
Multiple Choice
1. b
2. c
3. b
4. a
5. d

Glossary

acetone A major ketone compound that results from fat breakdown for energy in uncontrolled diabetes; persons with diabetes periodically do urinary acetone tests to monitor status of their diabetes control.

adipose (L. *adeps*, fat; *adiposus*, fatty) Fat present in cells of adipose (fatty) tissue.

aerobic capacity (Gr. *aer*, air or gas) Requiring oxygen to proceed. Milliliters of oxygen consumed per kilogram of body weight per minute, as influenced by body composition.

agrogenetics Application of the science of genetic engineering to agriculture to produce hardier plant species that are more resistant to pests and disease.

albumin (L. *albus*, white) A major protein in many animal and plant tissues; specialized plasma protein maintaining normal blood pressure.

aldosterone A potent hormone of the outside layer of the adrenal glands that acts on the distal nephron tubule to cause reabsorption of sodium in an ion exchange with potassium. The aldosterone mechanism is essentially a sodium-conserving mechanism but also indirectly conserves water because water absorption follows the sodium resorption.

allergy (Gr. *allos*, other; *ergon*, work) A state of hypersensitivity to particular substances in the environment that work on the body tissues to produce problems in functions of affected tissues; the agent involved (allergen) may be a certain food eaten or a substance such as pollen inhaled.

amino acids Nitrogen-bearing compounds that form the structural units of protein. The various food proteins, when digested, yield their specific constituent amino acids, which are then available for use by the cells to synthesize specific tissue proteins.

aminopeptidase Specific protein-splitting enzyme secreted by small glands in the walls of the small intestine that breaks off the nitrogen-containing amino ($-NH_2$) end of the peptide chain forming protein, producing smaller chained peptides and free amino acids.

anaerobic (Gr. *an-*, without; *aer*, air; *bios*, life) A microorganism that can live and grow in an oxygen-free environment.

anemia (Gr. *an-*, negative prefix; *haima*, blood) Blood condition characterized by a decreased number of circulating red blood cells hemoglobin or both.

angina pectoris (L. *angina*, severe pain; *pectus*, breast) Spasmodic, choking chest pain due to lack of oxygen to the heart muscle, symptom of a heart attack; may also be caused by severe effort or excitement.

anorexia nervosa (Gr. *an-*, negative prefix; *orexis*, appetite) Extreme psychophysiologic aversion to food resulting in life-threatening weight loss. A psychiatric eating disorder resulting from a morbid fear of fatness in which the person's distorted body image is reflected as fat when the body is actually malnourished and extremely thin from self-starvation.

antibody Any of numerous protein molecules produced by B-cells as a primary immune defense for attaching to specific related antigens.

antidiuretic hormone (ADH) A hormone of the pituitary gland that acts on the distal nephron tubule to conserve water by causing its reabsorption; also called *vasopressin*.

antigen (antibody + Gr. *gennan*, to produce) Any foreign or "nonself" substances, such as toxins, viruses, bacteria, and foreign proteins, that stimulate the production of antibodies specifically designed to counteract their activity.

anuria (Gr. *an-*, negative prefix; *ouron*, urine) An absence of urine, indicating kidney shutdown or failure.

ascites (Gr. *askites*, from; *askos*, bag) Outflow and accumulation of serous (blood and lymph serum) fluid in the abdominal cavity; also known as abdominal or peritoneal dropsy.

ascorbic acid Chemical name for vitamin C from its ability to cure scurvy.

atherosclerosis (Gr. *athere*, gruel; *skleros*, hard) The underlying pathology of coronary heart disease; a common form of artheriosclerosis, characterized by the formation, beginning in childhood in predisposed individuals, of yellow cheeselike fatty streaks containing cholesterol that develop into hardened plaques in the inner lining of major blood vessels such as the coronary arteries.

atrophy (Gr. *a-*, negative prefix; *trophē*, nourishment) A wasting away.

azotemia (Gr. *a-*, negative prefix; *zoe*, life; *azote*, nitrogen; *haima*, blood) An excess of urea and other nitrogenous substances in the blood.

basal metabolism (Gr. *basis*, base; *metabole*, change) The amount of energy needed by the body for maintenance of life when a person is at digestive, physical, and emotional rest. This basal metabolic rate (BMR) is reported as the percent of variation in the person above or below the normal number of kilocalories required for a person of like height, weight, sex, and age.

beriberi (Singhalese "I can't, I can't) A disease of the peripheral nerves caused by a deficiency of thiamin (vitamin B$_1$) that is characterized by pain (neuritis) and paralysis of legs and arms, cardiovascular changes, and edema.

bile (L. *bilis*, bile) A fluid secreted by the liver and transported to the gallbladder for concentration and storage; released into the duodenum with the entry of fat to facilitate enzymatic fat digestion by acting as an emulsifying agent.

blood urea nitrogen (BUN) A basic test of nephron function by measuring its ability to normally filter urea nitrogen, a product of protein metabolism, from the blood.

body composition The relative sizes of the four basic body compartments that make up the total body: lean body mass (muscle mass), fat, water, and bone.

bulimia nervosa (L. *bous*, ox; *limos*, hunger) A psychiatric eating disorder related to a person's fear of fatness, in which cycles of gorging on large quantities of food are followed by self-induced vomiting and use of diuretics and laxatives to maintain a "normal" body weight.

cachexia (Gr. *kakos*, bad; *hexis*, habit) A specific profound effect caused by malnutrition and a disturbance in glucose and fat metabolism usually seen in patients with terminal cancer or AIDS; general poor health indicated by an emaciated appearance.

cajun (Derivative, *Acadian*) Group of people with an enduring tradition whose French-Catholic ancestors established permanent communities in the southern Louisiana coastal waterways after being expelled from Acadia (now Nova Scotia, Canada) by the reigning English in the late 18th century; developed unique food pattern from blend of native French influence and mix of Creole cooking found in the new land.

calcitriol The activated hormone form of vitamin D.

callus (L. *callositis*, callus, bone) Unorganized meshwork of newly grown, woven bone developed on a pattern of original clot of fibrin, formed after fracture or surgery, and normally replaced in the healing process by hard adult bone.

calorie (L. *calor*, heat) A measure of heat. The *energy* required to do the work of the body is measured as the amount of *heat* produced by the body's work. The energy value of food is expressed as the number of kilocalories a specified portion of the food will yield when oxidized in the body.

carboxypeptidase (L. *carbo-*, carbon; *oxy*, oxygen) A specific protein-splitting enzyme secreted in inactive form in the pancreas that is activated by trypsin in the small intestine to break off the acid (*carboxyl*, COOH) end of the peptide chain forming protein, producing smaller chained peptides and free amino acids.

carotene A group name of three red and yellow pigments (alpha-, beta-, and gamma-carotene) found in dark green and yellow vegetables and fruits. The one found to be most important in human nutrition is beta-carotene because the body can convert it to vitamin A, thus making it a primary source of the vitamin.

catabolism (Gr. *katabole*, a throwing down) The process by which body tissues are broken down, the opposite of *anabolism*. Catabolism includes all the processes in which complex substances are progressively broken down into simpler ones, usually with the release of energy. Together, anabolism and catabolism constitute metabolism, which is the coordinated operation of anabolic (building up) and catabolic (breaking down) processes into a dynamic balance of energy and substance.

cellulitis Diffuse inflammation of soft or connective tissues (e.g., in the foot) from injury, bruises, or pressure sores that lead to infection; poor care may result in ulceration and abscess or gangrene.

cerebrovascular accident (L. *cerebrum*, brain; *vas*, vessel) A stroke, caused by arteriosclerosis in a blood vessel in the brain that cuts off oxygen supply to the affected portion of brain tissue, thus paralyzing body muscle actions controlled by the affected brain area.

cholecalciferol The chemical name for vitamin D in its inactive dietary form; often shortened to calciferol.

cholesterol (Gr. *chole*, bile; *steros*, solid) A fat-related compound, a sterol, synthesized only in animal tissues; a normal constituent of bile and a principal constituent of gallstones. In the body, cholesterol is synthesized mainly in the liver. In the diet, it is found only in animal food sources. In human body metabolism, cholesterol is important as a precursor of various steroid hormones, such as sex hormones and adrenal corticoids. In disordered lipid metabolism, however, it is a major factor in atherosclerosis, the underlying disease process in coronary arteries that leads to heart attacks.

chronic dieting syndrome The cyclic pattern of weight loss by dieting to achieve an unnatural but culturally ideal body thinness, then regaining weight by compulsive food binges in response to stress, anxiety, and hunger. This abnormal psychophysiologic food pattern becomes chronic, changing the person's natural body metabolism and relative body composition to the abnormal state of a "metabolically obese" person of normal weight.

chyme (Gr. *chymos*, juice) Semifluid food mass in the gastrointestinal tract following gastric digestion.

chymotrypsin (Gr. *chymos*, semifluid food mass from digestion; *trypein*, enzyme trypsin) One of the protein-splitting and milk-curdling pancreatic enzymes activated in the small intestine from the precursor chymotrypsinogen; breaks specific amino acid peptide linkages of protein.

cobalamin The chemical name for the B-complex vitamin B$_{12}$; found mainly in animal protein food sources so deficiencies seen mostly among strict vegetarians (vegans). It is closely related to amino acid metabolism and formation of the heme portion of hemoglobin. Absence of its necessary absorbing agent in the gastric secretions, intrinsic factor, leads to pernicious anemia and degenerative effects on the nervous system, which requires continuing monthly cobalamin injections, bypassing the intestinal absorption defect, to control.

collagen disease (Gr. *kolla*, glue; *gennan*, to produce) A disease attacking collagen tissues, the protein substance of the white fibers (collagenous fibers) of skin, tendon, bone, cartilage, and other connective tissues; any of a group of diseases that cause widespread changes in the connective tissue, such as rheumatoid arthritis, lupus erythematosus, scleroderma, and rheumatic fever.

colloidal osmotic pressure (COP) Fluid pressure produced by the protein molecules in the plasma and in the cell. Because proteins are large molecules, they do not pass through the separating membranes of the capillary cells. Thus they remain in their respective compartments exerting a constant osmotic pull that protects vital plasma and cell fluid volumes in these areas.

colostrum (L. *colostrum*, pre-milk) A thin, yellow fluid first secreted by the mammary gland a few days before and after childbirth, preceding the mature breast milk. It contains up to 20% protein including a large amount of lactalbumin, more minerals, and less lactose and fat than does milk, and immunoglobulins that represent the antibodies found in maternal blood.

complex carbohydrates Larger, more complex molecules of carbohydrates composed of many sugar units (polysaccharides). Complex forms of dietary carbohydrates are starch, which is digestible and provides a major energy source, and dietary fiber, which is nondigestible (humans lack the necessary enzymes) and thus provides important bulk in the diet.

congestive heart failure Chronic condition of gradually weakening heart muscle unable to pump normal blood flow through the heart-lung circulation, resulting in congestion of fluids in the lungs.

coronary heart disease Term designating the overall medical problem resulting from the underlying disease of atherosclerosis in the coronary arteries serving the heart muscle tissue with blood oxygen and nutrients.

creatinine Nitrogen-carrying product of tissue protein breakdown, excreted in the urine.

dehiscence (L. *dehiscere*, to gape) A splitting open; the separation of layers of a surgical wound, partial or superficial or complete, with total disruption requiring resuturing.

dialysis (Gr. *dia*, through; *lysis*, dissolution) The process of separating crystalloids (crystal-forming substances) and colloids (gluelike substances) in solution by the difference in their rates of diffusion through a semipermeable membrane; crystalloids (e.g., blood sugar and other simple metabolites), pass through readily and colloids (e.g., plasma proteins) pass through slowly or not at all.

dietetics Management of diet and the use of food; the science concerned with the nutritional planning and preparation of foods.

diverticulitis (L. *divertere*, to turn aside) inflammation of pockets of tissue (diverticuli) in the lining of the mucous membrane of the colon.

dysphagia (Gr. *dys-*, painful; *phagein*, to eat) Difficulty in swallowing.

edema (Gr. *oidema*, swelling) An unusual accumulation of fluid in the interstitial (small structural spaces between tissue parts) tissue spaces of the body.

elemental formula A nutrition-support formula composed of simple elemental nutrient components that require no further digestive breakdown and are thus readily absorbed; formulas with the protein as free amino acids and the carbohydrate as the simple sugar glucose.

emulsifier An agent that breaks down large fat globules into smaller, uniformly distributed particles; action accomplished in the intestine chiefly by bile acids, which lower the surface tension of the fat particles, breaking the fat into many smaller droplets, thus greatly increasing the surface area of fat and facilitating contact with the fat-digesting enzymes.

enteral (Gr. *enteron*, intestine) A mode of feeding that uses the gastrointestinal tract, oral, or tube feeding.

enzyme (Gr. *en*, in; *zyme*, leaven) Specific proteins produced in cells that digest or change specific nutrients in specific chemical reactions without being changed themselves in the process. Their action is therefore that of a *catalyst*. Digestive enzymes in the gastrointestinal secretions act on food substances to break them down into simpler compounds. An enzyme is usually named according to the substance (substrate) on which it acts, with common word ending of *-ase*; for example, sucrase is the specific enzyme for sucrose, which it breaks down into glucose and fructose.

ergogenic (Gr. *ergon*, work; *gennan*, to produce) Tendency to increase work output; various substances that increase work or exercise capacity and output.

essential hypertension An inherent form of high blood pressure with no specific discoverable cause, considered to be familial; also called primary hypertension.

exudate (L. *exsudare*, to sweat out) Various materials (e.g., cells, cellular debris, and fluids), usually resulting from inflammation, that have escaped from the blood vessels and are deposited in or on the surface tissues; protein content is high.

fatty acids The major structural components of fats.

food guide pyramid A visual pattern of the current basic five food groups (bread-cereal, 6-11 servings; vegetable, 3-5 servings; fruit, 2-4 servings; milk-cheese, 2-3 servings; meat-dry beans-egg, 2-3 servings), arranged in a pyramid shape to indicate proportionate amounts of daily food choices. The largest food group, breads-cereals, forms the entire base foundation. The next two narrowing tiers indicate relatively fewer daily portions of vegetables and fruits, and then of the milk-cheese and meat-egg groups. The small tip at the pyramid top indicates sparing use of fats, oils, and sweets.

glomerulus (L. *glomus*, ball, cluster) First section of the nephron, a cluster of capillary loops cupped in the nephron head that serves as an initial filter.

glucagon (Gr. *glykys*, sweet; *gonē*, seed) A hormone secreted by the A cells of the pancreatic islets of Langerhans in response to hyperglycemia; it has an opposite, balancing effect to that of insulin—raising the blood sugar, and thus is used as a quick-acting antidote for a low blood sugar reaction of insulin. It also counteracts the overnight fast during sleep hours by breaking down liver glycogen to keep blood-sugar levels normal and maintain an adequate energy supply for normal nerve and brain function.

glycerides Chemical group name for fats, from their base substance glycerol; formed from the glycerol base with one, two, or three fatty acids attached to make monoglycerides, diglycerides, and triglycerides. Glycerides are the principle constituents of adipose tissue and are found in animal and vegetable fats and oils.

glycogen (Gr. *glykys*, sweet; *gennan*, to produce) A polysaccharide, the main storage form of carbohydrate, largely stored in the liver and to a lesser extent in muscle tissue.

goiter (L. *gutter*, throat) An enlarged thyroid gland caused by lack of sufficient available iodine to produce the thyroid hormone thyroxine.

health A state of optimal well-being—physical, mental, and social; relative freedom from disease or disability.

health promotion (A.S. *hal*, hale, sound; L. *promovere*, to move forward) Active involvement in behaviors or programs that advance positive well-being.

Heimlich maneuver A first-aid maneuver to relieve a person who is choking from blockage of the breathing passageway by a swallowed foreign object or food particle. Standing behind the person, clasp the victim around the waist, placing one fist just under the sternum (breastbone) and grasping the fist with the other hand. Then make a quick, hard, thrusting movement inward and upward to dislodge the object.

hematuria (Gr. *haima*, blood; *ouron*, urine) The abnormal presence of blood in the urine.

hemoglobin (Gr. *haima*, blood; L. *globus*, globe) A conjugated protein in red blood cells; composed of a compact rounded mass of polypeptide chains forming *globin*, the protein portion, attached to an iron-containing red pigment called *heme*. Carries oxygen in the blood to cells.

homeostasis (Gr. *homoios*, like, unchanging; *stasis*, standing, stable) The state of relative dynamic equilibrium within the body's internal environment; a balance achieved through the operation of various interrelated physiologic mechanisms.

hyperglycemia (Gr. *hyper*, above; *glykys*, sweet) Elevated blood sugar above normal limits.

hypertension High blood pressure.

hypoglycemia (Gr. *hypo-*, below; *glykys*, sweet; *haima*, blood) An abnormally low blood-sugar level that may lead to muscle tremors, cold sweat, headache, and confusion; a serious condition in insulin-dependent diabetes management that requires immediate sugar intake to counteract, followed by a snack of complex carbohydrate food (e.g., bread or crackers) and a protein (e.g., lean meat, peanut butter, or cheese) to maintain the normal blood sugar.

immunocompetence (L. *immunis*, free, exempt) The ability or capacity to develop an immune response (i.e., antibody production or cell-mediated immunity) following exposure to an antigen.

ketoacidosis Excess production of ketones, a form of metabolic acidosis that occurs in uncontrolled diabetes or starvation from burning body fat for energy fuel; a continuing uncontrolled state can result in coma and death.

ketones Chemical name for a class of organic compounds, including three keto-acid bases (e.g., acetone) that occur as intermediate products of fat metabolism.

ketosis The accumulation of ketones, intermediate products of fat metabolism, in the blood.

kilocalorie (Fr. *chilioi*, thousand; L. *calor*, heat) The general term *calorie* refers to a unit of heat measure and is used alone to designate the *small calorie*. The calorie used in nutritional science and the study of metabolism is the *large calorie* (which equals 1000 calories) or kilocalorie, to be more accurate and avoid the use of very large numbers in calculations.

lactated Ringer's solution Sterile solution of calcium chloride, potassium chloride, sodium chloride, and sodium lactate in water given to replenish fluid and electrolytes; developed by English physiologist Sidney Ringer (1835-1910).

linoleic acid The ultimate essential fatty acid for humans.

lipectomy (Gr. *lipos*, fat; *ectomē*, excision) Surgical removal of subcutaneous fat by suction through a tube inserted into a surface incision, or by removing larger amounts of subcutaneous fat by major surgical incision.

lipids (Gr. *lipos*, fat) The chemical group name for organic substances of a fatty nature. The lipids include fats, oils, waxes, and other fat-related compounds such as cholesterol and lipoproteins.

lipoproteins Chemical complexes of fat with protein that serve as the major carriers of lipids in the plasma because most of the plasma fat is associated with them. They vary in density according to the size of the fat load being carried; the lower the density, the higher the fat load. The combination package with water-soluble protein makes possible the transport of non-water-soluble fatty substances in the water-based blood circulation.

macrosomia (Gr. *macro*, large; *sōma*, body) Excessive fetal growth resulting in an abnormally large infant carrying high risk of perinatal mortality.

major minerals The group of minerals, also called macronutrients, that are required by the body in amounts of more than 100 mg/day. The seven major minerals in the body are calcium, phosphorus, sodium, potassium, magnesium, chlorine, and sulfur.

metabolism (Gr. *metaballein*, to turn about, change, alter) The sum of all chemical changes that take place in the body by which it maintains itself and produces energy for its functioning. Products of the various reactions are called *metabolites*.

microvilli (Gr. *mikros*, small; L. *villus*, tuft of hair) Exceedingly small hairlike projections covering all villi on the surface of the small intestine that greatly extend the total absorbing surface area; visible through electron microscope.

mucosal folds (L. *mucus*, mucosa) Large visible folds of the mucous lining of the small intestine that increase the absorbing surface area.

mutation (L. *mutare*, to change) A permanent transmissible change in a gene.

myocardial infarction (Gr. *mys*, muscle; *kardia*, heart; L. *infarcire*, to stuff in) A heart attack; caused by failure of the heart muscle to maintain normal blood circulation due to blockage of coronary arteries with fatty cholesterol plaques that cut off delivery of oxygen to the affected part of the heart muscle.

neoplasm (Gr. *neos*, new; *plasma*, formation) Any new or abnormal cellular growth, specifically one that is uncontrolled and aggressive.

nephron (Gr. *nephros*, kidney) Microscopic anatomical and functional unit of the kidney that selectively filters and reabsorbs essential blood factors, secretes hydrogen ions as needed for maintaining acid-base balance, then reabsorbs water to protect body fluids and forms and excretes a concentrated urine for elimination of wastes. There are approximately 1 million nephrons in each kidney.

nephrosis (Gr. *nephros*, kidney) A nephrotic syndrome caused by degenerative lesions of the renal tubules of the nephrons, especially the thin basement membrane of the glomerulus that helps support the capillary loops; marked by edema, albuminuria, and decreased serum albumin.

niacin Chemical name for a B vitamin discovered in relation to the deficiency disease pellagra, largely a skin disorder; important as a co-enzyme factor in many cell reactions related to energy and protein metabolism.

nutrition (L. *nutritic*, nourishment) The sum of the processes involved in taking in nutrients and assimilating and using them to maintain body tissue and provide energy; a foundation for life and health.

nutritional science The body of science, developed through controlled research, that relates to the processes involved in nutrition—international, community, and clinical.

oliguria (Gr. *oligos*, little; *ouron*, urine) The secretion of small amounts of urine in relation to fluid intake.

organic farming Farming methods that use natural means of pest control by choosing hardy plant varieties that resist diseases and introduce beneficial insects to thrive and help control entrenched populations of destructive ones, thus avoiding dependence on stronger and stronger pesticides as resistant insects multiply; also uses time-tested natural means of enriching soil (e.g., crop rotation and cycling plant mulch and manure for a healthier soil and pesticide-free foods).

osmosis (Gr. *osmos*, a thrusting) Passage of a solvent such as water through a membrane that separates solutions of different concentrations, tending to equalize the concentration pressures of the solutions on both sides of the membrane.

osteodystrophy (Gr. *osteon*, bone; *dys*, painful, disordered, abnormal; *trephein*, to nourish) Bone disease resulting from defective bone formation. The general term *dystrophy* applies to any disorder arising from faulty nutrition.

osteoporosis (Gr. *osteon*, bone; *poros*, passage, pore) Abnormal thinning of the bone, producing a porous, fragile, latticelike bone tissue of enlarged spaces that is prone to fracture or deformity.

pancreatic amylase Major starch-splitting enzyme secreted by the pancreas and acting in the small intestine.

pancreatic lipase (Gr. *lipos*, fat) A major fat-splitting enzyme produced by the pancreas and secreted into the small intestine to digest fat.

pandemic (Gr. *pan*, all; *dēmos*, people) A widespread epidemic that is distributed through a region, a continent, or the world.

pantothenic acid (Gr. *pantothen*, from all sides, in every corner) A B-complex vitamin widely distributed in nature and occurring throughout the body tissues. Its one role, a major one, is as an essential constituent of the body's main activating agent, coenzyme A. This special compound has extensive metabolic responsibility in activating a number of compounds in many tissues; it is a key energy metabolism substance in every cell.

parasite (Gr. *para*, along side; *sitos*, food, grain; *parasitos*, one who eats at another's table; in ancient Greece, a term for a person who received free meals in return for amusing or flattering conversation) An organism that lives in or on an organism of another species known as the host, from whom all life-cycle nourishment is obtained.

parenteral (Gr. *para*, alongside, accessory, beyond; *enteron*, intestine) A mode of feeding that does not use the gastrointestinal tract but instead provides nutrition support by intravenous delivery of nutrient solutions.

parotid glands (Gr. *para*, beyond, beside; *ous*, ear) Gland situated near the ear; largest of three pairs of salivary glands. The parotid glands lie, one on each side, above the angle of the jaw, below and in front of the ear. They continually secrete saliva, which passes along the duct of the gland and into the mouth through an opening in the inner cheek, level with the second upper molar tooth. Normal saliva flow facilitates the chewing and swallowing of food and prevents dry mouth problems.

pellagra (L. *pelle*, skin; Gr. *agra*, seizure) Deficiency disease caused by a lack of dietary niacin and an inadequate amount of protein containing the amino acid tryptophan, a precursor of niacin. Pellagra is characterized by skin lesions that are aggravated by sunlight, and by gastrointestinal, mucosal, neurologic, and mental symptoms. The four Ds often associated with pellagra are dermatitis, diarrhea, dementia, and death.

pepsin (Gr. *pepsis*, digestion) The main gastric enzyme specific for proteins. Pepsin begins breaking large protein molecules into shorter chain polypeptides; gastric hydrochloric acid is necessary to activate.

peritoneal cavity (Gr. *per*, around; *teinein*, to stretch) A strong, smooth, serous membrane lining the abdominal and pelvic walls and undersurface of the diaphragm, forming a sac enclosing the body's vital visceral organs. *Peritoneal dialysis* is a form of dialysis through the peritoneum into and out of the peritoneal cavity.

pharynx (Gr. *pharynx*, throat) The muscular membranous passage between the mouth and the posterior nasal passages and the larynx and esophagus.

photosynthesis (Gr. *photos*, light; *synthesis*, putting together) Process by which plants containing chlorophyll are able to manufacture carbohydrate by combining CO_2 from air and water from soil. Sunlight is used as energy; chlorophyll is a ctalyist. $6 CO_2 + 6 H_2O + Energy \rightarrow Chlorophyl \rightarrow C_6H_{12}O_6 + 6 O_2$.

phylloquinone A fat-soluble vitamin of the K group found in green plants or prepared synthetically.

plasma protein Any of a number of protein substances carried in the circulating blood. A major one is *albumin*, which maintains the fluid volume of the blood through its colloidal osmotic pressure.

portal (L. *porta*, a portal or doorway) An entrance or gateway; for example, the portal blood circulation designates the entry of blood vessels from the intestines into the liver, carrying nutrients for major liver metabolism, then draining into the body's main systemic circulation to deliver metabolic products to body cells.

proenzyme An inactive precursor (forerunner substance from which another substance is made) converted to the active enzyme by the action of an acid, another enzyme, or other means. Also called zymogen.

prohormone A precursor substance that the body converts to a hormone; for example, a cholesterol compound in the skin is first irradiated by sunlight and then developed through successive enzyme actions in the liver and kidney into the vitamin D hormone,

which then regulates calcium absorption and bone development. Only a few food sources of vitamin D are found in food fats (e.g., cream, butter, egg yolks), but it occurs in other processed foods (e.g., breakfast cereals and milk(through enrichment.

proteinuria (Gr. *protos*, first, protein; *ouron*, urine) An abnormal excess of serum proteins such as albumin in the urine.

pulmonary edema (L. *pulmonis*, lung; Gr. *oidēma*, swelling) Accumulation of fluid in tissues of the lung.

purines (L. *purum*, pure; Gr. *ouron*, urine) Nitrogen-containing compounds that yield uric acid as a metabolic end product eliminated in the urine.

pyridoxine The chemical name of vitamin B_6. In its activated phosphate form, B_2-PO_4, pyridoxine functions as an important co-enzyme factor in many reactions in cell metabolism related to amino acids, glucose, and fatty acids. Clinically, pyridoxine deficiency produces a specific anemia and disturbances of the central nervous system.

ramadan (Ar. *ramadān*, the hot month) The ninth month of the Muslim year, a period of daily fasting from sunrise to sunset.

Recommended Dietary Allowances (RDAs) Recommended daily allowances of nutrients and energy intake for population groups according to age and sex, with defined weight and height that are established and reviewed periodically by a representative group of nutritional scientists, in relation to current research. These standards vary little among the developed countries.

registered dietitian (RD) A professional dietitian, accredited with academic degree course of university and graduate study and having passed required registration examinations administered by the American Dietetic Association.

rennin Milk-curdling enzyme of the gastric juice of human infants and young animals such as calves. Do not confuse with *renin*, an important enzyme produced by the kidney that plays a vital role in producing angiotensin, a potent vasoconstrictor and stimulant for release of the hormone aldosterone from the adjacent adrenal glands.

retinol (L. *retina*, from *rēte*, net, eye vision; suffix -*ol*, an alcohol) The chemical name of vitamin A; derived from its vision function relating to the retina of the eye, the back inner lining of the eyeball that "catches" the lens light refractions to form images interpreted by the optic nerve and brain and makes the necessary light-dark adaptations.

riboflavin   Chemical name of one of the early B vitamins, discovered in relation to an early vitamin-deficiency syndrome called "ariboflavinosis," evidenced mainly in breakdown of skin tissues and resulting infections; role as a coenzyme factor in many cell reactions related to energy and protein metabolism.

rickets   (Gr. *rhachitis*, a spinal complaint) A disease of childhood characterized by softening of the bones from an inadequate intake of vitamin D and insufficient exposure to sunlight; also associated with impaired calcium and phosphorus metabolism.

saccharide   (L. *saccharum*, sugar) Chemical name for sugar molecules. May occur as single molecules in monosaccharides (glucose, fructose, maltose), as two molecules in disaccharides (sucrose, lactose, maltose), or as multiple molecules in polysaccharides (starch, dietary fiber, glycogen).

salivary amylase   (Gr. *amylon*, starch) A starch-splitting enzyme in the mouth, sometimes called *ptyalin* (Gr. *ptyalon*, spittle) that is secreted by the salivary glands.

saturated   (L. *saturare*, to fill) State of being filled; state of fatty acid components of fats being filled in all their available carbon bonds with hydrogen, making the fat harder and more solid. Such solid food fats are from animal sources.

scurvy   A vitamin-deficiency disease caused by a lack of vitamin C. It is a hemorrhagic disease with diffuse tissue bleeding, painful limbs and joints, thickened bones, skin discoloration from tissue bleeding; bones fracture easily, wounds do not heal, gums are swollen and bleed, and teeth loosen.

senescence   (L. *senescere*, to grow old) The process or condition of growing old.

simple carbohydrates   Sugars with simple structure of one or two-single sugar (saccharide) units. A monosaccharide is composed of one sugar unit; a disaccharide is composed of two sugar units.

sorbitol   A sugar alcohol formed in mammals from glucose and converted to fructose. Named for its initial discovery in nature, it is found in ripe berries of the tree *Sorbus acuparia* and also occurs in small quantities in various other berries, cherries, plums, pears. Produced in food industry laboratories for use as a sweetener in candies, chewing gum, beverages, and other foodstuffs; side effect of diarrhea limits use.

Spina bifida   (L. *spina*, spine; *bifidus*, cleft into two parts or branches) Congenital defect in the embryonic-fetal closing of the neural tube to form a portion of the lower spine, leaving the spine unclosed and the spinal cord open in various degrees of exposure and damage.

steatorrhea   (Gr. *steatos*, fat; *rhoia*, flow) Fatty diarrhea; excessive amounts of fat in the feces often caused by malabsorption diseases.

steroids   (Gr. *stereos*, solid; L. *-ol*, *oleum*, oil) Group name for lipid-based sterols, including hormones, bile acids, and cholesterol.

stoma   (Gr. *stoma*, mouth, opening) The opening established in the abdominal wall, connecting with the ileum or colon, for elimination of intestinal wastes after surgical removal of diseased portions of the intestines.

sustainable agriculture   A system of agriculture that combines traditional conservation-minded farming techniques with modern technologies. Sustainable systems use modern equipment, certified seed, and soil and water conservation practices, with emphasis on rotating crops, building up the soil, diversifying crops and livestock, and controlling pests naturally. Major goals are safe soil preservation and avoiding heavy dependence on pesticides and chemical fertilizers.

thiamin   Chemical name of a major B-complex vitamin; formerly called vitamin B_1, discovered in relation to the classic deficiency disease beriberi; important in body metabolism as a co-enzyme factor in many cell reactions related to energy metabolism.

tocopherol   (Gr. *tokos*, childbirth; *pherein*, to carry) The chemical name for vitamin E, so named by early investigators because their initial work with rats indicated a reproductive functions, not true with humans. Instead, vitamin E functions as a strong antioxidant that preserves structural membranes (e.g., cell walls) in humans.

trace elements   The group of elements, also called micronutrients, that are required by the body in smaller amounts of less than 100 mg/day. The 10 trace elements in the body are iron, iodine, zinc, copper, manganese, chromium, cobalt, selenium, molybdenum, and fluoride.

triglycerides   Chemical name for fats in the body or in food; compound of three fatty acids attached to a glycerol base.

trypsin   A protein-splitting enzyme formed in the small intestine by action of enterokinase on the inactive precursor trypsinogen.

trypsin (Gr. *trypein*, to rub; *pepsis*, digestion) A protein-splitting enzyme, secreted as the inactive proenzyme *trypsinogen* in the pancreas, activated and acting in the small intestine to reduce proteins to shorter chain polypeptides and dipeptides.

urea Chief nitrogen-carrying product of dietary protein metabolism; appears in blood, lymph, and urine.

villi (L. *villus*, tuft of hair) Small protrusions from the surface of a membrane; fingerlike projections covering mucosal surfaces of the small intestine that further increase the absorbing surface area; visible through a regular microscope.

virus (L. *virus*, poison; *virion*, individual virus particle) A minute microscopic infectious organism characterized by lack of independent metabolism and by the ability to reproduce with genetic continuity only within a living host. Each particle (virion) consists basically of nucleic acids (genetic material) and a protein shell which protects and contains the genetic material and any enzymes present.

wean (Middle English, 1000 AD, *wenen*, to accustom) To gradually accustom a young child to food other than the mother's milk or a bottle-fed substitute formula as the child's natural need to suckle wanes.

xerostomia (Gr. *xeros*, dry; *stoma*; mouth) Dryness of the mouth from lack of normal secretions.

Index

NOTES

NOTES

NOTES

NOTES

NOTES

NOTES

NOTES

NOTES